S0-EPW-041

DISPLAY COPY
DO NOT REMOVE

Rigid Fixation of the Craniomaxillofacial Skeleton

Rigid Fixation of the Craniomaxillofacial Skeleton

Edited by
Michael J. Yaremchuk, M.D.
Joseph S. Gruss, M.B., F.R.C.S.
Paul N. Manson, M.D.

NO LONGER THE PROPERTY
OF THE
UNIVERSITY OF R. I. LIBRARY

Butterworth–Heinemann
Boston   London   Oxford   Singapore   Sydney   Toronto   Wellington

Copyright © 1992 by Butterworth–Heinemann, a division of Reed Publishing (USA) Inc.
All rights reserved.

No part of this publication may be reproduced, stored in a retrieval system, or transmitted, in any form or by any means, electronic, mechanical, photocopying, recording, or otherwise, without the prior written permission of the publisher.

Every effort has been made to ensure that the drug dosage schedules within this text are accurate and conform to standards accepted at time of publication. However, as treatment recommendations vary in the light of continuing research and clinical experience, the reader is advised to verify drug dosage schedules herein with information found on product information sheets. This is especially true in cases of new or infrequently used drugs.

∞ Recognizing the importance of preserving what has been written, it is the policy of Butterworth–Heinemann to have the books it publishes printed on acid-free paper, and we exert our best efforts to that end.

Library of Congress Cataloging-in-Publication Data

Rigid fixation of the craniomaxillofacial skeleton / edited by Joseph S. Gruss, Paul N. Manson, Michael J. Yaremchuk.
   p.   cm.
   Includes bibliographical references and index.
   ISBN 0-7506-9197-2 (case bound : alk. paper)
   1. Head—Surgery. 2. Face—Surgery. 3. Fracture fixation.
I. Gruss, Joseph S. II. Manson, Paul N. III. Yaremchuk, Michael J. [DNLM: 1. Facial Bones—surgery. 2. Fracture Fixation, Internal. 3. Jaw—surgery. 4. Skull—surgery. WE 705 R571]
RD521.R54 1992
617.5′1059—dc20
DNLM/DLC
for Library of Congress   91-20576
                                                                          CIP

British Library Cataloguing in Publication Data

Rigid fixation of the craniomaxillofacial skeleton.
   I. Gruss, Joseph S. II. Manson, Paul N.
   III. Yaremchuk, Michael J.
   617.510592

ISBN 0750691972

Butterworth–Heinemann
80 Montvale Avenue
Stoneham, MA 02180

10 9 8 7 6 5 4 3 2 1

Printed in the United States of America

Contents

Contributors ix
Preface xv

PART I BASIC CONCEPTS OF RIGID FIXATION 1

Chapter 1 Bone Healing 3
John H. Phillips, Berton Rahn

Chapter 2 Principles of Compression Osteosynthesis 7
John H. Phillips

Chapter 3 Principles of Monocortical Miniplate Osteosynthesis 15
Patrick Blez, Jean-Luc Kahn

Chapter 4 Principles and Technique of Lag Screw Osteosynthesis 22
Herbert Niederdellmann, Vivek Shetty

Chapter 5 Implant Materials in Rigid Fixation: Physical, Mechanical, Corrosion, and Biocompatibility Considerations 28
David E. Altobelli

Chapter 6 The Potential of Resorbable Biomaterials for Skeletal Fixation 57
Rudolf R.M. Bos, Frederik R. Rozema, Geert Boering, Albert J. Pennings

Chapter 7 The Effects of Mandibular Immobilization on the Masticatory System: A Review 63
Edward Ellis, III, David S. Carlson

PART II IMPLANT SYSTEMS FOR RIGID FIXATION OF THE CRANIOMAXILLOFACIAL SKELETON 77

Chapter 8 Specifications, Indications, and Clinical Applications of the Luhr Vitallium Maxillofacial Systems 79
Hans G. Luhr

Chapter 9 Champy's System 116
Jean Luc Kahn, Michael Khouri
Translated to English from French
by Patrick Blez

Chapter 10 The AO/ASIF Maxillofacial Implant System 124
Michael J. Yaremchuk, Joachim Prein

Chapter 11 The Würzburg Titanium System for Rigid Fixation of the Craniomaxillofacial Skeleton 134
Jürgen F. Reuther

Chapter 12 The ITI Dental Implant System™ (Bonefit®) 152
André Schroeder, Franz Sutter, Daniel Buser

Chapter 13 Osteointegration and Rigid Fixation 163
Rickard Brånemark, Richard Skalak, P-I Brånemark

Part III CLINICAL APPLICATIONS
Trauma — 177

Chapter 14 Rigid Internal Fixation of Mandibular Fractures — 179
Michael J. Yaremchuk, Paul N. Manson

Chapter 15 Lag Screws in Mandibular Fractures — 187
Herbert Niederdellmann, Vivek Shetty

Chapter 16 Rigid Fixation of Complex Mandibular Fractures — 195
Joseph S. Gruss

Chapter 17 Open Reduction and Rigid Fixation of Subcondylar Fractures — 209
Thomas S. Jeter, Fred L. Hackney

Chapter 18 Complications of Rigid Internal Fixation of the Mandible — 217
Joseph S. Gruss

Chapter 19 Management of Infected Fractures and Nonunions of the Mandible — 233
Roland R. Schmoker

Chapter 20 Rigid Fixation of Le Fort Maxillary Fractures — 245
Joseph S. Gruss, John H. Phillips

Chapter 21 Rigid Fixation of Zygomatic Fractures — 263
Joseph S. Gruss, John H. Phillips

Chapter 22 Rigid Fixation of Nasoethmoid-orbital Fractures — 283
Joseph S. Gruss

Chapter 23 Rigid Fixation of Orbital Fractures — 302
Oleh M. Antonyshyn

Chapter 24 Reconstruction of the Internal Orbit Using Rigid Fixation Techniques — 317
Michael J. Yaremchuk, Paul N. Manson

Chapter 25 Rigid Fixation of Frontal Bone Fractures — 323
Michael J. Yaremchuk, Paul N. Manson

Chapter 26 Rigid Fixation of Panfacial Injuries — 330
Bernard Markowitz

Chapter 27 Rigid Fixation of Complex Gunshot Wounds — 338
Joseph S. Gruss

Chapter 28 Complications in the Rigid Fixation of Midface Fractures — 351
Leon A. Assael

Chapter 29 Craniofacial Osteotomies and Rigid Fixation in the Correction of Post-Traumatic Craniofacial Deformities — 357
Joseph S. Gruss

Chapter 30 The Use of Rigid Fixation in Secondary Post-Traumatic Cranio-Orbital Reconstruction — 371
Ian T. Jackson

Chapter 31 The Use of Rigid Fixation in Post-Traumatic Maxillary and Mandibular Reconstruction — 379
Steven R. Cohen, Henry K. Kawamoto, Jr.

Chapter 32 The Role of Plate and Screw Fixation in the Treatment of Pediatric Facial Fractures — 396
Jeffrey C. Posnick

Part III CLINICAL APPLICATIONS
Orthognathic Surgery — 421

Chapter 33 Rigid Fixation of the Le Fort I and the Sagittal Split Ramus Osteotomies — 423
William H. Bell

Chapter 34 Rigid Fixation in Combined Surgery of the Maxilla and Mandible — 451
Joseph G. McCarthy, P. Craig Hobar, Barry H. Grayson

Chapter 35 Rigid Fixation and Bone Substitutes in Orthognathic Surgery: Stable Expansion of the Facial Skeleton — 461
Harvey M. Rosen

Chapter 36 The Role of Plate and Screw Fixation in the Treatment of Cleft Lip and Palate Jaw Deformities — 466
Jeffrey C. Posnick, Mark P. Ewing

Chapter 37 The Use of Rigid Fixation for Cleft Lip and Palate — 486
David S. Precious

Chapter 38 Orthodontic Considerations and
            Rigid Fixation   500
            James L. Ackerman, Harvey M. Rosen

PART III   CLINICAL APPLICATIONS
           Congenital Craniofacial Deformities   505

Chapter 39 Stability of Skeletal Fixation in
            Congenital Craniofacial Surgery   507
            Jean-Francois Tulasne, Paul Tessier

Chapter 40 The Role of Plate and Screw
            Fixation in the Treatment of Craniofacial
            Malformations   512
            Jeffrey C. Posnick

Chapter 41 Variations in Osteotomy Design
            to Facilitate Rigid Fixation in Craniofacial
            Surgery   527
            Craig R. Dufresne

Chapter 42 Rigid Fixation of Le Fort III
            Osteotomies   545
            *Joseph G. McCarthy, P. Craig Hobar,
            Barry H. Grayson*

Chapter 43 Rigid Fixation in Block
            Orbitofacial Advancement and Facial
            Bipartition Osteotomies   553
            Antonio Fuente del Campo

Chapter 44 Advantages of the Subcranial
            Approach in Craniofacial Surgery   561
            Joram Raveh, Thierry Vuillemin

Chapter 45 The Use of Rigid Fixation in the
            Treatment of Facial Asymmetries   582
            Bahman Guyuron

PART III   CLINICAL APPLICATIONS
           Tumors   593

Chapter 46 The Mandibular Reconstruction
            System (MRS) in Ablative Tumor
            Surgery   595
            Hans G. Luhr, Juergen Lentrodt

Chapter 47 Mandible Reconstruction for
            Tumor Defects Using AO Plates and the
            THORP   605
            Douglas Klotch

Chapter 48 Use of the Reconstruction Plate
            in Complex Tumor Reconstruction   612
            M. Jean Davidson, Patrick J. Gullane

Chapter 49 The Titanium Hollow-Screw
            Reconstruction Plate System (THORP)   620
            *Joram Raveh, Franz Sutter,
            Thierry Vuillemin*

Chapter 50 Three-Dimensional Mandibular
            Reconstruction with Vascularized Bone
            Grafts   637
            David A. Hidalgo

Chapter 51 Total Functional Mandibular
            Reconstruction Using Vascularized Bone
            Grafts, Osteointegrated Implants, and Rigid
            Fixation   648
            Frederick Lukash

Chapter 52 The Role of Plate and Screw
            Fixation in the Management of Pediatric
            Head and Neck Tumors   656
            Jeffrey C. Posnick

Chapter 53 Unusual Applications of Plating   671
            Joseph S. Gruss

Index   681

Contributors

James L. Ackerman, D.D.S.
Private Practice of Orthodontics
Bryn Mawr, PA

David E. Altobelli, D.M.D., M.D.
Instructor in Oral and Maxillofacial Surgery
Department of Oral and Maxillofacial Surgery
Harvard School of Dental Medicine
Boston, MA 02115
Craniofacial Centre
Children's Hospital
Boston, MA 02115

Oleh Antonyshyn, M.D., F.R.C.S. (C)
Assistant Professor
Division of Plastic Surgery
Dalhousie University
Halifax, Nova Scotia, Canada

Leon A. Assael, D.M.D.
Associate Professor and Residency Program Director
Department of Oral and Maxillofacial Surgery
University of Connecticut Health Center
Farmington, CT
Associate Chief of Staff
John Dempsey Hospital
Farmington, CT

William H. Bell, M.D., D.D.S.
Professor, University of Texas Southwestern Medical Center at Dallas

Patrick Blez, M.D.
Assistant
Department of Maxillofacial Surgery
University Hospital (Hopitel Civil)
Strasbourg France

G. Boering, D.D.S., Ph.D.
Professor and Chairman
Department of Oral and Maxillofacial Surgery
University of Groningen
Groningen / The Netherlands
Professor and Chairman
Department of Oral and Maxillofacial Surgery
University Hospital
Groningen / The Netherlands

Rudolf R.R.M. Bos, D.D.S., Ph.D.
Associate Professor
Department of Oral and Maxillofacial Surgery
University of Groningen
Groningen / The Netherlands
Chef de Clinique and Vice Chairman
Department of Oral and Maxillofacial Surgery
University Hospital
Groningen / The Netherlands

Per-Ingvar Brånemark, M.D., Ph.D., OD.hc, M.D.hc, Sc.D.hc.
Professor
The Institute for Applied Biotechnology
Göteborg Sweden

ix

Rickard Brånemark, M.D., M.Sc.
M.D.
The Institute for Applied Biotechnology
Gothenburg / Sweden

Laboratory of Exp Biology, Department of
   Anatomy
University of Göteborg
Göteborg Sweden

Daniel Buser, Dr. Med. Dent.
Associate Professor
Department of Oral Surgery
School of Dental Medicine, University of Berne
Berne, Switzerland

David S. Carlson, Ph.D.
Professor
Department of Orthodontics and Pediatric
   Dentistry
University of Michigan School of Dentistry
Ann Arbor, MI

Steven Cohen, M.D.
Service Chief, Pediatric Surgery
Director, Craniofacial Anomalies Program
University of Michigan Medical Center
Ann Arbor, Michigan

Assistant Professor
Section of Plastic and Reconstructive Surgery
University of Michigan Medical Center
Ann Arbor, Michigan

M. Jean Davidson, M.D., F.R.C.S.C.
Assistant Professor
Department of Otolaryngology
University of Toronto
Toronto, Ontario, Canada

Otolaryngologist
Department of Otolaryngology
St. Michael's Hospital
Toronto, Ontario, Canada

Graig R. Dufresne, M.D., F.A.C.S.
Clinical Assistant Professor
Department of Plastic Surgery, Neurosurgery
The Johns Hopkins Hospital
Baltimore, MD

Director, Center for Facial Rehabilitation
Department of Plastic Surgery
Fairfax Hospital
Falls Church, VA

Edward Ellis III, D.D.S., M.S.
Associate Professor
Department of Oral and Maxillofacial Surgery
University of Texas Southwestern Medical Center
Dallas, TX

Parkland Memorial Hospital
Dallas, Texas

Mark Ewing, M.D.
Former Orthodontic Fellow
Department of Dentistry
The Hospital for Sick Children
Toronto, Ontario, Canada

Private Practice
Hamilton, New Zealand

Antonio Fuente-del-Campo, M.D., F.A.C.S.
Professor of Craniomaxillofacial Surgery
Department of Plastic and Reconstructive Surgery
Universidad Nacional Autonoma de Mexico
Mexico City

Plastic and Reconstructive Surgeon
Department of Plastic and Reconstructive Surgery
Hospital General "De Manuel Gea Gonzalez," S.S.
Mexico City

Barry H. Grayson, D.D.S.
Associate Professor
Department of Orthodontics
New York University College of Dentistry
New York, NY

Associate Professor of Clinical Surgery
Department of Reconstructive Plastic Surgery
New York Medical Center
New York, NY

Joseph S. Gruss, MB., F.R.C.S. (C).
Professor of Surgery, Division of Plastic Surgery
Department of Surgery
University of Washington
Seattle, WA

Attending Plastic and Craniofacial Surgeon
Department of Surgery
Harbourview Medical Centre and
   Childrens Hospital and Medical Centre
Seattle, WA

Patrick J. Gullane, M.B., F.R.C.S. (C), F.A.C.S.
Associate Professor
Department of Otolaryngology,
Toronto General Hospital
University of Toronto
Toronto Ontario

Bahman Guyuron, M.D.
Associate Clinical Professor of Surgery
Department of Surgery
Case Western Reserve University
Cleveland, OH

Chief
Division of Plastic Surgery
The Mt. Sinai Medical Center
Cleveland, OH

Fred L. Hackney, D.D.S., M.D.
Resident
Department of Surgery
Vanderbilt University Medical Center
Nashville, TN

David A. Hidalgo, M.D.
Assistant Professor of Surgery
Department of Plastic and Reconstructive Surgery
Cornell Medical College
New York, NY

Assistant Attending Surgeon
Department of Plastic and Reconstructive Surgery
Memorial Sloan-Kettering Cancer Center
New York, NY

P. Craig Hobar, M.D.
Assistant Professor/Director of Pediatric Plastic
 Surgery and Craniofacial Surgery
Department of Surgery/Division of Plastic Surgery
University of Texas Southwestern Medical Center
 at Dallas
Dallas, TX

**Ian T. Jackson M.D., F.R.C.S., F.A.C.S.,
F.R.A.C.S. (Hon)**
Director
Institute of Craniofacial and Reconstructive Surgery
Providence Hospital
Southfield, MI

Thomas S. Jeter, D.D.S., M.D.
Clinical Professor
Department of Oral and Maxillofacial Surgery
University of Texas Health Science Center
San Antonio, TX

Private Practice
San Angelo, TX

Michael Khouri, M.D.
Department of Maxillofacial Surgery
Hopitol Univseritaire
Strousbourg France

Jean-Luc Kahn, M.D.
Maitre de Conférences
Department of Anatomy
University ULP
Strasbourg France

Praticien Hospitolier
Department of Maxillofacial Surgery
Hopitol Univseritaire
Strasbourg France

Henry K. Kawamoto Jr., M.D., D.D.S.
Clinical Professor, Division of Plastic Surgery
Department of Surgery
University of California at Los Angeles
Los Angeles, CA 90024

Douglas W. Klotch, M.D., F.A.C.S.
Associate Professor of Surgery
Department of Surgery/Otolaryngology
University of South Florida
Tampa, FL

Associate Professor of Surgery
Department of Surgery
H. Lee Moffitt Cancer Center
Tampa, FL

Hans G. Luhr, M.D., D.M.D.
Professor and Chairman
Department of Maxillofacial Surgery
University Hospital Goettingen
Goettingen, Germany

Frederick Neil Lukash, M.D.
Assistant Clinical Professor Surgery
Department of Plastic Surgery
Albert Einstein College of Medicine
New York, NY

Attending Surgeon
Department of Surgery, Division of Plastic Surgery
Long Island Jewish Medical Center
New Hyde Park, NY

Joseph J. McCarthy, M.D.
Lawrence D. Bell Professor of Plastic Surgery
Department of Surgery (Plastic Surgery)
New York University Medical Center
New York, NY

Director, Institute of Reconstructive Plastic Surgery
Department of Surgery (Plastic Surgery)
New York University Medical Center
New York, NY

Paul N. Manson, M.D.
Professor and Chairman of Plastic Surgery
The Johns Hopkins Medical Institutions
Baltimore, Maryland

Bernard L. Markowitz, M.D.
Assistant Professor
Department of Surgery
Division of Plastic and Reconstructive Surgery
UCLA Medical Center
Los Angeles, CA
Chief, Division of Plastic and Reconstructive Surgery
Department of Surgery
Olive View Medical Center
Sylmar, CA

Herbert Niederdellmann, M.D., D.M.D.
Professor and Chairman
Department of Oral, Maxillo and Facial Plastic Surgery
Regensburg University
Germany

Albert J. Pennings, M.S.C., Ph.D.
Professor and Chairman
Department of Polymer Chemistry
University of Groningen
Groningen / The Netherlands

John H. Phillips, M.D., F.R.C.S. (C)
Assistant Professor
Department of Surgery, Division of Plastic Surgery
University of Toronto
Toronto, Ontario, Canada
Active Staff
Division of Plastic Surgery
Sunnybrook Health Science Centre
Toronto, Ontario, Canada

Jeffrey C. Posnick, D.M.D., M.D., F.R.C.S. (C), F.A.C.S.
Assistant Professor
Department of Surgery
University of Toronto
Assistant Professor
Faculty of Dentistry
University of Toronto
Medical Director, Craniofacial Program
Division of Plastic Surgery
The Hospital for Sick Children
Toronto, Ontario, Canada

David S. Precious, D.D.S., M.Sc., F.R.C.D. (C) F.A.D.I., F.I.C.D.
Professor
Department of Maxillofacial Surgery
Dalhousie University
Halifax, Nova Scotia, Canada
Head of Department
Department of Maxillofacial Surgery
Victoria General Hospital
Halifax, Nova Scotia, Canada

Joachim Prein, M.D., D.D.S.
Professor of Maxillofacial Surgery
Head of Clinic for Plastic and Reconstructive Surgery
University Clinic of Basel
Basel, Switzerland

Burton A. Rahn, M.D., D.M.D.
Professor, University of Freiburg
Freiburg, West Germany
Director, Laboratory for Experimental Surgery
Swiss Research Institute
Davos, Switzerland

J. Raveh, M.D., D.M.D., Professor
Head of Department
Department of Maxillofacial Surgery
University Hospital, Inselspital
3010—Bern, Switzerland

Jürgen F. Reuther, M.D., D.M.D., Ph.D.
Full Professor and Head of Clinic for Cranio- and Maxillofacial Surgery
University of Würzburg
Würzburg, Germany

Harvey M. Rosen, M.D., D.M.D.
Associate Clinical Professor of Surgery
Department of Surgery
University of Pennsylvania
Philadelphia, PA
Chief, Division of Plastic Surgery
Department of Surgery
Pennsylvania Hospital
Philadelphia, PA

F.R. Rozema, D.D.S. Ph.D.
Resident
Department of Oral and Maxillofacial Surgery
University Hospital
Groningen / The Netherlands

Roland R. Schmoker, M.D., D.M.D.
Plastic and Reconstructive Surgeon
Department of Maxillofacial Surgery
Lindenhofspital
Berne, Switzerland

André Schroeder, Dr., Med. Dent., Dr.h.c.
Full Professor Emeritus
Former Head of Department of Operative Dentistry
School of Dental Medicine, University of Berne
Berne, Switzerland

Vivek Shetty, D.D.S., Dr. Med. Dent.
Assistant Professor
Department of Oral and Maxillofacial Surgery
UCLA School of Dentistry
Los Angeles, CA

Richard Skalak, Ph.D., Professor
Professor
Department of Applied Mechanics and Engineering Science
University of California
La Jolla, CA

Franz Sutter, Dr.h.c.
Dr.h.c./Affiliated to the University of Bern
Bern, Switzerland
Senior
Research Institute
Stratec Medical
Waldenburg, BL, Switzerland
Director of Engineering
Department of Technology
Straumann Research Institute
Ch-4437 Waldenburg, Switzerland

Paul Tessier, M.D.
Private Practice
Paris, France

Jean Francois Tulasne, M.D.
Private Practice
Paris, France

Thierry Vuillemin, M.D., D.M.D.
Lecturer
Department of Craniomaxillofacial Surgery
Msel Hospital, University of Bern
Bern, Switzerland
Senior Member of Staff
Department of Craniomaxillofacial Surgery
University Hospital, Inselspital
Bern, Switzerland

Michael J. Yaremchuk, M.D., F.A.C.S.
Assistant Professor of Plastic Surgery
Harvard Medical School
Cambridge, MA
Associate Plastic Surgeon
Department of Surgery
Massachusetts General Hospital
Boston, MA

Preface

The late 1960s and early 1970s marked the beginning of a revolution in the surgery of the facial skeleton. During that time, the European maxillofacial surgeons, Hans Luhr and Bernd Spiessl, working independently, performed the laboratory and clinical investigations to show the efficacy of plate and screw fixation of mandibular fractures. This method of fixation performed after open reduction provided, for the first time, a means of counteracting dynamic biomechanical forces to maintain anatomic alignment in function and allowed mobilization in the early phases of bone healing. The fixation was secure, obviating the need for external stabilization through maxillomandibular fixation with its attendant morbidity.

Later, miniaturized midface and microfixation systems were designed for the thinner bones of the mid and upper face. Here, plates and screws provide sufficient stability to counteract soft tissue deforming forces and allow precise, stable, three-dimensional restoration or rearrangement of the facial skeleton. Rigid internal fixation by plates and screws has redefined the treatment of traumatic, congenital, and ablative facial skeletal deformities.

The objective of *Rigid Fixation of the Craniomaxillofacial Skeleton* is to provide a comprehensive clinical reference for the use of plates and screws, as applied to all aspects of facial skeletal surgery. The book provides the biologic and biomechanical principles of the various implant systems as well as the nuances of their design and use. It provides an atlas of surgical procedures and diagnostic and clinical guidelines for their application. The book is written by many surgeons, from various disciplines, who are at the forefront of the development and refinement of plate and screw fixation techniques. Because implant systems and their applications continue to be refined daily, the reader will certainly note areas of controversy in addition to individual prejudice and preference.

It has been a privilege for us to work with this group of authors whose clinical insight and creativity have helped elevate surgery of the facial skeleton to its present level. We thank the editorial staff at Butterworth–Heinemann for their professionalism and attention to detail, Carmella Clifford for many of the illustrations, Barbara Parisi, RN and Margie Gallo for their tireless help in this project.

Michael J. Yaremchuk
Joseph S. Gruss
Paul N. Manson

PART I

Basic Concepts of Rigid Fixation

CHAPTER 1

Bone Healing

John H. Phillips
Berton A. Rahn

Bone is a dynamic tissue constantly undergoing both resorption and production. These processes are in a steady state that is regulated by many factors, both mechanical and physiologic.

MICROANATOMY

Bone is composed of cells, matrix, and mineral. The cells consist of osteoblasts, osteocytes, and osteoclasts. The organic matrix comprises 35% of bone and consists 95% as collagen and 5% as proteoglycans and low-molecular-weight proteins. The other 65% of bone exists as calcium-phosphate crystals laid down as hydroxyapatite.

Osteoblasts are derived from mesenchymal precursors. They deposit osteoid, the organic matrix of bone, which is converted into calcified bone at the calcification front. A layer of 1 micron of osteoid may be produced per day (bone apposition rate), followed by a maturation phase of 10 days prior to calcification. The mean width of an osteoid seam is, therefore, 10 microns. The two conditions necessary for bone formation and mineralization are ample vascular supply and mechanical rest.

Osteoclasts are multinucleated giant cells thought to originate from the fusion of mononuclear macrophages. The activity of the osteoclast is limited to Howship's lacunae (which are small subcellular chambers). Within this chamber a low pH is maintained by the production of hydrochloric acid, which dissolves the mineral. The organic matrix is degraded by the release of proteases and collagenase. Osteoclasts are able to resorb 50 to 100 microns of bone per day.

Osteocytes do not produce osteoid or multiply; however, they do take part in the calcium exchange between body fluids and bone.

The structure of bone is determined by its mechanical and metabolic function. The adaption to stress is reflected macroscopically by the shape and thickness of the cortex, as well as by the density and orientation of the trabeculae.

The basic building block of bone is the *osteon*, which is based on the vascular supply and on a network of canaliculi and lacunae, which extend from the surface into the deeper layers of the intercellular substance. The osteons are nutritional units consisting of a wall of concentric lamellae deposited around a vascular canal called a haversian canal. The osteocytes are lodged within these units and contact neighboring cells with their cytoplasmic processes, thereby forming an intercellular transport system. The reach of this transport system is 100 microns. This limits the diameter of the osteon to approximately 200 microns (Color Plate 1).

STRUCTURAL CHARACTERISTICS OF FACIAL BONE

Bones from different regions of the body show relatively small differences in their material properties when they are tested in small, standardized samples. The major difference is produced by the amount and the geometric distribution of the bone. The midface skeleton consists of thin lamina. The mechanics of the facial bones are determined by the arrangement of the thin bone layers in a three-dimensional structural frame. These are comparable to lightweight "honeycomb" constructions, in which a series of weak elements provides good mechanical properties, as long as the elements are loaded in the application for which they were designed and as long as their structure remains intact.

In the thin bone of the face, there is a relative increase in the surface area per unit of bone volume as compared to long bone. With this large surface, the bone tissue can react faster to a changing situation than can compact bone. On the level of cellular behavior, there are no principle differences.

Even though facial bone is of mesenchymal derivative—that is, facial bones undergo a direct bone formation without intervening cartilaginous formation, whereas long bone is of enchondral origin—there is no evident reason why after remodeling, or after replacement of primary bone to new bony tissue, there should be any significant difference in the material properties of one versus the other. The more obvious difference would relate to the surface area as related to the volume. In the thin facial bone, as in cancellous bone, the distance to the closest vessels and the surrounding soft tissue is shorter. The reconstitution to the circulatory system may occur faster. This may lead to the increased rate of healing of facial bone over some long bones.

The differences found in the mechanical and biological behavior of facial bones seem to be related to the geometric arrangement of the bone rather than to differences in the material itself.

INDIRECT BONE HEALING

The basic functions of bone are to carry load and to support and protect organs. The strength and rigidity of bone are, therefore, its prime qualities. After a fracture takes place, the continuity of the bone is destroyed and the normal force transmission through the bone is no longer possible. Any external dynamic forces of bending or torque will lead to displacement of the fracture ends. Due to these external dynamic forces, shortening as well as angular and rotational deviations may occur. Initially, fractions are immobilized by the patient who is in pain. Other factors, such as concomitant injuries to nerves overlying skin and soft tissue, may complicate the normal healing process of bone. This rupture of vessels in surrounding soft tissue, as well as in the bone itself, leads to hematoma that may add to the stability of the fracture. This vascular interruption of the larger vessels of the surrounding soft tissue may impede regional bone nutrition, which is also complicated by thrombosis of the vessels of the haversian and Volkmann's canals over a distance of a few millimeters from the fragment ends.

Bone does not necessarily need to be treated to unite, but function may be impaired as a result of any subsequent angulation or rotational deformity. The main aim of fracture treatment is to obtain a final function that is as close to the prefracture situation as possible. Different methods of treatment exist, which result in different degrees of fracture immobilization. The choice of method depends on the requirements of that local situation, as well as on expected outcome.

Biomechanical Aspects

An understanding of the biomechanics related to strain and tissue induction is essential to the understanding of direct and indirect bone healing. The elongation at rupture is a parameter that characterizes the tolerance of a tissue to deformation. It gives information on how much relative deformation a tissue can tolerate before breaking. Granulation tissue can act as a rubber band in elongating to twice its original length; however, because of its lack of rigidity it is unable to resist motion and will break under low tensile stress. Cortical bone will rupture when elongated only 2% (Perren 1979).

During the course of healing, different types of tissues can be seen in the fracture area, gradually substituting for one another. This leads to a gradual increase stiffness and strength and a gradual decrease in tolerance to deformation.

When external dynamic forces are applied across a fracture by the pull of muscles attached to the bone involved, the dynamic deformation of the interfragmentary tissue is many times greater than can be tolerated by bone. It is then understandable that the initial repair tissue to form is fibrous tissue, which can tolerate 100% of strain before rupture. The fibrous tissue formation and its replacement of the initial hematoma result in an increase in stiffness, thereby decreasing the amount of movement at the fracture site for the same external dynamic force. This results in less movement at the fracture site and a decrease in strain condition, which then allows for cartilage formation.

Fibrous tissue, tendon, and cartilage tolerate appreciably smaller amounts of elongation and have a nonlinear stress/strain relation. The strength of the tissue is its capacity to withstand force without rupture. Granulation in tissue can withstand 0.01 kg/mm^2, cartilage 1.5 kg/mm^2, and bone 13 kg/mm^2 (Schenk and Willenegger 1963). This is inversely related to their ability to tolerate strain (elongation). The rigidity of these repair tissues correlate to the strength of the tissue. The rigidity is the capacity to fight deformation and therefore motion. This nonlinear relation favors reduction of relative motion at the fracture site for the same amount of external dynamic force (Color Plates 2 and 3).

In spontaneously healing bone and in healing under relative fixation (for example, casting), fragment-end shortening due to resorption is a common phenomenon (see Color Plate 2). If the reduction of interfragmentary strain is the goal or prerequisite for the progression of fibrous tissue to cartilage to bone formation and fracture healing, then fragment-end resorption is adaptive. It reduces the interfragmentary strain for a given amount

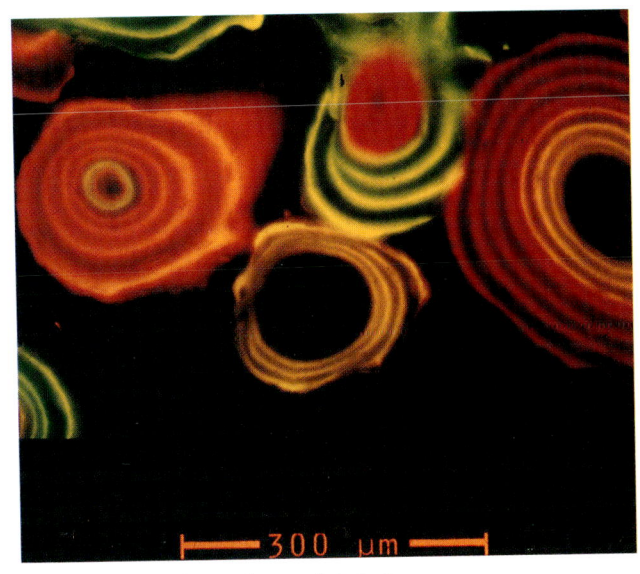

Color Plate 1 Fluorochrome-labeled osteons.

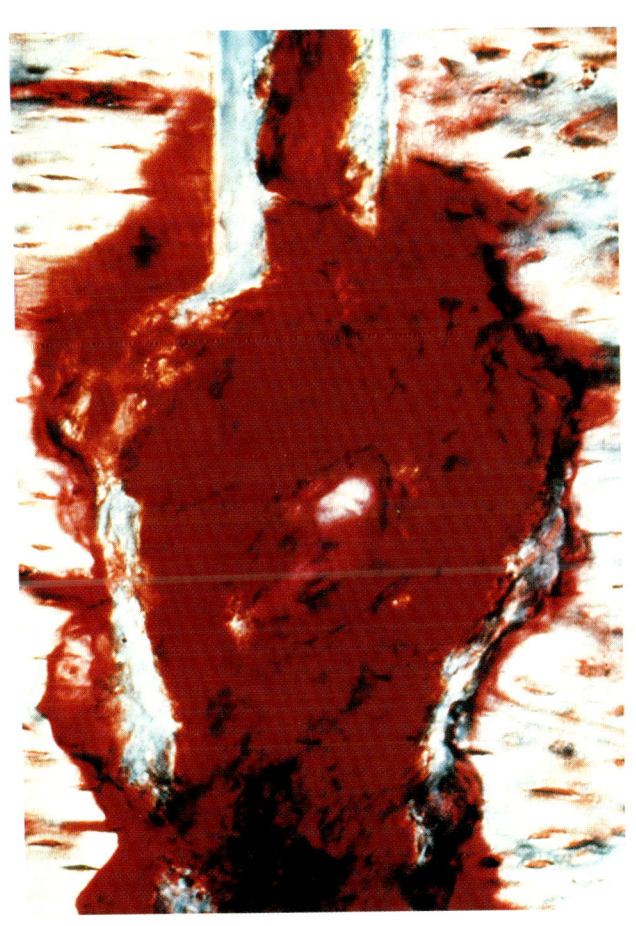

Color Plate 2 Fragment end resorption in an osteotomy where movement was allowed. This results in the reduction of interfragmentary strain.

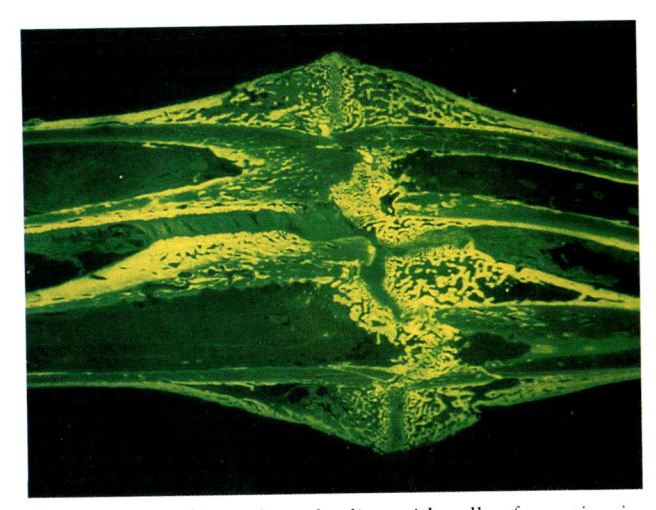

Color Plate 3 Indirect bone healing with callus formation in long bone. The rigidity of the tissue increases with the fourth power of the distance from the center of rotation or bending.

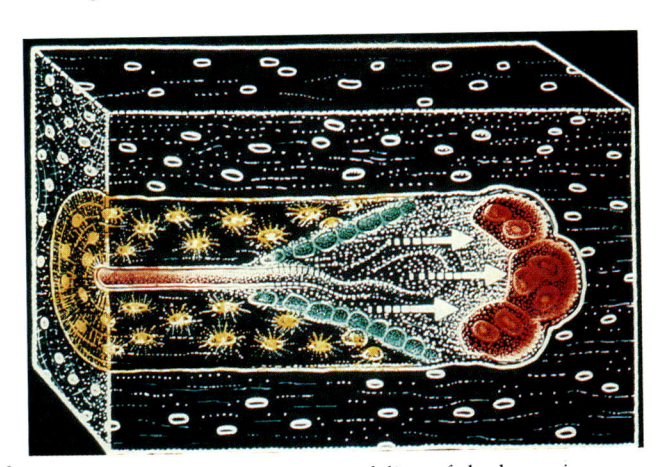

Color Plate 4 Cutting cone remodeling of the haversian canal. These contain osteoclasts and a conical surface of osteoblasts, which lay down new bone.

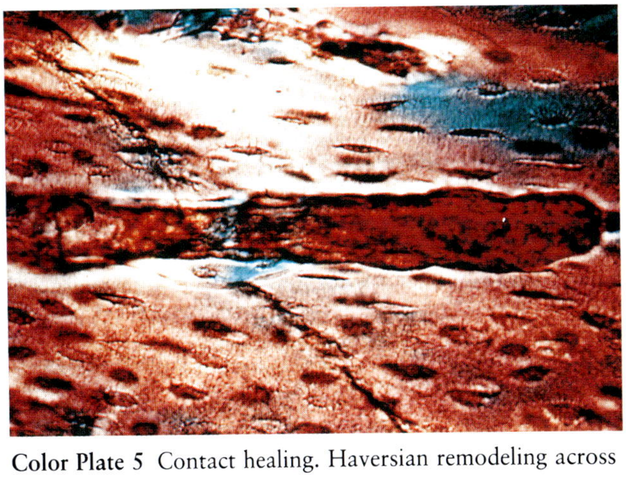

Color Plate 5 Contact healing. Haversian remodeling across a bony osteotomy.

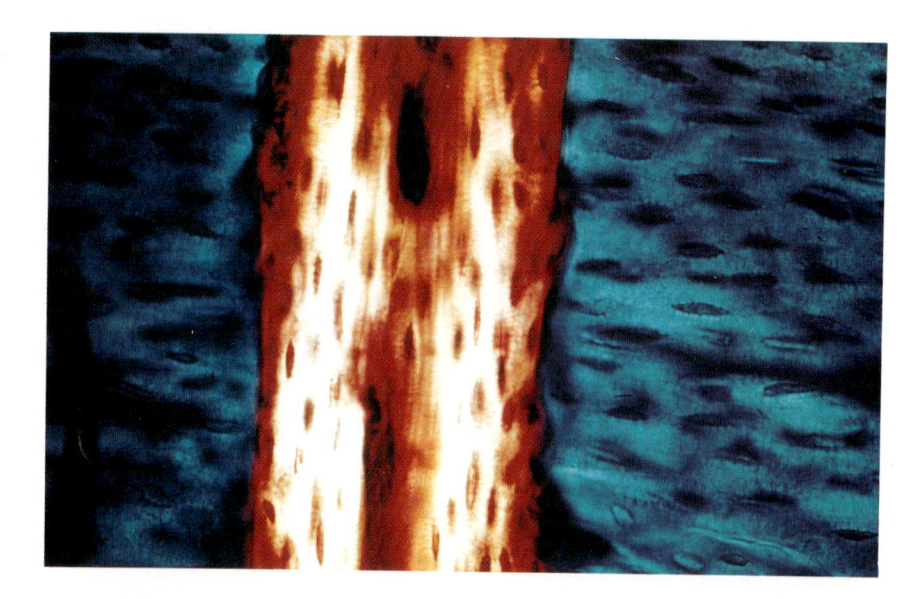

Color Plate 6 Gap healing. Sagittal bone deposition (red) in a gap between two fragment ends under the condition of absolute stability. This bone is deposited at right angles to its normal direction within the cortex.

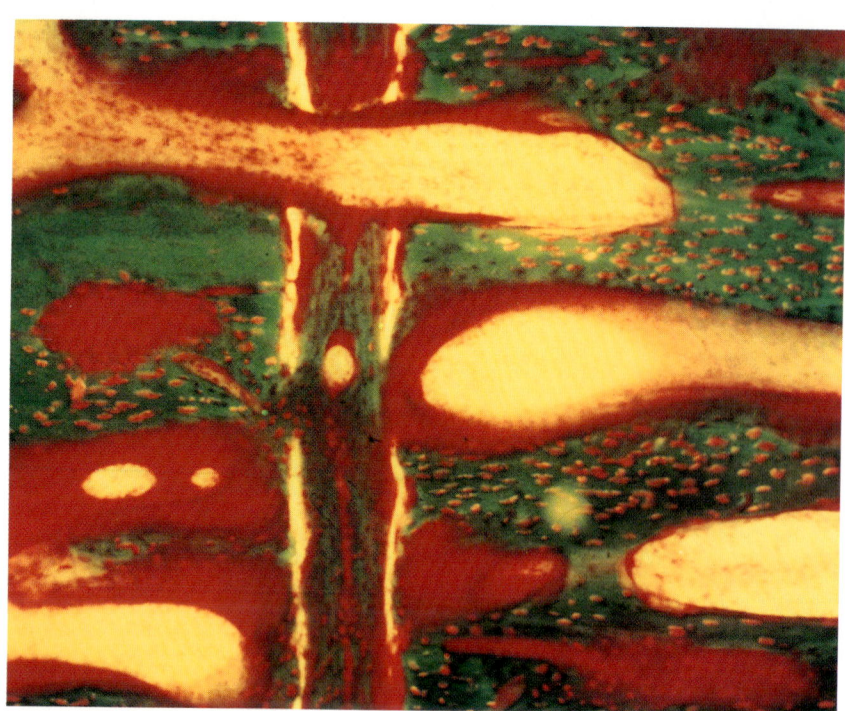

Color Plate 7 Gap healing. In a second stage, the sagittal bone is replaced by cutting cone remodeling of the haversian system along the axis of the bone.

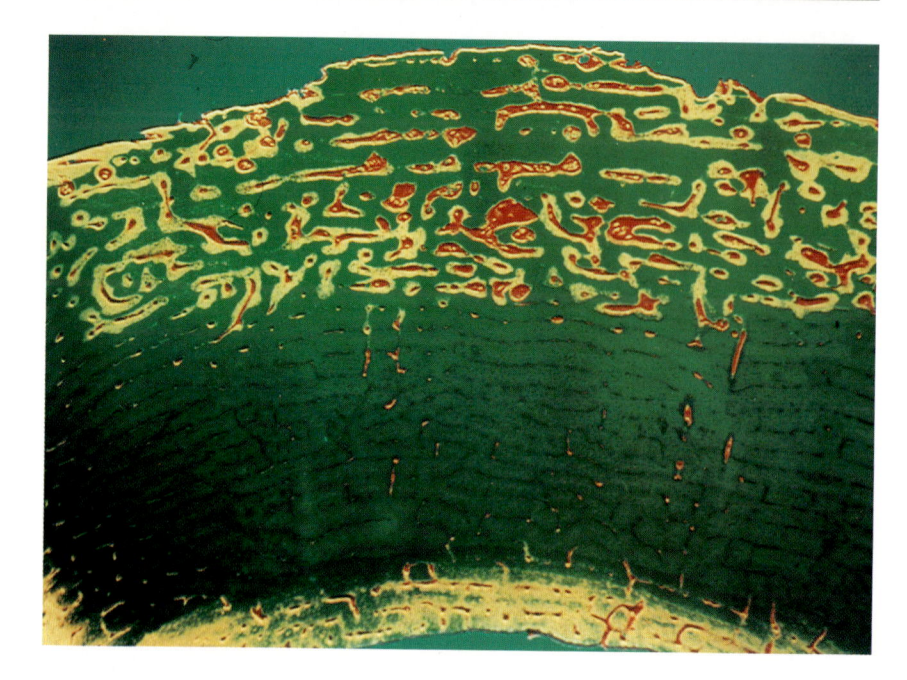

Color Plate 8 Plate-induced porosis. The plate interferes with circulation at the bone surface, leading to retrograde vessel thrombosis and subsequent bone resorption.

of motion because it depends on motion and gap width [strain = (gap length/change in gap length) × 100]. In a small gap, the ratio of the change in width to the total width is high (strain condition is high). The cells in the gap undergo high deformation. For the same angular deformation in an initially wider gap, the deformation of the cellular elements is much smaller, because the change in width is distributed over a larger distance, and therefore the single elements have to take over only part of the total change. The occurrence of surface resorption makes sense in secondary bone healing.

Another mechanism found to decrease interfragmentary strain in a spontaneously healing bone fracture is that of increasing the cross-sectional diameter at the fracture site due to the formation of callus. This increase in diameter provides the tissue with better leverage in respect to external dynamic forces of bending and torque. The rigidity of the tissue increases to the fourth power at the distance from the center of rotation or bending. Internal (endosteal) callus is less efficient than interfragmentary bone, which is less efficient than external (periosteal) callus (see Color Plate 3).

A tissue can be formed in the fracture gap only if the tissue formed tolerates the strain present. Once a tissue is formed, it will, in turn, due to its increased rigidity, decrease the motion in gap due to external dynamic loading and will reduce strain. Thus, the next step of tissue differentiation may be made possible. The deformation of fibrous tissue may reduce the strain to a level where cartilage formation is possible; and the formation of cartilage, which is more rigid than fibrous tissue, may further drop the strain condition to a level conducive to bone formation. If the biological stabilization is not able to prevent the interfragmentary motion caused by muscle contraction or external load, then delayed union or nonunion will result. This fracture healing by callus formation has been called *indirect bone healing*.

After the fracture site is bridged by fibrous bone, stability is obtained and some function is possible. Haversian remodeling then begins to reconstruct the lamellar direction of the bone, parallel to the long axis of the limb. The diameter of the callus is thereby reduced and in areas of the medullary cavity of the bone becomes less dense.

Mechanical Principles Associated with Fracture Fixation

The oldest type of fracture fixation is the use of wood splints. Due to its rigidity, the wood splint decreases the motion at the fracture site but does not completely abolish it. This is also true for plaster casts, which, if applied above and below the joints of the bone involved, may decrease torsion but still allow for axial movement.

Internal fixation devices, such as K wires and plates, applied without compression provide similar support but do not abolish all movement. Splintage using these methods relies on the rigidity of the splint. A pure splint fixation will always permit some motion that is proportional to the load and inversely proportional to the overall stiffness of the device. Increasing the stiffness of an implant reduces, but does not completely abolish, motion and strain. If the external dynamic load is low and the gap width appropriate, bony union can take place. This, however, may be complicated by nonunion and fatigue of the implant (Figure 1.1).

Compression, when applied to fractured surfaces, results in preload and friction. The compression preloads the contact surfaces such that, under a functional bending load at the convex side of the bend, tension results and tries to pull the contact surfaces apart. The preload prevents such dislocation as long as the static compression is greater than the dynamic external forces that are applying the bending force. Compression also results in friction that stabilizes against shearing forces produced by torsion.

Compression may produce a condition called *absolute stability*, indicating that no relative motion is occurring at the location of interfragmentary contact. This happens if the dynamic external load does not exceed the level of preload or friction. If no movement occurs, the strain condition is zero in the gap. There is, then, a condition conducive to direct bone healing.

DIRECT BONE HEALING

When discussing direct bone healing, two areas must be addressed: (1) areas where the bone fragments are in contact and (2) areas where there are gaps between the bony fragment ends.

Contact Healing

Schenk and Willenegger (1963) have discussed the histological aspects of direct fracture healing. Direct fracture healing consists of direct bone formation with-

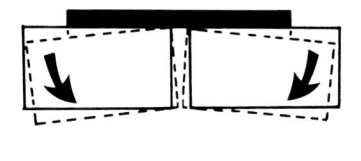

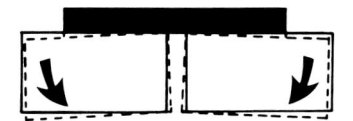

Figure 1.1 Without compression, the amount of movement in a fracture gap is proportional to the external load and inversely proportional to the stiffness of the implant.

out the classical multistage differentiation of connective tissue and cartilage. The direct union of the fragments in contact and under compression occurs by the remodeling of the haversian canals by *cutting cones* (Color Plate 4). These cutting cones contain osteoclasts and a conical surface of osteoblasts, which produce new osteons with incorporated new living osteocytes. These osteocytes are connected among themselves and to the vascular supply in the haversian canal by a network of canaliculi.

Haversian remodeling occurs in all fracture healing to achieve restoration of the original integrity. It is the only step needed in fracture healing under absolute stability (Color Plate 5).

Gap Healing

In closely adapted and compressed fracture surfaces, not all parts of the surface are in contact. Due to the nearby contact areas that are under load from compression, the gap areas are also under low strain. In the areas of gaps, sagittal bone is formed directly, deposited at right angles to its normal direction within the cortex. Final healing, therefore, takes place in two stages. First, sagittal bone is formed, then this bone is remodeled along the axis of the bone through haversian remodeling (Color Plates 6 and 7).

Although direct bone healing does not involve the intermediate stages of tissue differentiation, it is not faster than indirect bone healing with callus formation. Per unit of material, direct bone healing is more efficient than callus.

PLATE-INDUCED POROSIS

A plate interferes with the circulation of the underlying bone cortex (Gunst 1980). The reason for this locally disturbed circulation is not from compression of intracortical vessels, because bone tolerates only minimal deformation, but rather from a blockage in flow at the bone surface and eventual retrograde thrombosis (Color Plate 8).

Porosis found under plates contacting the bone has been called *stress protection*. The area of early porosis underneath the plate shows a relationship with the area of vascular damage (Gunst 1980). Many of the findings attributed to stress protection may be explained as sequelae of disturbed circulation.

PROBLEMS IN HEALING

The normal course of fracture healing may be complicated by infection. In the presence of instability and bacterial contamination, a part of the devitalized bone will not undergo remodeling. Intense bone resorption takes place at the border between supplied and nonsupplied bone, which leads to a sequestration of the nonsupplied parts.

The treatment of an infection is more efficient under stable conditions than in areas under continuing motion. It has been shown by Rittman and Perren (1974) that bony union can take place even in the presence of infection if stability of the fracture is provided. In the clinical situation, if an infected nonunion occurs in the area of open reduction and internal fixation of a fracture, most commonly the surgeon will find that the implant is loose. The appropriate treatment in this situation is a repeat of open reduction and internal fixation to assure stability.

Pseudarthrosis, or nonunion, is a second problem not uncommonly seen in fracture healing. It represents a standstill in the process of tissue differentiation. This may happen in the use of splints where the external dynamic forces are such that progressive tissue differentiation cannot occur, or in cases where the implant has not provided stability such as in the case of a loose implant. In these cases, additional stabilization is required for the resumption of the differentiation process and its continuation to the formation of bony union.

SUMMARY

The pattern of fracture healing depends on the mechanical situation at the fracture site. In cases of healing under nonrigid conditions, the healing process passes through different tissue stages with decreasing deformability and increasing stiffness and strength. Rigid internal fixation, on the other hand, provides preload and friction of fracture segments to counteract external dynamic forces and to allow direct bone formation to occur.

REFERENCES

Gunst MA: Interference with bone blood supply through plating of intact bone. In Current Concepts of Internal Fixation of Fractures. Uhtoff, HK (ed), Springer: Berlin, Heidelberg, New York, 1980.

Perren SM: Physical and biological aspects of fracture healing with special references to internal fixation. Clin Orthop 138:175–196, 1979.

Rittman WW, Perren SM: Cortical Bone Healing after Internal Fixation and Infection. Springer: Berlin, Heidelberg, New York, 1974.

Schenk R, Willenegger H: Histologie der primaren knocken heilung. Arch Klin Chir 19:593, 1963.

Spiessl B: Internal Fixation of the Mandible. Springer-Verlag: Berlin, Heidelberg, New York, 1989.

CHAPTER 2

Principles of Compression Osteosynthesis

John H. Phillips

There are two fundamentally different implant systems that are advocated for the treatment of mandibular fractures. One system extrapolates the AO principles originally developed for long bone fractures. It employs implants which substitute for the fractured bone during the healing process and assume the external strain placed on the bone. The system is designed for compression of fracture segments is a central feature of the system design. The biomechanical concepts in its design are the subject of this chapter. The other system is one derived from the work of Michelet (1973). It employs smaller plates and screws which are designed to neutralize unfavorable traction strains while at the same time allowing transmission of favorable compression forces. Screws purchase one cortex of the mandible. The biomechanical concepts of this system are presented in Chapter 3.

Bicortical internal fixation ensures stability by interfragmentary compression, which eliminates movements between the fracture surfaces, produces bony end contact, and reduces interfragmentary strain between the areas of contact to levels that allow for direct bone healing. This will occur as long as the stabilization that results from the use of the fixation devices is greater than the external dynamic forces generated by function. Stabilization is achieved by the use of plates and screws.

SCREWS

Compressive clamping of plate to bone (or bone to bone, in lag screw fixation) is the basis of fixation. The level of screw compression that is achieved before stripping of the bone thread or screw failure (fracture of the screw) determines the amount of functional load that is permitted while still preserving the rigid fixation for undisturbed bone healing. Stripping of the bone thread is the problem most often encountered during the insertion of a screw at surgery. This is especially a problem when working in thin cortical bone, as is found in the midfacial area.

The ability of the screw to provide this holding power is dependent on screw design, the changes in the bone as a result of screw insertion, reaction of the bone to the implant material, the resorption and remodeling of bone during fracture healing, and the reaction of bone to loading as a result of muscle forces.

Figure 2.1 demonstrates various screw parts. An essential element in the understanding of the use of

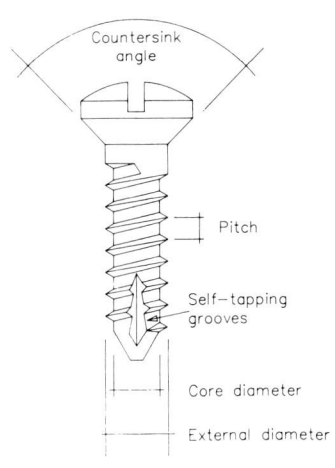

Figure 2.1 Basic screw design.

screws of the appropriate drill size is the core diameter, which is the internal diameter exclusive of the width of the threads. In general, the pilot hole drilled is slightly larger than the core diameter of the screw. The external diameter of the screw is the diameter from the tip of thread crest to the next thread crest. With the use of pretapped screws, the external diameter of the screw is the same as the size of the tap to be used. The pitch angle of the screw relates to the distance between threads. Pitch angle may vary from screw to screw of different external diameters.

The tensile stress in the screw is derived from the torque applied to the screw head by the screwdriver. The efficiency of the system may be regarded as the ease with which this applied torque is converted into tension in the screw.

There are two basic screw designs, pretapped and self-tapping screws. Pretapped screws have threads that are continuous all the way to the tip. The insertion of a pretapped screw requires two steps in hole preparation. Initially, a pilot hole is made with a drill that has a diameter slightly larger than the core diameter of the screw. Threads are then cut on the inside of this hole to accept the threads of the screw. This thread-cutting procedure is performed using a bone tap that usually has one to three large cutting channels (flutes) machined along a portion of its length. These flutes are wide enough to allow the bony debris generated in cutting the threads to fall through the channels to prevent binding.

The second type of screw, the self-tapping screw, comes in many varieties. Some have one to three cutting flutes machined in the tip; others may have conical tips or trocar tips; and others have a tip not significantly different from that of a pretapped screw. Insertion of a self-tapping screw requires the creation of a pilot hole that is drilled slightly larger than the core diameter of the screw. The screw is then inserted and cuts its own bone threads on the inner surface of the pilot hole.

Some controversies have arisen over the use of self-tapping screws. A 17–30% decrease in holding power of the fluted portion as compared to the fully threaded portion has been demonstrated. To avoid this loss, the screw must be inserted such that the cutting flutes extrude through the bone to maintain contact in only the area without flutes. This is a problem in hand and orthopedic surgery, where screw-tip protrusion may interfere with tendon gliding or extrude into soft tissue, causing pain. In maxillofacial surgery, this is not a problem because the screw tip can protrude safely into the maxillary antrum, frontal sinus, and nasal cavity.

More torque is required to insert a self-tapping screw than a pretapped screw due to cutting of the bone threads. It has been shown that tapping decreases insertional torque by 35–40%. This increased torque increases the stress placed on the screw, which can lead to screw failure (fracturing), as well as to increased stress on the surrounding bone, which may result in microfractures and subsequent screw loosening.

If a screw must be removed and then reinserted in the same hole at surgery, some authors have suggested that, due to their cutting ability, the risk of cross threading is increased with self-tapping screws.

It has been demonstrated that increased torque is required to remove self-tapping screws after healing has occurred, due to bone ingrowth into the fluted portion of the screw.

The literature shows little experimental evidence demonstrating any improved holding power or decrease in tissue damage using either type of screw in orthopedic surgery.

Recent research has demonstrated that for 1- and 2-millimeter bone thicknesses use of self-tapping screws resulted in the highest compression values (Phillips and Rahn 1989). This was thought to be due to the improved contact between the screw thread crest and the bone as compared to pretapped screws, where a gap of up to 150 micron exists. In thin bone only 1 to 3 thread crests may be in contact with bone. In 3- and 4-mm bone thicknesses, pretapped screws offered the highest compression values.

Whether the maximal compression values of one screw type versus another are significant in the clinical situation of maxillofacial surgery is unknown, as there has been little work looking at the functional forces in these areas. For these reasons, virtually all bone fixation of the facial skeleton outside of the mandible is done with self-tapping screws.

Other factors that may influence screw dynamics are materials from which the screw is made, surface finish, size, thread, head countersink, and screw orientation. It has been shown that the surface finish of a screw is an important factor in screw removal. Removal torque of screws with rough surfaces was approximately $8\times$ higher than that of polished screws (Claes, Hutzschenreuter and Pohier 1976).

External screw diameter has a direct relationship with holding power. This has been demonstrated theoretically as well as in long bone studies (Schatzker, Horne and Sumner-Smith 1975). Research in thin (1- and 2-mm) bone has not shown that increasing the screw diameter above 2 millimeters results in increased holding power (Phillips and Rahn 1989).

Bone screws are available with either buttress threads, V-threads, or a European-style thread (Figure 2.2); however, the holding power of these three designs does not appear to be significantly different.

Screws are available with a single slot, a cruciate slot, a Phillips-head cross slot, and a hexagonal socket (Figure 2.3). Phillips-head screwdrivers have a tendency to back out of the screw slots. This means that increased axial pressure must be applied to the screwdriver to keep the screwdriver tip secure in the screw slot. This same feature also provides some protection

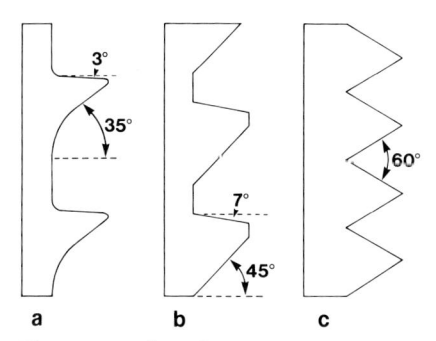

Figure 2.2 Thread types: (a) European thread, (b) buttress thread, (c) V thread.

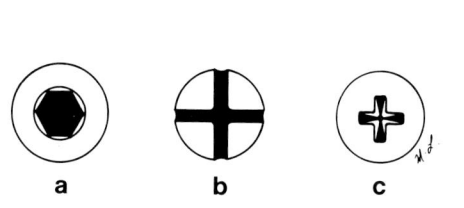

Figure 2.3 Head designs: (a) hexagonal socket, (b) cruciate head, (c) Phillips head.

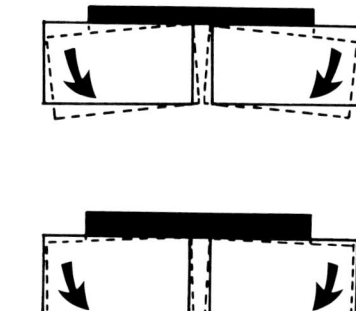

Figure 2.4 Implant stiffness in interfragmentary mobility. Stability of the system is dependent on the stiffness of the implant.

from overload and stripping. Hexagonal-shaped screwdrivers significantly decrease the axial pressure required to insert a screw; however, they also allow for increased torque application and possible stripping. The hexagonal-head design in small screw diameters (1.5 and 2.0 mm) has resulted in slot failure, with the screwdriver stripping the screw hexagonal slot into a circle. For this reason, the hexagonal-head screw is not commonly used in maxillofacial surgery. A cruciate slot allows better purchase on the screwhead than a single slot and does not have the backing-out tendencies of the Phillips-head screwdrivers.

The undersurface of the screw head may be flat or conical in shape. If a plate is not used, the bone surface should be countersunk to accept the undersurface of the screw to prevent bone splitting due to the increased pressure under the screw head.

BIOMECHANICS

Elasticity of bone is an important element in maintaining compression in internal fixation. The rigidity of bone is high compared to cartilage and fibrous tissue. This has been discussed on the relationship of strain to bone healing patterns.

Bone compressed by an internal fixation implant (screw or plate) will deform to about the thickness of one to two cell layers. Therefore, if fragmentation and shortening (resorption) of one to two cell layers occurs, the compression achieved will be lost.

COMPRESSION

R. Danis was the first to advocate the use of compression for stabilization of bone fractures. Without compression, the stability in the fracture or osteotomy site is dependent on the stiffness of the plate or screw and friction between the fragment ends. If a small gap exists between fragment ends, and if dynamic external forces result in plate bending, then movement in the gap and high strain result, with possible problems in bone healing (Figure 2.4).

Static compression can be used in the form of self-compressing plates or by the use of the lag screw technique. The use of compression results in both preload and friction. The compression preloads the contact surfaces and keeps them motionless. Under a functional load (for example, bending) at the convex side of the bend, traction (tension) tries to pull the contact surfaces apart. The preload will prevent any such distractions as long as the static compression is greater than the dynamic traction (Figure 2.5). Therefore, the contacting surfaces remain motionless. Absolute stability exists under these conditions, where the strain within the gap is zero (no change in size of the gap occurs under the influence of the dynamic force placed on the fragments).

Compression of any two surfaces also produces friction. The amount of friction produced is proportional to the force (preload) multiplied by the coefficient of friction. Friction is important to stabilize against shearing influences produced by torsional forces (Figure 2.6).

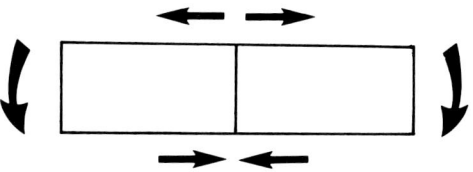

Figure 2.5 Preload. For any amount of bending moment caused by an external dynamic force on a bone, one side of the bone undergoes compression and the opposite side undergoes tensile force. Compression ($\rightarrow\leftarrow$) holds the fragments together; tension ($\leftarrow\longrightarrow$) pulls them apart. As long as the preload (compression) is greater than the external force that results in tension, the contacting surface remains motionless (absolute stability exists). The strain condition ($\Delta L/L = 0$) necessary for direct bone formation exists.

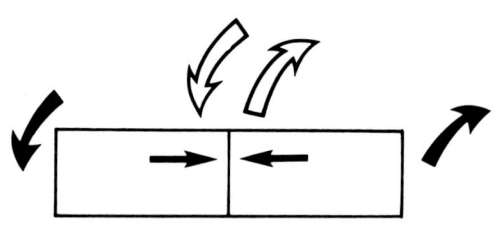

Figure 2.6 Friction results from compression of the contacting surfaces. As long as it is greater than the external shearing forces, friction prevents shearing displacement of the contact surfaces.

Compression, therefore, produces absolute stability as long as the dynamic external forces do not exceed the preload or friction. The lack of motion between the fragment ends results in no interfragmentary strain and therefore allows for direct bone formation.

Measurements of compression forces over time have demonstrated that applied compression decreases slowly and that the surfaces under compression do not show any fragment end shortening due to resorption. Compression drops to zero as bone remodeling occurs after direct bone formation and union have occurred.

In addition to providing compression, internal fixation allows for accurate contour restoration of fragments and the fixation of bone grafts for immediate reconstruction, decreases bone graft resorption, and allows for earlier function. The possibility of relapse is less than when wire osteosynthesis is used. These factors are important in trauma reconstruction and elective craniofacial procedures. Danis devised a plate with a built-in compression device; Muller developed a removable compression device.

Today, all the self-compressing plates on the market are based on the contact between a conical surface and edge. The dynamic compression plate (DCP) relies on a geometry of the spherical undersurface of the screw lying in a sloped or horizontal cylinder in the plate hole (Figure 2.7). The spherical gliding principle results in plate adaption and compression (Figures 2.8 and 2.9).

At the time of contouring the plate, controlled overbending is of great importance. The best position for achieving uniform compression force over a fracture is the point nearest the center of the fracture plane. This is not possible when compressive forces are produced from a plate positioned on one surface of the fracture fragments, the compressive forces are reduced the further they are away from the plate, with the result that

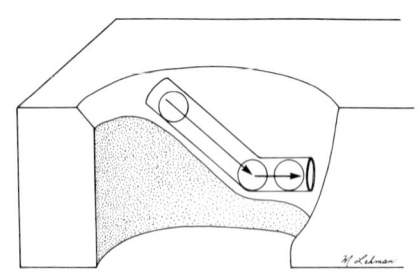

Figure 2.7 Spherical gliding principle with DCP (Algower et al. 1970). The course of a sphere in a bent cylinder results in downward movement being transformed into horizontal movement. The change in direction occurs at the point of intersection of the two cylinders (or at the bend). When a spherical screwhead is turned, it glides in a section of the inclined sphere. Therefore, the fragment grasped by the screw is moved horizontally. In the horizontal section of the cylinder, the screw is guided further toward the fracture gap.

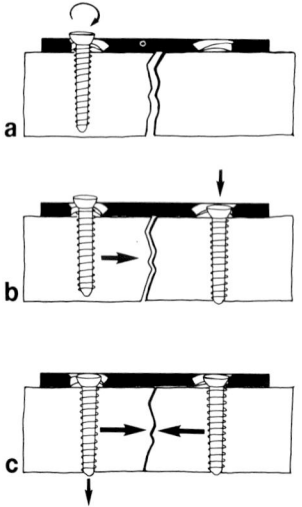

Figure 2.8 Action of the DCP. (a) The left screw is inserted but not tightened; (b) the right screw is inserted and tightened firmly, during which time the head of the screw moves on the gliding plane of the hole in the plate such that the plate moves in the direction of the arrow; (c) as the left screw is tightened, the plate is drawn to the left, in the direction of the arrow, and moves the fragment on the right toward the gap. The fragment is, therefore, compressed.

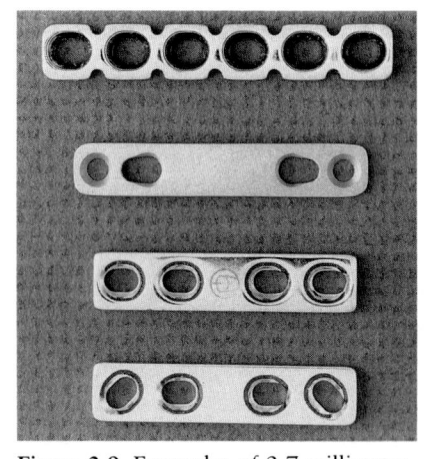

Figure 2.9 Examples of 2.7-millimeter plate systems used for mandibular reconstruction. From top to bottom: AO 2.7-millimeter reconstruction plate, Luhr 2.7-millimeter DCP, AO 2.7-millimeter DCP, AO 2.7-millimeter EDCP. All but the reconstruction plate are designed to use the spherical gliding principle.

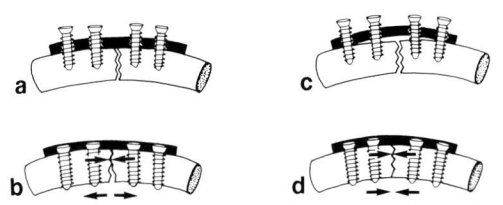

Figure 2.10 The effects of prebending: (a) and (b): If an unbent plate is tightened, the result is distraction of the fragment on the opposite side. Compression, therefore, acts on only part of the fracture area. (c) and (d): When the plate is over-bent and the screws are tightened, this results in compression over the whole fracture area.

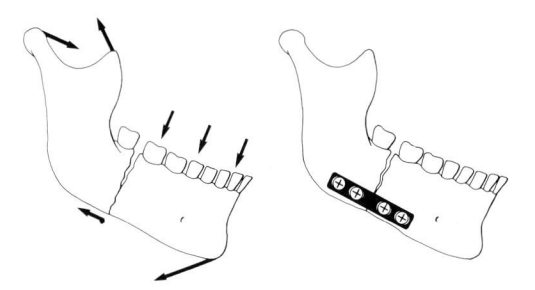

Figure 2.11 Distraction of the alveolar border when compression is applied to the lower border of the mandible.

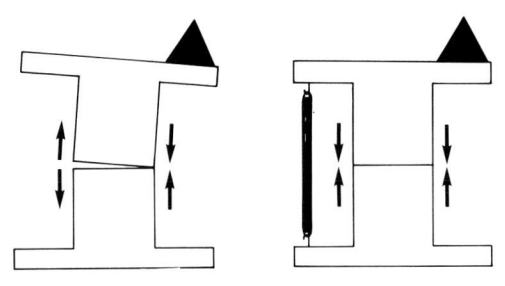

Figure 2.12 Tension band principle. (left) When a load is applied eccentrically, it results in compression on one side of the axis of the cylinder and distraction, or tensile effect, on the opposite side. (right) When a tension band is applied, the same eccentrically applied force results in compression across the whole contact surface.

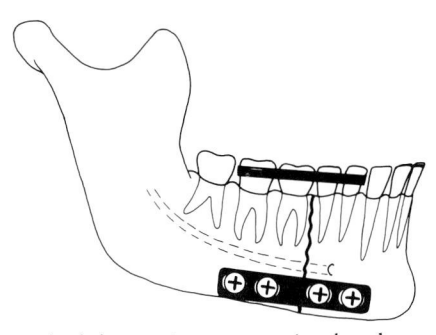

Figure 2.13 Arch bar acting as a tension band.

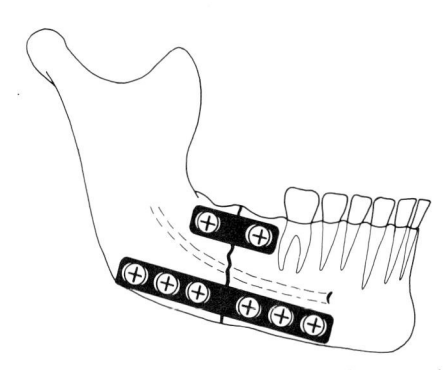

Figure 2.14 DCP acting as a tension band in an edentulous area.

opening in the fracture site on the opposite side may occur. An example is the fixation of a plate on the buccal side of the mandible, which may result in distraction on the lingual side of the fracture. This can be eliminated by slightly overbending the plate approximately 1 mm at the fracture site (Figure 2.10).

For fractures of the mandible, the plate cannot be placed centrally between the marginal and occlusal sides because the screws would penetrate the mandibular canal or tooth roots. The placement of the plate on the lower border may lead to gaps (distraction) at the alveolar (occlusal) border when compression is applied (Figure 2.11). This effect cannot be controlled by overbending. To overcome this effect, a tension-band principle and/or an eccentric dynamic compression plate (EDCP) can be utilized.

TENSION BAND

A tension band results in the transformation of tractional and compressive forces subjected to eccentric stress being transformed into symmetrical axial compression. If an eccentric force is applied to a column, the result is a compressive side and a tensile side, with opening of a gap on the tensile side. If a tension band is applied on the tensile side of the column, axial compression is distributed across the full width of the column (Figure 2.12).

The same is true for the mandible, where the alveolar side of the fracture is primarily exposed to tensile forces by the action of the muscles and is distracted by the eccentric position of the plate on the lower border. When a tension band is placed on the occlusal border of the mandible, compression across the mandible from occlusal to marginal border surfaces occurs, thereby preventing distraction at the occlusal border.

In areas where teeth are present, the tension band can take the form of an arch bar or wire ligature (Figure 2.13). In an area with no teeth on the occlusal surface, a DCP or minireconstruction plate may be used as a tension band (Figure 2.14).

ECCENTRIC DYNAMIC COMPRESSION PLATE

Another method, which can be used alone or in combination with a tension band to result in compression at the alveolar surface as well as at the marginal border, is the eccentric dynamic compression plate (EDCP). The compression at the alveolar surface is obtained from two oblique compression holes. As the screws in the outer oblique hole are tightened, the fragments are rotated about the screws nearest the fracture, which function as axes of rotation, and the fragments are consequently compressed at the alveolar border (Figure 2.15).

Once the compression between fragment ends has been achieved (after placing the first two screws in the fracture fragments in the case of the DCP, or after placing the first four screws in EDCP), all subsequent screws must be inserted centrically within the plate hole. This is important to prevent shearing forces across the screws.

In general, it is suggested that a minimum of two screws be placed on either side of a fracture for sufficient stability in the case of mandibular fractures, as well as for prevention of rotation in midface fractures.

It is imperative, even with the use of plates in both the mandible and midface, that the patient be held in the normal occlusion or newly determined occlusion using maxillo-mandibular fixation (MMF) prior to application of the plates. After placement of the plate, the MMF may be released to check for proper positioning.

LAG SCREW

A lag screw is not a special screw; rather, it is a technique of screw insertion when an oblique fracture or osteotomy exists. This technique results in compression between two bony fragments.

The proximal fragment is drilled using a drill bit having an external diameter that is the same as the screw to be inserted. This is called the *gliding hole*. The distal fragment is drilled with a drill bit that is slightly larger than the core diameter of the screw. This pilot hole is then tapped, in the use of pretapped screws, or the screw is directly inserted, in the case of self-tapping screws. Tightening of the screw results in compression between bone fragments (Figure 2.16).

A lag screw may be inserted by itself or through a plate. In the case of a sagittal fracture or osteotomy,

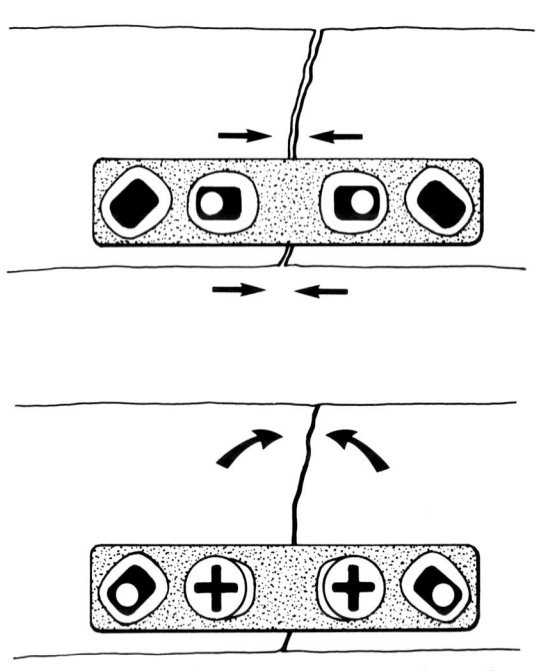

Figure 2.15 Eccentric dynamic compression plate. The outer hole is transverse. When screws are fully tightened in the screw holes closest to the fracture, compression results at the lower margin of the jaw. When the screws are fully tightened in the transverse outer holes, the rotation of the fragments around the inner screws (these are the axis of rotation) results in compression in the alveolar or upper border.

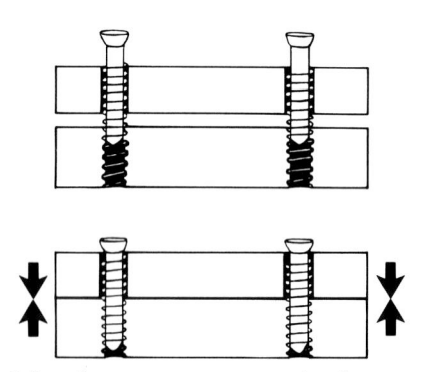

Figure 2.16 Interfragmentary compression between two bone surfaces by means of a lag screw. The gliding hole can be seen in the upper fragment and the threaded hole in the lower fragment. When the screw is tightened and the screwhead makes contact with the bone, interfragmentary compression results.

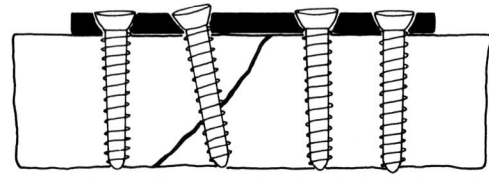

Figure 2.17 When a lag screw is placed through a plate, all subsequent screws must be placed neutrally to avoid shearing across the lag screw.

at least two screws must be inserted to prevent rotation. If a screw is placed as a lag screw through a plate, all the other screws in the plate must be placed in the centric position (middle of the hole) to prevent shearing across the lag screw (Figure 2.17).

FIXATION SCREW

In the case of osteotomies where asymmetric movements are occurring and gaps are created between the fracture fragments, the use of a lag screw may result in compression of the fragments and distortion in position of the proximal and distal fragments. An example of this is in a bilateral sagittal split osteotomy with crossbite. When the sagittal split is performed and the patient is then brought into normal occlusion, a gap may exist in the placement of the condylar segment with the distal segment in the upper or lower borders. If a lag screw were used in this case, displacement of the condyle could occur. To maintain this gap, a fixation screw alone or a fixation screw in combination with a interpositioned bone graft in the open gap may be used. When a fixation screw is used, a gliding hole is not used in the proximal fragment; therefore, both fragments are drilled with a pilot hole and then either tapped in the case of pretapped screws or the screw directly inserted in the case of self-tapping screws. This results in positioning the fragments with the gap open and therefore decreases the chance of malpositioning of the condyle (Figure 2.18). The principle and techniques of lag screw and fixation screw (also known as position screw) osteosynthesis are presented in detail in Chapter 4.)

RECONSTRUCTION PLATES (MINI AND MANDIBULAR)

In most situations, reconstruction plates are used as internal surgical splints. The reconstruction plate is designed to buttress fragments against displacement while absorbing all functional loads. Reconstruction plates do not come with holes designed to use the spherical gliding principle. Screw holes are designed for screws to be inserted neutrally (centrically). This method of stabilization, one in which interfragmentary compression does not play a role, is termed *fixation osteosynthesis*. In most areas of the thin boned mid- and upper face, where compression is not possible or desired, rigid stabilization is provided by fixation osteosynthesis.

Reconstruction plates are presently produced in four sizes: the micro system (0.8-mm screws), and 1.5, 2.0, and 2.7-millimeter systems (Figure 2.19). In general, as for the DCP and EDCP, the 2.7-millimeter system is recommended for the mandible. This is due to increased forces (preload) generated by these screws in thick bone. At present, investigations are looking at various fracture and osteotomy patterns and function loads to which they are subjected, to ascertain which patterns may be treated by smaller systems. This work is currently unavailable but suggests that there may be indications for the 2.0-mm system in certain mandibular fractures and osteotomies.

These plates may be used in the mandible that is segmentally fractured or has bony loss, such as in cancer resection, where the use of compression would result in bony collapse. In the case of segmental mandible fractures, the dentition is brought into normal occlusion. The fracture segments are then automatically reduced and held to each other with wires, miniplates, or lag screws. The reconstruction plate is then contoured

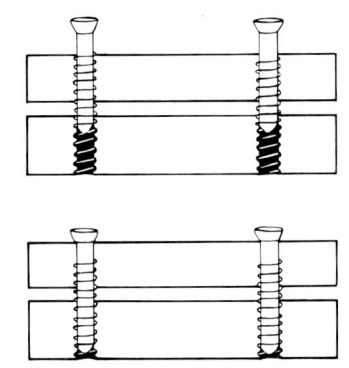

Figure 2.18 Positioning screw. Both outer and inner fragments are threaded so that on insertion of the screw, the gap between the fragments is maintained.

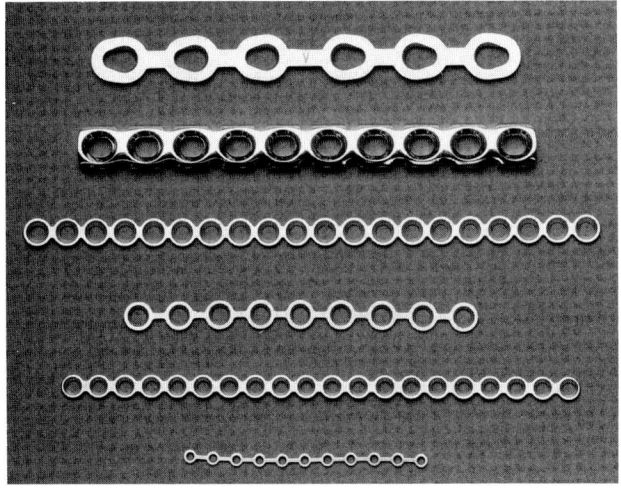

Figure 2.19 Various plate designs from top to bottom:
Luhr 2.7-millimeter reconstruction plate
AO 2.7-millimeter reconstruction plate
AO 2.0-millimeter reconstruction plate
Luhr 2.0-millimeter reconstruction plate
AO 1.5-millimeter reconstruction plate
Luhr microreconstruction plate

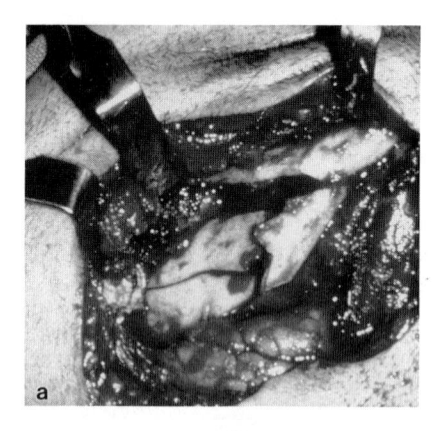

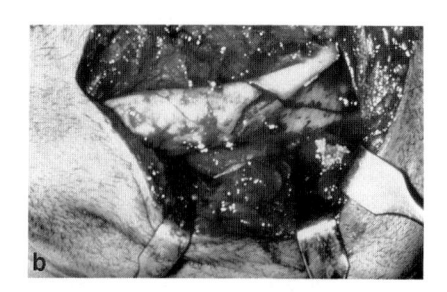

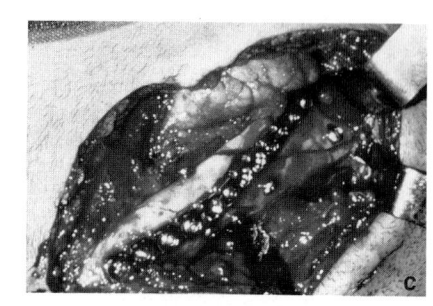

Figure 2.20 (a) Segmental mandibular fracture. (b) Various bony segments lagged to each other. (c) Reconstruction plate adapted and applied across all segments.

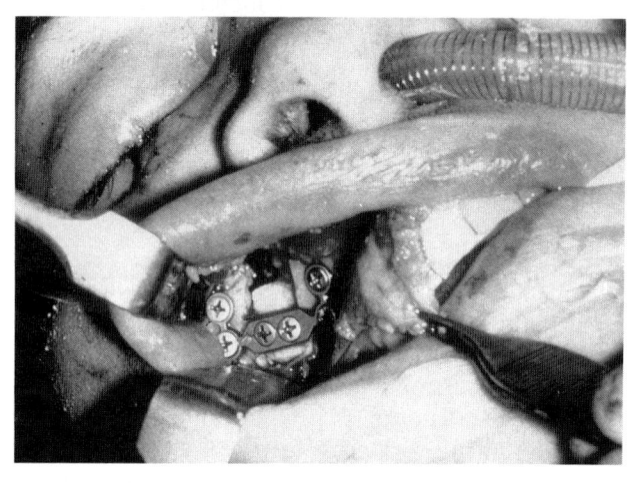

Figure 2.21 Bone graft lagged through mini reconstruction plate in right lateral buttress.

and fixed with a minimum of two screws to each stable lateral segment. The segmental fragments are then fixed to the reconstruction plates (Figure 2.20). In the case of cancer resection, the plate may be pre-bent to the mandible prior to resection to achieve accurate contour, then removed, the tumor resected with mandible, and the plate reapplied.

Minireconstruction plates may be used in the midface, orbital, and cranial areas. The functional load in these areas to be withstood by plate fixation is poorly understood. These reconstruction plates can be used to span segmental bone fractures and areas of segmental bone loss. The bony fractures or bone grafts can then be fixed to the plate for stability and primary contour reconstruction (Figure 2.21).

The understanding of the biomechanics of internal fixation is fundamental to the use of any of the systems available. Failure to adhere rigidly to basic principles can lead to disastrous results. Many areas of internal fixation of the facial area are poorly understood, as the basic understanding of the dynamic forces that apply in the various regions has not been fully determined.

REFERENCES

Algower M, Perron S, Matter P: A new plate for internal fixation—the dynamic compression plate [DCP]. Injury 2:40, 1970.

Claes L, Hutzschenreuter P, Pohier O: Losemonte von Cortical Iszugschrauben in Abhamgigkeit von Implantationszeit und Oberflachbeschaffenheit. Arch Orthop Unfall-Clir 85:115–159, 1976.

Michelet FX, Deymes J, Dessus B: Osteosynthesis with miniaturized screwed plates in maxillofacial surgery. J Max Fac Surg 1:79–84, 1973.

Phillips JH, Rahn BA: Comparison of compression and torque measurements of self-tapping and pre-tapped screws. Plast Reconstr Surg 83:447, 1989.

Schatzker J, Horne JG, Sumner-Smith G: The reaction of cortical bone to compression by screw threads. Clin Orthop 111:263, 1975.

CHAPTER

3

Principles of Monocortical Miniplate Osteosynthesis

Patrick Blez

Jean-Luc Kahn

"Monocortical miniplate osteosynthesis" derives from a concept of bone stabilization radically different from those designed for bicortical fixation. The use of plates that are malleable and miniaturized for maxillofacial reconstruction is based on precise anatomical considerations and extensive biological and mechanical experiments that have led to the development of a specific instrumentation.

The basic principles, resulting from research carried out between 1971 and 1974, have been progressively accepted and successfully applied by most maxillofacial surgeons. These principles have had no essential modification since their inception.

ANATOMICAL CONSIDERATIONS

In the Mandible

Experimental work has demonstrated that monocortical fixation by miniplates is strong enough to withstand the different strains created by masticatory forces. Because fixation is accomplished by anchoring the miniplates within the bone by means of screws, it is important to know

- the regions where the bone provides the screws with a firm fixation, and
- the topography of the dental apices and inferior alveolar nerve, in order to avoid damaging them when inserting the screws.

The outer cortex of the body of the mandible reaches an average thickness of 3.3 millimeters, is particularly strong, and offers a good anchorage for the osteosynthesis screws (see Figure 3.1). The cortical bone is thicker in the chin region and is reinforced laterally by the oblique line, which runs from the coronoid process to the molar region. In the symphysis region, cross sections of the mandible show the thickest cortex to be at the lower border; behind the third molar, it is stronger at the upper border.

Near the alveolar process, the thickness of the bone is variable; the anatomy of the tooth roots and the structure of the bone do not allow screw fixation in this region. To avoid damaging the root apices, it is safe to place the screws at least twice the length of the crown of the tooth from the alveolar process (see Figure 3.2).

The inferior alveolar nerve runs in the mandibular canal, from the lingula to the mental foramen, on a

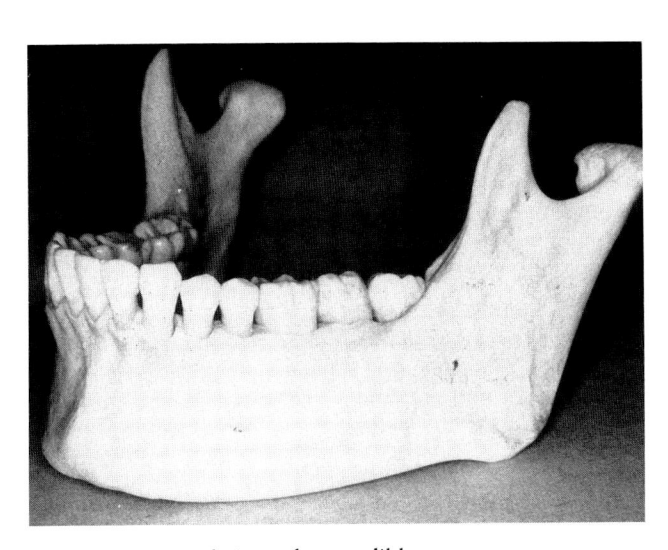

Figure 3.1 Lateral view of a mandible.

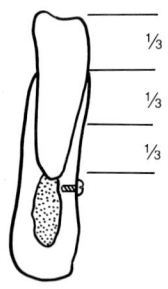

Figure 3.2 The screws should be placed at least twice the length of the crown from the alveolar process.

concave course. Measurements show that, from back to front, it runs ever closer to the outer cortex and to the lower border. At its lowest point, it is separated by 8–10 mm from the basilar border of the mandible. Although the average thickness of the cortex in that region is 5 millimeters, it may be less than 3 millimeters in some cases. About 1 centimeter before reaching the mental foramen, the canal turns upward and forward. The foramen lies approximately at the middle of the distance between the alveolar crest and the lower border of the mandible, on a vertical line corresponding to the first or second premolar. It is important to remember that the mental foramen lies higher than the canine apex. Therefore, osteosynthesis in this region involves a certain risk of apical injury.

In most cases, the mandibular canal surrounds the neurovascular bundle as a bony tunnel, but sometimes its bony structure is poorly developed. Repeated tests in freshly prepared mandibles have shown that the intrusion of a screw into the canal does not usually cause nerve injury, because the nerve moves away from the instrument. Drilling the holes appears certainly to be more dangerous for the nerve than tightening the screws.

It should be noted that, with ageing, the alveolar bone atrophies and the structure of the mandible is reduced to the two cortical layers. In edentulous patients, the flat upper border of the mandible is composed of sclerous bone, giving poor anchorage for the screws.

One should keep in mind that in children, the mandibular body is occupied by dental germs.

The alveolar bone is covered with the adherent gum. When a fracture occurs, the gum is lacerated, exposing the mandibular bone to the risk of infection from the oral cavity if treatment is not instituted within 12 hours.

During the first years of life, the blood supply of the mandible depends on the inferior dental artery. Later, periosteal vascularization increasingly takes over. In the adult subject, as demonstrated by Bradley, the blood supply relies entirely on the periosteum of the basilar border. This area should therefore be treated with care. This notion pleads in favor of buccal rather than cutaneous approaches, because it enables the avoidance of periosteal elevation in the basilar region.

In the Cranium and Upper Face

Only some parts of the craniofacial skeleton are constituted of compact and solid bone: the cranium, the nasal bone, the zygomatic bone, the orbital margin, the rim of the piriform aperture, and the zygomatic buttress. Apart from these areas are fragile zones of sagittal bone, constituting the walls of the various cavities, on which the fixation of osteosynthesis plates may be more hazardous (see Figure 3.3).

The frontal bone ranges from 4 to 9 mm in thickness. The upper orbital margins are particularly well suited for plate placement, but care should be taken to localize the contours of the frontal sinus. Bone thickness allows placement of 5-millimeter screws without risking dural penetration. The parietal bone also provides adequate thickness for screw fixation.

The fronto-zygomatic process, which resembles a triangular prism, is made of compact cortical bone and provides an area of excellent purchase for cortical screws. It is covered with a periosteum that is easily elevated, except at the frontomalar suture.

The lateral orbital rim passing to the zygomatic arch provides sufficient bone for screw purchase. The eye should be protected during the operation by using an appropriate retractor. The anterior cerebral fossa can be avoided; its deepest point is located 16 to 20 mm above the frontomalar suture, or 5 millimeters above a horizontal line tangential to the upper orbital margin.

The lower orbital rim is also an area of thick cortical bone. However, because neither muscular force nor any strain is exerted on it, its fixation with a plate seems unwarranted. If isolated fragments require immobilization, absorbable ligatures are mechanically sufficient.

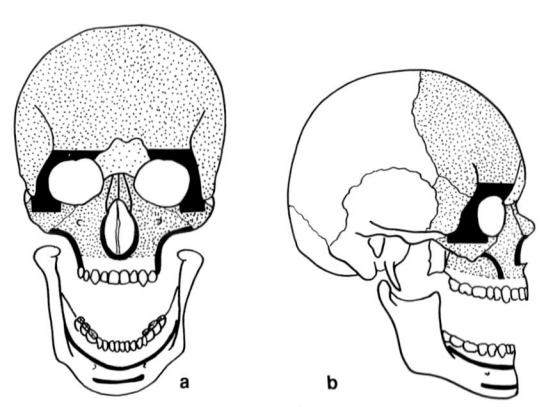

Figure 3.3 Elective zones of miniplate osteosynthesis: (a) frontal view, (b) lateral view. Favorable regions are colored black. Dotted zones are regions where osteosynthesis can be used. In our opinion, insertion of screws into the wall of the frontal sinus is controversial; bone plating along the inferior orbital rim is illogical in most cases; and the zygomatic arch is definitely an unfavorable zone because its transcutaneous approach is dangerous for the facial nerve, and even a very thin plate always becomes visible under the skin.

The maxilla has only two areas made of compact and strong bone: the lateral inferior aspect of the piriform aperture and the zygomatic buttress. The anterior wall of the maxillary sinus is thin and less ideal as a support for miniplates.

Finally, one must always keep in mind that many cavities exist in this area, some of which contain organs that must be preserved, such as the dura, the eyes, and the dental roots. The walls of the aerial cavities—such as the frontal sinus, the maxillary sinus, the ethmoid sinus, the nasal fossae, and the buccal cavity—are generally thin and fragile. Insertion of screws protruding through the mucosa results in putting their tips in communication with the underlying cavity, which, in our opinion, is in contradiction with the surgical imperatives of osteosynthesis and entails an infection hazard. Indeed, aerial cavities of the face, especially frontal sinus and nasal fossae, have little tolerance to any foreign body.

BIOMECHANICAL PRINCIPLES

The biomechanical principles of monocortical miniplate osteosynthesis are based on mathematical and experimental studies performed in Strasbourg, France, by the Groupe d'Etudes en Biomecanique Osseuse et Articulaire de Strasbourg (GEBOAS). This research work concerns the mandible only; its goal was to develop a tension banding osteosynthesis system, able to guarantee fracture healing with neither maxillomandibular fixation nor interfragmental compression. This was achieved as a result of the following considerations and experiments.

Goals

The ideal method of treatment of mandibular fractures is one that establishes a functional therapy by movement. Therefore, it should have the objectives of

- perfect anatomical reduction,
- complete and stable fixation, and
- painless mobilization of the injured region around its articulations.

Thus the biomechanical conditions of an ideal osteosynthesis are that

- the plates and screws must withstand the various stresses and tensile and torsional forces to which the mandibular bone is typically subject.
- the plates have to be malleable for easy adaptation to the bone surface, especially in the curved symphysis and molar region, in order to achieve anatomical reduction and restoration of perfect dental occlusion.
- the dimensions of the plates have to be adapted to the mandible, so as to minimize the amount of periosteal elevation and fracture site exposure necessary; furthermore, the oral mucosa must be able to cover the plate without any difficulty. Finally, the screws have to be appropriate for the thickness of the cortex.

Masticatory Stress Distribution into the Mandible

Knowledge of masticatory stresses exerted on the mandible is fundamental because these stresses determine the rational design and positioning of the osteosynthesis plates.

The activity of the masticatory jaw-closing muscles can be distributed into temporalis forces, masseter forces, and reactive biting force, which turn out to be most adverse to the immobilization of the fracture. These forces are variable from patient to patient. By means of strain gauges connected to a Wheatstone bridge, we measured maximal biting forces in young men with healthy teeth. The following values were obtained:

- incisor region: 29 DaN
- canine region: 30 DaN
- premolar region: 48 DaN
- molar region: 66 DaN

More important to understand is the repartition of the strains created into the mandibular bone as a result of these masticatory forces. Physiologically coordinated muscle function produces tension forces at the upper border of the mandible and compressive forces at the lower border (see Figure 3.4). In addition, torsion forces are produced anterior to the canines (see Figure 3.5).

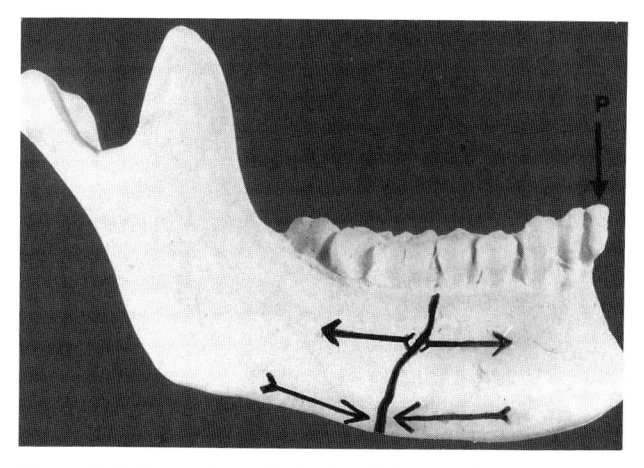

Figure 3.4 Throughout the body of the mandible, biting forces produce tension (←→) forces at the upper border and compressive (→←) forces at the lower border.

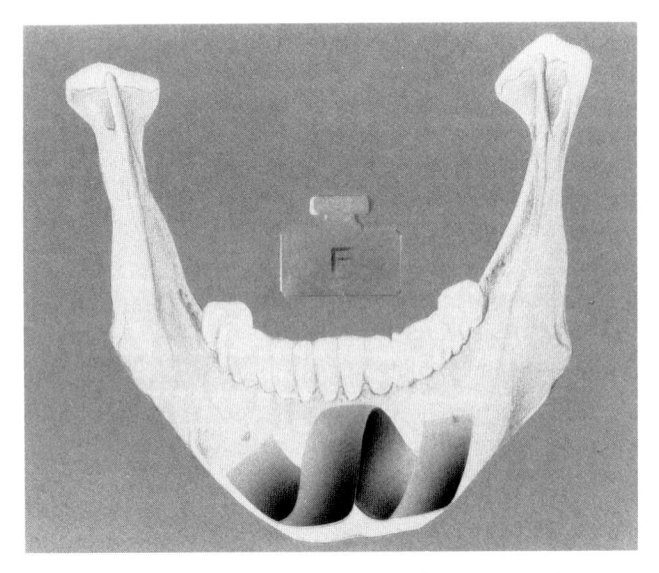

Figure 3.5 Torsion forces are produced anterior to the canines.

In every mandibular fracture, these forces cause distraction at the alveolar crest region, accentuated by trauma and by contraction of the muscles of the floor of the mouth. This can lead to displacement of the fragments. The compressive force at the lower border is a dynamic and physiological force, which is exerted permanently on the fractured fragments along their basilar border. This compression is due to the muscular tonus and increases during masticatory function. When the synthesis is adequately performed and provided there is no defect in the fracture site, this dynamic compression equals exactly the physiological strains that are exerted on an intact mandible (see Figure 3.6).

Using a very simple model, it was possible to simulate the anatomical and biomechanical characteristics of the undamaged mandible. First, the course of the tension lines was registered on a standardized mandibular model under the action of bending forces. A bar-shaped Araldit plate was fixed at one end, and the free end was loaded with a vertical force. By polarized light, isostatic tension lines were visible at the upper border and isostatic compression lines at the lower border. After transection of the Araldit bar, the continuity was restored by means of a miniplate osteosynthesis at various levels:

- When the miniplate was placed near the lower border, the vertical force caused distraction of the fracture at the upper border, preventing the transmission of tension forces; consequently, in this test model, the isostatic tension lines all ran through the plate and screws at the lower border.
- On the contrary, when the Araldit bar was reconstituted by an osteosynthesis plate at the upper border, the isostatic lines ran through the fracture in a relatively normal fashion. No distraction was observed at the upper border of the fracture site, and the course of the compression lines was similar to the intact experimental model (see Figure 3.7).

The value of tension and compression forces acting at the fracture site can be calculated by the following formula:

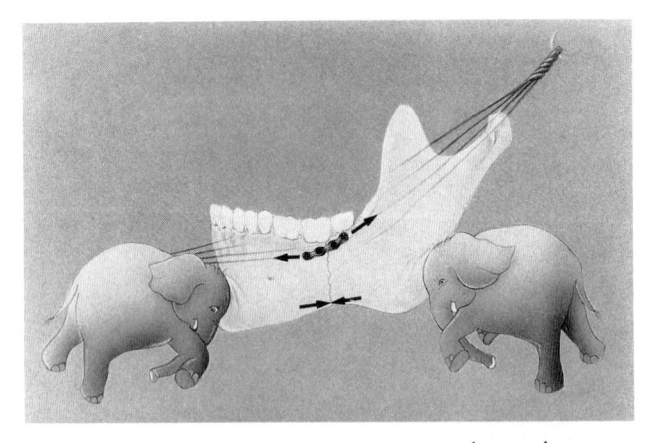

Figure 3.6 Provided that osteosynthesis is adequately performed, the miniplate neutralizes the distraction forces at the upper border and at the same time reestablishes the physiological strains of compressive forces at the lower border.

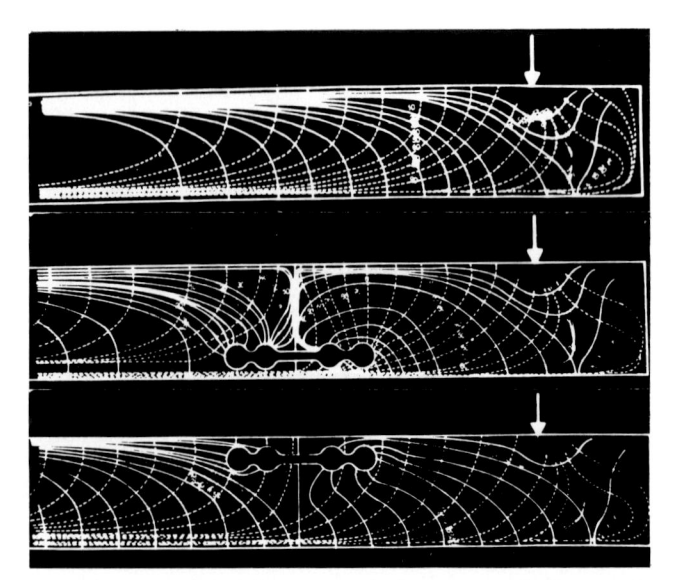

Figure 3.7 A vertical force is applied on one end of an Araldit bar. By polarized light, isostatic lines of tension (continuous lines) and compression (interrupted lines) are visible: (top) normal, (center) after synthesis at the lower border, (bottom) after synthesis at the upper border.

$$f_1 = f_2 = \frac{P \times L}{d},$$

where

> P = applied force,
> L = distance from chin to fracture, and
> d = distance from lower border to plate (see Figures 3.8–3.10).

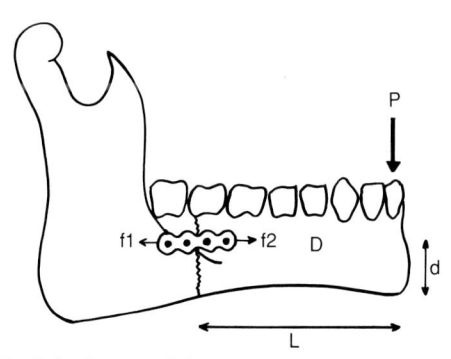

Figure 3.8 Calculation of the moments of traction, compression, and torsion permits the establishment of a mathematical model of the mandible.

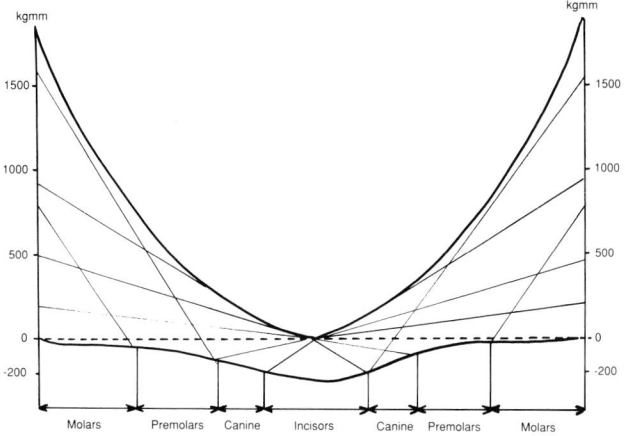

Figure 3.9 Representation of moments of flexion developed in the mandible. Their values increase from front to back.

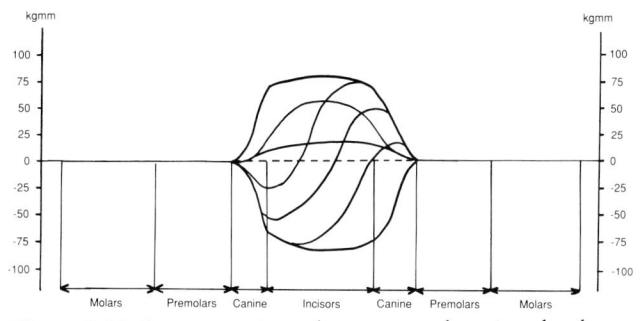

Figure 3.10 Representation of moments of torsion developed in the mandible. They are maximal in the symphysis region.

Definition of an Ideal Osteosynthesis Line on the Mandible

Given the unique anatomy of the mandible, this biomechanical study defines an ideal osteosynthesis line for the mandibular body (see Figure 3.11). It corresponds to the course of a tension line at the base of the alveolar process, just under the root apices. In that region, a plate can be fixed with monocortical screws:

- Behind the mental foramen, a plate is applied immediately below the dental roots and above the inferior alveolar nerve.
- At the angle of the jaw, the plate is most favorably placed on the broad surface of the external oblique line, as high as possible.
- In the anterior region, between the mental foramina, in addition to the subapical plate, another plate near the lower border of the mandible is necessary to neutralize the torsion forces (see Figure 3.12).

The result of such a monocortical tension banding osteosynthesis is the neutralization of the distraction and torsion strains exerted on the fracture site, while physiological self-compression strains are restored. Interfragmentary compression by means of bicortical screws does not permit this effect.

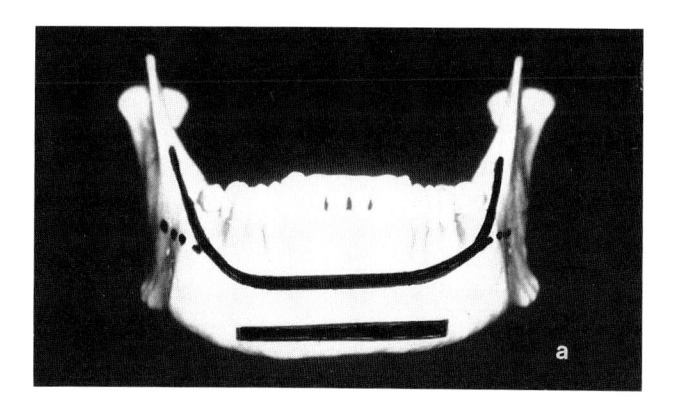

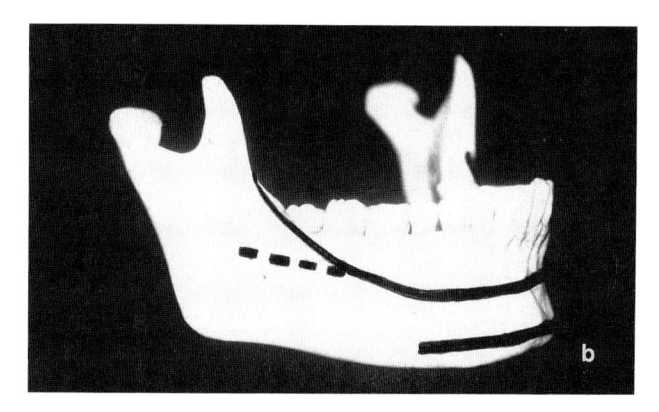

Figure 3.11 Ideal osteosynthesis line on the mandibular body: (a) frontal view, (b) lateral view.

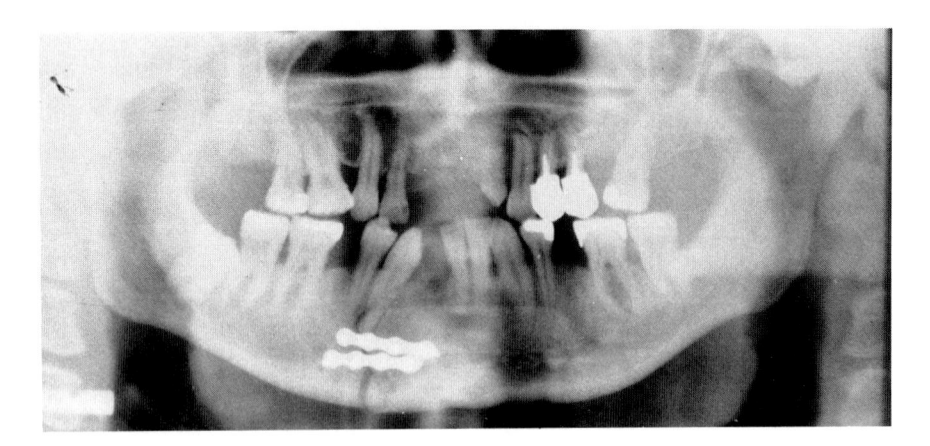

Figure 3.12 Osteosynthesis of a mandibular fracture in the right canine region.

Biomechanics in Cranium and Upper Part of the Face

The use of monocortical miniplate osteosynthesis in the cranium and upper part of the face is not based on experimental work but can be considered as a logical extension of this method, reflected by its excellent clinical results. For obvious reasons, it was impossible here to carry out the same biomechanical experiments as on the mandible. The forces exerted on the cranium and facial bones are numerous, tridimensional, and difficult to evaluate. They produce various strains on osteosynthesis plates in every direction, with a preponderance of bending and torsion stresses as opposed to compression forces. The first source of strain is the result of the masticatory forces, lingual pressure, and action of masseter and pterygoideus externus muscles. This strain is certainly less important and easier to neutralize than that on the mandible.

In orthopedic surgery of the face, consideration should also be given to other forces that appear in addition to the muscular actions, even if they do not compare in intensity with the biting forces. One should mention the external pressure on the zygoma or occiput, where the patient is lying. Scar retraction is a particularly harmful force because its action remains constant over a long period; it has a pulling effect on osteotomized fragments, especially when gaps are wide. In the specific case of facial osteotomies for cleft sequellae, the scar retraction exerts force not only backward along the line of the palatine cleft but also in a concentric way on the whole maxillomalar structure, on each side. As a result, the midface is forced backward and there is a tendency for the osseous banks to collapse toward the cleft. In other cases of midface osteotomy, the tendency of the fragment to be pushed backward can be explained by the pressure of the nasal septum in response to the displacement of the palatal bone. Monocortical miniplate osteosynthesis has been strong enough to withstand all these forces, and to ensure bone healing without interfragmentary compression.

CONCLUSION

Much biomechanical experimentation was performed to design a reliable system for maxillofacial skeletal stabilization. Its design evolved from an evaluation of biting forces during mastication, the application of miniaturized bone plates, and the response of the mandibular cortex to the shearing stresses transmitted by the screws. This research has also determined the positioning of the miniplates on the entire mandibular body, and the number of plates required to achieve a stable osteosynthesis for any fracture location.

As does every biomechanical study, this one has limitations:

- The values of flexion and torsion strains, although based on mathematical calculation, are not actual clinical measurements;
- furthermore, the masticatory stresses used for calculation are those of strong and healthy people rather than those with fractures.

Given these reservations, the Champy system has continued to provide consistent valuable experimental evidence, on the basis of which a successful clinical experience has accumulated.

BIBLIOGRAPHY

Bradley JC: A radiological investigation into the age changes of the inferior dental artery. Br J Oral Surg 13: 82, 1975.

Champy M, Wilk A, Schnebelen JM: Die Behandlung der Mandibularfrakturen mittels Osteosynthese ohne intermaxilläre Ruhigstellung nach der Technick von F.X. Michelet (Treatment of mandibular fractures through osteosynthesis without intermaxillary fixation according to Michelet's procedure). Dtsch Zahn Mund u Kieferheilk 63: 339, 1975.

Champy M, Lodde JP, Jaeger JH, Wilk A: Osteosynthèses mandibulaires selon la technique de Michelet. I—Bases biomécaniques. (Mandibular osteosynthesis according to Michelet's procedure. I—Biomechanical fundamentals). Rev Stomatol Chir Maxillofac (Paris) 77: 569–576, 1976.

Champy M, Lodde JP, Grasset D, Muster D, Mariano A: Ostéosynthèses mandibulaires et compression (Mandibular osteosynthesis and compression). Ann Chir Plast Esthet 22: 165–167, 1977.

Champy M, Lodde JP, Wilk A, Schmitt R, Muster D: Probleme und Resultate bei der Verwendung von Dehnungsmeßstreifen am präparierten Unterkiefer und bei Patienten mit Unterkieferfrakturen (Problems and results in the use of strain gauges with dissected mandibles and with patients with mandible fractures). Dtsch Z Mund- Kiefer- Gesichtschir 2: 41, 1978.

Champy M, Pape HD, Gerlach KL, Lodde JP: The Strasbourg miniplate osteosynthesis. In Oral and Maxillofacial Traumatology. Kruger E, Schilli W, Worthington P (eds). Quintessence, Chicago, 1986, 19–43.

Cohen L: Further studies into the vascular architecture of the mandible. J Dent Res 39: 936, 1960.

Lodde JP, Champy M: Justification biomécanique d'un nouveau matériel d'ostéosynthèse en chirurgie faciale (Biomechanical justification of a new facial osteosynthesis material). Ann Chir Plast 21: 115, 1976.

Schumacher G: Statik und Aufbau des Gesichtsschädels unter Berücksichttigung des Frakturmechanismus (Statics and structure of the facial skeleton with special respect to the fracture mechanism). Fortschr Kiefer Gesichtschir 19: 3, 1975.

CHAPTER 4

Principles and Technique of Lag Screw Osteosynthesis

Herbert Niederdellmann

Vivek Shetty

Lag screw osteosynthesis can be defined as the stable union of two bone fragments under pressure with the help of screws inserted in lag fashion. This entails preparing the screw holes in such a way that when a screw is inserted and tightened, it gains purchase only in the distal fragment—not in the fragment adjacent to the screwhead. The function of a lag screw is essentially to clamp bone fragments together by generating a tensile stress along the length of the screw. This tensile stress is produced by the torsional moment used to insert the lag screw into bone in a manner analogous to a nut on a bolt. Lag screws provide rigid internal fixation by preventing relative motion at the fracture site; thereby facilitating direct osseous healing while allowing early mobilization and functional loading of the fracture site.

Any osteosynthesis screw can be used as a lag screw; however, screws with a constant thread diameter along their entire length are ideal. A full thread also makes it easier for the operator to remove the screws from the bone, even after they are invested by new bone. To understand the concept of a lag screw it is necessary to understand the basic design of the cortical screw, the predominant type of screw used in the maxillofacial region. Each cortical screw consists of a head and a shank; the length of shank defines the screw length. Screwheads come with a variety of sockets; the popular ones have either a cruciform (Phillips) or a hexagonal slot. The shank has an inner diameter, also known as core diameter, and an outer diameter or thread diameter (see Figure 4.1). The cortical screw can act as a lag screw only if it can glide freely through the fragment adjacent to the screwhead and engage the opposite fragment. For this purpose, an oversized hole called the gliding hole is drilled through the near cortex. The diameter of the gliding hole is equal to or greater than the thread diameter of the screw. The diameter of the screw hole in the opposite fragment is smaller than the gliding hole and corresponds to the core diameter of the screw. Drilled coaxial to the gliding hole, it is described as the thread hole because a thread is cut into it to provide purchase for the screw.

A depression or counter-sink that corresponds to the screw head is created at the outer end of the gliding hole. Consequently, the spherical undersurface of the screwhead maintains a broad and even annular surface contact with the screw bed, be it in bone or bone plate hole, even if the screw is inserted at an angle. Annular contact between screwhead and bone precludes the development of pressure points, which could rupture the cortical bone during tightening of the lag screw. Additionally, a spherical design provides better axial compression than a conical design, which tends to produce high wedging forces, especially when the screw is placed eccentrically. With the distal end of the shank engaged in the thread hole, turning the screw pulls the fragments together once the spherical undersurface of the screwhead meets the countersunk surface of the bone bed or bone plate.

The anatomical and biomechanical characteristics of the facial bones, including the mandible, dictate the

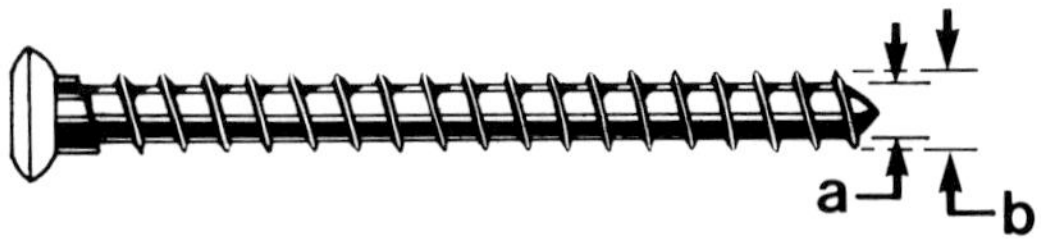

Figure 4.1 Cortical screw with hexagonal socket: (a) core diameter, (b) thread diameter.

Table 4.1 Details of cortical screws used for lag fixation (millimeters)

Screw Size	Drill Bit For Gliding Hole	Drill Bit For Thread Hole	Tap
1.5	1.5	1.1	1.5
2.0	2.0	1.5	2.0
2.7	2.7	2.0	2.7

use of cortical screws whose sizes are proportional to the bone fragments they fixate (see Table 4.1). Although smaller than those used in orthopedic surgery, the cortical screws devised for maxillofacial applications are remarkably strong and provide the degree of stability necessary for early postoperative mobilization. Lag screws depend on interfragmentary friction to hold the fragments together; additional stability is afforded by the intermeshing of the fractured bone surfaces. When lag screws are applied under sufficient primary tension, the interfragmentary compression converts potentially disruptive asymmetrical forces into symmetrical forces. This results in a high coefficient of fixation that is comparable to that achieved by compression bone plates.

As we alluded earlier, a lag effect can be achieved only if the screw can pass freely through the gliding hole and engage the thread hole in the opposite fragment (see Figure 4.2a). If the diameter of the gliding hole is smaller than the thread diameter of the screw, the screw will engage both the thread and the gliding hole. In this situation, similar to two nuts on the same bolt, the fracture gap will remain open, precluding any interfragmentary compression. Nonetheless, there are certain clinical situations where this transfixation effect is desired, in which case the cortical screw is referred to as a "position screw" (or a "fixation screw") (see Figure 4.2b). The position screw, which utilizes threaded holes in both the cortices, finds application in orthognathic procedures such as sagittal split ramus osteotomies when it helps maintain spatial relationships. The magnitude of the diastemata that develops between ramal cortices following mandibular mobilization depends on the inter-ramus angle, ramus curvature, and the amount of mandibular advancement or setback. Using lag screws would compress the cortices, leading to closure of these diastemata and change in condylar position. Although small distractions of the condyle from the glenoid fossa may be accommodated by the adaptive ability of the temporomandibular joints, larger displacements cause chronic compressive loading of the joints with its potential for temporomandibular dysfunction. In such situations position screws help maintain the interfragmentary diastemata and hold the osteotomized fragments in a rigid relationship to one another throughout the healing period.

INDICATIONS FOR LAG SCREW OSTEOSYNTHESIS

Lag screws have numerous applications in the mandible, but they have limited use in the midface region because of anatomical constraints (see Table 4.2). With the exception of oblique fractures in the periorbital or subnasal region, which can be reduced by lag screws, the bone in the other sites of the midface is too thin to permit placement of screws in lag fashion. The indication for lag screw osteosynthesis may manifest during preoperative planning or may become apparent during surgery.

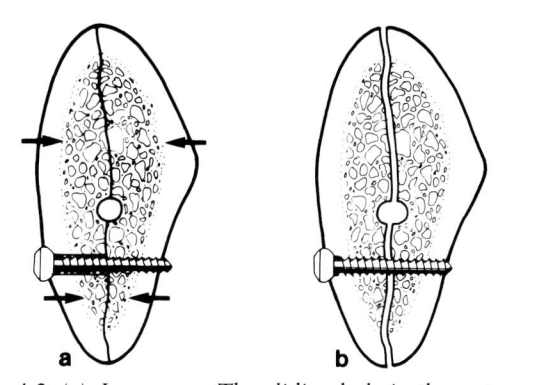

Figure 4.2 (a) Lag screw: The gliding hole in the outer fragment and the thread hole in the inner fragment facilitate interfragmentary compression. (b) Position screw: The threaded hole in both fragments keeps them apart.

Table 4.2 Indications for lag screw osteosynthesis

Procedure	2.7	2.0	1.5
Fracture Reduction			
• Sagittal mandible*	☐	—	—
midface	—	☐	☐
• Mandibular angle	☐	—	—
• Condylar	☐	—	—
• Comminuted mandible	☐	☐	☐
Orthognathic			
• Sagittal split ramus osteotomy	☐	—	—
• Genioplasty	☐	—	—
• Subapical osteotomy	—	☐	—
Graft Fixation			
• Mandible	☐	—	—
• Midface	—	☐	☐
Ridge Augmentation	☐	☐	—

*With or without compression plate
☐ Denotes screw application.

Sagittal fractures caused by a shearing of the cortical plates of the mandible are appropriate for lag screw fixation. Depending on the type of fracture, lag screws may be used exclusively or in combination with dynamic compression plates. Simple fixation with lag screws is ideal for wide sagittal fractures that have a large area of interfragmentary contact and hence sufficient friction between the lamellae. If two or even three lag screws are used, shearing and bending forces can be neutralized and optimal interfragmentary compression can be achieved. The composite structure resulting from lag screw fixation of the fragments can withstand functional loading of the mandible.

Short sagittal fractures may need additional stabilization by a dynamic compression plate used as a neutralization plate. In comminuted fractures, lag screws are used primarily to simplify the fracture situation. Several fragments can be transformed into a simple fracture with the aid of lag screws, and additional stabilization is achieved with a neutralization plate. Fractures of the mandibular angle may be reduced and fixated with a single lag screw, by applying the screw at the distraction zone to function as a tension band.

Screws placed in lag fashion are also used to reduce condylar fractures. Because the degree of fixation achieved by lag screws is far superior to that of wire fixation, lag screws are useful in the fixation of inlay and onlay bone grafts. This stable fixation is also used to advantage in various orthognathic procedures, such as genioplasties, subapical osteotomies, and sagittal split ramus osteotomies, as well as in alveolar ridge augmentation procedures.

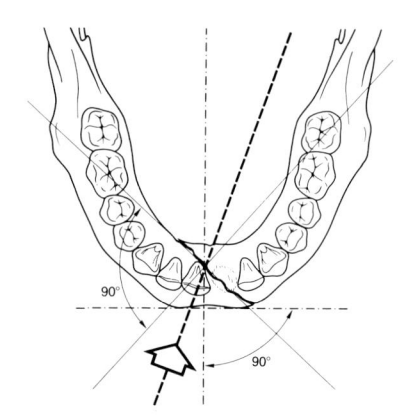

Figure 4.3 Schematic representation of orientation of lag screw axis. The screw bisects the angle between the perpendiculars to the fracture line and the bone surface.

surface (see Figure 4.3). However, this may not always be possible in practice, and lag screws are often placed perpendicular to the fracture surface. It must be emphasized that the use of lag screws demands technical precision, and limited exposure of the operative field often compounds the difficulty in evaluating their placement.

The standard armamenterium for carrying out lag screw osteosynthesis using the AO/ASIF system in the maxillofacial region includes (see Figure 4.4)

- trocar;
- drill bits, short and extra long, with external diameters of 1.5, 2.0, and 2.7 millimeters;
- corresponding drill sleeves for transcutaneous drilling;

TECHNIQUE OF LAG SCREW OSTEOSYNTHESIS

Lag screw osteosynthesis entails drilling a larger gliding hole in the outer fragment and a smaller thread hole in the inner cortical plate. Inserting and tightening an appropriate cortical screw causes interfragmentary compression. The diameter of the gliding hole must correspond to the thread diameter, and that of the thread hole must correspond to the core diameter of the screw used. Whenever possible, every screw crossing a fracture line should be inserted in a lag fashion. Because the orientation of the screw to the fracture line largely determines the stability achieved, careful attention should be given to the biomechanically correct placement of the screws in relation to the fracture line. This helps to distribute the compressive forces evenly across the fracture interfaces without distracting the fragments. To avoid shearing of the fragments, the screw holes for lag screws should be drilled so that the axis of the screw bisects the angle between the perpendicular to the fracture line and the perpendicular to the bone

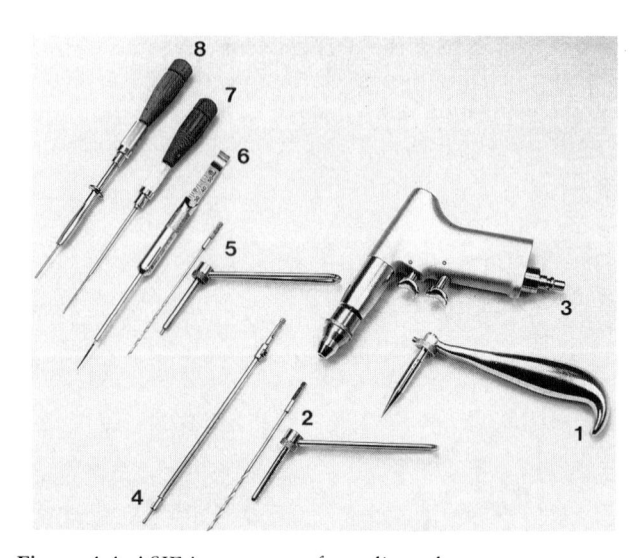

Figure 4.4 ASIF instruments for solitary lag screw osteosynthesis (from right to left): (1) trocar, (2) drill bit (2.7 millimeter) with corresponding sleeve, (3) universal air drill, (4) countersink, (5) drill bit (2.0 millimeter) with corresponding sleeve, (6) depth gauge, (7) tap (2.7 millimeter), and (8) screwdriver with screw.

- countersink;
- depth gauge;
- taps with diameters of 2.0 and 2.7 millimeters; and
- screwdriver.

Placement of any cortical screw in lag fashion is carried out in a series of coordinated steps and is best exemplified by the technique for lagging 2.7-millimeter screws (see Figure 4.5). The following description of the lag screw technique employs a pretapped screw system.

1. The fracture is accurately reduced and held in position with bone reduction forceps if possible.
2. The gliding hole is drilled first in the outer cortical plate. This is achieved with a 2.7-millimeter drill bit protected by a corresponding drill sleeve (see Figure 4.5a). It is advisable to pit the bone surface initially with a 2-millimeter drill bit to help center the 2.7-millimeter drill bit and prevent it from slipping.
3. For the spherical undersurface of the screwhead, a corresponding recess is created in the outer cortical plate over the gliding hole. This is achieved with a special countersink that has a small guide pin to help center it (see Figure 4.5b). To produce this countersink, 5-millimeter spherical burs that fit a dental handpiece can also be used. Excessive countersinking in the cortical bone with the aim of recessing the screwhead may cause the screwhead to break through, with subsequent loss of the compressive effect. In the case of thin cortices, small metal washers may be used to keep the screwhead from breaking through thin cortical bone; the head thereby distributing pressure more evenly.
4. Once the countersink in the outer fragment is completed, an insert sleeve with 2.7-millimeter outer diameter and 2-millimeter inner diameter is pushed through the gliding hole. A thread hole is drilled in the inner fragment with a 2-millimeter drill bit inserted through this sleeve (see Figure 4.5c). Using the insert sleeve ensures that the gliding hole and the thread hole are coaxial (see Figure 4.5d). Drilling the thread hole without the insert drill sleeve may cause the bit to skid when it encounters an oblique inner cortex, disturbing the coaxial arrangement of the gliding and thread holes. It is important that the fragments remain exactly reduced throughout this procedure.
5. Once drilling is complete, the length of the screw is determined by measuring the screw hole with a depth gauge (see Figure 4.5e). This is carried out prior to tapping the thread hole in order to prevent damage to the threads. Screw length must be adequate to ensure that the tip of the screw protrudes about 1 to 2 mm beyond the inner cortical plate. A short screw that partially engages the thread hole would damage the thread as the screw is tightened.
6. With a 2.7-millimeter tap, a thread hole is cut into the inner fragment (see Figures 4.5f and g). The threads may be stripped during screw insertion if the threads have not been cut by an appropriate tap. Because drill bits and taps have potential to traumatize the soft tissues, they must always be used within a drill sleeve. In addition to confining the drill bit and tap, the sleeve guides it along the predetermined axis of the gliding hole, ensuring

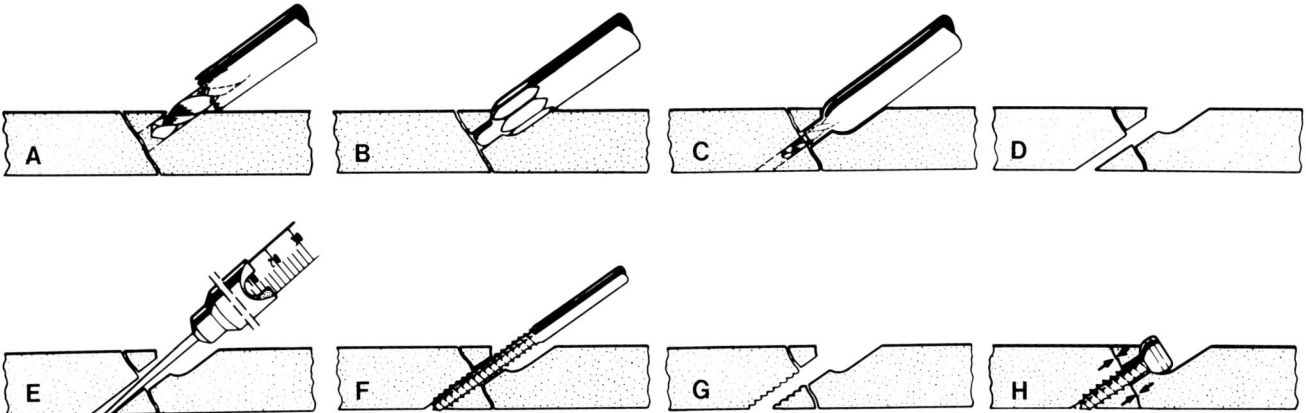

Figure 4.5 Step-by-step procedure in lag screw osteosynthesis: (a) preparation of gliding hole; (b) preparation of bed for screwhead; (c) drilling the thread hole via an insert drill sleeve; (d) prepared bed, gliding hole, and thread hole; (e) determination of screw length; (f) tapping of the thread hole; (g) completely prepared fragments; (h) lag screw in position.

concentricity of the thread and gliding hole. Tapping by hand provides a highly tactile sense of the thickness of the cortex; diminishing resistance implies that the thread has been completed. Tactile sense helps assess the screw hold that the inner cortex will afford and also prevents injury to the delicate soft tissue, a complication caused by driving the tap too far.

7. The 2.7-millimeter cortical bone screw can now slide through the hole in the outer fragment and obtain a firm hold in the thread of the inner cortical bone. When the screw is firmly tightened, the fracture surfaces are stabilized under pressure (see Figure 4.5h). The application of a second and, if needed, a third screw proceeds in a similar fashion.

As a rule, large, oblique fractures of the mandible should be rigidly fixed by at least two and preferably three lag screws placed in a staggered manner and with diverging axes. This form of fixation stabilizes the fracture surfaces uniformly and produces a composite structure that can resist bending and shear forces better than a single lag screw can. The position of the nerve canal as well as adjacent teeth may hinder placement of two or more lag screws in the case of short oblique fractures of the dentulous mandible with minimal overlap of fracture surfaces. In such fractures, which necessitate application of a compression plate, the screw placed in the plate hole crossing the oblique fracture line is inserted in lag fashion while the remaining screws are inserted in a neutral fashion (see Figure 4.6). The interfragmental compression produced at the fracture site by the lag screw augments the fixation afforded by the plate. Exceptions to the rule "two to three lag screws minimum" are mandibular angle fractures where the intermeshing fragments can be stabilized with a single lag screw due to the favorable biomechanical conditions in this region.

As indicated earlier, choice of appropriate screw size is dictated by the anatomy and biomechanics of the region. The screw size should be correlated to the size of the bone, and one must always begin with the smallest screw possible. Using large screws in small fragments can drastically weaken the fragment, leading to its fracture when the screw is tightened. In most cases 2.7-millimeter screws are adequate for mandible fractures; however, should the threads strip during screw insertion, an emergency screw (3.5 millimeters) can be placed after enlarging the gliding hole to 3.5 millimeters. If the fragments are very small, as is often found in the midface, miniscrews (1.1 millimeters) are used initially. If osteosynthesis is unsuccessful due to the threads stripping, it can be repeated with a 1.5-millimeter screw. In children and in elderly patients with atrophic mandibles, 2-millimeter screws are generally adequate. Care is taken that the screw hole is drilled at an adequate distance from the fracture line because placing it close to the edge will cause the bone to fragment when the screw is tightened.

Lag screw osteosynthesis is very sensitive to technique; any deviation from standard lag screw technique will affect the stability of the result. The thread hole in the far fragment should be drilled through a narrow insert sleeve placed in the gliding hole to ensure that the axes of the gliding and thread holes are coincident (see Figures 4.7a and b). An improperly centered thread hole will cause the fragments to displace as the screw is tightened (see Figure 4.7c). The holding power of a lag screw is determined to a large extent by the number of active threads (threads that grip the screw) in the thread hole. At least three active threads are needed to create a lag effect. Drilling a thread hole initially and then enlarging the outer hole to form a gliding hole carries the attendant danger of damaging the thread hole as the gliding hole is being prepared (see Figure 4.8). Overdrilling the gliding hole will result in a shortened thread hole that is weak and will strip when the screw is tightened. Besides preventing pressure resorption of adjoining bone, pretapping the thread hole also allows the

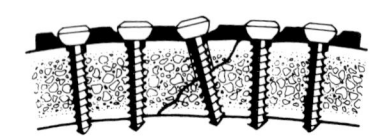

Figure 4.6 When used in conjunction with a compression plate, the screw placed in the plate hole crossing the oblique fracture line is inserted in lag fashion. The adjoining screws are inserted in neutral fashion to avoid shear stresses on the lag screw.

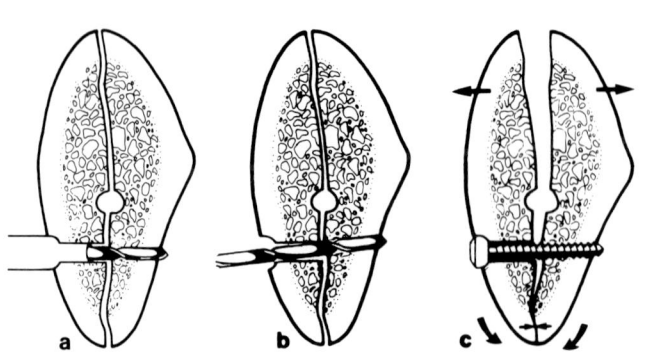

Figure 4.7 (a) A thread hole is drilled with the help of an insert drill sleeve. (b) Drilling without an insert sleeve results in a thread hole that is not coaxial with the gliding hole. (c) Noncoincident axes result in displacement and uneven compression of the fragments when the lag screw is tightened.

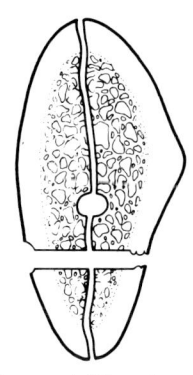

Figure 4.8 Overdrilling or drilling the gliding hole second damages the thread hole and jeopardizes the lag effect.

creation of maximal holding power. Screws must be inserted with care because they can exert great mechanical advantage during insertion. Application of too much torque with the screwdriver can easily strip the threads in bone.

SUMMARY

Lag screws are surgical bone screws used to clamp bone fragments together. A lag effect is achieved by preparing the screw holes so that the screw can glide through the hole in the outer fragment and engage the threaded hole in the opposite fragment. The torsional moment of screw insertion generates tensile forces along the length of the screw that draws the fragments together, resulting in interfragmentary compression. When used for the proper indications and applied correctly, lag screws provide a degree of fixation that equals or even surpasses that achieved with compression plates.

BIBLIOGRAPHY

Heim U, Pfeiffer KM: Internal Fixation of Small Fractures. 3rd ed. Berlin, Heidelberg, New York, London, Paris, Tokyo, 1987.

Muller ME, Allgower M, Schneider R, Willeneger H: Manual of Internal Fixation. Springer, Berlin, Heidelberg, New York, 1979.

Niederdellmann H: Rigid internal fixation by means of lag screws. In: Kruger E, Schilli W, eds. Oral and Maxillofacial Traumatology. Quintessence Publishing Co; Chicago, Berlin, Rio de Janeiro, Tokyo, 1982.

Niederdellmann H, Shetty V, Collins JVC: Controlled osteosynthesis with the position screw. Int J Adult Orthodont Orthognat Surg 2: 159–162, 1987.

CHAPTER 5

Implant Materials in Rigid Fixation: Physical, Mechanical, Corrosion, and Biocompatibility Considerations

David E. Altobelli

CLINICAL APPLICATIONS IN THE CRANIOMAXILLOFACIAL REGION

Utilization of biomaterials as components for medical devices in the craniomaxillofacial region has increased significantly. Previous treatment of fractures in the head and neck region used fixation techniques and devices predominantly in a transient fashion, with the hardware commonly removed within a short interval after completion of healing. With the current expanded use of these materials and devices for trauma and elective surgery, the hardware is often left in place indefinitely because removal of these devices would often require additional surgery.

In addition to the stabilization of fractured and osteotomized bone segments, other structural applications that employ metallic devices include osseointegrated fixtures for support of intraoral and extraoral prosthetics and temporomandibular joint replacements. With the extended clinical applications of these materials and devices, questions regarding the longevity of function and the effects of long-term exposures of these materials on the biologic system become of significant concern and must be evaluated.

PRINCIPLES AND REQUIREMENTS

Objectives of rigid fixation are to provide predictable healing, stability of bone fractures and osteotomies, and rapid return to function (Spiessl 1976, Prein 1987). The most important consideration for healing is stability of bone segments and/or the bone–implant interface. Relative motion, possibly at the level of a few microns, may modify the cellular response and differentiation at the healing interface.

The effect of forces and deformation on the response of bone has been studied since the law of bone remodeling was proposed by Wolff (1892) to relate function and structure. Although the mechanism/transducer in bone that results in a cellular response (that is, modeling, remodeling, repair) is still unknown, a concept of minimal effective strain (MES) has been proposed (Frost 1987). The MES for mammalian bone modeling is believed to be 1500 to 2000 microstrain (about 0.2% change in original length). For active bone remodeling, much less strain, 100 to 300 microstrain (about 0.025% change in length), is required. Although it is not currently known what level of tissue strain (micromotion) will promote primary bone healing without callus formation, it probably lies somewhere in this range.

Stability allows primary healing of bone segments (Schenk 1986) and osseointegration at the bone–implant interface of titanium fixtures (Brånemark 1983). In contrast, relative motion between fracture or osteotomy segments leads to callus formation and secondary healing. At the interface between bone and implant, instability leads to a less differentiated, fibrous tissue healing response. Because stability must be maintained in a dynamic functional environment, design must integrate biomaterial, biomechanical, and biologic parameters.

POLYMERS, CERAMICS, AND BIODEGRADABLE MATERIALS

The three basic classes of biomaterials are metals, ceramics, and polymers. Rigid fixation methods to date have relied almost exclusively on metallic components. This is because of their high strength and contourability.

Ceramics, including calcium phosphate preparations, bioglasses, and alumina have excellent biocompatibility profiles. They unfortunately tend to be brittle and cannot currently be sufficiently contoured or adapted to the anatomic site. Current polymeric materials do not have adequate strength and rigidity for all dynamic biomechanical conditions in the craniofacial skeleton. However, polylactic and polyglycolic acid preparations and other bioresorbable preparations are under development that may provide adequate fixation stabilities in areas of low stress (Getter 1972, Cutright 1971, Hollinger 1987, Bos 1987) (see Chapter 6).

In this chapter we will focus on metals currently used for rigid fixation. Much of information presented in regard to the development of standards, characteristics, and performance of materials, products, systems, and devices will be referenced from the American Society for Testing and Materials (ASTM). This scientific and technical organization, founded in 1898, is the largest source of consensus standards (ASTM 1986). In Table 5.1, composition, standards, and tradenames have been organized to provide some correlation with the various classification systems.

METALS CURRENTLY IN USE

Stainless steel(s), cobalt-chromium alloy(s), and titanium (commercially pure) and titanium alloy(s) are the metals most commonly used for rigid fixation and total joint replacement (see Table 5.2). Other biocompatible metals used clinically include tantalum and nitinol (nickel-titanium alloy). All preparations have the

Table 5.1 Surgical Metals: Classification Systems/Tradenames

Metal	Basic Composition	Preparation	ASTM	ISO	Trade names/Other
Ferrous Alloys (Stainless Steel)	Fe-Cr-Wi-Mo	Wrought	F55, F56, F138, F139	5832-1	AISI-316-L, AISI-316-LVW, 316L, Ortron 90®, 22-13-5®
Cobalt-Chromium	Co-Cr-Mo	Cast	F75	5834-4	Alivium® Endocast® Orthochrome®, Orthochome-Plus® Protasul®, Protasul-2® Vitallium-Cast® Zimaloy® Mediloy® Vinertia® Coballoy®
		Wrought Forged	F75		Endocast Hot Worked® Protasul-21WF® Vitallium FHS®
		Power Metallurgy	F75		Micrograin-Zimaloy®
	Co-Cr-W-Ni	Wrought	F90		H525
	Co-Ni-Cr-Mo	Vacuum Remelt Cast/Wrought	F562, F688	5832-6	Protasul-10® MP-35N® Biophase® AMS 5758
	Co-Ni-Cr-Mo-M-Fe	Wrought	F563		Syntacoben®
Titanium	Ti	Cast/Wrought	F67		Unalloyed Titanium CP (Commercially Pure) Grades 1, 2, 3, 4 (ASTM F67) T_{115}, T_{125}, T_{130}, T_{160}
Titanium Alloy	Ti-Al-V	Wrought	F136	5832-3	IMI-318A® Protasul-64WF® Tioxium® Tivaloy® Tivanium®

NOTE: This chart is provided to assist with classification of materials based on general categories or classification systems. Individual materials may have additional characteristics that make them different from others in the similar category.

Table 5.2 Composition of Ferrous, Cobalt, and Titanium Alloys

Composition, %		Ferrous Alloys				
		ASTM F55, F56		ASTM F138, F139		Cast ASTM F75
Element		A Grade 2	B Grade 1	A Grade 2	B Grade 1	
C	Carbon, max	0.03 max	0.08 max	0.03 max	0.08 max	0.35 max
Co	Cobalt	—	—	—	—	Balance
Cr	Chromium	17.00–20.00	17–20	17.00–19.00	17–19	27.0–30.0
Fe	Iron	Balance	Balance	Balance	Balance	0.75 max
Mo	Molybdenum	2.00–3.00	2.00–3.00	2.00–3.00	2–3	5.0–7.0
Mn	Manganese, max	2.00 max	2.0 max	2.00 max	2.00 max	1.00 max
Ni	Nickel	12–14	12–14	12–14	12–14	1.0 max
P	Phosphorous	0.025 max	—	0.03 max	0.03 max	—
S	Sulfur	0.010 max	—	0.03 max	0.03 max	—
Si	Silicon	0.75 max	—	0.75 max	0.75 max	1.00 max
Ti	Titanium	—	—	—	—	—
N	Nitrogen, max	—	—	—	—	—
H	Hydrogen, max	—	—	—	—	—
O	Oxygen, max	—	—	—	—	—
Al	Aluminum	—	—	—	—	—
V	Vanadium	—	—	—	—	—

basic mechanical, corrosion, and biocompatibility characteristics acceptable for clinical use as implantable materials.

The selection of a specific material for the specific application is often a balance of compromises: No one material possesses optimal characteristics in all categories. Material selection must take into account the specific biologic environment, the biomechanical structural requirements, and the length of required clinical usefulness. As a prerequisite to selection of the final design and material, comprehensive definition of the problem and approaches to a solution must be undertaken. In spite of an incomplete knowledge base, characteristic of interfacing biologic systems, reliable design solutions can be formulated.

History: Stainless Steel (Sutow 1981)

In 1821, Berthier found that iron alloyed with chromium demonstrated increased resistance to acid corrosion. It was not until 1926 that stainless steel (18Cr-8Ni) was introduced into orthopedic surgery. In 1947, the more corrosion resistant molybdenum-alloyed 18-8 stainless steel was recommended. Currently, the 316L alloy of stainless steels (ASTM F55, F56, F138, F139) are most commonly used. Iron comprises 60% to 68% of the stainless steel alloy, with 17% to 20% chromium, 12% to 14% nickel, and 2% to 4% molybdenum (see Figure 5.1).

History: Cobalt-chromium Alloys (Williams 1981)

The cobalt-chromium (Co-Cr) alloys have a significant role in the history of metallic implants. In the early 1900s Haynes did much of the pioneering work with cobalt-chromium alloys. Corrosion resistance and biological acceptance was demonstrated with stellite (Co-Cr alloys with starlike microstructures) during the 1920s and 1930s, leading to the introduction of Vitallium as a castable dental alloy. When used in medical applications, Co-Cr alloys demonstrate good overall balance of corrosion resistance, fatigue resistance, and

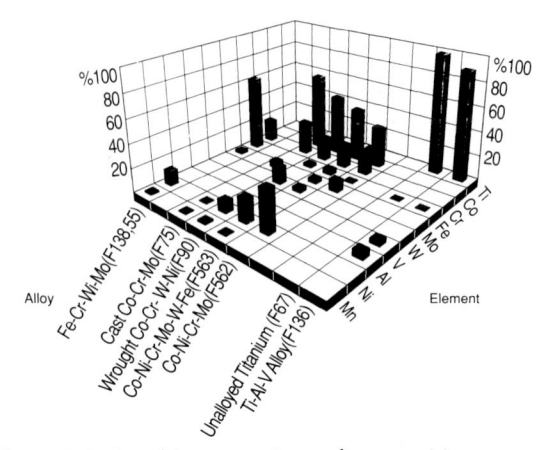

Figure 5.1 Graphic comparison of composition percentages of surgical metals.

Table 5.2 (continued)

	Co-Base Alloys		C.P. Titanium ASTM F67			Titanium Alloys ASTM F136	
Wrought ASTM F90	ASTM F563	ASTM F562	Grade 1	Grade 2	Grade 3	Grade 4	Ti6A14V
0.05–0.15	0.05 max	0.025 max	0.10	0.10	0.10	0.10	0.08
Balance	Balance	Balance	—	—	—	—	—
19.0–21.0	18.0–22.0	19.0–21.0	—	—	—	—	—
3.0 max	4.00–6.0	1.0 max	0.20	0.30	0.30	0.50	0.25
—	3.0–4.0	9.0–10.5	—	—	—	—	—
1.0–2.00	1.0 max	0.15 max	—	—	—	—	—
9.0–11.0	15.0–25.0	33.0–37.0	—	—	—	—	—
—	—	0.015 max	—	—	—	—	—
—	0.010 max	0.010 max	—	—	—	—	—
0.4 max	0.50 max	0.015 max	—	—	—	—	—
—	0.5–3.5	1.0 max	Balance	Balance	Balance	Balance	Balance
14–16	3–4	—	0.03	0.03	0.05	0.05	0.05
—	—	—	0.015	0.015	0.015	0.015	0.012
—	—	—	0.18	0.25	0.35	0.40	0.13
—	—	—	—	—	—	—	5.5–6.50
—	—	—	—	—	—	—	3.5–4.5

strength. Cobalt-chromium alloys are composed of 50% to 63% cobalt, 19% to 33% chromium, and depending on the specific alloy, can contain nickel 0% to 37%, molybdenum 0% to 10%, or tungsten 0% to 13% with additional small amounts of iron, carbon, manganese, or silicon (see Figure 5.1).

History: Titanium (Williams 1981)

The first reported discovery of titanium is attributed to Wilheim Gregor in 1791. The oxide of titanium, rutile, was isolated from the "black magnetic sand" at Menachan in Cornwall. Because the metal is so reactive at the temperatures needed for the extraction process, it took nearly 150 years for a method to be developed to extract the titanium with any significant degree of purity. The industrial process that is used today was developed by Kroll in the 1930s. The reduction of the rutile using magnesium is carried out in an argon atmosphere, and the metal is obtained in the form of a sponge. The sponge is consolidated in an electrode vacuum arc furnace. The titanium alloys were developed in the early 1950s.

Of the three major metallic implant systems, titanium and its alloys were the most recently introduced into the biomaterials field. Because of their combination of strength, light weight, corrosion resistance, and biocompatibility, titanium and its alloys are gaining widespread usage as implant materials.

The titanium (commercially pure) preparation is available in at least four grades, with titanium composing greater than 99%. Small amounts of oxygen can greatly modify the ductility and yield strength of the material. Titanium alloy, specifically Ti-6A1-4V (90% titanium, 6% aluminum, 4% vanadium) has been used most in clinical situations (see Figure 5.1).

ANATOMIC CONSIDERATIONS

Structural support and protection of vital organs of the human body is primarily served by bone. Bone is unique and quite different from any current biomaterials used to modulate or replace it. The most important distinction is that bone is self-repairing tissue that can adapt and respond to biomechanical demands. In contrast, a biomaterial placed into a biological and functional situation most often will have a finite period of clinical usefulness. A delicate balance must be considered in the design of devices for fixation, that being one of rigid structural support during healing and minimal interference with the biologic system during and at the completion of healing.

The craniomaxillary region is a complex structure composed largely of thin cortical bone. Conceptually, the structural elements are arranged in a series of columns, arches, and buttresses. The skull is comprised of many hollow regions (sinuses, cranial vault, nasal and oral cavities); thin plates of bone are common and provide lateral support to the primary structural members. Designing a fixation system to withstand large masticatory forces, to provide minimal profile above the bone surface, and to attach securely to thin plates of bone is a challenging problem. The fixation plates and screws must provide adequate strength to stabilize large bone segments from dynamic loads while capable of being contoured to very close tolerances that follow complex anatomic surface geometries. Ideally, biomaterials used for rigid fixation should satisfy the following basic requirements:

1. *Biocompatibility:* The material must be locally and systematically nontoxic, cause no form of immune response, and cause no dysplastic or malignant transformation.

2. *Mechanical:* Absolute stability of bone segments in a dynamic, functional environment with a device of minimal profile and geometry is essential. Strength must be adequate to allow the device to function in its elastic range and to provide the necessary stability for healing. In addition, the device must be contourable to allow close adaption to the anatomic surface geometry without significantly weakening the biomaterial. In situations with long-term function and many cycles of loading, the interface must remain intact and the device must not fracture secondary to fatigue.

3. *Corrosion:* The material must be highly resistant to corrosion to maintain its structural integrity and to avoid toxicity to local tissues and systemic sites. Biocompatibility and the nature of the interface are dependent on resistance to corrosion.

4. *Artifact:* There should be minimal distortion of currently used imaging modalities in the head and neck region; that is, CT and MRI are important. It is unacceptable to exclude the patient from these diagnostic studies.

5. *Remodeling and growth:* The interference of normal remodeling of bone or growth and development should be minimal.

The objectives of this chapter are to introduce definitions and general concepts used to characterize the physical, mechanical, corrosion, and biological properties of implant materials used for structural applications in the craniomaxillofacial region. We will discuss functional and biologic constraints important for the design, fabrication, and surgical use of the implant materials. We will supply specific properties of the most commonly used implant materials. Basic principles in relation to the handling and manipulation of the implant materials for surgical application will be outlined. Finally, future directions in methods and materials of fixation will be discussed.

MATERIAL AND PHYSICAL PROPERTIES

Metallic Structure

Metallic Bond

The atomic mechanism that determines the general behavior of metals is the metallic bond. This can be visualized as an array of metal *positive ions* in regular geometric patterns or crystallographic lattices. The positive ions' cores are surrounded by a relatively free electron cloud.

Unit Cell

The smallest unit to describe the arrangement or packing of the atoms is the unit cell. The three most simple unit cells are the body-centered cubic (BCC), the face-centered cubic (FCC), and the hexagonal close-packed (HCP) lattices (see Figure 5.2). The unit cells are arranged in lattices or planes to form crystals. Upon cooling of the molten metal, multiple sites of nucleation initiate crystalline formation. As they increase in size, their growth is impeded by their expanding neighbors. The crystals, now referred to as grains, are 10^{-2} to 10^{-6} m in length, with 10^9 to 10^{10} grains per cm^3. The interdigitating grains are of variable size, shape, and orientation. The grain structure greatly influences both mechanical and chemical properties of the bulk material.

Lattice Defects

Microdefects present in the cooled, solidified material are responsible for the disparity in the theoretical and actual strength of the materials. Postulated defects include (1) point defects, such as missing, substituted, and interstitially placed atoms; (2) line defects, or rows of missing atoms (dislocations); (3) area defects (grain

UNIT CELL		ATOMS PER UNIT CELL	% VOLUME OCCUPIED	EXAMPLES
Body Center Cubic (BCC)	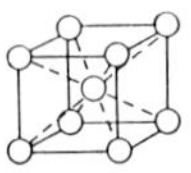	2	68%	Fe <916°C Ti(β) >1389°C Cr >900°C Mo Ta
Face Center Cubic (FCC)	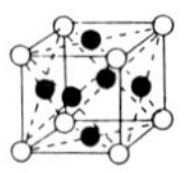	4	74%	Fe 916°–1389°C Al Co >460°C Ni SS Austenitic
Hexagonal Closed Packed (HCP)	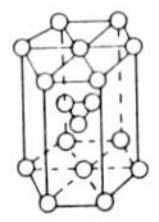	6	74%	Ti(α) Co

Figure 5.2 Unit cell configurations, properties, and examples.

boundaries); and (4) volume defects, such as cavities or voids.

Experiments have demonstrated that a material in its bulk, undeformed state contains 10^6 dislocations per cubic centimeter. After severe deformation, up to 10^{10} dislocations per cubic centimeter can be present. These sites of dislocation are points where internal stress is present. Although they do not influence the actual stiffness of the material, they are important in determining the ultimate strength of the material. Processing methods to strengthen materials must either minimize the incidence of these imperfections or modify the materials to immobilize dislocations. This prevents slip or shearing between closely packed atom planes.

Alloys and Phases

Alloys

In order to obtain desirable properties of strength and ductility, combinations of metals (that is, alloys) are often used. When two or more metallic elements are melted and cooled, they form intermetallic compounds, solid solutions, or combinations of both. The alloy can be single phase or multiphase, depending on the temperature and composition during crystallization.

Phase

A phase is defined as a physical homogeneous part of the material system. Foreign atoms of smaller size are accommodated interstitially, and those of similar size and properties are substituted into the parent lattice. If constituent metallic elements normally form different crystal structures or are of grossly dissimilar sizes, there will be a finite limit to the amount one element can dissolve into the other. This will effect the consistency of the crystal structure throughout the alloy. Multiple phases (areas of different composition and crystal structure) can also be present throughout the alloy. The crystal structure and solubility limits for a given alloy are strongly dependent on temperature and elemental proportions. Equilibrium diagrams map the various phase combinations.

Transition Temperature

The addition of elements in a solid solution of the metal will modify the transition temperature, or point where the metal can spontaneously change its lattice formation (that is, BCC to FCC). The addition of various elements to an alloy allows a specific lattice form with its characteristic properties to remain stable at room temperature. In contrast to the pure metal, the desired unit cell configuration would be present only at the elevated temperature.

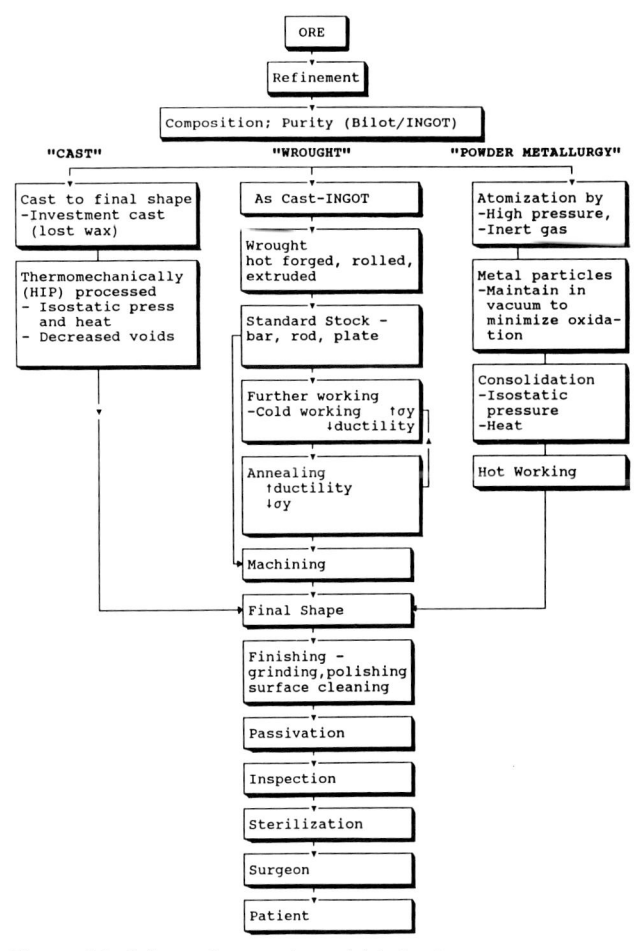

Figure 5.3 Schematic overview of fabrication process to prepare a medical device for application.

Material Modification and Manufacturing

Material Refinement

The fabrication of a medical device is an involved process (see Figure 5.3). After the materials are mined and refined from ores, they either remain single-element preparations or are combined in the form of alloys. At this point, the materials have often been melted into the form of an ingot or bilot. Material characteristics at this level of processing are a function of composition and methods of cooling.

Cast and Wrought Materials

The next leveling of processing involves either direct casting or further processing of the material. The material can be modified through several iterations of shaping and annealing (heat treatment) to modify its strength and ductility. A more recent technique initially forms the metal into small particles that are then formed into standardized forms using temperature and pressure (powder metallurgy). This approach minimizes some of the problems with imperfections in cast materials.

Investment casting is the easiest approach to manufacturing complex shapes. In applications with high strength requirements, "as cast" materials tend to have limited capability for plastic deformation or ductility secondary to small voids from the casting process. These defects can be minimized by careful techniques to control gas formation and the flow metal into the mold. The interdendritic porosity secondary to shrinkage on solidification can be minimized by hot isostatic pressing (HIP) of the cast part.

For critical load-bearing applications, wrought materials provide better mechanical properties. The process involves plastic mechanical deformation of the originally cast material to refine grain structure, close internal porosity, and, with subsequent annealing, to provide a more uniform phase composition.

Working and Annealing

Cold Working

Properties of bulk materials after solidification can be modified using techniques of cold working, hot working, and annealing. Cold working, or work hardening, involves the plastic deformation and/or shaping of the material below its transition temperature (the temperature at which atoms, by virtue of thermal energy, can rearrange themselves in the lattice to a less stressed, more normal position). These methods, performed typically at room temperature, include cold rolling, swagging, extrusion, and forging. This causes the atoms to shift within the bulk material, dislocation tangles to form, and potential sites for slip are eliminated. The final result is to strengthen (increase the proportional limit) and increase the hardness of the material, with the stiffness of the material remaining essentially unchanged. The materials now will have less ductility and toughness. With strength and ductility inversely related, cold working must be controlled to provide a satisfactory combination of properties.

Annealing

To allow materials to be elongated and shaped beyond the limits of cold working, a structure can be heat-treated, or annealed. Because the atoms are not rigidly fixed in their current cold-worked positions, thermal energy allows them to diffuse and rearrange themselves into less strained lattice positions. This internal adjustment of stress and strain occurs on a microscopic level; there are no macroscopic dimension changes. Thus, as the material softens with increasing temperature, new small grains of equal dimensions in all directions grow inside the old distorted grains and at the old grain boundaries. The higher the temperature is above the recrystallization temperature, the larger or more coarse the grain size. Hardness and strength decrease with increasing grain size, but elongation or ductility increases. It is generally desirable to have a fine grain size for an optimum combination of strength and ductility.

Hot Working

Instead of cold working and annealing, materials can be wrought or hot worked. When the temperature is increased above transition before the structure is deformed, the part can be worked or shaped with recrystallization occurring simultaneously with deformation. Suppliers use this approach to refine and modify the shape of the mill product into the form of bars, rods, and sheets for distribution. Hot forging may also be used as a final working operation with certain implant products that require very high yield strength and hardness. The disadvantages of hot working can be excessive oxidation of the metal surface and shorter life of the dies used to shape the material.

Isotropic and Anisotropic Materials

The physical and mechanical properties of the material may not be identical in all directions. This is predominantly a function of the method used to work the material. Materials with the same properties in all directions are classified isotropic, and materials with properties varying with direction are considered anisotropic.

Fabrication and Cleaning

Machining techniques, forging, and, more recently, laser cutting methods are commonly used to fabricate a medical device from the materials in stock preparations (bar, rod, or plate). ASTM carefully outlines recommended standards for composition, mechanical properties, biocompatibility testing, material preparation, and manufacturing of surgical implants.

After the surgical implant is formed, additional steps are required prior to implantation. The surface is inspected and must be free of imperfections (ASTM F86). The surface must then be cleaned of contaminants such as cutting fluid in ultrasonically agitated organic solvents and hot alkaline preparations. Titanium is chemically cleaned, passivated (ASTM F86-84); and with osseointegrated implants, special protocols using butinol are applied (Brånemark 1985).

Passivation

All surgical implants must have a passive surface condition. This surface spontaneously forms on most metals used for surgical implantation and can be increased in thickness using acid solutions or electrochemical techniques (ASTM F86). The implant surface energy can be modified and has been shown to influence the initial interaction and attraction of biomolecules and cells to the implant surface (Kasemo 1983, Baier 1988). Newer techniques using radiofrequency plasma glow discharge have been used to remove contaminants from the implant; a high-energy surface remains.

Sterilization

Heat, radiation, and chemical techniques are employed to sterilize implant materials. Each approach has specific advantages and disadvantages and is beyond the scope of this chapter. Autoclaving with steam under pressure is the most common technique used. Studies have shown (Baier 1982) that contaminants are introduced onto the surface of implants that are autoclaved, and that there is an increase in thickness of the oxide layer. These effects are probably of greater consequence in long-term applications like osseointegrated implant applications than they are in short-term applications with rigid fixation, where integrity of the bone–implant interface is not as crucial.

Surgical Handling

The final step before the device is introduced into function in the patient is the manipulation by the surgeon. The standardization and control of this step are the most tenuous in the entire process. Appropriate application of the device and patient selection are crucial for the implant to function as originally designed. Basic principles in handling the implant include the following:

1. Minimize handling and contamination of the implant.
2. Minimize the contouring of the implant.
3. Minimize damage and contamination to the implant surface with contouring instruments.
4. Minimize overbending and unbending—It is better to under-contour the implant and go through another iteration of fitting.
5. All screws must be stable. Any loose screw must be removed; otherwise, it will be a source of corrosion at the screw–plate interface.
6. Minimize trauma to bone. Use a slow cutting speed and irrigate copiously.
7. Try to minimize or eliminate use of dissimilar metals in near proximity, especially when they are in direct contact.
8. Antibiotic prophylaxis is suggested, especially in clean contaminated surgical sites, often encountered in the craniomaxillofacial-mandibular region.

More stringent requirements are required for implants that will require an osseointegrated interface:

1. The implant surface should be handled only with instruments of similar composition.
2. Any fixture that comes in contact with a patient, even if it is not used, cannot be adequately cleaned to be used in another patient (contamination of the oxide coating, requires special techniques to be reprepared).

Surface Properties

Behavior of a biomaterial in the biological environment is a function of properties of the bulk material, the structural form or geometry, and the interaction of the implant surface with the biological system. Although the first two considerations are important, it is behavior at the surface that is most complex and least understood.

The composition of the surface of surgical metals is quite different from that of the bulk material. The surface of passivated metals is often composed of the oxide of the metal; this surface thus has properties similar to those of ceramic materials. Alloys are composed of multiple elements in different percentages. However, the oxides of these constituent materials are not necessarily in the same proportion on the material surface (Kasemo 1983)

The surface layer primarily determines the resistance of the material to corrosion. The oxide surface layer must be continuous and tenaciously adherent to the surface of the bulk material and must possess a low solubility in the biological environment. It must have a self-limiting thickness, it must not break off into the adjacent tissues, and it must have the ability to regenerate rapidly if damaged.

The biocompatibility of the material is also determined essentially at the surface. Initial cell and biochemical interactions are largely determined by surface energy and surface chemistry. Corrosion products leaving the implant surface must be minimal in order that they will not adversely affect local or systemic tissues. The interaction at the surface is also an important consideration when dealing with infected tissues that have implants or "foreign bodies" present (Gustilo 1989).

Many mechanical properties are determined at the level of the implant surface. Surface imperfections can appear for many reasons, including improper material preparation, poor design and fabrication techniques, defects from contouring or manipulation, and sites of localized corrosion. These sites are often responsible for fatigue fracture from cyclic loading levels well below the yield strength of the material.

Details of surface energy and chemistry are beyond the scope of this chapter. The reader is referred to Baier (1982, 1988) and Kasemo (1983) for detailed discussion of surface energy and methods of modifying the surface (that is, radiofrequency glow discharge [plasma] techniques). The surface of titanium is probably the most extensively studied in relation to biocellular interaction in conjunction with osseointegration. The reader is referred to Brånemark (1983) for extended discussion of biological interaction at the bone–titanium interface.

Physical Properties of Implant Metals

Stainless Steel

Microstructure Stainless steels are produced in four primary categories: ferritic, martensitic, austenitic, and precipitation-hardened. Pure iron is allotropic and exists as a body-centered cubic ferrite. The recommended stainless steel for surgical implants is the American Iron and Steel Institute (AISI) type 316 L fully austenitic preparation. Austenitic stainless steels, with their good corrosion characteristics, have a face-centered cubic crystalline structure. Each of the alloying elements is included for specific purposes. A desirable addition to stainless steel is Ni (12% to 17%), which provides some corrosion resistance, controls the rate of work hardening, and maintains a fully austenitic crystal structure at room temperature. Carbon concentration is low to prevent carbide precipitation at grain boundaries, which would decrease corrosion resistance. Chromium, in a percentage of at least 12%, imparts significant resistance to corrosion of the bulk metal by the formation of a passive surface oxide. Molybdenum is added in small concentrations to prevent pitting and crevice corrosion. The molybdenum content must be limited to prevent ferrite and sigma phase formation (embrittlement). Manganese, present in small percentages of less than 2%, encourages austenite phase stability.

Fabrication Strict care is required in the manufacture of high-quality implant specimens. Stainless steels are perhaps the easiest metal implant and least expensive materials to fabricate. Although it is possible to cast these materials directly to their final shape, the impurity levels and internal imperfections produced by this technique lead to inferior corrosion and mechanical properties, especially when compared to forged and cold-worked production methods. Electric arc furnaces are used for melting, and subsequent vacuum arc remelting (VAR) techniques are often used to remove nonmetallic impurities such as sulfides, alumina, silicates, and globular oxides. Austenitic stainless steels can be hot worked readily in air within the appropriate temperature range for the alloy composition.

Cobalt-Chromium Alloys

Microstructure Cobalt has a polymorphic crystal structure, existing in the hexagonal close-packed (HCP) structure at room temperature and in the face-centered cubic (FCC) structure at temperatures greater than 460°C. Alloying elements will affect the crystal structure transition temperature of cobalt. Addition of chromium, molybdenum, and tungsten tends to increase the transition temperature, whereas addition of iron and nickel tends to lower the HCP-to-FCC transformation temperature. The addition of molybdenum, tungsten, chromium, manganese, and silicon to the alloy results in solid solution hardening. The alloys are toughened or increased in ductility by the addition of nickel.

Cast Alloys (ASTM F75 Co-Cr-Mo) Cast materials are essentially solid solutions of chromium in cobalt. Molybdenum aids in the reduction of grain size, which results in increased strength. The rate of cooling of the casting influences the grain size: If the casting is cooled too slowly, the grains are large, imparting decreased tensile properties; if it is cooled too rapidly, gases that evolve during solidification do not have time to bubble out of the mold, causing voids or porosities. These areas of imperfection are potential sites of corrosion and material failure. Vitallium is a common Co-Cr alloy used for casting surgical implants.

Forged Alloys To combat the problems with casting, new forms of Co-Cr alloy have been introduced. Alloys of Co-Cr with additional elements such as tungsten, nickel, molybdenum, and iron, create wrought preparations (ASTM F90, F563, F562) that are used mainly for joint prostheses. Forged cast Co-Cr alloys (alloys formed into shapes by both pressure and heat) have been developed to break up the structure into a smaller grain size and to obliterate and fuse any voids or imperfections in the structure. One example is forged high strength (FHS) Vitallium.

Powder Metallurgy/Hot Isostatic Pressing Recent developments in powder metallurgy that employ the hot isostatic pressing (HIP) technique have been used to produce Co-Cr metal implants. The implants that result from this technique have small grain size with virtually no porosity. This greatly enhances the mechanical properties, specifically the fatigue properties. The HIP process introduced in conjunction with improved powder metallurgy techniques has greatly improved the performance of Co-Cr alloy implants. In this procedure, alloy powder produced by argon atomization is loaded into vacuum containers to be consolidated into shape at 1100°C (2000°F) and 100 megapascals pressure for approximately one hour. This temperature is substantially below the melting point of the alloy (1240 to 1450°C). Bonding of the particles occurs by solid-state diffusion. The resulting product is fully dense with an ultrafine grain size.

Fabrication The major disadvantage of the cast Co-Cr alloy system is that these materials work harden rapidly and cannot be fabricated by conventional wrought metallurgy techniques. Control of the level of impurities and the rate of cooling to obtain the optimum grain size and mechanical properties of the alloy are important to maintain good quality castings. The materials are usually formed using casting techniques; however wrought preparations can also be machined using standard techniques.

Titanium and Titanium Alloys

Microstructure Commercially pure titanium and some titanium alloys exist in the α phase with an HCP crystal structure at room temperature. The α to β phase transformation, known as the β transus temperature, occurs at 882°C (1625°F). The β phase exists as BCC lattice structure only at temperatures above the β transus. The transition temperature is shifted by alloying with elements such as oxygen, carbon, nitrogen, and aluminum, which increase the transition temperature and stabilize the α (HCP) structure. Other elements—specifically chromium, copper, silicon, manganese, iron and nickel—stabilize the β phase by lowering the transition temperature.

The Ti-6A1-4V alloy has a two-phase (α+β) structure that results in dispersion hardening by inhibiting dislocation movements. Heat treatment influences the size, shape, and distribution of the second-phase particles in the matrix. The major advantage of Ti-Al-V alloy is its increased strength when compared to the unalloyed preparation. Annealing the alloys near their β transition temperature has greatly improved their endurance limit.

Fabrication Titanium and its alloys have excellent properties for use as implant materials. However, fabrication and processing of these materials are slightly more difficult than fabrication and processing of the stainless steel or Co-Cr alloys. Titanium has a very high melting point and is very reactive with the atmosphere. Control of environmental factors during fabrication is important.

Titanium can be cast using the lost wax process. Investment casting uses a water-cooled copper crucible in a vacuum-consumable electrode arc furnace. This process produces minimal contamination during melting, and the oxide-rich surface is removed prior to casting by etching with $HF-HNO_3$ solutions. A lost wax mold is used to produce a slightly oversized ceramic shell. The high-quality metal powder is placed in the shell and processed at 1000°C (1830°F) and 103 megapascals to produce full-density parts with fine grain size and mechanical properties approximating those of forged preparations, although their ductility is somewhat less than forged products.

Machining of titanium must be carefully controlled to minimize galling and seizing tendencies. Effective machining is achieved by using relatively slow cutting speeds; sharp, hard tools; and efficient coolants.

Effects of Implant Materials on Medical Imaging and Treatment

Radiographs and Computed Tomography

Although radiographic visualization of the implant is important to evaluate its position and integrity, it is also important not to preclude evaluation of surrounding structures. When an x-ray beam impinges on an object, only a portion of the energy will be transmitted in an unmodified form through the material. In addition, there will be unmodified scattered x-rays, modified scattered x-rays, fluorescent x-rays, scattered β x-rays, and other forms of radiation.

In the range of 60 to 110 kv (0.2×10^{-1} nanometers), diagnostic medical x-rays are attenuated as they pass through an object. This attenuation is a function of energy (wavelength) of the x-ray, thickness and density of the object, and atomic number of the constituents. The absorption of x-rays passing through a homogeneous material is an exponential relationship. The intensity, I, of x-rays passing through a material of thickness x is related to the initial intensity I_o,

$$I = I_o e^{-(\mu/p)px}$$

where μ is the absorption coefficient related to the specific material and the wavelength of the x-ray, and p is the density of the material.

The ratio μ/p at the wavelength of diagnostic x-rays is 0.15 for light elements, 1.5 for medium metals, and 15 for very dense materials. Thus the attenuation I/I_o through a 1-millimeter-thick section of material for the material density of stainless steel, $p = 7.9$, is 7.1×10^{-6}; for cobalt-chromium alloy, $p = 8.3$, it is 3.9×10^{-6}; for titanium, $p = 4.5$, it is 1.17×10^{-3}; for titanium alloy, $p = 4.45$, it is 1.26×10^{-3}; and for calcium, $p = 1.54$, it is 9.9×10^{-2}. The stainless steel and cobalt-chromium alloys, which have densities about twice that of titanium, decrease x-ray penetration by three orders of magnitude more than titanium and four orders of magnitude more than calcium.

Computed tomography generates a cross section, or slice, image based on a standard convolution–back-projection image-reconstruction process. The data are derived from multiple projections at a given slice level. With high-density materials, x-ray penetration is greatly attenuated, and minimal signal reaches the detector in that projection interval (hollow projection). Although techniques are available to compensate for this artifact, they require manual delineation of the object at all slice levels, linear interpolation of the missing data, and then back-projection recalculation of the modified data (Kalender 1987).

Magnetic Resonance Imaging

Due to the magnetic resonance effect described by Bloch and Purcell, magnetic resonance imaging is based on the response of substances to static and dynamic magnetic fields of significant magnitude (greater than 2 tesla). Two basic concerns arise with metallic objects in the vicinity and field of view of the study: (1) the introduction of artifact in the diagnostic image, and (2) the movement of the implant, or production of heat or electrical current at the site.

The effects of a magnetic field on a substance are greatly a function of their magnetic susceptibility. Ferromagnetic materials are of greatest concern. Not all materials with iron present are necessarily ferromagnetic. Although stainless steels with α phase (martensite) are strongly ferromagnetic, austenitic stainless steels (316L) are paramagnetic and do not cause imaging artifact or deflection. However, care must be taken with low-nickel austenitic preparations, because certain manipulations such as cold working (bending, cutting) can induce ferromagnetic domains in the material.

Other materials, including titanium, tantalum, Co-Ni-Cr-Mo, dental amalgam, and gold, cause minimal imaging artifact or deflection. Certain "stainless steels" used for dentures and orthodontic appliances produce large artifacts (New 1983, Shellock 1988, Bassett 1989).

Radiation Therapy

The dose distribution of radiation around plates and screws is of concern when postoperative radiation is required. The material parameters of atomic number, density, and thickness are of similar consideration as with radiographic imaging. External beam radiation therapy, whether by cobalt-60 or x-ray beam (5 megavolts), has much greater penetration than and different absorption characteristics from diagnostic x ray.

Studies have shown definite dose perturbation adjacent to fixation plates (Postlethwaite 1989). Backscatter causes elevated dose on the incident side of the plate by 25% with stainless steel and by 15% with titanium at the tissue–metal interface. On the side of the plate opposite the incident beam, the attenuated dose at the plate tissue interface was -10% for titanium and -15% for stainless steel. Although the authors do not recommend removal of the plate prior to radiotherapy, they suggest that materials of lower atomic number, closer to that of tissues, would be optimal and that an intervening layer of material (that is, 1-millimeter-thick silastic) would greatly decrease the areas of dose concentration and the possibility of breakdown of the overlying tissues.

Summary

Material properties are a function of composition, temperature, and methods of modifying the bulk material such as hot or cold working and annealing. After a material has undergone plastic deformation by cold working, the increased strength and decreased ductility can be changed by annealing. As the material is heated, microstructure recrystallization and grain growth can take place, to provide a specific balance of strength and ductility. Plates and screws used for rigid fixation have different requirements. The materials used for the plates must be ductile enough to allow adaption to the bone surface, while being strong enough to provide dynamic stability. In contrast, the screws do not require intraoperative modification and require less ductility. However, they must have high shear and yield strength to withstand the torsional forces required to introduce and tighten the screw. This balance is generally achieved by specifying the annealing condition for low-stress applications, and the cold-worked condition for high-stress applications.

MECHANICAL PROPERTIES

Introduction

Bulk Material Testing

The structural characteristics of devices used for fixation are a function of the properties and the geometric configuration of the material. To estimate the response of different materials to a given biomechanical application, the first approach is to test and evaluate the mechanical properties of the bulk materials in a standardized fashion. In this next section, terminology, testing methods, and mechanical parameters that characterize materials will be introduced.

Biofunctionality

Biofunctionality is the ability of a device to function predictably for the purpose for which it was designed. Devices used for rigid fixation are intended to stabilize bone until healing has occurred. In contrast, osseointegrated implants are designed to sustain long-term function. This requires direct contact of living bone with the implant surface on a microscopic level to allow physiologic transfer of biomechanical forces and long-term stability of the bone–implant interface. Finally, the functional demands placed on rigid fixation devices are immediate, whereas most osseointegrated fixtures are not routinely placed into biomechanical function for three to six months. Implants for fixation in the past were routinely removed. Now that we have biomaterials that are more compatible, implants in the craniomaxillofacial region are left in place indefinitely unless specific problems arise.

Basic Concepts

Units of Measure

The International System (SI) units will be used to describe both units and symbols. The fundamental base units are the kilogram (kg), meter (m), and second (sec). Derived units include force: $kg \cdot m/sec^2$ or newtons (N);

Base Units

Parameter	Unit	Comments
Length	meter(m)	Equals 1,650,763.73 wavelengths in vacuum transition $2p^{10}$ to $5d^5$ Krypton-86
Mass	kilogram(kg)	Mass of Int. protype of kilogram
Time	second(s)	Duration 9,192,631,770 periods Cesium-133
Temperature	kelvin (K)	1/273.16 of temperature of triple point of water

Derived Units

Force	Newtons(N)	mass times acceleration $(kg)(m)/s^2$
Pressure (Stress)	Pascal(Pa)	force per unit area N/m^2
Work	Joule(J)	force times distance (N)(m)

Prefixes

	Base	Exponent/Power
nano (n)	billionth	10^{-9}
micro (u)	millionth	10^{-6}
milli (m)	thousanth	10^{-3}
centi (c)	hundredth	10^{-2}
kilo (k)	thousand	10^{3}
mega (M)	million	10^{6}
giga (G)	billion	10^{9}

Figure 5.4 The SI Metric System: base units, derived units, and common prefixes.

Force (Conversions):

Start (A) \ Finish (B) →	Newtons(N)	kgf	lbf
Newton (N)	( ) 1.0	0.102	0.225
kgf (=kp)	9.81	1.0	2.21
lbf	4.45	0.454	1.0

Formula: Starting value to Finish (converted units) → A × ( ) = B

Stress/Pressure (Conversions)

Start (A) \ Finish (B)	Pa	MPa	lbf/in²	kgf/m²	kgf/mm²
Pa (=N/m²)	( ) 1.0	10^{-6}	1.45×10^{-4}	1.02×10^{-1}	1.02×10^{-7}
MPa (=N/mm²)	10^6	1.0	1.45×10^2	1.02×10^5	1.02×10^{-1}
lbf/in² (psi)	6.9×10^3	6.9×10^{-3}	1.0	7.0×10^{-4}	7.04×10^2
kgf/m²	9.81	9.8×10^{-3}	1.42×10^{-3}	1.0	10^{-6}
kgf/mm²	9.81×10^6	9.8×10^3	1.42×10^3	10^6	1.0

(conversions)

lbf= pound of force kgf= kilogram of force kp= kgf
Formula: Starting value to Finish (converted units) → A × ( ) = B

Figure 5.5 Conversion tables for force and stress (pressure) conversions. To convert a value with units in the form of (A), the left column, multiply this value by the conversion factor ( ) in the column that corresponds to your final desired units (B), for example, to convert 100 pounds per square inch to megapascals:

$$(100 \text{ psi}) \times 6.9 \times 10^{-3} \frac{\text{MPa}}{\text{psi}} = 0.69 \text{ MPa}$$

pressure or stress: force (N)/ unit area (m²) or pascals (Pa); and work: force (N) × distance (m) or Joules (J); see Figures 5.4 and 5.5.

Force, Moment

Force (F), a vector with magnitude and direction, is the product of mass (m) and acceleration (a):

$$F = m \times a.$$

Also commonly referred to as load, or weight, forces can be applied in the form of tension, compression, shear, and combinations thereof (that is, bending and torsion). Standard units are in newtons (N). One newton is approximately equivalent to the weight of one apple, or approximately one-fourth of a pound.

Moment (M), also a vector quantity, expresses the tendency of a force to cause an object to twist. This is commonly known as a torque or couple. Moment, defined as the product of the force (F) and the perpendicular distance (d) from the axis of rotation to the line of action of the force, is expressed in newton-meters:

$$M = F \times d.$$

Moments that tend to cause clockwise rotation are by convention positive, and those that cause counterclockwise rotation are negative.

Stress: Tension, Compression, Shear, and Combination

Stress (σ) is the resultant internal force that resists change in the size or shape of a body when that body is acted on by external forces. A change in size and shape begins when the load is applied and stops when the internal resisting stress holds the external forces in equilibrium. Stress, defined as the force per unit area

(a), has units of newtons per square meter or pascals, or as pounds per square inch (psi):

$$\sigma = F/a.$$

Tensile stress, or tension (see Figure 5.6), is the internal force that resists the action of external forces that tend to increase the length of a structure, with the cross-sectional area perpendicular to the force. On a microscopic level, tensile forces are acting to elongate the metallic bonds between the atoms.

Compressive stress, or compression (see Figure 5.6), is the internal force that resists the action of external forces that tend to decrease the length of a structure, again with the cross-sectional area perpendicular to the force. Microscopically, the atomic elements are being squeezed together.

Shear stress, or shear (see Figure 5.6), is the internal force acting along a plane between continuous sections of a structure, with the forces on each segment, tangential, parallel and in opposite directions. Shear resists the tendency of one part to slide or slip over the other part. Microscopically, the movement consists of slipping of interdigitating planes of packed, adjacent atomic elements with bending of the interatomic bonds.

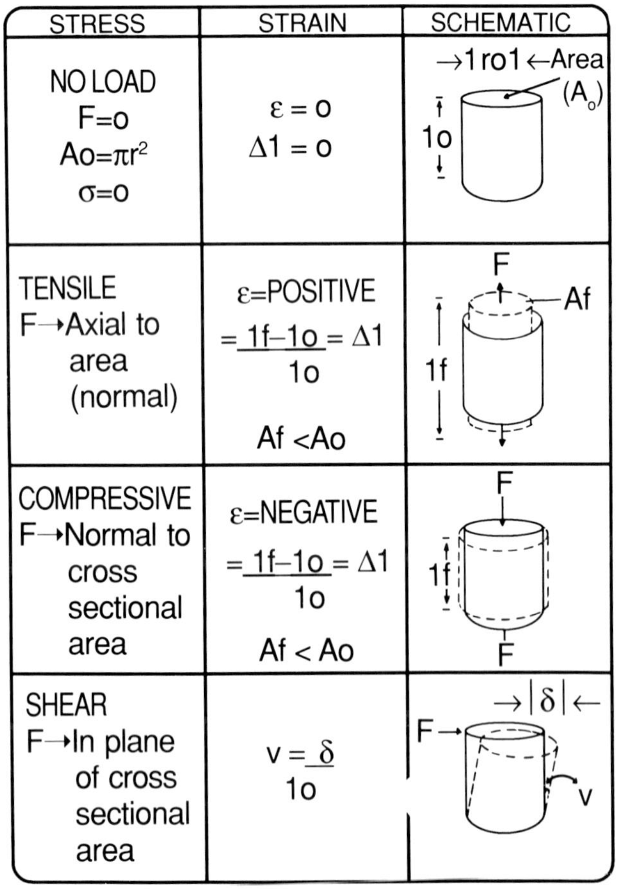

The majority of structural elements undergo a combination of tensile, compressive, and shear stresses. For example, in a bending beam, the material on the convex surface is in tension, that on the concave surface is in compression, and each imaginary cross section from the convex to the concave side is in shear with its upper and lower neighbors.

Strain: Elastic, Plastic, and Poisson's Ratio

Strain (ϵ) is the unit measure of deformation, or the change in size and shape, of a structure that occurs with application of external forces. Strain is defined as the difference of the deformed length (l_1) and the original length (l_0) divided by the original length (l_0):

$$\epsilon = (l_1 - l_0)/l_0.$$

Units are inches per inch or millimeters per millimeter. Elastic deformation of a material occurs when the stress-induced change in shape of the material is a totally reversible process; that is, the material returns to its original shape when the stress is removed. In contrast, plastic deformation of material occurs when the deformation exceeds a critical level, following which the material is permanently altered in dimension.

Poisson's ratio is the fractional change in lateral dimension from the original dimension of the material's cross section perpendicular to the tensile stress.

Percent elongation at failure (ϵ_f) is the difference in final length l_f and the original length l_o divided by the original length and multiplied by 100 to denote a percentage:

$$\epsilon_f = [(l_f - l_o)/l_o] \times 100.$$

This parameter provides some indication of the ductility, or plastic deformation, of the material before failure.

Elastic Modulus

The modulus of elasticity, or Young's modulus (E), a constant determined from the linear relationship (Hooke's law) between stress and strain in a material, represents the slope of the elastic region on the stress–strain curve:

$$E = \sigma/\epsilon.$$

The units of Young's modulus are the same as those for stress—pascals or pounds per square inch. It is actually a measure of the stiffness of the material; increasing magnitude of the modulus is a function of greater stiffness of the material.

Metals used for implants often have elastic moduli of 10^{10} pascals. To reduce the magnitude of the units, megapascals (MPa) is often used, where 10^6 pascals is equal to 1 megapascal.

STRESS	STRAIN	SCHEMATIC
NO LOAD F=o Ao=πr² σ=o	ε = o Δl = o	→1 ro1← Area (A$_o$) 1o
TENSILE F→Axial to area (normal)	ε=POSITIVE = 1f−1o / 1o = Δl / 1o Af < Ao	F — Af 1f
COMPRESSIVE F→Normal to cross sectional area	ε=NEGATIVE = 1f−1o / 1o = Δl / 1o Af < Ao	F 1f F
SHEAR F→In plane of cross sectional area	v = δ / 1o	→|δ|← F→ v

Figure 5.6 Basic configurations of stress (tension, compression, shear) with corresponding strain (F = force, A_o = initial cross-sectional area, A_f = final cross-sectional area, σ = stress, ϵ = strain, l_o = initial length, l_f = final length, δ = shear displacement, v = shear angle).

Material Testing

Stress: Mechanical Testing and the Strain Curve

Mechanical properties of materials are determined by standardized testing. These tests can compare different materials and provide the information necessary to estimate the mechanical behavior of a material in its final structural configuration. One testing method is four-point bending (ASTM E290), used for plate-shaped materials. Another, more common, test is tensile testing, where dumbbell-shaped materials are pulled by a mechanical testing machine at a fixed rate (ASTM E8).

Materials to be tested are prepared in a fixed shape, usually cylinder with threads at the ends. ASTM E8 carefully outlines the procedure: (1) Specimens are 0.25 inches, or 6.35 millimeters, in diameter at the middle. The threaded ends have a larger diameter, producing an overall dumbbell shape (see Figure 5.7). (2) The surface has a ground finish. (3) The strain rate is 0.003 to 0.007 mm/mm per minute through yield strength, after which the rate is increased to produce failure within the next minute. The applied force that maintains the constant strain rate and the total change in length are simultaneously measured. Because the original cross-sectional area and displacements are known, the stress versus strain can be plotted. Several characteristics of a material can be determined from this curve (see Figure 5.8):

1. *Young's modulus (E):* The initial linear portion of the curve demonstrates the elastic behavior of the material. The slope (stress versus strain) is the modulus of elasticity, or Young's modulus. This slope is a function of the stiffness of the material. At any point along this portion of the curve, the material will return to its original dimension when the stress is returned to zero (see Figure 5.8).

2. *The proportional limit:* The proportional limit marks the end of a linear material response to deformation. Beyond this point, stress is no longer proportional to strain, and the material will experience plastic deformation. Because of this deformation, for design considerations, the proportional limit—and not the ultimate tensile strength—is the maximum stress to which a material may be subjected without permanent deformation.

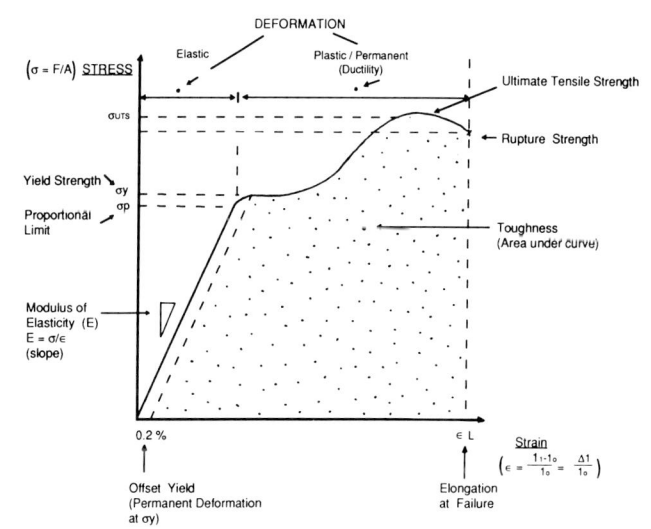

Figure 5.7 Schematic representation of a stress–strain curve for a metallic material. The configuration of the curve allows determination of the stiffness and strength of the material.

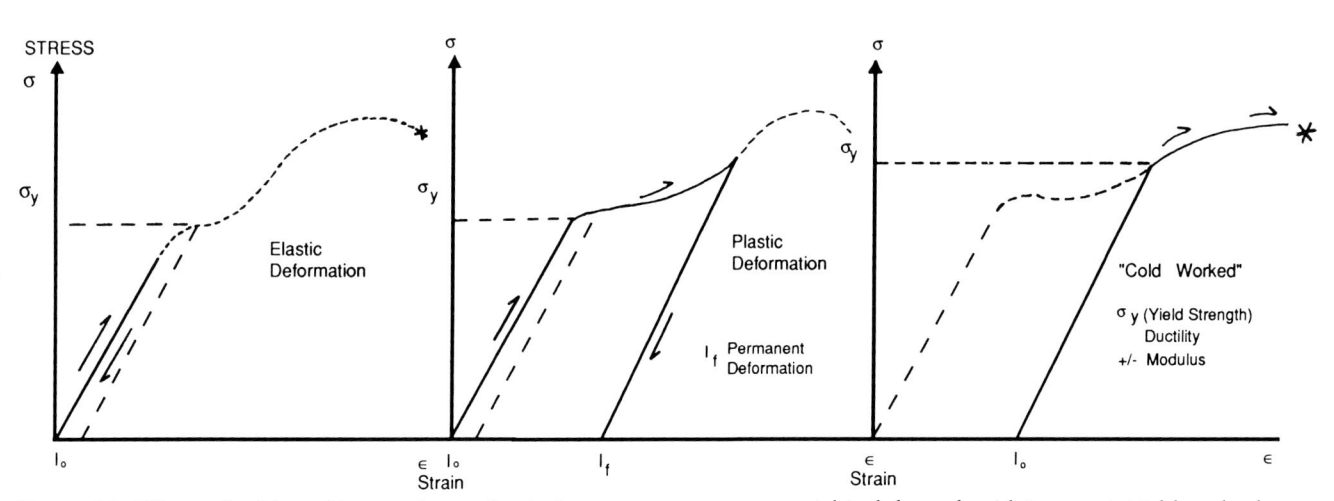

Figure 5.8 Effects of cold working on the mechanical properties of metals. If a material is deformed within its elastic range, it returns to its original shape/size l_o (left). If the material is deformed beyond its proportional limit, permanent plastic deformation (l_f) has occurred (middle). Now, if the same material is deformed, with its new initial length, the elastic range will be perceived as greater, with an increased yield strength and decreased ductility. Usually, the elastic modulus or stiffness is the same (right).

3. *Yield strength* (σ_y): The yield point is usually found at the beginning of the curve's plateau, where appreciable elongation of the material can be noted without increasing stress. The yield strength is closely related to the yield point. The yield strength, determined by drawing a line from an arbitrary offset strain of 0.2% parallel to the initial tangent to the stress–strain curve, is the stress at the point of intersection of the curve (see Figure 5.8). This point on the stress–strain curve represents a 0.2% permanent change in length of the material when the extrinsic load is removed.

4. *The length of the plateau beyond the linear region:* Beyond the linear region, the length of the plateau is a function of the toughness of the material. A material that fractures with no apparent plastic deformation is considered brittle. A material that can undergo large amounts of plastic deformation is considered ductile. A ductile material will demonstrate a large plateau on the stress–strain curve. Strictly speaking, *ductility* refers to the plasticity of a material under tensile forces, and *malleability* describes plasticity under compressive forces.

"Toughness" and "ductility" have slightly different meanings. Ductility describes only the ability of a material to deform. Toughness describes both the ability to deform and the level of stress developed during the deformation. Toughness, a function of the total energy that can be absorbed by the material before failure, is determined from the integral, or area under the stress–strain curve.

Cold working, or plastic deformation of a material below its transition temperature, effectively increases a material's yield strength and decreases its apparent ductility. Notice in Figure 5.8 (c) that the stiffness, or slope of the elastic portion of the curve, is essentially unchanged.

5. *Ultimate tensile strength* (σ_{UTS}): The ultimate tensile strength (UTS) is the maximum stress a material can bear before it fails. The rupture strength, the stress at failure, is often less than the UTS because of the rapid decrease in a material's cross-sectional area at the time of failure. For fracture to occur, a crack must form and then propagate across the structure. The reason for difference between UTS and rupture strength is that the calculated stress based on bond strengths (as opposed to based on actual strengths) lies in the phenomenon of stress concentration that occurs at surface imperfections, voids, sites of nonuniformity, and internal stresses.

Most imperfections are on the surface, produced by fabrication or handling. In brittle materials, a crack propagates quickly once it is initiated. In ductile materials, a crack propagates much more slowly; and in some cases, the atoms ahead of the moving crack are capable of rearranging themselves to prevent continuation of the crack. Because significant plastic deformation has often occurred before reaching these points, these parameters are of much less significance than the proportional limit in design applications.

6. *The percent elongation at failure:* A commonly measured parameter, the percent elongation at failure provides some indication of the ductility of the material before failure. It is defined as the difference between length at failure (l_f) and original length (l_o), divided by original length and multiplied by 100:

$$(l_f - l_o)/l_o \times 100.$$

Stress versus the Number of Cycles

The behavior of a material subjected to repeated or cyclic stresses is called *fatigue*. This mechanism of fracture occurs in a material in spite of the fact that it has been functioning well within its elastic range. The cause of fracture is often related to the condition of the surface. Nucleation and crack propagation initiate at sites of imperfection. This is related to intrinsic material defects, fabrication, handling, or corrosion. Materials are evaluated for fatigue by being subjected to cyclic rotational bending stresses at various amplitudes. The number of cycles to failure is noted in each case. These values are plotted as stress versus the number of cycles on the S–N curve (see Figure 5.9). A fatigue or endurance limit is present in some materials; this is defined as the stress at which the material can function and withstand cyclic loading. Typically, implant materials are fatigue tested with 10^6 to 10^7 cycles.

Mechanical Properties of Implant Metals

In this section, we discuss mechanical properties as they apply to the specific surgical metals. Specific details of all preparations in each class are beyond the scope of this chapter. Readers are referred to excellent discussions in Williams (1981, a–f).

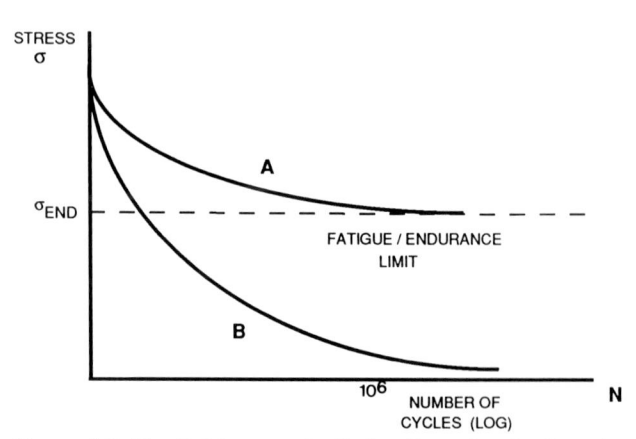

Figure 5.9 The S–N curve. Cyclic loading often leads to fatigue/fracture of materials even though the material functions in its elastic range. σ_{End} is the endurance limit, or maximum stress that would allow greater than 10^6 to 10^7 cycles of loading without failure.

Table 5.3 Mechanical Properties of Metallic Biomaterials

	σ_y (MPa) Yield Strength	σ_{uts} (MPa) Ultimate Tensile Strength	σ_{END} (MPa) Endurance Limit	$\epsilon L\%$ Elongation at Failure	(MPa) Compression Strength	E (GPa) Elastic Modulus	(GPa) Shear Modulus	Possion's Ratio	(VPN) Hardness	P Density gm/cm³
Ferrous Alloys										
FeCrNiMo (F138)						(200–210)	(8.4)	(0.283)	(190–325)	(7.9)
Annealed	211–380	517–700	190–269	46–68	550					
Cold Worked	689–1160	860–1256	345–700	6–12	965					
Cobalt-Chromium Alloys										
CoCrMo (F75)					(700)	(213–248)	—	—	(300–450)	(8.3)
Cast	450–600	665–1000	190–400	8–25	—					
Wrought	500–800	1000–1200	500–860	10–15	—					
Cast-Forged	860–930	1200–1280	500–750	15	—					
P-M	825–920	1200–1300	620–790	15	—					
Titanium (F67)			(150–300)		(620)	(100–120)	(4.6)	(0.361)	(220–300)	(4.5)
Grade 1	170	240	—	24	—					
Grade 2	275	345	—	20	—					
Grade 3	380	450	—	18	—					
Grade 4	485	550	—	15	—					
Titanium Alloy										
Ti-Al-V (F136)	838–1036	948–1147	440–670	10–15	(900)	(100–120)	—	(0.361)	—	(4.45)
Bone-Cortical	(130)	(140)	—	1	130	(18)				

( ) - Approximate values for category/class of materials.
Sources: ASTM (1986), Von Recum (1986), Semlitsch, in Ducheyne (1984).

Stainless Steel

The 316L stainless steels used for medical implants have an excellent combination of mechanical properties. Fully annealed (softened) stainless steels exhibit a fairly high ultimate tensile stress; however, the proof (yield) stress is low, and the ductility is high. As a result, plastic deformation occurs quite readily with these materials. Only few implants, such as small-diameter suture and wire, are produced from annealed 316L.

These alloys can be strengthened by cold working. Cold working does not change the elastic modulus, but it does increase the yield, ultimate, and fatigue strengths. Some newer austenitic stainless steels contain a relatively high nitrogen content, which significantly increases the strength properties while apparently sacrificing none of the alloy's corrosion resistance.

Stainless steels have an elastic modulus of approximately 200 gigapascals. Other mechanical parameters can vary significantly, depending on the working of the metal. Comparison of fully annealed and cold-worked preparations reveals significant differences in yield and ultimate tensile strengths (see Table 5.3). Cold-worked preparations have much higher yield and ultimate tensile stresses but lower ductility or elongation at failure than annealed preparations have.

Co-Cr Alloys

Cast and wrought Co-Cr alloys demonstrate a wide range of strength and ductility, which depends largely on the annealing and cold-working treatments employed. Of particular concern are the high elastic modulus and limited ductility demonstrated by the cast materials. These alloys exhibit adequate resistance to abrasion and corrosion. The rapid work hardening demonstrated by these alloys limits implant fabrication primarily to investment casting methods, however.

The wrought alloys have a much lower work-hardening rate, with a concomitant increase in strength, ductility, and toughness when fully annealed. Wrought Co-Cr alloys can be cold worked to achieve good balance of mechanical properties. Extremely high fatigue strengths can be obtained by use of carefully controlled thermomechanical processing, such as hot forging.

Product forms fabricated by powder metallurgy and the HIP technique exhibit properties superior to those of cast Co-Cr alloys and comparable to cold-worked 316L stainless steel. In particular, the fatigue strength of certain wrought Co-Cr alloys is considerably enhanced by this new processing technology.

Co-Cr alloys have an elastic modulus of 210 to 240 GPa and a stiffness similar to that of stainless steel. Yield strength and ultimate tensile strength vary significantly as a function of material fabrication or working.

Titanium and Titanium Alloy

The mechanical properties of titanium are strongly related to the degree of purity and the alloying elements. Increased oxygen content in unalloyed titanium will increase the tensile strength, with a corresponding decrease in ductility.

In addition to titanium's excellent corrosion resistance and biocompatibility, one of the major advantages of titanium has centered on its modulus of elasticity, 100 to 120 GPa. The current theory is that a material used for replacement of bony structures should have an elastic modulus that closely approximates that of bone. Of the three basic metal implant systems, titanium has the lowest modulus—approximately one-half that of stainless steel and the Co-Cr alloys. However, it is still about five times greater than that of bone. This may be important for minimizing stress concentration or stress shielding in certain applications. However, to provide the required stability of rigid fixation, which is a function of material stiffness and geometric configuration, more material cross section (thickness) is required to match the stiffness of materials with a higher modulus.

The yield and ultimate tensile strength of the titanium alloys are about twice those of CP titanium. Although mechanical indices for the unalloyed preparation are lower, its superior corrosion and biocompatibility properties are often given greater significance in the balance of risk and benefit when compared to the titanium alloy and other implant metals.

Summary

For orthopedic rigid fixation applications, moduli of elasticity of 100 to 200 GPa and yield strengths of 200 to 1000 MPa are recommended (Williams 1973). This can be extrapolated to craniomaxillofacial applications, where smaller fixation devices balance the reduced loading conditions. Requirements for total hip replacement are more stringent, where recommendations are yield strength of 450 megapascals, ultimate strength of 800 megapascals, and endurance strength of 400 megapascals. The elongation at failure should be greater than 8% (Semlitsch 1984).

The three types of metallic materials—316L stainless steel (SS), Co-Cr alloys, and titanium, unalloyed and alloyed—have been used extensively for fracture fixation. All these materials have characteristics that fulfill minimum criteria for fixation. The differences in stiffness, yield strength, and ductility can be chosen to work to the advantage of the specific design application. The data in Table 5.3 and Figure 5.10 provide a comparison of the mechanical parameters of the surgical metals currently in use. Other considerations, including corrosion resistance, biocompatibility, medical imaging artifact, and potential toxic reactions, are important parameters in the design of a medical device and are covered in their respective sections.

CORROSION PROPERTIES

Introduction

Corrosion is the slow disintegration or wearing away of a substance by an environmental agent. Metals corrode in air by combining to form oxides; they corrode in aqueous media by going into solution as ions or by reacting with nonmetallic elements and precipitating as ceramiclike by-products. The driving force that makes metals reactive lies with their original configuration as combinations of elements in unrefined ores. This configuration is often quite similar to their configuration in corrosion products. The natural tendency is for the higher-energy, synthetically produced, or extracted materials to revert to their original lower-energy form, as they are found naturally in the environment. Thus metals are susceptible to environmental attack, where they are transformed from the elemental to the combined state. The combined state can be an oxide, a sulphide, or a chloride. Metal's corroding to produce a ceramic-type structure demonstrates one reason that ceramic materials possess excellent environmental chemical resistance. It is unfortunate that the mechanical properties of ceramics are not entirely satisfactory for most structural applications in rigid fixation.

The application of metals as structural components in a biologic system adds additional constraints. First, in order to maintain an implant's integrity and function, the biomaterial must remain relatively inert in a highly corrosive environment. Second, the release of corrosion products into the biologic system may disrupt the normal homeostasis. Corrosion products cause significant toxicity to the host in both local and systemic sites.

The process of corrosion is driven by differences in electrochemical potential. Current, or the movement of charged particles, takes the form of cations (positive ions) and electrons. The oxidation of metal (M) at the anode results in the production of positively charged metal cations (M^{+n}), which dissolve in the electrolyte solution. The accumulating electrons (e) at this site of oxidation are what render the anode negative:

$$M \rightarrow M^{n+} + ne^-$$

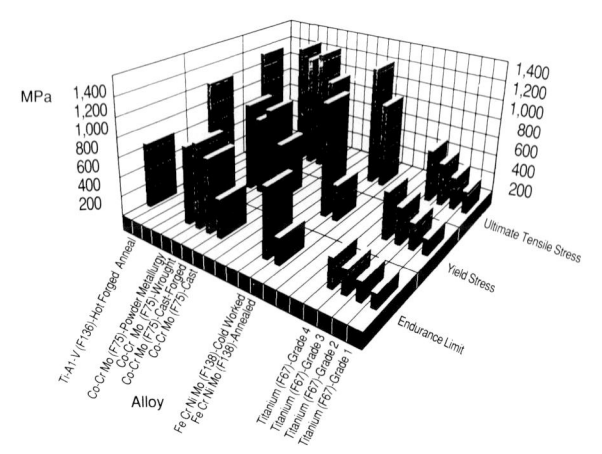

Figure 5.10 Graphic comparison of endurance limit (σ_{End}), yield strength (σ_y) and ultimate tensile strength (σ_{UTS}) of selected metallic biomaterials.

Metals that are more electronegative (more reactive than hydrogen—arbitrarily defined as 0.0 volts) tend to act as the anodic site.

The electrons exit the anode as current to the less electronegative site, the cathode. At the cathode, or positive pole, the electrons are consumed in a reduction reaction. The specific reaction—whether the deposition of metal from solution, the production of hydrogen gas, or the formation of hydroxide ion or water—is determined by the environment at the cathode:

$2H^+ + 2e^- \rightarrow 2H^\circ \rightarrow H_2$	acid solutions;
$O_2 + 2H_2O + 4e^- \rightarrow 4OH^-$,	neutral/alkaline solutions;
$O_2 + 4H^+ + 4e^- \rightarrow 2H_2O$,	dissolved O_2, acid solution;
$M^{3+} + e^- \rightarrow M^{2+}$,	dissolved metals;
$M^{2+} + 2e^- \rightarrow M^\circ$,	dissolved metals (electroplating).

The cathode is electropositive, or more noble, with respect to the anode. To maintain electrical neutrality, the rates of reaction at the anode and the cathode must be equivalent. These data and the galvanic series are summarized in Figure 5.11.

The magnitude of the current flow, or the actual rate of corrosion, is a function of the potential difference between the anode and the cathode, of electrolyte concentrations at each electrode, of the presence of inhibitors, and of temperature. For example, a battery is a controlled form of corrosion. Although corrosion most commonly occurs between materials of differing electrochemical potentials, corrosion can also occur in adjacent areas of the same material that have slight differences in composition, in geometry, or in the surrounding electrochemical environment. Rates of corrosion are usually given in units of weight per unit area lost per unit of time.

Forms of Corrosion

The mechanisms of corrosion that follow are the most common in association with implant materials.

General Corrosion

Steady-state dissolution of the bulk material or of the protective passive film is responsible for a small but measurable amount of metallic release from components. The bulk material and the film can be isolated from local tissues and organ systems in the biologic host. Loss of material from the bulk metal is independent of galvanic or localized corrosion. There is often no sign of degradation due to corrosive process associated with an implant.

Galvanic Corrosion

When two metals with different electrochemical potentials are present in a conducting electrolyte, the more anionic, or electronegative, metal usually suffers metal loss from galvanic corrosion. Although measures of differences in electrochemical potential are often used, these measures are taken on bare, nonpassivated metal surfaces in a standard solution containing their own ions in unit concentration. This is not a reliable guide to the actual rate of corrosion in the biologic environment. Even if one uses a practical series of galvanic potentials on passivated metals in biologic environments, this provides only a measure of corrosion tendency, and not the important parameter of corrosion rate. Corrosion rate can be determined by polarization testing methods. It is a function of the relative surface areas of the anode and the cathode. In most circumstances, it is still generally accepted that metallic components should be of the same metallic composition when used in conjunction at adjacent biological sites.

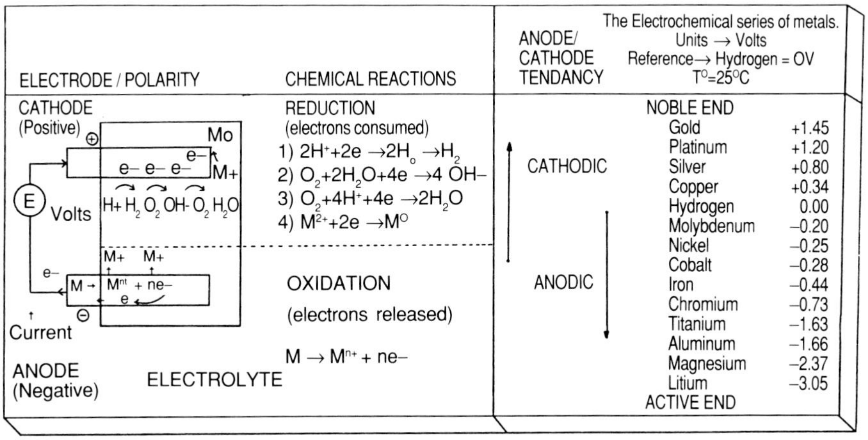

NOTE: Potential (Half Cell) varies with:
1) Electrolyte concentration (Nernest relationship)
2) Saline environment
3) Passive vs. active surface
4) e = electron n = number of electrons M = metal

Figure 5.11 Schematic representation and summary of basic corrosion cell.

Localized Corrosion

1. *Crevice corrosion:* Crevices are unavoidable with such implants as plates and screws in contact with bone. Because a crevice has limited access to the surrounding electrolyte, there are often increased concentrations of chloride and hydrogen ion (with decreased pH). In addition, an increased concentration of the metal cation and decreased concentration of oxygen (which normally facilitates passivation) gradually develop in this microenvironment. Thus, even though the crevice is composed of similar metals, concentration gradients establish potential differences at adjacent sites, with subsequent formation of a corrosion cell. This results in oxidation of the metal at the more anodic, or electronegative, site.

2. *Pitting corrosion:* A pit begins when a chemical breakdown process exposes a discrete site on the implant surface to chloride ions. The sites where pits originate are unclear; however, areas of inhomogeneity, scratches, or places where environmental variations are present are often suspect. If the rate of passivation at the affected site is unable to keep up with corrosion at the site, the continued build-up of corrosion products covers the pit, thus enabling selective entry or exit of ions. This leads to increased concentrations of chloride and hydrogen in the microenvironment of the pit and hence to rapid deterioration of the area. The prevalence of chloride ions in the biological environment makes pitting corrosion a significant concern.

3. *Fretting corrosion:* Abrasion between metallic components can disrupt the protective, passive layer and expose the underlying, more reactive metallic substrate. Normally, the surface passivates rapidly to reestablish the corrosion-resistant surface barrier. However, the repeated removal of the oxide films produces corrosion-product debris in the adjacent tissues, which can be detrimental to biologic tissues.

Stress-Corrosion Cracking and Corrosion Fatigue

Sustained tensile stress and simultaneous action of a corrodent can produce cracks in the passive layers on the metal surface, thus exposing the underlying metallic substrate. The tip of the crack becomes the anionic, or more electronegative, region in relation to the walls of the crack, based on the concentration gradients in the surrounding electrolytic medium. Thus the depth of the crack can increase secondary to metallic oxidation.

Corrosion Testing

Methods used to evaluate the corrosion of materials in biological applications must take into account several variables: the composition and methods of processing of the material; the nature of the surface; and the biological environment, including concentrations and concentration gradients of oxygen, hydrogen, and chloride. Of less predictable nature is the method of handling the implant material, the biomechanical function, and other materials that may be present at the surgical site.

Potentiostatic and potentiodynamic in vitro methods are used to evaluate an implant system's tendency for corrosion. The potentiostatic polarization method is used most commonly for testing. The polarization curve of voltage versus current demonstrates the important constants—the corrosion and breakdown potential, the corrosion current, and the passivation characteristics of the material (see Figure 5.12).

The corrosion tendency in vitro tends to be greater than that in actual in vivo applications. Although the in vitro environment reproduces the electrolyte environment seen in the biological system, it has been shown that protein and other organic substances modify the environmental factors. For a detailed description of methods used to evaluate corrosion, readers are referred to excellent discussions by Hoar and Mears (1966), Champion (1964), and Lemons (1986).

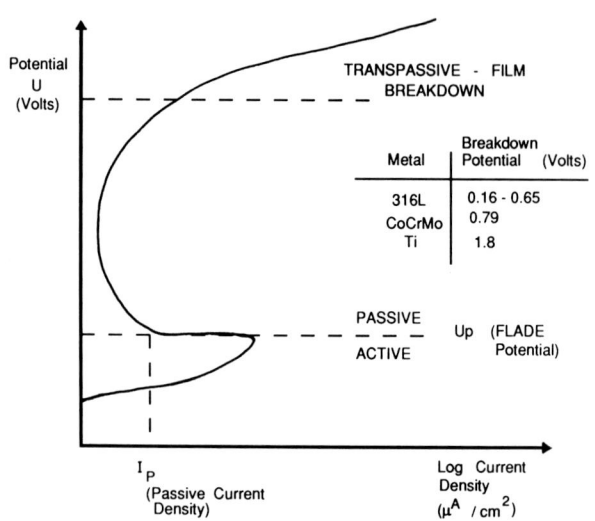

Figure 5.12 The anodic polarization curve. Within the active range, there is increased current density and subsequent corrosion. If the corrosion product is adherent to the substrate surface, is relatively insoluble, and has a relatively high dielectric constant, it will reach an equilibrium thickness and provide a "barrier" to subsequent corrosion. Even with increased potential (v) in the "passive range," minimum current flow or corrosion will occur. The behavior is characteristic of a passivated surface.

Metal	Breakdown Potential (Volts)
316L	0.16 – 0.65
CoCrMo	0.79
Ti	1.8

Passivation Methods

Resistance to corrosion of metallic implants often results from a protective film that spontaneously forms on the implant surface. Although the corrosion potential remains the same, the rate of corrosion is significantly inhibited or decreased. To bring the potential of the metal surface to a value in the passive range, deposition of a passive film on the surface is necessary. The passivated surface of a metal can be enhanced by several methods, including anodic protection and chemical treatment by oxidative solutions. The film must adhere tenaciously to the underlying metal substrate and must resist breakdown by mechanical or chemical means. If the film is violated, it must be capable of repassivation at a rate sufficient to minimize exposure of the metallic surface to the corrosive environment. For example, the titanium surface re-forms its oxide surface to 30 to 50 A in a time on the order of milliseconds.

Corrosion Properties of Implant Materials

Stainless Steel

Stainless steel forms a passive layer that has greatest resistant to corrosion when between 10 and 50 angstroms in thickness. The surface is often passivated by treatment in a 50% HNO_3 solution. The principle surface component is chromium oxide, which has a dielectric constant of 15.6. The corrosion resistance of stainless steel is afforded by this adherent oxide film. The film is a form of the bulk composition enriched with chromium, molybdenum, and silicon. The final composition of the passive surface layer is a function of the surface treatment and the nature of the corrosive environment.

Although austenitic stainless steels are highly resistant to corrosion in comparison to most other metals and alloys, they are often susceptible to localized corrosion, such as crevice and fretting corrosion, in the biological environment. Stainless steel shows a greater tendency to corrosion than do Co-Cr alloys and titanium.

Co-Cr Alloys

Co-Cr alloys are highly resistant to corrosion in the biological environment. Chromium oxide is the dominant surface constituent; its concentration in the surface is far greater at the surface than throughout the bulk of the implant. Even though all the metallic elements found in Co-Cr alloys are potentially toxic if present in relatively high concentrations in their elemental form, when present in the alloy form they demonstrate minimal toxicity. It would seem that the tissue levels of elemental constituents around implants are sufficiently small to preclude toxic effects on tissues. Their potential for toxic effects are more suspect in situations with potential for high wear or in unusual corrosion situations.

Titanium and Alloys

Titanium is one of the most corrosion-resistant engineering materials available. It is virtually uncorrodable at near neutral pH and is especially resistant to chloride ion, which is detrimental to most other metals and alloys. Paradoxically, titanium is a highly reactive metal that is unstable in comparison to its oxide in air and in aqueous environments. It is the rapidly forming, tenaciously adherent oxide that forms from the reactive titanium substrate that imparts its superior resistance to corrosion. Titanium dioxide is the primary oxide on the metal surface, forming spontaneously in air to a thickness of about 30 to 50 A. The high dielectric constant of the oxide (50 to 117) allows increased van der Waals bonding and facilitates attachment of water and biomolecules (Kasemo 1983). Because the oxide is stable in the physiological environment little reaction takes place, and the material is extremely well tolerated.

Systemic Considerations

Even with the most corrosion resistant metallic preparations, ionization of the metal occurs causing both local and systemic increases in metal concentration, despite the fact that there is no detectable corrosion of the implant system.

Experimental evidence has shown that ionization occurs around all metallic alloys currently used clinically, regardless of how resistant to corrosion these preparations are as determined by standardized testing methods (Ferguson 1960). To determine the extent of this effect Ferguson et al. (1960, 1962) implanted metallic preparations in the back muscles of rabbits. Using spectrochemical methods, controls were obtained in rabbits without implants to profile trace ion concentrations of chromium, cobalt, nickel, titanium, molybdenum, aluminum, and iron in the muscle, spleen, kidney, lung, and liver. Several metal specimens, including stainless steel, Co-Cr, titanium, and aluminum were implanted; the surrounding muscle and systemic organs were analyzed at 6 and 16 weeks.

Stainless steel (316L) demonstrated increases in chromium, nickel, and iron in the surrounding muscle, with notable increases in nickel concentration in lung tissue. Co-Cr (Vitallium) demonstrated significant increases in cobalt and chromium in the surrounding muscle tissue; and systematically, increased amounts of cobalt were found in kidney, spleen, and liver preparations. Titanium was also found in increased concentration in the surrounding muscle and in spleen and lung.

Thus, although the process of corrosion is minimal in these metallic preparations—stainless steel, 0.05 micrograms per square centimeter; Co-Cr alloys, 0.05 micrograms per square centimeter; and titanium and titanium alloy, 0.01 micrograms per square centimeter per day in vitro (Steinemann 1984)—notable increases in amounts of constituent elements are found in the surrounding tissue and systematically. Localized accumulation will be a function of the solubility of the corrosion products of the metals. The implications of these increased concentrations are not known. The increased concentrations may be of significance with regard to sensitive biological responses such as hypersensitivity reactions.

Conclusion

In conclusion, titanium and titanium alloys demonstrate excellent resistance to corrosion. Cobalt-chromium alloys are resistant to corrosion; only rarely does significant corrosion occur. Stainless steels, although demonstrating good corrosion properties, are susceptible to crevice and pitting corrosion. Laing et al. (1967) observed that, in general, the degree of tissue reaction is proportional to the amounts of constituent elements released by the corrosion of a pure metal or alloy. Thus, to maintain structural integrity of the material and to minimize unfavorable tissue response, optimal corrosion properties are essential.

BIOCOMPATIBILITY

Definitions

Biomaterials are substances of either natural or synthetic origin used as components of a medical device. In general, the role of a biomaterial is to substitute or augment a biological component in a controlled, predictable fashion. This substitution must be accomplished with a margin of benefit that significantly outweighs potential or known risk.

"Biocompatibility" is a general term that describes a compatible, nonharmful interaction of a foreign material or device with the biological host. Although this term is often used in an objective manner, the determination of biologic acceptance is the result of a battery of testing methods and is not an absolute condition. The overall response is a function of two considerations: (1) the effect of the biomaterial on the biologic host, and (2) the effects of the biologic system on the material or device. The objectives of in vitro and in vivo testing methods are to identify potential toxicity of a biomaterial or device in the biologic host and to detect the potential for premature failure of the device in its specific application. Because metallic implants are currently the primary materials used for rigid fixation, corrosion and surface properties of these materials are often closely related to the biologic response.

The objectives of this section are to introduce approaches to biocompatibility testing, to review immune-system-related response to biomaterials, to discuss the role of biomaterials in infections, and to review the current risks of malignant transformation related to implant materials.

Biologic Response

The initial response to an implant material cannot be distinguished from the normal inflammatory response that results from tissue damage due to placement of the implant. There is an initial accumulation of polymorphonuclear leukocytes (PMN) in the vicinity of the implant. This is soon followed by invasion by monocytes and macrophages. The macrophages can go on to form foreign body giant cells (large multinuclear cells) if the implant material is identified as a foreign material. With physically and chemically inert biocompatible materials, no foreign body giant cells are formed, and the sites heal with normal scar or fibrous tissue characteristic to the site. In soft tissue sites, a thin layer of fibrous-tissue encapsulation seems to wall off the material from the biologic environment. This fibrous encapsulation is not mandatory; for example, titanium and hydroxyapatites in bone have no other tissues between their surface and bone.

Early Testing Methods

Early biocompatibility testing methods measured thickness of the fibrous-tissue interface around the implant; this thickness was considered one index of biocompatibility (Laing 1967). This measure is valid in a majority of cases; however, a fibrous-tissue interface also results when there is relative motion between a biocompatible implant and bone. The thickness of the resulting fibrous-tissue encapsulation can be totally independent of the material's biocompatibility. For example, a stable titanium fixture in bone will develop a bone–implant interface without interposed fibrous tissue (osseointegration). If there is significant micromotion during the healing interval, however, a fibrous-tissue interface will result (Brånemark 1983).

Current Testing Methods

Several sources are available for detailed review of biocompatibility testing protocols. In the section to follow, we give generalized overview of testing methods. Readers should consult appropriate references for more detail (ASTM 1986, von Recum 1986, ADA/ANSI 1979, US Pharmacopeia 1980).

Currently, there is no single, standardized, mandatory approach to biocompatibility testing. In addition, because several parameters—such as processing, fabrication, handling, sterilization, and various surface preparations—can greatly modify the response to a specific material's composition, a collated database with all the biocompatibility data on currently used materials is not available.

Evaluation of the biocompatibility of new materials and devices is approached by use of four levels of testing. These include the following.

1. In vitro cell culture methods, which are used for initial screening of newly developed materials. These techniques provide a rapid, inexpensive way to identify potential problems

and to allow processing of large numbers of formulations.
2. In vitro and in vivo testing of the biomaterial or device is the second level of testing. Tests can be focused on the individual biomaterial constituents as well as on the final configuration of the material or device. This level of testing includes assessment for cytotoxicity in vitro, for acute local and systemic toxicity, and for mutagenic and carcinogenic activity. The bulk material as a substrate, as well as extracts from the material, are tested.
3. Use of the material or device in the intended anatomic site and functional environment constitutes the next phase of evaluation. These procedures try to duplicate closely the entire clinical procedure, from implant processing and sterilization to surgical placement of the device. In cases where the medical device plays a structural role, demands of normal and excessive function will be placed on the system. Testing at this level provides information about both the biocompatibility and the biofunctionality of the material or device.
4. Clinical trials in human patients are considered last. Careful experimental and statistical design of the studies is needed to provide accurate, conclusive data with the minimum number of test subjects.

The effects, either systemic or local, of an implant material on the biologic site are frequently caused by constituents actually leaving the bulk material—for example, unreacted monomers leeching out of plastic materials or metallic ions and corrosion products leeching out of metals. Thus both the bulk material and extract preparations must be evaluated. Cell culture preparations using mouse fibroblasts provide a sensitive method for detecting toxic substances in short intervals. Cytotoxicity can be determined, and newer techniques that monitor cell metabolism can be used to study the response to bulk materials and extracts. Cell culture techniques are limited; immunologic and systemic responses to the materials require assessment in vivo.

The battery of testing methods selected is based on the anatomic environment of proposed use, for example, external contact with skin or mucosal surfaces; percutaneous or permucosal location; and specific sites interfacing soft tissue, hard tissue, or blood. Cell culture studies provide high sensitivity to cytotoxicity to bulk material or leechable substances in extracts. Hypersensitivity and potential systemic responses are evaluated by implantation of materials in subcutaneous and intramuscular sites in rodents or rabbits; or by intravascular, intraperitoneal, or intracutaneous injection of extracts. Carcinogenic potential is assessed by in vitro determination of the mutagenic potential of the bulk material or extract using the Ames test (Ames 1971, 1975) or the Styles test (Styles 1977) or by long-term animal studies (over 6 to 24 months) (ASTM F469). Evaluation of results is largely subjective; the response can be compared to that of a control material, or a grading system with definable criteria can be used.

Immunology

Immune Response

Immunologic reactions to biomaterials are of concern because they may warrant premature removal of the device. With increased knowledge of the immune response, the potential for sensitivity reactions has been greatly decreased. In this section we briefly discuss the properties of an antigen, humoral and cell-mediated response, and the four types of hypersensitivity reactions.

The basic role of the immune system is to prevent foreign substances from establishing themselves in the body. Thus infectious agents, such as bacteria and viruses, and foreign tissues are neutralized or killed by the immunologic system. In addition, cells that have changed their characteristics, becoming precancerous cells, can be eliminated in a similar manner.

Antigens

An antigen is a substance that stimulates the immune system to respond and react in a specific manner. By strict definition, the term "immunogen" refers to the substance that stimulates the immune response; the antigen is the substance that reacts. The immune response is generated by the immunogen. Although which substances will be antigenic cannot be predicted with certainty, common characteristics include

1. substances with a large molecular weight, 10,000 or larger;
2. haptens, or substances of smaller size that combine with substances of larger size (for example, metal salts combining with host proteins and host cells); and
3. chemical composition—proteins are highly immunogenic; carbohydrates are weakly immunogenic; and lipids are nonimmunogenic.

Types of Immune Response

The immune system has two separate arms. One arm is humoral immunity; the end product of this response is antibody. The other is cell-mediated immunity; the end product of this response is the accumulation and action of T-cells.

Humoral Response The humoral response leads to the proliferation of B lymphocytes and the production and circulation of antibody. Haptens, which can be derived from foreign materials (biomaterials) placed in the biologic environment, can attach to host cells, combine with antibody, and activate the complement system. The humoral response initially causes local inflammation with capillary leakage, chemotactic factors attracting polymorphonuclear leukocytes (PMN), degradation products of phagocytic cell activity, and (often) nonspecific tissue damage.

Cellular Response Cell-mediated immunity involves direct interaction with antigens of specific receptors on the leukocytes. This results in production of soluble factors, *lymphokines,* and leads to the accumulation at the antigen site of T-cells and other white cells, such as monocytes and macrophages. Foreign substances are neutralized at the site by either chemical substances released from these cells or by ingestion of foreign particles by phagocytosis.

Hypersensitivity

Inadvertent damage to host tissue is a consequence of a hypersensitivity immune reaction. The terms "sensitivity," "allergy," and "hypersensitivity" are often used synonymously, and can be grouped into four types of reactions (see Figure 5.13).

Type I: Immediate Hypersensitivity The reaction of cell surface IgE immunoglobulin with antigen results in the release of histamine or other vasoactive substances from the cells to which the IgE is attached, that is, mast cells. The response can be similar to that seen with allergies like hay fever, or it can be life threatening, as with anaphylactic reaction to penicillin. Type I response to biomaterials is virtually unknown. Type I responses due to chromium salts and nickel salts have been documented, but these have not come directly from implanted biomaterials.

Type II: Antibody Mediated The end result of a Type II hypersensitivity reaction is similar to that of a Type I reaction; histamine and other vasoactive substances are released. In contrast, the antigen is part of or attached to the cells—such as mast cells, platelets, basophils, and eosinophils—that contain vasoactive substances. The antibody, usually IgE or IgM, will react with a surface antigen, cause damage to the cell membrane, and release the vasoactive substances. This response can be in reaction to foreign substances that have adhered to cell membranes, or it can be associated with autoimmune type responses. In some patients, reactions to drugs of small molecular weight cause the drug to adhere to the membrane. At this point, there are no reports of response caused by adherence to cell surfaces of products of biomaterial corrosion or degradation.

Type III: Immune Complex This response results from the precipitation of antigen–antibody complexes. The response is usually self-limited, and there are often no long-term sequelae or life-threatening symptoms. With prolonged exposure, organs such as the kidney, lung, heart, and joints can be permanently affected. Precipitates can occlude small vessels, causing subsequent complement activation and nonspecific inflammatory response, which can lead to damage at the site.

Types I, II, and III hypersensitivity are mediated by antibody, and they can occur within minutes or hours of the reaction. These are classified as humoral or immediate hypersensitivity reactions.

Type IV This is cell-mediated sensitivity involving T-cells and does not involve antibody or B-cells. Many of the associated symptoms are related to the soluble lymphokines released by T-cells. The reaction, which often takes days to develop, is known as *delayed hypersensitivity.* Involving the accumulation of T-cells, monocytes, and macrophages at the site, this reaction is commonly associated with sensitivity to biomaterials. It is well known that some individuals develop contact sensitivity to components of biomaterials. Skin rashes can develop, caused by materials, by direct contact with the surface of the skin, and by materials implanted deep in tissues in the region. Although systemic responses are rare, often there can be a localized subcutaneous or muscular response, causing palpable increase in tissue mass.

Hypersensitivity (Type)	Clinical Examples	Schematic
I Immediate	- Allergic Asthma - Hay Fever - Excema - Anaphylaxis	Activation by Antigen → Mast Cell → Degranulation → Inflammation (IgE)
II Antibody Mediated	- Transfusion Reaction - Hemolytic Disease of Newborn	IgG, K-Cell, Target Cell, Cell Surface Antigens, Cytotoxic, Complement, Activated C₃, Cell Membrane Damage/Lysis
III Immune Complex Mediated	- Persistent Infections - Inhaled Antigens - Autoimmune (High Antigen Load)	Antigen, Antibody, Complex, Complement Activation (C3), Immune Complex Deposition, Local Damage, Blockage Small Vessels
IV Delayed	- Skin Contact Reactions - Chronic Pathogens - Biomaterials	Antigens, Antigen Sensitizer T-Cell, Lymphokines, Macrophages, Tissue Damage, Chronic Granulomatous Reactions

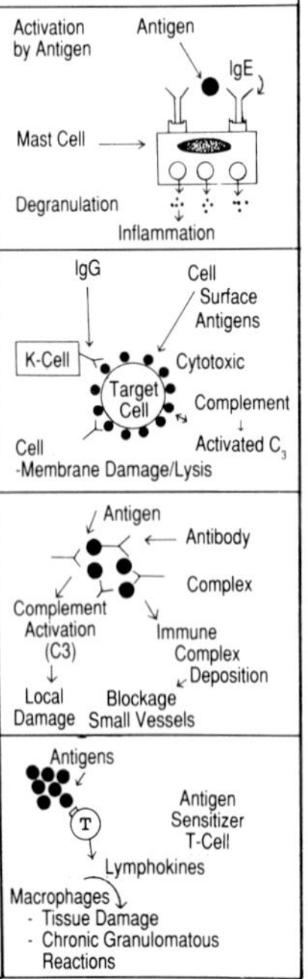

Figure 5.13 Summary of hypersensivity reactions.

Testing for Hypersensitivity

Tests of the potential of a biomaterial to induce hypersensitivity must be performed with an intact biomaterial and with products that the host could encounter from in vivo degradation and wear. The material is often placed in fluids that simulate the wear or degradative environment, and then the materials are injected into a living system for evaluation (ASTM F719, F720, F749). Briefly, the methods include (1) injection of substances into animals with and without adjuvants to induce sensitivity, and (2) injection of substances into animals that have already been sensitized to the substances with salts of the components in order to elicit a response.

Clinical Response

Most sensitivity reactions to biomaterials have been of the cell-mediated type. Humoral responses to biomaterials probably occur, but adequate testing has not been undertaken to document this. Approaches include skin testing; in vitro responses; observations of agglutination, precipitation, and complement fixation; or immunosorbant assays. Testing for cell-mediated immunity using in vitro responses is not well defined.

A major problem is recognizing whether or not a hypersensitivity reaction is occurring. Many of these reactions are occult. They cause no signs or symptoms. Clinically, it is known that a large percentage of the population is sensitive to nickel, cobalt, and chromium. At least one of these components is present in stainless steel and cobalt chromium alloys. Alloys or devices containing these materials have elicited only a small percentage of reactions in patients. No hypersensitivity reactions have yet to be reported with titanium and titanium alloy. The benefits of utilizing these elements as components in alloys must be contrasted to the rare risk of hypersensitivity that would require removal of the device. High-quality alloys are now available, which have a greatly reduced potential for corrosion or degradation. The minimal concentrations of metal salts in the surrounding tissues have greatly reduced subsequent immune responses. In addition, techniques that minimize wear between articulating devices have reduced the unfavorable cellular response.

Carcinogenicity

Introduction

The subject of implant-related carcinogenicity is of significant concern now that biologic systems are exposed to biomaterials over indefinite intervals. Material-induced malignant tumors have been well documented in experimental animals, particularly in rodents. However, only a limited number of clinical cases have been reported in the literature.

Theories

Malignant transformation can be related to four basic theories (Lawrence 1986):

1. With polymers, chemical leachable agents can leave the material. With metals, corrosion products or metal oxides can separate from the surface of the bulk material.
2. Implant materials can biodegrade. The substance can be made to biodegrade intentionally; the substance can degrade as a function of the biological environment; or the substance can functionally break down.
3. Physical contact with a material can cause formation of reactive centers and barriers to the metabolism of adjacent cells.
4. Existing preneoplastic cells can occur. This is also known as solid-state (Brand 1975) or foreign-body carcinogenesis. The implant induces cellular proliferation and encapsulation, where cells with neoplastic determination may be present in normal tissue.

Mechanical irritation from implant materials does not seem to induce tumor formation. In one study (Salyamon 1961) it was even found that nonspecific inflammation had an anticarcinogenic effect.

Material Testing

Experimental evaluation of the tumorigenicity of a biomaterial has been approached by in vitro and in vivo methods. Carcinogenicity may be evaluated in vitro with the Ames mutagenicity test (Ames 1971, 1975), the Styles cell transformation test (Styles 1977), or the dominant lethal test (ICPEMC 1983). The Ames test, the most commonly used test, uses genetically altered bacteria. When these bacteria are grown in the presence of a mutagenic substance, the bacteria exhibit an increased rate of reversion back to the normal nutrient requirements of the initial strain. The rate of reversal is related to the mutagenic potential of the compound. This test, frequently used as a preliminary screening method for chemical carcinogens, provides low-cost, rapid results. The main purpose of the Ames test is to detect mutagenic leachable substances in the bulk material.

The other approach, which uses animal models to study the cellular response to implanted materials, is of uncertain validity (ASTM F361, F469–78). Tumors are easily induced in the rat; however, there has been little to show that responses or tumor formation are similar in humans. To evaluate biomaterials for tumor production, their response in rats is compared to materials that have proven clinically safe.

Studies in animals (ASTM F748) involve placing the implant metal in muscle tissue. The results in rats indicate that the risks of malignant transformation are very low with the commonly used alloys. However, experiments with nickel, chromates, cobalt, and cobalt-chromium have produced tumors in various animal models (Tayton 1980).

Clinical Cases

Eleven cases of induced local malignancies were cited in a literature review by Waalkes et al. (1987). At least two of the cases involved corrosion at sites where dissimilar alloys were used. Tumors are usually soft-tissue sarcomas, although two cases of lymphoma have been reported. Although tumor type and the form of medical device are identified, it is often unclear what specific metal alloy was present. Table 5.4 lists some of these reported cases.

In studies of implants, malignant transformation has been seen in association with stainless steel, Co-Cr alloy (Vitallium), and titanium alloy. In certain cases with dissimilar metals, corrosion debris was noted; in other cases, the cause-and-effect relationship was unclear.

Conclusions

The clinical decision to use a prosthetic replacement is often a function of the demonstrated benefits compared to the potential risks. The very low incidence of reports of malignant transformation associated with materials currently used for rigid fixation (stainless steels, cobalt-chromium alloys, and titanium materials) justifies their application as safe. Although constituents in the stainless and cobalt alloys, including nickel and cobalt, are potentially carcinogenic, the tissue response appears much different when these constituents are in the alloy form. Unalloyed titanium has not been associated in the literature with malignant transformation.

Infection

Foreign Bodies

The presence of infection at a fracture site raises questions regarding the effects of a foreign body on healing at the site. The primary approach to treatment should address the stability of the fracture site and the possible impediment to healing caused by the "protected or inaccessible environment" around the implant. The microbiology of infection is beyond the scope of this chapter; readers are referred to Gustilo (1989) for detailed discussion of microbial adhesion and pathogenesis of biomaterial-centered infections. The production of a glycocalyx, or slime layer, is an important factor that limits the effectiveness of host defenses and approaches to antiobiotic treatment. The best approach is to ensure that the race to the high-energy surface of the implant material is won by host cells and biomolecules instead of by bacteria that would tenaciously secure the surface of the implant (Gristina 1989).

Animal Studies

Rittmann and Perren (1974) studied fracture healing prospectively in the presence of local infection in the sheep tibia. Transverse tibial osteotomies were stabilized with plate fixation and then were infected with human pathologic staphylococci. After eight weeks, 18 of 19 osteotomies showed patterns of bone union, with

Table 5.4 Malignancies Associated with Implant Devices

Tumor	Device	Material	Reference
Squamous cell carcinoma	Mandibular staple bone plate	?Ti-Al-V	Friedman (1983)
Ewing's sarcoma	Sherman plate/screws	Vitallium	Tayton (1980)
Malignant tumor	Bone plate	Stainless steel; two different alloys	McDougall (1956)
Sarcoma	? plate (tibia)	?	Delgado (1958)
Malignant fibrous histocytoma	Total hip arthroplasty	?	Bago-Granell (1984)
Hemangioendothelioma	Sherman plate; screws of different alloy	Stainless steel; 316, 304	Dube and Fisher (1972)

areas of primary bone healing. Conclusions from this study were as follows:

1. Rigid fixation of fragments offers favorable conditions for healing of the fracture. It is advantageous to leave stabilizing implant material in situ when an infection is present, and to repeat osteosynthesis if the infected fracture becomes unstable.
2. Primary bone healing is of great advantage where an infection is present.
3. The advantage of the stabilizing effect of the implants outweighs the disadvantages of a foreign body effect.
4. An implant that is not providing stabilization or that is, in fact, loose, should be removed.

Although this study demonstrated that hard tissue will heal in the presence of infection with a foreign body, the animals were not treated with antibiotics during the eight weeks. Details of final resolution of infection at the site are therefore unclear. Additional basic principles to consider with clinical infection are as follows:

1. Stability of the fracture, osteotomy, or bone graft site takes absolute priority in the choice of treatment approach (Prein 1987).
2. Loose fixation devices must be removed (Spiessl 1976).
3. In a grossly infected site that has necrotic tissue, debridement and stability must be achieved. Fixation of external pins in noninfected sites and/or intermaxillary fixation may be a better alternative in this situation to internal fixation. When the necrotic tissue has been debrided and/or when gross infection is more under control, internal fixation techniques can be employed.
4. Antibiotic prophylaxis, careful attention to aseptic technique, and minimal contamination of the implant are essential (Dougherty 1988).

Stress Shielding

Demineralization, or perceived disuse osteoporosis, associated with rigid fixation was at first attributed to stress shielding. Intuitively, based on the theories of Wolff (1892, 1986) and others, the bone underlying the plate was thought to experience significant decrease in biomechanical function, making it unable to respond appropriately by resorption. Although studies (Kennady 1989) have clearly demonstrated osteoporosis histologically, this has not been correlated to the state of stress in the bone as a structural unit. Recent work by Perren (1988) proposes that this effect is largely the outcome of a compromised circulation in the bone underlying the plate, and that porosity is a function of the remodeling of the necrotic underlying bone. Modification of the fixation plates that have less contact with the bone surface, or techniques that use an expanding screwhead to engage the plate and minimize pressure directed against the surface of the bone, may (Sutter 1988) alleviate some of these problems.

Conclusions

All current surgical metals fall into the three basic classes: ferrous alloys, or stainless steel (ASTM F55, F56, F138, 139), cobalt-chromium alloys (F75, F90, F562, F688, F563), and titanium (F67) and titanium alloy (F136). These preparations all demonstrate satisfactory mechanical, corrosion, and biocompatibility properties that can be applied to clinical applications. Yield strength, ultimate tensile strength, and hardness tend to be greater in the Co-Cr alloys and stainless steel alloys than they are in the commercially pure titanium preparation. Titanium alloys have comparable strengths to the Co-Cr and stainless steel alloys, but they still are not as hard and have a potential for wear in articulating applications. The titanium preparations have the advantage of superior corrosion and biocompatibility properties, and no clinical cases have been reported of hypersensitivity or malignant transformation.

In specific rigid fixation applications, one must consider the minimum structural requirements of the application. Materials are also selected to minimize the risks of a compromised biological response. Until one material is developed with superior properties in all categories, the balance of biofunctionally and biocompatibility, and of risk and benefit, will continue to be a significant part of the design criteria.

All current methods of rigid fixation are based on metallic biomaterials, with a residual or artifact remaining well after the fracture or osteotomy has healed. It is still unclear to what extent these devices compromise growth in the developing skeleton, in the remodeling of mature bone, and in the healing of bone graft preparations.

Ideally, a bioresorbable preparation that could provide stabilization during healing and then would gradually disappear to allow normal growth and/or remodeling would address these concerns. Although plates and screws are the predominant means of internal fixation, development of new approaches that use bioresorbable components—adhesives, light-cured plastics, and laminate materials—may provide an alternative approach. Additional factors that could enhance healing—such as a substrate for cell proliferation and a delivery system for growth enhancement factors—could be incorporated into the basic design requirements for stability. Although currently available biomaterials have excellent properties and provide predictable healing, the task they serve is ephemeral; the ultimate solution is one that demonstrates no evidence of prior intervention.

REFERENCES

American Dental Association: American National Standards Institute (ANSI/ADA) Document No. 41 for recommended standard practices for biological evaluation of dental materials (1979).

Ames BN: The detection of chemical mutagens with enteric bacteria. In Chemical Mutagens: Principles and Methods for Their Detection, Vol 1. Hollaender A. Plenum Press, New York, 1971, 267–282.

Ames BN, McCann J, Yamasaki E: Methods for Detecting Carcinogens and Mutagens with Saknibekka/Mammalian Microsome Mutagenicity Test. Mutat Res 31:347–364, 1975.

ASTM Annual Book of ASTM Standards—Medical Devices, Vol 13.01. ASTM Philadelphia, 1986.

Bago-Granell J, Aguirre-Canyadell M, Nardi J, et al: Malignant fibrous histocytoma of bone at site of total hip arthroplasty: A case report. J Bone Joint Surg 66: 30–40, 1984.

Baier RE: Conditioning surfaces to suit the biomedical environment: Recent progress. J Biomed Eng 104: 257–271, 1982.

Baier RE, Meyer AE: Implant surface preparation. Int J Oral Maxillofac Implants 3:1 9–20, 1988.

Baier RE, Meyer AE, Akers CK, Natiella JR, Meenaghan M, Carter JM: Degradative effects of conventional steam sterilization on biomaterial surfaces. Biomaterials 3: 241–245, 1982.

Bassett LW, Golf RH: Magnetic resonance imaging of the musculoskeletal system: An overview. Clin Orthop Rel Res 244: 17–28, 1989.

Bos RM, Boering G, Rozema FR, Leenslag JW: Resorbable poly (L-lactide) plates and screws for the fixation of zygomatic fractures. J Oral Maxillofac Surg 45:751–753, 1987.

Brand KG, Brand I: Risk assessment of carcinogenesis at implantation sites. Plast Reconstr Surg 66:591–595, 1980.

Brand KG, Buoen LC, Johnson KH, et al: Etiological factors, stages, and role of the foreign body tumorigenesis: A review. Cancer Res 35:279–286, 1975.

Brånemark PI: Osseointegration and its experimental background. J Prosth Dent 3:50, 399–410, 1983.

Brånemark PI, Zarb GA, Albrektsson T: Tissue Integrated Prosthesis: Osseointegration in Clinical Dentistry. Chicago, Quintessence, 1985.

Champion FA: Corrosion Testing Procedures. London, Chapman and Hall, 1964.

Cutright DE, Hunsuck EE, Beasley JD: Fracture reduction using a biodegradable material, polylactic acid. J Oral Surg 29:393, 1971.

Delgado ER: Sarcoma following a surgically treated fractured tibia. Clin Orthop 12:315, 1958.

Dougherty SH: Chart 24, Implant Infections: 276. In Handbook of Biomaterials Evaluation, von Recum 1988.

Dube VE, Fisher DE: Hemangioendothelioma of the leg following metallic fixation of the tibia. Cancer 30:1260, 1972.

Dube VE: Hemangioendothelioma of the lung following metallic fixation of the tibia. Cancer 30:1260, 1975.

Ducheyne P, Hastings GW: Metal and Ceramic Biomaterials, Vol 1 Structure. Boca Raton, FL, CRC Press, 1984.

Ducheyne P, Hastings GW: Metal and Ceramic Biomaterials, Vol 2 Strength and Surface. Boca Raton, FL, CRC Press, 1984.

Dumbleton JH, Black J: An Introduction to Orthopaedic Materials. Springfield, Charles C Thomas, 1975.

Ferguson AB, Akahoshi Y, Laing PG, Hodge ES: Characteristics of trace ions released from embedded metal implants in the rabbit. J Bone Joint Surg 44-a:2, 323–336, 1962a.

Ferguson AB, Akahoshi Y, Laing PG, Hodge ES: Trace metal ion concentration in the liver, kidney, spleen, and lung of normal rabbits. J Bone Joint Surg 44-a; 2, 317–322, 1962b.

Ferguson AB, Laing PG, Hodge ES: The ionization of metal implants in living tissues. J Bone Joint Surg 42-A:1, 77–90, 1960.

Friedman KE, Vernon SE: Squamous cell carcinoma developing in conjunction with a mandibular staple bone plate. J Oral Maxillofac Surg 41:265–266, 1983.

Frost HN: The mechanostat: Aproposed pathogenic mechanism of osteoporosis and the bone mass effects of mechanical and nonmechanical agents. Bone Mineral 2:73, 1987.

Getter L, Cutright DE, Bhaskar SN, Augsburg JK: A biodegradable intraosseous appliance in the treatment of mandibular fractures. J Oral Surg 30: 344, 1972.

Gristina GG, Barth E, Webb LX: Microbial Adhesion and the Pathogenesis of Biomaterial-Centered Infections. In Orthopaedic Infections: Diagnosis and Treatment, Gustilo RB. Philadelphia, W.B. Saunders, 1989.

Guidelines for Evaluating the Safety of Materials Used in Medical Devices, HIMA Report. Health Industry Manufacturing Assoc., Washington, D.C. 1978.

Gustilo RB: Orthopaedic Infections: Diagnosis and Treatment. Philadelphia, W.B. Saunders, 1989.

Harris B: Corrosion of stainless steel surgical implants. J Med Eng Technol 3:3, 117–122, 1979.

Hoar TP, Mears DC: Corrosion resistant alloys in chloride solutions: Materials for surgical implants. Proc R Soc A294, 486, 1966.

Hollinger JO, Schmitz JP: Restoration of bone discontinuities in dogs using a biodegradable implant. J Oral Maxillofac surg 45:594–600, 1987.

ICPEMC, Committee 4 final report: Estimation of genetic risks and increased incidence of genetic disease due to environmental mutagens. Mutat Res 115323, 1983.

Kalender WA, Hebel R, Ebersberger J: Reduction of CT artifacts caused by metallic implants. Radiology 164:2, 576–577, 1987.

Kasemo B: Biocompatibility of titanium implants: Surface science aspects. J Prosthet Dent 49:832, 1983.

Kennady MC, Tucker MR, Lester GE, Bucklye MJ: Stress shielding effect of rigid fixation plates on mandibular bone grafts. J Oral Maxillofac Surg 18:307–310, 1989.

Laing PG, Ferguson AB, Hodge ES: Tissue reaction in rabbit muscle exposed to metallic implants. J Biomed Mater Res 1:135–149, 1967.

Lawrence WH: Tumor induction. In Handbook of Biomaterials Evaluation: Scientific, Technical, and Clinical Testing of Implant Materials. von Recum AF. 188 New York, Macmillian, 1986.

Lemons JE: Corrosion and biodegradation. In Handbook of Biomaterials Evaluation, von Recum AF (ed). New York, Macmillan, 1986.

McDougall A: Malignant tumour at site of bone plating. J Bone Joint Surg [Br] Vol 38:709, 1956.

New PFJ, Rosen BR, Brady TJ, Buonanno ES, Kistler JP, et al: Potential hazards and artifacts of ferromagnetic and nonferromagnetic surgical devices in nuclear magnetic resonance imaging. Radiology 147:139–148, 1983.

Park JB: Biomaterials: An Introduction. New York, Plenum, 1979.

Perren SM, Cordey JC, Rahn BA, Gautier E, Schneider E: Early temporary porosity of bone induced by internal fixation implants. Clin Ortho Rel Res 232:139–151, 1988.

Postlehwaite KR, Philips JG, Booth S, Shaw J, Slater A: The effects of small plate osteosynthesis on postoperative radiotherapy. Brit J Oral Maxillofac Surg 27:375–378, 1989.

Prein J, Kellman RM: Rigid internal fixation of mandibular fracture: Basics of AO technique. Otolaryngol Clin of North Am 20:3, 441, 1987.

Rittmann WW, Perren SM: Cortical Bone Healing after Internal Fixation and Infection: Biomechanics and Biology. New York, Springer-Verlag, 1974.

Salyamon LS: The role of inflammation in the mechanism of carcinogenic, co-carcinogenic and certain anti-carcinogenic effects. Probl Oncol 7:44–50, 1961.

Schenk RK: Histophysiology of Bone Remodelling and Bone Repair. In Perspectives on Biomaterials. Lin O, Chao E (eds). Netherlands, Elsevier, 1986.

Semlitsch M: Mechanical properties of selected implant metals used for artificial hip joints. In Metal and Ceramic Biomaterials. Vol. II, Chart 1. Ducheyne P, Hastings S U (eds). Boca Raton, FL, CRC Press, 1–20, 1984.

Shellock FG: MR imaging of metallic implants and materials: A compilation of the literature. AJR 151: 811–814, 1988.

Shellock FG, Crues JV: High-field strength MR imaging and metallic biomedical implants: An ex vivo evaluation of deflection forces. AJR 151: 389–392, 1988.

Spiessl B: New Concepts in Maxillofacial Bone Fixation. Berlin, New York, Springer-Verlag, 1976.

Spiessl B: New Concepts in Maxillofacial Bone Surgery. New York, Springer-Verlag, 1976.

Steinemann SG: Corrosion of titanium and titanium alloys for surgical implants. In Titanium: Science and Technology. Lutjering G, Zwicker U, Bunk W (eds). Proc Fifth Int Conf on Titanium, 1984. Vol 1–4 Munich, Germany.

Sutter F, Raveh J: Titanium-coated hollow screw and reconstruction plate system for bridging of lower jaw defects: Biomechanical aspects. Int J Oral Maxillofac Surg 17: 267–274, 1988.

Styles JA: A method for detecting carcinogenic organic chemicals using mammalian cells in culture. Br J Cancer 36:558, 1977.

Sutow EJ, Pollaack SR: The biocompatibility of certain stainless steels. In Biocompatibility of Clinical Implant Materials, Vol 2. Williams DF. Boca Raton, FL, CRC Press, 1981.

Tayton KJJ: Ewing's sarcoma at the site of a metal plate. Cancer 45:413–415, 1980.

The United States Pharmacopeia, 20th revised ed. Rockville, Md. United States Pharmacopeial Convention, 1980.

von Recum AF: Handbook of Biomaterials Evaluation-Scientific, Technical and Clinical Testing of Implant Materials. New York, Macmillian, 1986.

Waalkes MP, Rehm S, Kaspreak KS, Issaq HJ: Inflammatory proliferating and neoplastic lesions at the site of metallic identification ear tags in wistar rats. Cancer Research 47: 2445–2450, 1987.

Walker PS: Human Joints and their Artificial Replacements. Springfield, Charles C Thomas, 1977.

Wapner KL, Morris DM, Black J: Release of corrosion products by F-75 cobalt base alloy in the rat. II: Morbidity apparently associated with chromium release in vivo: A 120-day study. J Biomed Mater Res 20: 219–233, 1986.

Williams DF: Biocompatibility of Clinical Implant Materials, Vol 1. Boca Raton, FL, CRC Press, 1981a.

Williams DF: Biocompatibility of Clinical Implant Materials, Vol 2. Boca Raton, FL, CRC Press, 1981b.

Williams DF: Systemic Aspects of Biocompatibility, Vol 1. Boca Raton, FL, CRC Press, 1981c.

Williams DF: Systemic Aspects of Biocompatibility, Vol 2. Boca Raton, FL, CRC Press, 1981d.

Williams DF: The properties and clinical uses of cobalt-chromium alloys. In Biocompatibility of Clinical Implant Materials, Vol 2. Williams DF. Boca Raton, FL, CRC Press, 1981e.

Williams DF: Titanium and titanium alloys. In Biocompatibility of Clinical Implant Materials, Vol 2. Williams DF, Boca Raton, FL, CRC Press, 1981f.

Williams DF, Roaf R: Implants in Surgery. Philadelphia, W.B. Saunders, 1973.

Wolff J: Über die Theorie des Knocheusch windes durch ver mehrte Druck und der Knochenan bild ung durch Drucken las tung. Arch Klin Chir 42: 302, 1892.

Woodman JL, Jacobs JJ, Galante JO, Urban RM: Metal ion release from titanium-based prosthetic segmental replacements of long bones in baboons: A long-term study. J Orthopaedic Res 1: 421–430, 1984.

CHAPTER 6

The Potential of Resorbable Biomaterials for Skeletal Fixation

Rudolf R.M. Bos
Frederik R. Rozema
Geert Boering
Albert J. Pennings

INTRODUCTION

The internal fixation of facial bones with metallic plates and screws is a reliable method of achieving osteosynthesis while, at the same time, usually allowing the patient passive or even functional loading of the fractured or osteotomized bone. These metal devices are not without certain real or theoretic disadvantages. Depending on the location and the type of replacement it may be necessary to remove plates and screws after bone healing because of the potential risk of stress-protection-induced osteopenia in the cortex directly underlying the plate and a reduction of the shaft caliber, which is obvious on radiographs (Uhthoff 1971, Akeson 1975, Paavolainen 1978, Simon 1978, Szivek 1981, Christel 1982, Uhthoff 1983, Woo 1983, Katz 1984, Terjesen 1986, Vert 1984, Zimmerman 1987). This, however, has not yet been proven for the maxillofacial skeleton. In addition, it is possible that, in the future, loosening or corrosion of these metallic devices will cause inflammatory reactions (Winter 1974, Danzig 1980, Clark 1982, Tarr 1983, French 1984, Koegel 1984, Wapner 1986, McAuley 1987).

In those patients in whom reconstruction plates have been used for mandibular reconstruction after tumor extirpation, the backscatter caused by the metallic implants during radiation treatment must be considered in the treatment planning (Castillo 1988, Scher 1988). Metal in the human body also produces artifacts in computer tomography and magnetic resonance imaging.

Another problem in the use of metallic osteosynthetic devices is the possibility of the patients becoming sensitized. This applies to alloys that bear nickel, cobalt, and chromium. Titanium and molybdenum are not believed to be haptens, whereas the immune role played by vanadium remains unclear (Merrit 1985, Black 1988).

The carcinogenic potential of metallic osteosynthesis devices cannot be ignored. Chromium and nickel and some of their compounds, as well as cobalt, are potent carcinogens in animals. Titanium is not known to be oncogenic in animals; the evidence concerning vanadium is inconclusive (Weber 1986, Bauer 1987, Black 1988). Finally, patients may request removal of their metallic implants because of visibility, palpability, or cold sensitivity.

Plates and screws that are made of biocompatible, bioresorbable material and that have appropriate load bearing properties and a sufficient rate of degradation could obviate the necessity to remove plates and screws used in the internal fixation of maxillofacial fractures or in orthognathic surgery. The avoidance of a second operation, with its concomitant morbidity and expenses, would be attractive to both the patient and the health care providers.

BIORESORBABLE MATERIALS

Resorbable polymers have been used for biomedical application, especially for surgical sutures, for many years. In 1962, polyglycolic acid was developed by the American Cyanamid Company as the first absorbable synthetic suture, Dexon® (Davis and Geck, Inc., Manati, Puerto Rico) (Frazza 1971). It has been commercially available since 1970. A copolymer of 92% polyglycolic acid and 8% polylactic acid came onto the market in 1975 as a competitive resorbable suture, Vicryl® (Ethicon, Somerville, N.J.) (Gilding 1979).

Biocompatible and resorbable poly (a-hydroxy acids) like poly(L-lactide) (PLLA), polyglycolide (PGA), and polydioxanon (PDA) have been proposed as potential orthopedic repair materials. However, only a few experimental studies concerning this form of application have appeared in the literature (Cutright 1972, Getter 1972, Alexander 1981, Vert 1981, Christel 1982, Christel 1984, Vert 1984, Tunc 1985, Ewers 1985, Gerlach 1986). In the majority of these studies, compression-molded devices have been evaluated. It has been reported that compression-molded PLLA composites, reinforced with fibers of PGA and carbon, revealed promising load-bearing properties when tested as bone plate candidates (Alexander 1981, Christel 1982, Vert 1984, Zimmerman 1987). It is likely that only composites may lead to resorbable bone fixation parts that will be suitable for human application (Vert 1984). Of the available biodegradable polymers, PLLA seems to have the best potential for use as base material in the manufacture of bone plates and screws. PLLA, a semicrystalline, biodegradable thermoplastic material, is available from renewable resources. The starting compound L-lactic acid (2-hydroxy-propanoic acid) can be produced in high yields by many fermentation and chemical derivation treatments of cheap biomass materials, such as molasses and potato starch (Waksman 1937, Pan 1940, Schindler 1977, Kalb 1979, Wehrenberg 1981, Eling 1982).

The L-lactic acid polymer eventually returns to L-lactic acid after gradually being hydrolyzed in the environment. In cases where high molecular weight is described, L-lactic acid usually is first converted into L-lactide (3, 6-dimethyl-1, 4-dioxane-2, 5-dione), followed by ring-opening polymerization of this crystalline compound, either in the bulk or in solution. In addition, L-lactide can easily be copolymerized with other environmentally compatible compounds, such as glycolide, caprolactone, and o-valerolactone. Copolymers of this type can replicate the physical properties of many of today's petrochemical thermoplastics (Waksman 1937, Pan 1940, Schindler 1977, Kalb 1979, Wehrenberg 1981, Eling 1982). In view of increasing problems with environmental waste, PLLA or related copolymers may finally substitute for some of the conventional, relatively biostable plastics.

The literature shows that L-lactic acid, the apparently nonallergic, noncarcinogenic and nontoxic product of hydrolysis, can leave the body by normal excretory routes. L-lactic acid is a normal intermediate in the carbohydrate metabolism and shows up the end of the anaerobic metabolism of glucose and glycogen.

The preparation of PLLA is well described by Leenslag (1987a, 1987b). Polymerizations of L-lactide were performed after purification of the monomer (peak of melting 98° C) by recrystallization from toluene under N_2 atmosphere. Polymerizations were carried out in vacuum-sealed (10^{-7} torr), silanized glass ampules at different temperatures (100 to 130° C).

Table 6.1 Typical mechanical properties of poly(L-lactide) (PLLA) as found by Leenslag (1987b).

Tensile Strength	Bending Modulus	Impact Resilience
75 MPa	5 GPa	47 kJ/m²

N = newton, MPa = megapascal (= 10^6 N/m²), GPa = gigapascal (= 10^9 N/m²), kJ/m² = kilojoule per square meter (= 10^3 Nm^{-1}).

Stannous-2-ethylhexanoate was used as a catalyst (0.015 wt%). At the lowest temperature investigated (100° C), samples of PLLA with the highest intrinsic viscosities—up to 13 deciliters per gram as measured in chloroform—were synthesized (polymerization time 190 hours). This method resulted in the synthesis of high-molecular-weight poly(L-lactide), which has very promising mechanical properties for use as internal fixation (see Table 6.1).

EXPERIENCE WITH BIORESORBABLE MATERIALS

Only a few studies on resorbable plates and screws for internal fixation of fractures or osteotomies have appeared in literature. Getter (1972) reported the internal fixation of mandibular fractures in six adult beagle dogs with plates and screws of polylactic acid (PLA). All fractures healed well, with secondary callus formation. The plates and screws were almost completely degraded after 40 weeks. No appliance was rejected. Niederdellmann (1983) used a screw of polydioxanon (PDA) for the fixation of a fracture of the mandibular angle in one patient. This screw was shaped like an AO-screw with a core diameter of 3.2 millimeters and a thread diameter of 4.5 millimeters. This fracture healed well. Vert (1984) used six-hole PLA plates reinforced with two-dimensional woven fabrics of polyglycolic acid (PGA) threads (0.1 millimeter in diameter) for the internal fixation of two osteotomized tibiae in sheep. They used stainless steel screws instead of biodegradable screws. One plate broke after one month in spite of use of a plaster cast. The second plate was found to be broken at sacrifice, but the osteotomy had healed, although it showed a large amount of callus. They also used small-size PLA/PGA composite plates (2 millimeters thick) in combination with stainless steel screws for the repair of mandibular and skull fractures in 25 patients. All of the fractures healed without inflammatory reactions. Partial degradation of retrieved bone plates was found. Tunc (1985) used specifically designed plates and screws of high molecular weight PLA for reduction of radial osteotomies in a series of dogs. The healing was uneventful. However, abundant callus formation was observed. In the longest follow-up period, of two years, 93% of the PLA was resorbed. Ewers (1985) used plates and screws of polydioxanon (PDA) for the fixa-

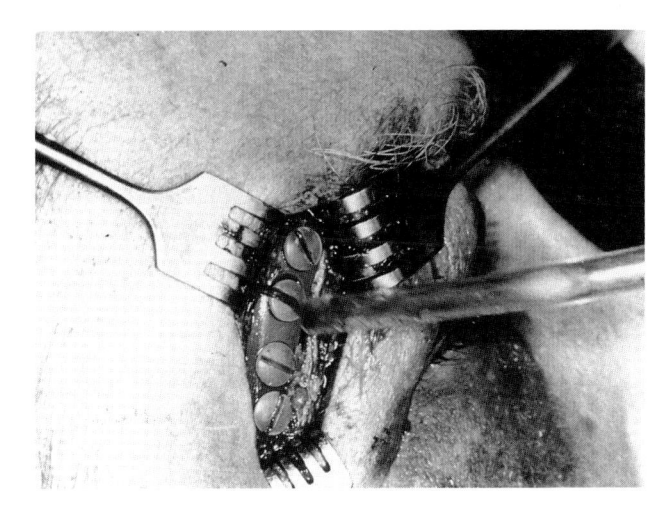

Figure 6.1 Fixation of an unstable zygomatic fracture with a PLLA plate and PLLA screws in the lateral orbital rim (Bos et al. 1987).

Table 6.2 Mechanical properties of a four-hole PLLA bone plate and a four-hole stainless steel Champy mini bone plate (Bos 1989).

	Tensile Strength	Bending Modulus
PLLA plates	650 N	5 GPa
Champy plates	1300 N	5–7 GPa

N = newton, GPa = gigapascal (= 10^9 N/m^2)

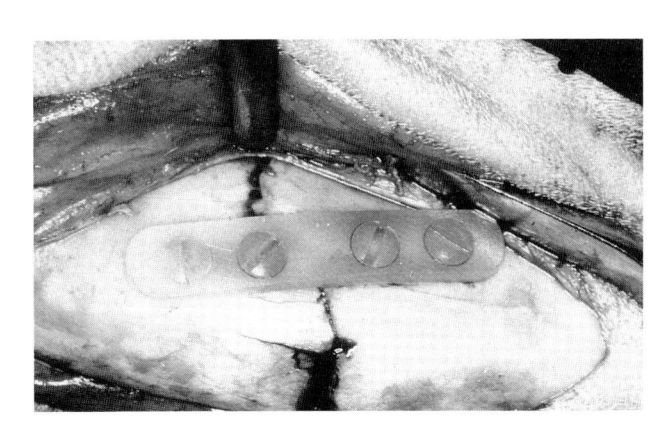

Figure 6.2 In a sheep, fixation of a fracture with a four-hole PLLA plate and screws half the height of the mandible (Bos 1989b).

tion of six osteotomized ribs in five Beagle dogs. The plates and screws were compression molded. Five osteotomies healed through primary bone healing. One osteotomy, which had been infected artificially, healed through secondary bone healing and showed marked callus formation. Premature resorption of the polydioxanon was found in the case that had been infected artificially.

Bos (1987) treated ten patients who had unstable zygomatic fractures with resorbable poly (L-lactide) (PLLA) plates and screws (see Figure 6.1). Their results showed that this method of fixation gave good stability over a sufficiently long period to enable undisturbed fracture healing.

Gerlach (1988) reported on the internal fixation of 15 mandibular fractures in 12 beagle dogs. PLA plates and screws were used for fixation of three contralateral fractures made in 3 of the 12 dogs six months later. The fracture healing was uneventful. Callus formation, however, was observed. Bos (1989a) described the use of poly (L-lactide) plates and screws for internal fixation of eight artificially created mandibular fractures in two sheep (Bos et al. 1989b) and six dogs (Bos et al. 1989c). The plates and screws used had dimensions similar to those of AO plates and screws. Plates and screws were inserted in accordance with Champy's principles of internal fixation (see Figure 6.2) (Champy 1986). All fractures healed without callus and without any complications. The plates and screws did not fail, despite the lesser tensile strength of the PLLA as compared to that of metallic implants (see Table 6.2).

Rozema (1990a) reported the use of poly (l-lactide) plates and screws with dimensions similar to those of AO plates and screws for internal fixation of paramedial osteotomies of the mandible in five patients. Two plates were inserted parallel to each other, according to Champy's principles for medial and paramedial fractures of the mandible (see Figure 6.3). These patients

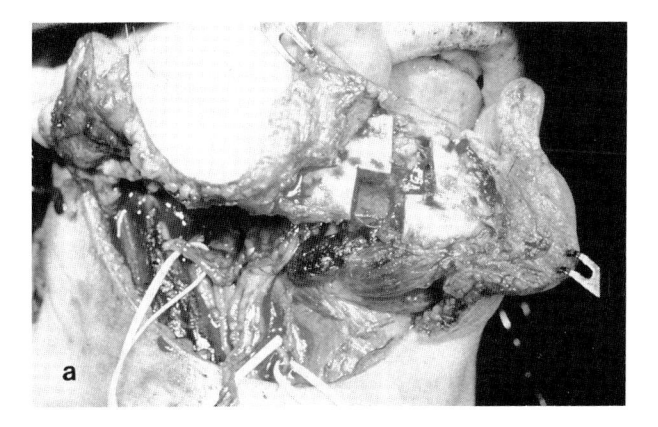

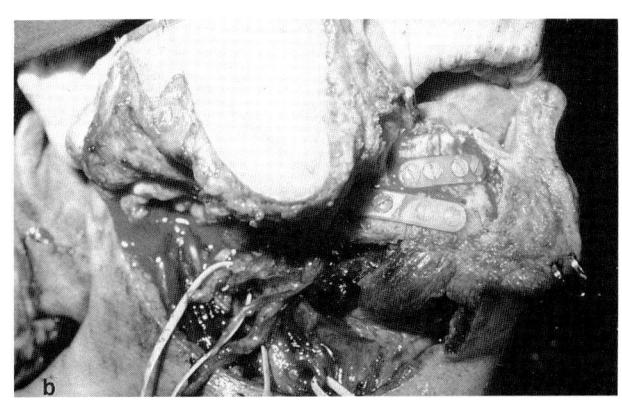

Figure 6.3 (a) Z-shaped osteotomy of the mandible in a case of a lateral swing approach to an oropharyngeal tumor. (b) Fixation of this osteotomy with insertion of two parallel AO shaped polylactide plates and screws. (Rozema 1990a).

were operated on for the treatment of oropharyngeal tumors. A lateral swing procedure was chosen to get better access to the tumor region. All the patients were irradiated four to six weeks postoperatively. The authors claim that PLLA plates and screws caused no backscattering effects (Rozema 1990b). All osteotomies healed without any complication. Callus formation was not observed.

SUMMARY

Although resorbable plates and screws have been investigated for almost 20 years, no system is commercially available. Unfortunately, the composition and the mechanical characteristics of the polymers used in these studies are often poorly characterized. The dimensions of plates and screws used in these studies are often coarse compared with those of miniplates. This restricts their usage in the maxillofacial area. Plates and screws of smaller scale have less strength, which will probably limit their potential use for the functionally stable fixation of the mandible or for the functionally loaded midface. Furthermore, the required strength of plates and screws has to be determined not only by the loading forces a patient can develop but also by the nature and pattern of a fracture. Particularly, in cases of oblique, complex, or comminuted fractures, or when bridging of a defect is needed, loading on plates and screws is much greater than in the case of simple fractures, such as those employed in experimental studies. It is likely that the higher loading forces the resorbable plates and screws have to withstand, the more rapidly the material will decrease in tensile strength. This decrease is due to a stress cracking process, a phenomenon that is well known in loaded polymers (Christel 1982). This cracking process may result in premature failure of the osteosynthesis and thus in disturbed bone healing. Despite the limitations of bioresorbable plates and screws, the currently available resorbable plates and screws can be used for many fractures and osteotomies of the craniomaxillofacial skeleton, including the mandible. Future investigations should look for resorbable materials that have greater strength and that remain stable for a longer period during fracture healing. Such plates and screws will be able to withstand more loading and will be suitable for other types of fractures of the human skeleton as well. Dimensions of resorbable plates and screws can be reduced; this makes it possible to apply them to smaller bones and to sites where the anatomical situation demands smaller plates and screws. Reinforcement of plates and screws with strong biodegradable fibers might provide the solution. Ideally, the strength and rates of degradation of the plates and screws would align the osteosynthesis and strengthen the healing fracture sufficiently to prevent redislocation and to make bone healing possible. The strength of the plate fixation could be lowered to zero as soon as the normal load-bearing properties of the fractured bone segment have been replaced. The plates and screws would then be resorbed in a short period of time.

The polymer chemist and the clinician will have to find ways to improve and evaluate biodegradable, biocompatible materials that meet these requirements. The clinical potential for the use of biodegradable osteosynthetic implants makes their development worthwhile.

REFERENCES

Akeson WH, Woo SL-Y, Coutts RD, Matthews JV, Gonsalves M, Amiel D: Quantitative histological evaluation of early fracture healing of cortical bones immobilized by stainless steel and composite plates. Calcif Tiss Res 19:27–37, 1975.

Alexander H, Corcoran S, Parsons JR, Weiss AB: Internal fracture fixation with partially degradable plates. J Bioengineering 9:115–118, 1981.

Bauer TW, Manley MT, Stern LS: Osteosarcoma at the site of total hip replacement. Trans Soc Biomater 10:36, 1987.

Black J: Orthopedic Biomaterials in Research and Practice, Churchill Livingstone, New York, Edinburgh, London, Melbourne, 1988, 292–302.

Bos RRM, Boering G, Rozema FR, Leenslag JW, Pennings AJ, Verwey AB: Resorbable poly(L-lactide) plates and screws for the fixation of zygomatic fractures. J Oral Maxillofac Surg 45:751–753, 1987.

Bos RRM: Poly(L-lactide) osteosynthesis: Development of bioresorbable bone plates and screws. PhD thesis, University of Groningen, ISBN 90-73152-01-1, 7–16, 1989a.

Bos RRM, Rozema FR, Boering G, Nijenhuis AJ, Pennings AJ, Jansen HWB: Bone plates and screws of bioabsorbable poly(L-lactide): An animal pilot study. Br J Oral Maxillofac Surg 27:467–476, 1989b.

Bos RRM, Rozema FR, Boering G, Nijenhuis AJ, Pennings AJ, Verwey AB: Bioabsorbable plates and screws for internal fixation of mandibular fractures: A study in six dogs. Int J Oral Maxillofac Surg 18:365–369, 1989c.

Bos RRM, Rozema FR, Boering G, Nijenhuis AJ, Pennings AJ, Verwey AB, Nieuwenhuis P, Jansen HWB: Degradation of and tissue reaction to biodegradable poly(L-lactide) for use as internal fixation of fractures. A study in rats. Biomaterials, 1990, in press.

Castillo MH, Button TM, Homs MI, Pruett CW, Doerr R: Effects of radiation therapy on mandibular reconstruction plates. In Transactions of the forty-first annual cancer symposium. The Society of Surgical Oncology, 114. New Orleans, LA, 1988.

Champy M, Pape HD, Gerlach KL, Loddé JP: The strassbourg miniplate osteosynthesis. In Oral and

Maxillofacial Traumatology. Krüger E, Schilli W, Worthington P (eds). 2:19–43. Chicago, London, Berlin, Rio de Janeiro, Tokyo, Quintessence 1986.

Christel P, Chabot F, Leray JL, Morin C, Vert M: Biodegradable composites for internal fixation. In Biomaterials 1980. Winter GD, Gibbons DF, Plenk H (eds). 271–280. New York, Wiley 1982.

Christel P, Vert M, Chabot F, Abolts F, Leray J: Polylactic acid for intramedullary plugging. In Advances in Biomaterials. Ducheyne P, Perre G vd, Aubert AE (eds). 6:1- Amsterdam, The Netherlands, Elsevier, 1984.

Clark GCF, Williams DF: The effects of protein on metallic corrosion. J Biomed Mater Res 16:125–134, 1982.

Cutright DE, Hunsuck EE: The repair of fractures of the orbital floor using biodegradable polylactic acid. Oral Surg 33:28–34, 1972.

Danzig LA, Woo SL-Y, Akeson WH, Jemmott GF, Wickham MG: Internal fixation plates after fifty-six years of implantation: Report of a case. Clin Orthop Rel Res 149:201–206, 1980.

Eling B, Gogolewski S, Pennings AJ: Biodegradable materials of poly(L-lactide) acid. I. Melt-spun and solution-spun fibers. Polymer 23:1587–1593, 1982.

Ewers R, Förster H: Resorbierbare Osteosynthesematerialien. Eine tierexperimentelle Studie. Dtsch Z Mund Kiefer GesichtsChir 9:196–201, 1985.

Frazza EJ, Schmitt EE: A new absorbable suture. J Biomed Mater Res Symposium 1:43–58, 1971.

French HG, Cook SD, Haddad RJ: Correlation of tissue reaction to corrosion in osteosynthetic devices. J Biomed Mater Res 18:817–828, 1984.

Gerlach KL: Biologisch abbaubare Polymere in der Mund- Kiefer- und Gesichtschirurgie. Tierexperimentelle Untersuchungen. PhD thesis, University of Cologne 1986, Carl Hanser Verlag, München, Wien, 1988.

Getter L, Cutright DE, Bhaskar SN, Augsburg JK: A biodegradable intraosseous appliance in the treatment of mandibular fractures. J Oral Surg 30:344–348, 1972.

Gilding DK, Reed AM: Biodegradable polymers for use in surgery: Polyglycolic/poly(lactid acid) homo- and copolymers:1. Polymer 20:1459–1464, 1979.

Kalb B, Pennings AJ: General crystallization behavior of poly(L-lactic acid). Polymer 21:607–612, 1979.

Katz JL, Yoon HS, Lipson S, Maharidge R, Meunier A, Christel P: The effects of remodelling on the elastic properties of bone. Calcif Tiss Int 36:31–36, 1984.

Koegel A, Black J: Release of corrosion products by F-75 cobalt base alloy in the rat. I. Acute serum elevations. J. Biomed Mater Res 18:513–522, 1984.

Leenslag JW, Pennings AJ: Synthesis and morphology of high-molecular weight poly(L-Lactide) with tin-2-ethylhexanoate. Makromol Chem 188:1809–1814, 1987a.

Leenslag JW, Pennings AJ, Bos RRM, Rozema FR, Boering G: Resorbable materials of poly(L-lactide). VI. Plates and screws for internal fixation. Biomaterials 8:70–73, 1987b.

McAuley JP, Gow KV, Covert A, McDermott AG, Yabsley RH: Analysis of a Lane-plate internal fixation device after 64 years in vivo. Can J Surg 30(6):424–427, 1987.

Merritt K, Brown SA: Biological effects of corrosion products from metals. In Corrosion and degradation of implant materials. ASTM STP. Fraker AC, Griffin CD (eds). 859:195–206. American Society for Testing Materials. Philadelphia, 1985.

Niederdellmann H, Buhrmann K: Resorbierbare Osteosyntheseschrauben aus Polydioxanon (PDS). Dtsch Z Mund Kiefer Gesichts Chir 7:399–400, 1983.

Paavolaine P, Karaharju E, Slatis P, Ahonen J, Holmstorm T: Effect of rigid plate fixation on structure and mineral content of cortical bone. Clin Orthop Rel Res 136:287–293, 1978.

Pan SC, Petersen WH, Johnson MJ: Acceleration of lactic acid fermentation by heat-labile substances. Ind Eng Chem 32:709–714, 1940.

Rozema FR, Bos RRM, Boering G, Pennings AJ: Resorbable poly(L-lactide) plates and screws for internal fixation in case of postoperative irradiation in cancer patients: 1990a, submitted.

Rozema FR, Levendag PC, Bos RRM, Boering G, Pennings AJ: The influence of resorbable poly(L-lactide) bone plates and screws on the dose distributions of radiotherapy beams. Int J Oral Maxillofac Surg: 19:374–376, 1990.

Scher N, Poe D, Kuchmir F, Reft C, Weichselbaum R, Panje WR: Radiotherapy of the resected mandible following stainless steel plate fixation. Laryngoscope 98:561–563, 1988.

Schilli W, Luhr HG: Rigid internal fixation by means of compression plates. In Oral and Maxillofacial Traumatology. Krüger E, Schilli W (eds). 1:308–370. Chicago, London, Berlin, Rio de Janeiro, Tokyo, Quintessence, 1982.

Schindler A, Jeffcoat R, Kimmel GL, Pitt CG, Wall ME, Zweidinger R: Biodegradable polymers for sustained drug delivery. In Contemporary Topics in Polymer Science. Pierce EM, Schaeger JR (eds). 2:251–289. New York, Plenum, 1977.

Simon BR, Woo SL-Y, McCarthy MP, Lee S, Akeson WH: Parametric study of bone remodelling beneath internal fixation plates of varying stiffness. J Bioengineering 2:543–556, 1978.

Szivek JA, Weatherly GC, Pilliar RM, Cameron HU: A study of bone remodelling using metal-polymer laminates. J Biomed Mater Res 15:853–865, 1981.

Tarr RR, Jorge R, Latta L, Ghandur-Mnaymneh L: Histopathology and metallurgical analysis of a removed Lane plate at 53 years post-implantation: a case report. J Biomed Mater Res 17:785–792, 1983.

Terjesen T, Nordby A, Arnulf V: The extent of stress protection after plate osteosynthesis in the human tibia. Clin Orthop Rel Res 207:108–112, 1986.

Tunc DC, Rohovski MW, Lehman WB, Strongwater A, Kummer F: Evaluation of body absorbable bone fixation devices. Proc. 31st Ann Orthop Res Soc, 165. Las Vegas, NV, 1985.

Uhthoff HK, Dubuc F: Bone structure changes in the dog under rigid fixation. Clin Orthop 81:165–170, 1971.

Uhthoff HK, Finnegan M: The effects of metal plates on post-traumatic remodelling and bone mass. J Bone Joint Surg 65B(1):66–71, 1983.

Vert M, Chabot F, Leray J, Christel P: Stereo regular bioresorbable polyesters for orthopaedic surgery. Makromol Chem Suppl 5:30–41, 1981.

Vert M, Christel P, Chabot F, Leray J: Bioresorbable plastic materials for bone surgery. In Macromolecular Biomaterials. Hastings GW, Ducheyne P (eds). 120–142, Boca Raton, FL, CRC Press, 1984.

Waksman SA, Hutchings IJ: Lactic acid production by species or rhizopus. J Am Chem Soc 59:545–547, 1937.

Wapner KL, Morris DM, Black J: Release of corrosion products by F-75 cobalt base alloy in the rat. II. Morbidity apparently associated with chromium release in vivo: a 120 day rat study. J Biomed Mater Res 20:219–233, 1986.

Weber PC: Epithelioid sarcoma in association with total knee displacement: A case report. J Bone Joint Surg 68B:824–825, 1986.

Wehrenberg RH: Lactic acid polymers: Strong degradable thermoplastics. Mater Eng 13:63–66, 1981.

Winter GD: Tissue reactions to metallic wear and corrosion products in human patients. J Biomed Mater Res 8:11–26, 1974.

Woo SL-Y, Simon BR, Akeson WH, Gomez MA, Seguchi Y: A new approach to the design of internal fixation plates. J Biomed Mater Res 17:427–439, 1983.

Woo SL-Y, Lothringer KS, Akeson WH, Coutts RD, Woo YK, Simon B, Gomez MA: Less rigid internal fixation plates: historical perspectives and new concepts. J Orthop Res 1:431–449, 1984.

Zimmerman M, Parsons JL, Alexander H: The design and analysis of a laminated partially degradable composite bone plate for fracture fixation. J Biomed Mater Res 21:345–361, 1987.

CHAPTER 7

The Effects of Mandibular Immobilization on the Masticatory System: A Review

Edward Ellis, III
David S. Carlson

Maxillomandibular fixation (MMF), also called intermaxillary fixation (IMF), is the standard method of postsurgical immobilization of the osseous segments following either traumatically induced or surgically created fractures of the jaws. The purpose of MMF is to immobilize the skeletal segments until osseous healing is accomplished, usually within a period of from six to eight weeks. MMF is by no means a new procedure. Writings from the time of Hippocrates indicate that wiring the upper and lower teeth together was an accepted form of treatment of fractures of the jaw as early as 2000 years ago.

Although there are various methods by which to secure MMF, most of them use the dentition, and all rely on immobilization of the mandible. However, mandibular immobilization, although employed extensively as part of MMF, has not been thoroughly evaluated in terms of its effects on the masticatory system. The probable reason for this is that MMF has been accepted as a benign technique whose use is necessary in order to accomplish orthognathic surgical objectives. Only recently, with the advent of alternative techniques of postsurgical immobilization of the skeletal segments (for example, rigid internal fixation), has examination of MMF begun with a more critical eye.

Preliminary studies have shown that MMF may not be as benign a procedure as commonly thought. Indeed, several of the problems encountered in the clinical practice of orthognathic surgery may be the result not of the type of surgery performed, but of the method of postsurgical immobilization employed. For instance, the technique of securing mandibular immobilization may play a significant role in relapse of the skeletal segments following mandibular advancement, in decreases in mandibular range of motion and bite force, and in internal derangements of the temporomandibular joints.

To bring into focus the pathophysiological effects of mandibular immobilization on the masticatory system, in this chapter we review what is currently known regarding this topic. Because the literature contains a surprising paucity of information on this subject, much of our review is taken from the orthopedic surgery literature, where the effects of immobilization on extremities has been the subject of investigation for many years. Because of the many problems encountered by extremity immobilization, orthopedic surgeons have pioneered methods to allow fracture healing without immobilization across a joint. This research spawned the beginnings of rigid internal fixation, which is now being adapted for use in orthognathic surgery and maxillofacial trauma. Although there are many differences between structure and function of the extremities and those of the masticatory system, there are also many parallels. The purpose of this chapter is not to advocate any particular method of treatment, but to evaluate critically the effects of immobilization on the masticatory system so that fixation methods can be selected rationally.

THE EFFECT OF IMMOBILIZATION ON BONE

The clinical phenomenon of disuse osteoporosis has been recognized for years. Briefly, when a bone is not used, it progressively loses mineral content. In 1936,

Rieder proposed that disuse osteoporosis may be the result of circulatory stasis and acidosis. Since then, numerous experimental studies have been performed on the structural and physiological changes that occur in immobilized limbs (Geiser 1958, Burkhart 1967, Sundén 1967). The structural changes that characteristically occur following joint immobilization include cortical and trabecular thinning, vascular distention, and increased osteoclastic activity (Geiser 1958). The physiological parameters measured during the period of bone resorption have revealed decreased blood flow (Sundén 1967), increased venous Pco_2 and decreased venous Po_2 and pH in nutrient veins (Burkhart 1967), an apparent increase in the effectiveness on the immobilized bone of circulating parathormone (Burkhart 1967), and an increase in the loss of administered ^{3}H-tetracycline (as compared to control) (Klein 1982). As a result of this evidence, hypotheses have been advanced that bone loss in an immobilized limb is the result of a change in the local environment involving either reduced blood flow (Geiser 1958, Sundén 1967) or the induction of changes in cell metabolism (Burkhart 1967).

Although no studies are available which address disuse osteoporosis of the jaw, there is no reason to believe that disuse osteoporosis should not occur at that location as well. The clinical significance of disuse osteoporosis in the jaw, even if it occurs, is questionable, however. Even though cortical and trabecular thinning may occur during a period of mandibular immobilization, with time and function this thinning should rapidly reverse.

THE EFFECT OF IMMOBILIZATION ON MUSCLES

The anatomical effects of immobilization on muscle has been known for years and are most obvious to anyone who has had an arm or a leg immobilized in a cast. Muscle atrophy, which can be marked, is an obvious finding and is associated with weakness of the involved muscle(s) for several weeks or even months following immobilization. A wealth of information has accumulated in recent years concerning nerve–muscle characteristics and interactions. This information has prompted experimentation regarding the effects of immobilization on muscular (and neural) tissue. It has been found that skeletal muscle, the body's largest mass of tissue devoted to a common purpose, is perhaps the most responsive in terms of adaptation to changes in patterns of activity. Muscle possesses a tremendous capacity to adapt to stresses that are imposed upon it by shortening, lengthening, exercise, and disuse. Much attention has been directed to the problem of disuse of the appendicular skeletal musculature. Helander (1957) showed that encasing the hindlimb of a rabbit in a plaster cast resulted in considerable atrophy of the calf muscles. This atrophy was associated with a marked decrease in the diameter of muscle fiber and reduction in the number of blood vessels. Also noted was a marked decrease in the amount of contractile protein within the muscle. Wells (1969) found a great reduction in tetanic tension and muscle weights after immobilizing the ankle joints.

Immobilization of the muscles during growth also has an inhibitory effect on their longitudinal growth (Goldspink 1972). Several investigations of animals have shown a decrease in the size of both Type II and Type I fibers, albeit to varying extents (Boyes 1979, Herbison 1979, Edgerton 1975, Lindboe 1982). Electrophysical studies have shown a significant impairment of contractile function (force-generating capacity) of both fast and slow muscles following immobilization (Wells 1969, Fischbach 1969, Witzman 1982). Animal studies have also demonstrated that the *total number* of muscle fibers does not change during immobilization, although the size and configuration of the fibers (fiber architecture) are affected (Cardenas 1977). However, the effects of immobilization on the musculature have also been found to be temporary and reversible (Witzman 1982). The exact mechanisms responsible for the atrophic response seen during immobilization remain elusive. It has been documented, however, that the atrophic response involves a loss of both contractile and metabolic proteins (Jokl 1983) and that these alterations begin very early after immobilization, within the first few hours.

The amount of myofibrillar protein loss has been shown to have some dependency on the position (or length) of the muscle during immobilization. Jokl (1983) found that stretching a muscle during the immobilization period causes a reactive production of protein, which can balance what is usually lost. Conversely, immobilization of *shortened* muscle causes a marked loss of myofibrillar protein content—more so than would be expected from the effects of immobilization alone. Contractile properties of the involved muscles reflected the same findings as protein content: A severe loss of contractile force was found with a shortened muscle.

Little information is available in the literature regarding the adaptations of masticatory muscles to changes in length or activity. We recently reported the histochemical characteristics of masseter and temporalis muscles in four juvenile rhesus monkeys (*Macaca mulatta*) following five weeks of MMF (Mayo 1988). Biopsies of the masseter and temporalis muscles were obtained on these animals, which were processed for histochemical analysis. The muscle fiber types and areas were calculated and compared to controls published previously by our laboratory (Maxwell 1979). Decreases in mean cross-sectional area in both Type I and Type II fibers were clearly observed (Table 7.1); with the mean fiber areas following five weeks of immobilization were less than half found in controls (see Figure 7.1). The percent composition of Type I and II fibers remained unchanged from control percentages, how-

Table 7.1 Cross-sectional area of masseter and temporalis muscle fibers after five weeks of MMF

	Type I (μ^2)		Type II (μ^2)	
	mean	s.d.	mean	s.d.
Masseter				
Exper. ($n = 2$)	793	191	290	50
Contr. ($n = 12$)	2090	1603	688	618
sig.*				
Temporalis				
Exper. ($n = 4$)	1033	227	465	104
Contr. ($n = 12$)	2255	810	1810	750
sig.	0.05		0.01	

*Statistics were not obtained due to small sample size (two specimens were lost in processing).

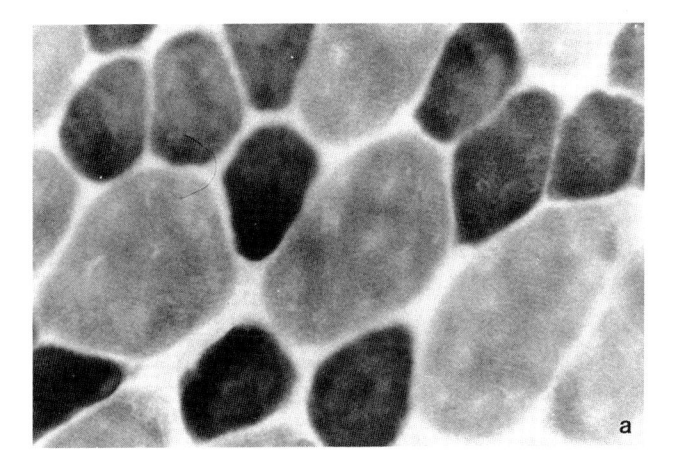

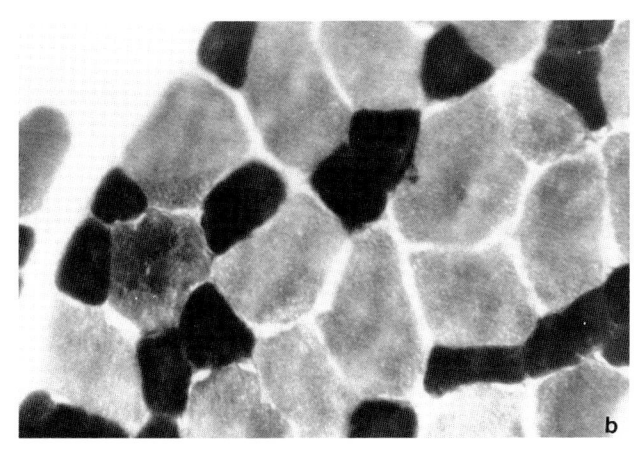

Figure 7.1 (a) Photomicrograph of the normal histochemical appearance (stained with ATPase) of masseter muscle from a rhesus monkey. The large, pale cells are Type I (slow twitch) fibers; the smaller, darker, cells are Type II (fast twitch) fibers. (b) Photomicrograph of masseter muscle sample after five weeks of maxillomandibular fixation (same magnification as sample above). Note the decrease in size of both Type I and Type II fibers.

ever. This indicates that overall recruitment of the muscle, and not just of one type of motor unit, was affected by immobilization.

Several studies have reported procedures that are beneficial for the recovery of muscle function following surgery of the lower extremity in humans. Improvement in the vascularity of muscle (Salmons 1981), increased muscle mass and protein metabolism (Sargeant 1977), decreased muscle fatigability and increased strength (Muller 1970), and restoration of the normal anatomy of the internal fibrous structure (Allbrook 1981) are all proven benefits of physical exercise after limb surgery and immobilization. Simple measures—such as isometric exercise of the quadriceps muscle within a plaster cast during the period of immobilization—have been shown to reduce the amount of muscle atrophy (Wolf 1971). It has been demonstrated that if a moveable cast and brace unit is used instead of a rigid cast for surgical repair of knee injury, there is minimal reduction in cross-sectional fiber areas (Haggmark 1979). Further, full range of motion was obtained by 4 weeks in patients with moveable casts, but it took 16 weeks in patients with rigid casts.

Eriksson (1979) found that percutaneous electrical stimulation prevented the reduction in aerobic capacity following anterior cruciate ligament repair when compared to isometrically trained control muscle. Gould (1983) found that patients who underwent transcutaneous electrical stimulation of the leg muscles following meniscectomy had a significantly smaller loss in leg volume and muscle strength. They also were able to ambulate sooner and had a greater range of knee motion, less edema, and less pain than a comparable group without electrical stimulation. Another study, by Sherman (1983), demonstrated that patients recovered remarkably early after meniscectomy when they undertook a rehabilitation program that involved range-of-motion exercises; toe-touch weight bearing; and progressive, active, resistive exercise the day of knee surgery when compared to individuals immobilized for two weeks after surgery.

Given these results, one might hypothesize that the use of rigid internal fixation following surgery in the maxillomandibular complex may prevent the severe atrophy of masticatory muscles that has been demonstrated when mandibular immobilization is used for fixation (Mayo 1988). In order to test this hypothesis, a recent investigation in our laboratory compared stimulated molar bite force in two groups of adult female rhesus monkeys (*Macaca mulatta*) before and after mandibular advancement surgery using MMF in one group of animals and rigid internal fixation (without MMF) in another (Ellis 1988). Stimulated molar bite is that force which can be generated between the teeth when the elevator muscles of mastication are maximally depolarized with electrical stimulation (Dechow 1979, 1986). The results showed that at 6 weeks postsurgery,

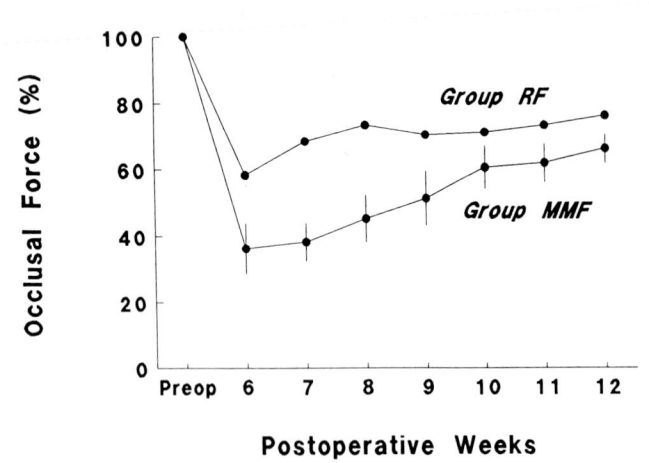

Figure 7.2 Mean change in stimulated molar bite force following mandibular advancement surgery in two groups of adult female rhesus monkeys. Group MMF ($n = 6$) underwent 6 weeks of maxillomandibular fixation; Group RF ($n = 11$) underwent rigid internal fixation without immobilization of the mandible. Note that at 6 weeks postsurgery, Group RF animals had significantly more bite force than did those in Group MMF. At 12 weeks postsurgery, however, there was no longer any significant difference between them.

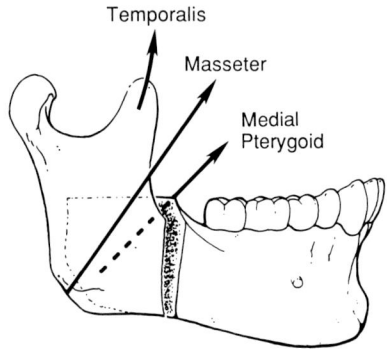

Figure 7.3 Illustration demonstrating the mean force vector of the mandibular elevators on the mandibular ramus. With inadequate fixation of the proximal and distal segments following sagittal ramus osteotomy, the proximal segment will rotate up and forward, effectively shortening the mandibular elevator muscles.

when the first postsurgical bite force recording was made, the maximum bite force was significantly less than presurgical values in both groups (see Figure 7.2). However, the animals that had MMF had significantly less maximum bite force at 6 weeks postsurgery than did the animals that had rigid fixation without MMF. By the ninth postsurgical week, the bite force in the MMF animals had recovered so that there was no longer any significant difference between the rigid and MMF groups. Neither group, however, regained maximum bite force to the level of the presurgical recordings, possibly indicating some permanent reduction in maximal muscle activity following mandibular advancement. Histochemical analysis of masseter and temporalis muscle samples taken at 12 weeks postsurgery verified a significant decrease in the size of muscle fibers in the animals who underwent MMF when compared to those who did not or to controls (Mayo 1989).

Implications for Maxillofacial Surgery

This brief review of the literature points out several important implications for oral and maxillofacial surgical procedures. The overriding message is that any time a muscle is immobilized, atrophic changes will occur. This will be especially evident if the muscle has undergone any surgical insult. Therefore, the less the mandible is immobilized, the better off our patients may be (from a muscular standpoint). A point of equal importance, perhaps, is the finding that immobilizing a *shortened* muscle causes more severe changes than are found normally during immobilization (Jokl 1983). This finding indicates that one should strive to maintain the preoperative position of the proximal segment when performing the sagittal ramus osteotomy. Any upward and forward rotation of the proximal segment after mandibular osteotomy will shorten the elevator muscles of mastication (see Figure 7.3). This not only diminishes the mechanical advantage of these muscles, but also the immobilization of these *shortened* muscles during the period of MMF may cause more extensive irreversible changes within the muscle fibers. When the proximal segments are allowed to rotate upward and forward (see Figure 7.4), not only will there be an esthetic problem from loss of the gonial angle prominence, but also the patient may complain of an inability to masticate even soft foods. Although some strength may return with proper physiotherapy, an irreversible loss of bite force will probably be assured. When MMF is to be employed, any technique that will allow placement of the proximal segment in its preoperative position should therefore help minimize myatrophy.

Summary

It is clear that muscles (and nerves) rapidly atrophy from disuse caused by immobilization. It is thought that the earlier a patient can resume active motion of the joint following surgery, the more rapid will be the recovery of muscle function. Avoiding or decreasing the immobilization period, using electrical stimulation and, active motion, and/or exercising isometrically have been found to prevent or diminish these changes. The use of rigid internal fixation has the advantage of allowing the surgeon to place the proximal segment in any position and to securing it there reliably. Additionally, when the mandible is allowed to function throughout the period of osseous healing, there may be less myatrophy. This

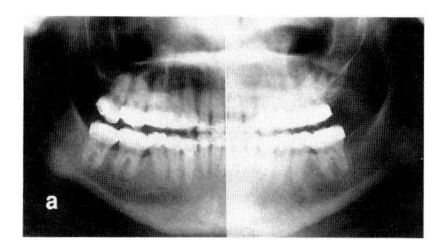

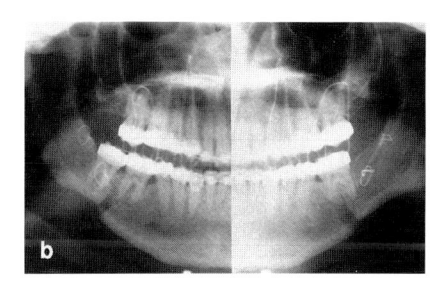

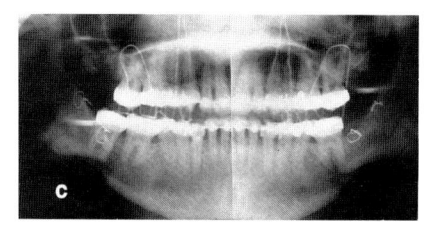

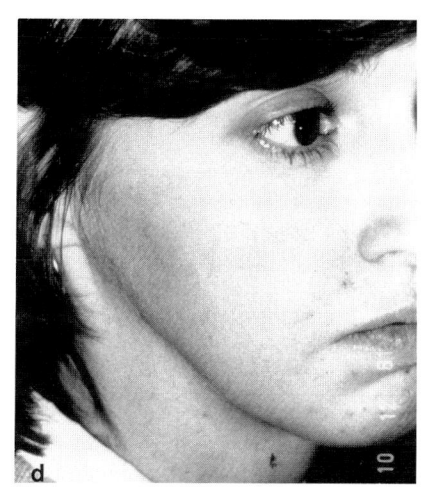

Figure 7.4 Radiographs of a patient who underwent maxillary intrusion and mandibular advancement osteotomies: (a) presurgery, (b) immediately postsurgery, and (c) following removal of MMF at eight weeks postsurgery. Note that the proximal segment was allowed to rotate up and forward during surgery, and even though wired in two locations, it continued to rotate during the period of mandibular immobilization. This resulted in poor esthetics with loss of the gonial angle prominence (d) and a dramatic loss of bite force.

should be manifest clinically as a smaller reduction in bite force. Perhaps the greatest advantage of rigid internal fixation is permitting the institution of physiotherapy earlier postsurgically than in patients who undergo MMF: Just as muscle atrophies rapidly from disuse, it can rapidly regain bulk and strength from exercise.

THE EFFECTS OF IMMOBILIZATION ON SYNOVIAL JOINTS

Orthopedists have studied extensively the intra-articular changes that take place following immobilization of synovial joints. In this section, we present the results of orthopedic immobilization studies, followed by a review of what is known about the effects of immobilization on the TMJ. However, note that there are obvious histological differences between the synovial joints (which have received greatest attention in the orthopedic literature) and the temporomandibular joint (TMJ). These differences are discussed later and should be borne in mind when relating the results of immobilization of these synovial joints to the TMJ.

Orthopedic Immobilization Studies

The knee is the most common synovial joint that has been examined by immobilization studies on animals and humans. The knee joints of rats (Evans 1960, Thaxter 1965), dogs (Ely 1933), rabbits (Finsterbush 1973, Candolin 1980), and monkeys (Ginsberg 1969) have been subjected to immobilization by plaster casts, internal splints, neurectomy, compression devices, and combinations of these. Irrespective of the method of immobilization and of whether weight bearing was permitted, the morphological alterations were strikingly similar. When a knee joint is immobilized for a period of time, a series of degenerative changes appears in the articular cartilage and the synovial membrane. The intra-articular effect of immobilization appears histologically similar to osteoarthritis.

Following immobilization, there is a progressive contracture of the capsule and pericapsular structures of the joint; this contracture increases with time (see Figure 7.5). A synovial proliferation begins, and a fibrofatty connective tissue (pannus), which encroaches on the articular surfaces of the joint, with time completely obliterates the entire intra-articular cavity. Initially, the interface between the fibrofatty tissue and articular cartilage is quite distinct, but with time this interface is replaced by mature fibrous connective tissue, which becomes confluent with the articular cartilage. The fibrofatty tissue matures and forms fibrous adhesions between opposing articular surfaces. A synovitis may or may not be apparent. When there is any compression of the articular surfaces—either by positioning or be mechanical means—a synovitis seems to be more frequent. In areas where the articular surfaces are in apposition, various changes are noted; these changes depend on the rigidity of the immobilization,

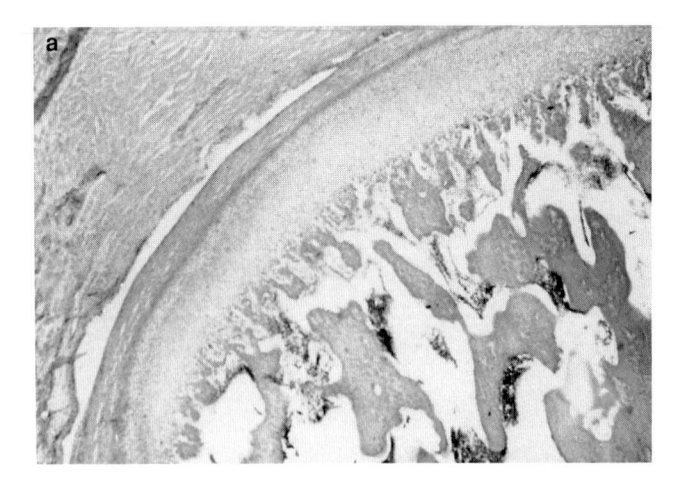

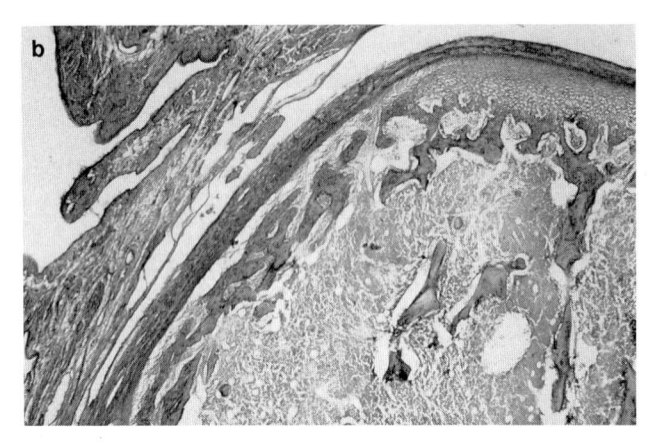

Figure 7.5 (a) Posterior–superior aspect of a normal right mandibular condyle in a juvenile rhesus monkey.
(b) Posterior–superior aspect of the right mandibular condyle following several weeks of immobilization of the mandible by MMF. Note the replacement of the condylar cartilage with sagittal bone and the thinning of the cartilage present more anteriorly.

the position of the immobilized bones, and, most importantly, the degree of compression of the articular surfaces. Mild changes consist of loss of intensity of staining of the matrix. In areas of greater compression, pressure necrosis and liquefaction of the articular cartilage, "fibrillation and cartilage erosion," and "intracartilaginous cysts" (Evans 1960; Thaxter 1965) are found. Finally, the subchondral bone may become invaded by primitive mesenchymal tissue proliferating from the marrow spaces; this will destroy and replace the deep layers of the articular cartilage (Evans 1960). The same sequence of events was also shown to occur in humans following immobilization of the knee joint (Enneking 1972) and interphalangeal joints (Field 1970).

The amount of damage produced in synovial joints by immobilization seems directly related to the duration and frequency of immobilization. Videman and co-workers (1981) found that short, repetitive periods of immobilization are just as detrimental as is a long period in rabbits. He found that either periodic or continuous immobilization for more than 30 days will lead to progressive osteoarthritis in the rabbit knee. The range of motion after periodic immobilization depends more on the total immobilization time than on the duration of either the immobilization or mobilization periods. Even an immobilization period of 4 days had a cumulative effect in producing osteoarthritis. An interval of 4 weeks between immobilization periods did not prevent immobilization from causing osteoarthritis.

Several investigators have applied compression to articular surfaces in addition to immobilization of the joints through either a forced position of the bones (such as extreme extension of the knee) or through the application of external compression apparati (Trueta 1956). Their findings indicate that the combination of compression *and* immobilization is more devastating to the health of the joint than is immobilization alone. This seems to be more true in mature animals than in immature ones. The articular cartilage undergoes progressive cell death in the area of the apposed surfaces; this results in lesions that may vary from superficial necrosis to loss of the full thickness of the articular cartilage. The articular cartilage may slough into the joint space. The extent of the lesions seems to vary with the duration of compressed immobilization.

TMJ Immobilization Studies

The effects of immobilization on the TMJ have been studied recently in rabbits (Lydiatt 1985) and in monkeys (Carlson 1980; Glineburg 1982). These studies have shown thinning of *actively growing* condylar cartilage, a disorganization of the cartilaginous layers, and even destructive changes. These effects, however, seem to be less severe than those described above for the knee joint (see Figure 7.5). No fibrofatty synovial proliferation or joint adhesions were noted in any of these TMJ studies.

Although the available TMJ studies show the ill effects of immobilization on the growing mandibular condyle, an important point regarding these studies is that the animals used were all skeletally immature—significant amounts of hyaline growth cartilage were still present. When studies are performed on growing animals, confounding factors come into play. Actively growing mandibular condylar cartilages have a richer blood supply than does an adult condylar head. How this affects the regenerative capacity of tissue damaged from immobilization is unknown. It is well known, however, that younger individuals (and tissues) have a markedly enhanced recuperative capacity over older individuals. It is not surprising, therefore, that the severity of the changes demonstrated in the TMJ studies was less than that of the knee studies. Based on the age of the animals, changes found in TMJ immobilization studies might be expected to be less disruptive than those in the knee.

MMF is performed much more frequently in individuals who are not growing than in those who are. Most of these patients have almost no appreciable condylar growth cartilage remaining and probably have a much reduced capacity for repair of articular tissue. Therefore, the results of those TMJ immobilization studies just cited may not be analogous to changes occurring when immobilization is instituted in an adult TMJ. Given these considerations, we still know very little regarding the effects of immobilization on the adult TMJ.

Nutrition of Articular Surfaces in Synovial Joints

All of the aforementioned studies, which have demonstrated changes in the articular cartilage after joint immobilization, have failed to elucidate the mechanisms by which these changes occur. Why does immobilization of a joint cause the observed degenerative changes? Most investigators have hypothesized that an interference in nutrition of the articular cartilage is responsible. The hypothesis that still prevails is that the continuous contact *and any pressure* on the articular surfaces due to immobilization prevent diffusion of nutritive materials from the synovial fluid into the areas of contacting cartilage, and that any pressure on the articular cartilage prevents diffusion of nutritive fluids through the intercellular substance of the cartilage in and around this area (see Figure 7.6) (Maroudas 1968). As a result, the chondrocytes die, the intercellular substance becomes disorganized, and, finally, both components of the articular cartilage liquefy and disappear. Most investigators feel that mobility *and exercise* allow a pumping action of synovial fluid and articular cartilage, aiding the diffusion of nutrients into the articular cartilage. Without this action, the health of the articular cartilage is jeopardized.

Repair of Articular Cartilage

Numerous orthopedic studies have evaluated the ability of articular cartilage in synovial joints of the extremities to heal following lacerative injury. Most have shown a weak and ineffectual response to such injuries, especially in mature animals (Calandruccio 1962, Campbell 1969, Meachim 1971, Fuller 1972). A better response is seen with immature animals. In injuries confined to the substance of the cartilage of adult animals (that is, not extending into the underlying bone) the response lacks an inflammatory response because the tissue is avascular. The reaction consists of an attempt on the part of the cartilage cells to repair the defect; however, they are almost never effective. The first response is a relatively intense burst of mitotic activity in the cartilage adjacent to the margins of the defect (Mankin 1962, DePalma 1966). This activity is associated with a concomitant increase in the synthesis of cartilage matrix components. By the end of the first week, however, the levels return to normal. Lacerations into the cartilage do not usually heal, and the defects may appear unaltered a year later.

In lacerations extending through the cartilage into the subchondral bone, a much different response is seen (Mankin 1962, Calandruccio 1962, Meachim 1971). Initially, the defect fills with blood derived from the subchondral vessels. With time, granulation tissue grows into the area and fibroblasts begin to organize the tissue. At the base of the lesion, bone formation begins but does not usually extend beyond the original bone–cartilage junction. The fibrous tissue with the articular defect undergoes progressive hyalinization and chondrification to produce a fibrocartilagenous mass, firmly securing the wound edges together.

It has been stated that one cannot expect much healing by the deposition of *hyaline* cartilage in articular defects that extend into subchondral bone (full-thickness defects). A recent investigation in adolescent and adult rabbits by Salter (1980), however, has shown that articular cartilage has the *capacity* to heal full-thickness defects by formation of hyaline cartilage. Defects extending through the articular cartilage and subchondral bone of the rabbit knee joints were created in three groups of rabbits (both adult and juveniles were

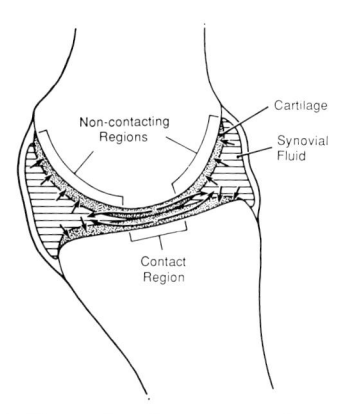

Figure 7.6 This illustration demonstrates how normal joint motion helps "pump" nutrients from the synovial fluid into the articular cartilage. Where the articular surfaces are in contact, extracellular fluid is "squeezed" out of the cartilage. In those areas where the cartilage is not in contact, synovial fluid is drawn into the cartilage. With joint motion, different regions of the cartilage alternate between contact and loss of contact, "pumping" synovial fluid into the cartilage. When a joint is immobilized, the same areas of cartilage stay in perpetual contact, which inhibits the diffusion of nutrients from the synovial fluid into these contacting areas. The cartilage undergoes degenerative changes as a result of lack of nutrition from the synovial fluid.

in each group). In one group, each animal's leg was immobilized; in another group, each animal's leg was not immobilized, and the animals were allowed to use the legs for normal activities. In the third group, each animal's leg was constantly moved in a physiological range of motion by an apparatus while healing progressed. The results showed that this "continued passive motion" allowed healing with hyaline articular cartilage in a significant number of defects (approximately 50%). The defects treated with immobilization showed very poor results, with adhesions and fibrous connective tissue filling the intra-articular space. The animals allowed to use the leg for normal activities showed better results than those who were immobilized; however, the results were significantly poorer than those legs placed into continuous passive motion.

A review of the literature shows a striking paucity of information concerning the capacity of the mandibular condyle to repair either surgically created or traumatically induced defects of the articular surface. Hochman and Laskin (1965) published a paper that directly explored this question. Using skeletally immature rabbits, full-thickness incisions were created in the articular tissue of the mandibular condyle and examined histologically at various post-injury periods. The results showed that defects in the skeletally immature articular surface can undergo complete repair in 12 weeks. Some of the repair came from cells that were derived from the subchondral bone; however, proliferation of the prechondroblastic cells within the articular cartilage contributed greatly to the repair process.

Another study, designed to evaluate the effect of microtraumatic injury on the TMJ, was reported by Misawa and colleagues (1985). Using 12 adult monkeys, a #700 fissure bur under sterile coolant was used to score the lateral (nonarticulating) surface of the mandibular condyle. They found that this defect healed in a manner similar to any bony wound. After initial replacement of the blood clot with fibrous tissue, new bone formed along the margin of the drill hole, beginning at two weeks. Later remodeling resulted in a fibrous—not fibrocartilagenous—covering to the condylar surface. Poswillo (1970) showed similar findings after performing high condylectomies in skeletally mature monkeys.

The results of these studies may indicate that the skeletally immature TMJ can repair articular defects in an excellent manner using cells derived from both the subchondral bone and the prechondroblastic layer of cartilage. When skeletally mature, however, little cartilage is present in the mandibular condyle, and therefore no prechondroblastic cells are available to aid in the reparative/regenerative process. This may be the reason the studies by Misawa and colleagues (1985) and Poswillo (1970) showed a bony/fibrous healing process. In these studies, the animals were skeletally mature, and at maturity the condylar surface is generally a bony cap with a fibrous covering. Of interest is the fact that the animals in each of these experiments were permitted the active use of their TMJs following injury. On the basis of Salter's work (1980), this is thought to assist the reparative process. One can only speculate on the changes that may have occurred had the TMJs been immobilized following injury.

Implications for Maxillofacial Surgery

Without histological studies on the *adult* TMJ, it is difficult to know how this joint reacts to immobilization. However, if any parallels between the TMJ and the synovial joints of the extremities can be drawn, one can clearly see from the above reviews that immobilization interferes with the nutrition of the articular tissues. Whether this will adversely affect the structure and function of the adult TMJ is unknown. We also do not know whether traumatic lesions on the articular surfaces of the TMJ occur during surgery around the mouth. It is conceivable, however, that microfractures of the condylar head appear during the manipulations associated with mandibular osteotomies. Similarly, following traumatically induced fractures of the mandible, small fractures through the articular surface of the condylar head not visible on radiographs probably occur more frequently than one might think. If these patients are immobilized, there is a chance that intra-articular adhesions will form, the functional implications of which are unknown. If these patients are allowed to function, however, the joint may be much more able to deal satisfactorily with any defect present.

EFFECT OF IMMOBILIZATION ON PERIARTICULAR CONNECTIVE TISSUES

Periarticular connective tissues* connect the bones and add structural support to them. Although their gross size and shape vary considerably, all periarticular connective tissues share a remarkably simple and similar structure consisting of a woven mesh of collagen fibers bunched together into parallel arrays along the principle axis of the ligament or fascia. The bundles are further arranged into meshed layers for added strength. The cells responsible for synthesis and maintenance of these connective tissues are spindle-shaped fibroblasts. These cells reside in an extremely hypovascular envi-

---

*The periarticular connective tissues consist of all those connective tissue elements which comprise the structural and functional framework of a joint and mobility about that joint, with the exception of the bone and articular cartilage as these were defined in the previous section. Included in this definition are the joint and muscular ligaments and tendons, the joint capsule, surrounding fascia, aconnective tissue within the muscle (that is, endo-, peri- and epimysium), periosteum, and Sharpey's fibers inserting into the osseous tissues.

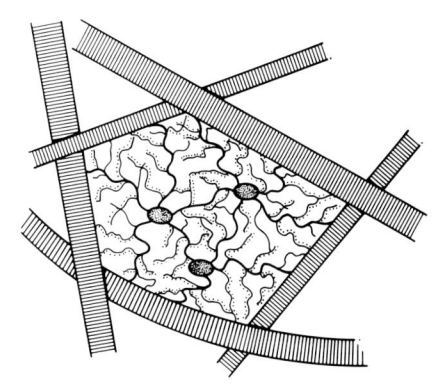

Figure 7.7 Illustration showing the intricate interaction between proteoglycan (center) and collagen fibers. The proteoglycan gives structural support to the collagen fibers, separates them, serves as a lubricant between them, and permits smooth motion of the fibers past one another.

ronment within the connective tissue and rely on diffusion of nutrients from distant capillaries to meet their minute-by-minute metabolic needs.

The composition of these tissues is a simple mixture, which consists of 20% cellular material and 80% extracellular material by volume (Amiel 1984). By far the largest component is water, which makes up 70% of the total structure. The remaining 30% is organic solids, of which 80% is collagen, 18% is proteoglycan, and 2% is noncollagen protein, elastin, and minerals.

Collagen is the predominant tensile-resistant protein in these tissues. Proteoglycans act as a cementlike substance, filling in between the collagen microfibril struts (Comper 1978) (see Figure 7.7). The name *proteoglycan* reflects their structure, in that they are part protein and part *glycan* or sugars of large molecular weights. Their importance far outweighs their minority status in composition. Primarily, proteoglycans bind most of the extracellular water of the connective tissue, making the matrix a highly structured gel-like material rather than an amorphous solution. Second, as the cementing substance, they contribute to the overall strength of the composite connective tissue.

The structure of proteoglycans consists of sulfated polysaccharide chains called glycosaminoglycans, which are bonded to a core protein forming the basic proteoglycan (see Figure 7.8). These individual proteoglycan units bind to a long hyaluronic acid chain to form the proteoglycan aggregates, which are of extremely large molecular weight. Together, the water and proteoglycan create a gel-like material, which acts as a lubricant and spacing buffer system between the collagen fibers (see Figure 7.9a). The water and proteoglycan impart very important viscoelastic properties to the composite.

Various studies have shown that the physical properties and composition of ligaments and periarticular connective tissues change with activity, adapting to the functional demands placed on them (Noyes 1974,

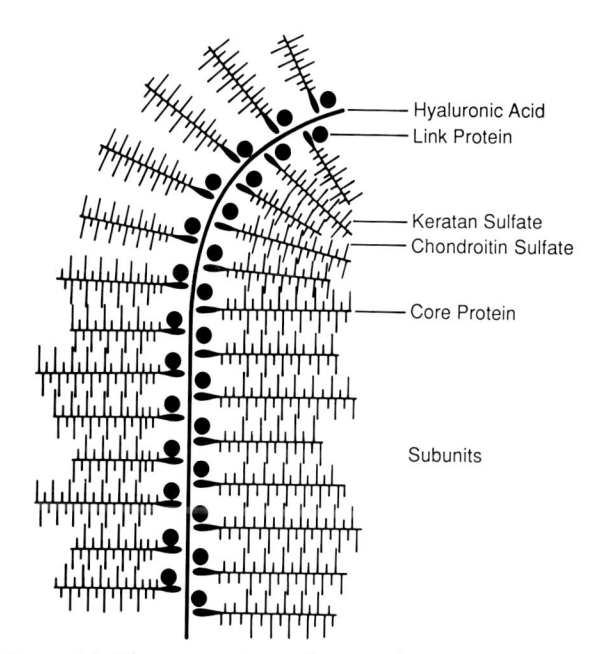

Figure 7.8 The composition of a typical macromolecule of proteoglycan. Most of the glycosaminoglycans composing this molecule are highly negatively charged, binding a considerable amount of extracellular water, which imparts very important viscoelastic properties to these tissues.

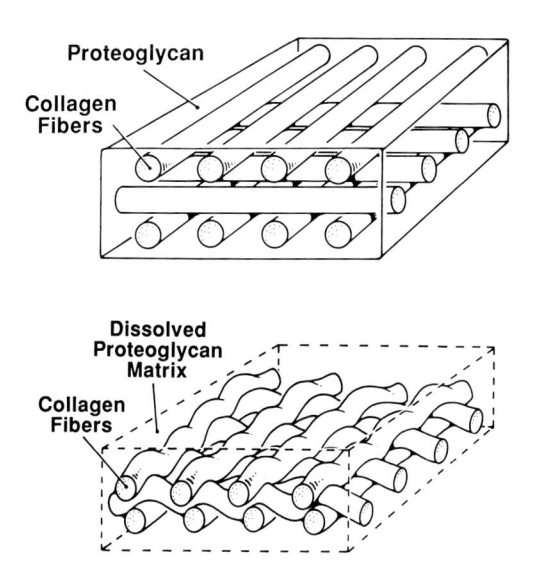

Figure 7.9 (a) This illustration shows how proteoglycan separates the collagen fibers in a healthy state. (b) With immobilization, proteoglycan and extracellular water are depleted. This disrupts the normal separating and lubricating activity of proteoglycans. The collagen fibers thus lose their interfiber support and become closely apposed. This apposition, along with a stationary attitude due to immobilization, allows aberrant cross-linkages between adjacent collagen fibers.

1977). It has been demonstrated, for instance, that inactivity in dogs as a result of cage confinement results in premature failure of certain ligaments in the leg (Laros 1971). A study by Woo (1975) showed significant decreases in range of motion of the knee joint of rabbits from immobilization of the hind leg. Noyes (1974), in an extensive study on adult rhesus monkeys, showed that eight weeks of immobilization of one leg caused a statistically significant decrease in strength of the anterior cruciate ligament on the immobilized side. It took 12 months of normal activity following the eight weeks of immobilization before the ultimate strength of the ligament returned. These effects are presumably due to disuse changes within the tendons or at the tendon–bone interfaces in the confined or immobilized animals.

Biochemical investigations have shed light on the nature of the changes within the extracellular elements of the connective tissues. Because both elements of the structure of connective tissue (collagen and proteoglycan) are affected by stress deprivation, it is useful to divide a discussion of this subject between the effects of immobilization on (1) collagen, and (2) proteoglycans (glycosaminoglycans).

Collagen

Studies have shown that the biochemical composition of collagen changes when synovial joints are immobilized (Akeson 1977, Amiel 1982). These investigations have found alterations in collagen crosslinking, an increase in concentration of some of the precursors of collagen with no change in collagen type (Amiel 1980), and no change in collagen mass (Akeson 1968, 1973). The aberrant cross-links between adjacent collagen fibers during immobilization create an effective "shortening" of the tendon or fascia if the tendon was immobilized in a shortened position (see Figures 7.10 and 7.11). This makes it difficult to regain normal range of motion following a period of immobilization.

Proteoglycans

Extracellular Fluid Volume Changes

The water content of fibrous connective tissues is in the range of 65% to 70%. The population of cells is relatively sparse in this tissue, so the majority of this water is within the extracellular space. Water content of fibrous tissue decreases to a statistically significant degree with immobilization (Akeson 1961, Akeson 1973, 1980). It appears that this amount of water loss is functionally significant. Fluid movement, which plays such an important role in articular cartilage load bearing and lubrication, is probably equally important in performing this role in fibrous connective tissue. It has recently been established that hyaluronic acid and its attracted or entrapped water is the principal lubricant of fibrous connective tissue (Swann 1974).

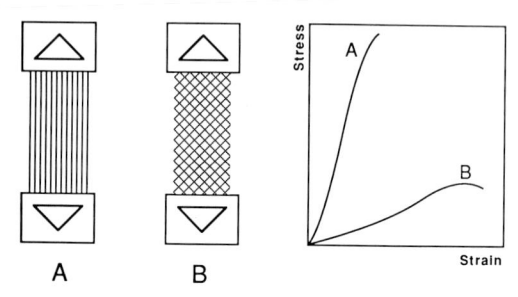

Figure 7.10 This illustration demonstrates how the physical arrangement of collagen fibers can alter the characteristics of the tissue. On the left (a), the fibers are oriented in a parallel manner. When the tissue is stretched (as indicated by the boxed arrows), the intramolecular bonds must be broken to provide any laxity. Thus, it takes large amounts of stress to provide any strain (right). Most collagen fibers in the body are arranged in alternating waves, or at angles to one another (b). When stretching occurs, the first thing that happens is rearrangement of the collagen fibers to a more parallel attitude. Thus, much strain is provided without the breaking of intramolecular bonds.

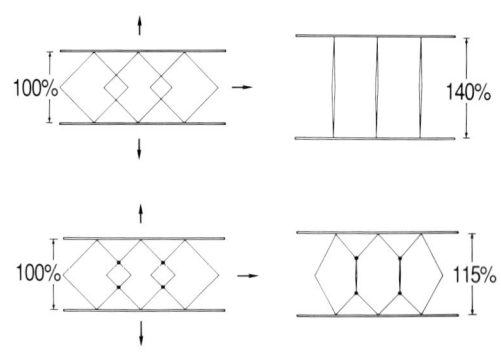

Figure 7.11 This illustration demonstrates the effect of intermolecular cross-links between adjacent collagen fibers on connective tissue mobility. (above) When fibers are oriented at angles to one another, mobility is readily provided by a reorientation into a more parallel arrangement. (below) When cross-linking of adjacent fibers occurs at the small black nodes, less mobility is allowed in the tissue due to the mechanism demonstrated. Adapted with permission from *Biorheology* 17:95–110. WH Akeson, D Amiel, and S Woo, Immobility effects on synovial joints: The pathomechanics of joint contracture. © 1980, Pergamon Press plc.

Glycosaminoglycan Changes

The largest change found in the composition of stress-deprived periarticular connective tissue is reduction in the concentration of glycosaminoglycans (Akeson 1967, 1973, 1980, Amiel 1982). A significant decrease in several of the component materials of glycosaminoglycans (Chondroitin-4 and -6 sulfate, hyaluronic acid) are noted with joint immobilization. Decreased concentrations of glycosaminoglycans and water can be expected to alter the plasticity and pliability of connective tissue matrices, and to reduce lubrication efficiency. It is presumed that the lubricating and volume-separating effects provided by hyaluronic acid and water permit the independent gliding of collagen microfibrils past one another, facilitating the tissue's adaptation to motion permitted by the particular connective tissue's weave pattern (see Figure 7.9a). Loss of this separating and lubricating property provides for collagen fibril–fibril friction as well as the potential for adhesions or cross-linking between adjacent collagen fibrils (see Figure 7.9b). Any newly synthesized collagen is apt to be randomly dispersed and to create interference with the functional gliding between fibers necessary for normal mobility.

Overview

The above studies can be synthesized to form an overall picture of connective tissue homeostasis. Physical forces of normal stress and motion modulate synthesis of proteoglycans and collagen in normal joints by fibroblasts. The proteoglycans—which loosely bind and entrap water, creating a "gel"—lubricate the connective tissue–fiber interface and minimize the number of anomalous cross-linkings of collagen fibers by maintaining a critical interfiber distance. Flexibility is preserved, the joint moves easily, and the applied physical forces further stimulate cellular synthesis. At the same time, stress and motion influence the deposition of *newly* synthesized collagen fibers in such a manner as to resist tensile stresses while preserving joint motion. Furthermore, motion of collagen fibers precludes the development of anomalous cross-links, the formation of which requires a stationary attitude over a period of time.

If a joint is immobilized, loss of connective tissue, water, and proteoglycan allows collagen fibers to become more closely apposed. The combination of this approximation and the immobility allows the development of anomalous interfiber cross-links. These cross-links inhibit joint mobility by the mechanism shown in Figure 7.11. To make matters much worse, *newly* synthesized collagen is laid down in a haphazard manner due to lack of functional stimulation from normal joint use. Many of these fibers will be laid down in a manner that will not be conducive to joint mobility. The net effect of these processes is *joint stiffness*.

Implications for Maxillofacial Surgery

To understand the nature of these changes as they apply to orthognathic surgery, it helps to consider a common orthognathic surgical procedure as an example. Recent investigations have found decreases in range of mandibular motion after mandibular sagittal advancement osteotomy (Aragon 1984, Storum 1984, 1986). If we consider this osteotomy, those technical aspects of this procedure that are potentially detrimental to range of mandibular motion can be examined in light of the information just presented.

An incision is made through oral mucosa, submucosa, buccinator muscle, buccopharyngeal fascia, and periosteum to gain access to the mandibular ramus and posterior body area. Several muscles of mastication are stripped from their bony insertions to some extent during this procedure, and subperiosteal dissection is necessary to expose the mandible for the surgical cuts.

The importance of these procedures becomes obvious when one understands the biological processes of the healing process. With the exception of epithelium, an incision in all soft tissues in the body heals, not with native tissues (such as muscle, salivary glands, and so on), but instead by deposition of fibrous connective tissue (that is, scar). During the normal sequence of wound repair, fibroblasts produce collagen and proteoglycan to give structural integrity to the disrupted tissue. An overabundance of collagen is usually deposited to provide the necessary strength to the healing wound. Because the deposition of collagen is normally regulated by functional stresses placed on it, immobilization of the mandible by MMF during this healing period allows the *newly* synthesized collagen to be laid down in a haphazard manner. Many of these collagen fibers will inevitably be oriented in a manner antagonistic to future mobility of the mandible. When allowed to mature over the six- to eight-week immobilization period, the mandible contracts and stiffens from continued cross-linking of the collagen molecules (both newly synthesized and that present in periarticular connective tissues preoperatively), further restricting mandibular mobility. When the mandible is remobilized and functional movements commence, the collagen deposited during the healing phase and that formerly present—which now may contain numerous cross-links—will begin the long process of functional remodeling. If one considers the time it takes a surgical scar on the skin surface of the body to soften, one gets a feel for the enormous problem established by the healing process in the immobilized mandible.

A recent investigation in our laboratory (Ellis 1988) tested the presumption that mandibular range of motion will be better following advancement using rigid internal fixation, than it is following advancement using MMF. Seventeen adult rhesus monkeys who underwent sagittal advancement osteotomy were placed in either MMF ($n = 6$) or rigid internal fixation *without* MMF ($n = 11$). Range of mandibular motion, using forced gape, was calculated preoperatively and at weekly intervals postoperatively for 12 weeks. The results showed that animals who underwent rigid internal fixation maintained a greater range of motion in the early postsurgery period and obtained preoperative mobility by 12 weeks postsurgery (see Figure 7.12). At each period of time post surgery, the animals who underwent 6 weeks of MMF showed statistically significant decreases in range of motion when compared to the group

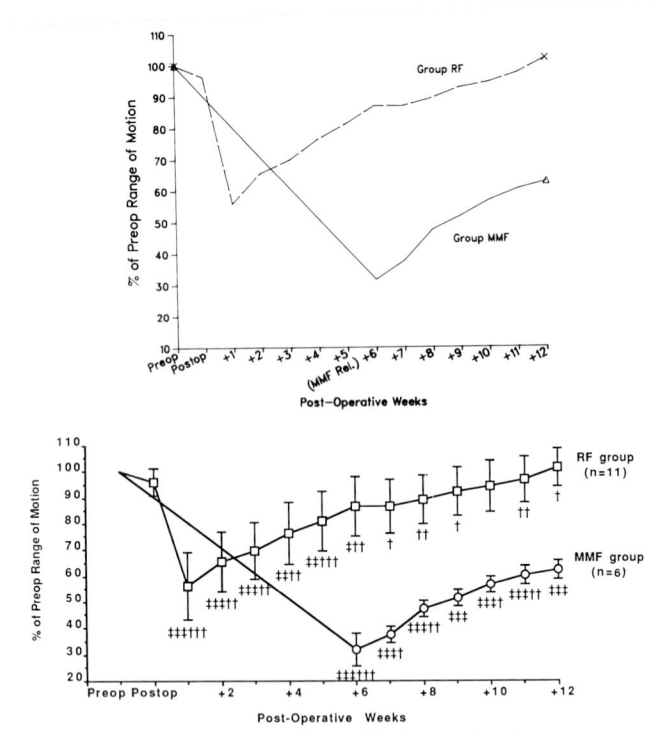

Figure 7.12 Mean range of mandibular motion in two groups of adult rhesus monkeys who underwent mandibular advancement. Group MMF ($n = 6$) underwent six weeks of maxillomandibular fixation. Group RF ($n = 11$) underwent rigid internal fixation without mandibular immobilization. Note the significant difference in mandibular mobility between the groups at all time periods. [Error bars indicate ± 2 SE. † = significant difference from one time period to the next († = 0.05, †† = 0.01, ††† = 0.001 level of confidence). ‡ = significant difference from preoperative value (‡ = 0.05, ‡‡ = 0.01, ‡‡‡ = 0.001 level of confidence).]

who underwent rigid fixation. They also had significant reductions from preoperative values at 12 weeks postsurgery. This study supports the hypothesis that if the mandible is not *immobilized* during the healing process, newly synthesized collagen will be laid down in a manner that will promote functional movements of the mandible. Therefore, the initial wound-healing process will not inhibit joint motion to the point it would when the mandible is immobilized. Further, with the ability of the mandible to function, postoperative physiotherapy can be instituted at a much earlier time, thereby hastening the remodeling process of the connective tissue.

The effects of immobilization on the periarticular connective tissues are perhaps more detrimental to mandibular mobility than to any tissue type yet discussed. The reason for this is that the connective tissues are relatively hypocellular and hypovascular. This is why they appear "white" on gross examination. Because of the hypocellularity, the poor blood supply, and the extracellular nature of most of the products composing these tissues, the periarticular connective tissues adapt very slowly to changes in functional demands. For instance, when functional stimulation changes in either quantity or quality, the fibroblasts must both break down the connective tissues that do not meet these new demands, and produce new connective tissues that do. Both of these processes are performed inefficiently (in comparison to a tissue like muscle) due to the extracellular nature of the components of the connective tissues.

SUMMARY

It is clear from this review that mandibular immobilization is not as benign a procedure as once thought. Detrimental effects on several tissues within the masticatory apparatus have been observed following mandibular immobilization. Atrophy of the muscles of mastication, degenerative changes within the mandibular condyle, and decreases in range of passive bite opening are all consistent findings following several weeks of mandibular immobilization. The use of fixation procedures that avoid the use of mandibular immobilization (that is, rigid internal fixation) has been shown to minimize these problems. As with any procedure, however, the risks and benefits of rigid internal fixation must be weighed against the time-honored standard (that is, MMF). Future research and clinical experience will direct the surgeon to select whichever technique is in the best interest of the patient.

REFERENCES

Akeson WH: An experimental study of joint stiffness. J Bone Joint Surg 43-A:1022, 1961.

Akeson WH, Amiel D, La Violette D: The connective tissue response to immobility: An accelerated aging responses? Exp Gerontol 3:289–301, 1968.

Akeson WH, Amiel D, La Violette D: The connective tissue response to immobility. A study of chondroitin 4 and 6 sulfate and dermatan sulfate changes in periarticular connective tissue of control and immobilized knees of dogs. Clin Orthop 51:183–197, 1967.

Akeson WH, Woo S, Amiel D, et al: The connective tissue response to immobility: Biochemical changes in periarticular connective tissue of the immobilized rabbit knee. Clin Orthop 93:356–362, 1973.

Akeson WH, Amiel D, Mechanic GL, et al: Collagen cross-linking alterations in joint contractures: Changes in the reducible cross-links in periarticular connective tissue collagen after nine weeks of immobilization. Conn Tiss Res 5:15, 1977.

Akeson WH, Amiel D, Woo S: Immobility effects on synovial joints. The pathomechanics of joint contracture. Biorheol 17:95–110, 1980.

Allbrook D: Skeletal muscle regeneration. Muscle and Nerve 4:234, 1981.

Amiel D, Akeson WH, Harwood FL, et al: Effect of nine weeks of immobilization of the types of collagen synthesized in periarticular connective tissue

from rabbit knees. Trans Orthop Res Soc 5:1, 1980.
Amiel D, Savio LW, Harwood FL, et al: The effect of immobilization on collagen turnover in connective tissue: A biochemical-biomechanical correlation. Acta Ortho Scand 53:325–332, 1982.
Amiel D, Frank C, Harwood FL, et al: Tendons and ligaments. A morphological and biochemical comparison. J Orthop Res 1:257, 1984.
Aragon SB, Van Sickels JE, Dolwick MF, et al: The effects of orthognathic surgery on mandibular range of motion. J Oral Maxillofac Surg 43:938–943, 1985.
Boyes G, Johnston I: Muscle fibre composition of rat vastus intermedius following immobilization at different muscle lengths. Pflügers Arch 381:195–200, 1979.
Burkhart JM, Jowsey J: Parathyroid and thyroid hormones in the development of immobilization osteoporosis. Endocrinology 81:1053–1062, 1967.
Calandruccio RA, Gilmer WS: Proliferation, regeneration, and repair of articular cartilage of immature animals. J Bone Joint Surg 44-A:431–455, 1962.
Campbell CJ: The healing of cartilage defects. Clin Orthop 64:45–63, 1969.
Candolin T, Videman T: Surface changes in the articular cartilage of rabbit knee during immobilization. A scanning electron microscopic study of experimental osteoarthritis. Acta Pathol Microbiol Immunol Scand 88:291–297, 1980.
Cardenas DD, Stolow WC, Hardy R: Muscle fiber number in immobilization atrophy. Arch Phys Med Rehab 58:423–426, 1977.
Carlson DS, McNamara JA, Graber LW, et al: Experimental studies of growth and adaptation of TMJ. In Current Advances in Oral Surgery, Vol. III. Irby WB (ed), St. Louis, Mosby, 1980.
Comper WD, Laurent TC: Physiological function of connective tissue polysaccharide. Physiol Rev 58:255, 1978.
Dechow PC, Carlson DS: A method of bite force measurement in primates. J Biomech 16:797, 1979.
Dechow PC, Carlson DS: Occlusal force after mandibular advancement in adult rhesus monkeys. J Oral Maxillofac Surg 44:887, 1986.
DePalma AF, McKeever CD, Subin DK: Process of repair of articular cartilage demonstrated by histology and autoradiography with tritiated thymidine. Clin Orthop 48:229–242, 1966.
Edgerton VR, Barnard RJ, Peter JB, et al: Properties of immobilized hind-limb muscles of the Galago senegalensis. Exp Neurol 46:115–131, 1975.
Ellis E: Mobility of the mandible following advancement using maxillomandibular fixation and rigid internal fixation—An experimental investigation in *Macaca mulatta*. J Oral Maxillofac Surg 46:118, 1988.
Ellis E, Dechow PC, Carlson DS: A comparison of stimulated bite force after mandibular advancement using rigid and non-rigid fixation. J Oral Maxillofac Surg 46:26, 1988.
Ely LW, Mensor MC: Studies on the immobilization of the normal joints. Surg Gynecol Obstr 57:212–215, 1933.
Enneking WF, Horowitz M: The intra-articular effects of immobilization on the human knee. J Bone Joint Surg 54-A:973–985, 1972.
Eriksson E, Haggmark T: A comparison of isometric muscle training and electrical stimulation in the recovery after knee ligament surgery. Am J Sports Med 7:48–56, 1979.
Evans EB, Eggers GWN, Butler JK, et al: Experimental immobilization and remobilization of rat knee joints. J Bone Joint Surg 42-A:737–758, 1960.
Field PL, Hueston JT: Articular cartilage loss in long-standing immobilization of interphalangeal joints. J Plast Surg 23:186–191, 1970.
Finsterbush A, Friedman B: Early changes in immobilized rabbits knee joints: A light and electron microscopic study. Clin Orthop 92:305–319, 1973.
Fischbach GD, Robbins N: Changes in contractile properties of disused soleus muscles. J Physiol London 201:305–320, 1969.
Fuller JA, Ghadialy FN: Ultrastructural observations on surgically produced full-thickness defects in articular cartilage. Clin Orthop 86:193–205, 1972.
Geiser M, Trueta J: Muscle action, bone rarefaction and bone formation. An experimental study. J Bone Joint Surg 40-B:282–311, 1958.
Ginsberg JM, Eyring EJ, Curtiss PH: Continuous compression of rabbit articular cartilage producing loss of hydroxyproline before loss of hexosamine. J Bone Joint Surg 51-A:467–474, 1969.
Glineburg RW, Laskin DM, Blaustein DI: The effects of immobilization on the primate temporomandibular joint: A histological and histochemical study. J Oral Maxillofac Surg 40:3–8, 1982.
Goldspink G: Postembryonic growth and differentiation of striated muscle. In The Structure and Function of Muscle, Vol I, Bourne GH (ed), Academic Press, New York, 2nd ed., 1972.
Gould N, Donnermeyer D, Gammon GG, et al: Transcutaneous muscle stimulation to retard disuse atrophy after open meniscectomy. Clin Orthop 178:190–197, 1983.
Haggmark T, Eriksson E: Hypotrophy of the soleus muscle in man after achilles tendon rupture: Discussion of findings by computed tomography and morphological studies. Am J Sports Med 7:121–126, 1979.
Helander E: One quantitative muscle protein determination. Acta Physiol Scand [41-Suppl]:141, 1957.
Herbison GJ, Jaweed MM, Ditunno JF: Muscle atrophy in rats following denervation, casting, inflammation and tenotomy. Arch Phys Med Rehab 60:401–404, 1979.

Hochman LS, Laskin DM: Repair of surgical defects in the articular surface of the rabbit mandibular condyle. Oral Surg 19:534–542, 1965.

Jokl P, Konstadt S: The effect of limb immobilization on muscle function and protein composition. Clin Orthop 174:222–229, 1983.

Klein L, Player JS, Heiple KG, et al: Isotopic evidence for resorption of soft tissues and bone in immobilized dogs. J Bone Joint Surg 64-A:225–230, 1982.

Laros GS, Tipton CM, Cooper RR: Influence of physical activity on ligament insertions in the knees of dogs. J Bone Joint Surg 53-A:275, 1971.

Lindboe CF, Platou CS: Disuse atrophy of human skeletal muscle. An enzyme histochemical study. Acta Neuropathol [Berl] 56:241–244, 1982.

Lydiatt DD, Davis LF: The effects of immobilization on the rabbit temporomandibular joint. J Oral Maxillofac Surg 43:188–193, 1985.

Mankin HJ: Localization of tritiated thymidine in articular cartilage of rabbits. II. Repair in immature cartilage. J Bone Joint Surg 44-A:688–698, 1962.

Maroudas A, Bullough P, Swanson SAV, et al: The permeability of articular cartilage. J Bone Joint Surg 50-B:166–177, 1968.

Maxwell LC, Carlson DS, McNamara JA, et al: Histochemical characteristics of the masseter and temporalis muscles of the rhesus monkey *Macaca mulatta*. Anat Rec 193:389–401, 1979.

Mayo KH, Ellis E, Carlson DS: Histochemical characteristics of masseter and temporalis muscles after 5 weeks of maxillomandibular fixation: An investigation in *Macaca mulatta*. Oral Surg 66:421, 1988.

Mayo KH, Ellis E, Carlson DS: Histochemical analysis of the masseter and temporalis muscle 12 weeks after mandibular advancement using rigid and nonrigid fixation. J Oral Maxillofac Surg 48:381–384, 1990.

Meachim G, Roberts C: Repair of the joint surface from subarticular tissue in the rabbit knee. J Anat 109:317–327, 1971.

Misawa T, Ohnishi M, Kino K, et al: Experimental study on microtraumatic injury to the temporomandibular joint. In Oral and Maxillofacial Surgery: Proceedings from the 8th International Conference on Oral and Maxillofacial Surgery, Hjørting-Hansen E (ed.), Chicago, Quintessence, 1985, 236–238.

Muller EA: Influence of training and of inactivity on muscle strength. Arch Phys Med Rehab 51:449, 1970.

Noyes FR: Functional properties of knee ligaments and alterations induced by immobilization. A correlative biomechanical and histological study in primates. Clin Orthop 123:210–242, 1977.

Noyes FR, Delucas JL, Hyde WB, et al: Biomechanics of ligament failure. II. An analysis of immobilization, exercise, and reconditioning effects in primates. J Bone Joint Surg 56-A:1406, 1974.

Poswillo D: Experimental investigation of the effects of intra-articular hydrocortisone and high condylectomy on the mandibular condyle. Oral Surg 30:161, 1970.

Salmons S, Hendricksson J: The adaptive response of skeletal muscles to increased use. Muscle and Nerve 4:94, 1981.

Salter RB, Simmonds DF, Malcolm BW, et al: The biological effects of continuous passive motion on the healing of full-thickness defects in articular cartilage: an experimental investigation in the rabbit. J Bone Joint Surg 62:1232–1251, 1980.

Sargeant AJ, Davies CTM: The effect of disuse muscular atrophy on the forces generated in dynamic exercise. Clin Sci Mol Med 53:183–188, 1977.

Sherman WM, Plyley MJ, Pearson DR, et al: Isokinetic rehabilitation following meniscectomy: A comparison of two methods of training describing strength changes during and following release from rehabilitation. Am J Sports Med 10:155–161, 1983.

Storum KA, Bell WH: Hypomobility after maxillary and mandibular osteotomies. Oral Surg 57:7–12, 1984.

Storum KA, Bell WH: The effect of physical rehabilitation on mandibular function after ramus osteotomies. J Oral Maxillofac Surg 44:94–99, 1986.

Sundén G: Some aspects of longitudinal bone growth. An experimental study of the rabbit tibia. Acta Orthop Scand Suppl 103, 1967.

Swann DA, Radin EL, Nazimiec M: Role of hyaluronic acid in joint lubrication. Ann Rheum Dis 33:318, 1974.

Thaxter TH, Mann RA, Anderson CE: Degeneration of immobilized knee joints in rats. Histological and autoradiographic study. J Bone Joint Surg 47-A:567–585, 1965.

Trueta J: Osteo-arthritis: An approach to surgical treatment. Lancet 1:585–589, 1956.

Videman T, Eronen I, Friman C: Glycosaminoglycan metabolism in experimental osteoarthritis caused by immobilization. Acta Orthop Scand 52:11–21, 1981.

Wells JB: Functional integrity of rat muscle after isometric immobilization. Exp Neurol 24:514, 1969.

Witzman FA, Kim DH, Fitts RH: Recovery time course in contractile function of fast and slow skeletal muscle after hindlimb immobilization. J Appl Physiol 52:677, 1982.

Wolf E, Magora A, Gonen B: Disuse atrophy of the quadriceps muscle. Electromyography 11:479–490, 1971.

Woo SLY, Matthews JV, Akeson WH, et al: Connective tissue response to immobilization. Correlation study of biomechanical and biochemical measurements of normal and immobilized rabbit knees. Arthritis Rheum 18:257, 1975.

PART II

Implant Systems for Rigid Fixation of the Craniomaxillofacial Skeleton

CHAPTER 8

Specifications, Indications, and Clinical Applications of the Luhr Vitallium Maxillofacial Systems

Hans G. Luhr

INTRODUCTION AND HISTORY OF RIGID FIXATION

Simple bone plates have been in use for a century, since the Hamburg surgeon Hansmann (1886) and the British surgeon Sir William A. Lane (1893) published their ideas on rigid fixation of long-bone fractures using plates and bone screws (see Figure 8.1). Nevertheless, only during the past 25 years has their use been widened to include every aspect of skeletal surgery. In maxillofacial surgery, the interest in rigid fixation began with the treatment of fractures of the edentulous mandible. Fractures located in dentulous mandibular segments were easier to manage; they could be treated with dental splints and MMF. Unfortunately, the patient had to undergo four to five weeks of discomfort and exclusion from most professional activities and social events.

However, management of fractures of the edentulous or partly edentulous mandible using conservative treatment procedures was even less satisfactory: Realignment of the fracture ends was difficult and often resulted in poor reduction; immobilization of the mandible might require complex intraoral or extraoral appliances (for example, gunning splints, monoblocs, plaster of Paris head caps combined with chin caps; see Figure 8.2), which were uncomfortable for long-term use. Furthermore, the poor reduction and relative instability often extended the healing period to six or seven weeks. Most of the surgical fixation methods used in maxillofacial surgery (for example, interosseous wiring) were unstable clinically, leading to the use of additional MMF. Investigations into the properties of wire connections confirmed this clinical experience.

Simple bone plates were not generally accepted because of the high rate of complications, that is, delayed healing or nonunion and osteomyelitis. Outcomes were unsatisfactory, for example, when adaptation of the fragments was less than ideal and screws were inserted slightly off center. This may cause distraction of the fracture ends, enlarging the fracture gap and significantly decreasing the primary stability. These conditions are unfavorable for fast and safe bone healing. Some authors attempted to reduce these problems by using additional MMF with use of plates and screws, but many surgeons did not favor such a solution. Furthermore, despite antibiotic prophylaxis there was a high rate of infection. Thus, for many years, most surgeons strongly resisted using any procedures involving bone screws or plates.

The two keys to fast and economic bone healing are optimal reduction of the fracture ends and maxi-

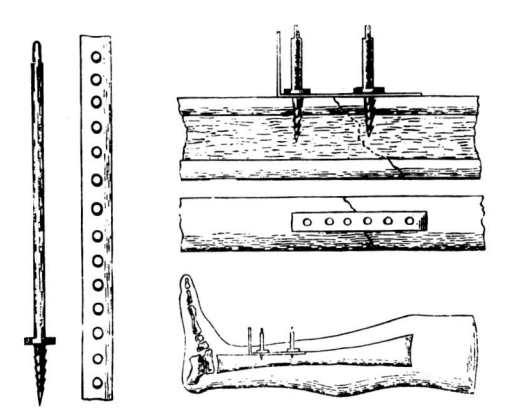

Figure 8.1 The first use of plates and screws in fractures of the long bones (Hansmann 1886).

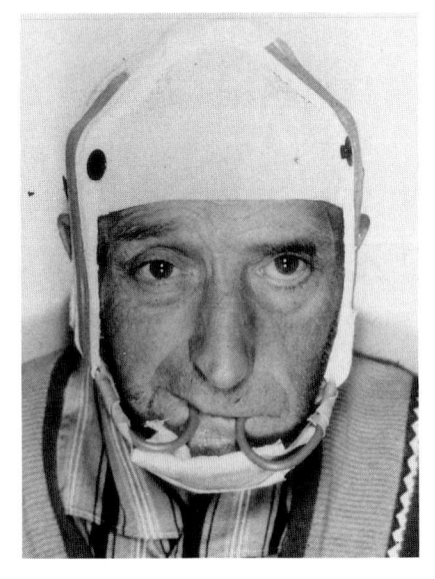

Figure 8.2 Fractures of the edentulous mandible. The immobilization of the mandible required intraoral gunning splints connected by intra/extraoral bars to a head cap. A chin cap was also required.

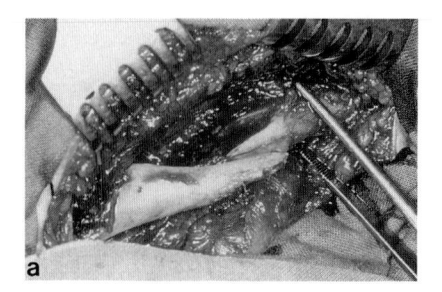

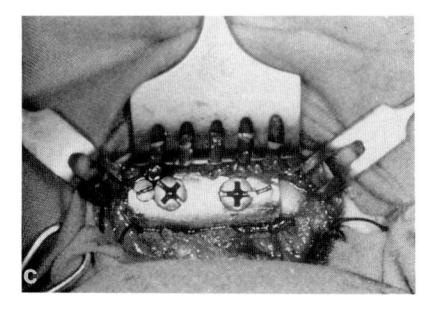

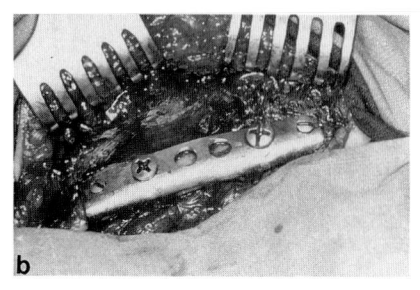

Figure 8.4 The first compression osteosynthesis, performed in maxillofacial surgery in 1967. (a) Exposure of the fracture of the edentulous mandible. (b) Rigid fixation was performed by a long mandibular compression screw plate because an oblique fracture was present. (c) The second fracture in the same patient at the mandibular angle was stabilized by a shorter MCS plate. These first MCS plates were custom made (cast in a dental laboratory). The alloy was Vitallium, and screws were self-tapping.

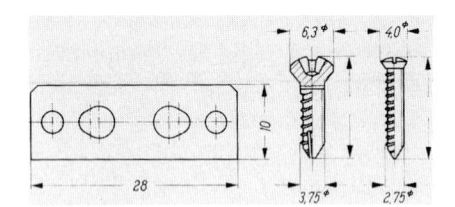

Figure 8.3 Technical drawing of the first Mandibular Compression Screw plate (MCS plate) that allows automatic axial compression of the fracture ends by means of eccentric compression holes and screws with conical screw heads. The standard type was 28 millimeters long. Two types of screws were used originally: 3.75-millimeter diameter "compression screws" and 2.75-millimeter diameter "retention screws" (inserted in the outermost neutral plate holes). The screws were self-tapping with a cutting flute (Luhr 1968).

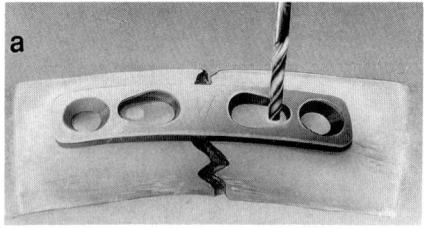

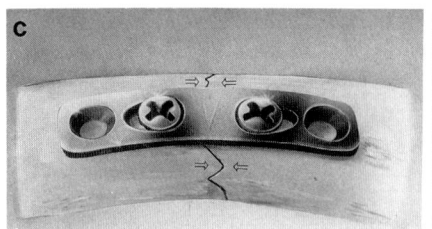

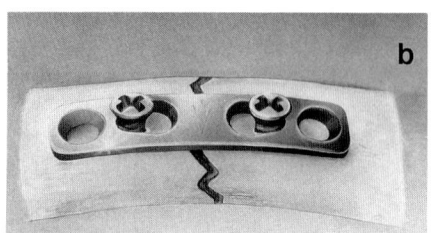

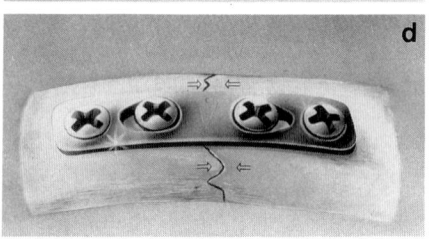

Figure 8.5 Principle and function of axial compression of the mandibular compression screw plate (MCS plate). (a) Within the small diameter of the eccentric plate holes, the bone is predrilled. Both the cortices are perforated. (b) Two screws with conical screwheads are inserted. Only when the conical screwheads touch the eccentric plate holes do they start to be pulled toward the larger diameter. Both fragments are thereby moved against each other. Note that the fracture gap is already smaller than in (a). (c) When the screws are completely tightened, they have moved further toward the fracture line, having been pulled into the great diameter of the eccentric plate holes. The fracture line is completely closed, and both fragments have been impacted by axial compression. The arrows indicate the axial compression. (d) Only when axial compression is achieved are two additional screws inserted at the outermost plateholes. These screws increase the degree of rigidity.

mum stabilization of the fracture area. The simplest way to meet these goals is to apply the principle of axial compression of the fracture ends. This principle, first advocated by the Belgian surgeon Danis in 1949, has undoubtedly brought the greatest progress in bone surgery in this century. The idea was adopted and brought into wider clinical use in surgery on extremities by the Swiss Association for the Study of Internal Fixation (ASIF). However, the traction devices used to create axial pressure in the extremities were not anatomically suitable for the mandible. Thus, the self-tightening, or automatic, Mandibular Compression Screw (MCS) plate was developed (Luhr 1968) (see Figure 8.3).

In 1967, using the MCS plate we performed the first compression osteosynthesis in the field of maxillofacial surgery in a case of an edentulous fractured mandible (see Figure 8.4). The MCS plate is an automatic compression device that guarantees axial compression of the fracture ends by using eccentric plate holes and screws with conical screw heads (see Figure 8.5). From the onset we have used self-tapping screws exclusively and have not seen any disadvantages in their use during several thousand clinical cases.

Later, other types of "dynamic" plates were advocated by various authors, primarily for surgery of the long bones and for subsequent application in mandibular fractures and later adapted for mandibular fracture therapy.

THE MANDIBULAR COMPRESSION SCREW SYSTEM AND THE TREATMENT OF MANDIBULAR FRACTURES

When the MCS system was introduced in 1968, we and many other surgeons were still frequently using an extraoral approach, in accordance with the principles of strict asepsis practiced in general surgery to control high infection rates. Gradually, we came to prefer the intraoral approach, and we adapted the MCS system for intraoral use by adding straight plates without the basal rim. During the next 15 years we gradually modified the plates and screws, without affecting the principles of function. Eccentric plateholes, self-tapping screws, and the alloy, Vitallium, remain unchanged.

Specifications of the Mandibular Compression Screw System

The MCS System* now consists of a sterilizable box (see Figure 8.6), the upper tray of which contains plates, screws, and templates [with additional space for the Mandibular Reconstruction System (MRS)]. The lower tray holds the instruments: clamps for plates and screws, forceps to bend the plates, a protective sleeve for transbuccal insertion of the surgical drill, and screwdriver.

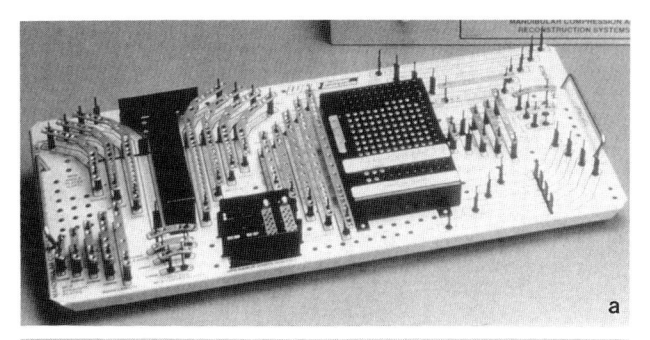

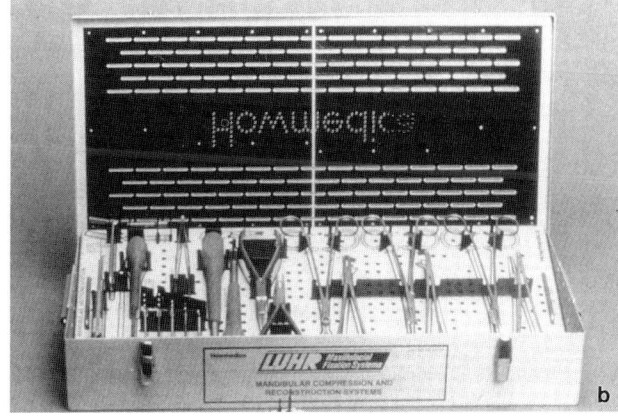

Figure 8.6 This sterilizable box contains the Mandibular-Compression-Screw System (MCS System) and the plates of the Mandibular Reconstruction System (MRS). (a) The upper tray contains both MCS plates and MRS plates and provides space for the corresponding templates. (b) The lower tray holds the instruments for both systems. Types and lengths of screws are the same in both systems.

The Screws

The screws are self-tapping with a conical head and a Phillips slot (see Figure 8.7), which optimizes the transfer of power from screwdriver to screw. Two cutting flutes near the tip of the screw facilitate screw insertion and the self-cutting of threads into the bone. The diameter of the screws is 2.7 millimeters; the bone is predrilled with a 2.1-millimeter-diameter surgical drill.

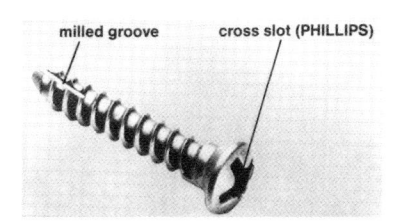

Figure 8.7 This Vitallium self-tapping screw shows one of the two milled grooves (cutting flutes) and the conical screwhead with the Phillips slot.

---
*Manufactured by Howmedica, Inc., of Rutherford, N.J.

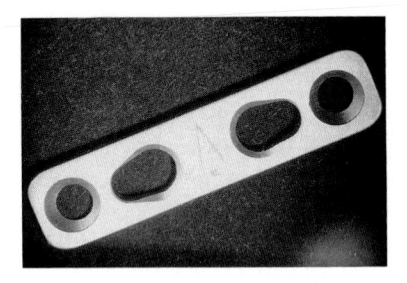

Figure 8.8 Standard MCS plate with eccentric compression holes and two neutral holes (at the outer ends of the plate).

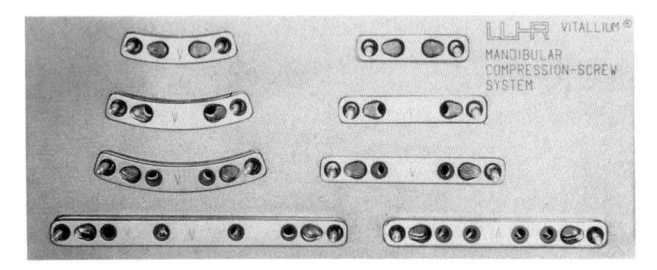

Figure 8.9 Straight and curved plates of the MCS System.

The 2.7-millimeter-diameter standard screws come in lengths of 6, 8, 10, 12, 14, 16, 20, 24, and 28 millimeters. If a screw is stripped in the bone, it can be exchanged for an "emergency screw" with a larger diameter (3.0 millimeters). The emergency screw cuts new threads in the stripped hole, ensuring a safe support. The emergency screw is easily distinguished from the standard screw by its highly polished head. Emergency screws come in lengths of 10, 12, and 14 millimeters. Physical tests using extremely high torque forces under experimental conditions in fresh bone suggest that the maximum torque of the emergency screw is about 75% of the torque that was needed to strip the first screw.

The Mandibular Compression Screw Plates

Due to the excellent stability properties of Vitallium the plates can be kept relatively thin; they are only 1.25 millimeters in thickness.* Optimal fitting of screws to the countersunk plate holes keeps the surface of implants very flat without interference of soft-tissue contour. Each plate is provided with two of the characteristic eccentric compression holes (see Figure 8.8) to achieve

---
*Sixty- and 80-millimeter plates are 1.5 millimeters thick.

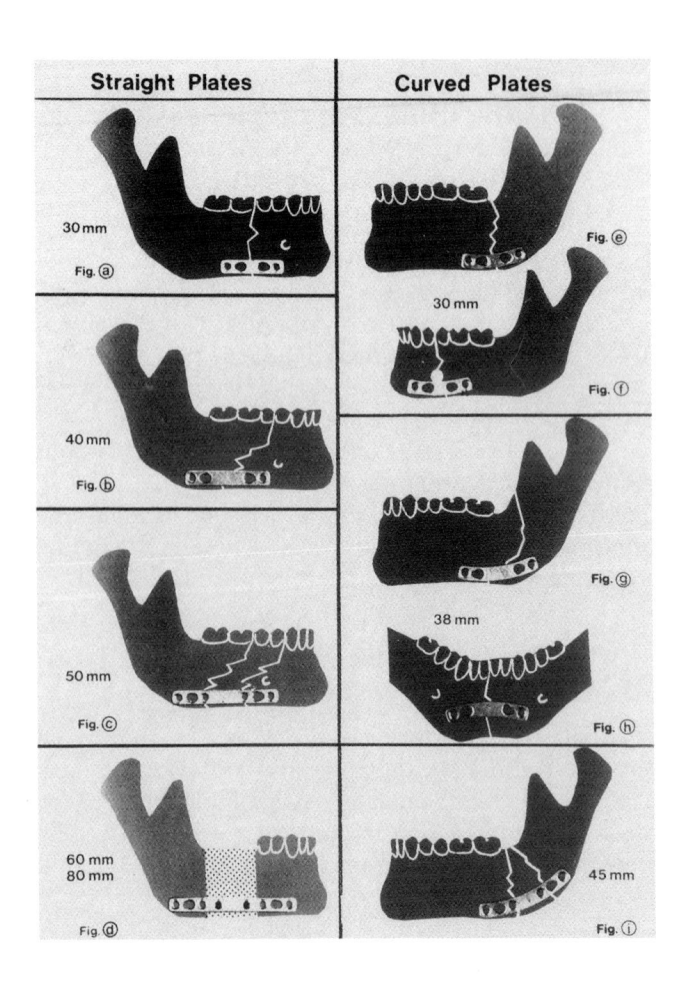

Figure 8.10 Application of different types of plates in various fracture types. (a) Simple vertical fractures in the horizontal ramus of the mandible. (b) Oblique fractures in the horizontal ramus of the mandible. Oblique fractures always need a larger distance between the two compression screws to the fracture gap and therefore a greater length of plate. (c) Extreme oblique fractures, or sagittal fractures (these fractures sometimes appear as two fracture lines on an x ray). The 50-millimeter plate is suitable for these fractures. (d) Fixation of bone grafts by axial compression (this length of plate may also be used in comminuted fractures). For fixation of larger bone grafts in mandibular reconstruction procedures the Mandibular Reconstruction System (MRS) is recommended. (e) Simple vertical fractures in the region of the mandibular angle. (f) Fractures in the region of the mental foramen. The curved plates are easily applied below the nerve without irritation of the nerve structures. (g) Oblique fractures at the mandibular angle. Oblique fractures always require a larger distance between the compression screws and the fracture line and therefore a greater length of plate. (h) Fractures in the chin region. The slightly curved 38-millimeter plate has proved especially suitable for fractures of the medial and lateral chin region. In the upside-down position (concavity of the plate downward) this type of plate can be contoured easily to the bony mental protuberance. (i) Multiple fractures of the mandibular angle. The application of the three-dimensional MCS plate is recommended in severely comminuted fractures.

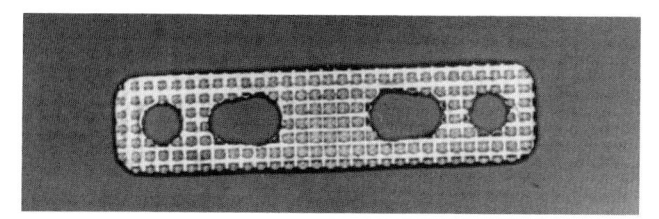

Clinical Applications of the Luhr Vitallium Maxillofacial Systems

Figure 8.11 A trial template made from a soft malleable tin alloy. For ease of identification, the templates have a gridded surface.

axial compression of the fracture ends when the screws are tightened. Straight plates are 30, 40, 50, 60, and 80 millimeters in length, and the three types of slightly curved plates are 30, 38, and 45 millimeters in length (see Figure 8.9). Figure 8.10 shows the recommended application for the different types of plates in different types of fractures. For each type of plate, a corresponding trial template (see Figure 8.11) consisting of a soft, malleable tin alloy is provided to facilitate optimal contouring to the bone surface. These templates are easily adapted to any bone surface by placing them over the bone and applying light pressure with the fingers. Tin, as opposed to aluminium, does not show any "backspring effect"; so these templates exactly reproduce the contour of the individual bone surface. Away from the surgical field, the corresponding Vitallium plate is then contoured to duplicate the shape of the template.

A supplementary three-dimensional MCS plate, recently introduced, can be contoured in all three dimensions with use of a special three-prong bending pliers (see Figure 8.12). This type of plate comes in various lengths (see Figure 8.13). When plates of different lengths are needed, they can be cut off from any of the longer ones by means of a heavy plate cutter. Three-dimensional MCS plates are particularly useful in rigid fixation of comminuted mandibular fractures.

Instruments

Figure 8.14 shows the standard instruments of the MCS system: plate- and screw-holding clamps with different angulations, the screw depth gauge, bending pliers with Vitallium-plated jaws, and the tissue protectors. A tissue protector is a protective sleeve that has a removable mandrel for transbuccal drilling and screw insertion. A special clamp holds this instrument when it is inserted transbuccally.

Principles of Rigid Fixation Using Plates and Screws

Today's standard of rigid skeletal fixation is the result of yesterday's research and the long-term experience of pioneers of modern bone surgery. To transfer this standard to an everyday procedure, every surgeon must respect some basic principles. Most often failures are not those of the system but of the surgeon. The following list should help the surgeon to avoid the most frequent errors in technique:

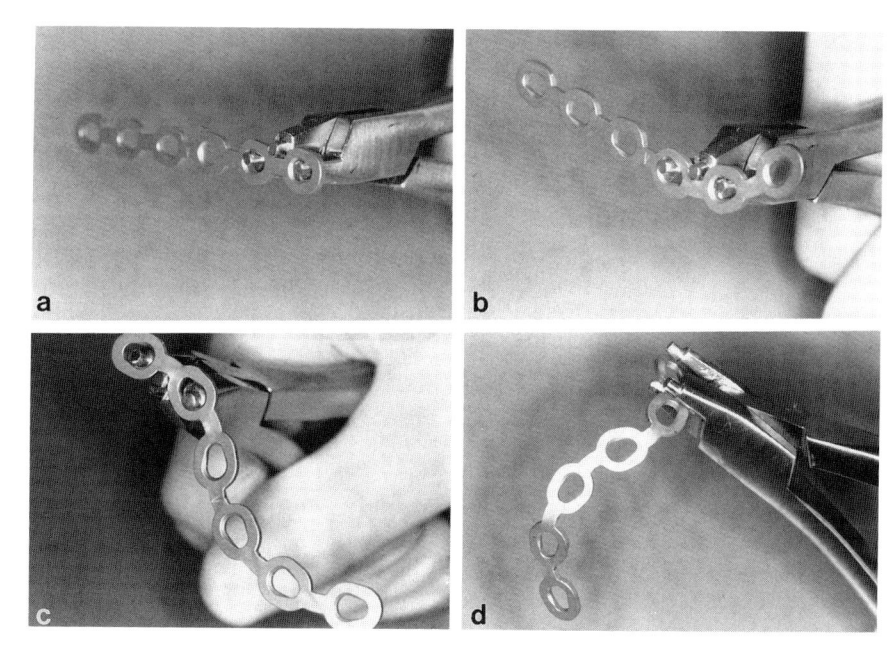

Figure 8.12 A supplementary three-dimensional MCS plate, which can be contoured in all three dimensions. (a) A three-prong bending pliers is inserted. (b) and (c) The plate can be contoured in different directions in the horizontal plane by closing the branches of the bending pliers. The plate holes are not deformed. (d) The plate can be further contoured in any direction with the three-prong bending pliers.

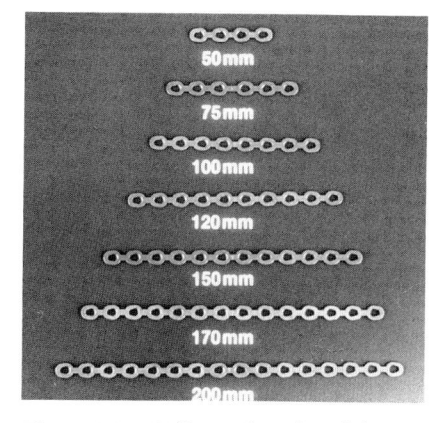

Figure 8.13 Different lengths of three-dimensional MCS plates, which can be used in mandibular fracture treatment as well as in reconstructive procedures of the mandible. Because of their eccentric plate holes, axial compression in fractures and bone graft fixation are possible. Individual lengths can be cut from one of the longer plates with a heavy plate cutter.

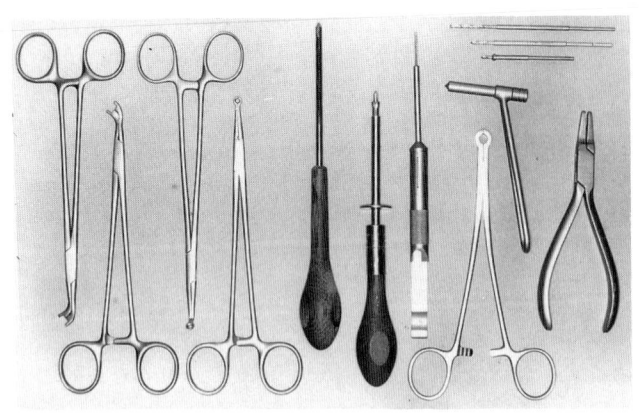

Figure 8.14 Instrumentation of the MCS System. (left to right) Plate-holding clamps with different angulations, screw-holding clamps, standard screwdriver, self-retaining screwdriver, depth gauge, protective sleeve with special clamp for transbuccal drilling and screw insertion, and plate-bending pliers. Drills of different lengths are available. The lower one is the lag screw drill that has a larger diameter than the usual ones. It can be identified by the countersinker at the drill bit.

1. *Securing occlusion.* If tooth-bearing segments are involved (in the mandible or the maxilla), the occlusion must be secured by rigid MMF during application of the plates. Otherwise, there is always the risk of an error in the occlusion. At the end of the surgery, however, the MMF can be immediately released. If the fracture is located within a tooth-bearing segment of the mandible, the lower arch bar should be left in place for three to four weeks, thus acting as tension band and providing additional stabilization. This does not mean any major discomfort for the patient and is easily tolerated.

2. *Drilling characteristics.* The use of excessive drill speed is a common error in bone surgery, and the usual cause of stripping of screws. It is most common when high-speed air-driven equipment is used. One possible solution is to reduce the air pressure to 40 pounds per square inch. Even a normal electrical power unit needs a reduction handpiece to decrease the drill speed to less than 1000 revolutions per minute. High-speed drilling may cause necrosis of the bone and undesirable enlargement of the drill hole because of centrifugal forces. Although continuous cooling with physiologic saline solution is mandatory in every kind of bone drilling, it cannot compensate for the unfavorable effect of high-speed drilling. Because the coolant will not reach the depth of the drill hole, in high-speed drilling the critical temperature for bone necrosis (47° C applied for one minute only) may easily be exceeded.

Additional factors that may cause necrosis of the bone adjacent to the screw are the use of dull drill bits and the application of excessive pressure while inserting the drill.

3. *Choice of bone plate and its optimal contouring.* To treat mandibular fractures, we recommend a rigid plate with bicortical screw fixation. These stronger plates, especially designed for the mandible, together with axial compression provide a high degree of rigidity, producing a very high rate of success (see also Complications). The forces of muscle traction acting on the fracture area in the midfacial skeleton are much lower than in the mandible. Therefore, plates and screws can be kept much thinner.

After the fracture ends are repositioned, the plate must be contoured until it fits perfectly. Imperfect contouring will cause fragments to dislocate when the screws are tightened and will disturb occlusion when tooth-bearing segments are involved. It is essential to insert at least two screws in every fragment. The plates should be applied intraorally. Although this procedure is more difficult in the area of the mandibular angle, its optimal results convince us to recommend this technique.

4. *Choice of implant material.* To avoid later implant removal and a second surgical intervention, implant materials resistant to corrosion should be used (for example, Vitallium or titanium).

5. *Use of antibiotics.* It is generally agreed that antibiotic prophylaxis should be used in open-reduction bone surgery. However, this will not compensate for failures of surgical technique. Optimal reduction and maximal stability are the most important factors in preventing infection of the fracture line.

Indications and Surgical Technique

The indications for compression plating in mandibular fractures are reliably established. They are summarized in Table 8.1. In addition, most of the patients with simple fractures of the fully dentured mandible (which could be treated nonsurgically using arch bars and MMF for a period of four to five weeks) today prefer rigid fixation. The avoidance of any MMF postoperatively makes this kind of treatment more comfortable for the patient. The period of morbidity decreases significantly, which means earlier return to work and social activities.

Surgical Technique

The main principles of surgical technique are the following:

1. axial compression of the fracture ends
2. bicortical screw fixation
3. intraoral approach.

Axial compression of the fracture ends is the simplest way to achieve maximum rigidity and optimum reduction of a fracture, thus providing optimal conditions for a fast and economic bone healing.

For bicortical screw fixation, the screw must sit firmly in the outer and inner cortical bone of the man-

Clinical Applications of the Luhr Vitallium Maxillofacial Systems

Table 8.1 Indications of compression osteosynthesis of mandibular fractures

I Fractures of edentulous or insufficiently dentulous mandible (also if maxilla is edentulous)

II Fractures of fully dentulous mandible:
  1. displaced fractures of mandibular angle
  2. fractures of the body of the mandible combined with fractures of TMJ (requiring early functional therapy)
  3. comminuted mandibular fractures
  4. mandibular fractures in patients with polytrauma
  5. when maxillomandibular fixation is not desirable (epilepsia, travel by sea or air, etc.)
  6. delayed fracture healing and pseudarthrosis
  7. fixation of bone grafts in fractures with defect

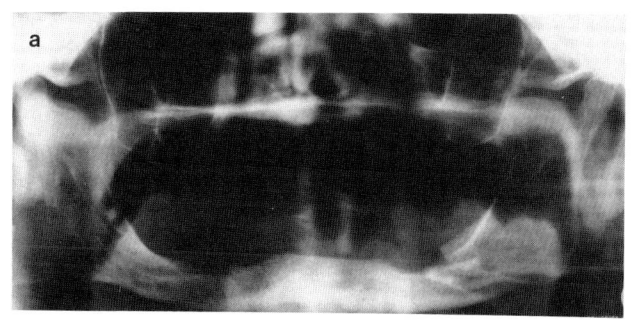

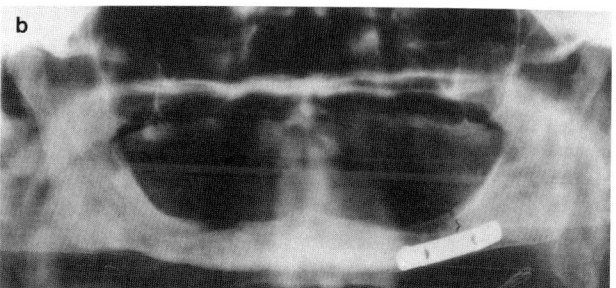

Figure 8.16 (a) Fracture of the edentulous mandible. (b) After fracture reduction, an MCS plate was placed intraorally with bicortical screw fixation and axial compression of the fracture ends. This is the standard treatment. (Only in extremely atrophic mandibles are the smaller Mini-Compression plates recommended.)

dible (see Figures 8.15a–c) to achieve a maximum anchorage. The holding power of a screw in the spongiosa is poor. Plates and screws must be placed near the lower border of the mandible to avoid the roots of the teeth and the neurovascular bundle.

For the past eight years the intraoral approach has been our unit's principal method for rigid fixation of mandibular fractures. This approach has the advantage of producing no outer scar and avoiding any risk of damage to facial nerves. However, there are a few exceptions to this standard procedure, where an extraoral approach should be preferred. These are rigid plate fixation of severely comminuted mandibular fractures, plate fixation of bone grafts, and fractures of the condylar neck and of the extremely atrophic mandible. The intraoral incision is first placed deep in the vestibule in a vertical direction (see Figure 8.15). At a depth of about 5 millimeters, the cut is directed more horizontally toward the bone surface. This technique preserves a broad gingival soft-tissue pedicle, which later facilitates wound closure with a wide soft-tissue contact (see Figure 8.15c). This technique effectively prevents wound dehiscence.

The standard intraoral technique is simple in compression plating of fractures of the edentulous mandible (see Figure 8.16). A soft solid diet is recommended for a period of about three weeks. After this time the pros-

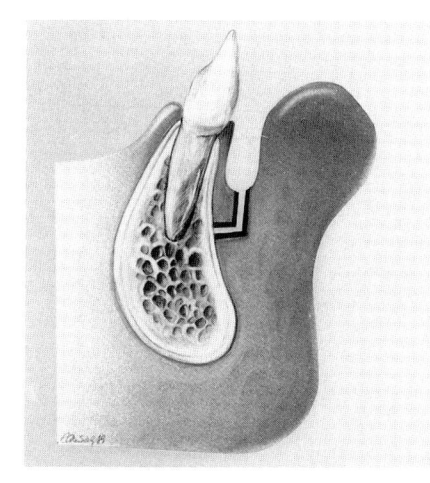

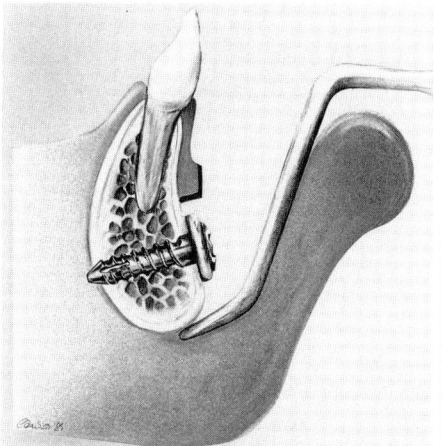

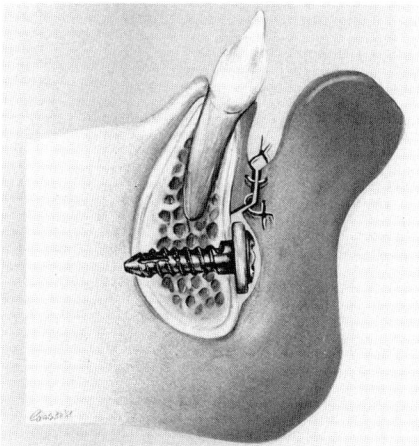

Figure 8.15 Intraoral technique of bicortical plate and screw fixation in mandibular fractures. (a) An intraoral vertical incision, 4 to 5 mm deep, is made in the vestibule. Only then is the incision directed more horizontally, thus preserving a broad gingival soft-tissue pedicle. (b) The plate and screws are placed near the lower border of the mandible. To achieve a firm anchorage, the screw should sit firmly in the outer and inner cortex of the mandible. (c) The plate and screws are covered by a thick soft-tissue layer. Some resorbable sutures should be placed at the muscle layer just above the plate. This technique helps to prevent wound dehiscence and exposure of the plate.

thodontist may perform minor corrections of the fitting of the lower dentures, if required. Although usually there is no need to remove Vitallium implants later on, this may be different in the edentulous mandible, because the plate and screws in some cases can interfere with the lower denture. In these cases the implants should be removed (about three months after surgery) at the earliest. In rigid fixation of fractures of the fully dentured mandible, the patient must be put in MMF during surgery. The occlusion must be restored and ensured by arch bars and MMF while the fracture is stabilized by a compression plate. The technique is easily performed in fractures of the anterior part of the mandible, holes can be drilled and screws can be inserted after retracting the lips (see Figure 8.17).

After the fracture has been stabilized by fixation of an MCS plate and bicortical screws, the maxillomandibular fixation is released at the end of surgery. The lower arch bar, which is left in situ for about four weeks, provides additional stabilization by acting as a tension band. The intraoral technique is more difficult in fractures of the posterior region of the mandible toward the mandibular angle. In this area, besides the common intraoral exposure of the fracture line, a transbuccal technique is required for drilling and screw insertion (see Figure 8.18). In displaced fractures of the mandibular angle, keeping the mobile proximal segment in place during application of the MCS plate can occasionally be difficult. Because instruments, such as clamps and forceps, have proved to be unsatisfactory with the intraoral technique—particularly at the posterior part of the mandible—we use a small plate from the Mini-System as an auxilliary repositioning device.

A small Mini-Compression plate (preferably a five-hole plate of the slightly curved type) is first fixed with two monocortical screws (6 or 8 millimeters in length) at the anterior border of the proximal fracture end (see Figure 8.19a). The free anterior end of the miniplate then serves as a handle to guide the proximal segment back to its original position. The free end of the plate is then contoured by means of a bending pliers until it fits to the bone surface beneath the third molar at the distal segment. The miniplate is fixed by two additional screws, 6 millimeters in length, which are inserted in a slightly oblique vertical direction (see Figure 8.19b). This monocortically fixed miniplate keeps both the segments in position during the application of the stronger MCS plate, which is placed beneath the first plate near the mandibular border (see Figure 8.19c).

The miniplate can be left in place; acting as a tension band, it provides even more rigidity. We do not use this tension band principle routinely; we use it only when the fracture pattern is such that an arch bar will not function as a tension band. Although the intraoral technique is more demanding in the posterior mandible, the optimal results of several hundred cases we treated in the last eight years have convinced us to prefer it to the extraoral approach. However, there are a few exceptions; and in these cases the extraoral approach still has some advantages. One of these is the treatment of comminuted fractures that need a wide exposure to identify a complex fracture pattern and to achieve a proper reduction of fragments and placement of plates (see Figure 8.20). The extraoral approach is favored also when bone grafts are placed to bridge mandibular defects (see Figure 8.21).

Figure 8.17 Compression plating of a mandibular fracture at the right parasymphyseal area by an intraoral approach. (a) After arch bars are applied and the occlusion is ensured by intermaxillary fixation, the fracture area is exposed. Note that the mental nerve has been dissected. The MCS plate is carefully contoured to the bone surfaces. (b) The bone can be drilled easily under direct visualization. (c) The same applies to screw insertion. (d) The fracture is stabilized by axial compression. At least two screws are required in each segment.

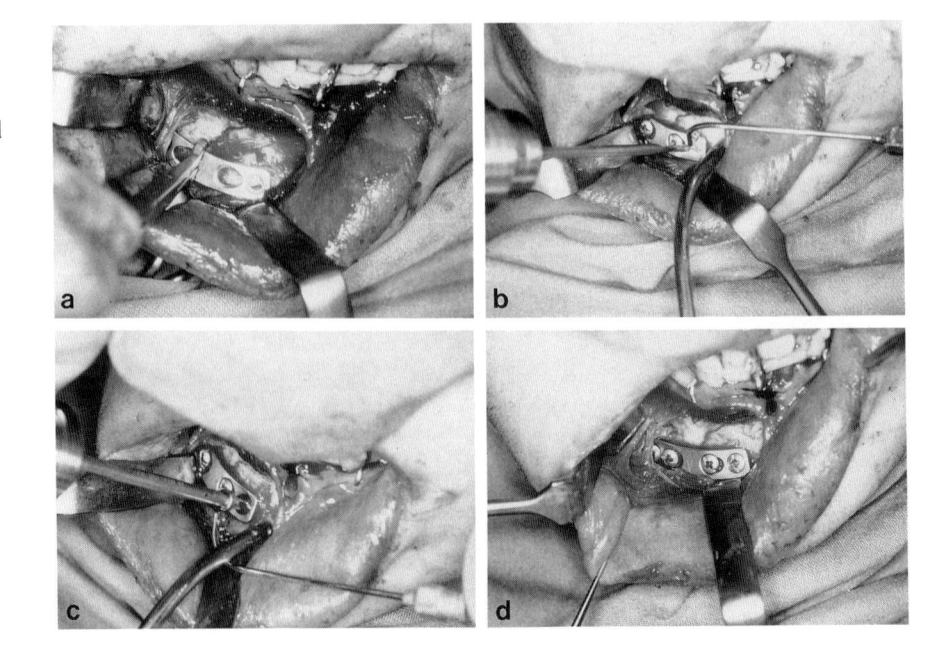

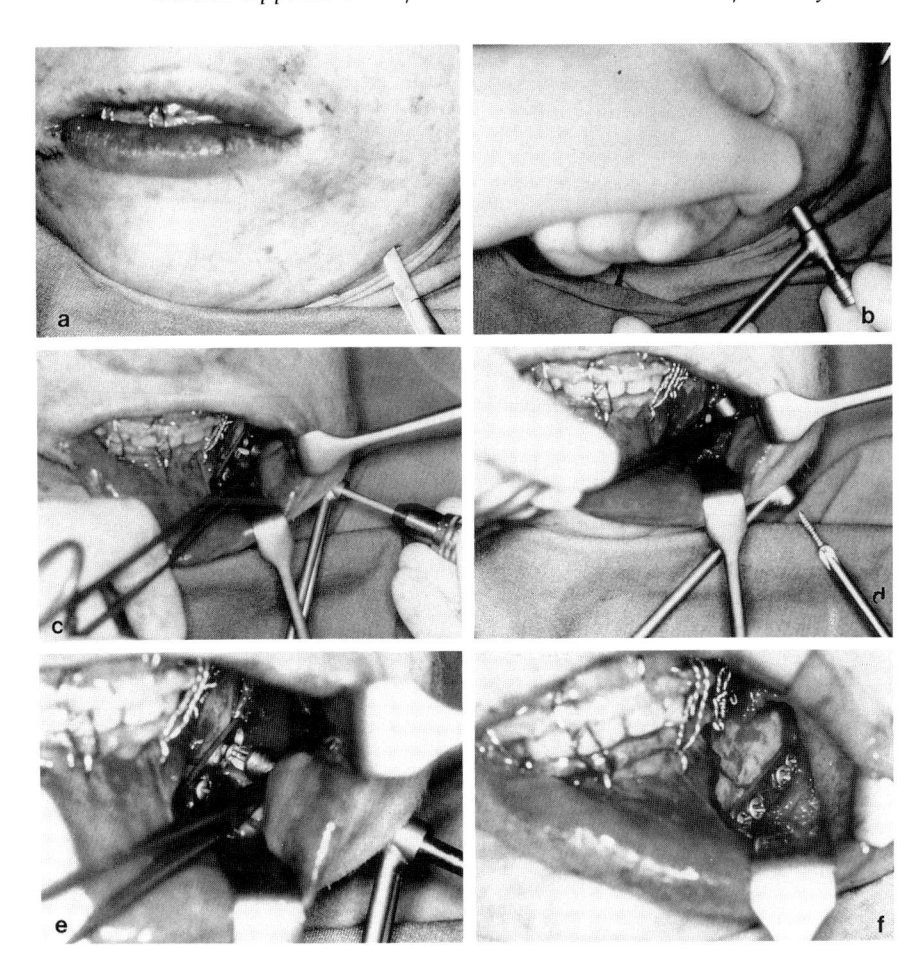

Clinical Applications of the Luhr Vitallium Maxillofacial Systems 87

Figure 8.18 Intraoral technique of compression plating with the transbuccal approach in fractures of the mandibular angle. (a) A 4-millimeter stab incision is made in the skin. This incision corresponds to the intraoral exposed fracture. (b) The protection sleeve with mandrel is inserted into the soft-tissue canal, which has been opened by blunt dissection. The intraorally visible end of the protection sleeve is fixed by means of a special holding clamp. The mandrel is taken out. (c) The drill is inserted intraorally through the bore sleeve, and the desired part of the mandible is drilled. (d) The screw of the desired length (the length can be measured by means of the depth gauge transbuccally via the bore sleeve) is attached to the screwdriver and inserted through the bore sleeve. (e) The screw is inserted transbuccally into the predrilled bone, cutting its own thread. (f) After both compression screws in the compression holes have been tightened, two outer retention screws are inserted through the same approach (the bore sleeve is moved medially or distally). The fracture is stabilized by axial compression and bicortical screw fixation. MMF can be released.

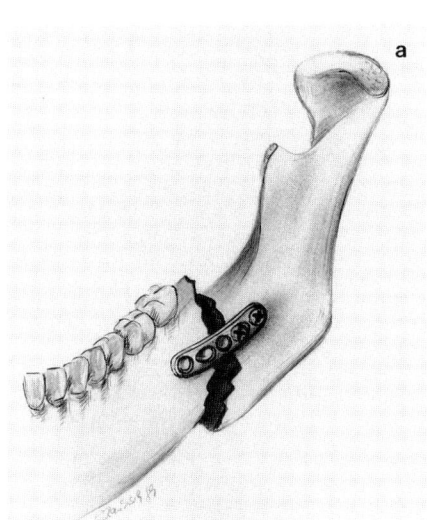

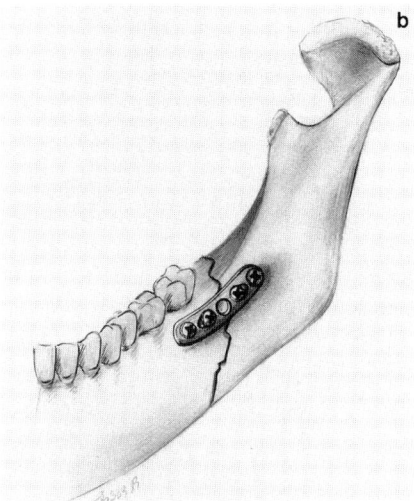

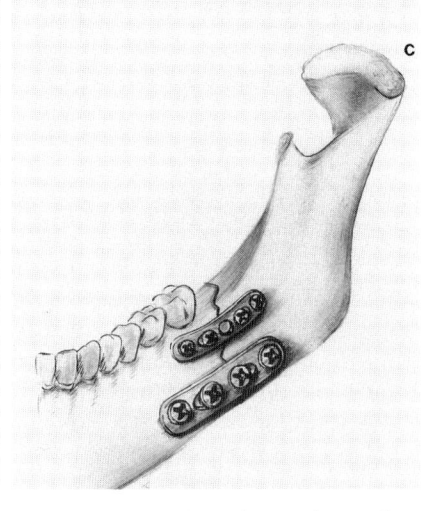

Figure 8.19 Plating technique in displaced fractures of the mandibular angle. (a) A small plate from the Mini-Compression System is first fixed by two monocortical screws at the anterior border of the proximal fragment. The free anterior end of this miniplate serves as a handle to guide the proximal segment back to its original position. (b) When fracture reduction is achieved the plate is fixed to the distal segment by two more monocortical screws. This fixation keeps both the segment in place during the application of the actual MCS plate, which is placed near the lower border of the mandible. (c) Both plates are in place. The upper, smaller miniplate can be left in place to act as a tension band. Note that the tension-band configuration at the anterior border of the mandible is not a routine procedure. It is used only in those cases where fracture reduction is difficult.

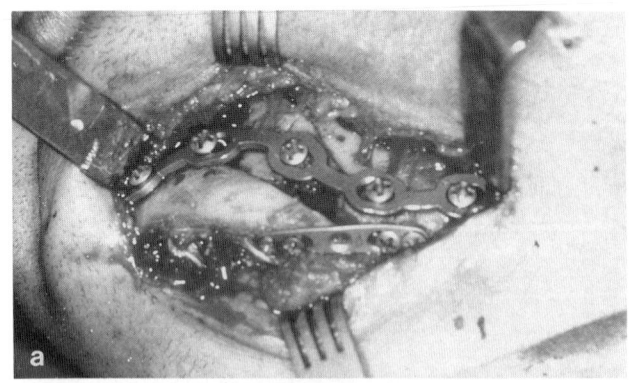

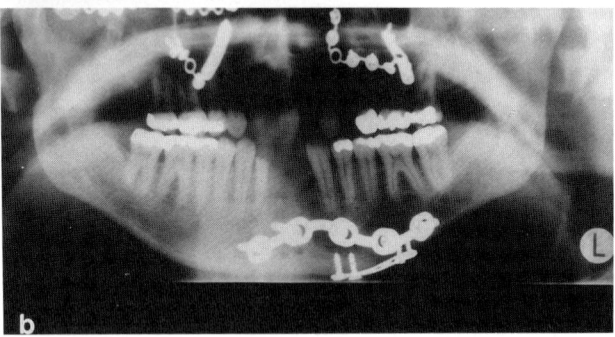

Figure 8.20 Treatment of a comminuted mandibular fracture at the parasymphyseal area. Comminuted fractures are one of the exceptions where the extraoral approach is preferred. (a) After the occlusion was ensured with arch bars and MMF, the fracture area was exposed by an extraoral incision. An auxiliary miniplate was placed at the lower border of the mandible to keep the fragments in place while the three-dimensional MCS plate was contoured and fixed by multiple screws. Because of the special design of the connecting bars between the plate holes, the three-dimensional MCS plate can be contoured to the requirements of the individual fracture pattern. (b) The postoperative x-ray shows the strong three-dimensional MCS plate with bicortical screw fixation spanning the comminuted fracture area.

The Lag Screw Principle

The lag screw principle is used whenever two wide contact surfaces of bone should be pressed together (for example, in oblique sagittal fractures of the mandible or for the fixation of onlay bone grafts). A hole is drilled through the outer cortex or onlay graft with a diameter identical to that of the screw, so that the screw will slip through the outer cortex. The lag screw drill, which is of the same outside diameter as the screw, will simultaneously create a conical countersink to provide an optimal fitting of the screwhead. The inner cortex is then perforated with the normal surgical drill, and the screw is inserted. It grips the inner cortex and, when tightened, exerts great force to pull the outer segment into close contact with the inner one. This principle can be used in oblique sagittal mandibular fractures, with the placement of at least three screws; or in combination with a plate, lagging only one or two of the total number of screws. We prefer the latter technique for extremely oblique sagittal mandibular fractures (see Figure 8.22).

Variations of the Standard Surgical Technique

Special types of fractures require some variations of the standard surgical technique and a different kind of plating system. Because of the small size of certain skeletal areas of the mandible, the common MCS plates are too large. The areas where we prefer the smaller Mini-Compression plates are the condylar neck, the atrophic mandible, and the mandible in children.

a) *Condylar neck fractures*. The majority of condylar fractures are treated nonsurgically using dental splints with a few days of MMF, followed by early function with support of guiding elastics. There are limited indications for surgery, however. These are mainly fractures of the condylar neck with severe dislocation of the proximal fragment (more than 45° angulation). This is particularly true when both the condyles are involved and pan-facial fractures are present. Then open reduction and rigid fixation is the only way to reestab-

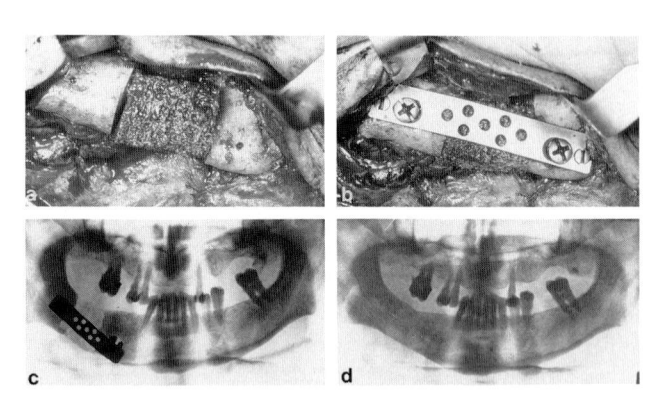

Figure 8.21 The extraoral approach is favored when bone grafts are placed to bridge mandibular defects. (a) An autogenous cancellous bone graft is placed between the bony stumps after part of the mandible has been resected because of a chronic osteomyelitis. (b) The graft is fixed between the two resection stumps by axial compression using an MCS plate (shown is the older type of MCS plate). Note that in smaller bone grafts there is no need to fix the graft by separate screws. (c) This x-ray shows graft and MCS plate in place. There was no need for MMF postoperatively. The plate was removed after four months to expose the graft to functional stress during the phase of bone remodeling. This is to prevent atrophy of the graft. (d) One year after removal of the plate, an x-ray shows complete integration of the graft without any significant graft resorption.

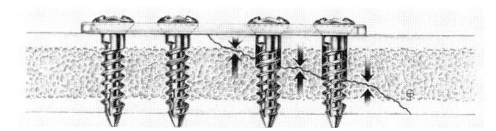

Clinical Applications of the Luhr Vitallium Maxillofacial Systems

Figure 8.22 Application of the lag screw principle in rigid plate fixation of an extremely oblique fracture. The two screws on the right act as lag screws. The outer cortex was predrilled with a lag screw drill having exactly the outside diameter of the screws. When these screws are inserted, the fracture ends are pulled together (the arrows indicate the pressure in the oblique fracture line). Additional screws are placed at the other plate holes. By combining plate fixation with the lag screw principle, a maximum of rigidity is achieved. Note that when this principle is applied the bone has to be predrilled within the large diameter of the compression holes, because in this technique the usual axial compression is not possible.

lish the vertical dimension of the facial skeleton. In condylar neck fractures the small Mini-Compression plates are preferred with bicortical screw fixation using an extraoral approach.

b) *Fractures of the extremely atrophic mandible.* Fracture treatment of the edentulous mandible when excessive atrophy is present (height of the mandible less than 10 millimeters) involves some substantial difficulties. This applies to all the various methods—circumferential wiring, interosseous wiring, and even bone plating. The fracture ends consists of a dense, sclerotic, and poorly vascularized bone; and the cross section of the fracture site is distinctly decreased. These elements combined significantly decrease the osteogenetic potential in this type of fracture. Because in extremely atrophied mandibles the central mandibular artery may be absent, the blood supply depends on the periosteum only. Treatment planning has to consider these conditions. We therefore recommend the extraoral approach in rigid plate fixation of fractures of the atrophic mandible (as one of the exceptions to the standard procedure). Extensive periosteal stripping when exposing the fracture should be avoided. (The salvage of the periosteum and its blood supply is much easier by an extraoral exposure than with an intraoral procedure in those particular cases.) Whenever possible the plate should be placed epiperiosteally. Rigid fixation should be performed using a compression Miniplate with bicortical screw fixation (see Figure 8.23).

Particularly difficult is the treatment when multiple fractures are present in an atrophic mandible. Because the patient's dentures are frequently broken or do not fit perfectly because of traumatic edema and hematoma, any reference to the individual curvature of the mandibular arch is missing. When only one of the fracture sites is exposed first and a plate is contoured to the bone, this contour might be incorrect (note that the fracture line at the inner surface of the mandible is not visualized). When the screws are tightened, this may result in a severe dislocation of the other segments (see Figure 8.24a). To avoid this error, we strongly recommend exposure of all the fractures first. Then the plates can be manually reduced and contoured to the bone surfaces. The compression miniscrews should then be inserted only partially in each of the plates (see Figure 8.24b). When the alternating screws are finally tightened, the opposite fracture line should be observed. If a tendency of displacement of the other fragments is seen, the first plate must be removed and recontoured before it is placed again. Compression plating is the treatment of choice even in fractures of the atrophic mandible, which are generally regarded as problematic. In 31 consecutive cases of fractures of the atrophic mandible treated in our unit, there was only one failure that resulted in a nonunion following a fracture line infection.

c) *Mandibular fractures in children.* For mandibular fractures in children, we prefer the small com-

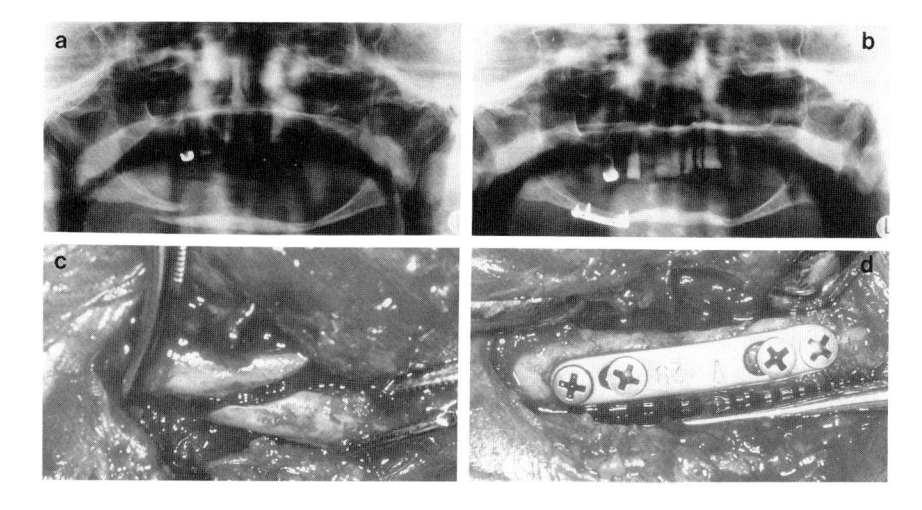

Figure 8.23 (a) Rigid plate fixation of a fracture of an extremely atrophic mandible. (b) Rigid fixation was achieved with a mini-compression plate. Because of the reduced height of the atrophic mandible, the smaller miniplates are preferred; MCS plates are too large. (c) Fractures of the atrophic mandible are a further indication for an extraoral exposure. (d) By applying axial compression, a mini-compression plate stabilizes the fracture.

pression plates of the Mini-System together with monocortical screw fixation (see Figure 8.25). Short screws in lengths of 3, 4, and 6 millimeters are available; these lengths avoid any lesion of the tooth buds. MMF is released immediately at the end of surgery; we found this method particularly useful in children because it avoids major discomfort. The lower arch bar is left in situ for about four weeks. Although as of now there is no evidence of inhibition of growth and development following rigid fixation in children, we tend to remove plates and screws (at least in the mandible) four to five weeks after surgery. Because in children the removal of the lower arch bar generally requires general anesthesia, both procedures can be performed in one intervention.

There is virtually no indication for open reduction of condylar fractures in young children (less than 10 years of age). Because of the potential of adaptation and bone remodeling at this age, a functional, nonsurgical treatment using arch bars and guiding elastics usually produces satisfactory results.

Complications of Compression Plating in Mandibular Fractures

In the eight years that we have used the intraoral approach exclusively in compression plating of mandibular fractures, our infection rate has dropped significantly. This was shown by a study where two nonselected groups of patients were compared retrospectively: 105 had undergone the extraoral technique and 255 the intraoral approach (Luhr 1985b). Serious complications, such as osteomyelitis or nonunion, were relatively rare, particularly for the intraoral group (see Table 8.2). The extremely low incidence of osteomyelitis—0.8% in patients in the intraoral group (compared with 2.8% in the extraoral group)—was similar to the

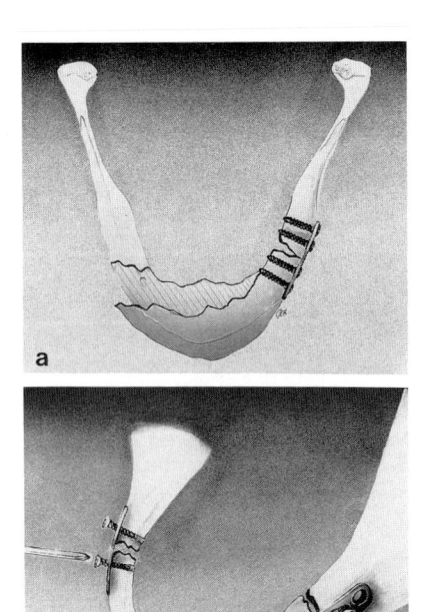

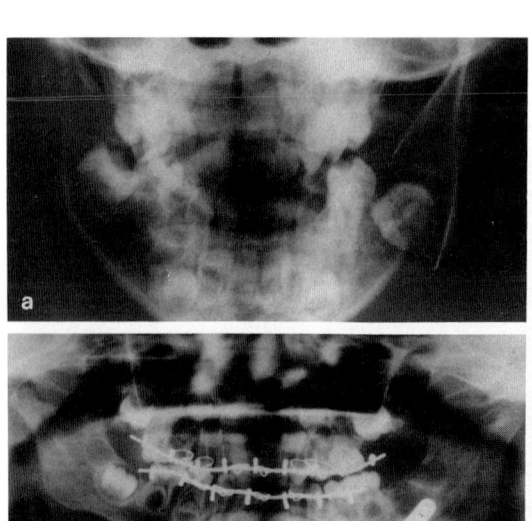

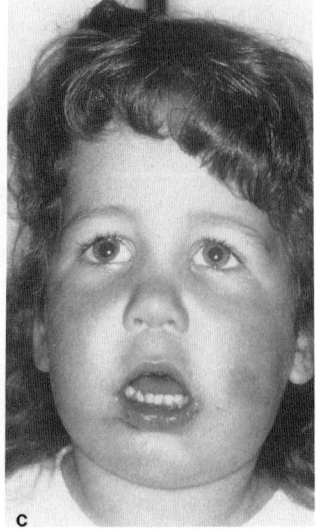

Figure 8.24 Technique of rigid fixation in multiple fractures of the edentulous mandible. (a) If only one of the fractures is exposed first and plated, the fragments may become severely dislocated. Because teeth are missing and an MMF usually is not possible, it is difficult to identify the original curvature of the mandible. Any error in plate contouring will displace the opposite fracture when the screws are tightened. (b) All the fracture areas should be exposed first, so the surgeon can perform reduction and then contour the plates. While the screws on one side of the mandible are tightened, the other fracture line must be observed. If a displacement of the fracture at the opposite side of the mandible is seen at that time, the plate must be recontoured. The screws should be tightened alternately at both the fracture areas.

Figure 8.25 Rigid plate fixation in mandibular fractures of children. (a) Displaced fracture of the left mandibular angle in a child 2½ years of age. (b) The fracture was stabilized with a mini-compression plate and monocortical screw fixation via an intraoral approach. Short screws, 4 or 6 millimeters in length, were used, and the plate was placed near the lower border of the mandible to avoid injury to the tooth buds. MMF is required during surgery. In children, plates should be removed after four or five weeks. (c) The condition of the child a few days after surgery. No MMF is needed postoperatively.

Table 8.2 (Luhr 1985b)

Rate of Serious Complications (= Osteomyelitis) in a Total Number of 360 Cases of Compression Plating

105 cases *extraoral* approach 3 cases of osteomyelitis	= 2.8%
255 cases *intraoral* approach 2 cases of osteomyelitis	= 0.8%

Rate of Serious Complications (= Osteomyelitis) in a Total Number of 1614 Cases of Mandibular Fractures with Conservative Treatment (Dental Splints, Prosthetic Appliances etc., and Maxillomandibular Fixation)

11 cases of osteomyelitis	= 0.7%

rate (0.7%) found in 1634 cases that had been treated using only the conservative nonsurgical methods of dental splints and additional MMF. The finding that the risk of infection in intraoral bicortical mandibular compression plating is not significantly higher than in conservative nonsurgical treatment may help increase the use of this technique and influence legal considerations.

Conclusions

The Vitallium MCS system is based on 20 years of clinical experience and extensive basic research. The system has the following advantages:

1. Axial compression of the fracture ends, which is achieved using eccentric holes of the MCS plate and screws with conical heads, results in an optimal reduction and maximum rigidity of the fracture site.
2. Because the compression plates provide extreme stabilization of the fracture, there is no need for any additional MMF postoperatively. Therefore this technique provides greater comfort for the patient and facilitates oral hygiene, particularly in polytraumatized patients who need complex treatment in intensive care units.
3. The overall time of morbidity is significantly reduced, and the patient may return quickly to work and social activities. Thus the procedure is cost effective.
4. Because Vitallium is corrosion resistant, usually it is not necessary to remove the plates and screws, thus avoiding a second surgical intervention. Because of Vitallium's excellent mechanical properties the implants can be kept relatively small and do not interfere with soft-tissue cover.
5. Self-tapping screws make the surgery fast and simple. Specially developed implants and instruments permit use of intraoral approach, which avoids a visible scar and the risk of facial nerve damage and decreases the frequency of complications.

THE MINI-SYSTEM

Based on our experiences with the treatment of mandibular fractures, the use of rigid fixation was gradually extended to the midfacial skeleton and the skull. To adapt these techniques to the smaller and thinner bones of the midface, miniaturized boneplates (miniplates) of different shapes and lengths were developed. The Vitallium Mini-System offers both compression plates and the noncompressive fixation plates. The technical design and perfection in manufacturing, the very low plate thickness and screwhead profile, along with the superior mechanical strength of the well known alloy Vitallium, provide the surgeon with a most versatile bone fixation system for a wide range of indications in trauma, orthognathic surgery, and craniofacial reconstruction.

Specifications of the Mini-System

The Mini-System* consists of a sterilizable box, the upper tray of which (see Figure 8.26) contains 2.0-millimeter-diameter self-tapping screws of different lengths, both the different types of minicompression plates, and the noncompressive minifixation plates. The corresponding templates are arranged in a separate section. The lower tray holds the instruments.

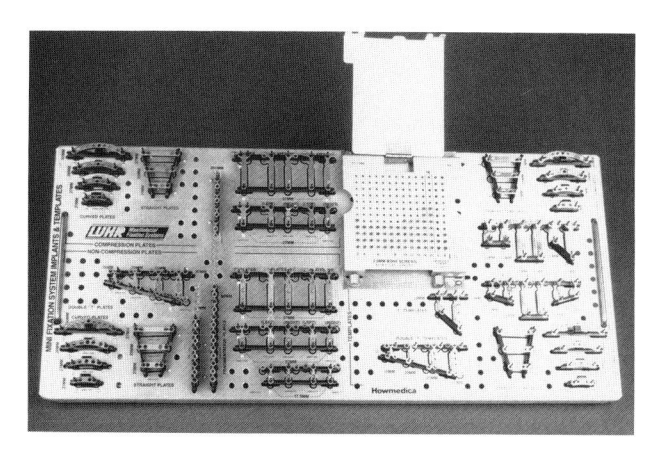

Figure 8.26 The upper tray of this sterilizable box contains plates and screws of the Mini-Compression and the Mini-Fixation Systems. The right side of the tray holds the trial templates.

---

*Manufactured by Howmedica, Inc., of Rutherford, N.J.

The Screws

The diameter of the screws is 2.0 millimeters. The screws are self-tapping, which is the key for a safe anchorage, particularly in the thin bones of the midfacial skeleton. The screwhead is kept flat and fits exactly to the countersink of the plate holes. The fit results in a very low plate–screwhead profile. The Phillips slot optimizes the transfer of power from screwdriver to screw. Two cutting flutes near the tip of the screw facilitate screw insertion and the cutting of threads into the bone.

The bone is predrilled with a 1.5-millimeter-diameter surgical drill. Low drill speed is essential to avoid enlargement of the drill hole as well as necrosis of the adjacent bone. The drill speed recommended is less than 1000 revolutions per minute. Excessive drill speed is the usual cause of stripping of screws. However, if a screw has been stripped, so-called "emergency screws" are available; their diameter, 2.4 millimeters, is slightly larger. The emergency screws come in lengths of 6 and 8 millimeters and can be identified easily by their highly polished heads.

The Instruments

Figure 8.27 shows the standard instrumentation: plate- and screw-holding clamps with different angulations, standard screwdriver and bending pliers, the protective sleeve for the transbuccal approach, and the drillbits of various length. Some special instruments, however, need a more detailed description.

Self-Retaining Screwdriver The screws can be picked up from the screw rack with the self-retaining screwdriver (see Figure 8.28) and then directly inserted into the bone. This speeds up the surgical procedure.

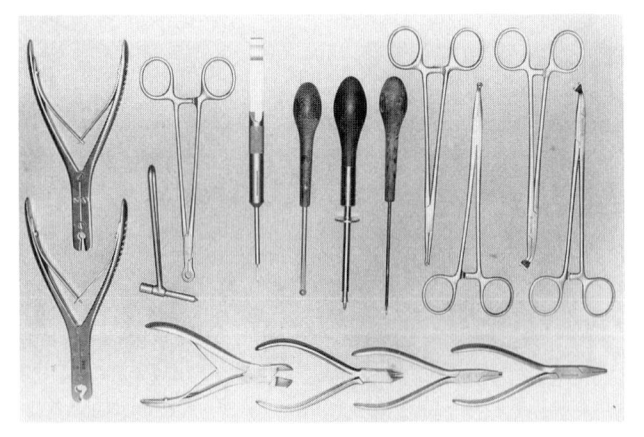

Figure 8.27 The instrumentation of the Mini-System. (top, left to right): Plate-bending pliers, bending pliers with post, three-prong bending pliers, and plate cutter. (bottom, left to right): Plate-holding clamps, screw-holding clamps, standard screwdriver, self-retaining screwdriver, centric drill guide, depth gauge, protective sleeve with special clamp for transbuccal drilling and screw insertion. (right) Right-angle and tubular bending pliers.

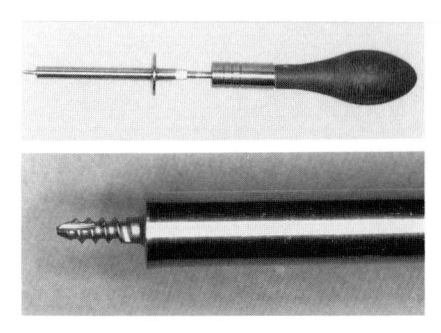

Figure 8.28 The self-retaining screwdriver allows the screws to be picked up from the screw rack and directly transferred to the surgical site. The sleeve that holds the screwhead must be retracted before the screw is completely tightened.

90° Bending Pliers The 90° bending pliers facilitates bending of the plates, particularly in those stronger sections where no holes are present. When simple pliers are used, the plate always tends to bend in areas where holes are situated. Every desired angle up to 90° can be formed (see Figure 8.29).

Tubular Bending Pliers Miniplates are sometimes used on fractures of tubular bones, for example, in hand surgery. A miniplate can be adapted to the rounded surface of tubular bones with tubular bending pliers (see Figure 8.30).

Bending Pliers with Post and Three-Prong Bending Pliers Bending pliers with post require plates to be stabilized with another pliers during three-dimensional bending. By inserting the post of this pliers into a hole of one of the segmented minifixation plates then closing the pliers the adjacent connection bar to the next hole can be bent in the horizontal plane without deforming the plate holes (see Figure 8.31).

Centric Drill Guide The centric drill guide places the tip of the drill exactly within the center of the plate hole (see Figure 8.32), avoiding any drilling off center (and thereby preventing any dislocation of the bone segments when the screw is finally tightened). Centric placement of screws is particularly important in orthognathic surgery to avoid any shifting of toothbearing segments.

Mini-Compression Plates

The excellent mechanical properties of Vitallium provide plates of superior strength with a thickness of only 0.7 millimeter. Although of a limited number, the various types of straight, curved, L-type, and T-plates (see Figure 8.33) provide a wide range of application.

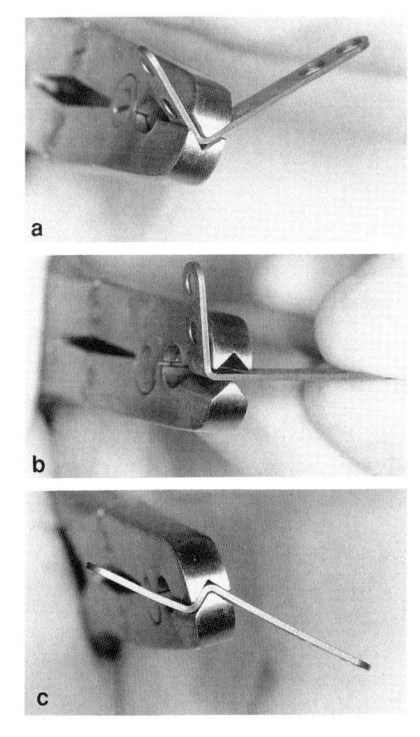

Clinical Applications of the Luhr Vitallium Maxillofacial Systems 93

Figure 8.29 The right-angle bending pliers facilitates plate contouring. The instrument is particularly useful in orthognathic surgery when an exact, steplike plate contouring is required.

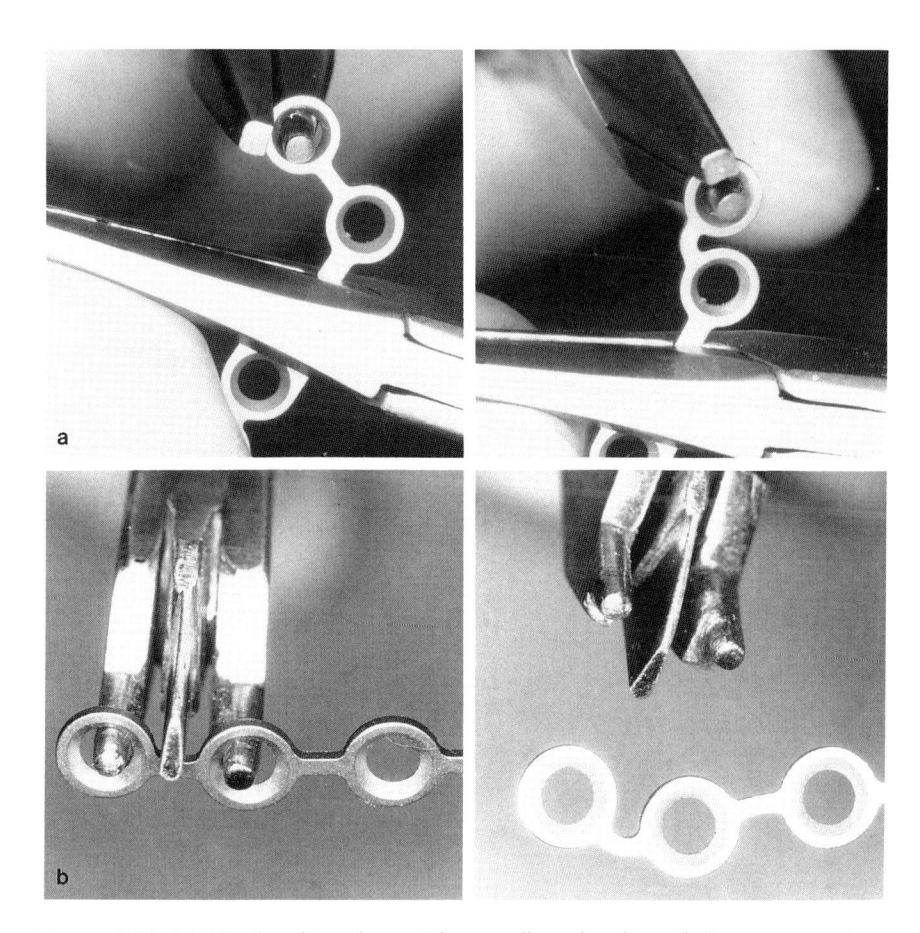

Figure 8.31 (a) The bending pliers with post allows bending of plate segments in the horizontal plate without deforming the plate holes. (b) The same procedure can be carried out with a three-prong bending pliers. However, the extent of bending with this instrument is limited.

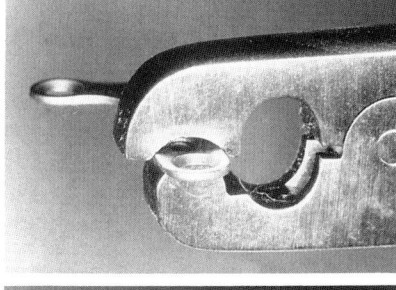

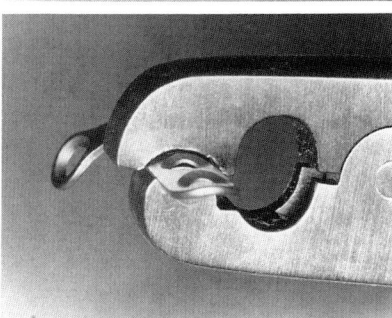

Figure 8.30 This special bending pliers facilitates tubular plate contouring, which is particularly required in hand surgery.

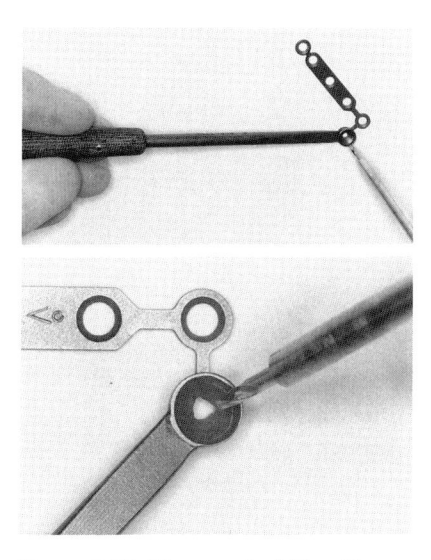

Figure 8.32 The centric drill guide places the drill hole exactly in the center of the plate hole. The triangular shape of the drill guide hole (bottom) allows irrigation while drilling.

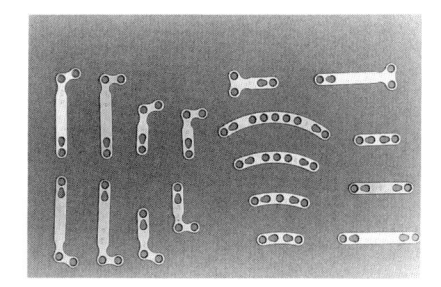

Figure 8.33 This selection of Mini-Compression plates shows various types of straight, curved, L-shaped and T-shaped plates. These plates are equipped with one or two eccentric compression holes, which allow axial compression in the fracture line.

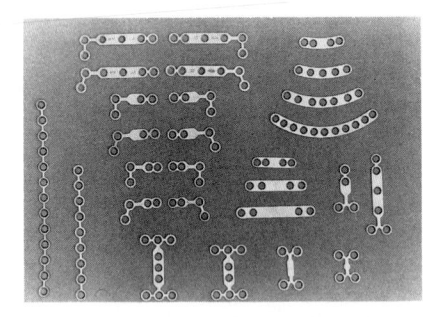

Figure 8.34 Mini-Fixation plates (non-compressive plates). The L-shaped plates and, in particular, the fragmentation plates are equipped with smaller connection bars to facilitate three-dimensional plate contouring.

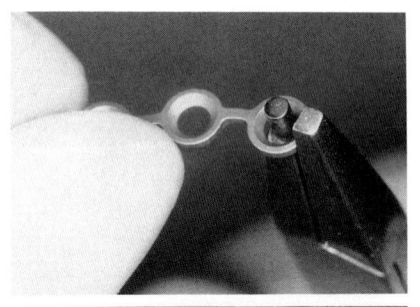

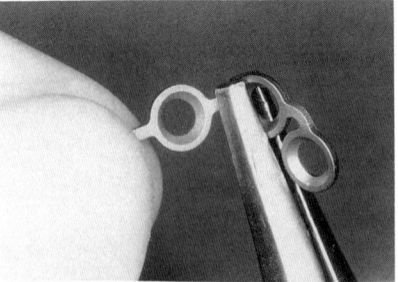

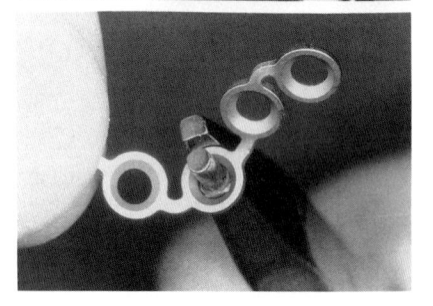

Figure 8.35 Due to its specially designed connection bar, the fragmentation plate can be bent in all three dimensions without deforming the plate holes. The bending pliers with post is used for this bending procedure. The plates can be bent in the horizontal plane with the three-prong bending pliers.

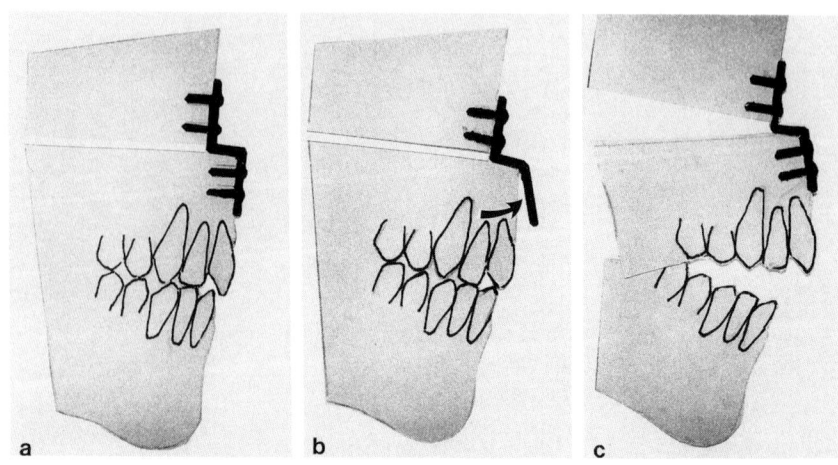

Figure 8.36 (a) When tooth-bearing segments are involved, the plates must be contoured to lie flat against the bone because the shape of the plate will always determine the position of the bone. This is true for fractures of the maxilla and for osteotomies in orthognathic surgery. (b) If the plate is inadequately contoured, the tooth-bearing segment will be pulled toward the plate when the screws are tightened. (c) This will result in an error of the occlusion. This error can also happen when, during plate fixation, the occlusion is ensured by MMF. The whole mandibular–maxillary bloc will be pulled toward the plate and the condyles will be distracted out of the fossa. When IMF is released, the condyles will slip back into their original position. The result is an occlusal error—commonly a frontal open bite.

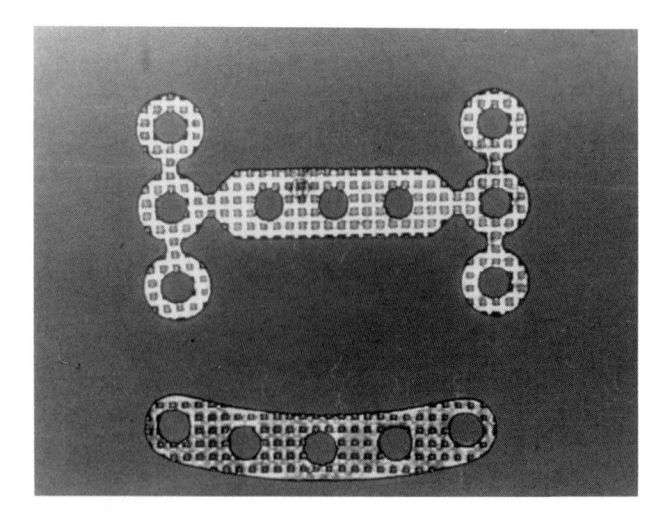

Figure 8.37 Trial templates which are useful in plate contouring. Templates are made of a soft, malleable tin alloy, which can be contoured to the individual bone surface by light finger pressure. The template's shape can be reduplicated on the instrument table.

All these plates show at least one eccentric compression hole, which allows axial compression of the fracture ends (the principle of function is described in Figure 8.5).

Mini-Fixation Plates (Noncompressive Plates)

The Mini-fixation plates were developed for skeletal fixation of maxillary fractures and for orthognathic surgery where axial compression is not desired. The plate thickness of 0.7 millimeter corresponds to the thickness of the Mini-compression plates. Various types of plates (see Figure 8.34), including straight and curved ones, L-type, T-type, and double T-plates, as well as fragmentation plates, provide a wide range of application in craniomaxillofacial surgery. A specially designed connection bar between the plate holes facilitates contouring of the plate in all three dimensions (see Figure 8.35). This allows an optimal adaptation of the plates to the complex structures of the midfacial skeleton.

Principles of Rigid Fixation with the Mini-System

Some of the general principles of rigid fixation have already been mentioned. These principles apply also to rigid fixation in the midfacial skeleton, so we repeat them briefly here and add some remarks of particular importance to midfacial surgery.

Securing the Occlusion When teeth-bearing segments are involved in midfacial trauma, as well as in all cases of orthognathic surgery, the occlusion must be secured during surgery. However, MMF can be released at the end of surgery.

Low-Speed Drilling Because high-speed drilling will cause heat necroses of the bone and—particularly in the thin bones of the midface—may result in an enlargement of the drill hole (due to wobbling of the drill bit), the speed must be reduced to less than 1000 revolutions per minute. We prefer electrically driven power units and reduction dental handpieces.

Selection of the Adequate Plate and Plate Contouring Compression miniplates—as opposed to the noncompressive fixation plates—have a limited, although well established, indication in midfacial surgery. Because of the high degree of rigidity achieved by axial compression of the fracture ends, compression miniplates are preferred in stabilizing the zygoma complex, which is exposed to strong muscle forces. This applies to isolated zygoma fractures as well as to the fixation of the frontozygomatic suture line in complex midfacial fractures. (Further indications are fractures of the condylar neck, the atrophic mandible, and mandibular fractures in children. See the section on variations of the standard surgical technique.)

When tooth-bearing segments are involved in midfacial fractures, and in general in orthognathic surgery, the noncompressive mini-fixation plates should be used in order to avoid errors in the occlusion. The wide range of different types of fixation plates allows the selection of appropriate shape and length to fit the individual situation.

The plate must lay flat against the bone in order to avoid any displacement of segments when the screws are tightened. This is particularly important when tooth-bearing, dentoalveolar segments are involved. Inadequate plate contouring in such a case will result in errors of the occlusion (see Figure 8.36). Trial templates (see Figure 8.37) are available to facilitate this plate contouring. They consist of a soft tin alloy and can be adapted to the bone surface by light digital pressure. The actual osteosynthesis plate then is contoured by means of bending pliers outside the operation field so that it will duplicate the configuration of the template.

When the plate lies flat to bone across the fracture line, the drill holes must be placed in the center of plate holes. This is achieved using the center-drill guide (see Instrumentation). Any drilling off center will result in a shifting of the underlying bone segment, which can cause another error in the occlusion. Every plate should be fixed to each segment by two screws to exclude any rotational movement.

Choice of Implant Material To avoid later implant removal and a second surgical intervention, the implant materials used should be resistant to corrosion. Vitallium and titanium are good choices of implant material.

Indications and Surgical Technique of Rigid Fixation with Miniplates

Craniomaxillofacial Trauma

In the treatment of facial fractures, miniplates offer some substantial advantages over use of wire suspension and interosseous wiring. Miniplates allow a rigid three-dimensional fixation of the skeleton, thus reestablishing the skeletal frame as the basis for facial projection, symmetry, and vertical dimensions. With miniplate fixation, MMF postoperatively can usually be avoided, thus facilitating oral hygiene and being more comfortable for the patient. The renunciation of long-term MMF significantly reduces the overall time of morbidity, making rigid fixation a cost-effective technique. However, there are some disadvantages. Miniplate fixation is more time-consuming and technically more demanding than wire suspension. Additionally, the avoidance of errors in the occlusion in maxillary fractures is more difficult with rigid fixation than with internal wire suspension and long-term MMF.

Zygoma Fractures

Because the zygoma fracture is a quadrapod fracture, at least two (of the total number of four) fracture areas must be exposed when reduction is performed. These are the frontozygomatic suture and the zygomatic buttress. When the fracture lines at these two areas show an exact realignment, the zygoma usually is correctly repositioned. (Note that the correct reduction cannot be recognized when only one fracture line—for example, the frontozygomatic suture—is exposed.) In certain cases a third fracture area at the infraorbital rim needs exposure. This is when comminuted fractures are present or the repair of an orbital floor defect is indicated.

Although we recommend the exposure of the above mentioned areas, this does not mean that all the fracture areas need plate fixation. In common zygoma fractures, a single-point plate fixation at the frontozygomatic suture has proved to be sufficient, presuming that a mini-compression is used (see Figure 8.38). This type of plate results in a much higher degree of rigidity than does a noncompressive fixation plate. In rare cases—mainly when the buttress area is comminuted or the surgeon has doubt concerning the rigidity of a single-point fixation—a second miniplate is placed at the buttress (see Figure 8.39). In cases where an exposure of the orbital floor is indicated or when multiple fragments at the infraorbital rim are present, the second noncompressive mini-fixation plate can be placed infraorbitally (see Figure 8.40). Although these plates are relatively thin, they might be palpable by the patient later on beneath the lower eyelid. Therefore we now prefer a plate of the Micro-Systems in this area (see also the section on the Micro-System in craniomaxillofacial surgery).

Periorbital and Complex Zygoma Fractures

When multiple fragments are present around the orbit, the mini-fragmentation plate is particularly useful. Because it can be contoured three-dimensionally, it can be placed circular around the orbit, thus restoring the outer orbital frame (see Figure 8.41). In complex fractures of the zygoma and the periorbit, an exposure of the arch is required, with realignment of the multiple fragments. Mini-fragmentation plates are placed at the arch and the lateral orbital wall as well as at the lower orbit (see Figure 8.42). The wide exposure and anatomically correct reduction of all the fractures followed by

Figure 8.38 Single point plate fixation of a zygoma fracture. (a) Preoperative x-ray. (b) Postoperative result. The single-point plate fixation at the frontozygomatic suture line is standard procedure today. We prefer a Mini-Compression plate for this technique.

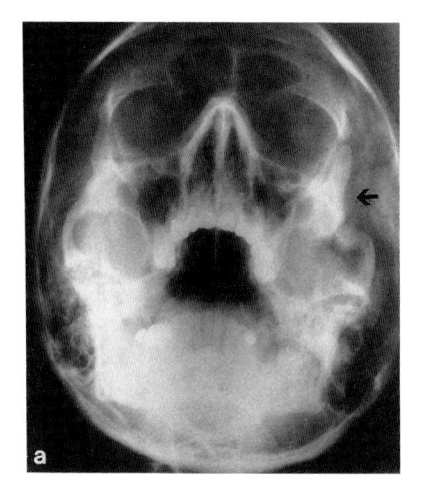

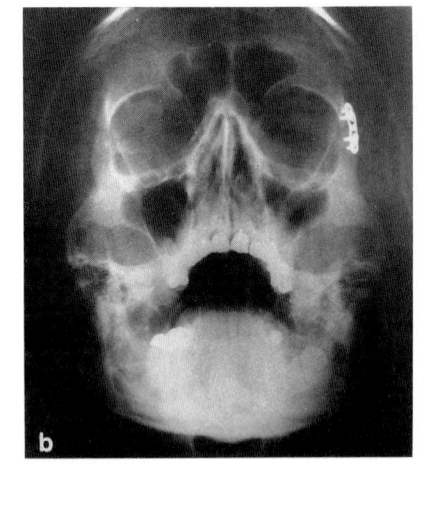

Figure 8.39 Two-point fixation at the frontozygomatic suture line and at the buttress. (a) Displaced zygoma fracture. (b) In addition to the plate at the frontozygomatic suture line, a second plate was placed intraorally at the zygomatic buttress. A two-point fixation is performed when there is any doubt concerning the rigidity achieved by the plate at the lateral orbit.

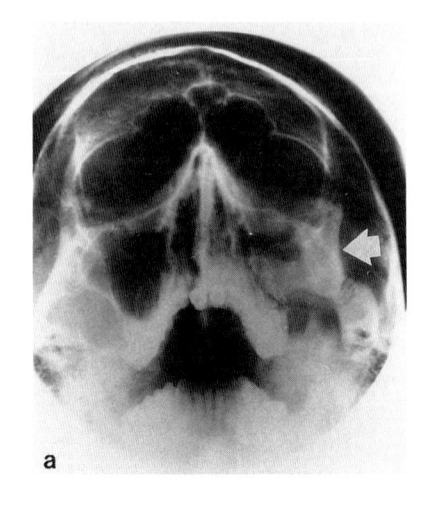

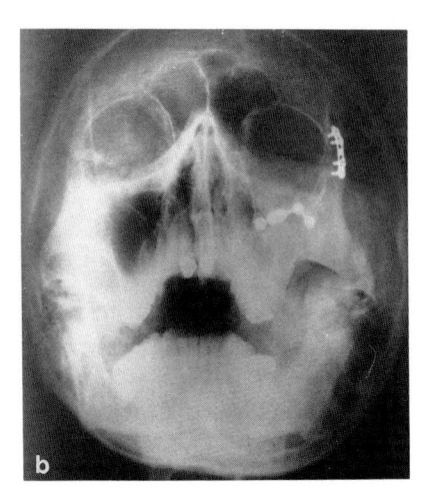

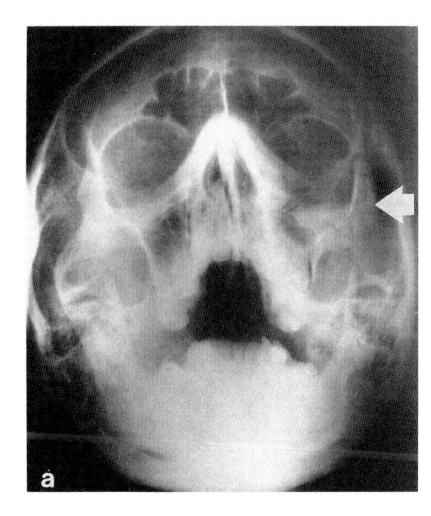

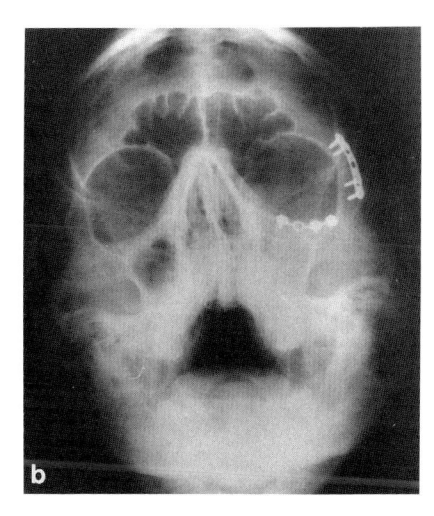

Figure 8.40 (a) Severely displaced fracture of the left zygoma. There was an indication for revision of the orbital floor. (b) In this case, three areas were exposed: the lateral orbit, the infraorbital rim, and the buttress area via an intraoral incision. When the reduction of the displaced zygoma was achieved, the fixation was performed by means of two plates. A compression miniplate was placed at the fronto-zygomatic suture, and a second noncompressive fragmentation miniplate was placed at the infraorbital rim. In the latter area a Microplate could be used instead of a Miniplate.

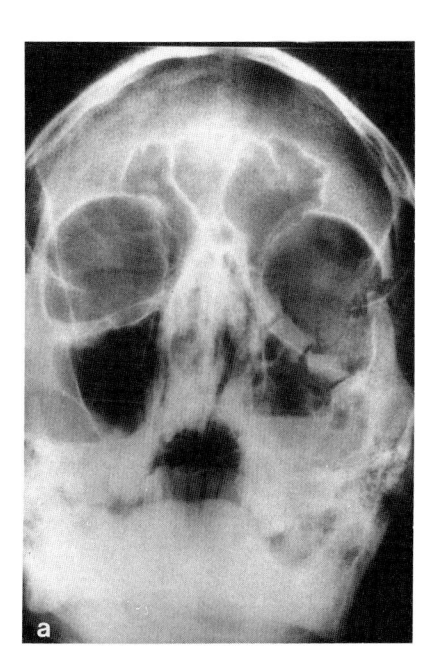

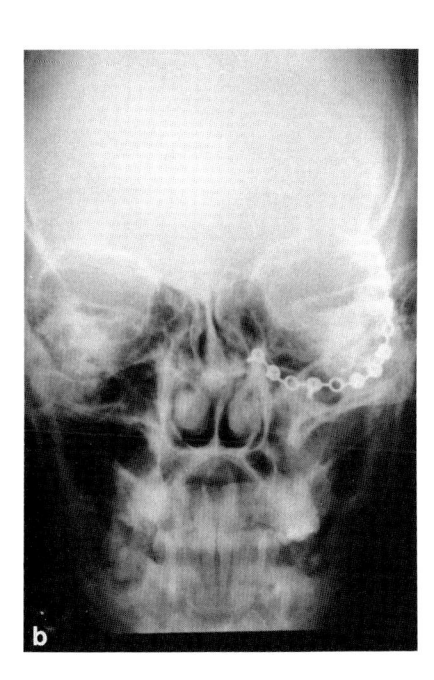

Figure 8.41 (a) Comminuted periorbital and zygomatic fracture. (b) Reconstruction of the outer orbital frame by one minifragmentation plate, which was contoured circularly around the orbit.

rigid plate fixation in all three dimensions of the space are the keys to a normal facial appearance (see Figure 8.42f).

Le Fort Type Fractures

The pattern of midfacial fractures usually does not correspond exactly to the Le Fort classification. Nevertheless, this scheme has proved useful for clinical application. The occlusion is involved in all Le Fort type fractures. It has to be restored and ensured by MMF when rigid plate fixation of the fractures is performed. In Le Fort I fractures, there are four areas where the bone is strong enough to provide a safe anchorage for the screws. These are at both the zygomatic buttresses and along the piriform apertures. L-shaped or slightly curved noncompressive Mini-fixation plates are preferred (see Figure 8.43). During plate fixation, while the mandibular-maxillary complex is rotated upward until bony contact in the fracture lines is achieved, the mandibular condyles should be seated in the fossa (see Figure 8.44). In particular, a distraction of the condyles out of the fossa during rigid fixation—usually unnoticed by the surgeon—will result in an error of the occlusion. When MMF is released at the end of surgery, the displaced condyles will slip back into their normal positions. This will result in a backward and downward rotation of the mandible creating a frontal open bite. To avoid further errors of the occlusion, the plates must be passively laid flat against the bone when crossing the fracture line, and the bone must be predrilled exactly within the centers of the plate holes.

98 RIGID FIXATION OF THE CRANIOMAXILLOFACIAL SKELETON

Figure 8.42 Rigid fixation of complex fractures of the zygoma and the periorbit requires exposure of the zygomatic arch with subsequent plate fixation of all the fragments. (a) X-ray shows severely comminuted fractures of the right zygomatic complex. (b) Postoperative x-ray demonstrates the fixation of the zygomatic arch and the lateral orbit by one long fragmentation plate. Another fragmentation plate stabilizes the lower orbit. There is another plate at the buttress area, and two lag screws were placed at the thicker bones of the central zygoma. (c) After the arch was exposed by a coronal incision, the multiple segments were fixed to the lateral orbit by a long fragmentation plate. (d) An L-shaped minifixation plate stabilizes the buttress area. (e) Another fragmentation plate was placed at the infraorbital rim. The defect of the orbital floor was bridged by a lyophilized dura (any other type of graft or implant may be used). (f) Condition of the patient one year after the accident demonstrates the symmetry of the zygomatic area.

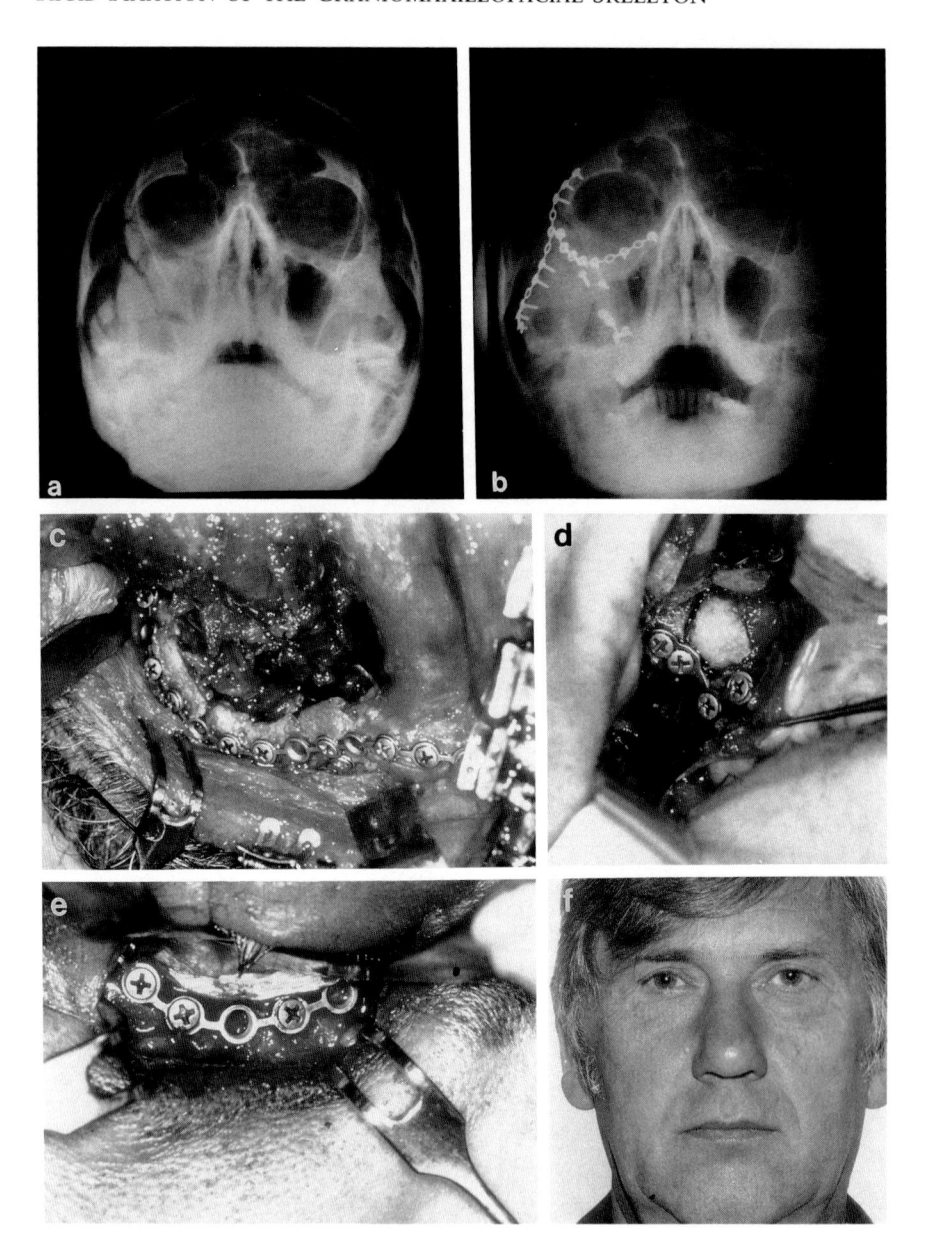

Figure 8.43 Rigid fixation and placement of plates in Le Fort I fractures. (a) L-shaped noncompressive minifixation plates are most frequently used in this type of fracture. Four plates are always needed; they should be placed beside the piriform aperture and at the zygomatic buttresses, where the bone is strong enough to provide safe anchorage for the screws. (b) Slightly curved plates may be used as an alternative for this type of plate fixation.

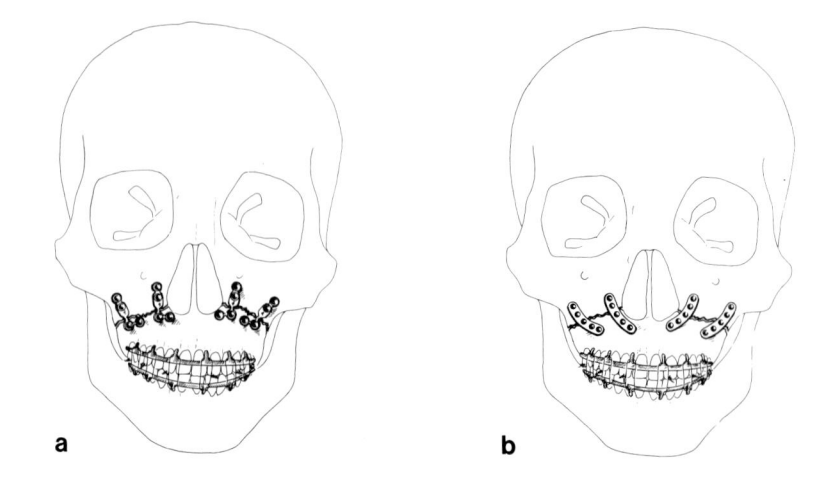

Clinical Applications of the Luhr Vitallium Maxillofacial Systems

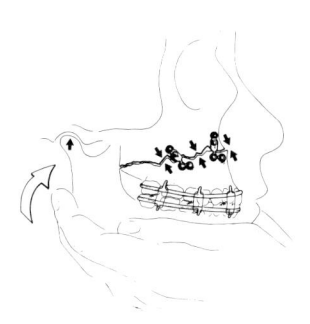

Figure 8.44 During plate fixation of Le Fort type fractures (or Le Fort type osteotomies in orthognathic surgery), any displacement of the TMJ condyles must be avoided. Condyles should be passively seated in the fossa. The application of a light upward and forward pressure on the mandibular angles may be helpful in avoiding condylar displacement during upward rotation of the mandibular–maxillary complex and plate fixation.

In severely comminuted Le Fort I fractures, the fracture line may run so close to the apices of the teeth that it is not possible to place screws in this area. A solution then is to fix the lower end of a plate directly to the upper arch bar (see Figure 8.45). The lower end of the plate is pushed through a stab incision in the gingival flap, thus appearing in the oral cavity. A small platform made of self-curing acrylic resin is placed at the upper arch bar. When the acrylic is hardened, it is predrilled and the plate is fixed there with two common self-tapping screws. Those plates penetrating into the oral cavity, however, will be removed later under local anesthesia when fracture healing is completed (six to eight weeks following surgery). There is usually no need for MMF postoperatively in rigid fixation of Le Fort type fractures. Light guiding elastics only may be useful during a period of eight to ten days.

When additional sagittal fractures of the maxilla are present those miniplates at the buttresses cannot provide sufficient rigidity to maintain the transverse dimension of the hard palate. An additional miniplate placed horizontally beneath the anterior nasal spine adds stability but does not address the stabilization of the posterior aspect of the maxilla. This can be accompanied by a two-hole segment (cut off from the mini-fragmentation plate) and two screws after having the fracture line exposed by dissection of an edge of mucoperiosteum off the fracture margin (Manson 1988). This solution is preferable when immediate treatment of the facial fractures is performed and the services of a dental laboratory are not available. In other cases of delayed treatment (two to four days after an accident), impressions of the jaws are taken and an acrylic palatal splint is manufactured in the lab when the correct occlusion has been established by model surgery. This palatal splint should stay in situ for about six weeks. It is particularly useful in comminuted fractures of the hard palate when plate fixation in this area would be too difficult.

In Le Fort II fractures, the areas of plate application are different. After arch bars are applied in both jaws, the fractures are exposed at both the zygomatic buttresses intraorally and at the infraorbital rims via incisions in the lower eyelid. The reduction of the Le Fort II complex is performed, and the occlusion is ensured by intermaxillary wires. The maxillomandibular complex is rotated upward with close contact at the fracture lines. Noncompressive miniplates are placed at the zygomatic buttresses (L-shaped or slightly curved plates). Finally, miniplates are placed across the fracture line at the infraorbital rims (see Figure 8.46). MMF is

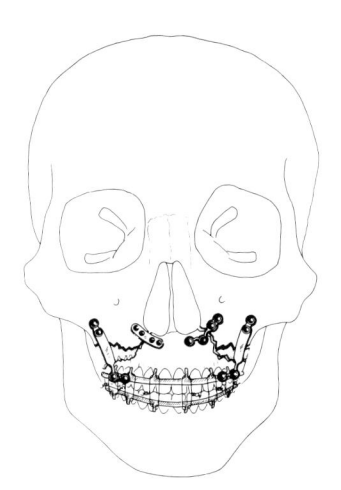

Figure 8.45 When the fracture lines in Le Fort type fractures run close to the apices of the teeth, sometimes it is not possible to place screws at the alveolar segment. In these cases, the lower end of the plate can be pushed through a stab incision in the gingival flap. It can then be fixed directly to a small platform made from self-curing acrylic resin at the upper arch bar. Although those plates are penetrating into the oral cavity, we have not seen any infection. After the fracture heals, plates exposed intraorally must be removed.

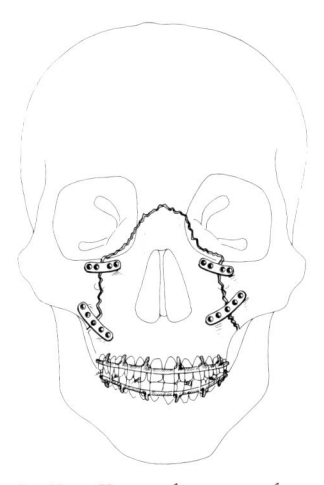

Figure 8.46 In Le Fort II type fractures, four miniplates are placed at the infraorbital rims and the buttress areas.

released and the occlusion is checked. Because classical Le Fort III fractures are extremely rare, we mention only briefly the principle of plate fixation. Miniplates are placed at both the frontozygomatic sutures and across the nasofrontal suture line (presuming the nasal skeleton itself is intact). Additional plate fixation may be required when multiple fractures of the zygomatic arches are present.

Complex Midfacial Fractures

Rigid plate fixation is preferred in the treatment of complex midfacial fractures. These are a combination of different Le Fort type fractures that usually are associated with comminuted fractures of various areas of the facial skeleton. Miniplates allow the three-dimensional reconstruction of the skeleton which is the precondition for an uneventful healing of associated soft-tissue lesions. Wire suspension techniques cannot do this. Wide exposure of all the fracture areas, anatomically exact reduction of the fragments, and their rigid fixation help to achieve the forward projection of the face, to maintain the vertical facial height, and avoid an increase of the facial width. Note that arch bars and MMF must be applied during plate fixation whenever tooth bearing segments of the maxilla are involved. Different types of plates may be used for rigid fixation of those complex fractures (see Figure 8.47).

The sequence of treatment in a case of complex midfacial fractures (with an associated mandibular fracture) is shown in Figure 8.48. After all the fractures are exposed and the mandible is plated, the plate fixation starts with the zygoma and the arch (see Figure 8.48c) followed by the stabilization of the left lower orbit and naso-ethmoidal area. Only when the upper third of the facial skeleton is completely stabilized is the maxilla rigidly fixed by four mini-fixation plates (see Figure 8.48d). At the end of surgery MMF is released (see Figure 8.48e), which is of a great advantage particularly in polytraumatized patients. A soft solid diet is recommended for a couple of weeks. Figures 8.48f and g demonstrate the final result of treatment.

Miniplates in Orthognathic Surgery

Rigid fixation has gained increasing popularity for use in orthognathic surgery in the last ten years. The advantages of plate and screw fixation of osteotomized segments are obvious. The benefits for the patient consist of the avoidance of postoperative maxillomandibular immobilization including free movement of the mandible, avoidance of airway problems in the acute phase after surgery, the maintenance of oral hygiene, the possibility of uptake of a soft solid diet, a reduced hospital stay, and a shorter time of overall morbidity. Postsurgical orthodontic treatment can start earlier—usually four weeks after surgery. These factors may positively influence the patients decision to undergo this kind of elective surgery.

In orthognathic surgery the use of plates and screws, however, demands a greater precision than do wiring techniques. Because in all cases of orthognathic surgery toothbearing segments are involved, any errors in rigid plate fixation will result in errors of the occlusion, which are difficult (if not impossible) to correct by orthodontic procedures later on. To avoid these errors the following principles should be regarded:

1. Axial compression in orthognathic surgery is not indicated. It may lead to an uncontrolled shortening at the osteotomy site and result in an undesired shifting or tilting of the toothbearing segments. Therefore the use of noncompressive mini-fixation plates is recommended.

2. In orthognathic surgery usually toothbearing segments need to be moved in a three-dimensional direction. This results in steps, and frequently gaps, at the osteotomy site. It is essential to contour the plate until it fits passively to the bone surface of both the segments when bridging the osteotomy line, thus maintaining these gaps and steps. When the plate is not lying flush to the bone, the toothbearing segment will be pulled toward the plate when the screws are tightened. This uncontrolled movement will result in an error of the occlusion (see Figure 8.36). To facilitate this exact plate contouring, the use of trial templates is recommended (see Figure 8.37).

3. It is mandatory to ensure the occlusion by MMF during the placement of plates and screws. The use of occlusal splints is recommended.

4. The maintenance of the TMJ condyle position is another key point in orthognathic surgery, particu-

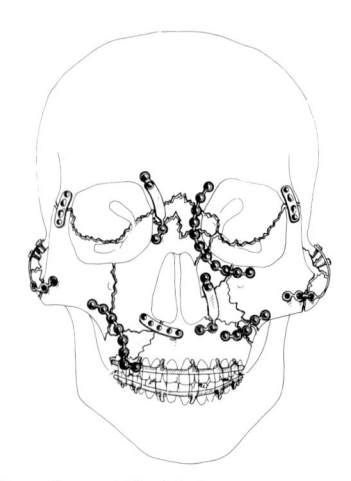

Figure 8.47 Complex midfacial fractures require a wide exposure of each fracture. The fractures are fixed by different types of miniplates. Note that the only areas where mini-compression plates are used are the frontozygomatic sutures. All the other fractures are stabilized by noncompressive fixation plates.

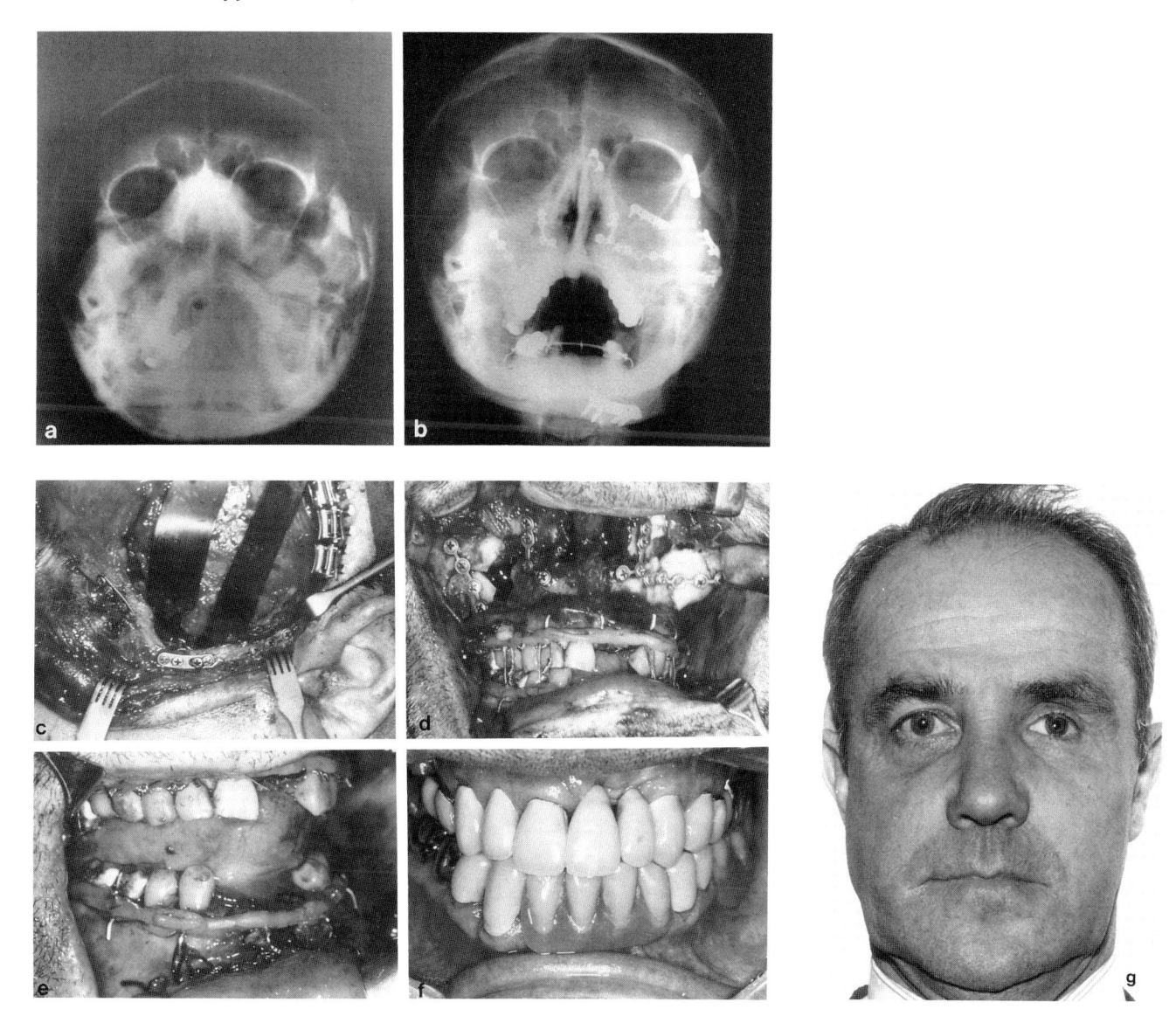

larly when rigid fixation is used. Any displacement of the condylar head during surgery, as well as the fixation of the proximal segment in a wrong position, will result in an error of the occlusion. This happens when the condyles slip back to their original position after MMF has been released. To avoid these errors, the condylar positioning technique for sagittal split ramus osteotomies described by Luhr (1985a, 1989) and the position control technique in maxillary osteotomies (Luhr and Kubein-Meesenburg 1989) is recommended.

Sagittal Split Ramus Osteotomy of the Mandible

Although most surgeons today use a fixation of the sagittal split ramus osteotomy (SSRO) with bicortical screws (usually three screws applied in a noncompressive mode—that is, not as lag screws), we prefer

Figure 8.48 Rigid fixation of complex midfacial fractures. (a) Complex midfacial fractures (comminuted Le Fort I type fracture with comminuted fractures of the left zygomatic area and periorbit). (b) Postoperative x-ray demonstrates the different types of plates in various areas (an additional mandibular fracture was stabilized by an MCS plate). (c) After all fractures have been exposed, the reduction of the zygoma and the arch was performed, followed by plate fixation. Further plates were placed around the lower orbit and at the naso-ethmoidal area. (d) Only when the upper part of the face was rigidly fixed is the maxilla stabilized by various fixation plates. By reduction of multiple displaced small bone fragments and subsequent plate fixation, the supporting pillars of the maxilla are reconstructed. Note that during plate fixation the occlusion is ensured by arch bars and intermaxillary fixation. (e) At the end of surgery, when rigid fixation is achieved, MMF can be released and the occlusion can be checked. (f) Final result after a prosthodontic rehabiliation. (g) Condition of the patient one year after the accident. The patient, who lost his left eye, has to wear an artificial one.

Figure 8.49 Fixation of a sagittal split ramus osteotomy with a noncompressive miniplate and monocortical screws. Note that in SSRO, because of the parabolic shape of the mandible, steps and gaps frequently arise between the two segments. To avoid displacement of the condyle, these steps and gaps should be maintained. Note that the miniplate is bent to follow the steplike bone contour. A prefabricated acrylic wafer and guiding, or training, elastics are used. The elastics and the wafer can be removed by the patient during meals. A soft solid diet is recommended for the first three to four weeks.

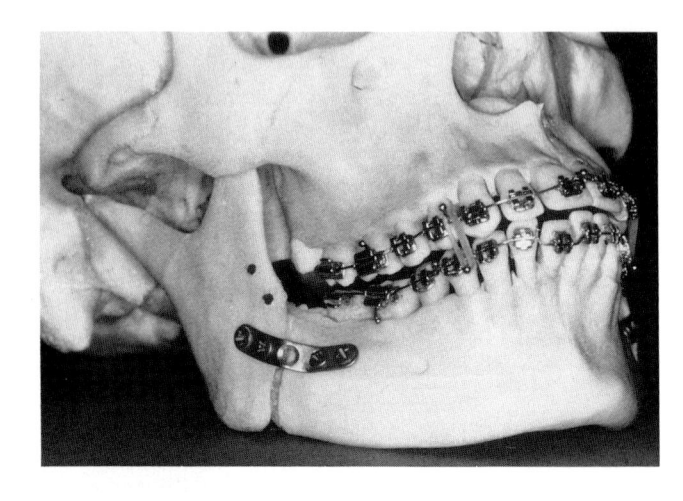

Figure 8.50 Correction of a mandibular prognathism by sagittal split ramus osteotomy and plate fixation.
(a) Preoperative occlusion (multiple teeth had been extracted previously elsewhere). (b) Final occlusion following SSRO, orthodontic treatment, and prosthodontic rehabilitation. (c and d) Preoperative and postoperative profiles of the patient. (e and f) The intraoperative pictures show the positioning plates (upper L-shaped plates) connecting the ascending ramus with the platform of the occlusal splint. Because the occlusal splint will not change its position with regard to the maxilla, the connection of the splint to the ascending ramus maintains the exact preoperative position of both condyles. The lower plates are bridging the osteotomy. These plates are carefully contoured to the sometimes steplike configuration of the bone surfaces and are fixed by monocortical screws. Note that during plate fixation, the occlusion is ensured by MMF and an additional occlusal splint. (g and h) The positioning plates are removed, and MMF is released. The occlusion can be checked. (For further details see Luhr 1989a.)

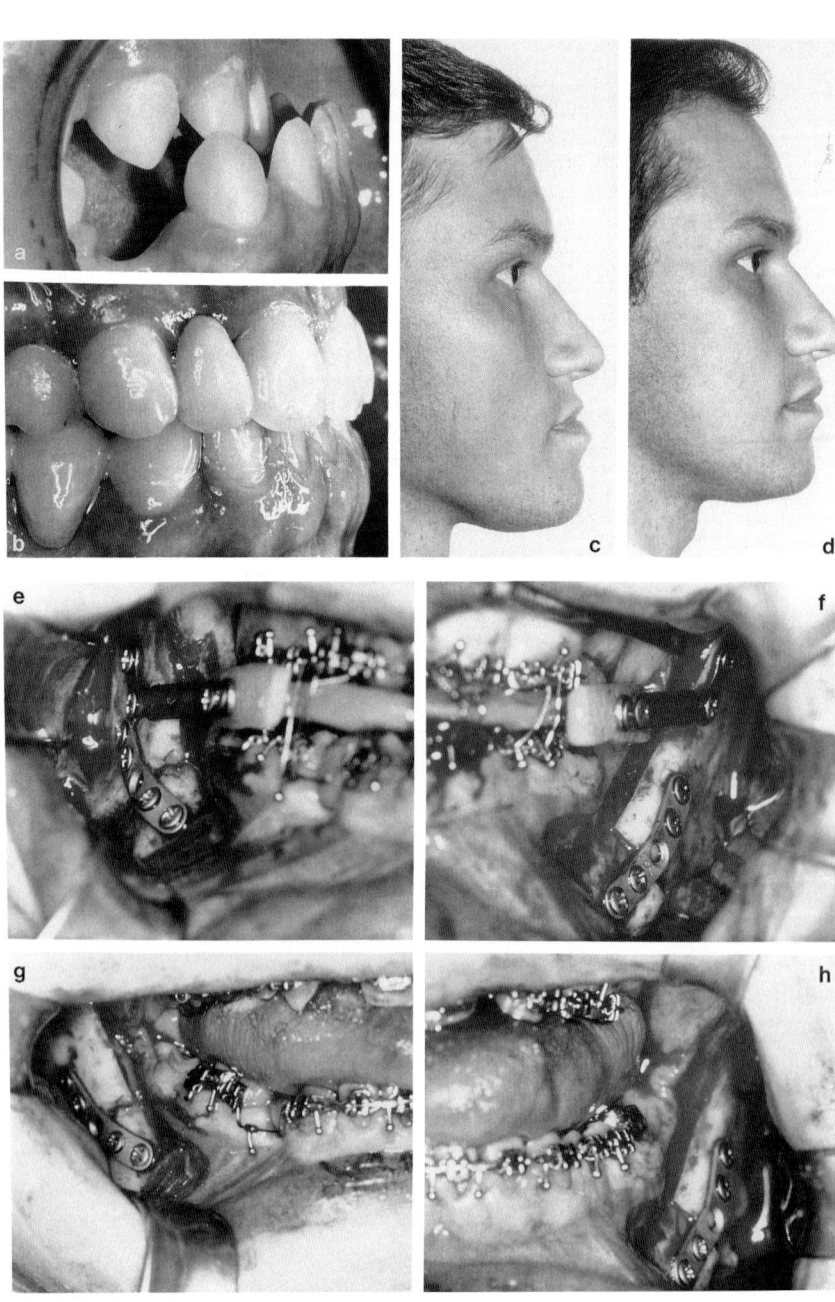

plate fixation with monocortical screws (see Figure 8.49). Using an exactly contoured and passively applied noncompressive miniplate, it is easier to avoid any displacement of the proximal segment and the condyle. Although this technique seems not to be as rigid as bicortical screw fixation is, we have never observed a delayed healing or a nonunion in our series. The sagittal split osteotomy offers completely different conditions for bone healing from those offered by mandibular fractures, where we strongly recommended the stronger compression plates and bicortical screw fixation. In the SSRO two broad spongious bone surfaces are present with an enormous osteogenetic potential resulting in a very fast bone healing. Furthermore the majority of orthognatic surgery patients are young adults, in whom bone regeneration is rapid. The use of an occlusal splint (wafer) and guiding elastics postoperatively prevents uncontrolled stress to the osteotomy site. Last but not least, orthognathic surgery patients usually have a much better compliance than mandibular fracture patients have. These factors together make even a monocortical plate fixation successful in SSRO.

A case of a combined orthodontic and surgical treatment of a mandibular prognathism illustrates this technique (see Figure 8.50). To facilitate screw insertion at the posterior part of the mandible, and in order to avoid a transbuccal approach, a 90° screwdriver was developed (see Figure 8.51). The bone is predrilled with a common, right-angle dental handpiece, the 90° screwdriver serves for screw insertion.

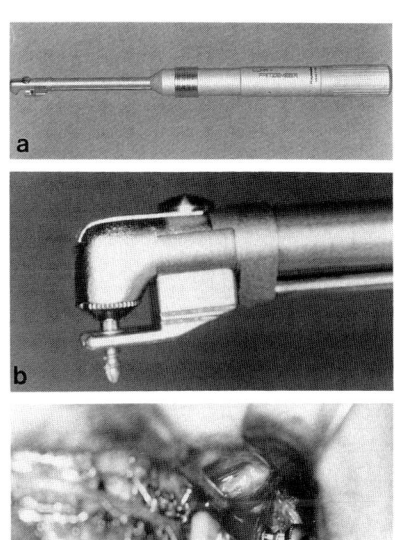

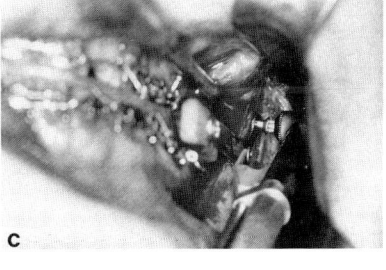

Figure 8.51 The 90° screwdriver issued to insert screws in the posterior parts of the oral cavity. (a) The screwdriver consists of a turnable handle (right part of the instrument) and the screwdriver head, which holds a very short screwblade. A screw-holding device can be shifted forward (when it holds the screw) and must be retracted before the screw is finally tightened. (b) Detail of the screwdriver head with the screw-holding device and a miniscrew. (c) A screw is inserted at the ascending ramus of the mandible. The screw-holding device is retracted before the screw is tightened.

Mini-Fixation Plates in Maxillary Osteotomies

The Mini-Fixation System is particularly useful in rigid fixation of Le Fort I osteotomies. Self-tapping screws are the key to plate fixation in the thin bones of the maxilla. Plates and screws should be placed beside the piriform apertures and at the zygomatic buttresses, where the bone is strong enough to provide a safe anchorage. Low-speed drilling is essential to avoid wobbling of the drill bit. Wobbling might enlarge the drill hole and risks stripping the screw. If a screw is stripped, a so-called "emergency screw," with its greater diameter (see the section on screws), will provide a safe anchorage. In Le Fort I osteotomies the application of four plates is recommended (each plate is fixed by four screws). L-shaped fixation plates with 90° or 110° angles are particularly useful in the maxilla. Because of their thinner connecting bars between the holes they can be more easily adapted to the irregular bone surfaces that result from three-dimensional movements of maxillary segments. Another type of fixation plate, the slightly curved one, is frequently used. During plate fixation MMF is mandatory, and the use of prefabricated occlusal splints is recommended. In maxillary osteotomies, the TMJ condyles may be displaced when the mandibular-maxillary bloc is rotated upward until optimal contact is achieved at the osteotomy site. During this maneuver and when the plates are applied it is important to make sure that both the condyles are passively seated in the fossa by applying a light upward and forward pressure to both of the mandibular angles (see Figure 8.44). Because the condyle's position is not easily controlled, we use the "position control technique"; for further details refer to the article by Luhr and Kubein-Meesenburg (1989). A typical case illustrates rigid plate fixation of a Le Fort I osteotomy (see Figure 8.52). With similar techniques any type of midfacial osteotomy can be stabilized by mini-fixation plates. According to the fixation techniques described above, these techniques are applied also in bimaxillary surgery. An example is shown in Figure 8.53.

In genioplasty, rigid fixation by plates and screws is favored. There are some variations in fixation techniques of the smaller distal segment, which has to be moved in a certain direction depending on the requirements of the individual case. We prefer either the lag

Figure 8.52 Rigid fixation of Le Fort I osteotomy for correction of an open bite and a long face deformity. (a) Preoperative cephalometric x-ray shows the typical soft-tissue contour of a long face. (b) Postoperative cephalometric x ray following Le Fort I osteotomy with intrusion of the maxilla and genioplasty (vertical reduction and advancement). (c and d) Preoperative and postoperative views of the patient demonstrating the harmonization of the facial proportions. (e) Drawing of the osteotomy lines. The intermediate section (posteriorly 6 millimeters, anteriorly 4 millimeters) will be removed. (f) Rigid plate fixation after intrusion of the maxilla. An over-intrusion of the maxilla can be avoided, with this technique; it cannot be avoided with use of internal wiring. There is no need for bone grafts. (g and h) Preoperative and postoperative occlusion.

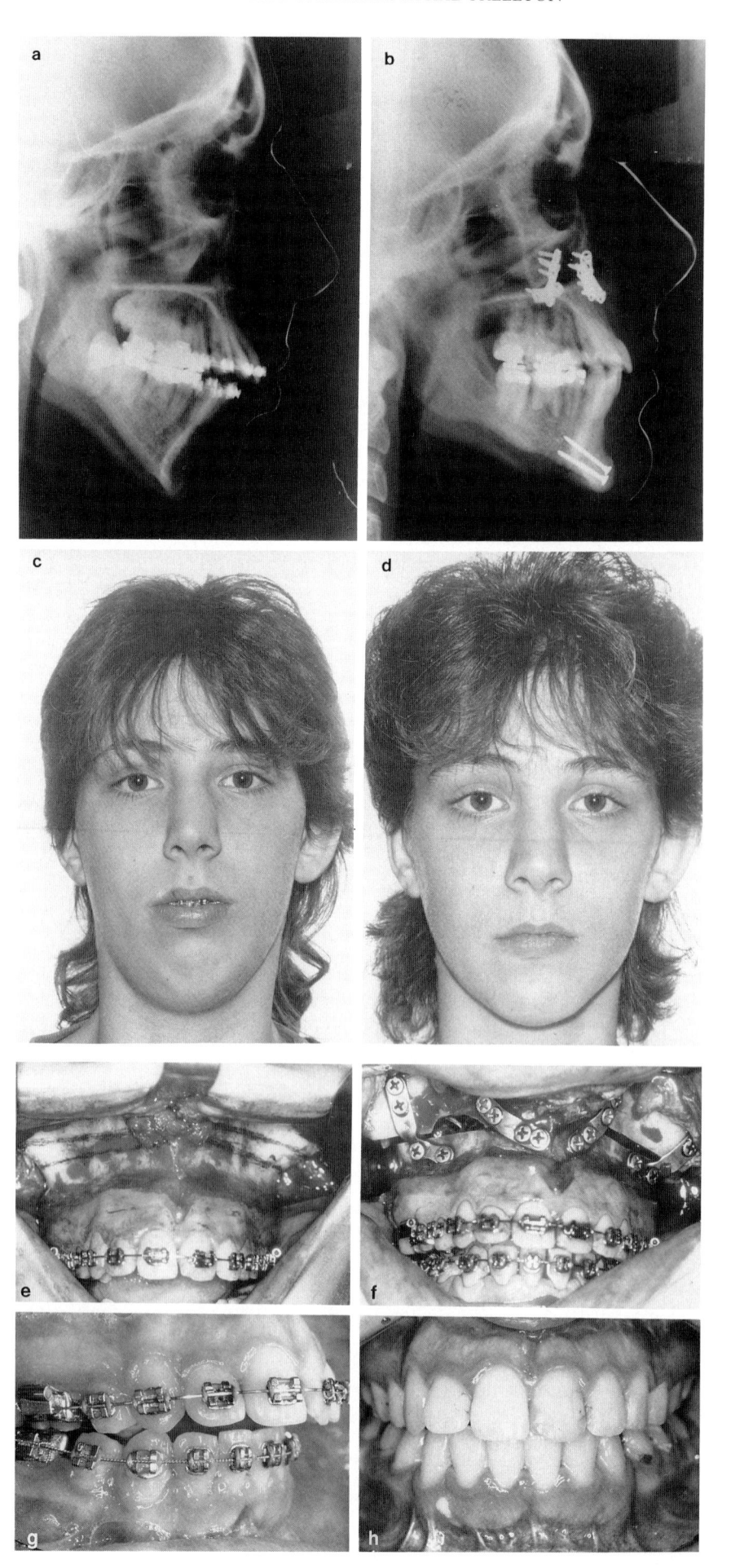

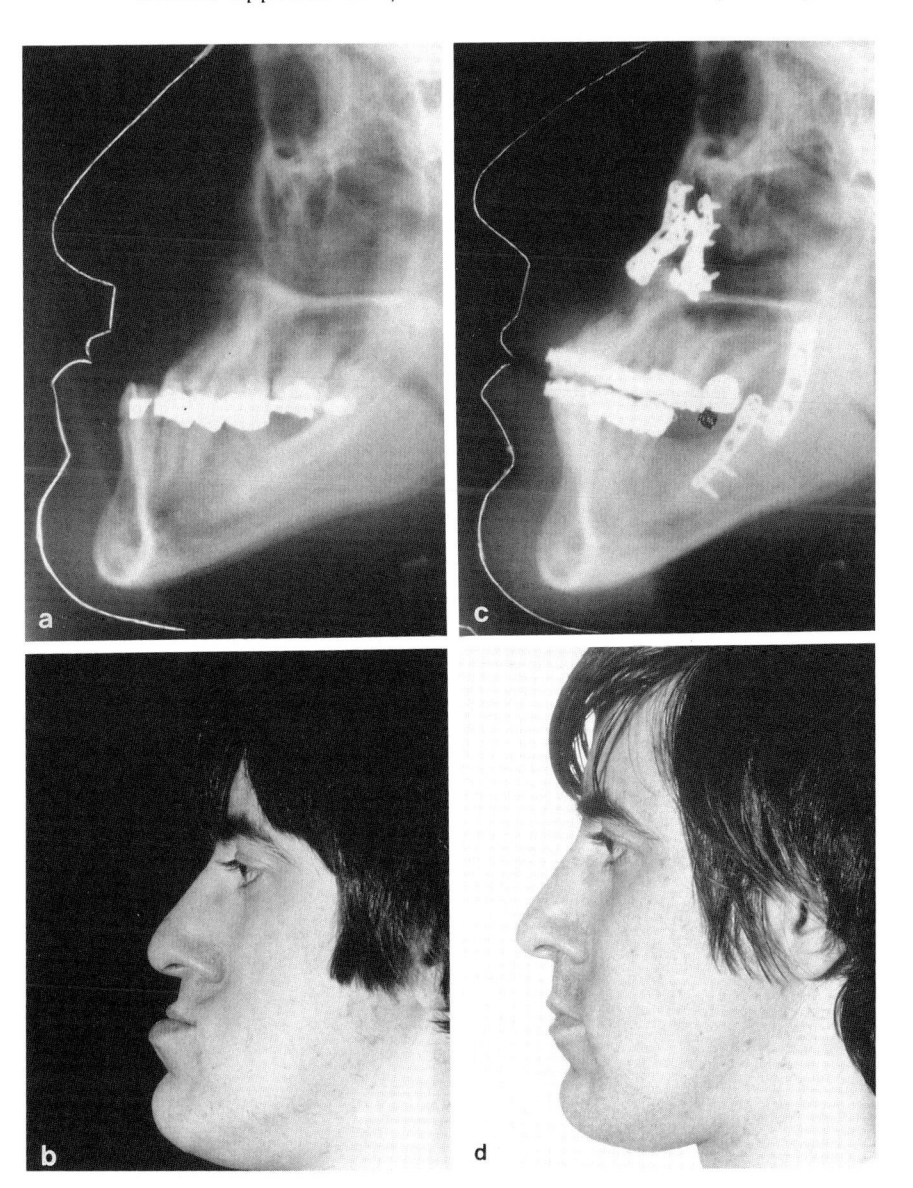

Figure 8.53 Rigid plate fixation in bimaxillary osteotomies. (a) Cephalometric x-ray showing maxillary retrusion and a mandibular prognathism. (b) Postoperative cephalometric x-ray after advancement of the maxilla and mandibular setback. Plate fixation of the Le Fort I osteotomy and the SSRO. No MMF was needed postoperatively. (c and d) Preoperative and postoperative profiles of the patient. (e) The preoperative occlusion with a sagittal step of 12 millimeters. (f) Occlusion after surgery and final orthodontic treatment.

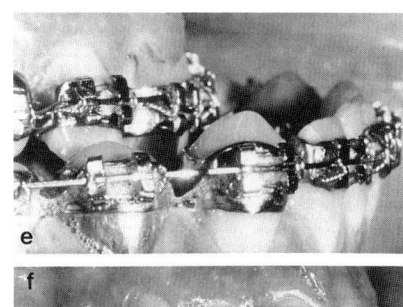

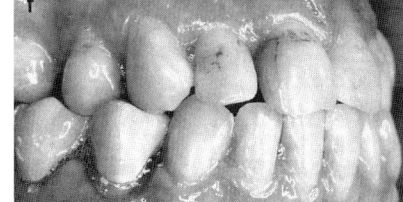

screw technique (see Figure 8.54a) or plate and screw fixation in the manner shown in Figure 8.54e–f.

In particular, the fixation with two 2-hole plates cut off from a longer fragmentation plate (see Figure 8.55) is a very fast and simple technique. When vertical lengthening of the chin with an interpositional graft is required, plate sections of three or more holes are used. The technique can easily be modified according to the requirements of the individual case. The versatility of this fixation technique is demonstrated in a case of a major advancement genioplasty (see Figure 8.56).

In orthognathic surgery, rigid fixation by minifixation plates has advantages over wiring techniques. These are (1) stabilization of moved skeletal segments in a three-dimensional manner with a significantly reduced need for bone grafts, (2) the renunciation of maxillomandibular fixation postoperatively (only training or guiding elastics are recommended, together with an orthodontic wafer), and (3) a reduced period of hospital stay and overall morbidity. However, rigid fixation in orthognathic surgery is technically more demanding and less forgiving than internal wiring is. It requires careful preoperative planning in close cooperation with an experienced orthodontist, the realization of the relationship between the TMJ and the occlusion, and, last but not least, some experience with plate and screw fixation.

THE MICRO SYSTEM IN CRANIOMAXILLOFACIAL SURGERY

Relatively large plates and screws are needed to stabilize those bones of the facial skeleton which are exposed to remarkable muscle traction and masticatory forces. This applies mainly to fractures and osteotomies of the mandible, the zygoma, and the maxilla. Numerous areas of the complex craniofacial skeleton, how-

Figure 8.54 (a) Different fixation techniques in genioplasty. The lag screw technique for the fixation of the distal segment in genioplasty. The distal segment has to be predrilled with a lag screw drill that shows the exact outside diameter of the screw. The proximal (tooth-bearing) segment is predrilled in the usual manner. Make sure that the inner cortex of this segment is perforated by the drill and that the screw sits firmly within this cortical bone. Depth gauging is required to determine the length of the screw. Screws of 16 or 19 millimeters length are usually required. (b) The lag screw technique is not suitable when interpositional hydroxy-apatite (HA) blocs are required for lengthening of the chin in the vertical dimension. When the screw is tightened, the hydroxy-apatite block frequently cracks. (c) Plate fixation of the genioplasty segment. A miniplate is contoured to form a double right angle, and it is fixed by monocortical screws. Because one end of the plate is fixed to the prominence of the chin, screws and plate may be palpable by the patient later on. This may require plate removal and a second intervention. (d) Example of an advancement genioplasty fixed by this type of plate fixation. (e) Fixation of the genioplasty segment by two-hole plates. The profile drawing shows that the upper screw is a short monocortical one. The screw in the distal segment must be long enough to be anchored in the cortical basis of the small segment. Because screw anchorage within the spongious part of the small segment is impossible, make sure that your screw sits firmly in the basal cortical bone. Depth gauging is required. Usually screws of 12 or 14 millimeters length are needed in this area. (f) Two of the two-hole plates are placed symmetrically left and right about 1.5 to 2 cm beside the midline in advancement genioplasty. The two-link plates are cut off from the mini-fragmentation plate (see Figure 8.55). This technique of fixation is fast and simple and does not have the disadvantage of palpating any plate or screws later on at the prominence of the chin.

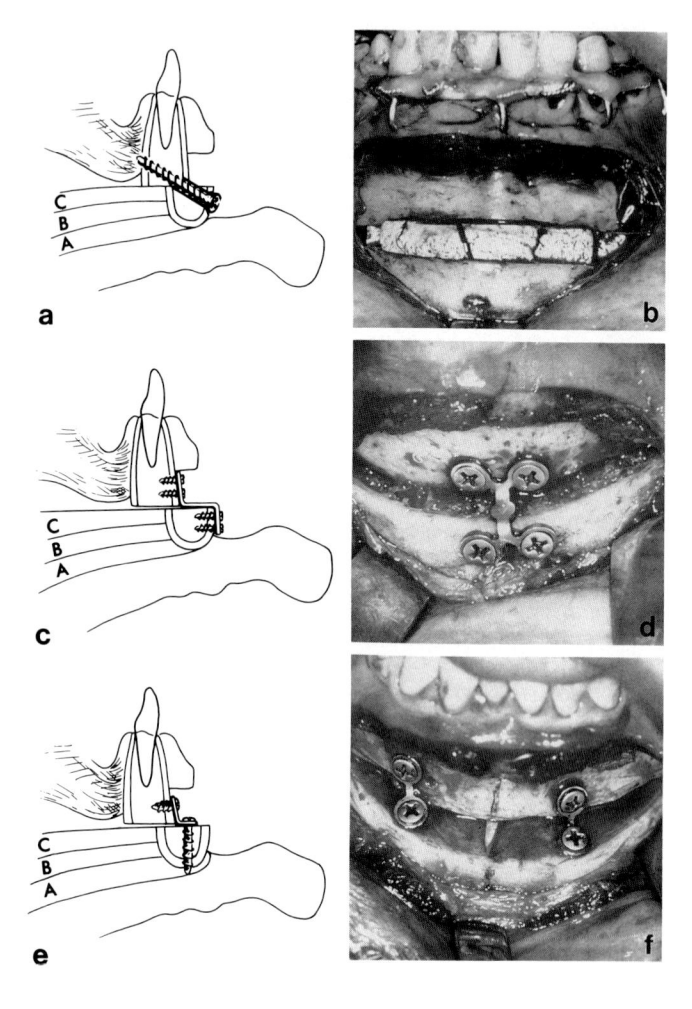

Figure 8.55 (a) Two links (or more if necessary) are cut from the mini-fragmentation plate using a plate cutter. (b) The plate is bent to a right angle and then placed as described in Figure 8.54 (e and f).

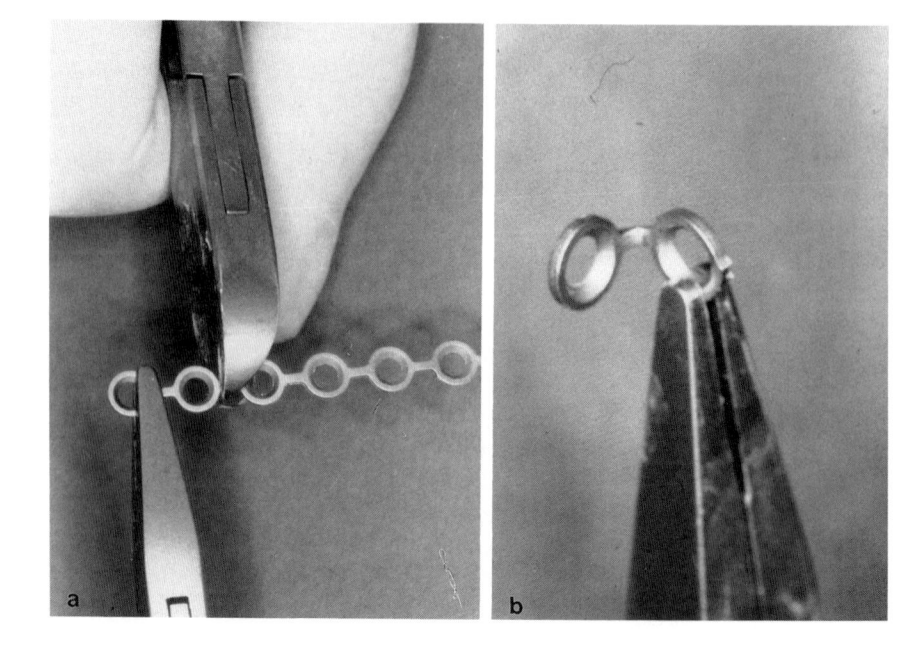

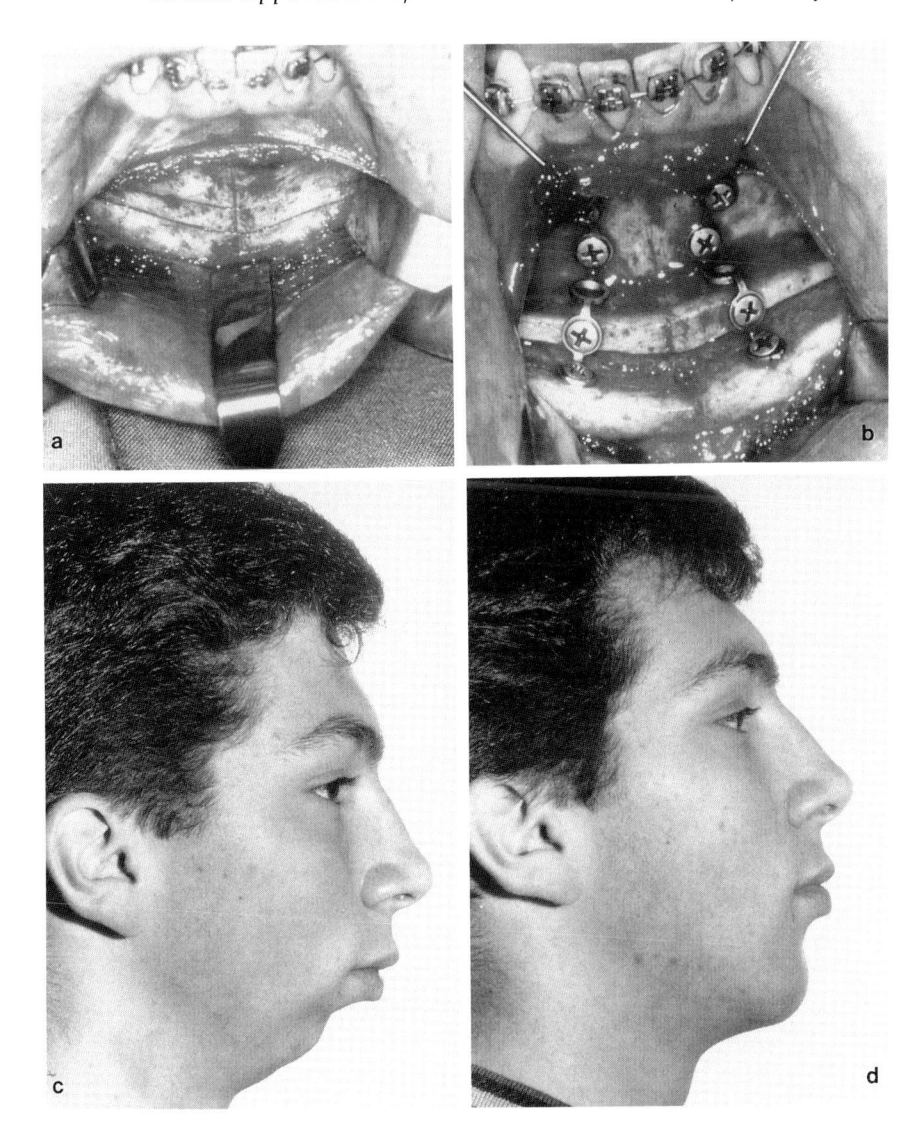

Figure 8.56 The versatility of rigid fixation using the fragmentation plate is demonstrated in a two-step advancement genioplasty of 2 centimeters. (a) Two segments are precisely cut by a reciprocating saw. (b) Each of the two broad, pedicled segments is advanced. The intermediate segment was moved forward 10 millimeters, the lower segment 20 millimeters. Using a trial template, a section of five holes was cut from a longer fragmentation plate and carefully contoured, following the double steplike configuration. Both the anterior screws in the lower segment required a length of 14 millimeters to be safely anchored in the basal cortical bone. All the other screws are monocortical screws 6 millimeters in length. In spite of the remarkable muscle traction acting on the lower segment, the fixation was solid. (c and d) Preoperative view and result after correction of a significant chin deficiency and advancement genioplasty of 2 centimeters.

ever, consist of very thin bones that are not exposed to any of these muscle actions or masticatory forces. In these areas the scale of miniplates is too great.

In particular, when placed under the thin skin of the naso-ethmoidal area or used in infant craniofacial surgery, the miniplates can be palpated by the patient (or the parents) later on. This has frequently caused complaints. These facts led to the development of a Micro-System with plates and screws of markedly smaller dimensions than the common plating systems (see Figure 8.57).

Specifications of the Micro-System

Because of its superior physical properties and its resistance to corrosion, Vitallium, a cobalt-chromium-molybdenum alloy, is particularly suitable for the manufacturing of very small but remarkably strong implants. Thus the Microplates are only 0.5 millimeter thick. The flat screw heads fit the countersink of the plate holes, resulting in a very low plate–screw profile.

Due to the special design of the connecting bars between the plate holes and the ductility of the alloy itself, the plates can be contoured in all three dimensions without the plate holes becoming deformed (see Figure 8.58). Thus the plates can be adapted to virtually all of the most irregular bone surfaces of the facial skeleton.

Microplates and Micromesh

The different types and lengths of Microplates are shown in Figure 8.59. The straight plates come in lengths of 14, 22, 30, 40, 60, and 90 millimeters. If plates of different length are required during surgery, they can be cut off from any of the longer ones by means of a special plate cutter. T-shaped plates are available in lengths of 14 and 22 millimeters. L-shaped plates with the plate holes countersunk on both sides can be used as either left or right ones. They come in lengths of 14 and 22 millimeters. H-shaped plates of 7, 10, and 18 millimeters have proved to be particularly useful in fixation of bone grafts in infant craniofacial surgery. Soft,

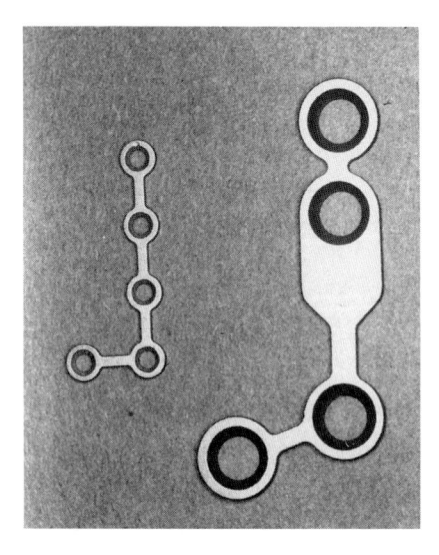

Figure 8.57 Microplates (left) are remarkably smaller than the common miniplates (right).

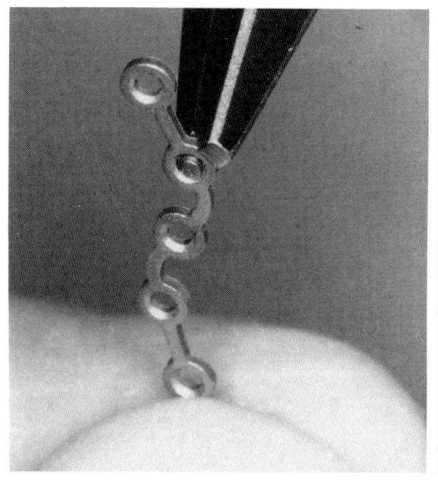

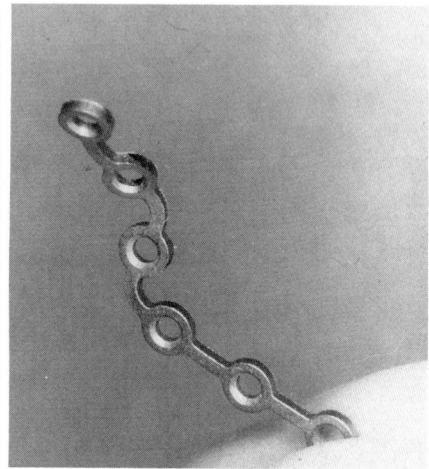

Figure 8.58 Due to the special design of the connecting bars between the plate holes, microplates can be contoured in the horizontal plane. Micro-bending pliers with a post is used to facilitate bending in the horizontal plane. Microplates can be contoured to any of the irregular bone structures of the midfacial skeleton without deforming the plate holes.

malleable templates (see Figure 8.60) made of a tin alloy can be adapted to any individual bone surface merely by light finger pressure. They serve as a model for contouring of the actual Vitallium Microplate outside the surgical site on the instrument table. The selection of plates is completed by a Micromesh (see Figure 8.61). In spite of its reduced thickness—only 0.3 millimeter—the Micromesh is remarkably strong. To keep the mesh–screw profile as low as possible, the holes at the cross points of the connection bars are countersunk. The Micromesh is available in sizes of 40 by 60 and 60 by 100 millimeters. Templates made of a soft, malleable tin alloy come in corresponding sizes. The template is cut to the shape and size required in the individual case. Then it is contoured to the bone surface (at the margins of the defect when bridging is required) merely by light finger pressure. The actual Vitallium Micromesh is then cut out with a wire cutter and contoured on the instrument table, reduplicating the individual shape of the template. A special bending pliers helps to contour the mesh to a concave shape (see Figure 8.62).

Screws and Drill Bits

The screws are self-tapping ones of 0.8-millimeter diameter. Two cutting flutes (see Figure 8.63) facilitate screw insertion. Although Microscrews show a significantly smaller torque load than the common 2.0-millimeter-diameter screws, tests have demonstrated a remarkable holding power (see Figure 8.64). The Microscrews come in lengths of 2, 3, 4, 5, 6, and 8 millimeters. An emergency screw of a slightly larger diameter (1.0 millimeter) can be used when one of the 0.8-millimeter standard screws has been stripped in the bone. The bone is usually predrilled with a 0.5-millimeter-diameter drill when screws of 2 or 3 millimeters in length

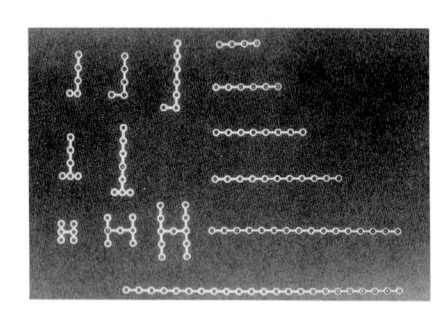

Figure 8.59 Different types and lengths of microplates.

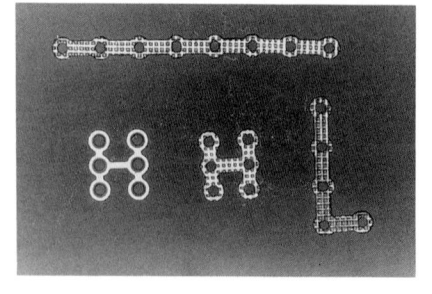

Figure 8.60 Templates made of a soft, malleable tin alloy have a gridded surface. The surface structure makes it easy to distinguish the templates from the original Vitallium plates (lower left).

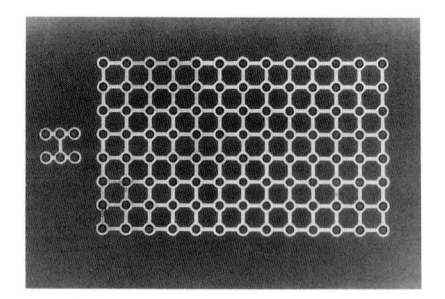

Figure 8.61 The micromesh of 0.3 millimeter thickness. The micromesh is compared to the size of the smallest micro H-plate.

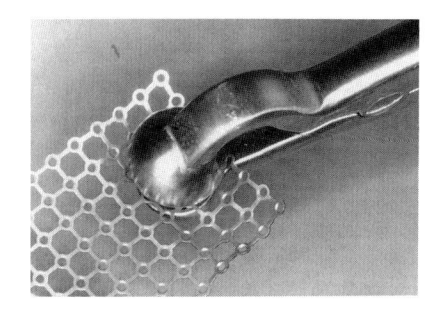

Figure 8.62 The micromesh can be contoured to a concave shape with a special bending pliers.

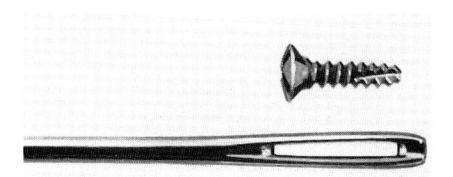

Figure 8.63 Self-tapping microscrew (0.8-millimeter diameter) compared to the size of the eye of a needle. One of the two cutting flutes is visible.

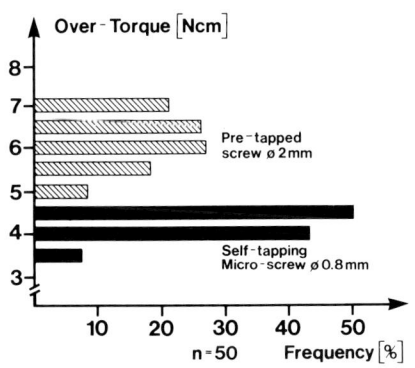

Figure 8.64 This diagram shows the over-torque (Ncm) of the 0.8-millimeter microscrews compared to pretapped common 2-millimeter diameter screws. The over-torque is a parameter for the holding power of a screw. The test was performed with a test sheet of 1 millimeter thickness (PVC test material) and 50 screws from each type. The mean holding power of the microscrews—about 4.5 Ncm—is remarkably high compared to the mean holding power of the large pretapped 2-centimeter screw (mean value about 6.5 Ncm).

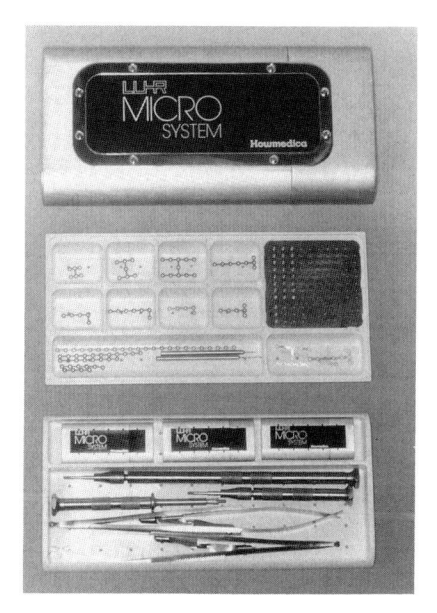

Figure 8.66 The sterilizable box for microplates and screws contains two trays. The upper tray (middle) holds the different types of plates, the templates, and the screws. The other tray houses the standard instruments.

are used. The length of this drill bit is 3 millimeters; it has a stop at the shaft to prevent penetration of the underlying tissue structures. The use of a slightly larger drill, of 0.6-millimeter diameter, is recommended when longer screws (4, 5, 6, or 8 millimeters in length) are used, particularly when cortical bone is present. This larger drill hole will reduce the strong friction forces (which increase with the length of the screw), thus facilitating screw insertion and preventing screw breakage. These 0.6-millimeter-diameter drills come in lengths of 5 and 11 millimeters. Another drill, with diameter of 0.8 millimeter (which corresponds exactly to the outside diameter of the Microscrews), is used for drilling a larger hole through the outer cortex or through an onlay bone graft when applying the lag screw technique. All of these drill bits are available for straight handpieces (drill shafts with the international standard diameter of 2.35 millimeters) as well as for 90° dental handpieces. To facilitate identification of the different drill diameters, the drill shafts are color coded: Red is for 0.5 millimeter, blue for 0.6 millimeter, and green for 0.8 millimeter (this is the lag screw drill). In clinical practice, both the straight and the 90° handpiece are needed. When there is a wide exposure (for example, in infant craniofacial surgery) we prefer the 90° handpiece, which gives a better balance. The straight handpiece usually is required at the naso-ethmoidal area, the infraorbital rim, and the lateral sinus walls.

Instrumentation

Miniaturized instruments, such as plate-bending pliers, plate- and screw-holding clamps, screwdrivers of different lengths, and a plate cutter, were developed to fit the special requirements of the small dimensions of the implants. A self-retaining screwdriver (see Figure 8.65) picks up the Microscrews from the screw rack and inserts them directly into the drill hole, thus speeding up the surgical procedure. Plates and screws, drill bits, and the basic instruments are housed in two trays of a sterilizable box (see Figure 8.66).

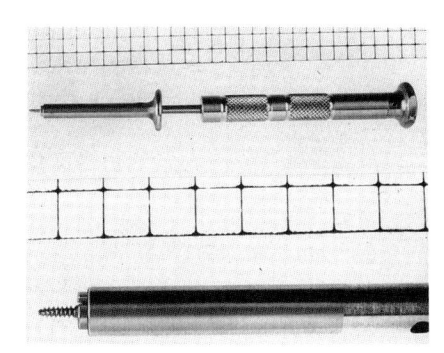

Figure 8.65 The self-retaining micro-screwdriver allows one to pick up a screw from the screw rack and insert it directly into the screw hole.

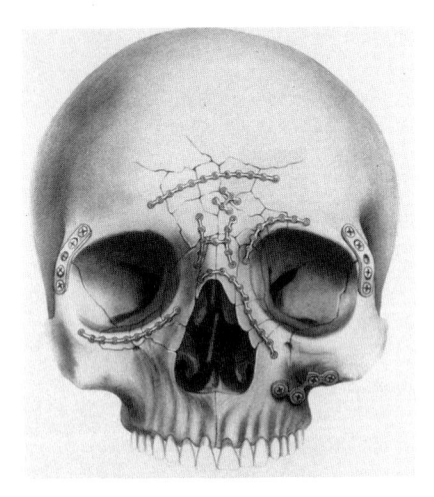

Figure 8.67 Indications for microplates are fractures of the thin bones of the naso-ethmoidal, the lower orbital, and the frontal area. Note that the stronger bones—such as the maxilla and the zygoma—which are exposed to remarkable muscle forces, should be stabilized by the larger and stronger miniplates.

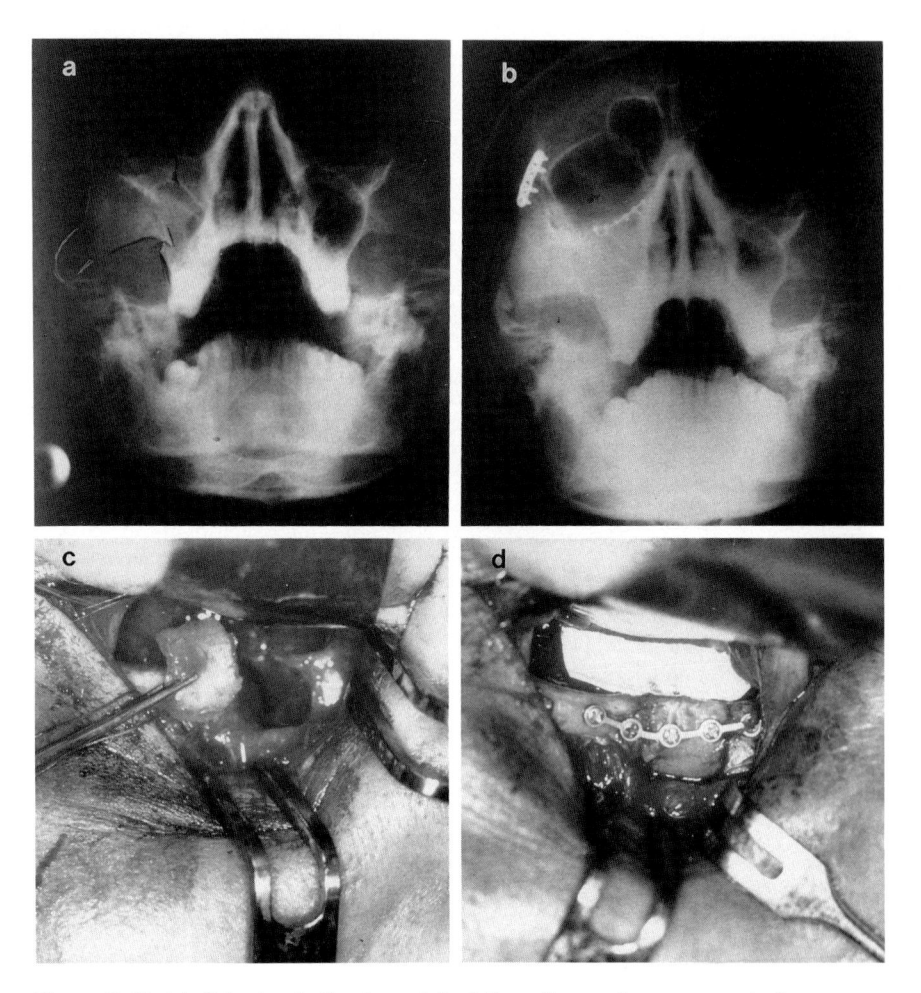

Figure 8.68 (a) Selective indication of the Micro-System in a zygomatic fracture. (b) After reduction, the zygoma was stabilized by a mini-compression plate at the frontal zygomatic suture. A microplate was placed at the infraorbital rim to keep small bone segments in place. (c) A small bone segment was present at the infraorbital rim. (d) Fixation of the small bone segment at the infraorbital rim by a microplate. The defect in the anterior part of the orbital floor was bridged by a lyophilized dura graft (any other type of graft or implant may be used).

Indications and Surgical Technique

Microplates are generally not a substitute for the larger plating systems but a preferred supplement in selected indications of midfacial trauma, in those areas of thin bones where no substantial muscle forces are present (see Figure 8.67). After two years of clinical experience with the Microsystem, the following indications can be recommended:

1. naso-ethmoidal fractures,
2. fractures of the infraorbital area,
3. fractures of the frontal sinus walls,
4. reconstruction of the skull, and
5. infant craniofacial surgery.

Selected cases will demonstrate the clinical application. Because the microplates are very thin and can be contoured in three dimensions, they are particularly suitable for the naso-ethmoidal area with its thin soft-tissue cover. Another region where the larger miniplates frequently caused complaints when the patient could palpate the plate is the infraorbital area (see Figure 8.68). The microplates are preferred, because they are barely palpable. It should be mentioned, however, that in severely comminuted complex midfacial fractures, when a greater rigidity may be required even in the infraorbital area, the stronger miniplates should be preferred. Fractures of the frontal sinus walls are another indication for use of microplates. Compared to wiring techniques, microplate fixation is much faster and more effective because with just one plate multiple fragments can be stabilized, thus reestablishing the convex shape of the frontal area (see Figure 8.69). In the past, relatively large miniplates were used for the fixation of bone grafts in reconstruction of the skull. More recently, in these cases we prefer microplates for graft fixation; these have proved to provide sufficient stability in this area (see Figure 8.70).

Clinical Applications of the Luhr Vitallium Maxillofacial Systems 111

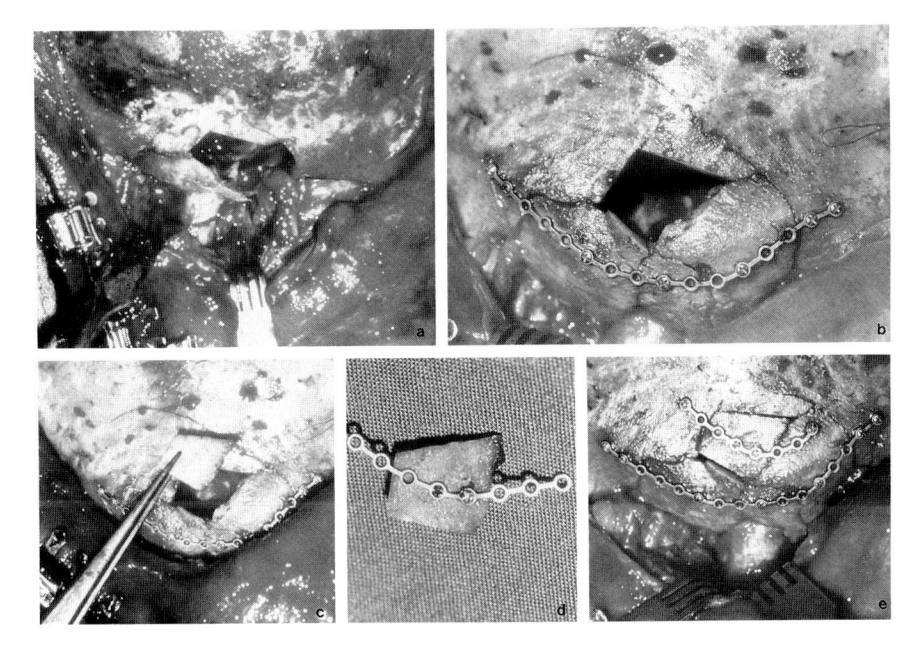

Figure 8.69 Fixation of comminuted fractures of the frontal sinus wall by microplates. (a) Fracture area is exposed by a bicoronal incision. The mucosa is removed from the sinus under microscopic view, and the sinus is drained to the nasal cavity. (b) Multiple fragments are reduced and firmly kept in place by only one microplate. (c) The last segment should not be replaced until it is fixed to a second microplate to avoid "pushing" this fragment into the frontal sinus. Those small bone fragments should be fixed to a microplate on the instrument table (d), after which both the segment and the plate can be transferred to the surgical site. (e) The concave contour of the frontal area is reestablished by means of two microplates.

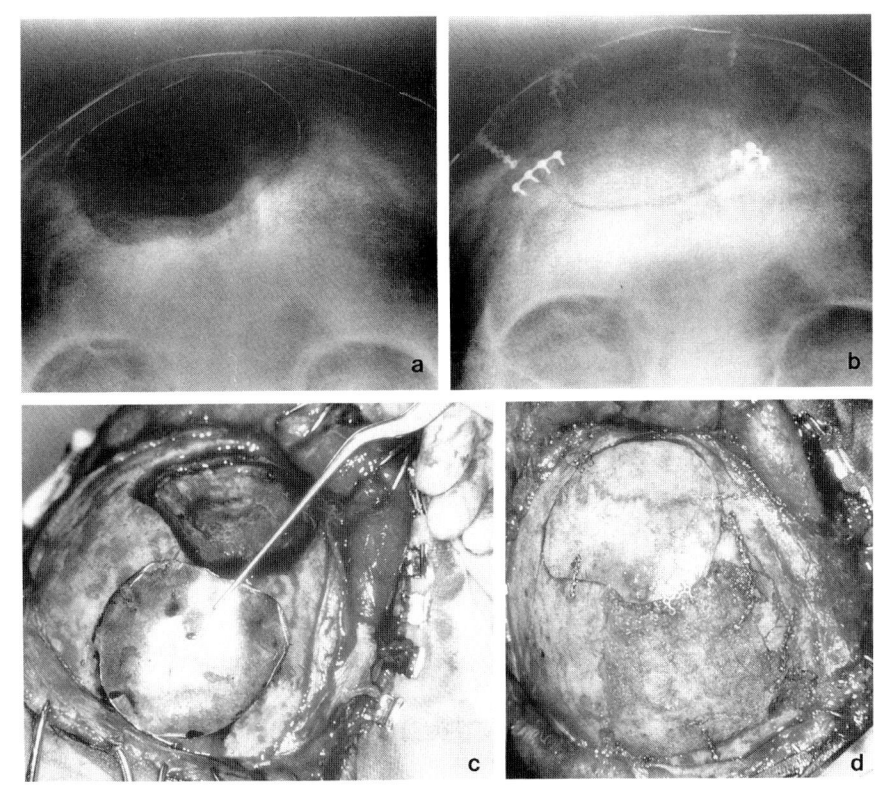

Figure 8.70 Fixation of bone grafts by microplate in reconstructive surgery of the skull. (a) Defect of the frontal area of the skull due to a gunshot injury. (b) Postoperative x-ray of graft fixation by microplates and screws. (c) When the skull defect was exposed, a template of exactly the shape and size was made from a sheet of lead. A full-thickness graft was cut out from the adjacent skull bone by the neurosurgeon (E. Markakis, M.D., Director of the Department of Neurosurgery, University of Goettingen). The graft was split between the inner and outer cortex. (d) The outer cortex of the graft was placed exactly to cover the original defect and fixed by microplates. The inner cortex serves for covering the donor side defect. Various microplates keep all the grafts in place. (e) Preoperative view of the skull defect. (f) Condition of the patient one week after surgery. Healing was uneventful.

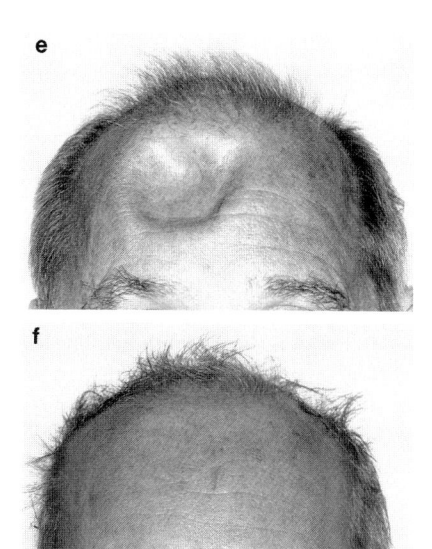

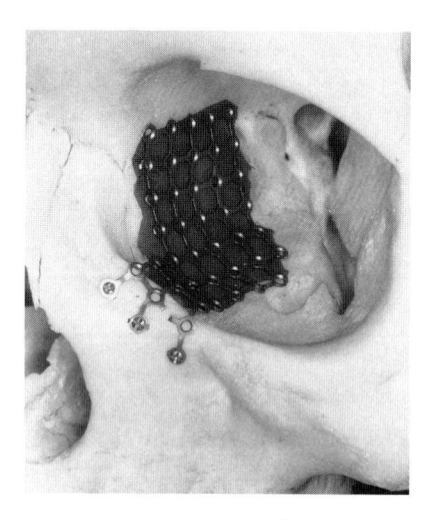

Figure 8.71 A defect of the orbital floor and the medial wall is bridged by a Micromesh, which is cut from the standard sheet according to the size of the defect. Some of the connection bars are cut off so that the remaining bars can be bent easily in any desired direction and can be contoured around the orbital rim. Screws are fixed at the infraorbital rim.

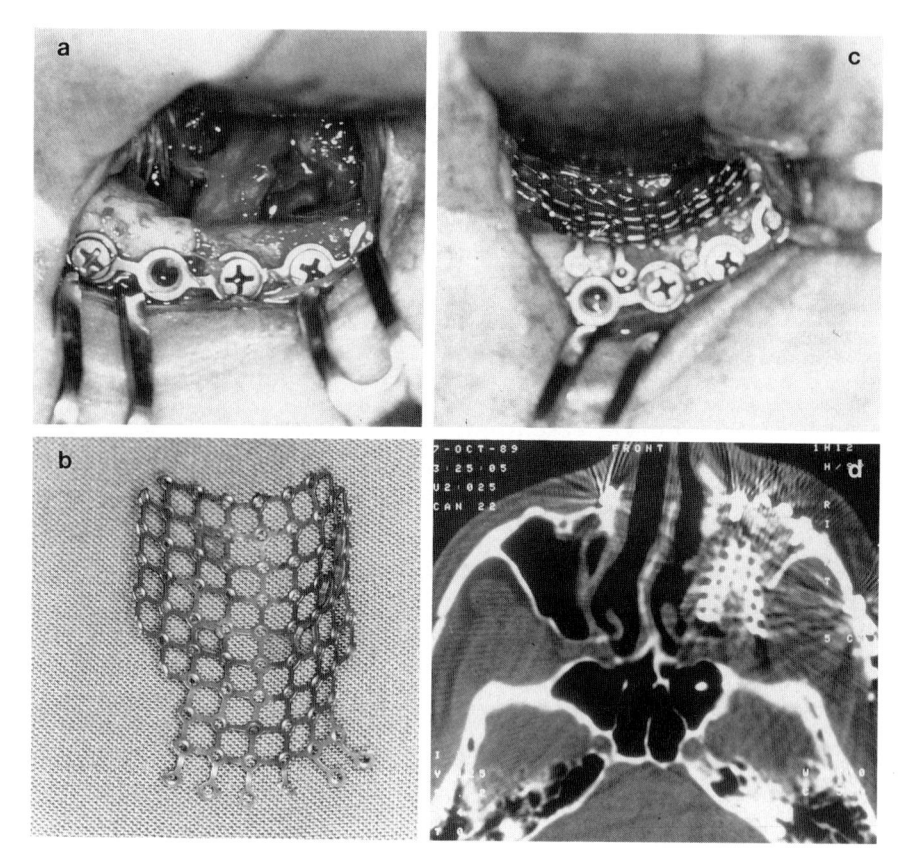

Figure 8.72 Reconstruction of the orbital floor and medial wall by Micromesh. (a) In a panfacial fracture, an extensive defect of the floor and the medial wall of the right orbit is present. The outer orbital frame already was reestablished by a mini fragmentation plate. (b) The required individual size and shape was cut out from a sheet of Micromesh. The sharp edges were smoothed by a diamond burr. A template was used to determine size and contour. Note that the horizontal connecting bars between the holes at the lower border were cut off. The remaining vertical bars can be contoured easily around the infraorbital rim. (c) The Micromesh is fixed at the infraorbital rim by Microscrews just above the minifragmentation plate. (d) Postoperative computerized tomogram demonstrates the micromesh and multiple miniplates in fixation of a panfacial fracture.

The Micromesh is indicated in major defects of the orbital walls, particularly when a two-wall defect is present (see Figure 8.71). The clinical application is shown in Figures 8.72 and 8.73. In infant craniofacial surgery the Micro-System has a wide range of indications (see Figure 8.74) showing some advantages over wiring techniques. In the past, particularly in advancement procedures of skeletal segments, bone grafts were needed together with wires to maintain the required forward projection. With microplates, this forward projection can be achieved easily with a firm fixation of segments in a three-dimensional manner. Microplates are much less palpable later on by the patient (or the parents) compared to the larger miniplates, which frequently caused complaints in the past.

Selected clinical cases demonstrate the technique of microplate fixation. Figure 8.75 shows an orbital advancement and reshaping of the cranial vault in correction of a trigonocephaly.

The Micro-System has been used successfully within the last two years for internal skeletal fixation in traumatology of the midfacial skeleton as well as in infant craniofacial surgery.

SUMMARY

The craniofacial skeleton consists of bones that are unique with respect to size, thickness and exposure to functional loading, that is, muscle traction and masticatory forces. Only one type or size of plate cannot

Clinical Applications of the Luhr Vitallium Maxillofacial Systems

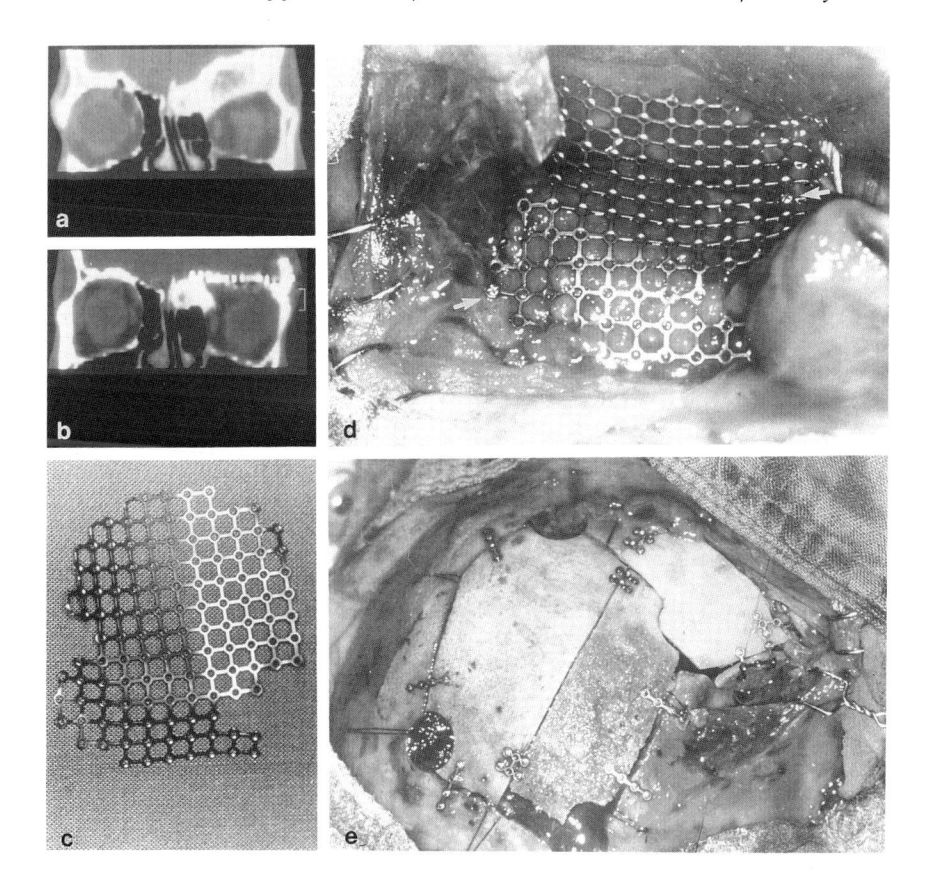

Figure 8.73 Reconstruction of the orbital roof by a Micromesh. (a) A fibrous dysplasia affecting the right orbital roof, anterior skull base, and frontal bones. (b) Postoperative computerized tomogram demonstrating the reconstruction of the orbital roof by a Micromesh after the affected bone had been resected by the neurosurgeon (W. Rama, M.D., Department of Neurosurgery, University of Goettingen). (c) The micromesh of the required size and shape was cut from a standard sheet with the aid of a template. (d) The mesh covers the defect in the anterior skull base and orbital roof. It is fixed by two microscrews. (e) The defect in the frontal bone resulting from the resection of the fibrous dysplasia is covered by the external table of a calvarial split graft; the internal table is used to restore the donor site. The grafts are fixed by multiple microplates and screws.

fulfil the requirements for rigid fixation of bones in all of these areas. Our goal, therefore, was to develop implant systems adequate in size and strength for those areas of the craniofacial skeleton. Based on research, biomechanical considerations, and, last but not least, clinical experience, the Vitallium Maxillofacial Fixation Systems were developed gradually over the last 20 years. The implants of all the systems consist of the well known alloy Vitallium, which is resistant to corrosion and shows excellent physical properties. All the different types of screws are self-tapping ones, which makes the surgery fast and simple.

The Mandibular Compression Screw System (MCS)

The MCS System is used for fractures of the mandible. The plates are equipped with eccentric compression holes. These holes allow axial compression of the fracture ends when the conical-head, 2.7-millimeter-diameter screws are tightened. The supplementary three-dimensional plates can be contoured in all three dimensions when this is required. Instrumentation is provided for the intraoral approach, which avoids any visible outer scar and facial nerve damage. Due to the rigidity of MCS plating with bicortical screw anchorage, there is no need of any postoperative MMF. Statistical data demonstrate that this technique has a minimal rate of complications.

The Mandibular Reconstruction System (MRS)

This system was developed for the reconstruction of the mandible, including the TMJ, following tumor resection. The self-tapping screws and instrumentation

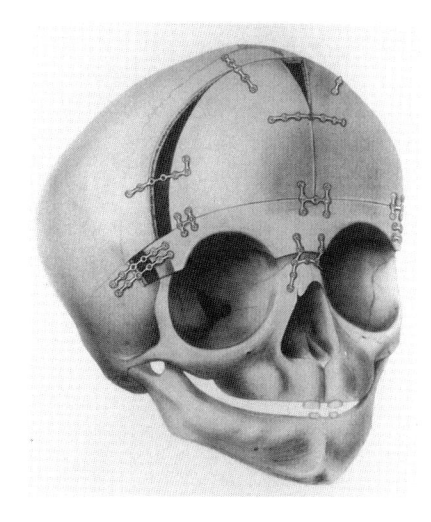

Figure 8.74 Microplates in infant craniofacial surgery. They are most useful in fixation of orbital advancement and in reshaping the cranial vault. Microplates can maintain gaps without the need for interpositional bone grafts; wires cannot.

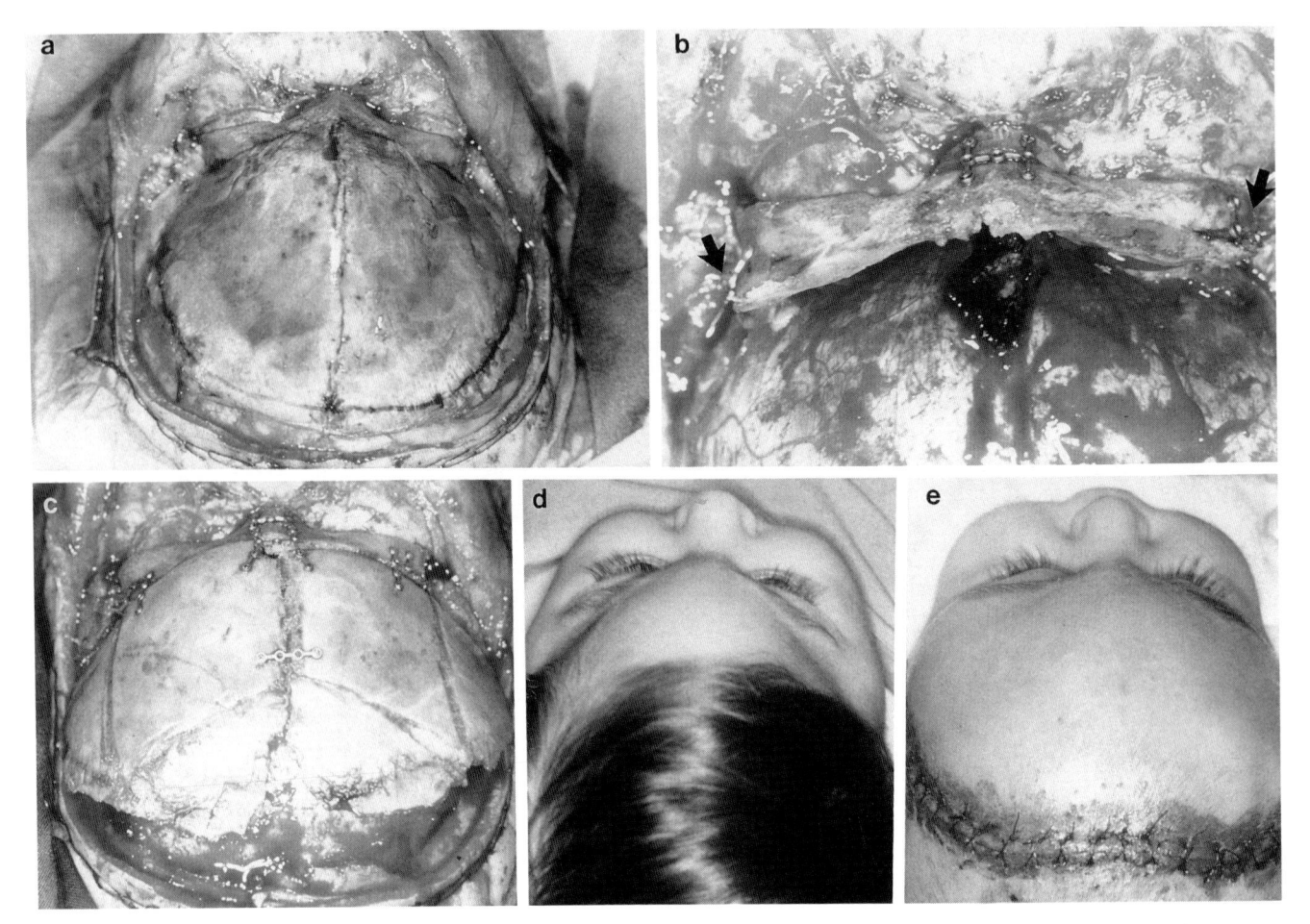

Figure 8.75 Surgical correction of a craniostenosis (trigonocephaly) (Neurosurgeon, E. Markakis, M.D., Department of Neurosurgery, University of Goettingen). (a) The typical V-shaped deformity of the supraorbital area and the skull. (b) The frontal bar (originally with its V-shaped configuration) was cut at its back side in the usual manner, infractured, and contoured to a normal shape. Frontal bar was fixed to the nasal skeleton by an H-type microplate. Two additional L-shaped microplates (on this photograph, only the upper end of the right one is visible) provide fixation of the advanced lateral orbits against the zygoma, bridging large gaps. There was no need for bone grafts in these areas (they would have been necessary if wires had been used). (c) Reshaping of the cranial vault after the frontal bone flap was separated in the midline and further contoured by infracturing. The bone flap was fixed to the frontal bar by three H-shaped microplates. (d) Preoperative photograph shows the typical deformity of a trigonocephalus. (e) Postoperatively, the reshaping of the cranial vault and the advancement of the lateral supraorbital rims are clearly recognized.

are interchangeable with those of the Mandibular Fractures System (MCS System). Different types of straight and angle plates and an adaptable condylar endoprosthesis make the system most versatile in alloplastic bridging of mandibular defects and joint replacement. Three-dimensional plates, which can be contoured in all three dimensions, increase the range of clinical application. Because all types of plates are equipped with eccentric compression holes, the MRS is further indicated for the fixation of bone grafts under axial compression between the resection stumps.

A detailed description of the MRS is given in Chapter 44.

The Mini-System

This system is a smaller plating system that has 2.0-millimeter-diameter self-tapping screws and two plate types:

1. The minicompression plates are provided with eccentric compression holes, which allow axial compression when the conical-head screws are tightened. Minicompression plates provide excellent rigidity and are indicated in fixation of zygoma fractures, fractures of the condylar neck and the atrophic mandible, and in mandibular fractures in children.

2. The minifixation plates are noncompressive plates with a wide range of indications in maxillary and midfacial fractures and orthognatic surgery. The plate thickness of 0.7 millimeter, the countersunk plate holes, and the very flat screwhead result in a remarkably low plate–screw profile. The special design of the connection bars between the plate holes allows three-dimensional plate contouring without the plate holes becoming deformed. Thus the plates can be adapted to any irregular bone surface; this gives them a wide range of clinical application.

The Micro System

This system is the smallest bone fixation system available. The self-tapping screws of only 0.8-millimeter diameter and their corresponding plates are significantly smaller than those in the common plating systems. In spite of their reduced size, Microscrews show a remarkably strong holding power in bones. Due to the special design of the connection bars, microplates can be contoured in all three dimensions; thus they can be adapted to virtually any of the most complex surfaces of the facial skeleton. The main indications for the Micro System are skeletal fixation in the area of the thin bones of the naso-ethmoidal and infraorbital area, in the skull, and in infant craniofacial surgery. Microplates provide a firm, three-dimensional fixation of segments, which wires cannot do. They cannot withstand greater muscle or masticatory forces. Therefore they are not a substitute, but rather a supplement, to the common plating system; indications for their use should be carefully selected. They have further indications in neurosurgery and hand surgery.

BIBLIOGRAPHY

Antonyshyn O, Gruss JS: Complex orbital trauma: The role of rigid fixation and primary bone grafting. Plast Reconstruct Surg 7:61, 1988.

Ardary WC: Plate and screw fixation in the management of mandible fractures. Clin Plast Surg 16:61, 1989.

Bell WH, Mannai C, Luhr HG: Art and science of Le Fort I downfracture. Int J Adult Orthod Orthognath Surg 3:23, 1988.

Danis R: Theorie et Prataque de L'Ostéosynthéses. Paris, Libraries de L'Academie de Medicine, 1949.

Gruss JS, Phillips JH: Complex facial trauma: The evolving role of rigid fixation and immediate bone graft reconstruction. Clin Plast Surg 16:42, 1989.

Gruss JS, Mackinnon SE: Complex maxillary fractures: Role of buttress reconstruction and immediate bone grafts. Plast Reconstr Surg 78:9, 1986.

Hansmann: A new method of fixation of fragments in complicated fractures. Verh D Deutseh Gesellsch F Chir 15:134, 1886.

Lane WA: On the advantage of steel screw in the treatment of ununited fractures. Lancet 2:1500, 1893.

Luhr HG: Skelettverlagernde Operationeu Zur Harmonisierung des Gesichtsprofils-Probleme der stabilen Fixation von Osteotomiesegmenten. In Pfeifer G (ed), Die Ästhetik von Form und Funktion in der Plastichen und Wiederherstellungschirurgie. Berlin, Springer-Verlag, 1985a, pp 87–92.

Luhr HG, Drommer R, Hölscher U, Schauer HW: Comparative studies between the extraoral and intraoral approach in compression ostesynthesis of mandibular fractures. In E. Hjorting-Hansen (ed), Oral and Maxillofacial Surgery. Proceedings from the 8th International Conference on Oral and Maxillofacial Surgery. Chicago, Berlin, Quintessence Publishing, 1985b.

Luhr HG: Vitallium Luhr Systems for reconstructive surgery of the facial skeleton. Otolaryngol Clin North Amer 20:573, 1987.

Luhr HG: A micro-system for cranio-maxillofacial skeletal fixation. J Cranio Max Fac Surg 16:312, 1988.

Luhr HG: The significance of condylar position using rigid fixation in orthognathic surgery. Clin Plast Surg 16:147, 1989a.

Luhr HG, Kubein-Meesenburg D: Rigid skeletal fixation in maxillary osteotomies. Clin Plast Surg 16:157, 1989b.

Luhr HG: Indications for use of a microsystem for internal fixation in craniofacial surgery. J Craniofac Surg 1:35, 1990.

Manson PN, Crawley WA, Yaremchuk M, et al: Midface fractures: Advantages of immediate extended open reduction and bone grafting. Plast Reconstr Surg 76:1, 1985.

Manson PN, Shack RB, Leonard LG, Su CT, Hoopes JE: Sagittal fractures of the maxilla and palate. Plast Reconstr Surg 72:484, 1983.

Manson PN: Management of facial fractures. Perspect Plast Surg 2:1, 1988.

Markowitz BL, Manson PN: Panfacial fractures: Organization of treatment. Clin Plast Surg 16:105, 1989.

Munro IR: The Luhr fixation system for the craniofacial skeleton. Clin Plast Surg 16:41, 1989.

Rosen HM: Miniplate fixation of Lefort I osteotomies. Plast Reconstr Surg 78:748, 1986.

Schilli W, Ewers R, Niederdellmann H: Bone fixation with screws and plates in the maxillofacial region. Int J Oral Surg 10 (Suppl 1):329, 1981.

Steinhäuser EW: Bone screws and plates in orthognathic surgery. Int J Oral Surg 11:209, 1982.

CHAPTER 9

Champy's System

Jean Luc Kahn
Michael Khouri
Translated to English from French
by Patrick Blez

HISTORY OF DEVELOPMENT

Much clinical and biomechanical research has examined the potential of miniaturized plates and screws designed for the fixture of the cranofacial skeleton. Two fundamentally different systems have been advocated for the treatment of mandibular fractures. One system extrapolates the AO principles, originally developed for long bone fractures, to treatment of the mandible. In this system the implant substitutes for the fractured bone during the healing process and assumes all external strains exerted on the bone. This system, which is popular in Switzerland and Germany, requires the use of rather bulky plates that often require a cutaneous approach which leave visible scars and may result in facial nerve damage.

The other system is derived from the work of Michelet (1973). Its design, a more physiological one, consists of neutralizing unfavorable traction strains while at the same time allowing transmission of favorable compression forces. As will be described, the experimental basis, surgical technique, and instrumentation are radically different in these systems.

In 1967, Michelet devised a monocortical osteosynthesis technique for the treatment of mandibular fractures. In this technique, miniaturized plates and screws, inserted by the extraoral (intraoral) approach, were placed in the juxta-alveolar position.

Although readily adopted by French surgeons, Michelet's techniques and principles were criticized by many. The biomechanical validity of Michelet's principles was confirmed in a series of multidisciplinary experiments performed in Strasbourg, France, between 1971 and 1974. These culminated to a practical clinical method that used a customized instrumentation.

SPECIFICATIONS OF OSTEOSYNTHESIS MATERIAL

Biophysical Characteristics

The material of the osteosynthesis implant was chosen for its various bending and torsional forces, its biocompatibility, and the anatomic requirements. This resulted in the selection of an alloy of known biotolerance; this alloy consists of chrome, nickel, and molybdenum with a trace (0.03%) amount of carbon to insure good flexibility. This alloy is very hard. It is strong enough to withstand breaking and straining to 100 decanewtons, and at the same time it is suitable for miniaturization.

Plates and screws are now available in pure titanium, a metal whose mechanical and physical properties are similar to that of stainless steel, but that has a higher degree of biocompatibility. Screws, plates, and instruments are all made of the same material, because variations in metal ions can lead to metallic contamination or oxidation-reduction phenomena, with detrimental tissue effects.

The miniplates were 2 centimeters long, 0.9 millimeter thick, and 6 millimeters wide. They had an elastic limit of flexibility between 70 and 80 per square millimeter, and their rupture point lay between 95 and 110 decanewtons per square millimeter. With this loading limit, one plate will guarantee the stability of a fracture in the cheek region near the teeth. Two plates are necessary in the symphyseal area; they must be applied

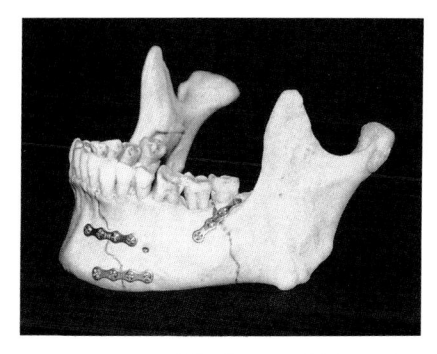

Figure 9.1 Model of a mandible with two miniplates at the symphysis and one miniplate in the angle region.

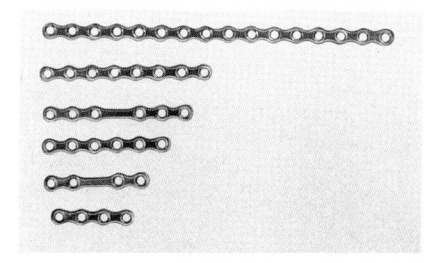

Figure 9.2 Different types of Champy's miniplates.

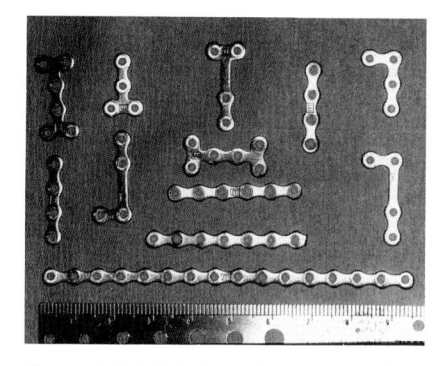

Figure 9.3 Miniplates for orthognathic and reconstructive surgery.

in parallel with a gap of 4 to 5 millimeters between them. This configuration resists torsion forces up to 220 decanewtons (see Figure 9.1).

Screws under stress give way first to shearing forces. When the tension forces in the plate reach the rupture point, 95 decanewtons, the shear force exerted on the screws is 40.27 decanewtons per square millimeter. At the maximal masticatory force, 60 decanewtons, a shear force of 20.35 decanewtons per square millimeter is expected. This value is one-fourth the rupture point of the material.

Experimental and Clinical Trial of the Miniplates

The loading capacity during mastication was investigated in three experiments (Champy 1977). In the first experiment, osteosynthesis of different fracture sites was performed on 13 freshly prepared mandibles. The mandibles were then load tested with increasing forces. In each instance, either the bone broke in the machine at the fracture site or the outer cortex was ripped off, but the osteosynthesis plate remained undamaged.

A second set of experiments employed strain gauges both in the laboratory and in volunteers (Champy 1978). Strain gauges were set up in the middle of the plate. Tension forces occurring in the plate were increased under load. This experiment showed that the force necessary to cause jaw fracture was substantially higher than the maximum masticatory force. In two consenting patients, strain gauges were fixed to osteosynthesis plates to show the actual strains developed within the plates during the postoperative period. Due to the involuntary limitation of masticatory forces in comparison with healthy patients, values of reactive biting forces between 13.5 and 30 decanewtons per square millimeter were measured during the first 15 postoperative days. About 30 days after the osteosynthesis, the plates still bore about 10% of the initially recorded strains.

REQUIRED EQUIPMENT

The Champy monocortical miniplate osteosynthesis system utilizes a precisely coordinated set of instruments that are conveniently stored in a special sterilizing container. The miniplates (see Figure 9.2) vary in length from 2 to 9 centimeters (4-hole, 6-hole and 8- to 16-hole plates), with a thickness of 0.9 millimeter. The 4- and 6-hole plates are available with intermediate spacing sections. In addition, a wide variety of preshaped plates (see Figure 9.3) are available to accommodate frequently used configurations (L-, T- and Y-shaped plates). The minimum diameter of the holes is 2.1 millimeters, and they have a bevel of 30°.

Recently, new types of plates have been designed, including mini orbital plates (Champy 1986b), miniplates for sagittal split osteotomy (McDonald 1987), and miniplates for jaw reconstruction (Pape 1989). These plate designs all use the same type of screw.

The high elasticity of the plate material allows easy deformation in all three planes, thereby allowing the exact adaptation of the plates to the bony surface. Special instruments have been designed to allow plate adaptation (See Figure 9.4): a plate-bending pliers, a plate-modeling pliers, and a plate-bending lever. The bending

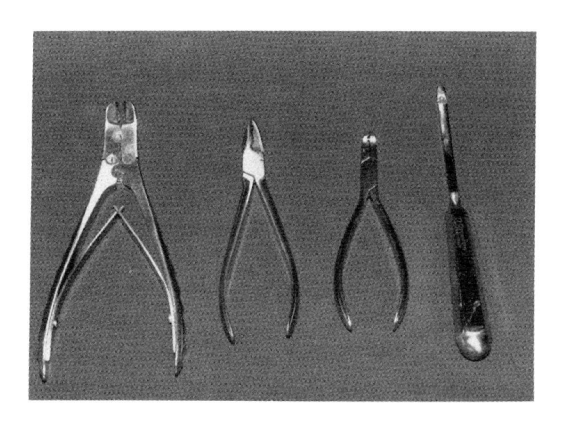

Figure 9.4 Plate-bending and plate-modeling pliers.

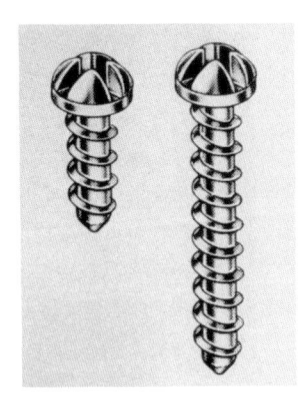

Figure 9.5 Champy's screws.

pliers allow the plate to be adapted over margins and surfaces by virtue of the indentation in the plate. Alternatively, the modeling pliers and the plate-modeling level may be used. With the side-cutting shears, the plates may be cut, if necessary, to a precise length.

All screws (see Figure 9.5) are cortical and self-tapping and have cruciate heads. They are available in lengths of: 5, 6, 7, 9, 11, 13, and 15 millimeters (head included). The screws have a diameter of 2 millimeters, with a thread core diameter of 1.6 millimeters. The screw thread is 10/10, so that one turn of the screw corresponds to 1 millimeter penetration into the bone. The screwhead has a diameter of 2.8 millimeters and is designed to allow insertion at a 30° angle with respect to the plate surface.

The drill has the same diameter as the core of the screws—1.6 millimeters. This ensures firm anchorage of the self-tapping screws (see Figure 9.6).

One screwdriver incorporates a spring-locking device, so that the screws may be easily withdrawn from the screw rack and screwed into the mandibular bone. A second screwdriver, of classical design, is used to complete the tightening of the screw. Screw-holding forceps and plate-holding forceps facilitate the handling of the materials during the operative procedure.

TECHNIQUE OF APPLICATION AND NUANCES

A previously discussed, the Champy system is designed to heal mandibular fractures by utilizing the biomechanical strains exerted on the fractured bone, as well as the ideal osteosynthesis line defined throughout the length of the horizontal ramus of the mandible.

Operative Procedure for Treatment of Mandibular Fracture

The operation is conducted under general anesthesia with nasal intubation. It is performed as early as possible after injury, preferably within 12 hours.

After meticulous preparation of the oral cavity with chlorhexidine, and after local infiltration with 1% lidocaine and adrenaline solution, the incision of the oral mucosa is performed 5 millimeters from the attached gingiva. This allows easy suturing at the time of closure. The fracture site is exposed by careful periosteal elevation. Care should be taken not to traumatize the surrounding soft tissues. An assistant placed at the head of the patient is responsible, during the entire operative procedure, for the exact anatomical restoration and maintenance of the dental occlusion.

The most suitable plate is selected and accurately adapted to the bone surface by means of modeling and bending pliers (see Figure 9.7). The plate is then placed onto the bone and held with a straight forceps while the first hole is drilled through the distal hole of the plate (see Figure 9.8). The first screw is inserted and gently tightened with the screwdriver (see Figure 9.9). The same procedure is used to insert each screw, one

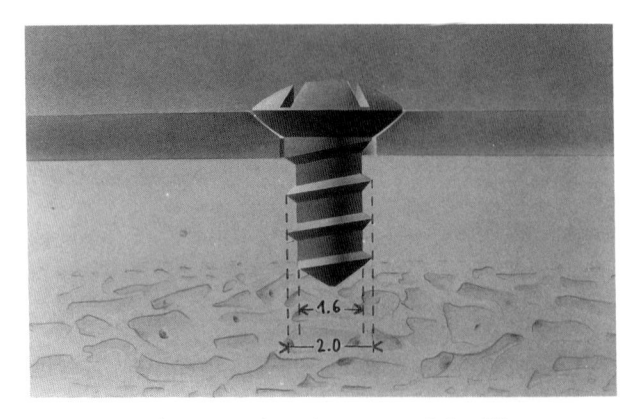

Figure 9.6 The screw thread measures 2.0 millimeters across. Drill diameter is 1.6 millimeters, which is the same as the core diameter of the screw.

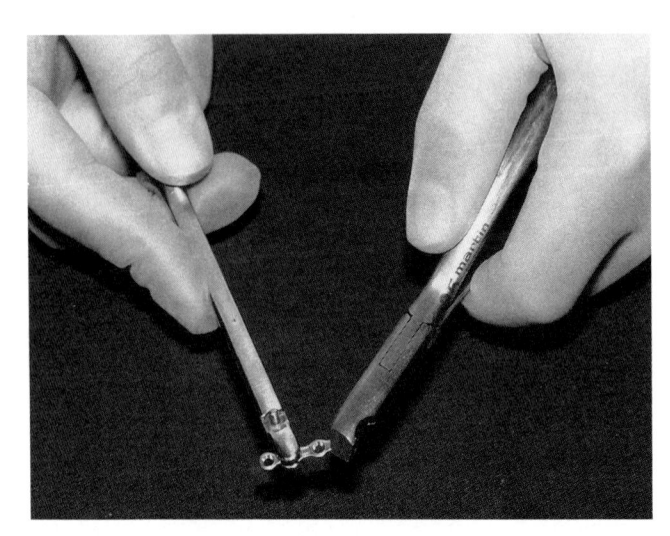

Figure 9.7 Adaptation of the plate to the bone surface. The instrument set allows accurate modeling of the plate in all directions.

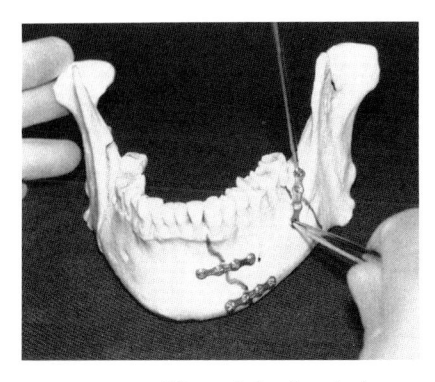

Figure 9.8 Drilling of the first hole through the distal hole of the miniplate; the plate is held onto the bone surface with a pair of straight forceps.

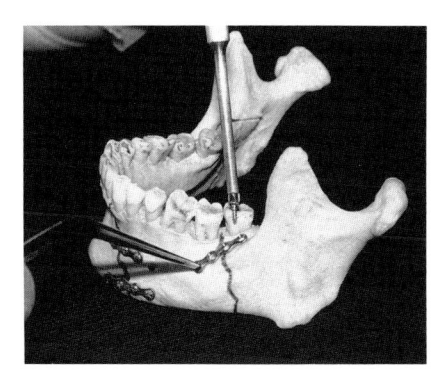

Figure 9.9 Insertion of the first screw.

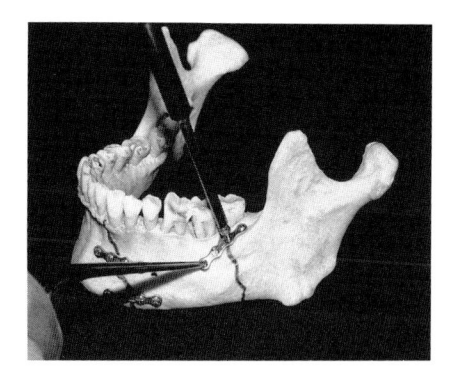

Figure 9.10 Each screw is inserted one after the other.

after the other (see Figure 9.10). Two screws must be placed on each fragment (see Figure 9.11).

A four-hole plate is usually sufficient, although some situations require a six-hole plate with an intermediate spacing section. In the symphyseal region, a second plate is placed in the basal position to counteract the torsional forces; this plate must be placed at least 4.5 millimeters lower than the other. Complex plate applications are sometimes necessary if a complicated fracture is present.

After the plate is applied, mechanical stability and adequacy of dental occlusion are checked. The buccal cavity is rinsed with an antiseptic solution, and the mucosa is closed with a firm, nonresorbable suture. Suction drainage may be helpful during the initial 24-hour postoperative period. A pressure bandage is applied last.

Antibiotics are administered postoperatively. A fluid diet is administered for the first 10 days, after which semisolids are given. On the 15th postoperative day, the patient may resume a normal diet. Sutures are removed on the tenth day. The plate is removed under local anesthesia two or three months after the operation.

Additional Technical Details

1. The strength of a monocortical osteosynthesis depends on adequate fixation of the screws into the cortical bone. Careful and accurate drilling is therefore crucial. Although the hole need not be perpendicular to the surface plate (an angle of up to 30° is acceptable), it must be monoaxial (see Figure 9.12). Inaccurate, eccentric drilling will invariably result in an imperfect conical hole that will lessen the ability of the screw to grip firmly (see Figure 9.13). Because the average thickness of the outer cortical layer is 3.3 millimeters, the fixation of the screws depends on three screw threads; a conical bur hole might reduce the grip of the screw to one or two threads.

After a hole of 3 or 4 millimeters is drilled into healthy bone, a decrease in resistance indicates that the cancellous bone layer, or dental canal, has been reached. At this point the drilling must be stopped and the screw should be inserted. During the entire drilling procedure, continuous liquid cooling will avoid thermal necrosis of the bone.

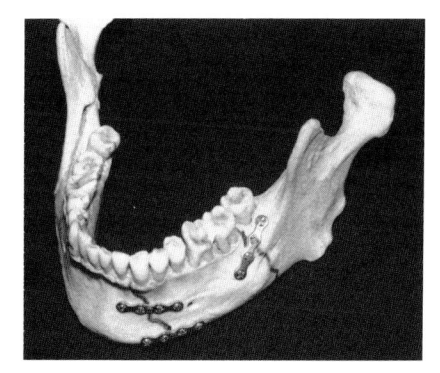

Figure 9.11 At least two screws are necessary on each fragment. A second plate should be placed in the anterior region.

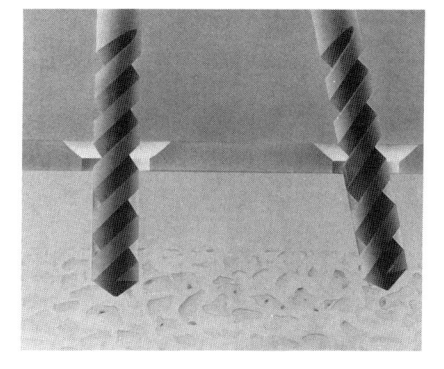

Figure 9.12 Accurate drilling is fundamental. It may be angulated with the plate surface up to 30° but must be strictly monoaxial.

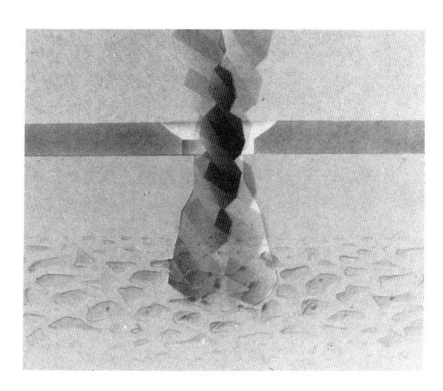

Figure 9.13 Any change in the drilling angle during the drilling procedure results in an inadequate conical hole.

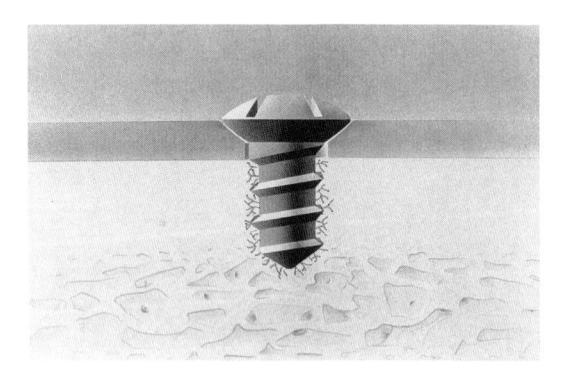

Figure 9.14 Excessive tightening of the screw produces microfractures within the bone hole.

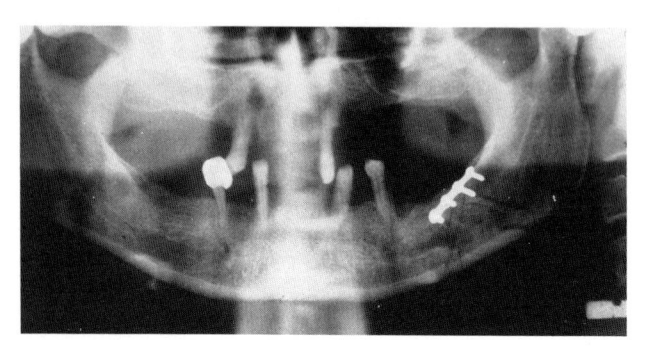

Figure 9.16 Miniplate osteosynthesis in an edentulous region of the mandible.

2. Seven millimeters is most often the appropriate length of screw for the thickness of the mandibular cortex. Solid fixation necessitates inserting two screws on each side of the fracture.

Excessive tightening of the screws produces microfractures within the bone hole (see Figure 9.14). If a screw fails to obtain a firm grip into the cortex, a better anchoring area, further from the fracture site, should be sought by exchanging the plate for a longer one or one with an intermediate spacing section.

3. The plate must be as congruent as possible to the bone surface before the screws are fixed. Once a screw has been inserted, no attempt should be made to adjust the shape of the plate. Such an attempt would result in a loosening of the screw already fastened.

If osteosynthesis has failed to restore normal occlusion or anatomical reduction, neither MMF nor elastic traction can modify the shape of the plate. In that case, the plate has to be removed, and a new osteosynthesis with a longer plate has to be performed.

4. Miniplate osteosynthesis in the subapical position is able to neutralize traction strains only if the fractured surfaces are perfectly adapted to each other. When there are bone defects or when the broken fragments are not in close contact, the plate is submitted to excessive strains. These strains may rupture the plate or loosen the screws (see Figure 9.15).

5. When there are multiple fractures of the body of the mandible, it is often useful to secure a perfect anatomical reduction by means of a temporary maxillomandibular wiring. The osteosynthesis should then be performed first in the tooth-bearing section of the mandible.

6. When fracture treatment is delayed, granulation tissue appears in the fracture site, making anatomical reduction and the reduction of dental occlusion less likely. The rate of postoperative malocclusion is therefore higher in these cases. In addition, bone demineralization occurring near the fracture site decreases the quality of the fixation of the screws.

For these reasons, where treatment is delayed it is often necessary to use longer plates or plates with spacing sections so as to assure screw insertion into healthy bone.

7. Miniplate osteosynthesis should not be performed on the superior aspect of an edentulous mandible, because the sclerotic alveolar bone does not offer a strong fixation for the screws (see Figure 9.16).

8. In children under 13 years of age, the plate must be placed at the lower border of the mandible to avoid damage to the tooth germs. From 6 years of age, osteosynthesis is possible at the basilar border in the incisor region. From the age of 9, it is possible on the entire horizontal body of the mandible. After 13, the anatomical conditions are similar to those of adults.

Complications

A series of more than 2000 mandibular fractures was treated by Champy's method in the hospitals of Cologne and Strasbourg between 1974 and 1986. This series shows that the complication rate, which is low, decreases as the surgical team acquires experience.

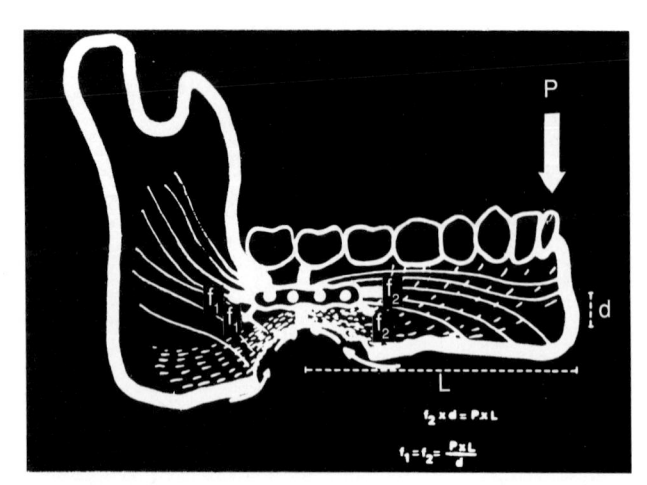

Figure 9.15 Strain concentration in an osteosynthesis plate in case of bone defect at the lower border of the mandible.

Suture dehiscence (3.9%) and postoperative infection (3.2%) were observed principally when there had been undue delay between the time of trauma and the time of the operation, as well as in patients who received no antibiotic treatment. Inadequate immobilization of the fractured fragments can also lead to secondary infection. Postoperative disturbances of the occlusion are always due to a failure of occlusal fixation during osteosynthesis.

CONCLUSION

The efficiency of Champy's miniplate osteosynthesis has been borne out over its 15 years of use in many areas of application. These include various simple or complex fractures (see Figure 9.17)—except for the fractures of the condyle neck, because intraoral exposure and reduction of the fragments are not sufficiently reliable—midface and upper face fractures (see Figures 9.18–9.20), fragments in orthognathic mandibular (see

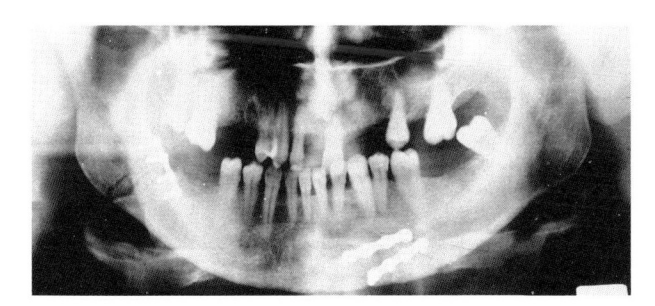

Figure 9.17 Miniplate osteosynthesis in a bifocal fracture of the mandible.

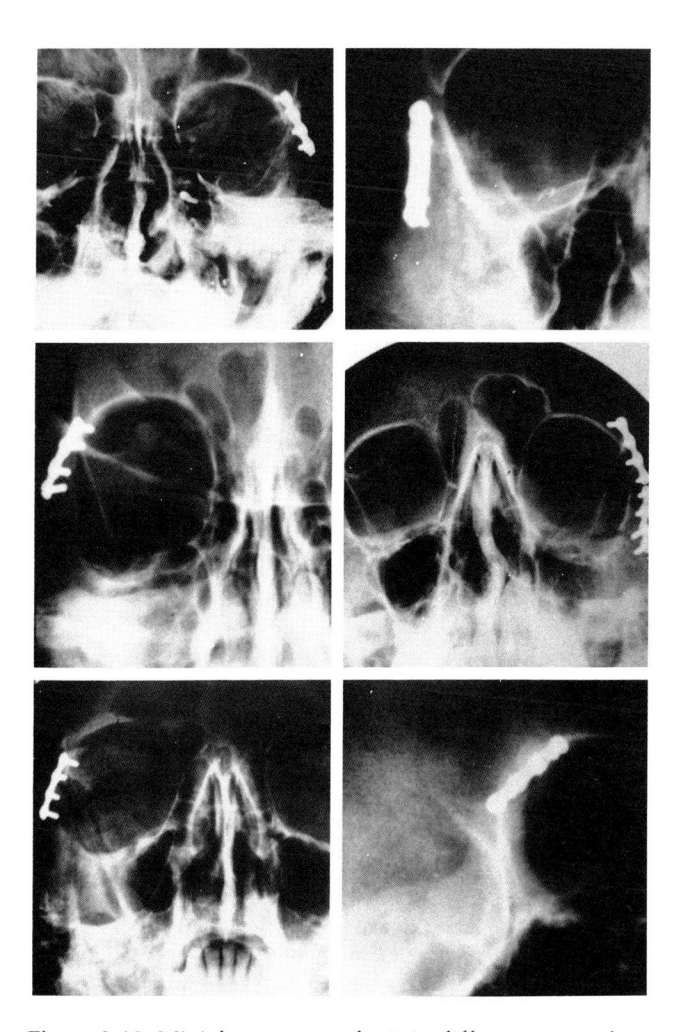

Figure 9.18 Miniplate osteosynthesis in different types of zygomatic bone fractures.

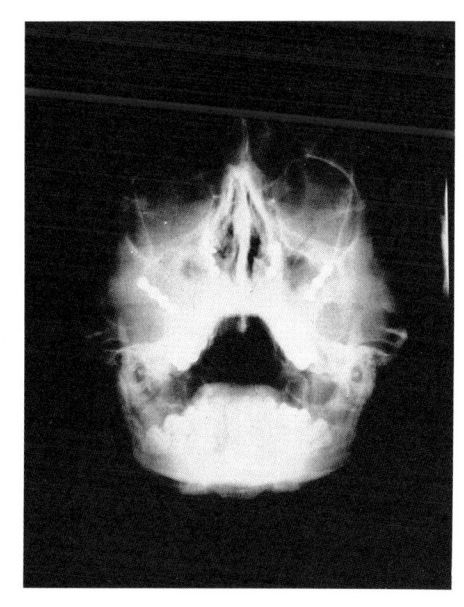

Figure 9.19 Miniplate osteosynthesis in a Le Fort II fracture.

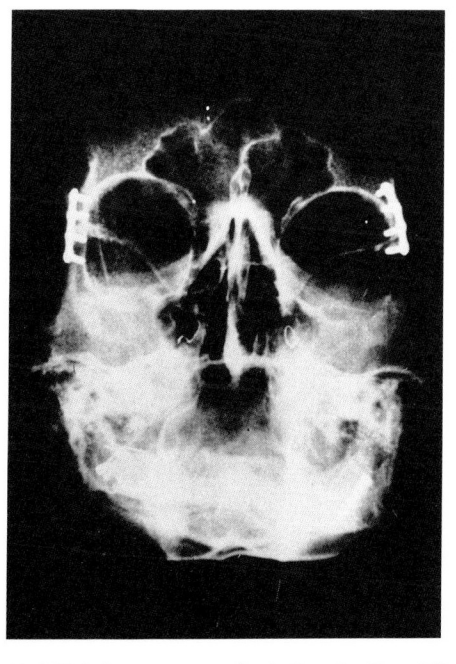

Figure 9.20 Miniplate osteosynthesis in a Le Fort III fracture.

Figures 9.21 and 9.22) and maxillary surgery (see Figure 9.23) or congenital procedures, transfacial osteotomy (see Figures 9.24 and 9.25), and for fixture of bone fragments in various procedures by genioplasty (see Figure 9.22).

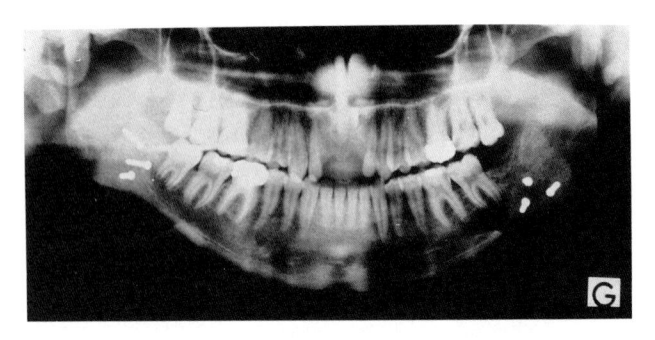

Figure 9.21 Fixation of a sagittal split osteotomy with three screws on each side.

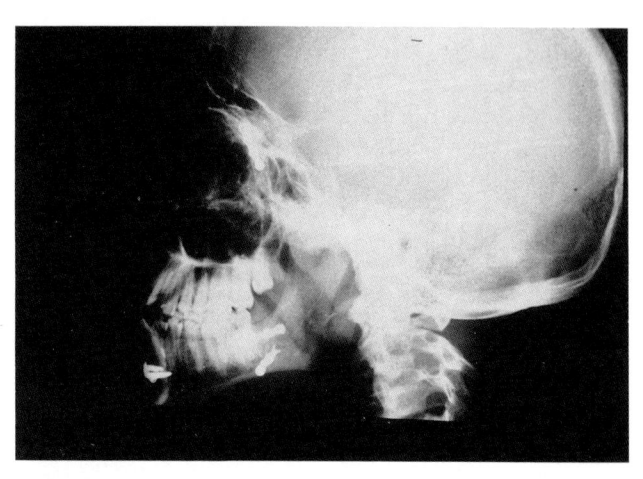

Figure 9.22 Sagittal split osteotomy stabilized by miniplates, and genioplasty using screws.

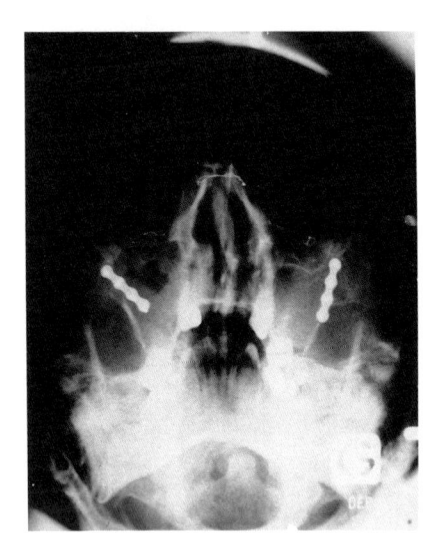

Figure 9.23 Le Fort I osteotomy stabilized with two miniplates.

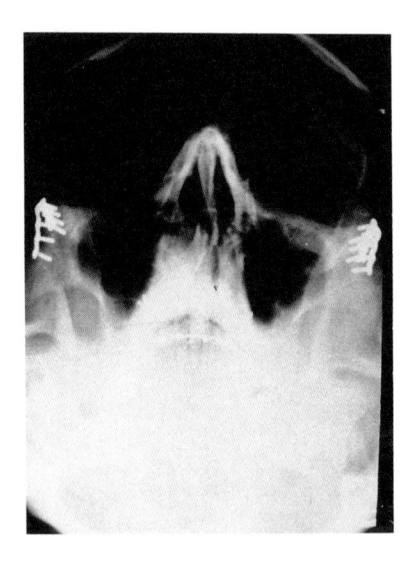

Figure 9.24 Transfacial intermediate osteotomy: Two plates are necessary on each side to achieve a long-term stabilization.

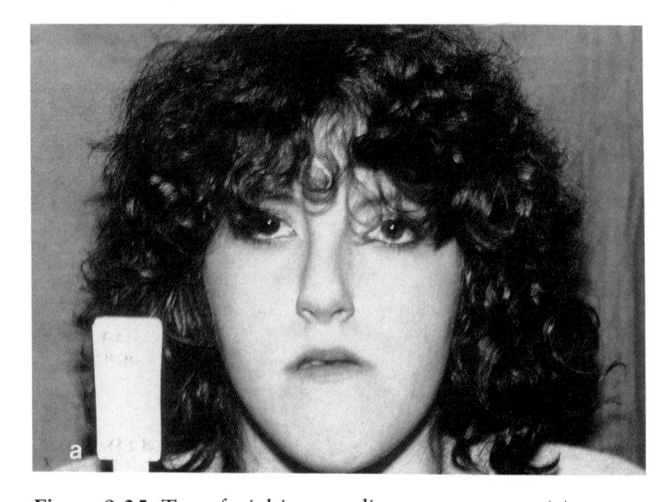

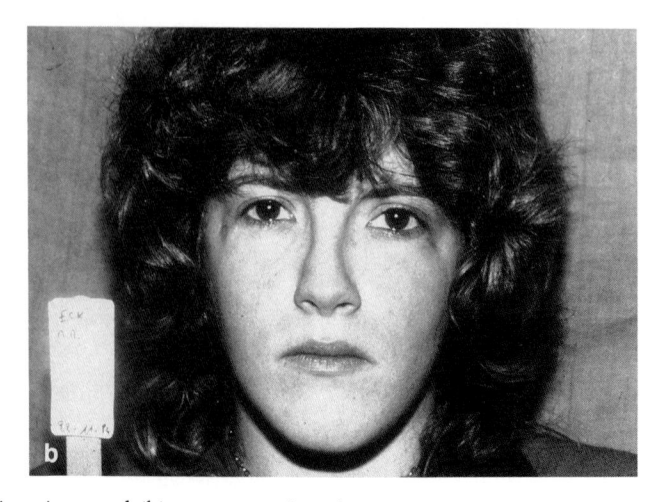

Figure 9.25 Transfacial intermediate osteotomy: (a) preoperative view, and (b) postoperative view.

BIBLIOGRAPHY

Champy M, Lodde JP, Jaeger JH, Wilk A, Gerber JC: Ostéosynthèses mandibulaires selon la technique de Michelet. II- Présentation d'un nouveau matériel. Résultats. (Mandibular osteosynthesis according to Michelet's procedure. II- Presentation of a new material. Results). Rev Stomat (Paris) 77: 577, 1976.

Champy M, Lodde JP: Synthèses mandibulaires. Localisation des synthèses en fonction des contraintes mandibulaires. (Mandibular osteosynthesis. Positioning of the miniplate according to mandibular stresses). Rev Stomat (Paris) 77: 971–976, 1976.

Champy M, Lodde JP: Etude des contraintes dans la mandibule fracturée chez l'homme. Mesures théoriques et vérification par jauges extensométriques in situ. (Study of the stresses in mandibular fractures in man. Theoretical measurements and confirmation by extensometric gauges in situ). Rev Stomat (Paris) 78: 545–551, 1977.

Champy M, Lodde JP, Muster D, Wilk A, Gastelo L: Les ostéosynthèses par plaques miniaturisées vissées en chirurgie faciale et crânienne. Indications. Résultats à propos de 400 cas. (Osteosynthesis by miniaturized screwed plates in facial and cranial surgery. Indications. Results in 400 cases). Ann Chir Plast 22: 261–264, 1977.

Champy M, Lodde JP, Schmitt R, Jaeger JH, Muster D: Mandibular osteosynthesis by miniature screwed plates via a buccal approach. J Max Fac Surg 6: 14–21, 1978.

Champy M: Surgical treatment of midface deformities. Head and Neck Surg 1980; 2: 451–465.

Champy M, Lodde JP, Kahn JL, Kielwasser P: Attempt at systematization in the treatment of isolated fractures of the zygomatic bone: Techniques and results. J Otolaryngol 15: 39–43, 1986a.

Champy M, Pape HD, Gerlach KL, Lodde JP: Mandibular fractures. Chap. 8: The Strasbourg miniplate osteosynthesis. In Oral and Maxillofacial Traumatology. Kruger E, Schilli W, Worthington P, (eds). Quintessence, Chicago 1986b; 19–43.

Hildebrand HF, Champy M: Biocompatibility of Co-Cr-Ni alloys. New York, Plenum, 1988.

Gerlach KL, Pape HD: Prinzip und Indikation der Miniplattenosteosynthese (Principle and indication of the miniplate osteosynthesis). Dtsch zahnärztl Z 35: 346, 1980.

Gerlach KL, Pape HD, Tuncer M: Funktionsanalytische Untersuchungen nach der Miniplattenosteosynthese von Unterkieferfrakturen (Clinical tests and function analyses after miniplate osteosynthesis of mandibular fractures). Dtsch Z Mund Kiefer Gesichtschir 6: 57, 1982.

Gerlach KL, Khouri M, Pape HD, Champy M: Ergebnisse der Miniplattenosteosynthese bei 1000 Unterkieferfrakturen aus der Kölner und Strasburger Klinik (Results of miniplate osteosynthesis with 1000 mandibular fractures from Cologne and Strasbourg hospitals). Dtsch zahnärztl Z 38: 363, 1983.

Horch HH, Gerlach KL, Pape HD: Indikationen und Grenzen der intraoralen Miniplattenosteosynthese bei Frakturen des aufsteigenden Unterkieferastes (Indications and limitations of the intraoral approach with fractures of the ascending ramus of the mandible). Dtsch zahnärztl Z 38: 447–452, 1983.

McDonald WR, Stoelinga PJW, Blijdorp PA, Schoenaers JHA: Champy bone plate fixation in sagittal split osteotomies for mandibular advancement. Int J Adult Orthod Orthognat Surg 2: 87, 1987.

Michelet FX, Deymes J, Dessus B: Osteosynthesis with miniaturized screwed plates in maxillofacial surgery. J Max Fac Surg 1: 79–84, 1973.

Pape HD, Gerlach KL: Le traitement des fractures des maxillaires chez l'enfant et l'adolescent (Treatment of maxillary fractures in children and adolescents). Rev Stomatol Chir Max Fac 81: 280–284, 1980.

Pape HD, Gerlach KL: The use of long miniplates in jaw reconstruction. Presented at the 10th International Conference on Oral and Maxillofacial Surgery, Jerusalem, Israel, May 22, 1989.

Pape HD, Herzog M, Gerlach KL: Der Wandel der Unterkieferfrakturversorgung von 1950 bis 1980 am Beispiel der Kölner Klinik (The change of mandibular fracture treatment from 1950 to 1980 on the example of the Cologne hospital). Dtsch zahnärztl Z 38: 301, 1983.

CHAPTER 10

The AO/ASIF Maxillofacial Implant System

Michael J. Yaremchuk

Joachim Prein

THE AO/ASIF

In 1958, a group of 15 Swiss surgeons founded the Arbeitsgemeinschaft für Osteosynthesefragen; Association of Osteosynthesis/Association for the Study of Internal Fixation (AO/ASIF). The AO set out to define the role of internal fixation in the treatment of skeletal fractures in an effort to improve upon the results of nonoperative treatment modalities prevalent at that time. The group was led by Maurice E. Muller, who had studied with and was deeply influenced by Danis, the Belgian surgeon who performed much of the basic scientific and clinical work on which the concepts of rigid internal fixation are based. Through the use of internal fixation, this Swiss group set out to achieve rapid recovery of form and function. They established four basic conditions that had to be met to accomplish this with their surgery:

1. anatomic reduction of the bone fragments,
2. functionally stable fixation of the fragments,
3. preservation of the blood supply to bone fragments by atraumatic operating technique, and
4. early, active, and pain-free mobilization.

To effect this new mode of fracture treatment, they realized that a commitment to the research of the basic biology of bone healing, the development and refinement of implant materials and instrumentation, as well as documentation of the results of treatment, were all critical parts of the program.

At the Laboratory for Experimental Surgery in Davos, Switzerland (see Figure 10.1), the Maurice E. Muller Institute for Biomechanics in Bern, Switzerland, and other collaborating laboratories, AO/ASIF investi-

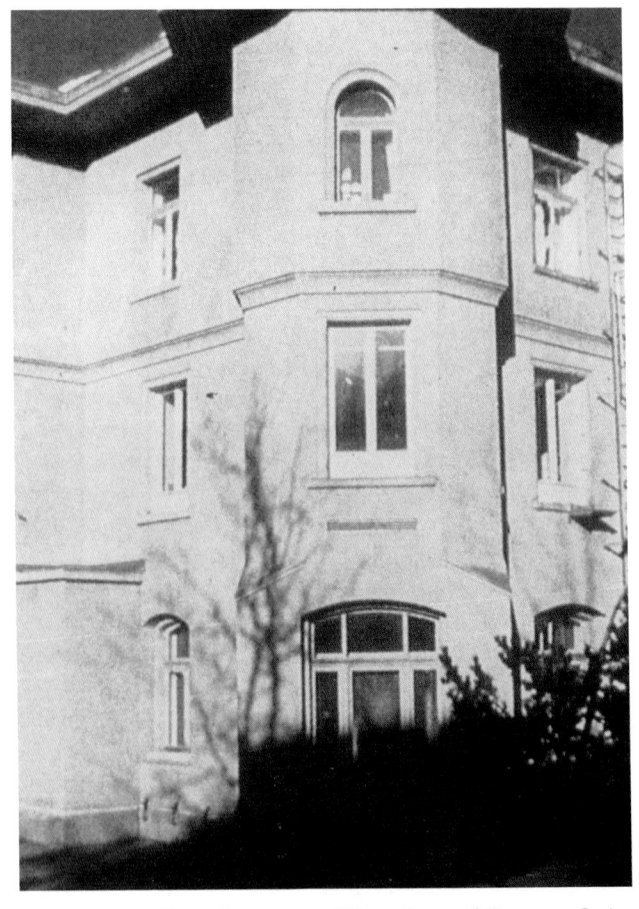

Figure 10.1 The Laboratory of Experimental Surgery, Swiss Research Institute, Davos, Switzerland.

gators have documented the biologic basis for the concepts on which rigid fixation techniques are based. Schenck and Willenegger (1967) solidified and confirmed the early work of Lane (1914), Krompecher (1934), and Danis (1949) showing that rigidly immobilized ends would heal primarily; that is, without a cartilage intermediate. Rittmann and Perren (1974) showed that infection did not interfere with the healing process as long as immobility and bone vascularity were maintained. Perren and others refined Danis' concept of compression osteosynthesis on bone healing. He and his associates showed that compression increased the stability of internal fixation systems and that the gradual decrease in compression that occurred over time was the result of bone remodeling and not the resorption seen with the osteolysis that accompanies the inevitable interfragmentary movement seen with nonrigid fixation techniques.

In the late 1960s and early 1970s, Spiessl applied the AO/ASIF concepts of long-bone healing and modified AO/ASIF instrumentation for use in the mandible. His early work showed the need for control of the tension generated at the alveolar level when the standard dynamic compression plate was placed at the inferior border. He showed that an arch bar could decrease the strain 100× and prevent separation at the alveolar level when the standard AO dynamic compression plate was used. The AO/ASIF investigators, Schmoker (1976, 1987) and Niederdellmann (1976), developed the concept of eccentric dynamic compression plates. They modified the terminal holes of the standard AO compression plate so that it was no longer parallel to the long axis of the mandible. The final holes were oriented eccentrically toward the alveolar tension portion of the plate, thereby compressing the alveolar portion, which otherwise tended toward distraction. Professor Berton Rahn at the Laboratory of Experimental Surgery in Davos continues to refine our knowledge of the biology of bone healing and biomechanics.

In addition to the basic biology of bone healing, basic investigations of biomechanics, stress shielding, metallurgy, and implant design have been carried out throughout the years in the various AO laboratories. The AO group enlisted the services of the metallurgist Fritz Straumann and the manufacturer Robert Mathys to develop implant materials and instrumentation. This collaboration continues and is strengthened by the Synthes Corporation working in North America. Working with these manufacturers, the AO/ASIF has formed technical committees to aid in instrument development and quality control. The Subcommittee for Maxillofacial Surgery has overseen the development of the instrumentation and implants for the mandibular and craniofacial implant systems we describe in this chapter.

At its inception, the AO/ASIF realized that the proper application of rigid fixation concepts and execution of surgical techniques requires pragmatic instruction. To this end, the AO/ASIF has continued a series of instructional courses, of which the first was held in Davos, Switzerland, in 1960. Today, an international program of continuing education is maintained.

TENETS OF THE AO/ASIF MANDIBULAR SYSTEM

The AO Mandibular System is designed to provide rigid fixation of the mandibular segments. This system is designed and implanted so that the plate and screw system can withstand and overcome any biomechanical deforming forces that may arise, thereby avoiding micromotion of the bone ends. This clinical concept of absolute immobilization of bone ends and the maintenance of the implant and bone within limits of physiologic loading has been given the term "absolute stability." Under conditions of absolute stability—that is, with the absence of micromotion between plate, screw, and bone—the condition of primary bone healing will occur; that is, new bone will form along the surface of the screw without intervening fibrous tissue. Furthermore, when the situation of absolute stability exists, vascularized bone ends may heal even in the presence of bacterial contamination. Most important is the fact that absolute stability allows immediate mobilization of the mandible and therefore frees the patient from MMF with its concomitant morbidity.

Its bone architecture, shape, and muscular attachments permit the mandible to be conceptualized as a structure that converts imposed stresses into either tension or compression. Compressive forces are generated along the basal border and tension forces along the alveolar border. An imaginary transverse axis that lies approximately along the mandibular canal separates the alveolar process (tension area) from the basal process (compression area) (see Figure 10.2). When the mandible is fractured, forces on both sides of this imaginary axis must be neutralized to achieve a functionally stable

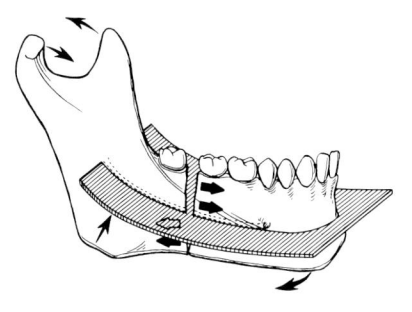

Figure 10.2 The muscular forces acting on the mandible produce pressure forces along the basilar border and tension forces along the alveolar border. Conceptually, the canal of the inferior alveolar nerve forms an arbitrary boundary between these two zones. With a body fracture, these forces tend to distract the fracture at the tension side, creating a gap.

reduction. This is accomplished by a plate and tension band system whose individual nuances are determined by the location and type of fracture. In general, the pressure trajectory of the mandible is restored with a plate and the tension trajectory with a tension band. The plate is of sufficient stability to neutralize shear and torsional stresses. The tension band minimizes bending stresses at the alveolar border, or buttresses, away from the plate.

In dentulous portions of the mandible, a splint is sufficient to neutralize tension forces; in the angle and ramus area, a small plate may perform this function (see Figure 10.3). In certain situations, the tension band cannot be used. In these cases, tension forces can be neutralized by a reconstruction plate, which is a much stronger implant. Reconstruction plates are designed to buttress fragments against displacement and angulation while absorbing all of the functional load.

When the plate and tension band principles are used for mandibular fracture fixation, plates designed to provide interfragmental compression are used. In the design of implant systems, compression is sought for the ability to produce large frictional forces to prevent motion between bone and the implant, which would otherwise lead to implant loosening and bone resorption. Compression can be achieved either through static

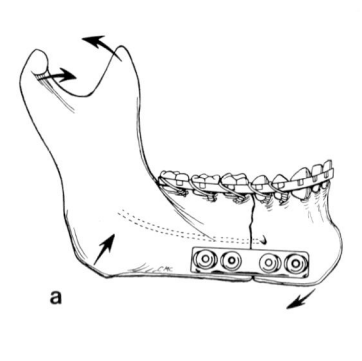

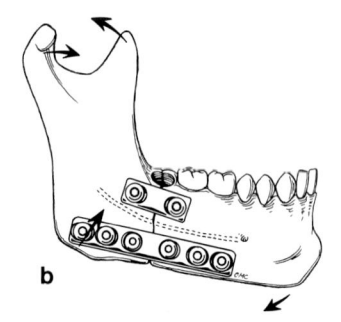

Figure 10.3 (a) In the horizontal portion of the mandible, the tension and pressure trajectories are neutralized by a plate placed at the basilar border and a tension band system placed at the alveolar border. In tooth-bearing areas of the mandible, an arch bar can function as a tension band.
(b) The tension band function outside of the tooth-bearing portion of the mandible can be furnished by a small mandibular plate (as shown) or a miniplate.

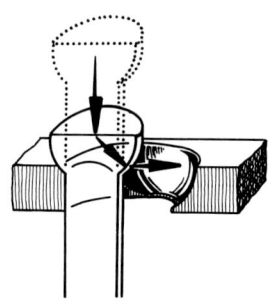

Figure 10.4 The spherical gliding principle involves a spherically shaped screw head that slides down an inclined plane as it is tightened. The bone grasped by the screw tip moves horizontally with the screw. This is the fundamental component of the dynamic compression plate that allows bone to be compressed across the fracture site by the movement of the screw.

or dynamic means. The two devices that produce static compression are the self-compressing plate and the lag screw.

The self-compressing plate designed by Perren for the ASIF has been called the dynamic compression plate (DCP). It generates interfragmentary compression by the spherical gliding principle. This principle causes the screw to move in both the vertical and horizontal directions, which compresses the fracture segments (see Figure 10.4).

The lag screw concept, which is extensively discussed in Chapters 2 and 4, uses the principle that a screw that glides through the cortex of one fragment and engages the cortex of the opposite fragment will compress surfaces when the screw is tightened.

The eccentric dynamic compression plate (EDCP) has longitudinal inner holes for producing interfragmental compression on the basal side and oblique outer holes for compression on the alveolar side (see Figure 10.5). The eccentric action of the plate obviates the need for a tension band. This plate has most utility for simple transverse fractures in the molar region when there are no teeth available for splinting.

The reconstruction plate is a larger, reinforced version of the basal stabilization plate designed for use without a tension band. It is malleable and can be adapted to local bony contours. It has two-way DC holes that enable compression to be applied in either longitudinal direction, depending on the placement of the drill hole (see Figure 10.6). In most situations, the reconstruction plate is used as an internal surgical splint. The reconstruction plate is designed to buttress fragments against displacement while absorbing all functional loads. The reconstruction plates are used for certain difficult fractures around the angle, and more commonly for those with comminution or bone loss where interfragmental compression is not a workable principle.

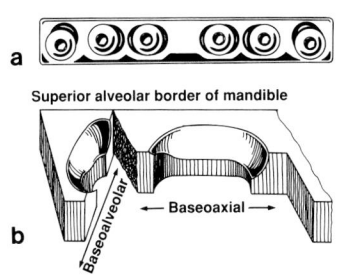

Figure 10.5 (a) The eccentric dynamic compression plate has inner holes that are transverse and outer holes that are oblique. The EDCP plate provides both axial (centric) and eccentric compression by having spherical gliding holes oriented in two different directions. (b) Driving the screws in the inner, horizontally oriented holes compresses the fracture at the basilar border. (c) Driving the screws in the outer, oblique holes causes the fracture to rotate along the inner screws and to compress the fracture along the alveolar border.

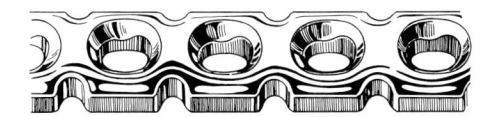

Figure 10.6 The reconstruction plate is a larger, reinforced version of the basilar stabilization plate. Its holes are designed so that dynamic compression can be applied in either longitudinal direction depending on where the hole is drilled.

ASIF INSTRUMENTATION

Mandibular Instrumentation

The ASIF mandibular instrumentation set is a modular one designed to supply sufficient implant instruments to deal with virtually any type of fracture. In addition, a set of transbuccal instruments are available for placement of 2.7- and 2.0-millimeter screws through the buccal tissues for fractures, sagittal split osteotomies, and plate osteosynthesis (see Figures 10.7 and 10.8).

Materials

ASIF implants are made from stainless steel (316L) or titanium in accordance with national and international standards. They are designed and manufactured for optimum mechanical strength, corrosion resistance, and tissue compatibility. The stainless steel implants are composed of 18% chromium, 14% nickel, 3% molybdenum, 1.5% manganese and silicon, and less than 0.03% carbon and iron. Special smelting processes are used to produce a crystalline structure of extremely high purity.

The titanium is a commercially pure grade of metal reworked to provide the desired strength and ductility. The yellow-gold color is produced by an oxide coating applied during the surface-treatment process. Color changes reflect changes in this oxide layer and have no significance. They may result from storage, sterilization,

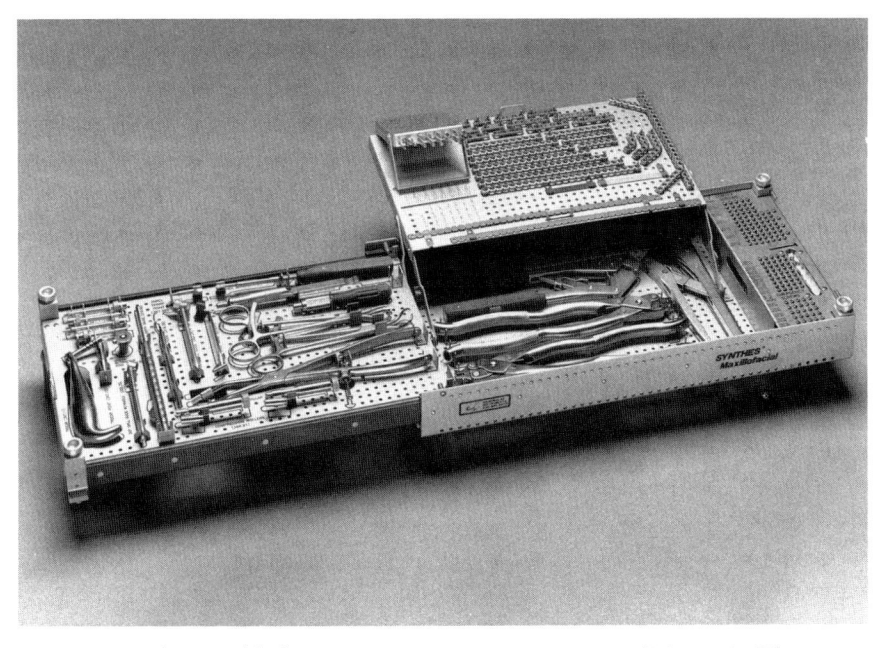

Figure 10.7 The mandibular system comes in a compact sterilizing unit. The case holds all of the instruments and implants in the mandibular set and is available for either stainless steel or titanium implants.

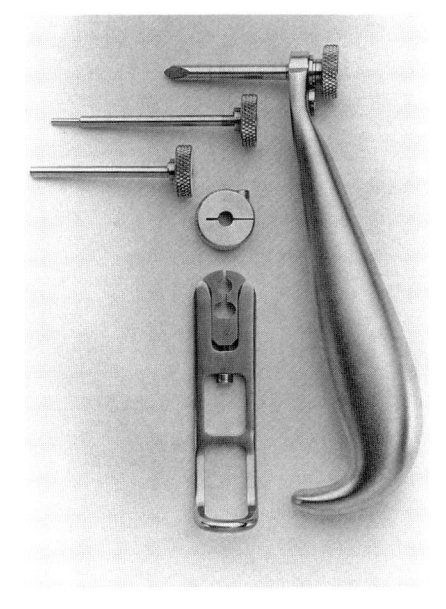

Figure 10.8 The transbuccal instrumentation set is available in two cannula sizes, for 2.7-millimeter and 2.0-millimeter screws.

or interaction with the biologic environment. Titanium has a density and elastic modulus approximately half that of stainless steel and cobalt-chromium alloys. X rays, MRI, and CT techniques can be used with titanium implants.

Mandibular Implants

Plates

Two types of plate systems are used for the basilar stabilization of the mandible: the linear system (compression plates) and the universal system (reconstruction plates). Linear plates are straight and can be deformed in only two dimensions. They consist of the DCP and the EDCP plates. These plates are available in 2-hole (20 millimeters) to 12-hole (100 millimeters) lengths (see Figures 10.9 and 10.10). Both the stainless steel and titanium plates are 8 millimeters wide. Plates with fewer than six holes are 2 millimeters thick when made of stainless steel and 2.2 millimeters thick when made of titanium. The stainless steel plates with greater than six holes are 2.5 millimeters thick, and those of titanium are 2.9 millimeters thick. Fundamental to the DCP plate, by nature of the gliding hole principle, is the ability to provide axial compression. The DCP plate is designed to withstand tensile loading force in the mandible. The DCP plate is indicated for fractures of the symphysis, body, or angle. It can be applied intraorally or through an extraoral incision. It should be used with a tension band (see Figure 10.10).

The EDCP plate produces a compressive force through a centric (axial) and eccentric arrangement of the plate holes (see Figure 10.5). EDCP plates are 8 millimeters wide and come in four-hole (36 millimeters long) and six-hole (42 millimeters long) lengths. The stainless steel plates are 2 millimeters thick, and the titanium plates are 2.2 millimeters thick. The 75° angulation has been found to provide optimal compression at the alveolar side of the fracture (see Figure 10.11). It is important to place the sloped edge of the angled hole at the inferior border of the mandible (if the plate is placed upside down, it will tend to distract bone edges at the alveolar border). For the EDCP, the central screws are inserted first (longitudinal holes, eccentrically away from the fracture), then screws are placed in the 75° oblique holes eccentrically toward the inferior border; and, finally, the remaining screws are inserted in a neutral position. The EDCP plate is used when a tension band splint or plate cannot be used, for example, in fractures in the region of the mandible from the canine teeth to the mandibular angle when no teeth are available for tension band splinting (see Figure 10.12). The reduction forceps with pressure splinting (see Figure 10.13) are useful initially to reduce and compress the fragments when applying the EDCP plate.

The Universal System: Reconstruction Plates

Reconstruction plates are deformable in three dimensions and can be applied at any site. They are designed to give the surgeon the maximum number of options in screw placement and plate contour. Straight plates, as well as plates with preformed angles, are available. The reconstruction plate is thicker than the standard DCP or EDCP plate so that it can be used without a tension band. The holes in the plate and the modified DCP design allow compression to be applied

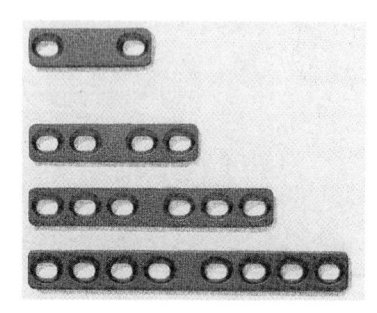

Figure 10.9 The dynamic compression plates are available in 2-hole (20 millimeter) to 12-hole (100 millimeter) lengths. Plates with 2, 4, 6, and 8 holes are shown.

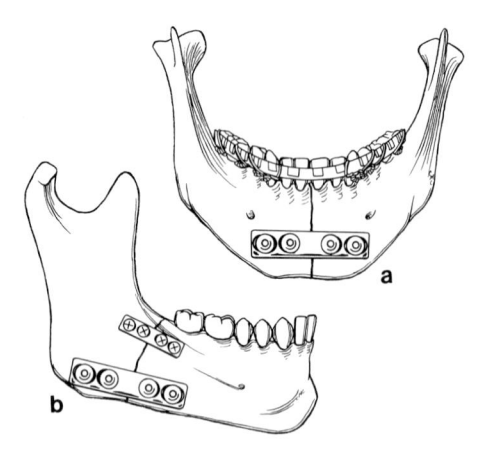

Figure 10.10 Use of the dynamic compression plate in the dentulous mandible. (a) Four-hole DCP used with a tension band arch bar for a symphyseal fracture. (b) Four-hole DCP plate used with a four-hole miniplate (as a tension band) for a posterior body fracture.

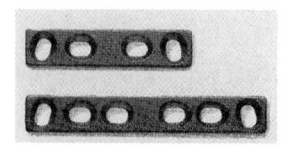

Figure 10.11 The EDCP has the outermost holes oriented at 75° to the long axis of the plate. It comes with four and six holes.

in either direction to stabilize fractures with multiple fragments or bone grafts. The plate can be contoured and bent between the screw holes of 15° without distortion of the plate hole. These plates are 8 millimeters in width. The stainless steel plates are 2.7 millimeters thick; and those of titanium are 2.7 and 3.2 millimeters thick, depending on length. Straight plates of 6 to 24 holes and mandibular angle plates of 4, 6, and 8 holes are available (see Figure 10.14).

Reconstruction plates can be used for fractures of the mandibular angle and comminuted fractures of the mandible. They are especially useful for stabilization of the mandible and subsequent bone grafting following tumor reconstruction (see Figure 10.15).

The key to a successful osteosynthesis is the proper adaptation of the plate to the mandible. After reduction of the fracture, the plate is adapted to the contours of the mandible. A template may be used as a guide. Bending is done with bending pliers (see Figure 10.16). The plate should always be bent between holes. Twisting is done with bending irons (see Figures 10.17 and 10.18). For the three-dimensional bending often required of reconstruction plates, two special pliers (see Figures 10.19 and 10.20) allow the plate to be bent edgewise. Bending irons designed for reconstruction plates are available (see Figure 10.21).

Overbending is done after precise contouring of the plate to the bone. A slight gap of 1 to 2 mm is created between the plate and the convex surface of the mandible to increase interfragmental compression and to improve the plate's distribution over the lingual side of the fracture (refer to Chapter 14).

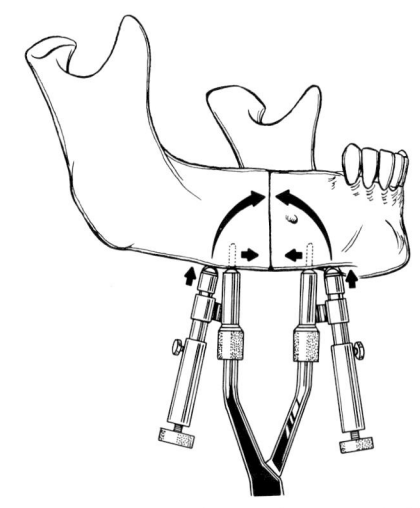

Figure 10.13 The reduction forceps have attachable pressure rollers that provide compression at both the basilar and alveolar borders. They can be cumbersome for the inexperienced operator.

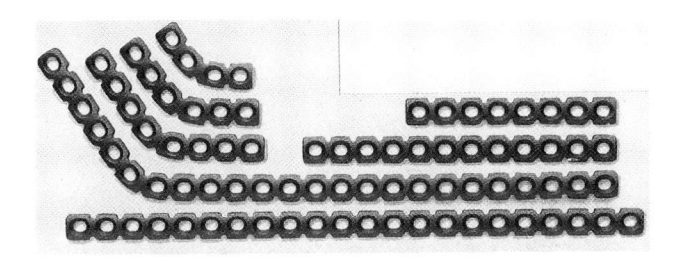

Figure 10.14 The reconstruction plates are thicker than the standard DCP plate and are designed to be bent in three dimensions. Multiple lengths are available.

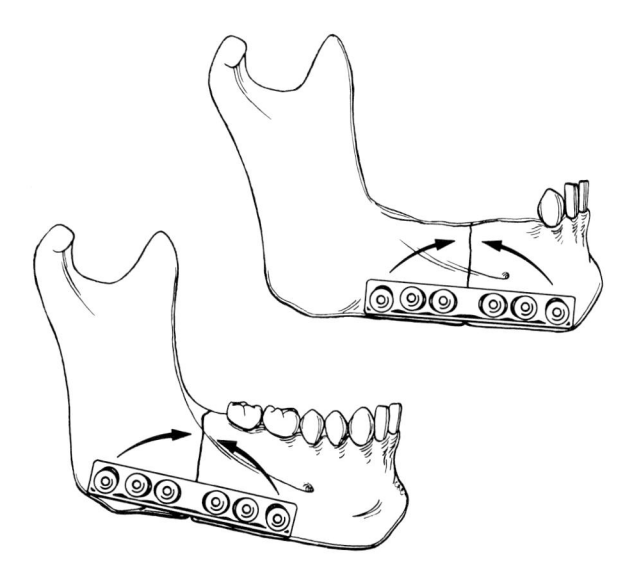

Figure 10.12 The EDCP plate can be useful in fractures of the mandible in the region from the canine teeth to the mandibular angle when no teeth are available for placement of a tension band splint.

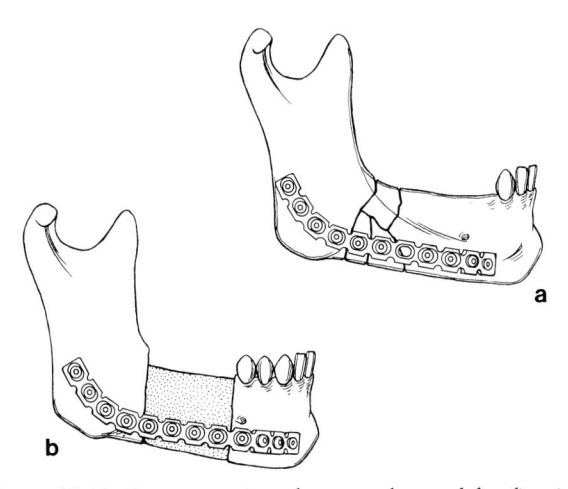

Figure 10.15 Reconstruction plates can be used for fixation of the mandibular angle and are particularly useful for comminuted fractures and the bridging of bone defects. (a) Reconstruction plate used to stabilize a comminuted fracture. (b) Reconstruction plate used to stabilize a defect bridged with a bone graft.

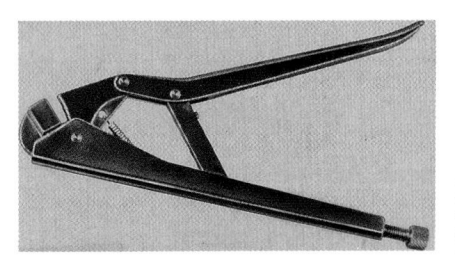

Figure 10.16 Plate-bending pliers.

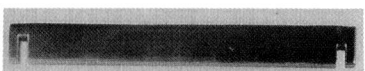

Figure 10.17 Plate-bending iron.

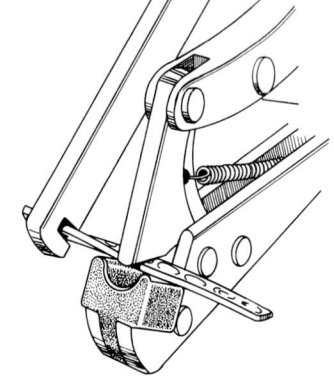

Figure 10.18 Plate being stabilized with pliers to allow bending with iron.

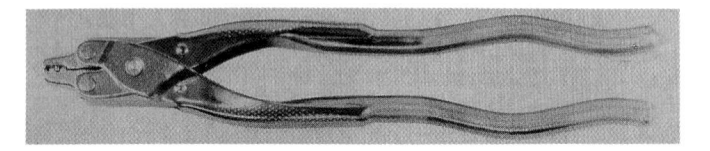

Figure 10.19 Bending pliers for reconstruction plates.

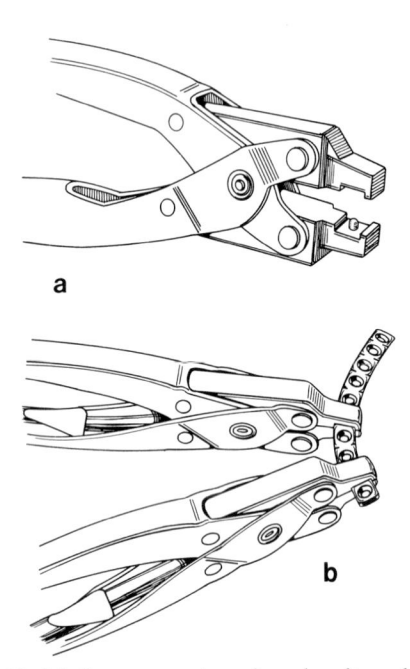

Figure 10.20 (a) Reconstruction-plate–bending pliers have jaws designed to hold the reconstruction plate securely for bending or twisting. (b) Two pliers are used for bending the reconstruction plate edgewise.

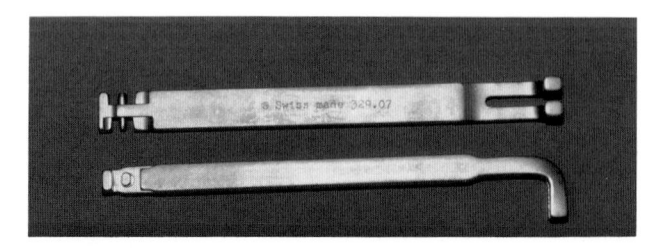

Figure 10.21 Bending irons for reconstruction plates.

Screws

The 2.7-millimeter cortex screw is used as both a fixation screw and a lag screw for mandibular surgery. This fully threaded screw has the same diameter from the head to the tip, permitting good purchase with the last thread. Its thread design requires pretapped holes. The thread has a saw-tooth profile, with flat load bearing surfaces at right angles to the screw axis. There are no flutes in the screw. (The flute in the tap collects and removes the bony debris.) The screw has a hemispherical screwhead with a hexagonal recess. The hemispherical shape allows the screw to be angled ± 25° axially and ± 7° transversely. This allows more flexibility in screw placement relative to the direction of the fracture line, to avoid anatomic structures or to allow placement of a lag screw across a fracture (see Figure 10.22). When the screwdriver is placed coaxial with the screw, the screw can be inserted and reinserted with axial pressure. These screws are available in lengths of 6 to 40 millimeters. The long screws may be necessary for certain lag screw applications (see Chapter 15).

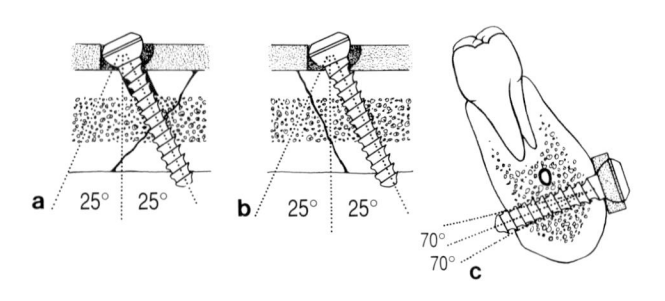

Figure 10.22 The hemispherical screwhead design allows flexibility in screw orientation. The screw can be angled longitudinally ± 25° (a) to allow it to be used as a lag screw or (b) to enable better positioning relative to the plane of fracture. (c) Transverse angulation of ± 7° may allow one to avoid anatomic structures (after Spiessl).

Emergency Screws Faulty technique occasionally causes a defective thread hole that does not allow good purchase of the 2.7-millimeter cortex screw. If this happens, an emergency screw whose thread profile matches that of a 3.2-millimeter cancellous screw can be used to gain a secure purchase by cutting its way through the stripped hole.

Technique of Screw Insertion Effective screw insertion requires a specific sequence of actions: drilling, length measurement, tapping, screw insertion, and tightening. The diameter of the thread hole matches the core diameter of the screw; therefore, a 2-millimeter drill bit is used to drill the hole for the 2.7-millimeter screw. A drill sleeve is used during drilling to avoid damage to adjacent soft tissue and widening of the drill channel by the unsteady shank of the drill bit. One should not reverse the drill as the bit is withdrawn; this leaves debris in the hole (forward motion removes debris).

To select the appropriate length of screw, the drill holes should be measured with a depth gauge. This should be done with one hand before tapping, to avoid damage to the edge of the drilled hole. In order to be sure that the screwheads fully engage the holes in the far cortex, two scale markers more than is indicated on the gauge should be used as the appropriate screw length. This will result in the tapered tip of the screw projecting 1 to 2 millimeters beyond the edge of the far cortex. (The screw length includes the height of the screwhead.) (See Figure 10.23.)

Tapping should be done in a clockwise direction manually, slowly, and with a tap sleeve. The operator will feel a marked lessening in resistance when the tap traverses the second cortex. To avoid damage to the intraosseous threads, the screw should be inserted and tightened coaxially with the drill hole and tightened to the point where significant resistance is met. The drill guide can be used to place screws centrically or eccentrically in the DCP, EDCP, and reconstruction plates. When fixating a compression plate, after reduction of the fragments and contouring of the plate, one screw is

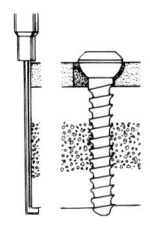

Figure 10.23 The length of the screw hole is measured to assure bicortical purchase of all screws. Depth is measured after drilling of the hole and before tapping. The screws should protrude at least 1 millimeter beyond the distal cortex.

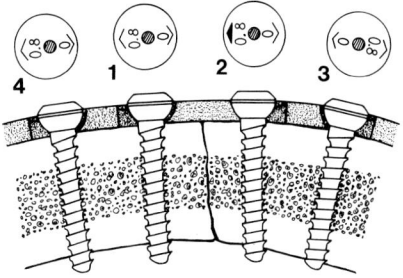

Figure 10.24 Use of the DCP plate drill guide to effect compression. The first screw (#1) should be placed in the neutral position on one side of the fracture to center the plate over the fracture line. The drill guide is oriented with the arrow marked 0 toward the fracture line (no compressive displacement). The second screw (#2) is drilled with the arrow marked 0.8 pointing to the fracture line (0.8-millimeter compressive displacement). The rest of the holes (#3, #4) are drilled in a neutral position (0 arrow pointing toward fracture).

fixed in the neutral position so that the center of the plate is over the fracture line. The arrow marked 0 on the drill guide is directed toward the fracture line to facilitate this. To effect compression, the next hole is drilled eccentrically on the opposite side, in the hole next to the fracture line. The arrow marked 0.8 (0.8 millimeter of compressive displacement will be produced by the DC hole of the plate) should be pointed toward the fracture line. The rest of the holes are drilled with a neutral position (arrow marked 0 pointed toward the fracture line) (see Figure 10.24).

Craniofacial Instrumentation

The craniofacial instrumentation is the result of collaboration within the AO/ASIF group of distinguished craniofacial surgeons from North America and Europe. It is a self-tapping system made of pure titanium designed for use in fractures, orthognathic surgery, and craniofacial reconstruction. A complete set of instruments and 37 different plate implants and screws with three different diameters are available. The plate sizes of 1.5 and 2 millimeters offer the flexibility of two systems in one set (see Figure 10.25).

Screws

The 1.5- and 2-millimeter screws for the craniofacial system are self-tapping with a conical tip. This tip design centers the screw and the drill hole for easy starting. A fine thread pitch coupled with a buttress-type thread provides excellent bone purchase and holding power even in the thin facial bones. The cruciform slot in the screwhead enables the screwdriver to remain engaged without the need for high axial forces, which can displace small bone fragments (see Figure 10.26).

Plates

Thirty-seven plates in eleven different patterns are provided in the system. This includes both 2-millimeter screws and the lower profile 1.5-millimeter screws. In most instances of application, craniofacial plates are used for the three-dimensional creation of a stable infrastructure where small gaps must be maintained. These plates are therefore contourable in three dimensions with a minimal of hole distortion. The plate design reduces the metal between the holes, which allows easier bending as well as little distortion of the holes (see Figure 10.27). A special pair of bending plates that preserve the shape of the hole during the bending operation are provided.

Plates with DCP holes are also provided for the situation where compression osteosynthesis may be appropriate. The complete range of 2-millimeter implants is shown in Figure 10.28. The 1.5-millimeter system is indicated when forces are low and a low-profile implant (pediatric, periorbital) is preferred (see Figure 10.29).

Templates

Each plate has a malleable blue anodized aluminum bending template to assist in the intraoperative contouring of the implants.

Orbital-Floor Plates

Orbital-floor plates are used with 1.5-millimeter screws and are designed to aid in the management or orbital-floor fractures or defects by providing support

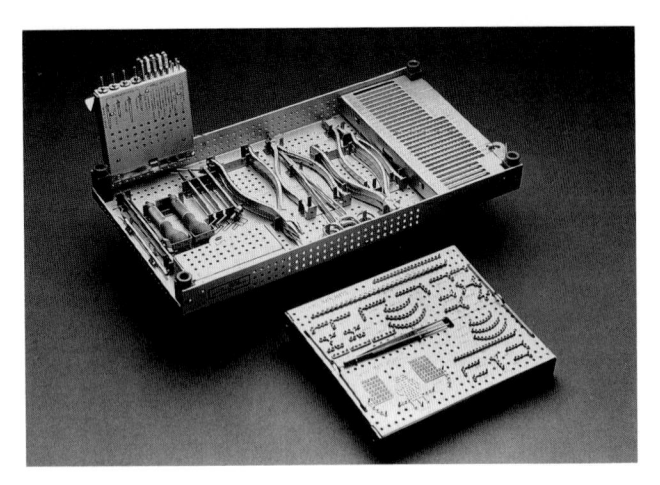

Figure 10.25 The craniofacial system comes in a compact sterilizing unit. The case holds all implants and instrumentation.

The head design is hemispherical with a low profile and an undercut surface to maximize the area of contact with the plate hole. This design allows a maximum of 20° of angulation within the plate while still maintaining a very low profile of screw to plate.

In certain thick areas of the craniofacial skeleton, such as the zygomatic frontal articulation, pretapping may be advantageous, and bone taps are included in the system for this purpose. A 2.4-millimeter emergency screw is provided in case the 2-millimeter screw is stripped during insertion.

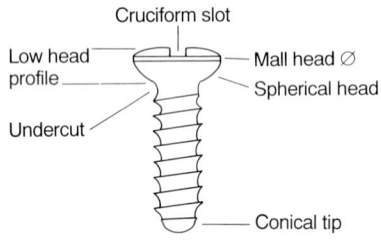

Figure 10.26 Design of the 1.5- and 2-millimeter craniofacial screw.

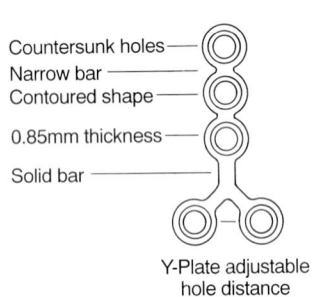

Figure 10.27 Design of the craniofacial system plate.

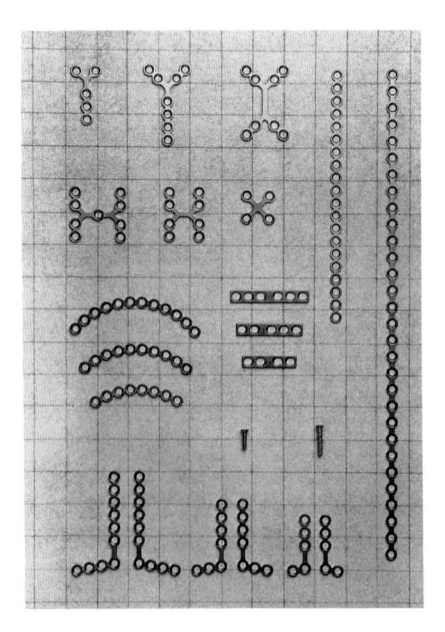

Figure 10.28 The 2.0-millimeter system.

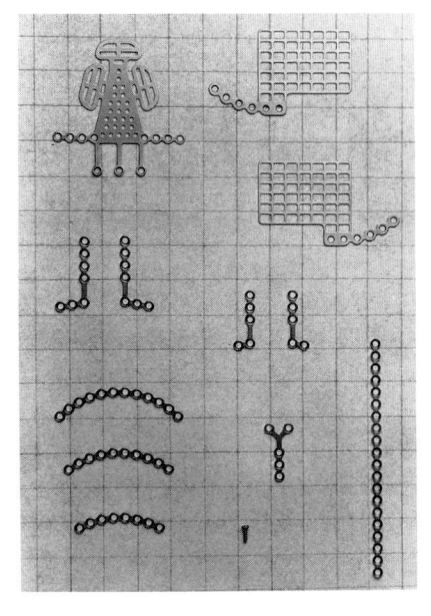

Figure 10.29 The 1.5-millimeter system. Orbital floor implants are located in the upper portion of the figure.

for grafts. A universal implant may be used in the right or left orbit. The implant is dramatically oversized, and the extensions are cut away as necessary for the particular defect. It may be attached to the lateral inferior border of a stable portion of the orbit. Left and right implants are designed for fractures of the medial wall and the floor of the orbit. Such an implant is attached to the intact bone at the lateral aspect of the orbit. Aluminum templates are provided for both types of plates (see Figure 10.29 and Chapter 24).

Instrumentation

The titanium craniofacial set has a complete set of uniquely designed instruments. The screwdriver has a cruciform tip for control during insertion and removal. It is designed with a holding sleeve to hold the screwhead gently without uneven force. Special bending pliers that have a pin placed within the screw hole in the plate are provided. This pin preserves the shape of the plate hole and prevents distortion of the plate during bending. The plate cutters cut the plate without leaving a burr along the cut edge of the plate.

SUMMARY

The AO/ASIF has applied many of the principles of the rigid fixation of long bones to the craniomaxillofacial skeleton and has designed unique systems for the mandible and another for the craniofacial skeleton. The mandibular system employs bicortical, pretapped screws with plates; these allow immediate function after surgery. This stability comes from the use of dynamic compression, the tension band principle, and the strength and design of the plates. It is well suited for the treatment of mandibular fractures, orthognathic surgery, and the reconstruction of post-ablative defects.

The titanium craniofacial system employs self-tapping screws and low-profile plates especially designed for the thin bones of the craniofacial skeleton. Plate design allows contouring in three dimensions to provide a three-dimensionally stable infrastructure for use in fractures, orthognathic and craniofacial reconstruction.

REFERENCES

Allgower M, Spiegel PG: Internal fixation of fractures: Evolution of concepts. Clin Orthop 138:26–29, 1979.

Danis R: Theorie et Prata que de L'Ostéosynthéses. Paris, Libraries de L'Academie de Medicine, 1949.

Krompecher I: Primary angiogenic bone formation. Magyar Orvosi Arch 35: 418, 1934.

Lane WA: The operative treatment of fractures, 2nd Ed. London, Med Publishing Co., 1914.

Luhr HG: Zur stabilen osteosynthese bei unterkieferfrakturen. Dtsch Zaharztl Z 23:754, 1968.

Luhr HG: The compression osteosynthesis of mandibular fractures in dogs. A histologic contribution to "primary bone healing." Europ Surg Res 1:3, 1969.

Muller ME, Allgower M, Willenegger H: Manual of Internal Fixation. New York, Springer-Verlag, 1970.

Niederdellman H, Schilli W, Duker J, et al: Osteosynthesis of mandibular fractures using lag screws. Int J Oral Surg 5:117, 1976.

Perren SM, Huggler A, Russenberger M, et al: The reaction of cortical bone to compression. Acta Orthop Scand [Suppl] 125:19, 1969.

Perren SM, Russenberger M, Steinemann S, et al: A dynamic compression plate. Acta Orthop Scand [Suppl] 125:31, 1969.

Rittmann WW, Perren SM: Corticale Knochenheilung nach Osteosyntheses und Infektion. Berlin, Springer-Verlag, 1974.

Schenck R, Willenegger H: Morphological findings in primary fracture healing. Symp Bio Hung 7:75, 1967.

Schilli W: Behandlungsmoglichkeiten bei unterkieferfrakturen. Therapiewoche 41:2005, 1969.

Schilli W, Ewers R, Niederdellman H: Bone fixation with screws and plates in the maxillofacial region. Int J Oral Surg 10:329, 1981.

Schmoker R: The eccentric dynamic compression plate. An experimental study as to its contribution to the functionally stable internal fixation of fractures of the lower jaw. AO Bulletin, 1976.

Schmoker R: Functional Reconstruction of the Mandible: Experimental Foundations and Clinical Experience, Berlin, Springer-Verlag, 1987.

Spiessl B: Erfahrungen mit dem AO-Besteck bei kieferbehhandlungen. Schweiz Mschr Zahnheilk 79:112, 1969.

Spiessl B: Rigid internal fixation of fractures of the lower jaw. Reconstr Surg Traumat 13:124, 1972.

Spiessl B: New Concepts in Maxillofacial Bone Surgery, Berlin, Springer-Verlag, 1976.

Spiessl B: Internal Fixation of the Mandible: A Manual of AO/ASIF Principles, Berlin, Springer-Verlag, 1989.

Texhammer R, Schmoker R: Stable Internal Fixation in Maxillofacial Bone Surgery: A Manual for Operating Room Personnel, Berlin, Springer-Verlag, 1984.

CHAPTER 11

The Würzburg Titanium System for Rigid Fixation of the Craniomaxillofacial Skeleton

Jürgen F. Reuther

In close collaboration with the Oswald Leibinger Gmbh, West Germany, we have developed an implant system for the various specific needs of craniomaxillofacial surgery. The system consists of a compression-plate system for use in specific mandibular fractures, a mandibular-reconstruction system, a miniplate system for general use in traumatology as well as in orthognathic surgery, and a dental implant system. The common denominator of all these systems is titanium, either in its pure form or as an alloy.

THE WÜRZBURG COMPRESSION-PLATE SYSTEM

In the early 1960s the Swiss Association for the Study of Internal Fixation (ASIF) started the modern evaluation of functionally stable fracture fixation. The main goal of this treatment was the restoration of full function as early as possible to enable active muscle and joint function. Absolute stability was achieved by rigid internal fixation together with axial pressure. Axial pressure in surgery of the extremities was produced by the use of traction devices. Because these devices could not be applied to the mandible, Luhr (1968) introduced a self-tightening compression plate. He was able to produce axial pressure with the use of conical screw heads and eccentric plate holes. The screws were placed in the distal position of the eccentric plate hole; tightening the screws put the plate under tension and pressed the underlying bone fragments against each other. Self-tightening compression plates have also been developed for surgery of the extremities (Mittelmeier 1968, Perren 1969, Allgöwer 1961) and have been modified and developed further, in part for the special needs of maxillofacial surgery (Spiessl 1971; Niederdellmann 1973; Becker 1973).

On the basis of background and our research (Reuther 1977a) (see Figure 11.1) we developed a compression-plate system for use in craniomaxillofacial surgery. Based on the consideration discussed later we chose titanium as the osteosynthesis material. Different grades of titanium for plates and screws were chosen for the compression-plate system.

The instruments necessary for the compression-plate system are contained in a special surgical case. They consist of two different types of bending pliers and two plate-bending tools for meticulous adaptation of the plates. In addition a drill guide, a tap, different twist drills, a depth gauge, and two screwdrivers are in-

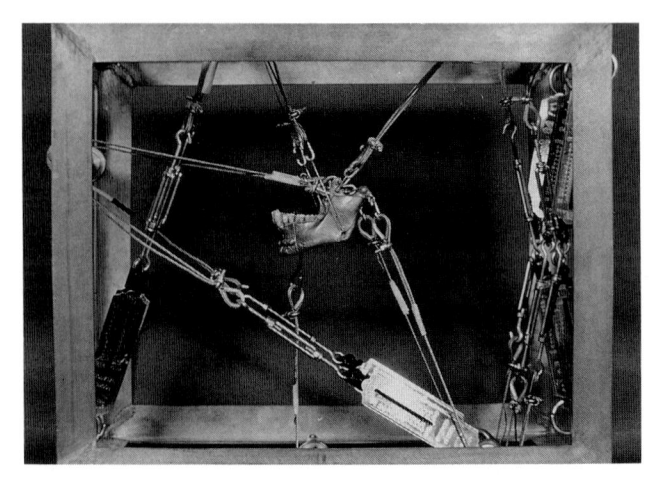

Figure 11.1 Experimental model for stress analysis to investigate the stability of internal fixation of the mandible.

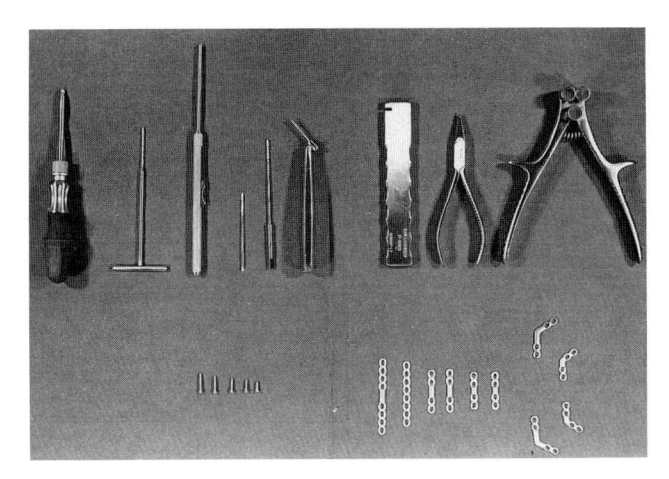

Figure 11.2 The Würzburg titanium compression plate system.

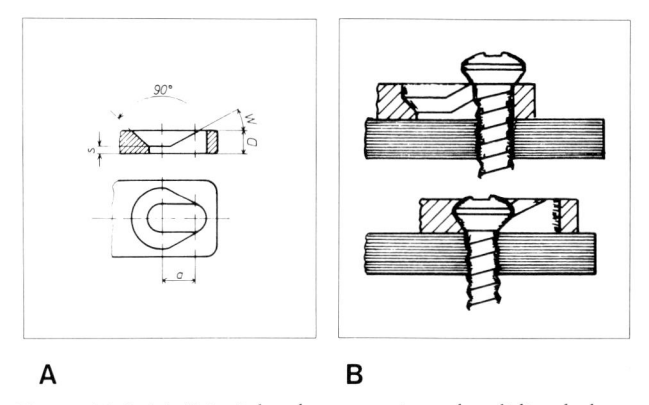

Figure 11.3 (a) Principle of construction of a gliding hole. (b) Development of axial compression by longitudinal shifting. In this case, the screw and the bone it has purchased move from right to left.

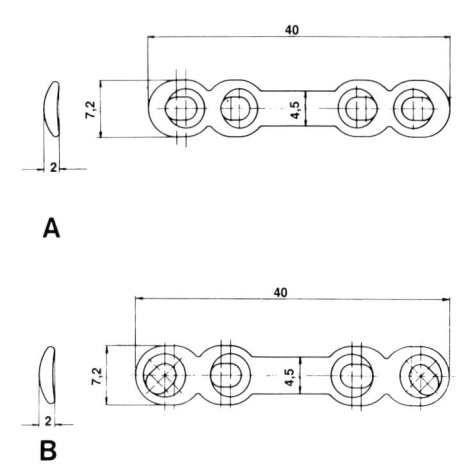

Figure 11.4 Principle of construction of the compression plates with (a) straight and (b) 45° (for holes) gliding holes.

cluded. One of the screwdrivers possesses a device for 2.7-millimeter screws. Use of a modified Spiessl repositioning forceps for reduction of fragments and a trocar and drill guide for transbuccal drilling and screwing is also advised (see Figure 11.2).

The cortex screws of the compression-plate system have a diameter of 2.7 mm. The screws used can be self-tapping or not, depending on the indication of their use. In cases of badly comminuted fractures, the main indication for this system, we recommend cutting a thread with the manual tap. A slow-running drill combined with meticulous sterile rinsing protects the bone against thermal damage. A drill guide protects the soft tissues. The borehole should extend through both cortical layers; its depth should be measured with the depth gauge. The thread is then cut with the manual tap, and the resulting bone chips are rinsed away carefully. This procedure minimizes bone damage and subsequent bone resorption. This procedure is recommended for all situations where the connection between bone and screw is needed for a longer period—such as in badly comminuted fractures—when the plate system is used in combination with a bone graft, or in cases where delayed bone healing is expected. In all other cases the self-drilling bone screws may be used, because in those cases the bone can be expected to heal before the screws become loose due to bone resorption.

The various plates, which are 2 millimeters thick and 7.2 millimeters broad, are all dynamic compression plates according to the principles of the ASIF technique. The plate holes follow the gliding principle described by Mittelmeier (1968) (see Figure 11.3), which allows axial compression. As first proposed by Niederdellmann (1973), plates are available with 45° oblique gliding holes to produce pressure in the alveolar crest area when the plates are placed on the border of the mandible (see Figure 11.4).

The drilled hole should be positioned in the distal end of the plate hole to create interfragmentary pressure. The conical head of the screw is applied to this hole, and it glides in the gliding hole toward the fracture when tightened further. The bone fragment is forced along with it, thus producing interfragmentary pressure. When reverse drilling is performed (with the drill hole on the end of the gliding hole near the fracture), the plate can be used as a neutral fixation plate without a pressure effect.

The plates can be applied to the mandible by the routine extraoral approach recommended by Spiessl (1971) and others. The plate system can be applied, however, via an intraoral approach. In most cases the transbuccal drill guide is necessary for drilling the screw holes and for inserting the screws. This can be performed using very tiny incisions not exceeding 5 millimeters.

In our opinion, this system has its main indication in badly comminuted fractures or when a small bone defect has to be bridged (see Figure 11.5). Another indication is situations where delayed bone healing is expected.

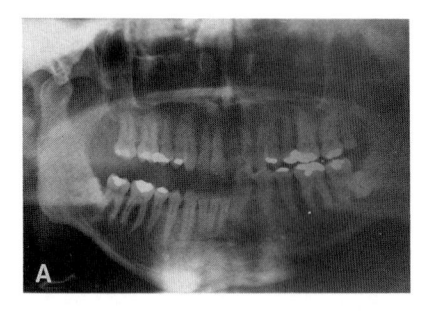

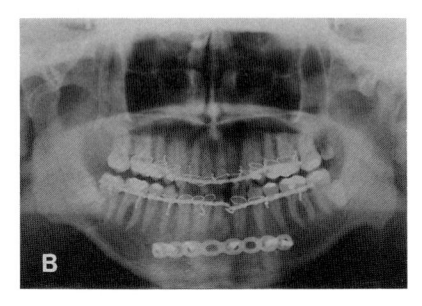

Figure 11.5 X-ray image of (a) a badly comminuted mandibular fracture in the chin area in combination with a condylar fracture and (b) the same patient after fixation and stabilization with a compression plate.

MANDIBULAR RECONSTRUCTION SYSTEM

The problem surrounding the reconstruction of the mandible after radical tumor ablation or after loss of continuity as a result of injuries has been discussed by specialists in oral and maxillofacial surgery for about a hundred years. The free bone graft is the standard method of reconstructing the mandible. Primary bone grafts are used for bridging defects of the mandible after resection of benign tumors. Defects resulting from the removal of benign tumors are usually reconstructed at the time of extirpation, while those resulting from the removal of malignant growth are reconstructed on a delayed basis.

The mandible is functionally integrated with mastication, swallowing, speaking, and breathing. Impairment of these functions to a various extent must therefore be an expected outcome of any operation that results in loss of mandible continuity caused by major bone defects. We have to differentiate between bone defects in the region of the mandibular body and those in the symphyseal region. Apart from the esthetic deformation, functional impairment in the region of the mandibular body is limited to an increased difficulty in chewing because of the displacement of the remaining part of the mandible from its normal position and the loss of its proper guide. The patient is frequently able to compensate for this functional impairment because the muscles become accustomed to the new situation and adapt accordingly. Consequences of central chin resection are far more significant. Loss of support from the muscles of the floor of the mouth and from the tongue may obstruct respiration. Without mandibular reconstruction, a tracheostomy is absolutely necessary in those cases. Scar shrinkage leads to a contraction of the soft tissues and collapse of the mandibular stumps. This results in a total loss of the chin contour and produces the typical "Andy Gump" defect. This scar tissue presents a major obstacle to later reconstructions.

It is therefore essential to reconstruct the mandible immediately after loss of the central chin section to preserve vital functions and to avoid tracheostomy. In order to prevent functional and esthetic impairment as a consequence of resections of the lateral mandible, primary reconstruction, even after resection caused by malignant growth, is desirable.

On the basis of knowledge gained from modern osteosynthesis we have developed a complete system for the functionally stable bridging of mandibular defects. In 1975 we described this system of various plates made of stainless steel. The results with this system were reported in many publications (Reuther 1977b, Reuther 1979, Weisser 1985). This system was redeveloped when new implant materials became available.

The new reconstruction plate system consists of straight as well as right and left angled plates of various lengths. To increase stability, the plate body, which is 9 millimeters wide and 2.8 millimeters thick, has a curvature corresponding to a tube section of 45°. The structure of the central section of the plates is arranged so that it is possible to fix bone grafts or implants. Reducing the plate width to 4.2 millimeters having straight connections between the screw holes results in improved bending characteristics and makes it easier to shape the plate without losing strength. For adaptation to the bone stumps, the plate ends are constructed with four holes on each side. Two holes follow the gliding principle described by Mittelmeier (1968) to facilitate the development of axial compression; and the other two holes are neutral fixation holes (see Figure 11.6). Because of their construction, the plates may be used as

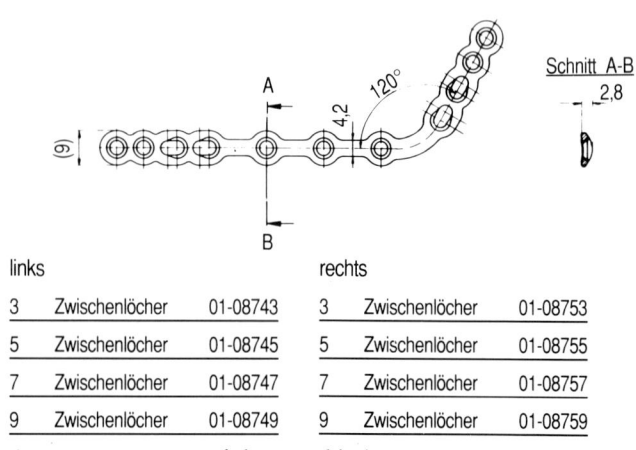

links			rechts		
3	Zwischenlöcher	01-08743	3	Zwischenlöcher	01-08753
5	Zwischenlöcher	01-08745	5	Zwischenlöcher	01-08755
7	Zwischenlöcher	01-08747	7	Zwischenlöcher	01-08757
9	Zwischenlöcher	01-08749	9	Zwischenlöcher	01-08759

Figure 11.6 Design of the mandibular reconstruction plate.

dynamic compression plates for the fixation of bone transplants as well as without a pressure effect for fixation of implants. For fixation of implants, the holes for the gliding screws must be placed medially, as described with the fracture plate system.

The material used for the plates permits cold forming both over the surface and over the edges with no significant loss of bending strength. It is a titanium-aluminium alloy with high strength, low density, and low modulus of elasticity. The stability of these plates was compared to that of our stainless steel implants, which we had used for more than 14 years in over 200 clinical cases. The comparison was undertaken with analogous conditions.

The tensile strength was similar to that of the old system (6700 newtons as opposed to 8500 newtons). The bending experiment demonstrated that the titanium alloy plates would bend at 510 newtons, whereas the stainless steel plates bent at 580 newtons. The backspring capacity of the steel plates was much larger due to their higher modulus of elasticity. Under physiological situations both plate systems are strong enough to withstand all conditions of a mandibular reconstruction.

The bone screws for fixation of the mandibular reconstruction plate system are non–self-tapping cortical bone screws with an outer diameter of 3.5 millimeters because the bone–screw connection for mandibular reconstructions is expected to last longer than that for the fracture system. They are available in various lengths. A thread should be cut so that there is no unpredictable pressure in the screw holes when the screws are screwed in. This guarantees the optimal adaptation of the screws and the most security and safety for the bone–screw connection without bone resorption.

The equipment of the Würzburg Titanium Mandibular-Reconstruction System consists of a newly developed plate bending pliers (with working parts made of titanium) and titanium plate-bending tools. Other instruments are the drill guide; the tap; a depth gauge; and two screwdrivers, one with a screw-holding device and one without. The plates and the instruments are stored in a sterilizing tray with teflon inlays and a teflon container (see Figure 11.7).

For functionally stable bridging, the essential principle of this system can be effective only if the plates can be anchored with at least three screws in each resection stump. The new design of the plate ends enables use of all four screw holes on each side. In our experience, problems arising from biomechanical stress cannot be expected if this requirement is observed.

For temporary bridging of defects, the system can be combined with an implant to facilitate the support of soft tissues in their original shape and to fix them to the implant. This is especially important for muscles of the tongue. In our clinical studies we have found implants of methyl-methacrylate in combination with gen-

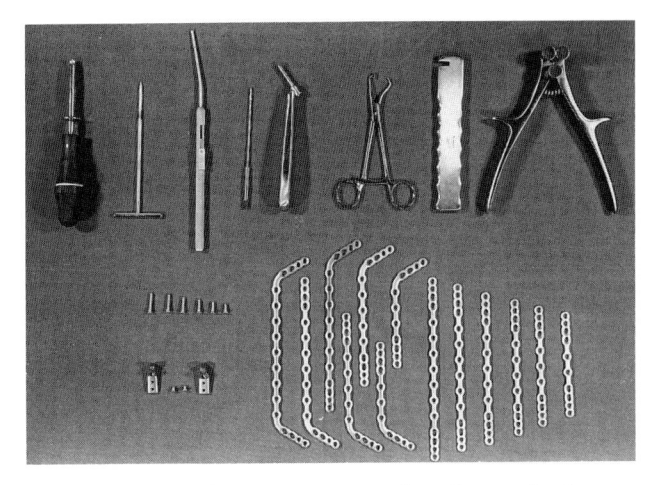

Figure 11.7 Würzburg Titanium Implant System for functionally stable mandibular reconstruction.

tamycin to be useful (see Figures 11.8 a and b). For definitive mandibular reconstruction, the plate system may be combined with a free nonrevascularized bone graft or with a microsurgically revascularized bone transplant.

A combined primary reconstruction using a functionally stable plate and an implant after extensive mandibular resections due to malignant growth has been perfomed in over 380 patients. This approach offers distinct advantages. The residual stumps of the mandible are firmly secured in their proper anatomical position, thus making it possible to maintain a normal occlusion. The mandibular functions are reestablished immediately after the operation, and the chewing is retained by virtue of the stabile bridging of the defect. The floor of the mouth and tongue soft tissues is easily attached to the implant in resections around the central section of the chin. Thus breathing problems can be avoided, and there is no necessity for a tracheostomy, which was generally necessary for operations of this kind. The filling of the bony defect, depending on the amount of soft tissue available for coverage or in combination with reconstruction of soft tissues—for example, with a microsurgically revascularized jejunal transfer (Reuther 1984)—allows restoration of the normal contour of the mandible and prevention of soft tissue contraction (see Figures 11.8 c–f). In addition, this method preserves a layer of soft tissue, which is useful for a secondary osteoplastic bridging operation. At that time the implant can be replaced by the bone graft material, while the same osteosynthesis plate can be used for osteoplastic surgery. An immediate reconstruction is less devastating for the patient. Elderly patients adopt much better to the changed chewing function, which is frequently very difficult for them.

Our radiation therapists state that the osteosynthesis material presents no contraindication for radiation therapy, should it become necessary later on. When accurate information regarding the shape, size, and lo-

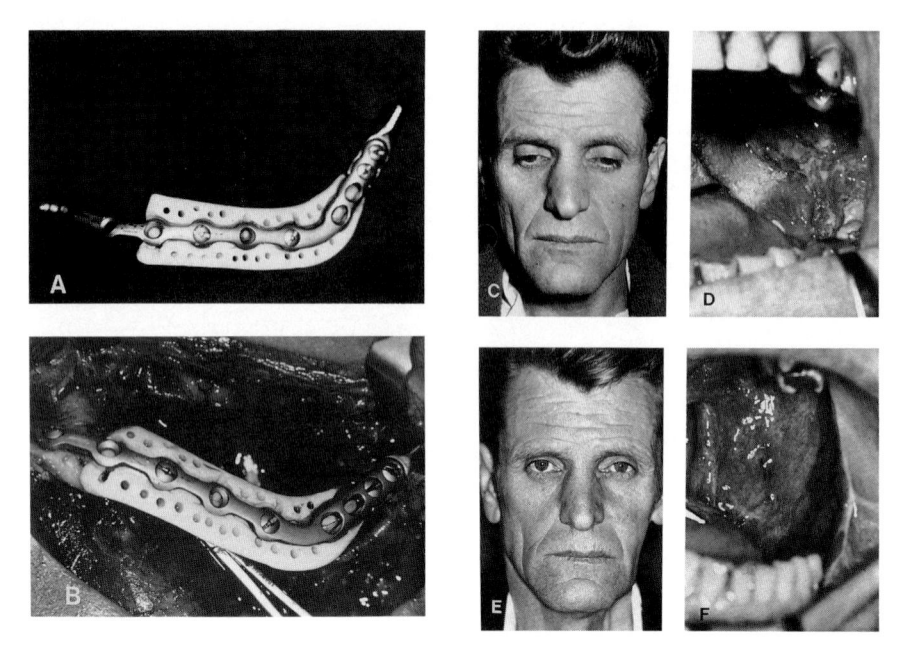

Figure 11.8 (a) Mandibular reconstruction plate in combination with a methyl-methacrylate implant for primary reconstruction. (b) Same plate system in situ for reconstruction of the mandible following radical tumor resection. (c) The patient, a 47-year-old male. (d) The patient's huge squamous cell carcinoma in the left pharyngeal wall. (e) The patient's appearance 18 months after radical tumor ablation together with left radical neck dissection and primary reconstruction of the mandibular defect. (f) Reconstruction of the intraoral soft tissue loss using a microsurgically revascularized jejunal transplant.

cation of the implants is available, the scatter radiation and the shadows the implants cause can be taken into account in the therapeutic strategy.

When the plate system is used in osteoplastic surgery (which we have performed in over 200 cases), the creation of axial compression makes possible optimum contact between the bony surface and the bone graft. This minimizes the functional dead space between the transplant and the bony surface and thereby optimizes vessel in growth (Reuther 1977) (see Figure 11.9).

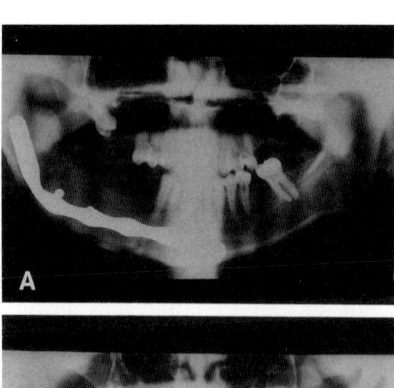

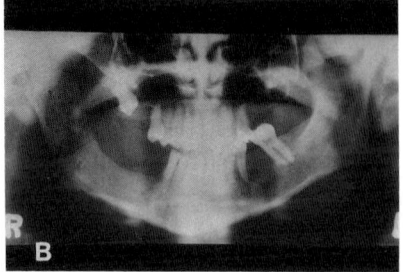

Figure 11.9 X-ray image of (a) a free iliac bone graft stabilized with a reconstruction plate in the right horizontal and ascending ramus, and (b) the same bone graft two years after removal of the plate. Note the significant bone resorption.

MINIPLATE SYSTEM

In collaboration with the company of Oswald Leibinger, we have developed a miniplate system that takes into account the experience of Michelet and Champy. In development of this system, we took into consideration biological and biomechanical aspects of fracture healing. As defined in 1941 by Böhler, these aspects are

1. uninterrupted mechanical immobilization of the fracture cleft,
2. adequate blood supply to the fragments, and
3. an intimate contact of the fracture ends.

Biological and Mechanical Considerations

The plate system was designed to provide stable repository of the fracture segments. The functional loading of the mandible and the force moments referred to by Champy (1977) play a crucial role in the establishment of stability. Wustrow (1919) classified the masticatory forces that act on the mandible and maxilla into a theoretically possible force, the force required physiologically, and the forces that are practically feasible. According to the investigations of Schumacher (1961), theoretically possible forces can be inferred from cross sections of the masticatory muscles. From this, roughly 1000 newtons can be calculated as a theoretically possible force for each side. Uhlig (1953) and Kraft (1962) found maximum values of 90–250 newtons as practically possible forces between antagonistic tooth pairs. Lower forces, however, would be sufficient in order to chew food. In the presence of a fracture, it can be assumed also that a protective posture due to pain is present with even lower values of loading. Schargus (1969) has determined the maximum force for forced opening of the mouth against a resistance to be 70–100 newtons.

Along with absolute level of the masticatory forces, knowledge of the direction of the masticatory forces is of crucial importance in understanding and appraising torsion and bending strain of the mandible. According to Motsch (1968), the mandible can be regarded as a general lever "with fulcrum in the area of mastication." The numerous resultants of the muscular forces concentrate masticatory pressure as economically as possible on the food bolus. This creates a complex cybernetic feedback regulation system (Graber 1982). Because this system is so complex, it is not possible to specify a constant, exactly defined point as a fulcrum for the mandible. The activated masticatory muscles always act via a certain force arm—that is, via the horizontal or the ascending mandibular branch of the masticating and the nonmasticating side—in accordance with their region of insertion. In the process of mastication, this leads to typical elastic deformations of the mandible, as described by Motsch (1968), Küppers (1971), Kessler (1980), Sonnenburg (1984), and Champy (1977) in photoelasticity experiments. It must be assumed that during biting, tensile stress occurs mainly in the alveolar crest region of the horizontal part of the mandible, whereas compressive stresses are developed at the lower edge. In the region between the canine teeth, overlapping tensile and compressive loads originate in both the craniocaudal and the caudocranial regions. Torsional forces are also significant.

On the basis of these considerations, Champy (1983) has described the treatment of mandibular fractures with monocortically anchored miniplates in the horizontal region of the upper margin of the mandible in the alveolar crest region. He has suggested placement of a second plate on the margin of the mandible in the premolar region to secure fixation. Our experience confirms these concepts (see Figure 11.10).

The Screws

Biophysical considerations and biological experiments provided data for the design of the self-cutting bone screws. The external diameter of the screws is 2 millimeters; their lengths vary from 5 to 15 millimeters. The extremely flat screwhead has a single slit and a centering hole to accommodate a screwdriver blade with a centering pin. The special design of the screwhead increases the load-carrying capacity, facilitates handling, and makes breaking out of the screw wing less likely. Because the maximum torque and the cranking torque in the very thin bone structures of the midface have such a low tolerance limit, an emergency screw with a diameter of 2.3 millimeters is available. This larger screw may be used cautiously when a previous screw is cranked.

The maximum torque of our osteosynthesis screws was studied in domestic pigs. After a hole with a diameter of 1.5 millimeters was drilled, a 7-millimeter long miniscrew was screwed in with a torque spanner with increasing tightening moment. The maximum cranking torque was found for the different bone thicknesses and compared with the data of Paulus (1986). This bone screw possesses adequate stability values in bone of 0.75 millimeter bone thickness. The fact that an appreciable increase of 2 millimeters in the torques cannot be observed is attributable to the introduction of two thread turns of our miniscrews. Further thread turns do not produce an appreciable increase in torque (see Table 11.1).

Based on these investigations and anatomic studies, which supported the findings of Ewers (1977), the Würzburg titanium miniplates can be fixed almost anywhere with adequate stability in the midface (see Figure 11.11). Plates should be applied in the longitudinal direction of the supporting columns of the midface in order to ensure a maximum force transfer. Because high

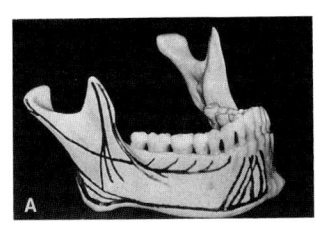

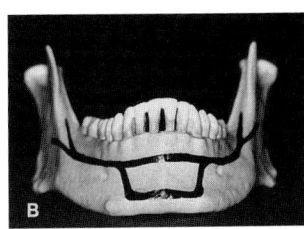

Figure 11.10 (a) Functional load of the mandible and (b) the ideal line for the position of miniplates as derived from functional load data suggested by Champy.

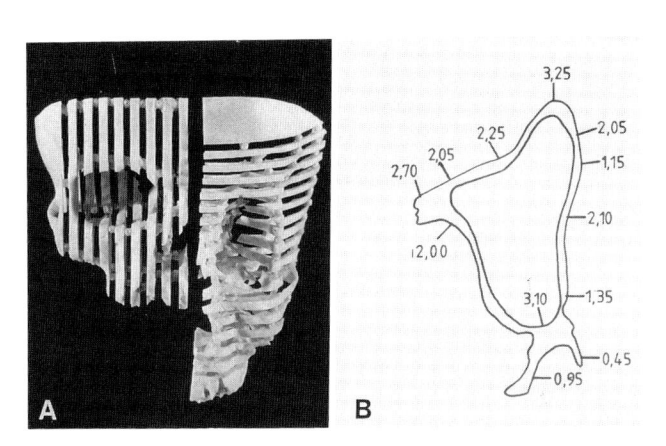

Figure 11.11 (a) Reconstructed skull following horizontal and longitudinal sectioning. (b) Example of measurement and documentation of the sectioned parts.

Table 11.1 Comparison of cranking torque for some biomaterials

Bone Thickness (mm)	2-mm Würzburg Titanium Screw (Nm)	2-mm AO Miniscrew (Nm) (Paulus 1986)
0.5	0.05	—
0.75	0.15	—
1	0.19	0.16
1.5	0.30	0.26
2	0.40	0.33
2.5	0.40	0.34
3	0.41	0.35
3.5	0.45	0.36
4	—	0.37

pulling forces do not normally act in the region of the skeleton of the maxillary sinus, excessive demands are not made on the stability of the plates in this area. This is also confirmed by the investigations of Paulus on plastic models (1986).

The Plates

The basic form of the Würzburg Titanium Miniplate System was optimized by computer calculation following experimental investigations and stability studies. The edge of the screw hole and the thickness of the connecting bridge were chosen in such a way that a deformation of the plate is mainly ensured in the region of the connection bridge without deformation of the screw edge (see Figure 11.12). The edge of the screw hole and the screwhead fit together in such a way that the plate level is exceeded to only a minor extent.

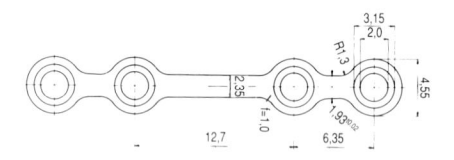

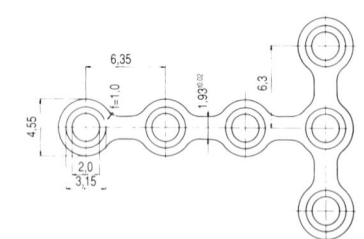

Because metals are stable only to the extent that their crystal structure is intact, we have attempted to prevent extreme plate deformations by making available a large variety of plates. The 20 plate variants ensure that adaptation of the plate is feasible without appreciable plate deformation.

Instrumentation

The Würzburg Titanium Miniplate System is based on a user-oriented harmonization of plates, screws, and instruments (see Figure 11.13). For adaptation of the plates, two pointed flat pliers and modified three-point bending pliers (Aderer pliers) are provided in the basic equipment. The core of the Aderer pliers is harmonized with the hole distance of the miniplates in such a way that deformation of the plates always occurs only in the region of the connecting bridges. The newly developed screwdriver fulfills several functions in one. The collet with socket ensures that the screw can be removed from the teflon bed, transported safely into the area of operation, and screwed axially into the borehole. The centering pin and the centering hole guarantee optimal hold

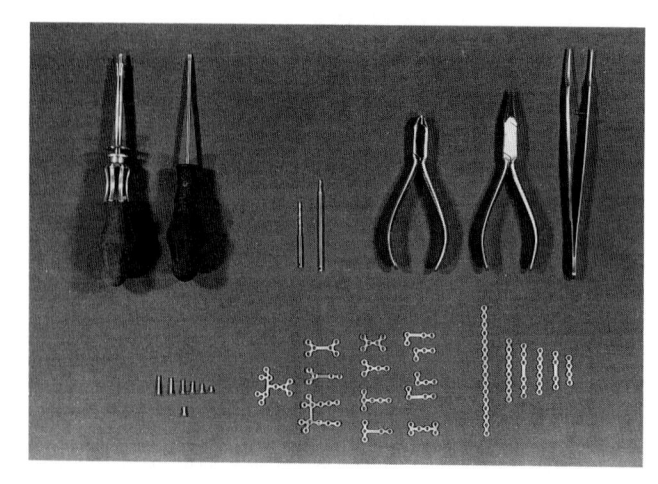

Figure 11.12 Principle of construction of the Würzburg titanium miniplate system: (a) straight and (b) with right angles.

Figure 11.13 The Würzburg titanium miniplate system.

of the screwdriver blade in the screw. For removal, the collet is put over the screwhead and drawn through the socket. The screw can thus be removed by the instrumentation nurse and given to the surgeon. With closed collet, the screw is turned axially; the socket is then drawn back and the screw is finally fixed with an open head. The handle of the screwdriver is shaped to the hand to ensure fatigue-free operation. The rotatory mechanism, which should be handled only with thumb and index finger, ensures sensitive adaptation of the screw (see Figure 11.13).

Titanium as the Material for the Würzburg System

The choice of osteosynthesis material was made on the basis of various considerations. First, the material has to display a biocompatibility and resistance to corrosion as high as possible. Second, the material should adapt easily, quickly, and accurately to the bone surface without excessive intrinsic elasticity. Third, the different masticatory forces have to be absorbed with sufficient certainty in various situations—such as in fracture cases or after mandibular resections.

After testing various materials, such as implant steels, cobalt-based alloys, niobium, tantalum, and titanium, we chose titanium. Several points support the selection of titanium:

1. As a pure metal, titanium is exceptionally well tolerated by human soft tissues and bone. It is resistant to corrosion in many media, especially in the biological environment. The chemical stability of titanium surfaces in the physiologic environment and the unique material/tissue compound are inherently connected with the passive oxide layer in the thermal equilibrium state. This oxide layer does not have a high shear strength. Shear forces arising from relative movements between implant and surrounding or underlying bone can lead to the destruction of the oxide layer. Surface properties change markedly when the oxide layer is destroyed. Mechanically activated surfaces, however, also repassivate spontaneously in the body environment. This process is supported by a local current between active and passive areas. The concentration of corrosion products depends on the size of the mechanically destroyed oxide layer and the velocity of repassivation. Small gaps, environmental stagnation, oxygen depletion, and acidification cause a delay in repassivation. However, even large amounts of titanium products can be stored in the surrounding tissue without producing known toxic effects (Thull 1986). However, the possible toxicity of titanium must be considered when titanium is used as a long-term implant under biomechanical load, for example, as an artificial tooth root. For these purposes we use titanium or titanium alloys whose oxide layers are improved by surface engineering.

2. With appropriate processing, titanium displays better deformability when compared to implant steels. Then lower modulus of elasticity allows titanium plates to be adapted very exactly and simply to the bone surface. Thus, after adaptation, titanium plates tend to spring back only to a very small extent, and so the strain on the bone–screw connection can be kept extremely small.

3. Compared with implant steels, titanium produces less artifact in x-ray examinations, computer tomograms, and in magnetic resonance imagings.

In addition to its biocompatibility, titanium was chosen for its physical properties. Titanium alloys, as well as the pure metal, possess a favorable combination of high strength, low density, and low modulus of elasticity. Like pure titanium, the alloys show a high resistance to corrosion and are proven to be nontoxic and biologically compatible with human bone and soft tissues (Semlitsch 1986).

Titanium and its alloys offer the opportunity to provide mechanical properties specific for the osteosynthesis or the implant material and they are much the same with regard to chemical stability. For example, for screws, a material can be chosen that is hard and has a high elasticity (low deformability), high tensile strength (high load-carrying capacity), and a low breaking factor. On the other hand, the material for miniplates can be chosen so that the elasticity is lower with a lower hardness in order to attain better deformability. Thus this material possesses stability adequate to compensate for the tensile load. In addition, the elongation at rupture can be chosen so that a deformation of the screw holes is largely avoided (compared to steels). This can be additionally supported by the individual form of the plates (see Table 11.2).

The modulus of elasticity of 108 to 105 kN/mm^2 is half that of corresponding implant steels. Therefore plastic deformations occur much earlier (that is, upon exposure to lower forces) than in steel alloys, so that lower load-carrying capacity can be expected for the bone–screw connection, which is responsible for the stability of the entire system. Because the modulus of elasticity of titanium is close to the elasticity of bone (see Table 11.3), the negative biological effects that occur in very rigid plate systems can be avoided. Finally, the damage of the passive oxide layer resulting from movements between implants and surrounding tissue can be minimized.

APPLICATION OF THE WÜRZBURG TITANIUM MINIPLATE SYSTEMS IN TRAUMATOLOGY

Since 1984 we have used our miniplate system for fixation of 394 midfacial fractures and 554 mandibular fractures. Miniplate osteosynthesis is indicated for all fractures of the mandibular body in the presence of full

Table 11.2 Comparison of the physical characteristics of some biomaterials

	Implant Material Champy System	Titanium (screw) Würzburg System	Titanium (plate) Würzburg System
Hardness (Brinell)	120–180	190	143
Elastic limit 1% (N/mm^2)	>235	410	270
Tensile strength (N/mm^2)	450–700	540–740	390–540
Elongation at rupture (%)	45	16	22
Transverse deformation (%)	60	16	22
Density (g/cm^3)	7.95	4.505	4.505
Specific heat (J/g · K)	0.50	0.54	0.52
Thermal conductivity (W/m · K)	15	18	17
Electrical resistance (ohm · mm^2/m)	0.75	0.55	0.48
Modulus of elasticity (kN/mm^2)	200	108	105

Table 11.3 Comparison of the cranking torque of the Würzburg titanium miniscrew and the AO miniscrew

Bone Thickness (mm)	2-mm Würzburg Titanium Screw (Nm)	2-mm AO Miniscrew (Nm) (Paulus 1986)
0.5	0.05	—
0.75	0.15	—
1	0.19	0.16
1.5	0.30	0.26
2	0.40	0.33
2.5	0.40	0.34
3	0.41	0.35
3.5	0.45	0.36
4	—	0.37

dentition, partial dentition, or no teeth. With regard to plate location, the criteria elaborated by Champy (1976, 1977) must be considered. In general, surgery is done through an intraoral approach. An accessory transbuccal incision is occasionally necessary in the region of the ascending mandibular ramus for insertion of the screws. In multiple fractures of the mandible, splinting should be employed to adjust the occlusion. In complicated fractures and poor mucosal conditions, we recommend additional maxillomandibular immobilization until the soft-tissue injuries have healed. In agreement with Horch (1983), joint fractures are treated operatively in our department only in special situations.

In our opinion, miniplate osteosynthesis is contraindicated in badly comminuted mandibular fractures as well as in patients in whom delayed fracture healing is expected. In those cases we recommend using the compression-plate system. This may also be considered when a severe infection of the fractured area is expected. Aside from these considerations, the general rules for operative treatment of mandibular fractures must be respected.

For the application of our miniplates we recommend the following procedure. After exact repositioning, the miniplate, which should be fixed with at least two holes in each fragment, is adapted meticulously to the bone surface (see Figure 11.14a). The wide selection of plates ensures that unnecessary bending and torsion are avoided. Special care should be taken with regard to passive adaptation of the plate to the bone surface. The plate is fixed on the bone surface with a holding instrument, the first borehole is predrilled centrally in the plate hole perpendicular to the plate surface with a 1.5-millimeter twist drill, and the screw is applied. The miniscrews of 5 millimeters or 7 millimeters length are appropriate in mandibular fractures. The remaining screws are inserted in the same way (see Figures 11.14b–d).

The ideal plate positions for various mandibular fractures are shown in Figure 11.15 in accordance with the specifications of Champy.

TREATMENT AND AVOIDANCE OF COMPLICATIONS

In our six-year experience with this miniplate system for mandibular fractures, we observed a soft-tissue infection in 4.1%, an abscess of the fracture cleft in 2.74%, and osteomyelitis of the fracture cleft in 2.74%. Altogether, infections could be observed in 9.58%; however, in no case did this lead to a pseudoarthrosis in the fracture cleft. These data are comparable with results after stabile osteosynthesis—there was no difference between the extraoral and the intraoral approaches; the rates of infection were between 1.25% and 14.1% (average 6.3%) (Börner 1977, Claudi 1975, Dunaevskij 1973, Härtel 1983, Höltje 1975, Joos 1983, Luhr 1972, Schettler 1983, Schmitz 1975, Wagner 1979). The data of Härtel and Sonnenburg (1977) reveal a similar infection rate of 4.4% to 19.4% (average 12.9%) in fractures treated purely conservatively. We have observed that infection decreases with the surgeon's increasing experience in the application of miniplate osteosynthesis. The use of MMF is also addressed for unrealistic patients who are likely to submit the reconstructed mandible to full masticatory loads immediately after the operation.

Wound dehiscence is managed by open wound treatment with H_2O_2 and chlorhexamed lavages. The bone is covered with a zinc-oxide–eugenol tamponade. This therapy enables complete healing of the soft-tissue wounds and an uncomplicated bone healing.

Postoperative soft-tissue infection, fracture cleft abscess, and osteomyelitis occurred mainly in patients whose fracture treatment had been delayed. In general, surgical treatment of the fracture proved to be free of complications within the first 12 hours after the accident. If treatment of the fracture is not possible within this period, we have found maxillomandibular immobilization in addition to miniplate osteosynthesis to be especially effective until the soft-tissue wound has healed. Perioperative chemoprophylaxis over 48 hours and meticulous oral hygiene are also of particular advantage. Careful readaption of the soft tissues, in some cases in combination with a fibrin tissue adhesive fixation, is especially effective in postoperative healing.

SURGICAL TREATMENT OF MIDFACE FRACTURES

For surgical treatment of midface fractures, the specific morphology and biomechanics of the maxilla are of crucial importance. Unlike in the mandible, dislocations of muscular origin in the maxilla occur only at the pterygoid process. In the midface, fracture dislocations are usually a manifestation of the intensity and direction of the action of force.

The maxilla, with its processes to the adjacent bones, is the predominant structure of the midface. Its

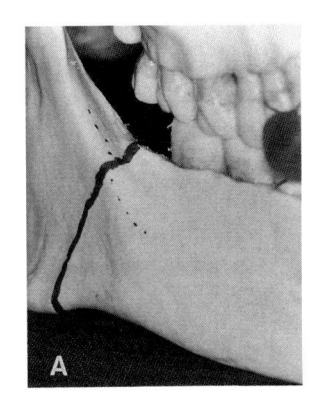

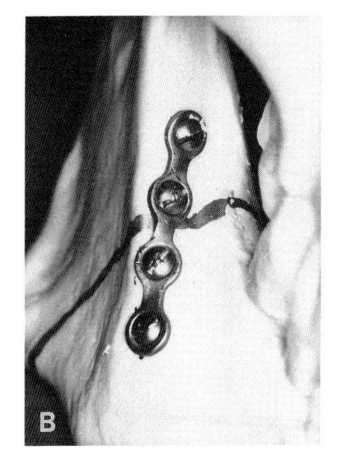

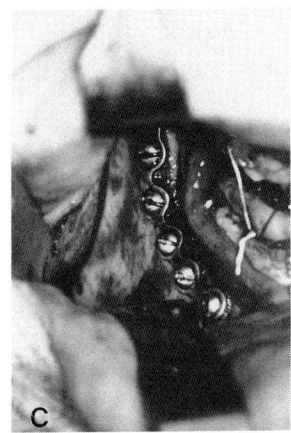

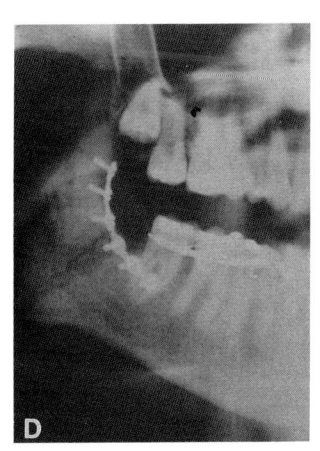

Figure 11.14 Mandibular fracture in the angulus. (a) Ideal osteosynthesis line for the position of a miniplate. (b) Fixation and stabilization of the fracture using a four-hole miniplate on the anatomical model. (c) Same situation in a clinical case using a six-hole miniplate. (d) X-ray image of this case.

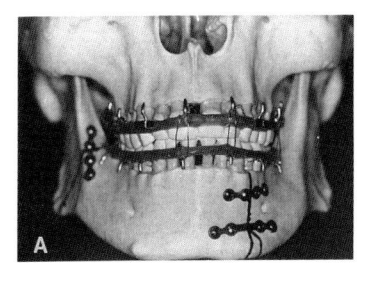

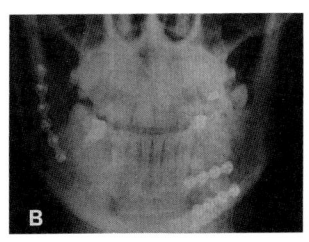

Figure 11.15 Typical positions of miniplates in different areas of the mandible: (a) anatomic model, and (b) x-ray image of a clinical case.

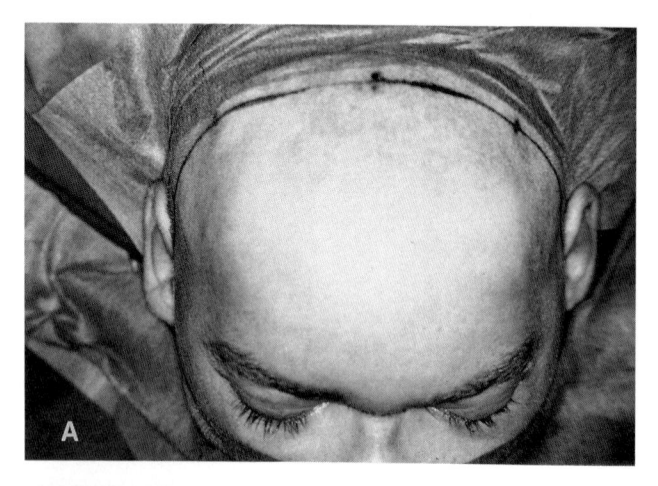

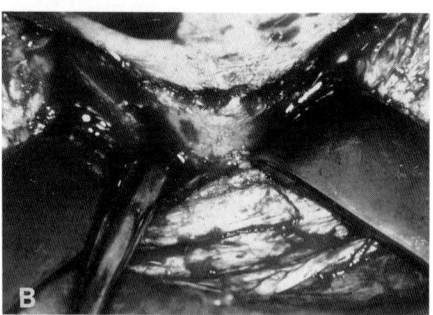

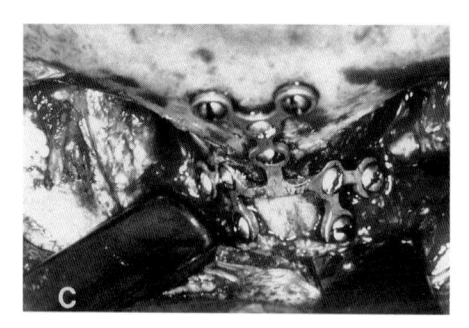

Figure 11.16 (a) Principle of the bicoronal incision for exposure of fractures in the midface area. (b) Exposure of the fracture on the basis of the nose. (c) Miniplate osteosynthesis of the fracture line together with fixation of the medial canthal tendon.

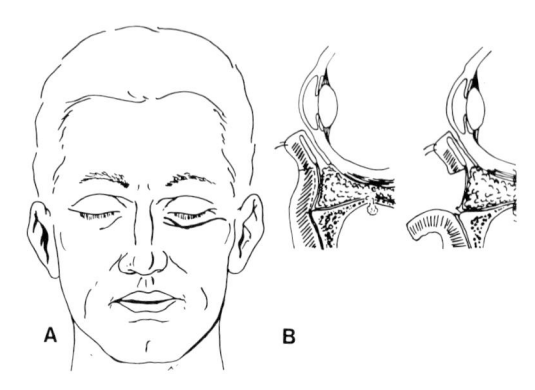

Figure 11.17 (a) Principle of the modified subciliary incision. (b) Exposure of the floor of the orbit via this route.

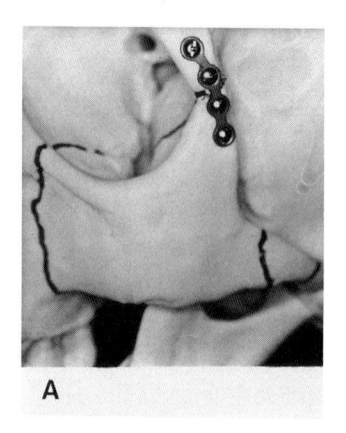

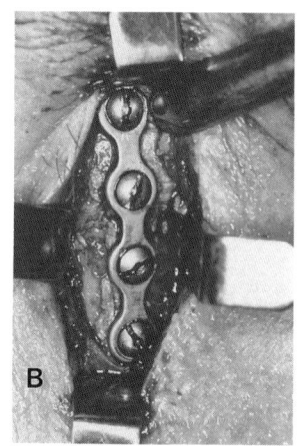

Figure 11.18 Fixation of an uncomplicated fracture of the zygoma with one miniplate on the zygomatic-frontal suture: (a) anatomic model and (b) clinical case.

thin bony walls are strengthened by basal arches, which form a frame (Sicher and De Bral, 1970). The course of functionally subdivided trajectories in the region of the jaws was demonstrated by Rohen (1958). The bony structures that bear the pressure of mastication are located on each side in the frontonasal, zygomatic, and sphenoid pillar buttresses (Wolff 1892, Pauwels 1965).

In the treatment of midface fractures, special attention must be paid to the restoration of the supporting pillars. The miniplates must be positioned parallel to these pillars to ensure appropriate transmission of forces. Measurements have demonstrated that these structures provide sufficient bone thickness for fixation of the miniscrews.

Various surgical incisions have been described to approach the midface and the upper face (Bull 1987, Casson 1974, Chuong 1986).

Over the last 6 years, in 72 cases, we have approached the supraorbital frontal and glabellar area through a bicoronal subperiosteal flap as described by Tessier (Figure 11.16). We have been exceedingly displeased with the aesthetic result of bilateral Kilian incisions linked with a transverse incision over the glabella (Dieckmann and Hackmann 1977). We use a modified subciliary incision to explore the orbital floor (Becker and Austermann 1977) (Figure 11.17). We have found that these approaches provide better exposure than the subciliary or transconjunctival approach (Tenzel and Miller 1971, Tessier 1973, Converse 1973).

In less severe midface fractures, the miniplate osteosynthesis can be carried out via the infraorbital approach and at the lateral orbit margin. The intraoral approach is used to approach fractures at the Le Fort I level.

In the treatment of lateral midface fractures the zygoma can be stabilized with a single osteosynthesis plate at the zygomatic frontal suture (see Figure 11.18)

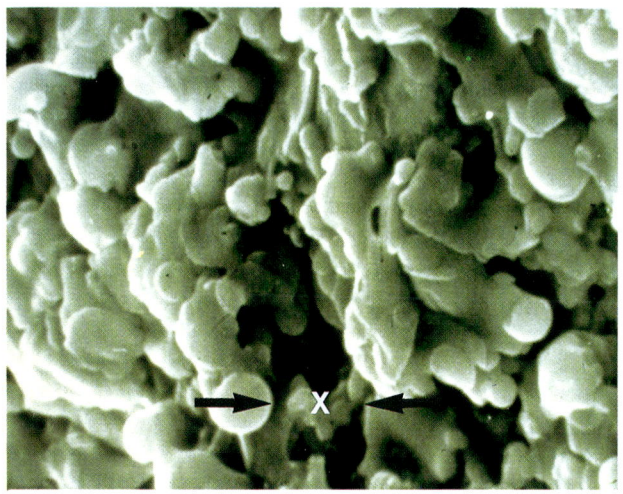

Color Plate 9 Surface of titanium plasma-coated implant (SEM; x = 20 to 40 µm).

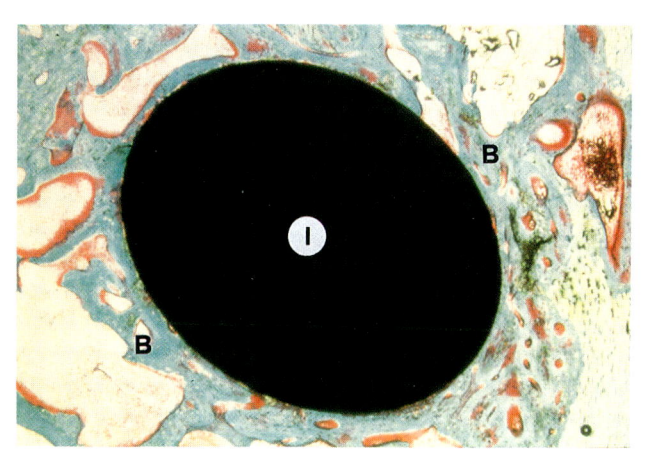

Color Plate 10 Ankylotic bond between the rough surface of a cylindrical titanium implant and the bone (monkey; I = implant, B = bone).

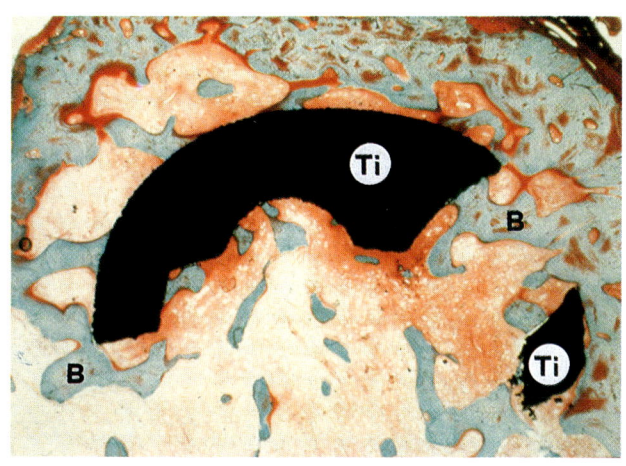

Color Plate 11 Histological section showing bone growth into and over the shoulder region of a HC implant (monkey; Ti = titanium with rough surface, B = bone).

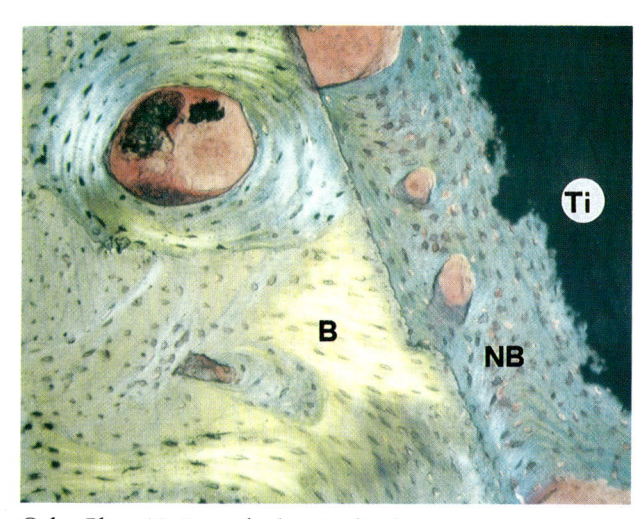

Color Plate 12 Part of a longitudinal section through a removed HC implant (HC outer side). New bone (NB) in direct contact with the rough implant surface. (B = old bone.)

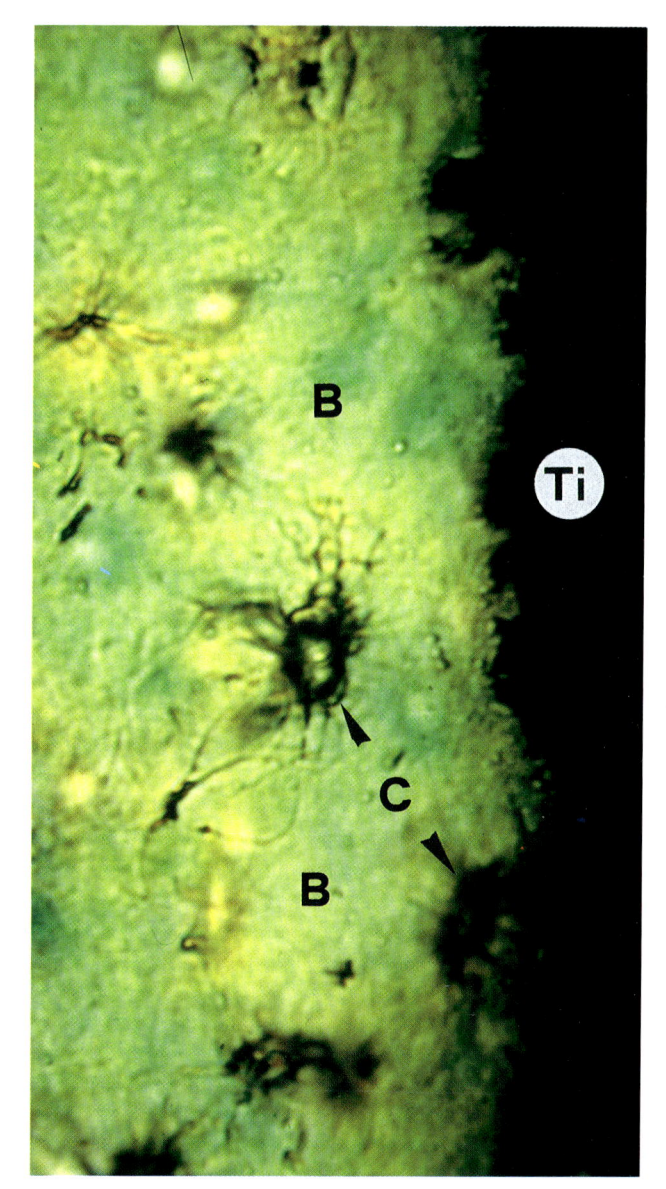

Color Plate 13 Inner surface of an osteointegrated HC implant. A compact cementum-like hard tissue (B) is deposited in all crevices of the titanium plasma-coated surface (Ti).

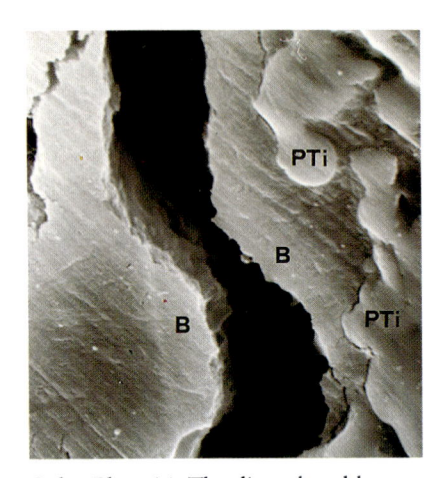

Color Plate 14 The direct bond between bone (B) and the titanium plasma layer (PTi) can also be demonstrated in SEM-micrographs. Extreme stresses may cause fissures in the bone rather than separation of the bone from the titanium-sprayed layer.

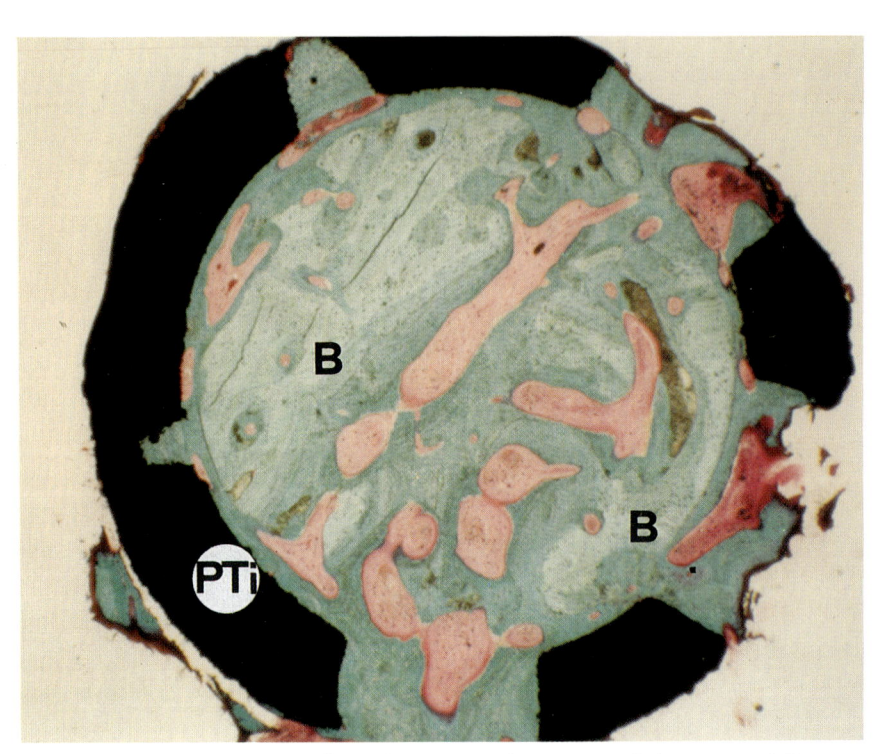

Color Plate 15 Cross section through a HC implant removed three years following implantation as a result of marginal "periimplantitis" (female patient, age 75). The interior space of the implant is completely filled with new bone (B), which is in direct (ankylotic) contact with the titanium surface (PTi).

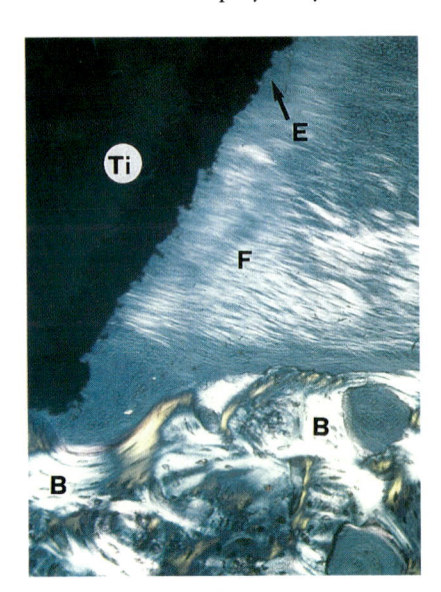

Color Plate 16 Light microscopy appearance of the marginal area of connective tissue between the bone (B) and the epithelium (E). Fibers (F) are attached perpendicular on the titanium-sprayed surface (PTi).

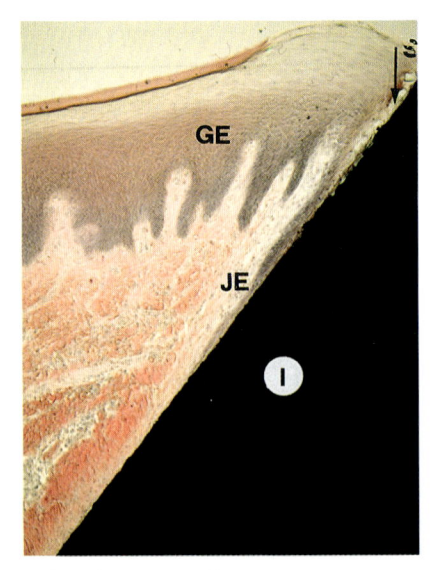

Color Plate 17 Light microscopy overview of junctional epithelium (JE) in close contact with the abutment of the implant (I). (GE = gingival epithelium, S = sulcus gingivae.)

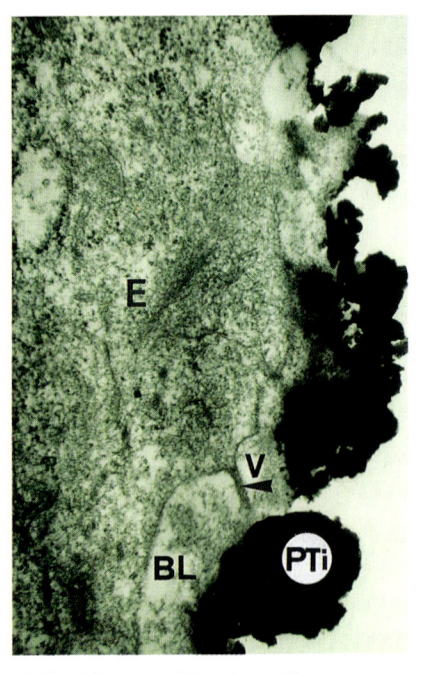

Color Plate 18 Titanium (flame-sprayed layer) in contact with regenerated epithelial tissue 83 days after implantation of a HC implant in a maccaca speciosa monkey. A finely granular substance that corresponds ultrastructurally to a basal lamina (BL) is situated between the titanium (PTi) and an epithelial cell (E). Microvilli (V) of the cell are buried in the basal lamina. Courtesy Prof. E. van der Zypen, Bern.)

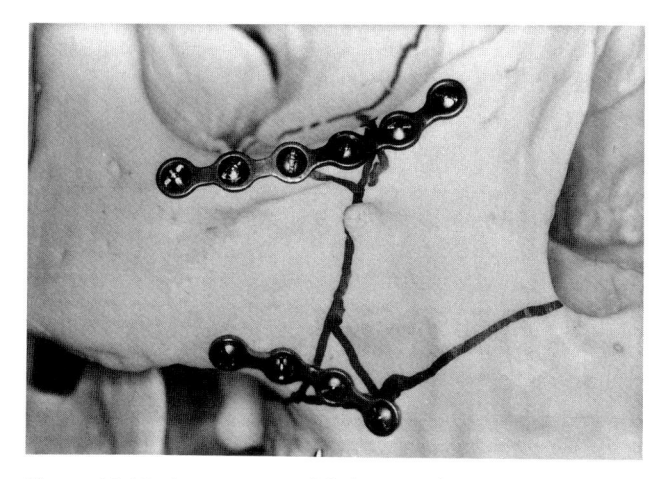

Figure 11.19 Anatomic model showing fixation of a badly comminuted fracture of the zygoma (a) at the zygomaticomaxillary suture and (b) at the infraorbital rim.

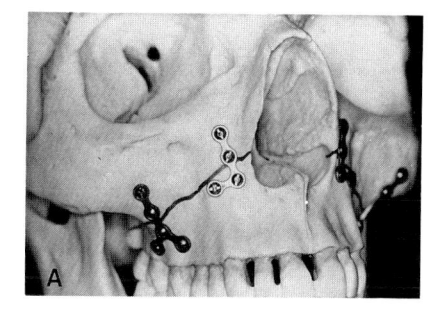

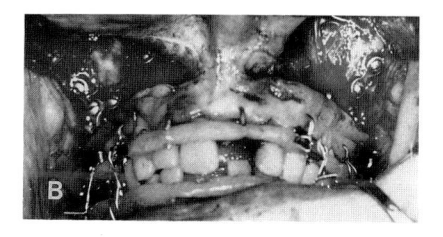

Figure 11.20 Stabilization of the Le Fort I fracture at the supporting pillars of the midface: (a) Anatomic model, and (b) clinical case.

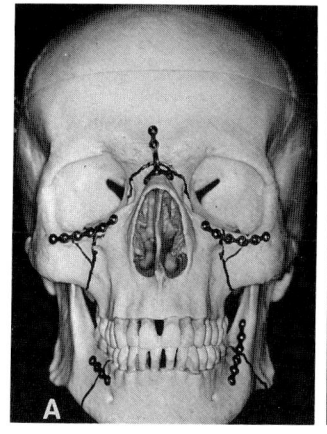

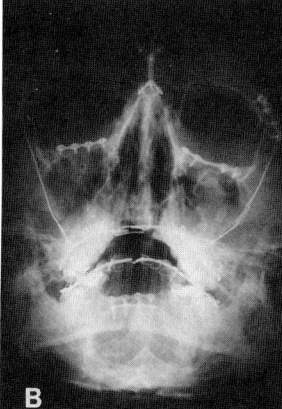

Figure 11.21 Typical fixation of the Le Fort II fracture: (a) anatomic model, and (b) x-ray image.

or at the zygomatico-maxillary suture (see Figure 11.19) via an intraoral approach. Additional fixation at the infraorbital rim is recommended for extensive comminuted fractures in the region of the infraorbital rim with involvement of the orbital floor.

Fractures of the Le Fort I type are stabilized in the region of the supporting pillars at the pyriform aperture and at the zygomatic alveolar process (see Figure 11.20).

In Le Fort II fractures, plates on the infraorbital margin frequently provide sufficient fixation. The need for additional osteosynthesis at the nasofrontal area is determined by the extent of involvement of the nasal skeleton. Various preformed nasal plates are especially suitable for this purpose (see Figure 11.21).

In badly comminuted midface fractures with skull and skull bone involvement, various combinations of the described plate positions may be necessary. Craniofacial suspension may be a careful adjunct in these situations (Figure 11.16). In those cases additional fixations of the midface by means of craniofacial suspension has also proved to be effective (see Figure 11.22).

Our experience with 394 midface fractures within the last six years using the Würzburg Titanium Miniplate System parallels the similar good results reported by Michelet (1971), Champy (1983) and many others (Gerlach 1980, Schilli 1986, Steinbauer 1986, Chuong 1986, Paulus 1986). We observed minimal complications. The infection rate, of only 5.8%, was effectively treated with a regimen of local lavages combined with antibiotics. There were no cases of pseudoarthrosis.

The plates can be adapted easily and exactly, enabling anatomic fixation of very small and thin bone fragments. In most cases the MMF can be avoided. In cases of very comminuted fractures, where stabilization cannot be achieved safely with miniplate osteosynthesis, additional MMF is required. Furthermore, in those cases,

it is our opinion that use of additional craniofacial suspension wires is essential. The miniplates in the midfacial area are stable only under compression forces. When tension forces due to the movements of the mandible are expected, these forces should be eliminated by suspension wires.

THE WÜRZBURG TITANIUM SYSTEM IN ORTHOGNATHIC AND CRANIOFACIAL SURGERY

The Würzburg system offers special equipment for fixation of elective osteotomies. For midfacial and craniofacial osteotomies, the system consists of our typical

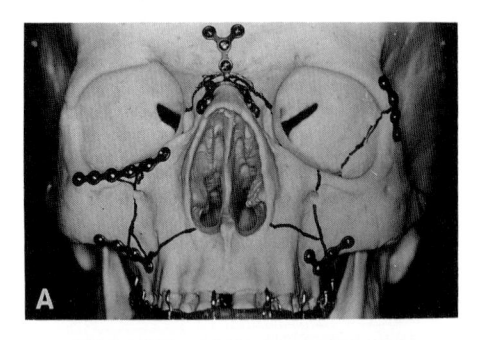

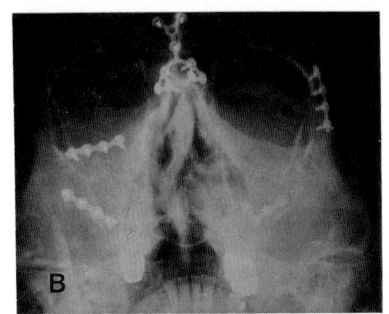

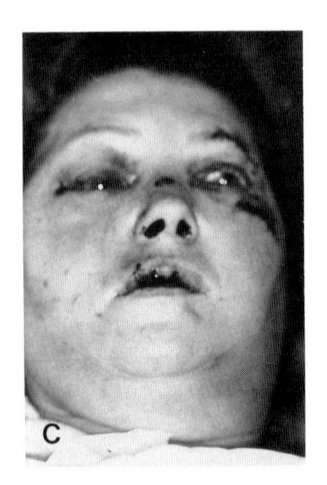

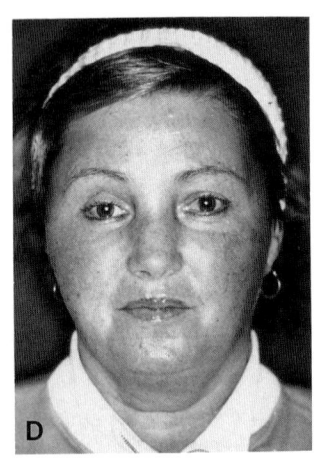

Figure 11.22 Fixation of comminuted fractures of the midface in various areas: (a) anatomic model, and (b) x-ray image. (c) The patient preoperatively and (d) the same patient one year after operation via bicoronal incision.

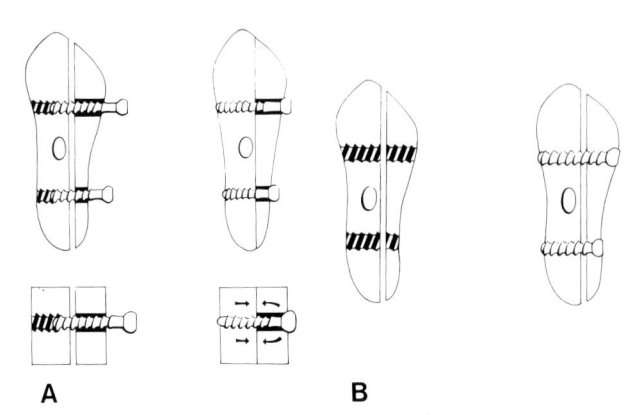

Figure 11.23 Schematic drawings of the functions of (a) lag screws and (b) positioning screws.

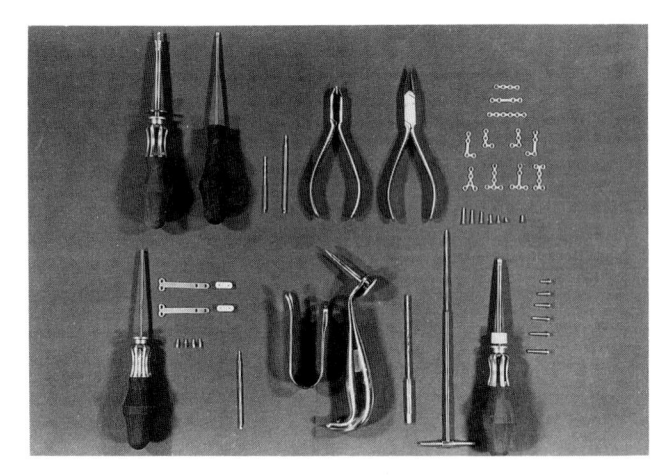

Figure 11.24 Würzburg titanium implant system for orthognathic surgery.

miniplate system whose use has been described in the section on traumatology.

For the rigid fixation of mandibular osteotomies, we offer special equipment consisting of positioning plates and self-cutting positioning screws. This combination was developed to enable the stabile fixation particularly after the sagittal split osteotomy of the ascending ramus without functional disturbances. We had found that stabile fixation of the ascending ramus after shifting of the segments was possible only with excessive rotation of the condyles when using the lag screw technique.

Therefore our system uses self-cutting positioning screws with a thread in the buccal and the lingual part of the ascending ramus (see Figure 11.23). This method maintains the gap between the osteotomized segments and avoids condylar dislocations. For this technique the positioning of the condyles is essential. Our positioning plates follow the proposals of Luhr (1985).

The system consists of a self-retaining cheek retractor combined with a transbuccal trocar, two T-shaped plates with labels for right and left use, miniscrews with hexagonal heads, acrylic blocs, 2.7-millimeter self-cutting positioning screws of various lengths, and two specialized screwdrivers. The equipment is stored in a sterilizing container together with a selection of the miniplate system (see Figure 11.24).

The preoperative planning of osteotomies is crucial when rigid fixation is used. The surgical planning is based upon the exact evaluation of the cephalometric films and extraoral photographs. The models for planning of the surgery must be mounted in a semiadjustable anatomic articulator. The maxillary cast is anatomically fixed by face–bow transfer. The mandibular cast can be fixed with common occlusal registration wax, or it can be fixed more exactly with Gerber's registration method. This prevents preoperative malpositions of the condyles, which would be maintained after the

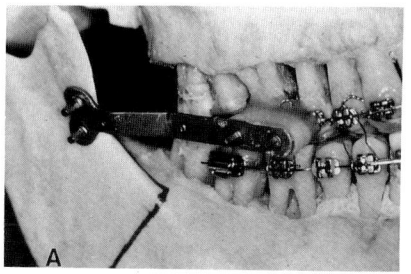

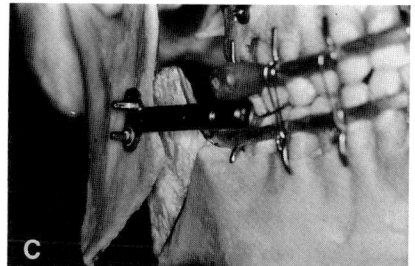

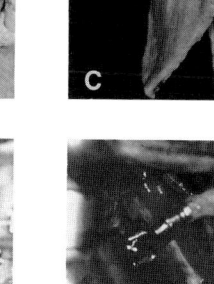

Figure 11.25 Reproduction of the condyle position during sagittal split osteotomy: fixation of the ascending ramus to the maxillary arch bar with two T-shaped plates and hexagonal-headed screws. (a) Anatomic model. (b) Clinical situation; readaptation of the plates after the sagittal split is completed. (c) Anatomic model. (d) Clinical situation; stabile fixation using positioning screws. (e) Anatomic model. (f) Clinical situation (notice the wide gap).

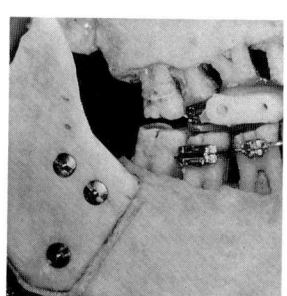

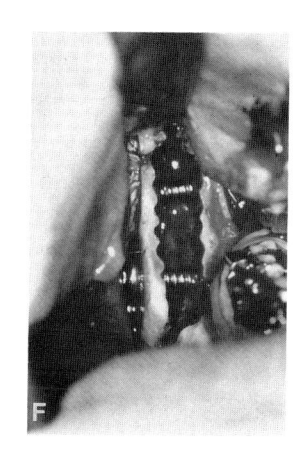

operation by rigid fixation. After cephalometric and soft-tissue analysis, the models are shifted in the articulator in all three dimensions. When surgery is planned with this method and the movements are accurately recorded, the movement of the dento-osseous segments at surgery accurately duplicate the movement planned on the articulated models. Splints for use at surgery are constructed on the articulated models prior to and after model surgery.

After the operation is started in the typical manner with exposure of the ascending ramus on both sides, the centric relationship is fixed using the preoperative interocclusal splint. To reproduce the condyle position, the two T-shaped positioning plates are fixed to the ascending ramus through a transbuccal incision on the anterior border of the masseter muscle using the self-retaining cheek retractor. The hexagonal head of our fixation screws provides the secure and easy fixation of the screws to the screwdriver. This facilitates substantially the use of this system during the operation. For tension-free adaptation, the positioning plates are fixed to the maxillary arch bar using self-curing methyl-methacrylate resin (see Figures 11.25 a and b). After the positioning plates are removed and the MMF is opened, the sagittal split osteotomy can be performed in the typical manner. Following this osteotomy, the positioning plates are readapted to the ascending ramus, and the acrylic bloc on the maxillary arch bar guarantees the preoperative position of the condyles (see Figures 11.25c and d).

The definitive occlusion is fixed using the splint made after model surgery. Sometimes when rotation of the mandible has to be performed some resection in the inner aspect of the ramus is necessary to achieve tension-free adaptation of the segments. In class III cases the typical resection in the buccal layer must be performed. Then rigid fixation of the ascending ramus is possible without dislocation of the condyles. The first positioning screw is inserted above the alveolar nerve after borehole is drilled with a 2-millimeter twist drill. After the hole's depth is measured with the special depth gauge, the screw is inserted through the transbuccal retractor. Care must be taken not to displace the segments; this is easy with the self-cutting titanium screws. The same procedure is followed below the alveolar nerve and a third screw is inserted above the first one (see Figures 11.25e and f). The positioning plates and the MMF are removed, and the new occlusion is checked very carefully. The additional time needed for this procedure in the operating theater may be about 15 minutes, but the rigid fixation method cuts down on wasted time. Over the last five years that we have used this method, we have surprisingly often found wide gaps in cases where we had not expected them. A cancellous bone graft may be necessary to bridge the gap. A follow-up study of our patients impressively demonstrates the efficacy of this technique, especially in class II cases. We observed less than 1% rates of relapse in over 140 cases.

Figure 11.26 Rigid fixation in a bimaxillary case without MMF. Front view: (a) x-ray image, (b) panorex, (c) preoperatively, (d) postoperatively. Side view of the same patient's occlusion: (e) preoperatively, (f) postoperatively. (g) preoperatively, (h) postoperatively.

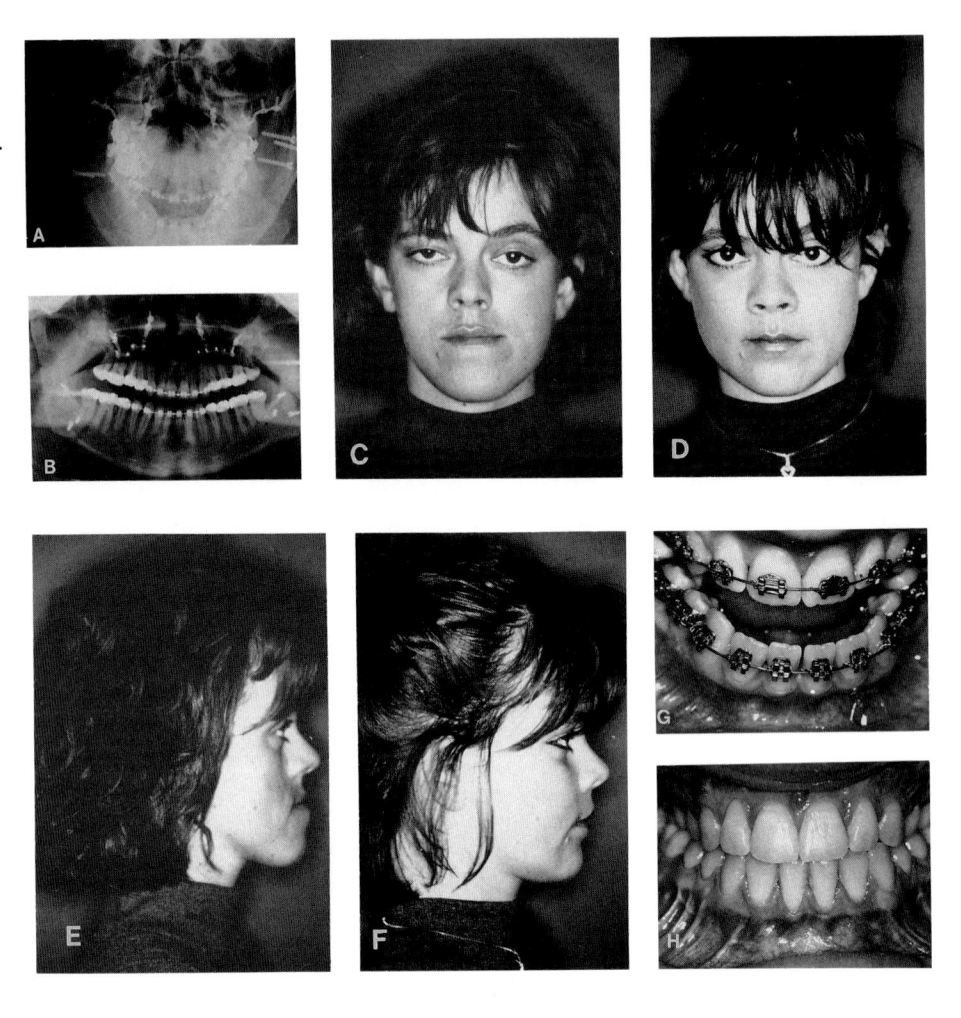

This technique also avoids the need for MMF in bimaxillary cases, which is a tremendous advantage to our patients. Using rigid fixation in mandibular and maxillary osteotomies enables optimum postoperative care and supervision of intraoral wounds and control of the adjusted occlusion (see Figure 11.26). In addition, elastics can be inserted early for functional adaptation of the musculature. The fixed preoperative joint position in combination with the early functional adaptation leads to better results.

WÜRZBURG DENTAL IMPLANTS

A dental implant system is available with conical screws in various lengths and in widths of 3.5 millimeters and 4.5 millimeters. Their development is based on principles of modern osteosynthesis and our experimental findings (Bossler 1981) as well as on the knowledge of modern biomaterials and biotechnology.

The functional incorporation of alloplastic materials for the fixation and support of dental prostheses is determined by the interaction of chemical processes and functional stresses induced by the implanted body in its biological environment. The extent and nature of the reaction is dependent on the one hand on the responsiveness of the surrounding tissue and on the other hand on the shape, material, and functional load of the implant. An additional factor is the operative technique employed.

In general, the responsiveness of the surrounding tissue and the dynamic stress of the implant must be assumed so that implantation of a dental prosthesis will be influenced only by the choice of material and the shape of the implant. No final judgment about the suitability of an implant material or about the shape of the implanted body should be made when considering one of these factors in isolation. On the contrary, these factors must be considered as a complete and integrated system.

The conical screw form of our dental implant (see Figure 11.27) is based on our stress analysis (see Figure 11.28). This screw design guarantees uniform distribution and transfer of the forces involved on the surrounding medium. Carving the thread with a manual tap provides maximum close adaptation of bone tissue and implant surface without resorption of the surrounding bone.

The choice of the material was based on several considerations. First, the material must be biocompatible and resistant to corrosion. Second, it must allow production of the implant in the desired shape. Third,

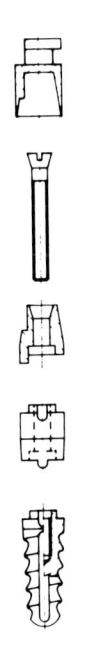

Figure 11.27 Construction drawing of the Würzburg Titanium Dental Implant System.

its modulus of elasticity should be as close as possible to that of bone, to ensure that movement between implant and surrounding bone tissue is minimal.

Pure titanium's modulus of elasticity is closer to that of bone than is Vitallium's (by a factor of 2) and ceramic's (by a factor of 4). The shear strength of the titanium-oxide layer, which provides the chemical stability of this material, is not very high. Therefore significant research has been performed in an attempt to improve the oxide layer by surface engineering. Today we use two different oxide layers. The first, applied to the intraosseous part of our screws, provides optimal stability to the oxide layer and an electrochemical stability that leads to the direct growth of bone cells onto the implant surface. A second oxide layer is applied to the supragingival parts of our implants to hinder the accumulation of plaques to an extent comparable to that of gold.

A more detailed discussion of this implant system and its clinical use is beyond the scope of this chapter.

The Würzburg system demonstrates the great versatility of titanium and its alloys in medicine.

REFERENCES

Allgöwer M: Osteosynthese und primäre Knochenheilung. Langenbecks Archiv klin Chir 308:423, 1967.

Bagby GW, Janes JM: The effect of compression on the rate of fracture healing using a special plate. Am J Surg 95:761, 1958.

Becker R, Austermann KH: Zur Wahl des Zugangsweges bei operativer Versorgung von Orbitafrakturen. Fortschr. Kiefer u Gesichtschir, 22:33–36, 1977.

Becker R, Machtens E: Druckplattenosteosynthese zur Frakturbehandlung und bei orthopädisch-chirurgischen Maßnahmen am Gesichtsschädel. Osteonews, 19, 1973.

Böhler L: Technik der Knochenbruchbehandlung im Frieden und im Kriege. Vol II Wien. W. Maudrich 49, 1941.

Börner K: Klinische Erfahrungen mit der Druckschienenosteosynthese nach Luhr. Bonn: 1979 (Med. Diss.).

Bossler L: Vergleichende spannungsoptische Untersuchung an verschiedenen blattförmigen und schraubenförmigen Dentalimplantaten. Mainz-Iserlohn: 1981 (Med. Diss.).

Bothe RT, Beaton KE, Davenport HA: Reaction of bone to multiple metallic implants. Surg Gynecol Obstet 71:598, 1940.

Bull HG, Ganzer U, Grüntzig J, Schirmer M: Der Schädelbruch. Urban u Schwarzenberg, 1987.

Casson PR, Bonanno PC, Converse JM: The midface degloving procedure. Plast Reconstr Surg 53:102–103, 1974.

Champy M, Lodde JP: Synthesis Mandibulaires-Localisation des syntheses en function des contraintex mandibulaires. Rev. Stoma. 77 (1976) 971.

Champy M: Biomechanische Grundlagen der Straßburger Miniplattenosteosynthese. Dtsch zahnärztl Z 38:358, 1983.

Champy M, Lodde JP: Etude des contraintes dans la mandibule fracturée chez l'homme. Mesures théoriques at vérification par jauges extensométriques in situ. Rev Stomat [Paris] 78:545, 1977.

Chuong R, Kaban LB: Fractures of the zygomatic complex. J Oral Maxillofac Surg 44,4:283–288, 1986.

Claudi B, Spiessl B: Ergebnisse bei konservativer und operativer Behandlung von Unterkieferfrakturen (ohne Kollumfrakturen). Fortschr Kiefer u Gesichtschir XIX:73, 1975.

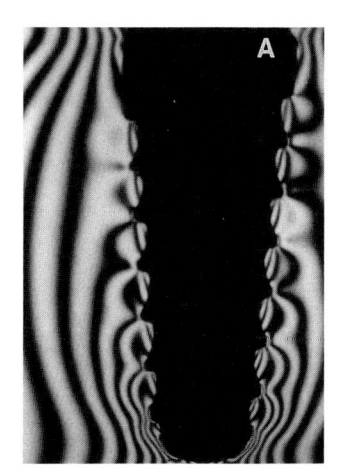

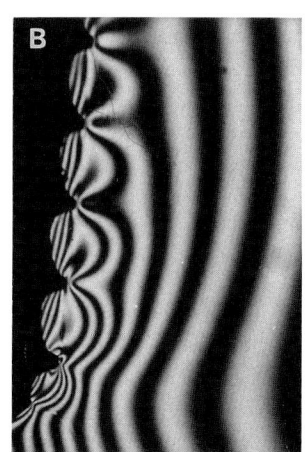

Figure 11.28 Stress analysis of our conical screw: (a) total view, (b) detailed view of the intraosseous part.

Converse JM, Furmin D, Wood-Smith D: The conjunctival approach in orbital fractures. Plast Reconstr Surg 52:656, 1973.

Danis R: Théorie et pratique des l'osteosynthése. Masson & Cie, Paris, 1949.

Dieckmann J, Hackmann G: Der operative Zugang zur Periorbita bei frontobasalen Frakturen. Fortschr Kiefer- u Gesichtschir 22:36–38, 1977.

Dunaevskij VA, Solovev MM, Pavlov BL, Magarill ES: Osteosintez pri Perelomach Niznej Celjusti. Leningrad, Medicina, 1973.

Emneus H, Stenram V, Backlund J: X-Ray spectrographic investigations of the soft tissue around titanium and cobalt alloy implants. Acta Orthop Scand 30:226, 1960.

Ewers R: Periorbitale Knochenstrukturen und ihre Bedeutung für die Osteosynthese. Fortschr Kiefer Gesichtschir 22:45, 1977.

Gerlach KL, Pape HD: Prinzip und Indikation der Miniplattenosteosynthese. Dtsch zahnärztl Z 35:346, 1980.

Graber G. Funktionelle Gebißanalyse. In Zahn-, Mund- und Kieferheilkunde. Prothetik und Werkstoffkunde. Schwenzer N (ed). Stuttgart, New York, Thieme, 1982;3.

Härtel J: Komplikationen nach funktionsstabiler Osteosynthese des Unterkiefers. Dtsch Z Mund-Kiefer-Gesichtschir 7:52; 1983.

Härtel J, Sonnenburg M: Methoden der stabilen Osteosynthese des Unterkiefers (Biomechanische, physikalisch-technische, histologische und klinische Untersuchungen). Rostock: 1977 (Med.Diss. Prom.B.).

Höltje WJ, Luhr HG, Holtfreter M: Untersuchungen über infektionsbedingte Komplikationen nach konservativer und operativer Versorgung von Unterkieferfrakturen. Fortschr. Kiefer- u. Gesichtschir., 19:122, 1975.

Horch HH, Gerlach KL, Pape HD: Indikationen und Grenzen der intraoralen Miniplattenosteosynthese bei Frakturen des aufsteigenden Unterkieferastes. Dtsch zahnärztl Z 38:447, 1983.

Joos U, Schilli W, Niederdellmann H, Scheibe B: Komplikationen und verzögerte Bruchheilung bei Kieferfrakturen. Dtsch zahnärztl Z 38:387, 1983.

Kessler W: Das spannungsoptische Oberflächenschichtverfahren zur mechanischen Spannungsmessung am menschlichen Unterkiefer unter physiologischer Belastung. München: 1980 (Med. Diss.).

Key JA: Positive pressure in arthrodesis for tuberculosis of the knee joint. South Med J 25:909, 1932.

König F: Über die Berechtigung frühzeitiger blutiger Eingriffe bei subcutanen Knochenbrüchen. Arch klin Chir 76:23, 1905.

Kraft E: Über die Bedeutung der Kaukraft für das Kaugeschehen. Zahnärztl Praxis 13:129, 1962.

Küppers K: Analyse der funktionellen Struktur des menschlichen Unterkiefers. Ergebnisse der Anatomie und Entwicklungsgeschichte, Berlin, Springer, 44:6, 1971.

Laing PG: Clinical experience with prosthetic materials; Historical perspectives, current problems and future directions. ASTM-STP 684:199–211, 1979.

Lambotte A: L'intervention operatoire dans les fractures. Paris, Maloine, 1907.

Lane WA: The operative treatment of fractures. London, The Medical Publisbury Co., 1914.

Luhr HG: Zur stabilen Osteosynthese bei Unterkieferfrakturen. Dtsch. zahnärztl. Z. 23:754, 1968.

Luhr HG: Die Kompressionsosteosynthese bei Unterkieferfrakturen. München, Hanser, 1972.

Luhr HG: Skelettverlagernde Operationen zur Harmonisierung des Gesichtsprofiles: Probleme der stabilen Fixation von Osteotomiesegmenten. In Die Ästhetik von Form und Funktion in der Plastischen und Wiederherstellungs- Chirurgie. Pfeifer G (ed). Berlin, Heidelberg, Springer, 1985;87.

Michelet FX, Benoit IP, Festal F, Despujols P, Bruchet P, Arvoir A: Fixation with blockage of sagittal osteotomy of the ascending branches of the mandible with endobuccal plates in the treatment of anteroposterior malformations. Rev Stomatol 72:531, 1971.

Mittelmeier H: Druckosteosynthese mit selbstspannenden Platten (Technik und Erfahrungsbericht). Homburg, Ref. Saarl. Westpfalz. Orthopädentreffen, 1968.

Motsch A: Kaufunktion und Kiefergelenkbeanspruchung. Dtsch zahnärztl Z 23:833, 1968.

Niederdellmann H, Schilli W: Zur Plattenosteosynthese bei Unterkieferfrakturen. Dtsch zahnärztl Z 28:638, 1973.

Paulus GW: Die Knochenbruchheilung am Oberkiefer bei Verwendung von Miniplatten. Erlangen, Med. Habil. Schr. 1986.

Pauwels F: Grundriss einer Biomechanik der Frakturheilung. Verh Dtsch Orthop Ges 34:62, 1940.

Pauwels F: Gesammelte Abhandlungen zur funktionellen Anatomie des Bewegungsapparates. Berlin, Heidelberg, New York, Springer, 1965.

Perren SM, Russenberger J, Steinemann S, Müller ME, Allgöwer M: A dynamic compression plate. Acta Orthop Scand [Suppl] 125:29, 1969.

Reuther JF: Druckplattenosteosynthese und freie Knochentransplantation zur Unterkieferrekonstruktion - Experimentelle und klinische Untersuchungen. Mainz, Med. Habil. Schr. 1977a.

Reuther J, Hausamen JE: System zur alloplastischen Überückung von Unterkieferdefekten. Dtsch zahnärztl Z 32:334, 1977b.

Reuther J: Druckplattenosteosynthese und freie Knochentransplantation zur Unterkieferrekonstruktion. Berlin, Quintessenz, 1979.

Reuther JF, Steinau HU, Wagner R: Reconstruction of

large defects in the oropharynx with a revascularized intestinal graft: An experimental and clinical report. Plast Reconstr Surg 73:3, 1984.

Rohen JW: Zur Anatomie deslrothesenträgers. Dtsch zahnärztl Z 20: 1161, 1958

Schargus G: Experimentelle Untersuchungen über den Halt verschiedener Schienungssysteme. Dtsch Zahn Mund u Kieferheilkd 53:378, 1969.

Schettler D, Vogeler E, Bringewald B: Therapiewandel bei Kieferwinkel-Frakturen. Dtsch zahnärztl Z 38:367, 1983.

Schilli W, Niederdellmann H: Internal fixation of zygomatic and midface fractures by means of miniplates and lag screws. In Oral and Maxillofacial Traumatology. Kruger E, Schilli W, Werthington P (eds). Chicago, London, Berlin, Rio de Janeiro, Tokyo, Qintessenz, 1986;2:177–196.

Schmitz R, Luhr HG, Schubert H: Indikation, Technik und klinische Ergebnisse der Kompressionsosteosynthese bei Unterkieferfrakturen. Fortschr Kiefer u. Gesichtschir 19:74, 1975.

Schumacher GH: Funktionelle Morphologie der Kaumuskulatur. Jena, G. Fischer, 1961.

Semlitsch M: Titanium alloys for hip joint replacements. In Designing with Titanium. The Institute of Metals (ed). Bristol: 1986 (Proceedings of Conference).

Semlitsch M, Staub F, Weber H: Titanium-aluminium-niobium alloy; development for biocompatible, high strength surgical implants. Biomed Technik 30:334–339, 1985.

Sicher H, De Bral E L: Oral Anatomy. 5th. ed. St. Louis, Mosby, 1970; 78.

Sonnenburg I, Fethke K, Sonnenburg M: Zur Druckbelastung des Kiefergelenkes; Eine experimentelle Studie. Anat Anz Jena 155:309, 1984.

Spiessl B, Schargus G, Schroll K: Die stabile Osteosynthese bei Frakturen des unbezahnten Kiefers. Schweiz Mschr Zahnheilk 81:39, 1971.

Steinbauer M: Mittelgesichtsfrakturen in den Jahren 1981 bis 1983; Ihre Ursachen, Diagnostik und Therapie sowie der Heilungsverlauf. Würzburg: 1986 (Inaug. Diss.).

Tamai T, Hoshiko W: A new compression plate for osteosynthesis. Clin Orth Surg 2:941, 1967.

Tessier P: The conjunctival approach to the orbital floor and maxilla in congenital malformations and trauma. J Max - Fac Surg 1:3, 1973.

Tenzel RR, Miller GR: Orbital blow-out fracture repair, conjunctival approach. Inaug Diss Amer J Ophthalmol 71:1141, 1971.

Uhlig H: Über die Kaukraft. Dtsch. Zahnṝztl Z 8:30, 1953

Wagner WF, Neal DC, Alpert B: Morbidity associated with extraoral open reduction of mandibular fractures. J Oral Surg 37:97, 1979.

Weisser J, Reuther J, Gutwerk W: Zwölfjährige Erfahrung bei der primären Unterkieferrekonstruktion mit funktionsstabiler Osteosyntheseplatte. In Die Ästhetik von Form und Funktion in der Plastischen und Wiederherstellungschirurgie. Pfeifer G (ed). Berlin, Heidelberg, New York, Tokyo, Springer, 1985.

Wolff J: Das Gesetz der Transformation der Knochen. Berlin, Hirschwald, 1982.

Wustrow P: Physikalische Grundlagen der zahnärztlichen Platte und Brückenprothese. vol 1. Berlin, Meusser, 1919.

CHAPTER 12

The ITI Dental Implant System™ (Bonefit®)

André Schroeder
Franz Sutter
Daniel Buser

The ITI (International Team for Oral Implantology) Dental Implant System (Bonefit) employs titanium plasma-sprayed implants to permanently osteointegrate into the human mandible and maxilla. These permanent implants are intended to support dental prostheses in fully and partially edentulous patients. This chapter describes biomaterial and biomechanic properties of titanium plasma-sprayed ITI implants and the rationale for the selection, the bone and soft tissue reactions to these implants, and the clinical procedures of their application in patients.

IMPLANT MATERIAL

The development of the ITI system began in 1974 with the investigation of tissue reactions to various implant materials and surfaces in experimental biological tests. Later, this work concentrated on titanium (commercially pure titanium) and the rough surface produced by the titanium plasma spraying.

Titanium, which has been in use since the 1960s in orthopedics and fracture treatment, is thought to be an ideal biomaterial for oral implants for the following reasons:

- An oxide forms on the surface of the metal in air, water, and any electrolyte; this oxide is one of the most resistant substances in the mineral world. It forms a thin film that protects the metal from chemical attack, even in aggressive body fluids.
- The oxide film in contact with tissue is practically insoluble. No ions are released which can react with organic molecules.
- The tensile strength of titanium is almost as high as that of the stainless steel used for load-bearing surgical implants. Furthermore, the metal is ductile such that it bends rather than breaks on overloading.
- Tissue or biomolecules attach to titanium or its oxidized surface probably by way of a true physicochemical bond; such a bond does not form on other metals used in bone surgery (stainless steel, for example) or on aluminium oxide ceramic.

IMPLANT SURFACE

The micromorphology of an implant's surface is important. Several studies have demonstrated that, compared to implants with polished surfaces, implants with rough surfaces produce faster bone apposition and more surface contact between implant and bone.

The bone anchorage section of ITI implants is titanium plasma-sprayed, giving a porous surface whose surface area is six times greater than that of a polished implant. This greater surface area ensures functional ankylotic anchoring of the implant in the bone (see Color Plate 9).

TISSUE REACTIONS

Data from animal experiments and human tissue sample preparations have demonstrated predictable bone and soft tissue reactions to the implants.

Bone Reaction

The bone reaction around the implant demonstrates true osteointegration; that is, the bone is in intimate contact with the implant surface. This situation has been repeatedly observed and can be consistently achieved under the following conditions:

- when extreme care is taken during preparation of the implant bed (low-speed drilling and milling, below 600 rounds per minute, under continuous intensive irrigation with chilled, physiological, and sterile saline for cooling);
- when a primary stability of the inserted implant is achieved due to a congruency between implant and implant bed; and
- when the implant is not loaded for at least three months.

Color Plates 10–13 clearly demonstrate that new bone is deposited directly on the implant surface, and that the shape of the implant is of secondary importance provided the above conditions have been strictly observed. The prepared sections seen at higher magnification clearly show that the bone follows every contour and pore of the titanium plasma-sprayed surface and that vital osteocytes are in direct contact with the implant surface. According to Albrektsson (1983), the distance between the oxide layer on the titanium and the mineralized bone tissue (the apatite crystals, to be exact) is no more than 100 angström (1 angström = 10^{-4} micrometers = 10^{-7} millimeter) and the gap is filled with matrix material (proteoglycans, or protein-polysaccharide complexes).

The scanning electron microscope (SEM) pictures confirm the conclusions reached from the light microscope studies. Direct contact between bone and the rough implant surface was observed on sections in the SEM. If cracks from internal stresses are present, they are on the tissue side (see Color Plate 14), another indication of the firm microanchorage of bone to the titanium plasma-sprayed surface.

The ankylotic bond is maintained on loaded implants. Remodeling to form a type of periodontal ligament does not take place even under the influence of occlusal forces. On the contrary, the impression is that with time the degree of osteointegration increases with the bone becoming denser and more compact (see Color Plate 15). It has thus been clearly demonstrated that ITI implants become directly anchored in bone tissue with no intervening connective tissue. The question remains as to how the absence of the periodontal ligament is to be judged in a purely functional sense. It has been shown—both histologically and, more significantly, clinically—that implants that transmit mastication forces directly to the bone are functionally as effective as natural teeth. This is true both for the magnitude of the masticatory forces supported and for the subjective experience of the patient. The patient's perception of the implant is no different from that of a natural tooth, despite the absence of the periodontal ligament and its proprioceptors.

Soft Tissue Reactions ("Gingival" Collar)

Oral implants are open implants and therefore are permanently exposed to the germ-laden oral cavity. The penetration of the mucosa by the implant is of fundamental importance; it could even be said that the whole future of oral implantology lies in the solution to this problem.

The Subepithelial Connective Tissue

Our experiments on rhesus monkeys and on beagle dogs showed that horizontal connective tissue fibers—that is, fibers perpendicular to the implant surface—are to be found on implants standing in nonmobile, keratinized mucosa. When studied by both light and scanning electron microscopy, these fibers are seen to be anchored onto the rough implant surface (see Color Plate 16). This fiber pattern was not observed around implants standing in mobile (nonkeratinized) mucosa; in this case the fibers were mainly oriented vertically, that is, parallel to the implant surface.

The Epithelium

It has been demonstrated repeatedly that epithelial cells attach to nonbiological materials. Basal lamina as well as hemidesmosomes have been observed electron-optically, despite the considerable technical difficulties posed by such studies. Firm attachment of the epithelial collar—or more exactly, of the junctional epithelium—around the post of ITI implants is possible when the subepithelial connective tissue has the aforementioned favorable structure. This may be suspected on macroscopic evaluation and can be demonstrated under the light microscope (see Color Plate 17). It has been observed in the transmission electron microscope (TEM) that epithelial cells are attached to the implant post even on rough surfaces through a basal layer in which occasional microvilli can be seen (see Color Plate 18). Hemidesmosomes have not yet been observed.

Conclusions Concerning Tissue Reactions

- Ankylotic bonding has been demonstrated between titanium plasma-sprayed ITI implants and bone (true osteointegration). The bond is maintained or renewed under loading. The achievement of an interface free of intervening connective tissue depends on several preconditions (primary stability of the implant, low-

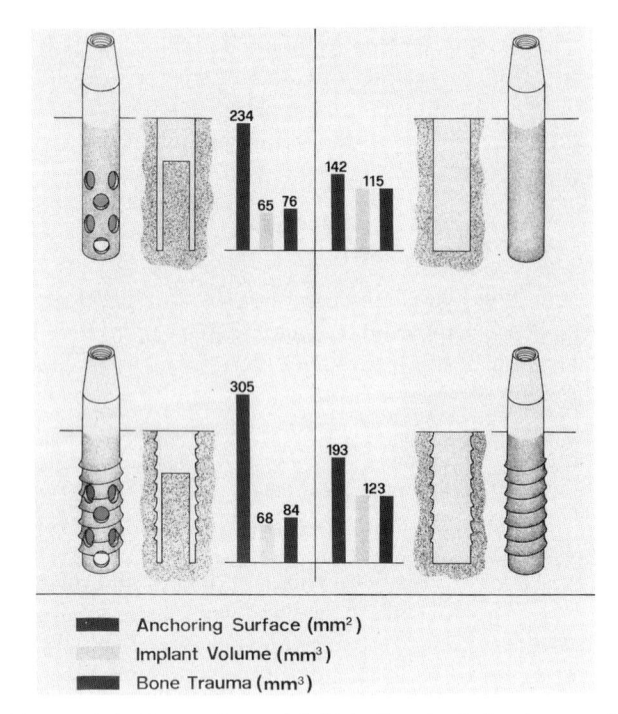

Figure 12.1 Comparison of (left) hollow-body implants and (right) corresponding full-body implants with respect to anchorage surface area, implant volume, and bone trauma.

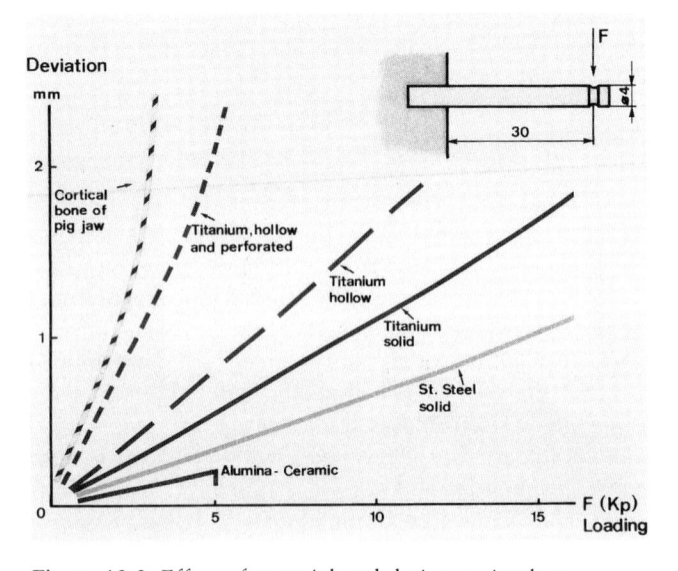

Figure 12.2 Effect of material and design on implant stiffness.

speed cutting procedures, sufficient cooling with sterile saline, no functional loading forces for at least three months).
- Under certain conditions (implant post in nonmobile, keratinized mucosa), it has been shown that collagen fibers attach themselves to the implant surface in the subepithelial connective tissue.
- A true epithelial attachment to the implant post is possible as long as these structures of connective tissue form and can be maintained.

CHARACTERISTICS AND PROPERTIES OF ITI IMPLANTS

The basic design concept of perforated hollow-body implants incorporates the following characteristics and properties.

Large Implant Anchorage Surface

A larger bone-contact surface area has been achieved with hollow-cylinder (HC) and hollow-screw (HS) implants than is possible with the corresponding solid bodies. This larger surface area also reduces specific pressure on the bone (see Figure 12.1).

Minimal Bone Trauma on Preparation of the Implant Bed

A smaller bone defect is produced when preparing the implant bed for the various hollow bodies than is necessary for the corresponding solid bodies (see Figure 12.1).

Smallest Possible Volume of the Implant Anchorage Section

The volume of the implant or foreign body is extremely modest because of the HC shape and the regularly spaced cylinder fenestrations; thus the biological acceptance of the implant is improved. The implant adapts to elastic deformations of the jaw better than a solid body would (see Figure 12.1).

Adaptation of Stiffness to That of Bone

Functional loading of the jaw produces tensile and compressional stresses, and the bone trabeculae orient themselves accordingly. Furthermore, it is known that the mandible possesses considerable flexibility to absorb mastication forces. When a foreign body in the form of an endosteal implant is placed in this flexible bone architecture, the bone defect must be as small as possible and the functional deformation of the mandible must not be compromised. The open, cagelike structure and the material of the hollow-body implants produce advantageous elastic properties. This means that the contact between bone tissue and the implant surface is maintained or always renewed under functional loading (see Figure 12.2).

Promotion of Biological Incorporation

The open implant form encourages good blood circulation and bone regeneration through the perforations, which connect the bone in the implant lumen

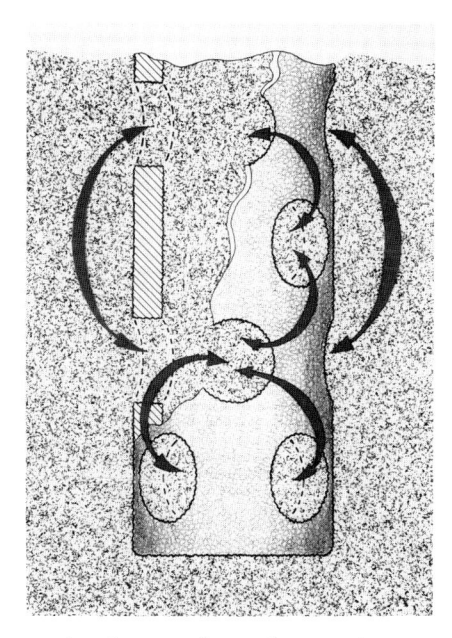

Figure 12.3 This drawing shows the most important design features of the HC form: reduction of stiffness, biologically advantageous conditions for healing, and bony incorporation.

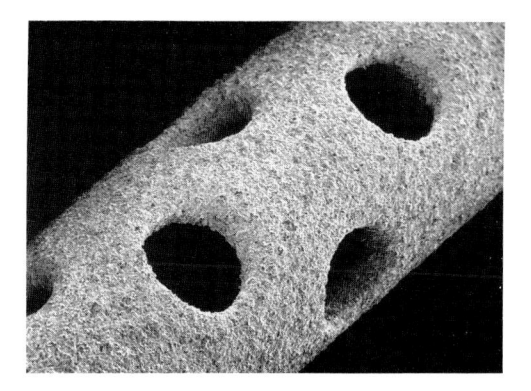

Figure 12.4 Implant section, characterized by the HC form and periodic wall perforations.

to the surrounding bone mass. The vitality of the bone in the lumen is retained, and the healing process is favored (see Figure 12.3).

Low Level of Stresses Between Bone and Implant

The bone that grows through the regularly spaced fenestrations acts as a kind of shock absorber on physiological loading and decreases the surface shear forces between bone and implant. The danger of pressure-related bone resorption after the healing phase is thus greatly reduced (see Color Plate 15 and Figure 12.4).

Primary Stability

Good primary stability of HC implants is achieved by slight precompression of the surrounding bone through a congruent implant bed. The open structure and reduced stiffness of these rotation-symmetrical implants (together with the degree of press fit established by experience) has proven to be effective with respect to transmission of physiological loads.

Preparation of the Implant Bed

The preparation of a congruent implant bed is not a problem for rotation-symmetrical ITI implants and requires only relatively simple instruments. Trauma to the jaw is minimal because a thin-walled trephine mill with outer flutes is used. The shape of the cutting teeth on the mill produces a vibration-free, clean cut in bone.

Another important factor for preparation of the implant bed in conjunction with the cutting quality is the cutting speed. The speed of the drill is reduced to approximately 600 rounds per minute by using a "double-reduction green contra-angle hand piece" (two green rings, reduction ratio 7,4:1). Continuous cooling with chilled, sterile, physiological saline is imperative.

One- and Two-Part Implants

Fundamentals

Theoretically, the two-stage procedure should always be the method of choice, as it ensures immobilization of the implant during the three-month healing phase, which in turn produces a pure bony anchoring of the implant. However, clinical experience and histological findings show that the achievement of an ankylotic bond between bone and implant was not purely the domain of the two-stage procedure.

For the wound-healing phase of two-part implants, there are essentially two design options:

- *The submerged, closed system.* The primary component, the anchorage part, is sunk to the level of the bone surface or at least deeply enough that the mucoperiosteal tissue can be sutured over the implant end without tension (see Figure 12.5 Var A and Var B).
- *The non-submerged, transmucosal system.* The primary component is implanted, leaving approximately 3 millimeters above the bone surface. The mucoperiosteal flap is not sutured over the implant but is closely adapted around the implant neck (see Figure 12.5 Var C).

The ITI prefers the nonsubmerged, transmucosal approach for the following reasons:

- In the case of a non-submerged implant, the microgap between the two implant parts, a potential site for plaque retention, is clearly

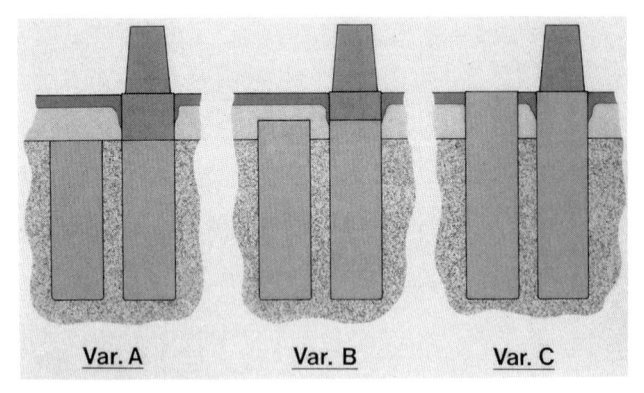

Figure 12.5 Options for two-part construction (procedures a, b, and c). In (a) and (b) the implant is beneath the periosteum (see text). In (c) the coronal end of the implant is at the gingival level.

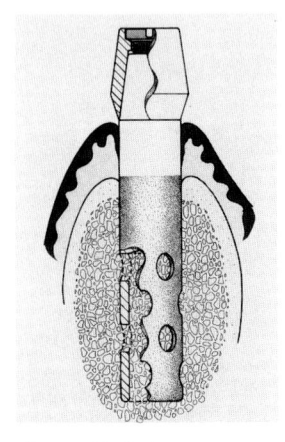

Figure 12.6 A one-part HC implant.

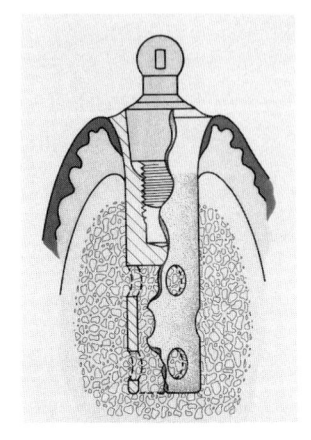

Figure 12.7 A two-part HC implant with a retentive anchor abutment.

outside the soft tissue; this presents an advantage from a microbiological point of view. If the gap were inside the tissue, a site for a peri-implant infection could be established.

- In contrast to submerged implants (see Figure 12.5 a and b), the transmucosal system does not involve a second surgical procedure to remove the temporary healing cap and to insert the abutment (see Figure 12.5 c).
- With the transmucosal system, insertion of the abutment part is simple and visibility is good.
- With the transmucosal procedure, the gingival seal is formed during the primary healing period and is not disturbed by the placement of abutments.
- Connecting the abutment to the implant at the gingival level allows a better mechanical joint adaptation between the two parts, as well as a more favorable "lever arm" condition on the connection than with separation at the bone surface level.

Hollow-Cylinder Implants

The basic shape of the HC implant (see Figures 12.6 and 12.7) is the same as that of the first single hollow-cylinder implant developed in 1974. The external diameter is 3.5 millimeters. The anchorage surface is plasma-sprayed titanium, following ITI principles. The cylinder is perforated to approximately 4 millimeters below the intended surface level of the bone. Primary stability is achieved by a slight press fit, which also promotes integration in the bone for secure and lasting secondary stability. The neck of the implants is highly polished to reduce plaque retention and to provide the most favorable conditions for formation of an epithelial attachment. Depending on the clinical indication, one- and two-part HC implants are available.

One-part HC implants (see Figure 12.6) are available in five lengths: 8-, 10-, 12-, 14-, and 16-millimeter sink depth in bone. The sink depth corresponds with the length of the plasma-sprayed section of the implant. The conical head is accurately manufactured with a cone angle of 8° and a height of 3.65 millimeters to accept a standardized gold cap. All the edges of the implant are rounded to prevent pressure-induced bone resorption. These one-part implants are particularly suited for overdenture retention in the edentulous mandible utilizing a multiple abutment system between the mental foramen.

Two-part HC implants (see Figure 12.1) were developed primarily for replacement of a single tooth, particularly in the anterior region of the maxilla. To improve performance in this application, the implant body widens at the shoulder to 5 millimeters in diameter, similar to a cervical preparation of a natural tooth for the placement of a jacket or veneer crown. The shoulder is buccally beveled to place the buccal crown margin slightly into the gingival sulcus for esthetic reasons. For situations having a slight maxillary alveolar protrusion, a variation with a 15° shoulder angle was developed (see Figure 12.8). Both implants are available in three lengths: 8-, 10-, and 12-millimeter sink depth (see Figure 12.9).

For the junction between the primary and secondary part, a cone–screw construction was chosen that guarantees an accurate marginal fit (see Figure 12.10) as well as an increased retention within the cone, against loosening of the secondary part. The angle of the cone is 8°, and the conical junctional surface is blasted by means of steel balls to increase retention for the abutments.

The outer cone of the crown-and-bridge abutment has three notches in the long axis to guarantee stabilization against rotation of a single crown. The cone angle of 5° and the blasted surface offer optimal prerequisites for retention and friction of the reconstruction, respec-

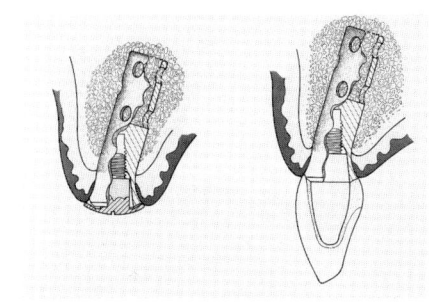

Figure 12.8 Diagram showing a 15°-angled two-part HC implant in the maxilla (left) during the healing phase and (right) with crown.

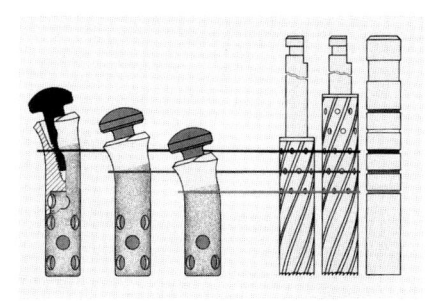

Figure 12.9 Relationship of the sink (anchorage) depth of 15° inclined two-part HC implants and markings on the trephine mill and depth gauge.

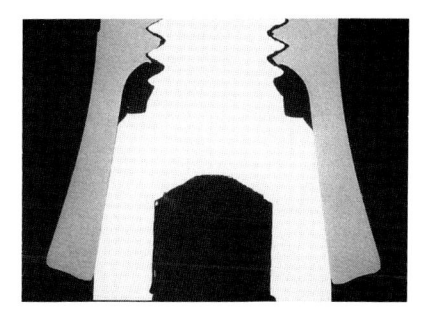

Figure 12.10 Cone–screw junction with its accurate marginal fit (SEM).

tively. The abutment, available with two cone heights of 4.0 millimeters and 5.5 millimeters, has an inner thread 2.0 millimeters in diameter.

Instruments and Implantation Procedure

The same instruments are used to prepare the implant beds for all HC variations—namely, a predrill, a trephine mill, and a depth gauge. The trephine mill has five rows of holes in its body; these holes correspond to the various lengths of the implants. The optimal implant length can be determined preoperatively with presurgical radiographs, and the bed can be prepared by sinking the mill to the corresponding markings. The surgeon should, however, check the prepared depth with the depth gauge. The gauge is marked with colored rings corresponding to the color codings on the implants. This aids in choosing the correct length—when the red groove corresponds to the level of the bone surface, a red-marked implant should be used (see Figure 12.11).

Hollow-Screw Implants

HS implants are a variation on the HC implants; they are identical except for a spiral screw thread. The head and neck region, pattern and size of the perforations, and the plasma-sprayed titanium anchorage region are also adapted from the HC implant. Both one- and two-part versions are available (see Figures 12.12 and 12.13). In addition to the previously described properties of HC implants, HS implants have the following characteristics:

- optimal primary stability even in low-density cancellous bone, and
- slight but even primary compression, achieved by preparing the bed with a thread tap 0.05 millimeter smaller than the implant profile.

The retention of the HC principles coupled with a suitable thread profile should produce improved stability of the implant anchorage with increasing implantation time. Axial pullout tests on threads with varying thread profiles have confirmed that the chosen thread geometry best fulfills the purpose (see Figure 12.14).

The one-part HS implants can be used in the mandible for overdenture retention in the same way as normal HC implants can. They are produced in the same standard lengths (8, 10, 12, 14, and 16 millimeters).

The main indications for two-part HS implants are distal extension situations in the mandible and in the maxilla, where they are used as abutments for fixed prostheses. This implant is also available in three lengths

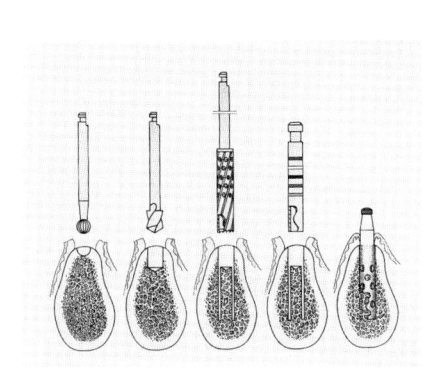

Figure 12.11 Implantation procedure of a one-part HC implant.

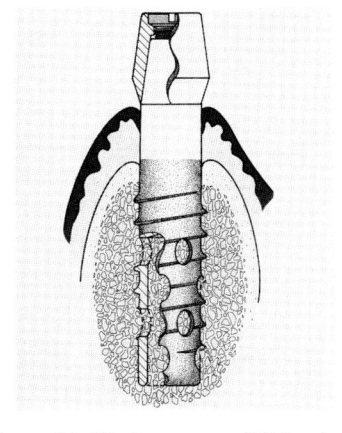

Figure 12.12 A one-part HS implant.

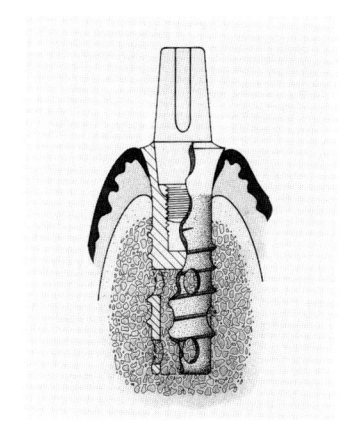

Figure 12.13 A two-part HS implant with a crown-and-bridge abutment.

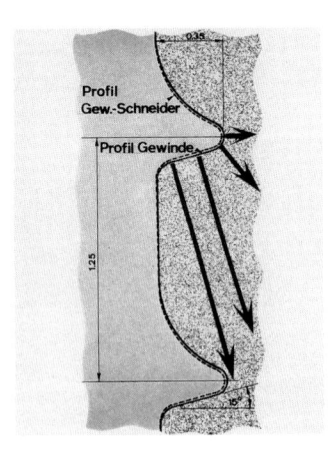

Figure 12.14 The 15° angle of the thread flank to the cross-sectional plane produces an even load distribution over the whole thread profile. On axial loading, the load is transmitted almost perpendicular to the load-bearing surface (arrows).

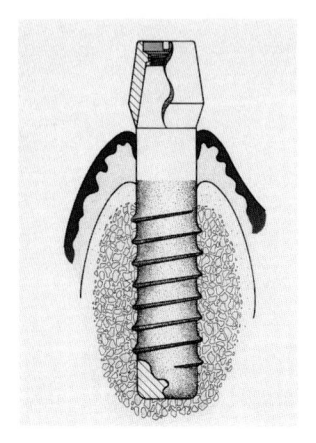

Figure 12.15 A one-part S implant.

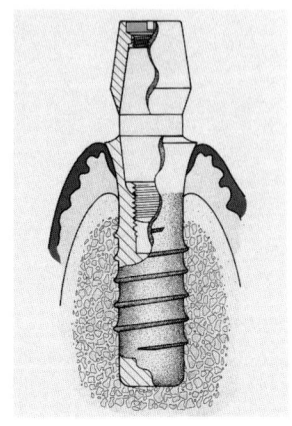

Figure 12.16 A two-part S implant with a bar abutment.

(8-, 10-, and 12-millimeter sink depth) and has the same abutments as the HC implants.

Screw Implants

Another classical ITI implant, the TPS screw, has been in clinical use since 1977 as an implant for the edentulous mandible. It was, therefore, an obvious step to integrate this implant into the new ITI Dental Implant System during the realization phase, and to take this opportunity to remedy certain minor faults in its design. The main improvement in the screw implant (S implant) is in the thread, which no longer is self-tapping but requires pretapping before insertion, just as the HS implants do. This greatly reduces the danger of thermal damage to the surrounding bone when the implant is screwed down. The external profile of both the one- and two-part S implants is now identical to that of the HS implants (see Figures 12.15 and 12.16), allowing the use of the same thread tap for both implant types. The main indication for S implants, according to previous experience, is in the edentulous mandible, where the S implants are used in combination with a bar-supported overdenture. The one-part S implant has the same head geometry as the one-part HC and HS implants; this is therefore a clear improvement on the old TPS implant from a hygienic point of view.

Instruments and Implantation Procedure

For the HC and the HS implants, the same instruments are used to prepare the implant bed (predrill, trephine mill, and depth gauge). The only difference is the use of a color-coded thread cutter for HS bed preparation. Figures 12.17 and 12.18 show the step-by-step implantation procedures for the HS and S implants. Instead of the predrill and the trephine mill, a twist drill is used. The one- and two-part HS and S implants, as well as the abutments, are inserted with the aid of a simple insertion device, which prevents damage to the neck and cone region.

Packaging and Presentation of ITI Implants

ITI implants are delivered in color-coded glass ampules (see Figure 12.19). The ampule caps are not airtight; they have a small slit, which is sufficient to allow preoperative sterilization (preferably in an auto-

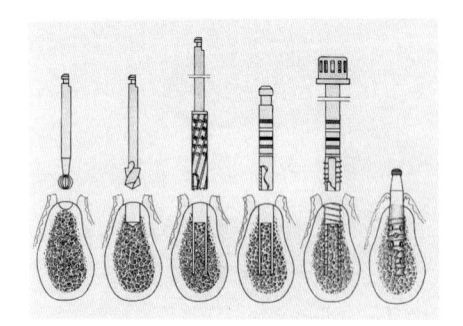

Figure 12.17 Implantation procedure of a one-part HS implant.

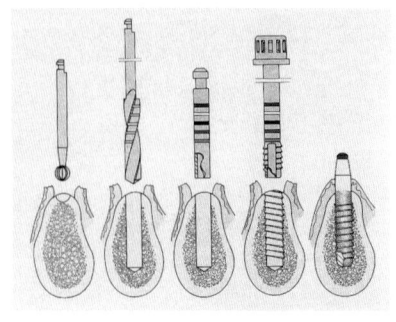

Figure 12.18 Implantation procedure of a one-part S implant.

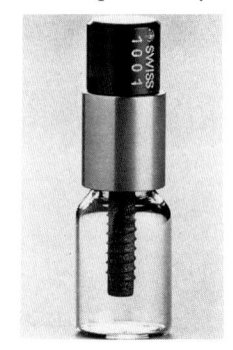

Figure 12.19 An ITI implant in a color-coded glass ampule.

The ITI Dental Implant System™ (Bonefit®)

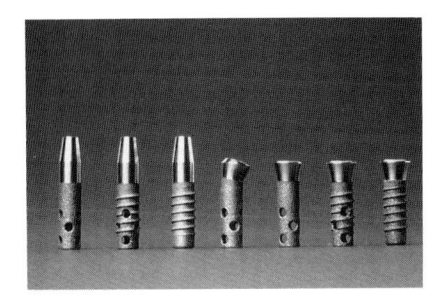

Figure 12.20 The ITI Dental Implants.

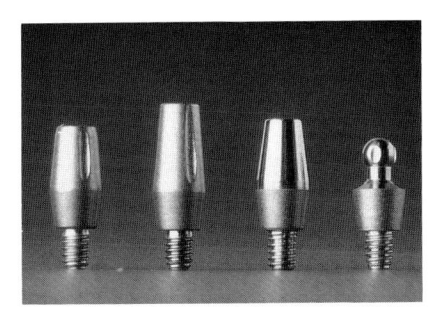

Figure 12.21 The standardized abutments: (left to right) the large and small crown-and-bridge abutments, the bar abutment, the retentive anchor abutment.

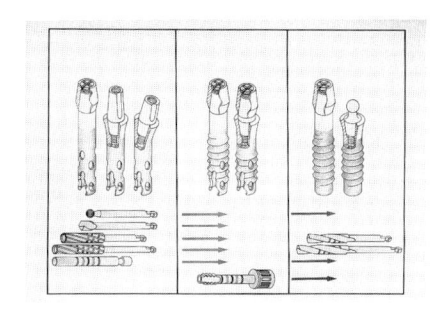

Figure 12.22 The complete ITI Dental Implant System, showing the seven implant types, and the corresponding standardized instruments.

clave) without the ampule being opened. This new storage and presentation system means that the implants can be stored in the implant cassette without fear of contamination and can be removed from the ampule and inserted without intra-operative contamination.

The ITI Dental Implant System as an Integrated Concept

An implant system concept is now available which possesses the following features:

- Choice between three different implant types. Depending on the clinical indications as well as personal preferences a choice can be made between HC, HS and S implant types (see Figures 12.20 and 12.21).
- Standardized instrument set, including a predrill, trephine mill, and depth gauge, which can be used for both the HC and HS implants. A fluted drill is used in place of the predrill and trephine mill for S implants. Both threaded implants require the use of the standard thread tap to complete preparation of the implant bed (see Figure 12.22).
- Standardized implant head shape to all one-part implant types. This allows the use of the same standard accessories—such as impression caps, transfer pins, gold caps, and occlusal screws (see Figure 12.23)—for the manufacture of the bar device.
- Standardized and interchangeable abutments for all two-part implant types (see Figure 12.21).
- Wide indication range. The range of different implant types available, along with implant heads optimized for prosthetic work (as shown in Figures 12.22 and 12.23), means that the full indication range in oral implantology is covered by this system (see Figure 12.24).

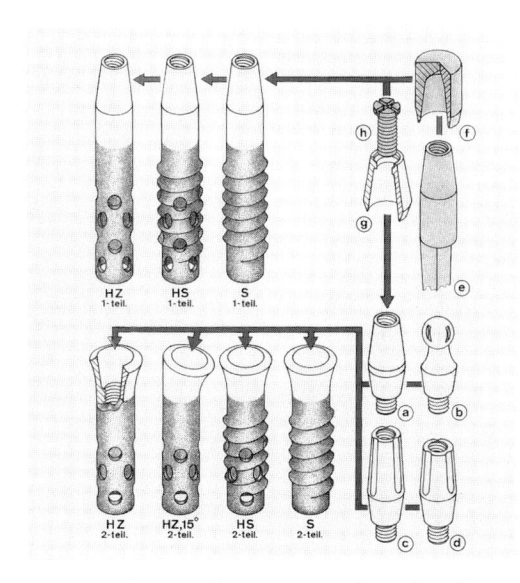

Figure 12.23 The complete ITI Dental Implant System and the available abutments.

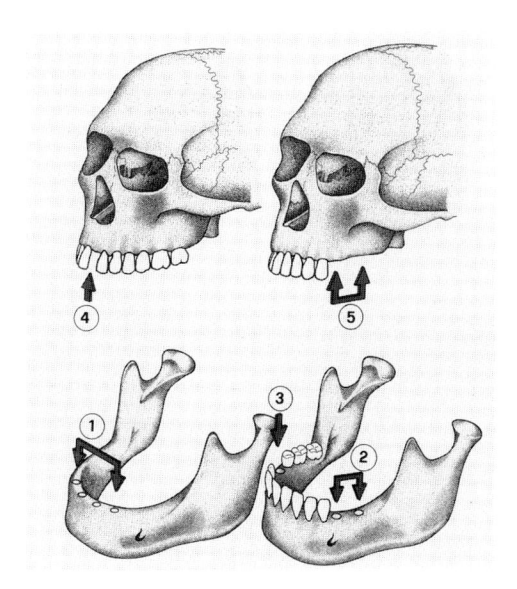

Figure 12.24 Indications for ITI abutments Implants.

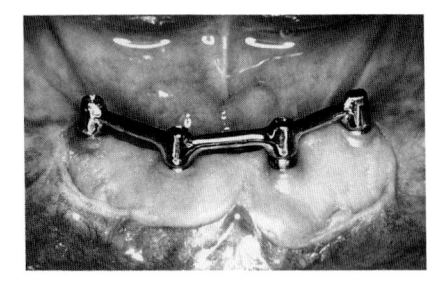

Figure 12.25 A 55-year-old male patient with an edentulous mandible. Clinical situation three years following implantation of one-part HC implants with a bar device.

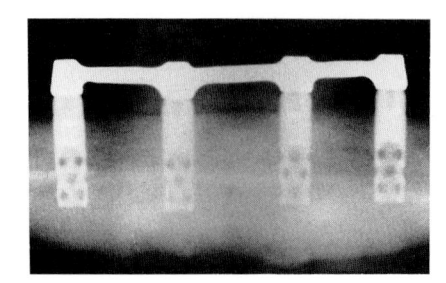

Figure 12.26 Detail of a panorex, three years following implantation.

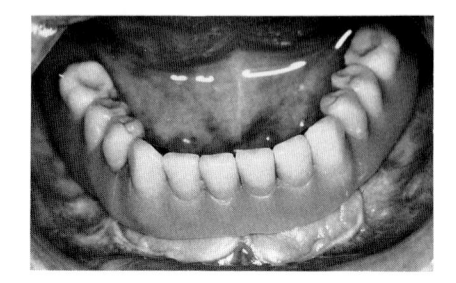

Figure 12.27 Implant supported overdenture in situ.

CLINICAL PROCEDURES FOR THE THREE MAIN INDICATIONS

The Edentulous Mandible

Many patients are unhappy with the lack of stability of their lower full dentures. In these cases, the placement of implants in the mandible between the mental foramen in combination with an implant-supported overdenture offers a beneficial treatment alternative to the patient. Two solutions are used with ITI implants:

- insertion of four one-part implants symmetrically distributed in combination with a bar-device, and
- insertion of two two-part implants in the canine region in combination with a retentive anchor system.

The first solution has been in clinical use since the late 1970s. In this situation, an impression with prefabricated transfer copings is taken directly after the surgical procedure. Then the technician can manufacture the bar device. The finished bar is attached to the implants with occlusal screws within 24 hours, thus it serves as external splint for the fixtures. Theoretically, the implants can be loaded at once, due to the splinting effect of the bar device. However, it is recommended to wait at least until the healing of the soft tissue is completed before integrating a denture. Then the denture can be temporarily relined and inserted, giving the patient some comfort, at least esthetically. Normally, new dentures should be made; this can be started at that time. A patient is shown in Figures 12.25–12.27.

The second solution, which has been in clinical use since 1986, needs two-part implants. In this situation, the tissue-integration period of at least three months has to be respected. After that period, the retentive anchors can be inserted and the overdenture can be manufactured (see Figures 12.28–12.30).

The Distal Extension Situation in the Mandible

This situation indicates very careful presurgical evaluation and reconstructive treatment planning. A width of the alveolar ridge of at least 5 to 6 mm is necessary. This width can be found in the mandible of most patients in the area of the first and second molar.

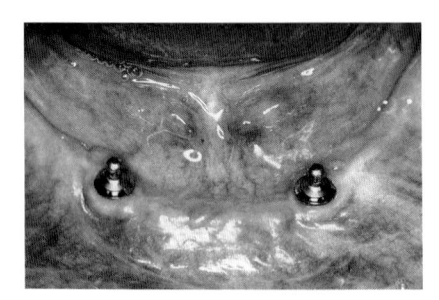

Figure 12.28 An 84-year-old male patient. Clinical situation 12 months following implantation of two-part HS implants in combination with retentive anchor abutments.

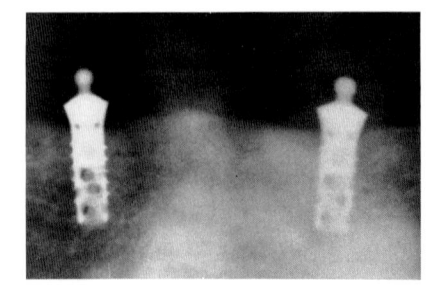

Figure 12.29 Detail of a panorex, 12 months following implantation.

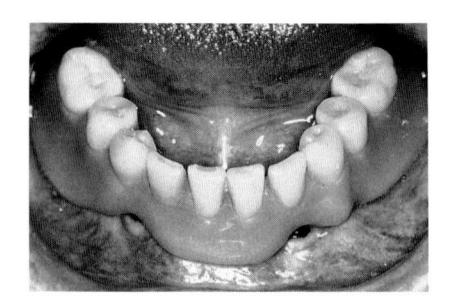

Figure 12.30 Implant supported overdenture in situ.

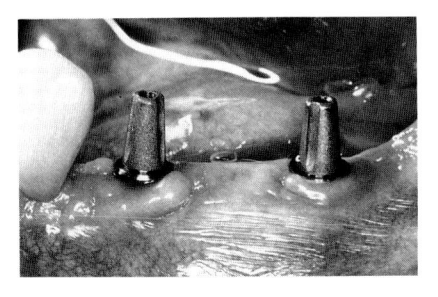

Figure 12.31 A 37-year-old male patient. Six months following implantation of two-part HS implants in a distal extension situation. The crown-and-bridge abutments are inserted.

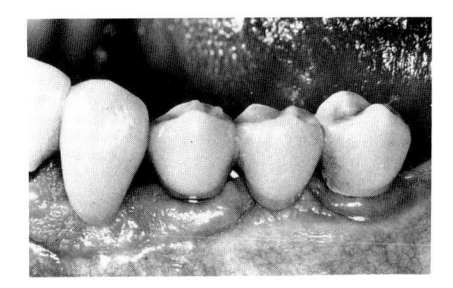

Figure 12.32 Clinical situation three years following implantation.

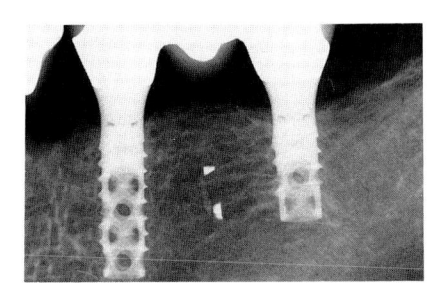

Figure 12.33 Periapical radiograph three years following implantation.

During the presurgical evaluation, the bone structure and the vertical bone height in the desirable area for an implant are analyzed in a panorex radiograph. A minimal bone height of 9 millimeters coronal to the mandibular canal should be present to avoid possible injuries to the mandibular nerve.

In this indication, two-part HS implants are preferred because they guarantee an optimal primary stability even in bone with a low density. If possible, superstructures supported by at least two HS implants are suggested. However, in situations where premolars are still present it is often impossible to place more than one implant, resulting in a reconstruction supported by a combination of a tooth and an implant.

The surgical procedures have been described previously (Buser et al, 1990a). After insertion of the implant, the large closure screw, slightly larger in diameter than the implant, prevents the wound margin from slipping over the implant shoulder, so that normally the preexisting width of keratinized mucosa can be maintained. Chemical plaque control (chlorhexidine-digluconate 0.12%) is used during soft-tissue healing, which takes about three weeks. After this time, large closure screw is replaced by a smaller one, and the patient can start to perform a normal hygiene procedure.

After the healing phase of three months, the closure screw will be removed and the crown-and-bridge abutment will be inserted into the implant, using the insertion device. After a direct impression is taken with a suitable material, the bridge is manufactured directly on the master cast and fixed with zinc-oxyphosphate luting cement. A clinical case is shown in Figures 12.31–12.33.

The Single Tooth Replacement in the Maxilla

It is mainly young patients who require a single tooth replacement in the maxilla. This is usually due to traumatic injuries or lack of development. The indication for an implant is elegant: if the neighbor teeth are free of caries, lesions, or fillings; if a neighbor tooth is already an abutment of a bridge reconstruction; or in the case of an upper front with diastemata. Two-part HC implants cannot be inserted immediately after traumatic loss of a tooth. For an implantation, a healing period of at least nine months is needed until bone regeneration is finished.

The preparation of the implant bed is done in the same way as for the one-part HC implant. After repositioning and suturing of the mucoperiosteal flap, the implant shoulder with the closure screw lies at the level of the mucosa. During the healing phase of three months, the patient usually wears a preexisting temporary partial denture. After three months the closure screw will be removed and the crown-and-bridge abutment will be inserted into the implant, with the aid of the insertion device and zinc-oxyphosphate luting cement. If necessary, the shape of the post may be changed quite easily—it can be prepared just as a regular abutment tooth would be. After a direct impression is taken with a suitable material (silicone, polyether), the crown is manufactured directly on the master cast and fixed with zinc-oxyphosphate luting cement onto the implant abutment (see Figures 12.34–12.36).

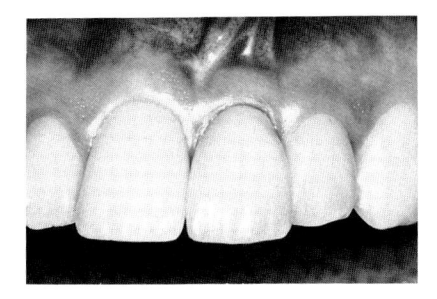

Figure 12.34 A 19-year-old female patient. Clinical situation two years following implantation of a two-part HC implant for a single tooth replacement.

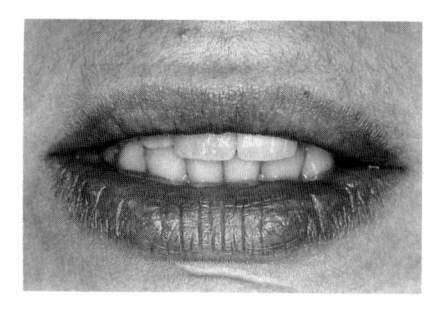

Figure 12.35 Esthetic result.

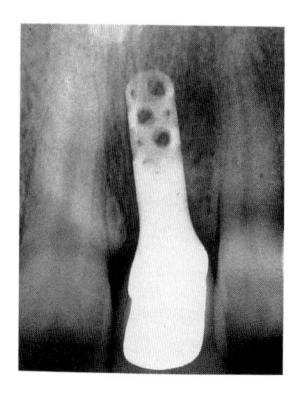

Figure 12.36 Periapical radiograph two years following implantation.

REFERENCES

Albrektsson, T., Brånemark P.I., Hansson B, Kanemo, K Larsson, I, Lundström, DM, McQueen, R Skalak: The interface zone of inorganic implants in vivo: Titanium implants in bone. Ann Biomed eng 11: 1–27, 1983.

Babbush CA, Kent JN, Misiek DJ: Titanium plasma-sprayed (TPS) screw implants for the reconstruction of the edentulous mandible. J Oral Maxillofac Surg 44: 274–282, 1986.

Buser D, Schroeder A, Sutter F, Lang NP: The new concept of ITI hollow cylinder and hollow screw implants. Part II: Clinical aspects, indications and early clinical results. Int J Oral Maxillofac Implants 3:173–181, 1988.

Buser D, Stich H, Krekeler G, Schroeder A: Faserstrukturen der periimplantären Mukosa bei Titanimplantaten: Eine tierexperimentelle Studie am Beagle-Hund. Z Zahnärztl Implantol V: 15–23, 1989.

Buser D, Weber HP, Brägger U: The treatment of partially edentulous patients with ITI hollow-screw implants: Presurgical evaluation and surgical procedures. Int J Oral Maxillofac Implants 5:165–174, 1990a.

Buser D, Weber HP, Lang NP: Tissue integration of non-submerged implants. 1-year results of a prospective study with 100 ITI hollow-cylinder and hollow-screw implants. Clin Oral Impl Res 1:33–40, 1990b.

Buser D, Schenk RK, Steinemann S, Fiorellini J, Fox C, Stich H: Influence of surface characteristics on bone integration of titanium implants. A histomorphometric study in miniature pigs. J Biomed Mat Res 25:898–902, 1991.

Buser D, Weber HP, Brägger U, Balsiger C: Tissue integration of one-stage ITI implants. 3-year results of a longitudinal study with hollow-cylinder and hollow-screw implants. Int J Oral Maxillofac Implants (in press).

Mericske-Stern R, Geering AH: Implantate in der Totalprothetik. Die Verankerung der Totalprothese im zahnlosen Unterkiefer durch zwei Implantate mit Einzelattachment. Schweiz Monatsschr Zahnmed 98:871–875, 1988.

Schroeder A, Pohler O, Sutter F: Gewebsreaktion auf ein Titan-Hohlzylinderimplantat mit Titan-Spritzschichtoberfläche. Schweiz Mschr Zahnheilk 86:713–727, 1976.

Schroeder A, Stich H, Straumann F, Sutter F: Ueber die Anlagerung von Osteozement an einen belasteten Implantatkörper. Schweiz Mschr ZahnheilK 88:1051–1058, 1978.

Schroeder A, van der Zypen F, Stich H, Sutter F: The reactions of bone, connective tissue and epithelium to endosteal implants with titanium-sprayed surfaces. J Maxillofac Surg 9:15–25, 1981.

Schroeder A, Maeglin B, Sutter F: Das ITI-Hohlzylinderimplantat Typ F zur Prothesenretention beim zahnlosen Unterkiefer. Schweiz Mschr Zahnheilk 93:720–733, 1983.

Schroeder A, Sutter F, Krekeler G: Oral Implantology. Basics—ITI Hollow Cylinder. Thieme Medical Publishers Inc., New York, 1991.

Steinemann S: The properties of titanium. In: Schroeder A, Sutter F, Krekeler G (eds.): Oral Implantology. Basics—ITI Hollow Cylinder, pp. 37–58. Thieme Medical Publishers Inc., New York, 1991.

Sutter F, Schroeder A, Buser D: The new concept of ITI hollow cylinder and hollow screw implants. Part I: Engineering and design. Int J Oral Maxillofac Implants 3:161–172, 1988.

CHAPTER 13

Osteointegration and Rigid Fixation

Rickard Brånemark
Richard Skalak
Per-Ingvar Brånemark

INTRODUCTION

There are many conditions of intraoral and extraoral defects in which long-term, stable anchorage of a synthetic component in the skeleton is a prerequisite for predictable, useful function. These defects involve not only major skeletal discontinuities and endoprosthetic joint replacement, in which the reconstruction is completely covered by biologic tissues, but also situations in which skin or mucous membrane must be penetrated in order to allow attachment of a prosthetic limb or, in craniomaxillofacial defects, a prosthetic replacement. The attachment of a bone-conduction hearing aid to the skull bone is another example requiring skin penetration. In all of these situations, a load-carrying prosthesis must become and remain connected to the skeleton in the defect region in such a manner that the bone tissue is not only capable of carrying the functional loads and shock loading, but also is able to react in a physiological manner to remodel according to the functional loads applied. Different philosophies have formed the basis for numerous methodological approaches to this problem. Most of these approaches provide adequate initial stability; but after shorter or longer periods of time, many end up suffering a loss of stability associated with ingrowth of fibrous connective tissue and with more or less severe local tissue damage as a consequence of the increasing mobility of the anchoring element. The predominant problem has been that it was considered an inevitable consequence of the presence of a synthetic component in living bone tissue to initiate formation of low-differentiated connective tissue in the biological interface due to the presence of the material itself or to the transferred dynamic load. However, contrary to popular opinion, it has been demonstrated that using a bioacceptable material, such as pure titanium with a specific surface microarchitecture, and a design of the anchorage element that allows controlled transfer of load to the adjacent bone in combination with extremely gentle surgical preparation of the bone site accommodating the titanium component and allowing adequate time for bone healing and remodeling, it is possible to create a situation where bone tissue incorporates the anchorage securely so it can accept functional demands without mechanical failure or rejection phenomena over very long periods (see Figures 13.1 and 13.2).

This principle, which we called osseointegration, was developed as a result of our experimental studies.

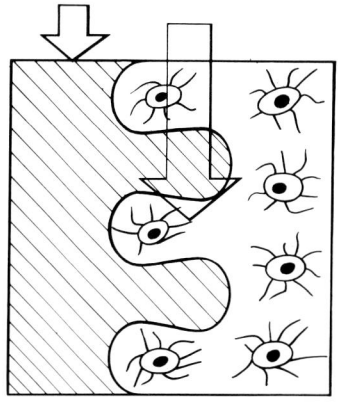

Figure 13.1 Direct connection between endoprosthesis and living bone, with adequate transfer of functional load. (From Brånemark et al., 1985.)

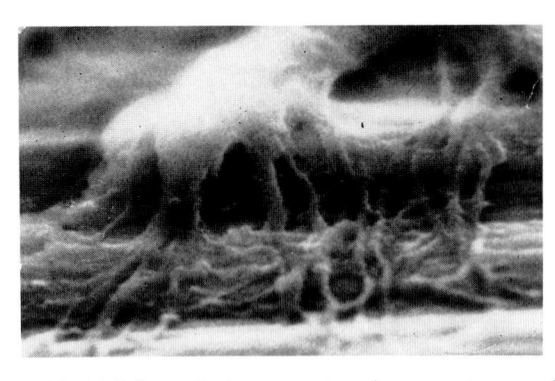

Figure 13.2 High-resolution scanning electron micrograph of a bone cell with its membrane processes adapted to the surface of a titanium endoprosthesis obtained from a clinical biopsy from the jaw bone. (From Brånemark et al., 1985.)

These started in 1952, when we focused on bone and marrow tissue response to injury, with microvascular disturbance as a sensitive identification factor. Later we performed a detailed evaluation of the interaction between titanium and hard and soft tissues in animals and humans. After the application of screw-shaped titanium components (fixtures) as anchorage elements for prosthetic teeth in dogs with a functional lifetime of up to 10 years, the procedure was first applied clinically in complete edentulism to provide permanent stable support of fixed dental prostheses. Since our clinical pilot cases in 1965, more than 100,000 edentulous patients have been treated to date, and 500,000 fixtures have been installed according to the osseointegration principle. In long-term, consecutive clinical studies, prosthetic stability without undue tissue reactions has been achieved in 99% of lower jaw prostheses and 95% of upper jaw prostheses (Adell 1989). Since 1976, craniomaxillofacial prostheses have been anchored to skull bone via osseointegrated titanium fixtures, and bone-conduction hearing aids have been similarly anchored in the mastoid bone. Titanium elements penetrating skin and mucous membrane following appropriate surgical procedures have functioned well and have not caused significant clinical problems (Tjellström 1989).

Starting in 1981, osseointegration was applied to endoprosthetic repair of finger joints with successive adjustments of designs and surgical procedures. The clinical results indicate that the long-term prognosis expected in hand surgery and orthopedic surgery can be similar to that found in oral and craniomaxillofacial reconstruction. Many publications have been devoted to the basic biology, physics, and chemistry—as well as the clinical procedure and results—of the osseointegration of titanium (Kasemo 1985, Albrektsson 1988).

Osseointegration as it applies to provision of permanent and stable connection of a synthetic component to the human skeleton can be defined as follows: A biological response resulting in a long-term coexistence of differentiated, remodeling bone tissue and strictly defined synthetic components, providing lasting, specific clinical functions without initiating rejection mechanisms. This long-term coexistence implies a time scale of decades, not merely a few years. Osseointegration as a means of incorporating a load-carrying endoprosthesis in the skeleton relies for prognostic predictability on three basic biologic concepts. First, the bone site for the anchoring element must be prepared with a careful and gentle surgical technique so that the wound that is created in the bone can heal with differentiated bone tissue, avoiding formation of any low-differentiated scar or fibrous tissue in the interface. Second, because in many situations the bone tissue is more or less deficient preoperatively because of long periods of inactivity, impaired circulation, and so on, it is important to allow adequate unloaded, undisturbed time for healing until remineralization has occurred. This avoids the risk that load could cause relative movement between prosthesis and adjacent bone. Third, that an immediate and direct contact is established between differentiated bone tissue and synthetic material, and the load transferred from the prosthesis via the interface to the anchoring bone can provide an adequate load-remodeling stimulus within the mechanical capacity of the bone at any particular time (see Figures 13.3 and 13.4). This requirement can be fulfilled only by careful attention to the micro as well as the macro aspects of the design of the fixtures.

In most orthopedic reconstructions, the prosthetic components are covered by skin. In craniomaxillofacial situations, however, the majority of cases require penetration of skin or mucous membrane in order to permit mechanical connection of intraoral or extraoral prostheses to the skeleton. That means that in addition to mechanical stability, long-term healthy conditions must be established at locations where the integumentum has been pierced by connectors supporting the prosthesis (see Figure 13.5).

In the osseointegration system that we have developed for the craniomaxillofacial region, the fixtures, which are made of commercially pure titanium, have specific geometry and surface characteristics (see Figure 13.6). This design provides to the synthetic components a combination of minimal volume and adequate surface area.

In situations where the skin or mucous membrane must be penetrated to accommodate the prosthesis, special surgical, prosthetic, and maintenance requirements should be considered in order to provide a safe, antiseptic clinical procedure and a stable, long-term result (see Figures 13.7 and 13.8). The stability and load-carrying capacity that can be achieved depend on the adaptation and continuous remodeling of the anchoring bone tissue during the early stage of bone healing and on the initial load-carrying period, when a dynamic

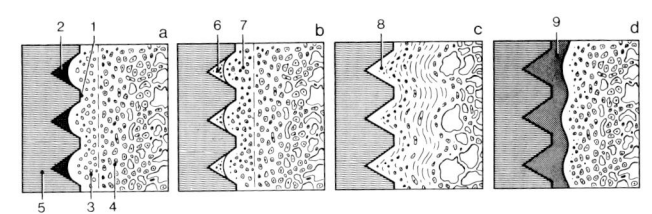

Figure 13.3 Diagrammatic representation of biology of osseointegration. (From Brånemark et al., 1985.) (a) The threaded bone site cannot be made perfectly congruent to the implant. The purpose of making a threaded socket in bone is to provide immobilization immediately after installation and during the initial healing period, but the threaded design is also favorable from a biomechanic point of view after the healing period when the fixture is loaded. The diagram illustrates relative dimensions of fixture and fixture site. [1 = contact between fixture and bone (immobilization); 2 = hematoma in closed cavity, bordered by fixture and bone; 3 = bone that was damaged by unavoidable thermal and mechanical trauma; 4 = original undamaged bone; and 5 = fixture.] (b) During the unloaded healing period, the hematoma becomes transformed into new bone through callus formation (6). Damaged bone, which also heals, undergoes revascularization, demineralization, and remineralization (7). (c) After the initial healing period, vital bone tissue is in close contact with the fixture surface, with no intermediate tissue. Border zone bone (8) remodels in response to the masticatory load applied. (d) In unsuccessful cases, nonmineralized connective tissue (9), constituting a kind of pseudoarthrosis, forms in the border zone at the implant. This development can be initiated by excessive preparation trauma, infection, loading too early in the healing period before adequate mineralization and organization of hard tissue has taken place, or supraliminal loading at any time, even many years after integration has been established. Connective tissue can become organized to a certain degree, but is not a proper anchoring tissue because of its inadequate mechanical and biologic capacities, resulting in creation of a locus minoris resistentiae.

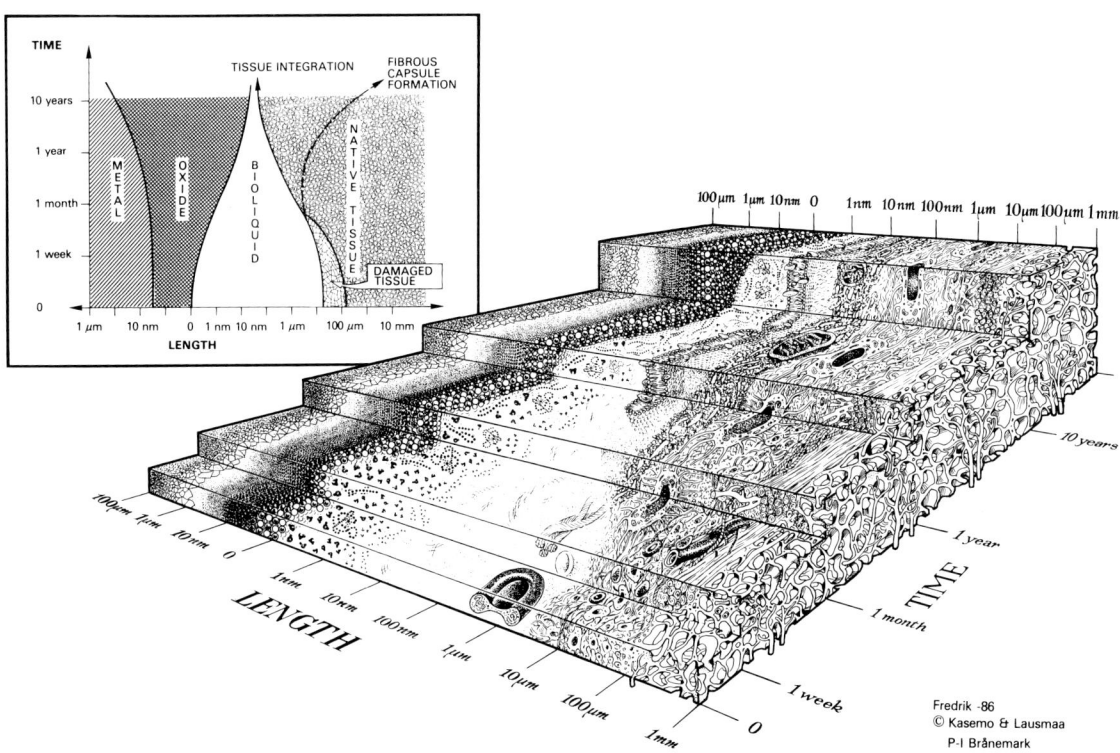

Figure 13.4 Tissue integration relies on a sequence of events at the molecular level occurring in the interface between tissue and titanium, where the dynamic events are located toward and in the titanium-oxide layer that covers the bulk metal. The interface is thus continuously remodeling and adapting, even after several years of function. This capacity of adequate response to physiological stimuli seems to be the fundamental basis for clinical application of osseointegration. The process of incorporation of the titanium component in the living tissue is strictly related to time and space. This process starts with the healing of a wound in the bone over a period of weeks, followed by regeneration of differentiating remineralizing tissue over a period of months. Subsequent and successive remodeling at functional load continues for decades. (From Brånemark, 1989.)

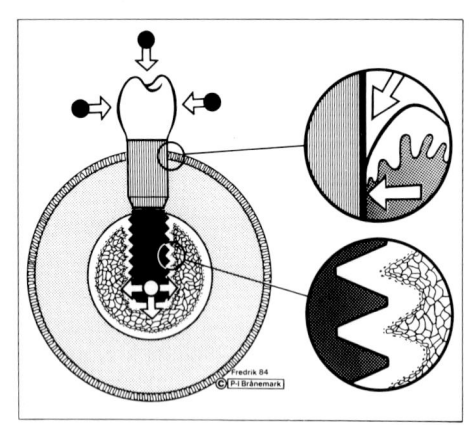

Figure 13.5 Diagrammatic summary of crucial problems in creating permanent tissue anchorage of prostheses penetrating skin or mucous membrane. Reliable stability must be achieved by incorporation of the anchorage element in normal bone tissue. This provides both adequate resistance to load and load distribution, which result in bone remodeling. Penetration through skin or mucous membrane to allow attachment of external prosthetic devices (for example, teeth) requires establishment of a biological barrier between the internal and external environment in the anchorage region. An anchorage unit consists of nonbiological anchoring elements together with its incorporating hard or soft tissues. (From Brånemark, et al., 1985.)

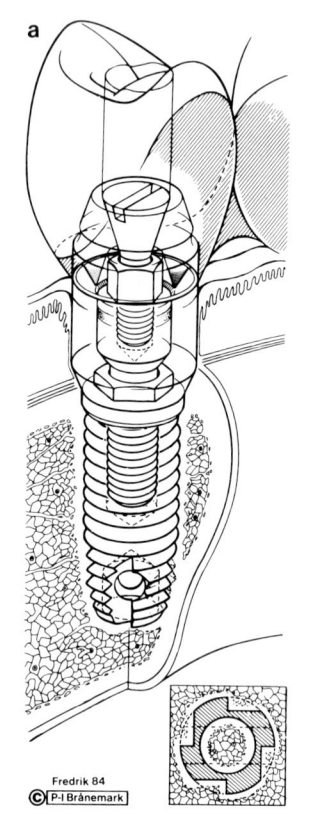

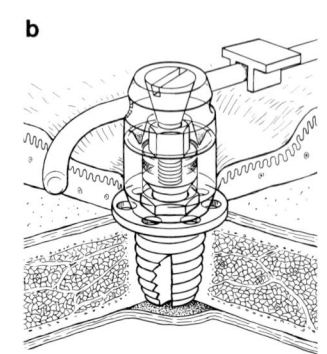

Figure 13.6 (a) The anchorage unit for oral rehabilitation using osseointegrated titanium fixtures as support for prosthetic substitutes for teeth. (From Adell et al., 1981.) (b) The modified fixture used for extraoral cranial anchorage.

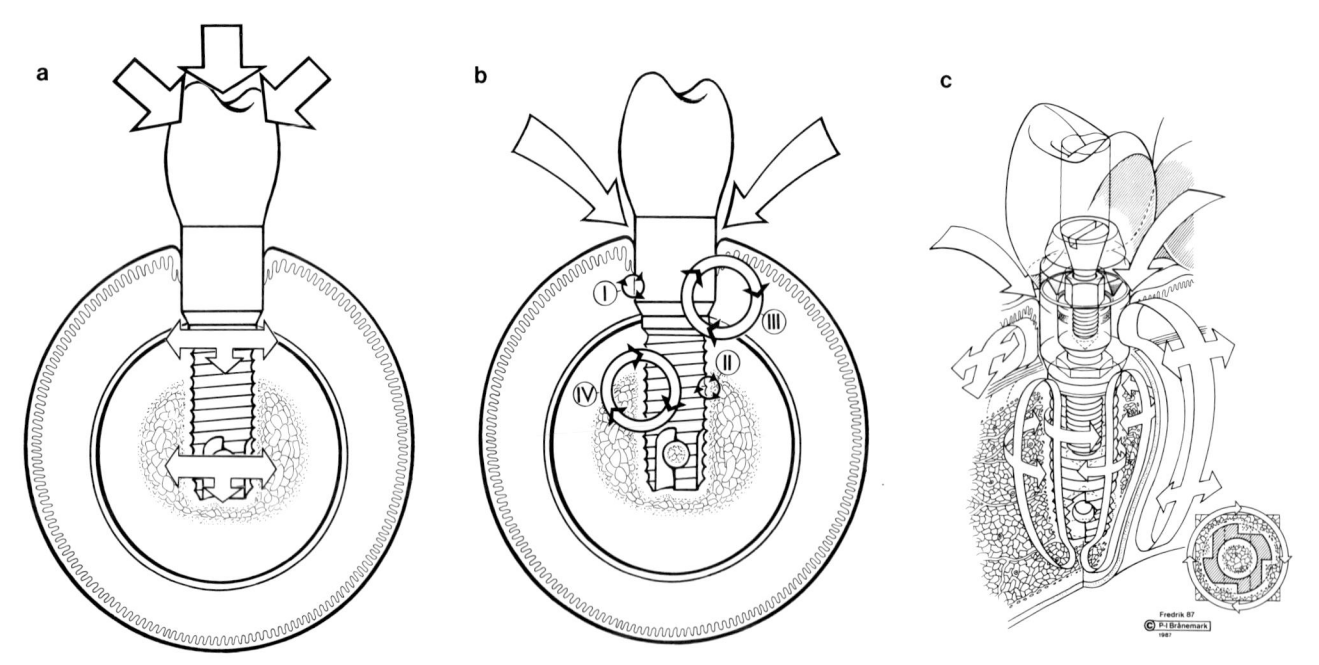

Figure 13.7 Biotechnological principles for permanent tissue integration of a prosthetic device that is attached via a component that penetrates skin or mucous membrane. (a) Primary mechanical stability requires sufficient load-bearing capacity of the anchoring bone. Long-term function is based on continuous bone remodeling according to adequate stimuli via controlled transfer of static and dynamic load to the anchoring bone tissue. (b) A predictable clinical prognosis presupposes that a dynamic interface relation and interaction between hard and soft tissues and the synthetic anchoring component can be established at the molecular level (I and II) and at the level of organized tissue (III and IV). (c) The continuing response to external and internal stimuli results in a complex three-dimensional network of remodeling and defense and reactive mechanisms in the hard and soft tissues protecting the anchoring region from mechanical, chemical, and bacterial attacks from the external environment. (From Brånemark, 1989.)

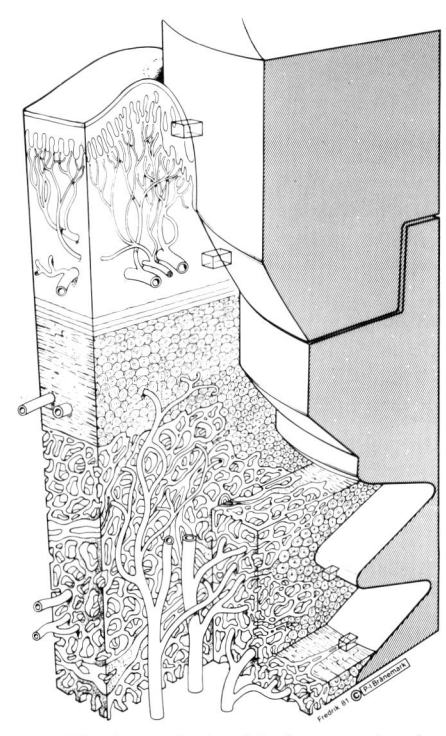

Figure 13.8 The interrelationship between hard and soft tissue and titanium is shown by this overall view of the intact remodeled interface zone around osseointegrated implants. (From Brånemark et al., 1985.)

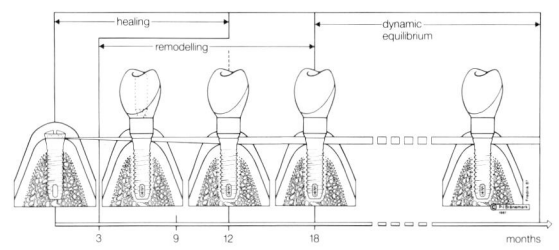

Figure 13.9 The sequence of events in tissues incorporating and integrating a titanium fixture. Osseointegration is a biotechnological phenomenon related to functional adaption in time and space.

equilibrium is created at the interface. This is a prerequisite for long-term prognostic predictability (see Figure 13.9).

Experimental studies and clinical documentation illustrate anatomical details of successful osseointegration (see Figures 13.10 and 13.11).

Osseointegration, in clinical dentistry and in reconstructive craniomaxillofacial surgery, has proven to be a reliable procedure for creating longterm mechanical stability. This includes single tooth replacement, treatment of complete edentulism, treatment of congenital or aquired defects, sometimes requiring bone grafting procedures and prosthetic substitution, as reprinted in our consecutive clinical materials for over two decades (see Figures 13.12 and 13.14).

The possibilities and limitations of permanent mechanical stability can be understood only when one regards bone as a complex biological tissue. Bone is composed of living cells and a mineralized ground substance in a special three-dimensional arrangement, with a microvascular system, necessary for the immediate coexistence with the hemopoietic marrow tissue (Figure 13.15). Accordingly, any application of osseointegration in clinical situations must consider, in addition to engineering and mechanical aspects, the biological dynamics and time perspectives involved.

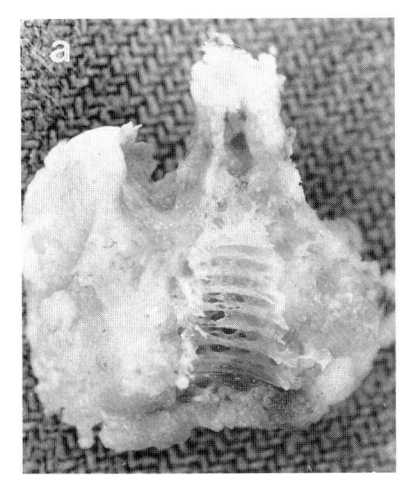

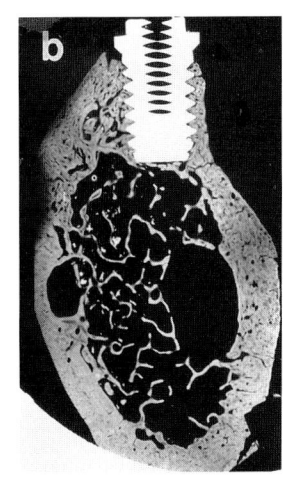

Figure 13.10 (a) Fixture removed from the upper jawbone of a dog to illustrate remodeling of bone with formation of a dense capsule in the trabecular bone after 32 months of function (b) Microradiogram of ground section shows the pattern of remodeling and density of the mineralized tissue on a fixture from the lower jawbone of a dog. (c) The typical encapsulation in compact bone follows exactly the anatomy of the fixture even at its apical part of a dog). (From Brånemark et al., 1985.)

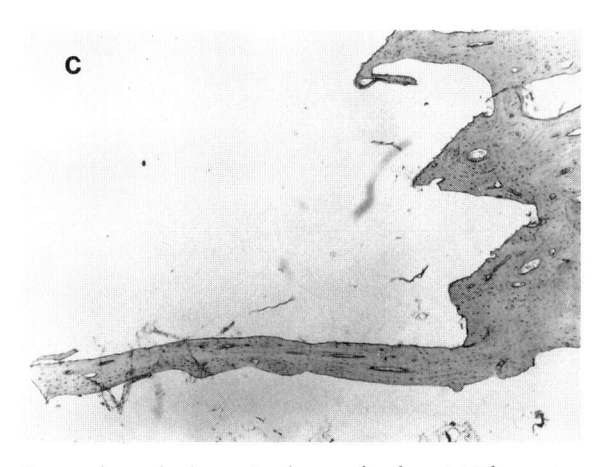

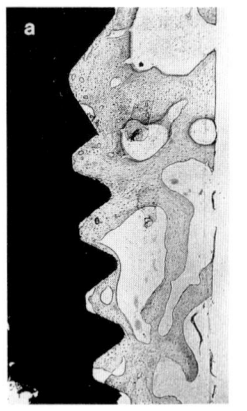

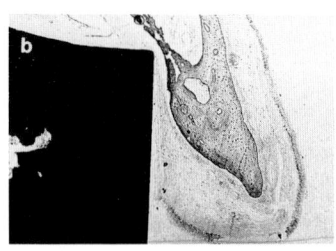

Figure 13.11 The behavior of jawbone and soft tissues are illustrated in this clinical specimen, obtained at autopsy from a case of a woman who had fixed bridges on fixtures in her upper and lower jaws. (a) Adequate adaptation and remodeling of the endosseous bone towards a mandibular fixture. (b) Reaction-free tissue at apex of fixture facing maxillary cavity. (Specimen obtained from and analyzed in collaboration with Professor Philip Worthington and Dr. T. Hall, Seattle, Washington, USA.)

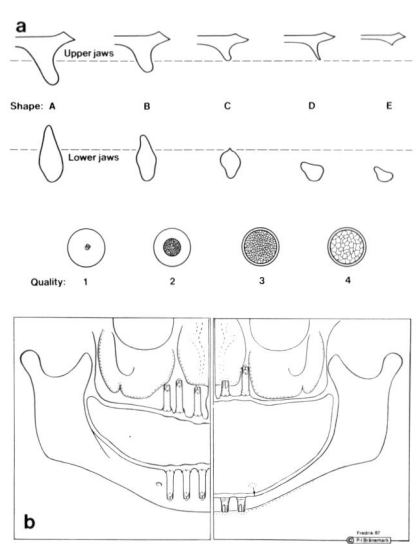

Figure 13.12 (a) Diagrammatic representation of range of jawbone defect anatomy and varying qualities of bone in edentulism. The reconstructive procedures must cover the entire range of defects. (b) Fixture positioning in edentulous jawbone with varying degree of resorption. Presurgical prosthetic planning of fixture topography provides optimal load-carrying capacity in the available jawbone. (From Brånemark et al., 1985).

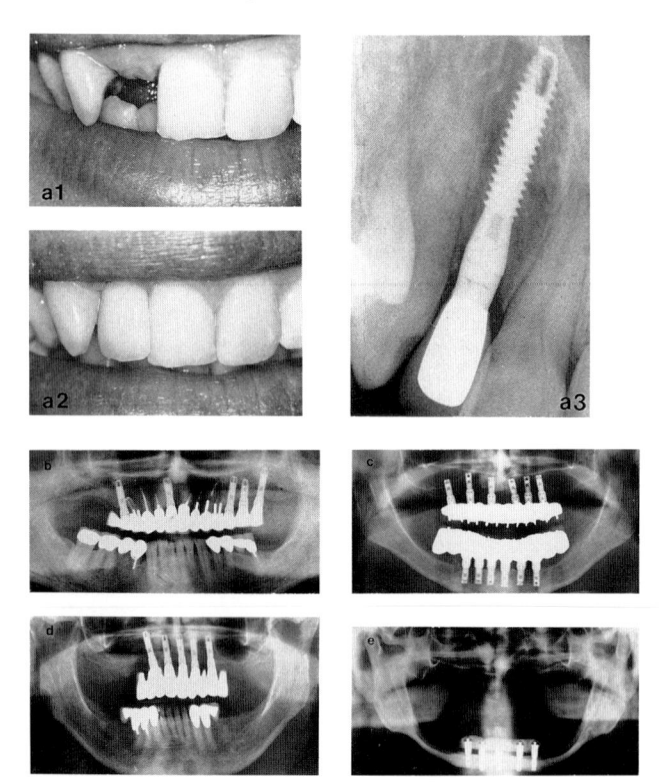

Figure 13.13 Clinical examples of bone-anchored dental prostheses: (a) Replacement of single tooth. (b) Replacement in partial edentulism. (c) Replacement in complete edentulism. (d) Replacement in a case of extreme jawbone resorption, requiring additional autologous bone grafting to ensure load-carrying capacity. (e) Replacement in a case of extreme lower-jaw resorption, where the continuous mandible almost always provides enough quantity and quality of bone for anchorage without grafting.

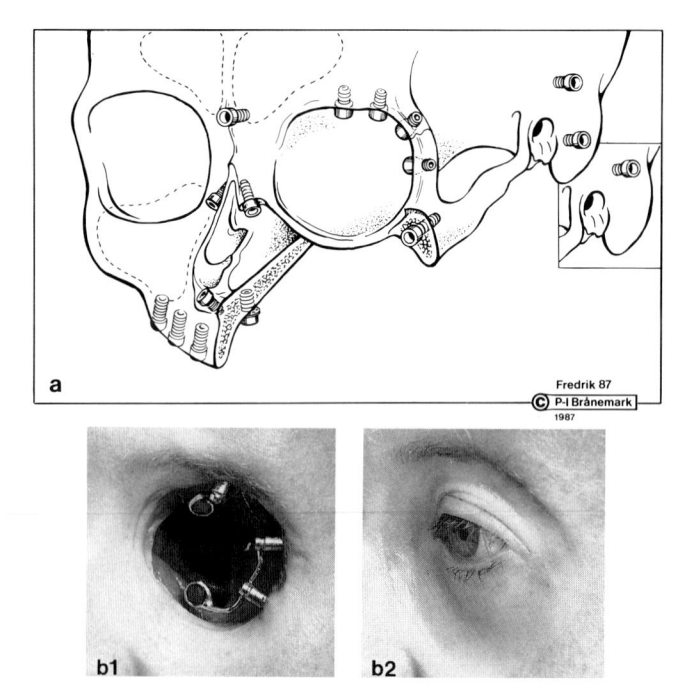

Figure 13.14 (a) Diagrammatic representation of topographical location of fixtures for retention of prostheses in craniomaxillofacial reconstruction: maxilla, nose, orbit, midface, and ear. (b) Orbital prosthesis supported by magnets connected to a splint attached to titanium fixtures in a 40-year-old patient. This case was treated in collaboration with Dr. S. Parel, prostodontist; G. Greg, prosthetist; and K. Jansson, anaplastologist. Fixtures were installed 16 years after radiation (3000 rads), with follow-up at 5 years. (From Brånemark, 1989.)

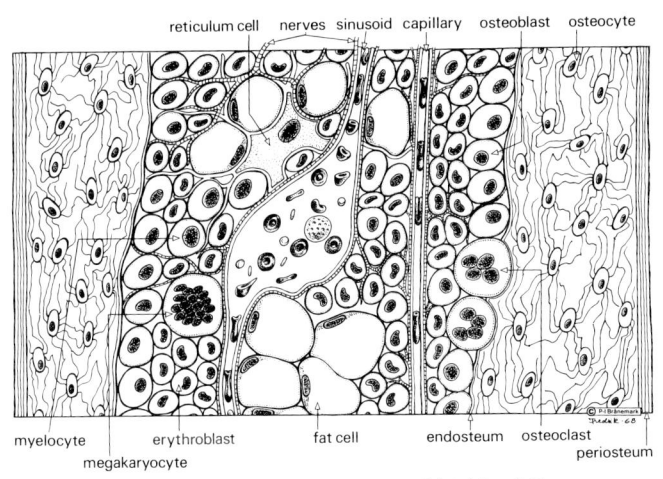

Figure 13.15 Diagrammatic summary of highly differentiated and potentially dynamic tissue components that constitute the biological aspect of the interface of osseointegrated prostheses.

EXPERIMENTAL INVESTIGATIONS

To supply quantitative data needed for sound clinical decisions concerning the feasibility and safety of osseointegrated fixtures in patients, an experimental (animal) model was developed in which various mechanical and histological parameters could be evaluated. Three different mechanical tests were performed: torque, pull-out, and lateral loading.

We used titanium fixtures with a shape identical to the Brånemark fixtures except for the bottom part, which had no transverse hole. Such a hole would interfere with interpretation and evaluation of the torque results. A set of three fixtures was inserted in a straight line in each animal's hind leg. On each set of three fixtures it was possible to perform torque and pull-out tests, or lateral loading tests. The animal chosen was the beagle dog. The unloaded healing time was at least three months.

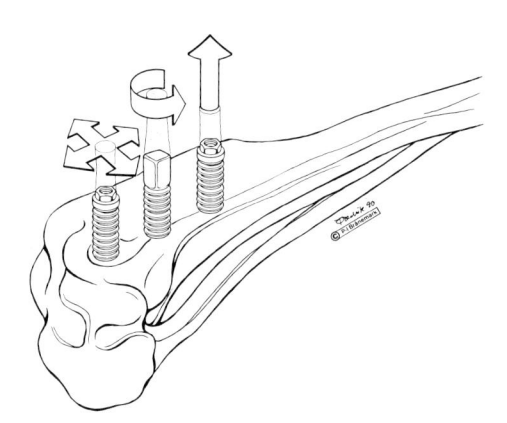

Figure 13.16 Schematic illustration of the different biomechanical tests performed on osseointegrated titanium fixtures.

The biomechanical testing (see Figure 13.16) consisted of computer-aided, in vivo registration of torque versus angle when torque was applied to the fixture to unscrew it, registration of applied force versus deformation (extension) when a pull-out test was performed in the axial direction of the fixture, and registration of applied force versus deformation when a lateral load test was performed. The lateral load test included loading in the axial direction of the bone as well as transversely to the axial direction of the long bone.

Results

Torque Experiments

Figure 13.17 shows the typical curve of torque versus angle of rotation. The curve begins sharply, showing a torque that rises almost linearly up to a maximum at a few degrees. After these few degrees of deformation there is a plastic deformation as indicated by the fact that after unloading the fixture the angle did not return to zero (see Figure 13.17). After the initial rising part, there was a second phase (plateau region) with almost constant torque, sometimes slightly, but then gradually declining toward zero for increasing angles. The initial, rising segment was nearly linear up to a small angle, at which the slope distinctly decreased. This breakpoint appears, on initial loading, to be similar to the elastic limit observed in tensile tests of metals. In this case, however, there is already some plastic (irrecoverable) deformation below the breakpoint, as shown by the unloading and reloading curves in Figure 13.17.

Pull-out Experiments

Figure 13.18 shows a typical curve of tensile force versus the extensional displacement measured in pull-out tests. The initial, more or less linear portion of the curve extended up to a relatively sharp breakpoint. The maximum load was reached shortly beyond this breakpoint, after which the load declined rapidly as the extension was increased. There was no plateau region in this case, and it was observed that the bone was splintered in a ring around the screw above the maximum load.

Lateral Load Experiments

Figure 13.19 shows a typical curve of lateral load versus deflection for a lateral load test. The general shape of the test curves was similar for axial and transverse directions of loading. Due to the different test arrangements required, only one kind of test was possible on each limb.

The typical test curve showed a distinctly linear initial portion up to a fairly well defined breakpoint. Thereafter, a plateau region followed, with slightly in-

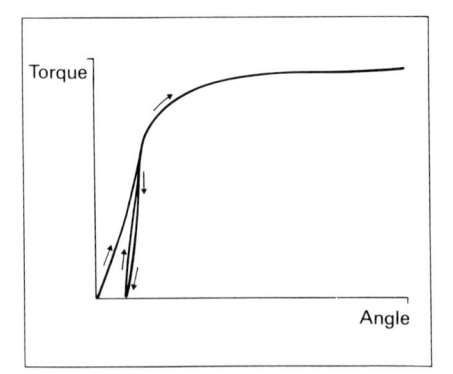

Figure 13.17 A typical curve plot of torque versus angle of rotation in the torque tests. Note that the initial part of the curve is approximately linear, but it is not reversible (elastic). There is some irreversible (plastic) deformation indicated by the unloading and reloading curves.

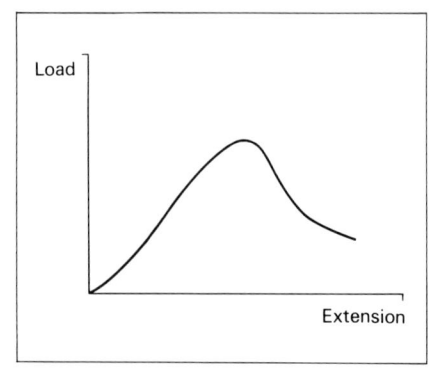

Figure 13.18 A typical curve plot of load versus extension in a pull-out test. Splintering of bone occurs soon after maximum load is reached.

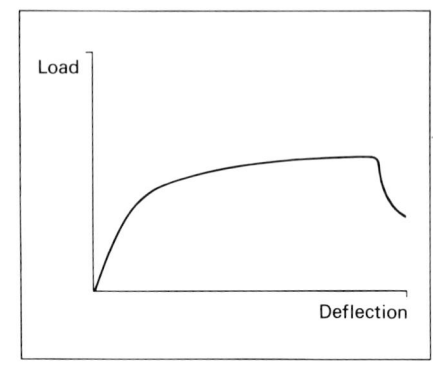

Figure 13.19 A typical curve plot of lateral load versus deflection in a lateral load test. In the plateau region, the bone is twisted and finally fractures.

creasing load and a sharp decline after the maximum load was reached. It appeared that the bone was split and/or splintered after the maximum load was exceeded.

Discussion and Implications

The several test results described above give some insights into how the interface of an osseointegrated fixture behaves under various types of stress. The torsional tests suggest that the screws are smoothly turning along the threads of osseointegrated bone without any indication of failure or cracking of the bone itself or of the implant. This indicates that it is the interface that is primarily tested. A surprising result was that at the resolution level of the equipment used, it was not possible to find a load range below which there was no plastic deformation. Such an elastic range should be expected if there were a direct bond between the implant and bone with a finite shear strength. The present tests imply that such shear bond strength is low, but the very considerable torques that are developed at small angles, below the breakpoint, are due to the close apposition of the bone to the implant. Due to close apposition, any small protrusion of titanium above the bone's mean surface must plastically deform the surrounding bone as the angle of deformation is increased. The breakpoint is then interpreted as the point where the maximum of the roughness is engaged. The plateau is interpreted as a region of steady plowing of the roughness along the surface of the bone. Some solid friction also may be involved during this stage. The ultimate decline of torque as the angle increases may indicate that the bone, when sufficiently abraded at the scale of the micro roughness, offers decreasing further resistance to sliding. These tests imply that the appropriate surface roughness is a key element in developing shear or torsional strength of the interfaces in osseointegrated fixtures.

It should be noted that any attempt at defining bone as an achieving biological material that uses only registration of the maximal torque required to create a relative movement between the synthetic component and adjacent bone tissue does not provide adequate and meaningful parameters for the understanding of bone as anchorage for endoprostheses in clinical reality. The maximum functional deformation may be reached long before the maximum load is found.

The present tests do not directly reveal the possibilities of tensile strength of bonds between titanium and osseointegrated bone. Previous researches have found appreciable tensile strength (Steinemann 1986). This indicates that the interface behavior might be different in tension and shear.

In contrast to the torsion tests, the results of pull-out and lateral loading tests appear to depend more on the properties of the bone surrounding the implant and less on the properties of the interface. This conclusion comes from the observations of the failure modes. The bone in the vicinity of the implant is obviously splintered and fractured in pull-out and lateral loading tests. The implants were not damaged in these tests; they appear to move as rigid bodies in deforming the surrounding bone. The fact that the pull-out and lateral loading tests primarily test the surrounding bone is partly due to the geometry of the implants. The threads are an efficient mechanism of load transfer.

While the present tests are reassuring in terms of the ultimate loads developed, to be able to relate these measured loads directly to the geometry of the test and the amount and distribution of the bone present would be desirable. This will require detailed computation of stress distributions, on one hand, and equally detailed histologic information about the density and distribution of the bone surrounding the fixtures in each case, on the other hand.

Some approximate average stress behavior may be definable by simplified models. This is most obvious for the torsion test. Assuming that sliding occurs at the interface, an average shear stress can be computed accurately for the screw as a whole. But to be a useful criterion, the fact that only a certain percentage of the implant area has a close apposition to bone must be taken into account. Careful histological analysis can measure this percentage. This is currently under way for the specimens described above and will be reported in a subsequent publication.

From the experimental side, tests are needed to determine whether the height, amount, and distribution of surface roughness affect the torque experimental results, as the current tests suggest.

For the pull-out and lateral loading tests, any approximate theory will probably be less realistic than the simple torsion case. For the pull-out test, an average shear stress can be computed readily using a cylinder with a diameter equal to the outer diameter of the threads and the axial length of screw integrated in the bone. To translate such a result to more basic properties of bone, the computation should incorporate the relative amount of bone present.

The lateral load test is the most difficult to reduce to quantitative predictive parameters. Derivation of an accurate stress distribution will require numerical methods such as the finite element method. Even with this analysis, various variables need exploration—for example, the influence of the length of the screw above and below the bone surface and the influence of anisotropy. Another variable is the direction of loading, either transverse, parallel, or at other angles to the axis of the bone. To be useful predictively for a patient, assessment of the extent and quality of the bone available is necessary.

In finite element modeling, an appropriate boundary condition on the contact surface between bone and implant must be specified to carry out the analysis. Brunski (1988) and Hipp (1985) have shown that the stress distribution computed in a two-dimensional model depends on whether a bonded or a slip surface is assumed at the interface. Although the present tests do not imply a bonded surface, they do not support the use of a slip surface. Because substantial shear can be generated with small slip motions, the bonded boundary condition is probably more realistic.

BIOMECHANICAL CONSIDERATIONS

Advantages of Screw Form

A primary consideration of the choice of an implant form is the reliability of load transfer from the prosthesis to the skeletal components. Connectors of many types have been developed in mechanical engineering, but the screw has been used in many applications because of its intrinsic advantages.

For dental implants, threads can be cut accurately with minimum trauma; and if the screw is manufactured accurately, it will give a close initial fit and immediate stability. Furthermore, it will not move or slip readily under small accidental forces during healing. After osseointegration, a screw offers a comparatively large surface for bonding and for transmission of stress. The screw interlocks the fixture and the bone. Even if bone is not grown entirely into the threads (see Figure 13.20a and b), there may be enough area of implant and bone in close contact to prevent relative motion in any direction, which is the primary requirement for long-term stability.

The fine roughness of a screw surface enables interlocking at the microscopic level similar to that provided by the screw threads at the macroscopic level. Bonding is an advantage: Computer models (Hipp 1985) show that a bonded screw generally has a lower peak stress for a given load than does a freely sliding unbonded screw. As discussed earlier, osseointegrated titanium screws develop a definite shear strength and do not slide freely.

Mechanics of a Single Screw

A single osseointegrated screw can resist forces from any direction at a level comparable to normal bite forces (Haraldsson 1977). A vertical force—that is, a force acting along the axis of the screw (see Figure 13.20a), such as a normal bite force—is resisted in an osseointegrated fixture by shear stress in the cylinder of bone surrounding the screw threads. Because titanium is about 10 times as stiff as bone, it will not deform appreciably under normal loading. This is an advantage in that the stress in the bone is likely to be more uniformly distributed than when a very flexible implant is used.

Because the ultimate strength of titanium in shear is also much higher than that of bone, testing a fixture in tension to failure will usually result in shearing in the bone in a cylindrical zone outside the screw rather than through the threads of the screw. It is possible that the shank of the screw in tension should fail first at the

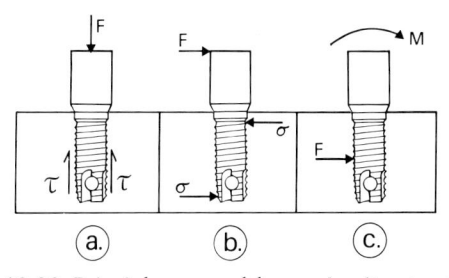

Figure 13.20 Principle types of fixture loading in vivo: (a) axial load by bite force, F; (b) lateral load by grinding force, F; (c) equivalent moment, M, plus lateral force, F, equivalent to (b).

level of threads just above the surface of the bone. This limits how thin a screw can be useful.

For lateral loads, such as those due to grinding of teeth, a primarily horizontal force is imposed at the level of the tooth surface (see Figure 13.20b). This kind of loading gives rise to a large compressive stress at the upper edge of the bone, counteracting the applied force as shown in Figure 13.20b. There is also a lesser compression on the opposite side near the base of the screw. In a brittle material the sharp edges at the base of the fixture and at the outer edges of the screw threads would give rise to stress concentrations and cracking. Such cracking is not observed either clinically or on the test specimens osseointegrated in vivo. Bone may fracture, acquiring a hairline crack, just as will a brittle material under impact loading. Such accidental fracture is obviously always a hazard.

The horizontal force at the upper surface of a tooth (see Figure 13.20b) is equivalent to a force at the level of screw threads in the osseointegrated region plus a bending moment, M, applied to the fixture (see Figure 13.20c). This bending moment causes the variation of stresses along the length of the screw. The high stress near the surface of the bone is most likely to damage the bone around a fixture used as a single tooth replacement.

Force Distribution to Fixtures: Rigid Prosthesis

If a rigid bridge, such as a gold casting, is mounted on four or more osseointegrated fixtures, a very stiff, unified total structure like that shown in Figure 13.21a is achieved. The upper horizontal bar represents the bridge structure. The vertical elements are the fixtures, and the lower horizontal element represents the mandible. Such a structure will distribute forces applied to the prosthesis so that all of the fixtures will share in carrying the load to some extent. The schematic is drawn as a single, unified structure to emphasize that each element and connection is capable of carrying bending moments as well as axial and shear forces. Such a construction reduces peak forces in any one fixture and reduces the bending moment that each anchorage must withstand.

An approximate theory for the distribution of forces applied to a prosthesis has been developed on the assumptions that the bridge is rigid and that the response of the fixtures and their supporting bony structures are elastic (Skalak 1983). In terms of the coordinates and distances shown in Figure 13.22a, the force on any one fixture due to a vertical bite force is

$$F_i = \frac{P}{N} + P(Ax_i + By_i), \quad (13.1)$$

where

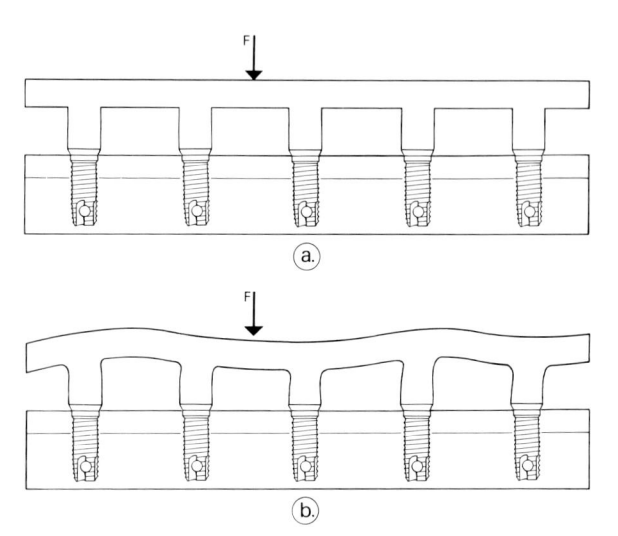

Figure 13.21 (a) Schematic illustration of the behavior of a rigid bridge. The bridge deflection is negligible and load distribution depends on elastic responses of fixtures. (b) Schematic illustration of the behavior of a flexible bridge. The bending of the bridge structure tends to increase loading of the fixtures adjacent to the applied load, F.

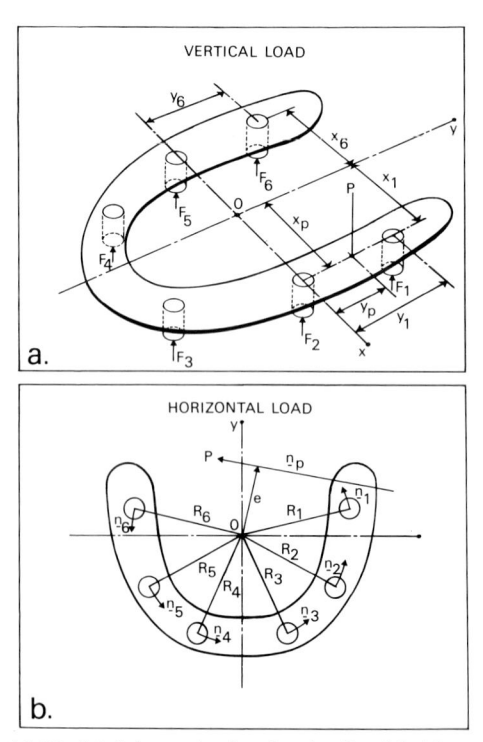

Figure 13.22 (a) Schematic sketch of a fixed bridge under vertical load, P. Center of gravity of the six fixtures is at 0. Eccentricity of the load is x_p with respect to the y axis and y_p with respect to the x axis. (b) Schematic plan of fixed denture bridge with horizontal load, P (grinding force) in the plane of the prosthesis. The load, P, has eccentricity e with respect to the centroid, 0, of the six fixtures. (From Skalak, 1983.)

i is the screw number, P is the applied force, N is the total number of screws, x_i and y_i are coordinates of the ith screw, and A and B are constant coefficients given by

$$A = (l_{xy}y_p - l_{xx}x_p)/(l_{xy}^2 - l_{xy}l_{yy}), \quad (13.2)$$

$$B = (l_{xy}x_p - l_{yy}y_p)/(l_{xy}^2 - l_{xx}l_{yy}), \quad (13.3)$$

where

$$l_{xx} = \Sigma y_i^2, \quad (13.4)$$

$$l_{yy} = \Sigma x_i^2, \quad (13.5)$$

$$l_{xy} = \Sigma x_i y_i. \quad (13.6)$$

The summations indicated in Equations (13.4–13.6) are over the N screws. The origin of the coordinates in Figure 13.22a is the centroid of the set of N screws. It follows from these equations that the forces on fixtures nearest the load will generally be greater than those on distant screws. It is possible that the force on a fixture F_i can be greater than the load P when the load is applied to the end of a cantilevered section, as will be illustrated below.

For horizontal (grinding) force P (as shown in Figure 13.22 b), the force, F_i on the ith fixture is given by the equation

$$\mathbf{F}_i = \frac{P}{N}\mathbf{n}_p + \frac{eP}{L^2}R_i\mathbf{n}_i, \quad (13.7)$$

where

$\mathbf{F}_i$ is the vector force.

The load due to the last term in Equation (13.7) acts in the direction of the unit vector $\mathbf{n}_i$, which is defined as the perpendicular directions to the radii R_i of each screw from the origin O. The eccentricity, e, of the load P is defined with respect to the centroid of the fixtures. The denominator L^2 in Eq. (13.7) is defined by

$$L^2 = \Sigma R_i^2 \quad (13.8)$$

where

the summation is over the N fixtures.

The results predicted by Equations (13.1) and (13.8) have not been verified in detail for any experimental or clinical situation. It is likely that actual forces will be different from the theoretical predictions because of the flexibility of the bridge in bending and twisting, as well as the flexibility of the mandible and the different behavior of the bone response around each fixture.

Force Distribution to Fixtures: Flexible Prosthesis

The effect of flexibility of a prosthesis, as compared to a rigid bridge, will generally be to increase the forces in the fixtures nearest to the loading point and to decrease the forces on more distant fixtures. These effects may be tolerable if the individual fixtures are sufficiently strong. In any case, it may be expected that the force on any one fixture, F_i, will be less than the applied force, P, except in the case of forces applied to cantilevered ends.

In the case of horizontal (grinding) forces (see Figure 13.22b), the distribution of forces is aided by the fact that even a comparatively thin bridge structure will be stiff in tension or compression along the tangential direction between any two fixtures. Then the components of force in the tangential direction will be transmitted and shared easily between adjacent fixtures.

A flexible bridge will usually result in significantly different force distribution due to its greater flexibility in bending. The influence of bending stiffness can be thought of as a continuous transition from no bridge at all (zero bending stiffness) to the extreme case of a rigid bridge (infinite bending stiffness). For the case of zero bending stiffness, the force applied to any fixture must be carried by the fixture itself. There is no load sharing, and each fixture acts independently, just as the natural teeth do. In the case of a rigid bridge, there will be a distribution of force applied to the prosthesis according to Equations (13.1–13.8). The results for a flexible bridge will generally lie between the two extremes of zero and infinite bending stiffness.

An exact analysis of stress distribution in a flexible bridge is possible using the theory of curved elastic beams on elastic supports. From a practical standpoint, however, this is not a useful procedure unless the stiffness of the fixtures and the bone in which they are integrated are accurately known. These factors are variable, and there has not been enough testing and measurements to allow accurate, reliable predictions.

Cantilever Action

A greater force can be applied to the fixture nearest to the cantilevered end when the bite (or grinding) force is located at the end of a cantilever. This can be readily understood in terms of the simple cantilevered bridge shown in Figure 13.23. In each case, it is assumed that there are supporting fixtures at A and B and that the force F is applied to the cantilevered end C. It is assumed that no bending moment is developed in the fixtures and that they resist only axial (vertical) forces. When the space between AB and BC is equal (see Figure 13.23a) the force exerted on the fixture at B is three times the bite force F, and the tension in the fixture at A is two times F. As the length of the cantilever increases, the force on the fixture at B increases; it may reach unacceptable values. The conclusion that may be drawn from these examples is that a cantilever of length up to the spacing of one or two teeth may be tolerated, but more than that is likely to be inimical to long-term stability.

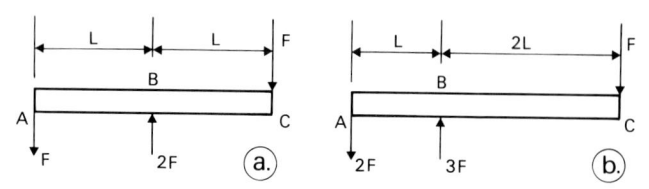

Figure 13.23 (a) Cantilever prosthesis with bite force, F, at cantilever end. Cantilever length, L, results in increased reaction ($2F$) on fixture at B. (b) Cantilever prosthesis with bite force, F, at cantilever end. Extended cantilever ($2L$) results in increased reaction ($3F$) on fixture at B.

The cantilever principles indicated in Figure 13.23 for vertical bite forces also apply to horizontal grinding forces. A long cantilever may cause failure in the fixture nearest to the cantilevered end by applying excessive forces and stresses of the type shown in Figure 13.23b.

Combined Supports: Natural Teeth and Fixtures

The basic consideration to keep in mind in relation to a prosthesis that is to be supported on a combination of natural teeth and osseointegrated fixtures is that a natural tooth has a range of movement made possible under moderate forces by the periodontal ligament but there can be no relative motion between an osseointegrated fixture and the encapsulating bone. In fact, the absence of a soft, fibrous tissue at the interface and the absence of any relative motion of the interface is characteristic of an osseointegrated fixture.

Due to the difference in stiffness of natural teeth and osseointegrated fixtures, there are various possibilities of overloading or underloading either the natural teeth or the fixtures. The clearest case is that of a stiff bridge spanning two fixtures between which there is a natural tooth, also connected to the bridge. In this situation, the natural tooth may be underloaded because the rigid bridge and stiff fixtures pick up the load before there is enough deflection of the bridge to load the natural tooth.

An overloading effect can occur if a bridge spanning two fixtures is extended by a cantilever to a natural tooth. This situation is shown in Figure 13.24, where the fixtures at A and B will be subject to excessive force. Both the underloading and the overloading that may occur can be avoided by the use of flexible prostheses. As mentioned above, flexibility in a bridge tends to increase the portion of the loading that is carried by the nearest support. The use of the appropriate flexibility of the bridge will increase the portion of the load carried by the natural teeth. The exact degree of flexibility required can be calculated by the theory of curved elastic beams on elastic supports. For this purpose, we need to know the stiffness of the fixtures and the natural teeth, although a wide range of bridge stiffness probably will give acceptable flexible performance.

Single Support

The mechanics of an isolated fixture—one not connected to any bridge—is direct and simple in principle: Any bite force that comes onto the fixture must be carried by the fixture itself, as illustrated in Figure 13.20. A rational decision to use an isolated fixture in a specific location in a particular patient could theoretically be made if sufficient data of prior test results were available. First, we need to know the ultimate strength of an isolated implant under axial and transverse loading (see Figure 13.20) and possible combinations of such loadings as a function of the bone cross section and density distribution. Next, we need an estimate of the peak bite, grinding, and accidental forces that are likely to be applied to the fixture. If these peak forces are less than some specified fraction (say, 50%) of the predicted strength, then we may assume that the use of such an isolated implant has a high probability of a long, fully functional, and trouble-free lifetime. At the present time, the test data and methods of prediction of strength in specific clinical situations are not sufficiently developed to allow such quantitative estimates to be made reliably. However, clinical experience is being accumulated using single fixtures to replace missing teeth with sufficient success that it can be said to be a practical, useful procedure in clinically favorable cases. Evidence to date must be regarded as incomplete and anecdotal, but sufficient to be optimistic.

SUMMARY

Osseointegration can provide fixation of prosthetic devices to the craniomaxillofacial human skeleton with long-term functional predictability and without untoward reactions by hard and soft tissue. Functional safety and efficacy have been proven in a large number of clinical studies. Clinical experience from intraoral and extraoral anchorage devices with varying degree of dynamic load demands has demonstrated that this kind of fixation provides, in addition to mechanical stability, adequate load-remodeling stimulus to the anchoring and surrounding bone tissue.

The character and composition of the interface, including titanium, titanium oxide, and the ground substance of bone tissue (possibly with a gradient of mineralization) have been analyzed in basic biologic, materials, and biomechanical tests.

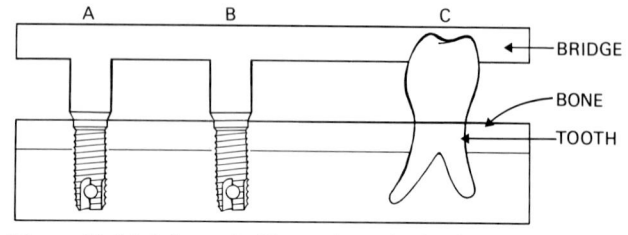

Figure 13.24 Schematic illustration of a bridge supported partially on fixtures and partially on natural tooth.

BIBLIOGRAPHY

Adell R, Eriksson B, Lekholm U, Brånemark P-I, Jemt T: A long-term follow-up study of osseointegrated implants in the treatment of the totally edentulous jaw. Int J Oral Maxillofac Impl 5:347–359 (1990).

Adell R, Lekholm U, Rockler, Brånemark P-I: A fifteen-year study of osseointegrated implants in the treatment of the edentulous jaw. Int J Oral Maxillofac Surg 10:387–416, 1981.

Albrektsson T, Albrektsson B: Implant fixation by direct bone anchorage, In Non-Cemented Total Hip Arthoplasty. Fitzgerald RH Jr (editor). New York, Raven Press, 1988.

Brånemark P-I, Breine U, Adell R, Hansson BO, Lindström J, Ohlsson Å: Intra-osseous anchorage of dental prostheses. I. Experimental studies. Scand J Plast Reconstr Surg 3: 81–100, 1969.

Brånemark P-I, Zarb G, Albrektsson T (eds.): Tissue-integrated prostheses—osseointegration in clinical dentistry. Chicago: Quintessence, 1985, Chapters 1, 11–76

Brånemark P-I: Tissue-integrated prostheses in oral and maxillofacial reconstruction. In Head and Neck Oncology Clinical Management, Kagan AR and Miles J (eds.). 121–141, 1989.

Brånemark P-I, Hansson BO, Adell R, Breine U, Lindström J, Öhman A: Osseointegrated implants in the treatment of the edentulous jaw. Experience from a 10-year period. Scand J Plast Reconstr Surg [Suppl] 11: 16, 1977.

Brunski JB: The influence of force, motion, and related quantities on the response of bone to implants. In Non-Cemented Total Hip Arthoplasty. R. Fitzgerald (ed). New York, Raven Press, 1988, 7–21.

Haraldsson T, Carlsson GE: Bite force and oral function in patients with osseointegrated oral implants. Scand J Dent Res 85: 200, 1977.

Hipp JA, Brunski JB, Shepard MS, Cochran GVB: Finite element models for implants in bone: Interfacial assumptions. In Biomechanics: Current Interdisciplinary Research. Perren SM, Schneider E (eds). Dordrecht, Martinus Nijhoff, 1985, 447 ff.

Kasemo BJ, Lausmaa J: Metal selection and surface characteristics. Reprinted from: "Tissue Integrated Prostheses—Osseointegration in Clinical Dentistry. Brånemark, Zarb, Albrektsson (eds.) Chicago: Quintessence, (1985).

Skalak R: Biomechanical considerations in osseointegrated prostheses. J Prosth Dent 49:843, 1983.

Skalak R: Aspects of biomechanical consideration. In Osseointegration in Clinical Dentistry, Brånemark P-I, Zarb G, Albrektsson T (eds). Chicago, Quintessence, 1985, 117.

Skalak R: Stress transfer at the implant interface. J Oral Implantology 4, 1988.

Steinemann SG, Eulenberger J, Maeusli PA, Schreoder A: Adhesion of bone to titanium. Adv Biomater 6:409, 1986.

Tjellström A: Osseointegrated systems and their applications in the head and neck. In Advances in Otolaryngology, 1989. In press.

PART III

Clinical Applications

Trauma

CHAPTER 14

Rigid Internal Fixation of Mandibular Fractures

Michael J. Yaremchuk
Paul N. Manson

The basic principles and concepts of rigid fixation as applied to the maxillofacial skeleton were presented in Part I. The indications, specifications, and nuances of the most commonly used maxillofacial plate and screw systems have been presented in Part II. In Part III, the clinical applications of these systems in the treatment of maxillofacial injuries are presented. The purpose of this chapter is to provide an overview for the treatment of mandibular fractures with rigid internal fixation using bicortical plate and screw systems.

INDICATIONS FOR RIGID INTERNAL FIXATION

The fundamental goal of mandibular fracture therapy is to restore the pre-injury anatomy. In so doing, the surgeon restores the pre-injury occlusion and facial aesthetics. The mode of therapy is determined by the nature of the mandibular injury in the context of the overall situation of the patient.

Plate and screw fixation techniques provide unparalleled stability when compared to other modes of fracture therapy. This stability may allow healing in complex situations where the time to bone union would otherwise be prolonged or complicated. For these reasons, multiple fractures; fractures with comminution, segmentation, defects, extensive displacement subject to rotation; and displaced fractures of the edentulous mandible are best treated with rigid fixation techniques.

In most cases, the stability inherent in plate and screw fixation makes postoperative MMF unnecessary or minimal. This avoids the morbidity associated with jaw immobilization necessary with other forms of fracture treatment. For this reason, simple fractures in patients with head injuries, cervical spine injuries, seizure disorders, and multiple systems injuries, as well as unstable midface fractures may be best treated with rigid fixation. The use of rigid fixation can avoid the need for tracheostomy in most of these patients. In certain patients with isolated simple mandibular fractures, the morbidity associated with the surgery necessary for rigid fixation is far outweighed by the shortened convalescence period and concomitant earlier return to pre-injury lifestyle. Finally, treatment with rigid fixation techniques makes postoperative compliance less critical and, for that reason, serves certain patient groups most effectively.

BASIC CONCEPTS

Mandibular plate and screw implant systems are designed and implanted to withstand and overcome any biomechanical deforming forces that may arise, thereby avoiding micromotion of the bone ends. This clinical concept of absolute immobilization of bone ends and of the implant and bone, within limits of physiologic loading, has been given the term *absolute stability*. Under conditions of absolute stability and perfect fracture reduction, the condition of primary bone healing will occur; that is, new bone will form along the surface of the fracture without intervening fibrous tissue. Furthermore, when the situation of absolute stability exists, vascularized bone ends may heal even in the presence of bacterial contamination. Most important, this stability allows immediate mobilization of the mandible and therefore frees the patient from postoperative MMF with its concomitant morbidity.

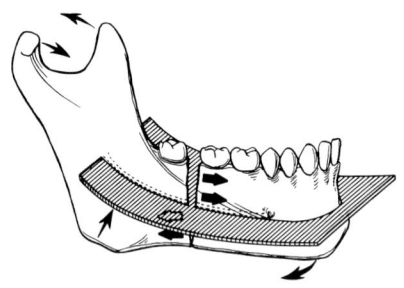

Figure 14.1 The muscular forces acting on the mandible produce pressure forces along the basilar border and tension forces along the alveolar border. Conceptually, the course of the inferior alveolar nerve forms an arbitrary boundary between these two zones. With a body fracture, these forces tend to distract the fracture at the tension side, creating a gap.

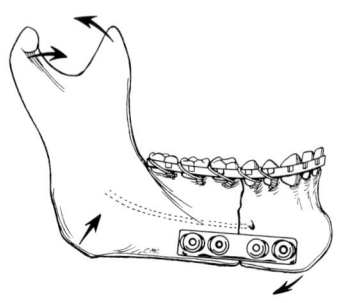

Figure 14.2 The positions of the inferior alveolar nerve canal and the tooth roots preclude placement of a bicortical plate above the inferior alveolar nerve. Therefore, these plates must be placed along the basilar border. Placement of these plates alone may cause a gap along the alveolar border due to the unbalanced tension forces. These are counteracted with a tension band. In tooth-bearing areas of the mandible, an arch bar can function as a tension band.

The bony architecture, shape, and muscular attachments of the mandible permit it to be conceptualized as a structure that converts imposed stresses into either tension or compression. Compressive forces are generated along the basal aspect; tension forces are generated along the alveolar process. An imaginary transverse axis that lies approximately along the mandibular canal separates the area of tension (alveolar process) from the area of compression (basal border). When the mandible is fractured, forces on both sides of this imaginary axis must be neutralized to achieve a functionally stable reduction (see Figure 14.1). From the standpoint of biomechanics, placement of a plate along the tension trajectory would provide the most stable fixation. However, the tooth apices and the inferior alveolar nerve restrict placement of a plate to the basal border. Neutralization of tension and pressure forces therefore is accomplished by a plate and tension band system whose individual nuances are determined by the location and type of fracture. In general, the pressure trajectory of the mandible is restored with a plate and the tension trajectory with a tension band. In dentulous portions of the mandible, an arch bar is sufficient to neutralize tension forces (see Figure 14.2), whereas in the angle and ramus area a small plate may perform this function (see Figure 14.3).

When the plate and tension band principle is used for fixation of a mandibular fracture, plates designed to provide interfragmental compression are used. In the design of implant systems, compression is sought for its ability to produce large frictional forces. These forces prevent motion between bone and the implant which would otherwise lead to implant loosening and bone resorption. The dynamic compression plate generates interfragmentary compression by the spherical gliding principle, causing the screw to move both vertically and horizontally along the plate. It is the horizontal movement that compresses the fracture segments (see Figure 14.4).

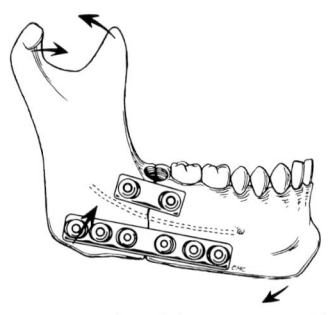

Figure 14.3 The tension band function outside of tooth-bearing portions of the mandible can be furnished by a small plate—in this case, a specially designed two-hole plate. A four-hole miniplate may also serve this function.

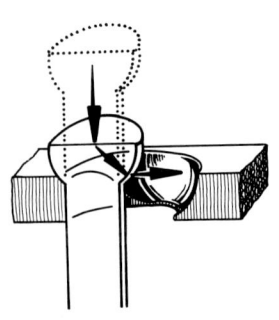

Figure 14.4 The spherical gliding principle involves a spherically shaped screwhead that slides down an inclined plane as it is tightened. The bone grasped by the screw tip moves horizontally with the screw. This is the fundamental component of the dynamic compression plate which allows bone to be compressed across the fracture site by the screw movement.

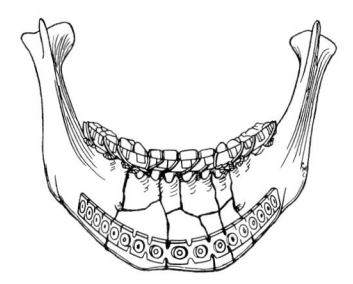

Figure 14.5 The reconstruction plate is a plate of large scale, and thus it is of sufficient strength to avoid the need for a tension band on the lingual side. When a reconstruction plate is used for extremely unstable fractures or those with bone loss, four screws should purchase stable bone on both sides of the fracture.

The lag screw concept, extensively discussed in Chapters 2 and 4, uses the principle that a screw that glides through the cortex of one fragment and engages the cortex of the opposite fragment will compress these surfaces when the screw is tightened. Lag screws may be used alone or in combination with plates and screws in mandibular fracture therapy.

The reconstruction plate is a larger, reinforced version of the basal stabilization plate; it is therefore strong enough to be used without a tension band. It is malleable and can be adapted to local bony contours. In most situations, the reconstruction plate is used as an internal surgical splint. The reconstruction plate is designed to buttress fragments against displacement while absorbing all functional loads. Reconstruction plates are used for fractures with comminution or bone loss, where interfragmental compression is not a workable principle (see Figure 14.5). The three-dimensional malleability of reconstruction plates makes them useful for certain angle fractures when curved plates are not available or are not applicable.

OPERATIVE SEQUENCE

Plate and screw fixation of mandibular fractures requires understanding of the concepts of rigid fixation and proper use of the fixation system. Because the commercially available plate and screw systems are so well designed, avoidable complications are most often a function of operator error. Because these systems are unyielding, the occlusion obtained at the end of operation is permanent. Unlike less rigid fixation systems, small discrepancies in occlusion cannot be corrected with postoperative traction and therefore leave little margin for error in fracture reduction and fixation. The preferred operative sequence for the rigid fixation of mandibular fractures is outlined below.

Upper Border Alignment: Restoring Occlusion

Arch Bars

Arch bars or their equivalent are fastened to the maxillary and mandibular dentition. Arch bars are necessary for the placement of MMF and, in most cases, to function as a tension band splint.

Maxillo-Mandibular Fixation

The pre-injury occlusion is restored and MMF established. This requires study of wear facets, especially when the pre-injury occlusion is abnormal. In complicated mandibular injuries, and particularly when sagittal fractures of the upper face are present, dental models and the use of intraoperative splints may be necessary to best determine the pre-injury status. If gaps exist in the occlusion, a splint will prevent segment overriding and collapse of the vertical space for the missing teeth. The condyles must be seated in the glenoid fossa after application of the MMF (as well as after plating of the maxilla and mandible).

Alignment of the Lower Border

Incision and Exposure

Fractures may be exposed through intraoral incisions, extraoral incisions, or the extension of pre-existing external lacerations. Although it avoids damage to the marginal mandibular branch of the facial nerve and scarring of the face, the intraoral approach significantly limits exposure. However, with considerable expertise and refinement in technique, the surgeon can treat most simple fractures through an intraoral approach. In the anterior mandible, the intraoral approach is relatively straightforward provided that the tooth roots and inferior alveolar nerve are avoided. Plate and screw fixation of the ramus, angle, and posterior body requires considerable expertise and the use of transbuccal instrumentation when approached via the mouth. In general, external incisions improve exposure and hence, the ability to understand and reduce the fracture, as well as to adapt the plate and fixate it to the mandible. For these reasons, it is suggested that the surgeon use an external approach until becoming well acquainted with rigid fixation techniques. Submental incisions are used to expose the central aspect of the mandible; Risdon or modified Risdon incisions are used to expose the posterior body, angle and ramus. Subcondylar fractures can be approached intraorally (see Chapter 17) but in most cases will require an external approach. Extension of the coronal incision, which affords excellent exposure of the condylar area, should be considered when upper facial injuries warrant its use.

Segmental fractures, comminuted fractures, and those with bone loss require external incisions to provide sufficient exposure for adequate reduction and fixation. The edentulous mandible should be exposed extraorally to minimize the amount of periosteal stripping and subsequent devascularization of this already compromised bone.

Fracture Reduction

Fracture ends are cleansed of debris (clot, soft tissue) and the fracture segments are reduced. This often requires temporary fixation with intraosseous wires, towel clips, miniplates, or compression forceps.

Plate Selection

General Rules

Plates and screws provide rigid fixation only if the strength of this fixation is greater than the functional forces acting on the mandible. Rigidity of fixation is determined by the strength of the plate, its length (number of screws), compression of the fixation, and the number of plates used.

Only bicortical compression and mandibular reconstruction plates have been designed to counteract the strong forces acting on the mandible. Miniplates may have an adjunctive role in certain fractures (for example, acting as a tension band at the upper border, temporary fixation), but they provide inadequate stability when used only on the pressure side of the mandible (see Chapter 18).

In order to control rotation and ensure adequate stability, a minimum of two screws on either side of the fracture, purchasing both anterior and posterior cortices, is required. If only two screws are engaged on each side of the fracture, compression is usually required across the fracture site to counteract functional forces. (As insurance for possible loosening of screws, three screws are used on each side of the fracture if their placement is relatively straightforward.)

When fractures are more complicated—with obliquity or sagittal splitting—a longer plate is necessary. Longer plates allow screws to be placed far enough from the fracture site to assure bicortical purchase and to increase the lever arm and mechanical advantage across the fracture site.

Fractures with segmentation or comminution should be treated with plates long enough to have three screws placed on either side of the fracture in case one screw should inadvertently loosen (this is the three-hole principle of Spiessl). With severely comminuted fractures or fractures with bone loss, a minimum of four screws is necessary (four-hole principle). For the horizontal portion of the mandible, when the fracture is treated with a bicortical compression plate, it should be placed at the lower border, and a tension band should be placed along the upper border.

Selection by Fracture Type and Location

The length and type of plate will be determined by the pattern and location of the fracture. Single fractures may have a transverse, oblique, or sagittal orientation. Multiple fractures may be comminuted or consist of a series of single fractures in one half (segmental fractures) or both halves (bilateral single) of the mandible, or they may be combinations thereof. Defect fractures are those with bone missing.

Single Fractures

Transverse Fractures In general, single transverse fractures in tooth-bearing segments are treated with dynamic compression plates placed at the basilar border in combination with a tension band placed at the occlusal border. Within the dental arch, tension banding is usually accomplished with an arch bar. Fractures in the angle region are also treated with a dynamic compression plate and a tension band plate. The tension band plate is a specially designed two hole plate in the AO system, or a miniplate may be used. A curved dynamic compression plate (Luhr system) or a pre-bent reconstruction plate (AO system) is preferred over the use of straight plates in the angle region. Straight plates of adequate length are difficult to position in this area. When plates are placed too low, they may protrude beyond the inferior border; when plates are placed too high, subsequent nerve damage is possible (see Figure 14.6).

In addition to problems with plate adaptation and positioning, fractures in the angle region are often complicated by the presence of a third molar. The erupted or nonerupted third molar is left intact if it is not involved in the fracture line. The erupted third molar is removed if the apex is exposed or if the root is fractured. Similarly, in other dentulous portions of the mandible, teeth in the line of fracture are preserved if they have secure attachments.

The eccentric dynamic compression plate (EDCP) can be used in place of the tension band in the edentulous jaw or in dentulous portions of the jaw where it is not desirable to use an upper-border tension band plate. This plate produces compression in two dimensions: The inner holes beveled horizontally compress the fracture at the inferior border; the outer, oblique holes tend to close the gap at the alveolar border (see Figure 14.7).

In the angle area, percutaneous fixation of a lag screw is possible for transverse fractures extending across the oblique line, retromolar fossa, and the vestibular and lingual expansion of the mandible. This is discussed

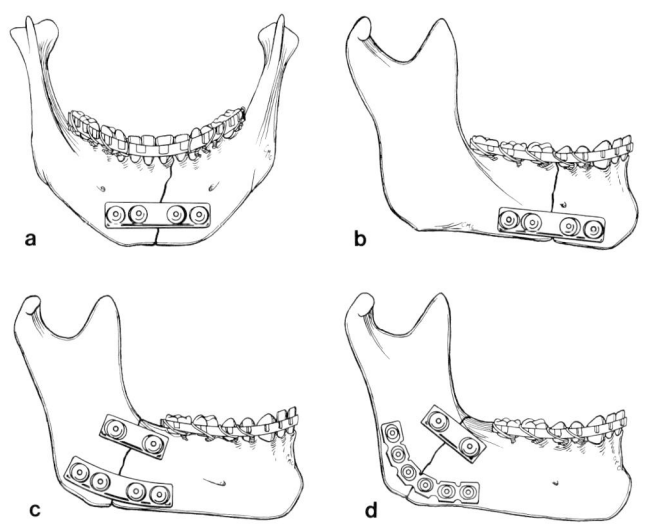

Figure 14.6 Simple transverse fractures of the horizontal portion of the mandible are usually treated by dynamic compression plates used together with a tension band. (a) A transverse fracture of the symphysis treated with a four-hole dynamic compression plate and an arch bar used as a tension band splint. (b) A simple transverse fracture of the body of the mandible treated with a straight dynamic compression plate and an arch bar used as a tension band splint. (c) A transverse fracture of the angle of the mandible treated with a curved dynamic compression plate and a miniplate used as a tension band splint. (d) A transverse fracture of the angle of the mandible treated with a six-hole reconstruction plate and a two-hole dynamic compression plate used as a tension band. Straight plates are usually avoided in the angle area.

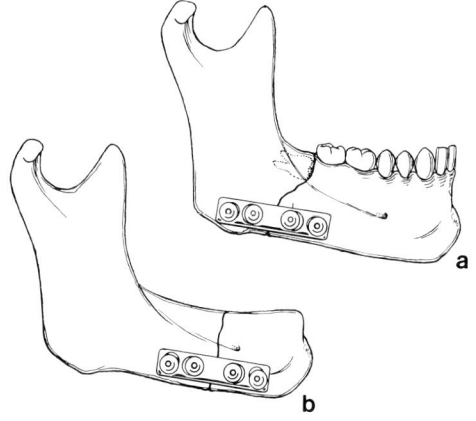

Figure 14.7 An eccentric dynamic compression plate (EDCP) may have application in certain situations. (a) The impacted molar precludes use of a tension band plate along the alveolar border, making this an ideal situation for the EDCP. (b) This transverse body fracture in the edentulous mandible is treated with an EDCP. If there is sufficient room above the inferior alveolar nerve, a tension band plate together with a standard dynamic compression plate would be adequate alternative therapy.

in Chapter 15. Transverse fractures of the ramus are the classic indication for a single plate placed at the tension side of the mandible.

With rare exception or unless associated with other local fractures, coronoid fractures are not treated. When indications for open reduction and internal fixation of subcondylar fractures exist, size limitations dictate they be treated with miniplates (see Chapter 17).

Oblique Fractures Oblique fractures are treated in the same manner as described for transverse fractures, with the exception that longer plates are necessary to assure bicortical purchase of at least two screws on each side of the fracture (see Figure 14.8).

Sagittal Fractures Sagittal fractures are shear fractures whose surfaces are oriented longitudinally to the bone axis. This results in a large surface area along the fracture line, which is the ideal situation for the use of lag screws. In general, three lag screws are sufficient to provide functional stability in all directions without a tension band. If space limitations preclude the placement of three screws, a neutralization plate may be used to protect the key lag screw (see Figure 14.9).

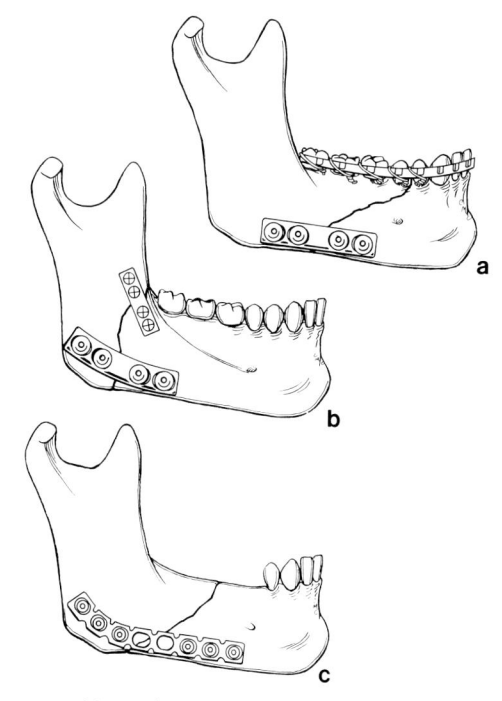

Figure 14.8 Oblique fractures require the use of longer plates to assure bicortical purchase of at least two screws on each side of the fracture. (a) Oblique fracture of mandibular body treated with long dynamic compression plate and arch bar used as a tension band splint. (b) Oblique fracture of the angle treated with a long curved plate and a miniplate used as a tension band plate. (c) Oblique fracture of the edentulous body of the mandible treated with a long reconstruction plate.

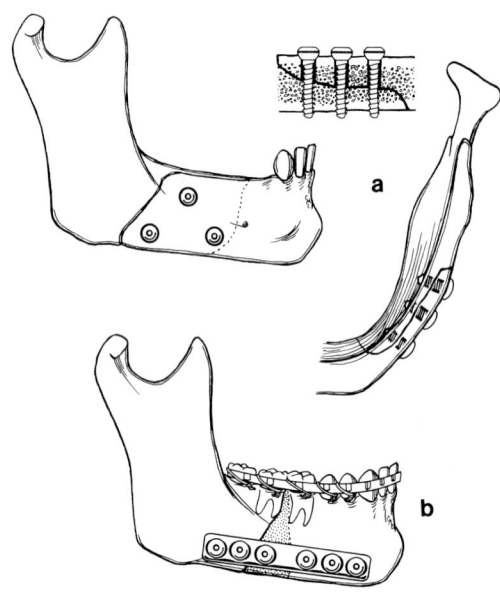

Figure 14.9 Sagittal fractures are ideally suited to the use of lag screws. (a) Sagittal fracture of the edentulous mandibular body treated with three screws. The cross section shows placement of lag screws. (b) Sagittal fracture of the body of the dentulous mandible. Tooth roots and inferior alveolar nerve preclude placement of more than one lag screw. This lag screw is protected by a long neutralization plate. The arch bar acts as a tension band.

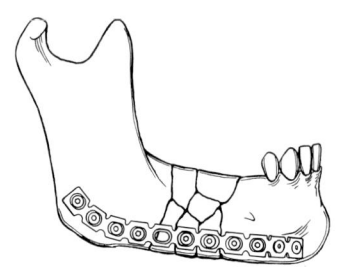

Figure 14.10 Reconstruction plates used to treat a comminuted fracture of the mandibular body. Large free segments are fixed to the plate. Note four-hole purchase on each major portion of the intact mandible.

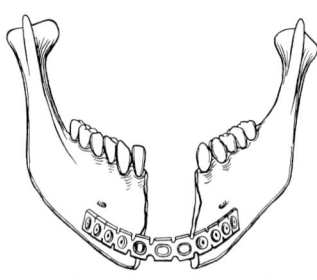

Figure 14.11 Defect fracture treated with a long reconstruction plate. Note four-hole fixation on each side of the defect.

Multiple Fractures

Multiple fractures usually arise in common patterns (see Chapter 16). In general, single fractures on each side of the mandible are treated as separate entities in terms of plate selection. However, reduction of all fractures is carried out before any fixation is applied.

Segmental Fractures Segmental fractures are two successive fractures occurring in the hemimandible. Such fractures cause an unstable intermediate segment. Restoration of the occlusion is particularly difficult and important in reduction of these fractures. The size of the intermediate fragment will determine whether it will be stabilized by a separate plate at each fracture line or included in a single neutralization plate. When a segmental fracture is associated with fractures in the other hemimandible, the mandible is particularly unstable. In general, the more stable fractures should be fixated first and used as a point of reference.

Comminuted Fractures A comminuted fracture may be thought of as a segmental fracture in which the large segment is further broken into smaller pieces. These fractures are usually managed by a combination of techniques that may include the use of lag screws, miniplates, and reconstructive plates (see Figure 14.10).

Defect Fractures

Bone loss may occur with open, very high energy fractures or missile injuries. These fractures are invariably associated with adjacent comminution. These injuries usually require reconstruction plates to bridge the defect. In general, four screws are attached to the main mandibular segments in these very unstable fractures (four-screw rule) (see Figure 14.11).

Plate Adaptation

The plate must be precisely contoured so that it passively adapts to the contour of the lower border of the mandible. A soft template may be used to guide adaptation of the plate. Plate-bending forceps and irons are used for plate contouring. The plate is positioned so that the inner holes are placed as far as possible from the fracture site to avoid extending the fracture while these holes are drilled and to assure bicortical screw purchase.

After the plate is passively adapted, it is slightly "overbent" (1 to 2 mm) to create a gap between the undersurface of the plate and the convex surface of the mandible and to assure maintenance of lingual reduction. This assures compression along the entire surface of the fracture site (see Figure 14.12). One should al-

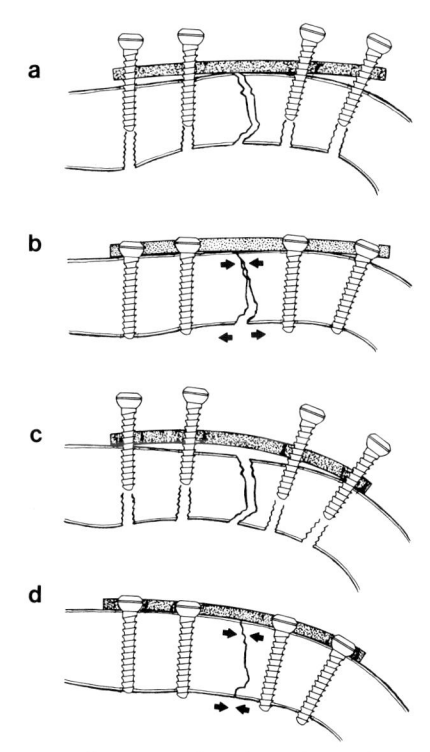

Figure 14.12 Plates must be adapted exactly to the contour of the mandible after fracture reduction. Failure of adequate plate reduction will result in distraction of the fracture segments. In addition to precise contouring, it is necessary to overbend the plate approximately 1 millimeter. The overbent plate will assure compression along the lingual surface of the fracture. (a) Plate with inadequate contour about to be applied to a fractured mandible. (b) Inadequate contouring and failure to overbend at the fracture site results in gapping at the lingual side. (c) Properly contoured plate overbent at the fracture site about to be applied. (d) Stabilization of properly contoured and overbent plate results in reduction along the entire surface of the fracture.

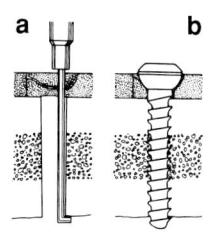

Figure 14.13 Screw length is measured to assure bicortical purchase of all screws. (a) Depth is measured after the hole is drilled and before it is tapped. (b) Screws protrude at least 1 millimeter beyond the distal cortex.

ways keep in mind that the shape of the plate always determines the position of the bone fragments and never vice versa.

Plate Fixation

Although axial compression of fractures increases stability and, through primary bone healing, may speed fracture healing, one has to be judicious in its use. Compression should be used only when there is good bone-to-bone contact. The inappropriate use of compression—when there is bone loss through comminution, delay in treatment, obliquity, or sagittal splitting—will shift bone segments. The bone segments' malformation will then be translated to the occlusal plane and/or to the condylar head.

When dynamic compression is appropriate, a lateral neutral hole should be drilled first, then a hole in the lateral aspect of a compression hole should be drilled adjacent to the fracture. The further away the lateral hole is drilled, the greater will be the amount of compression obtainable. The screw in the dynamic compression hole is then tightened. Drilling both compression holes first will maximize the amount of movement of fragments when the screw is tightened. When EDCP plates are placed, the innermost holes should be drilled first. This provides interfragmentary compression at the basilar border. Next, the most lateral oblique holes should be drilled. This provides compression at the lingual border. The remaining neutral holes should then be drilled.

To optimize the bone–screw interface, careful drilling is important. All drilling should be done under low speed (less than 1000 revolutions per minute), under irrigation, and using a sharp bit to avoid thermal damage to the bone. The hole is placed perpendicular to bone and plate and must purchase both cortices. The drill holes mimic the core diameter of the screw and are placed through both cortices using soft-tissue protection.

The depth gauge is used to measure the hole for screw length. Because the screw should protrude just beyond the posterior cortex to optimize purchase, a screw 1 to 2 mm longer than the depth measured should be employed (see Figure 14.13). With pretapped systems, tapping should be done after depth measurement to avoid thread damage, which is possible during depth measurement. When a defective thread hole does not allow good purchase of the screw, an emergency screw whose core diameter is the next size greater can be used to gain purchase by cutting through the stripped hole. For example, in the AO system a 3.2 millimeters cancellous screw is used if the hole does not allow purchase of the 2.7-millimeter screw.

When fixation is complete, MMF is released and the mandible is ranged. Occlusion and condylar position are checked. If the occlusion is incorrect, fixation must be removed and the procedure repeated. Because plate and screw osteosynthesis is unforgiving, occlusal discrepancies cannot be tolerated. Elastic traction will not improve the bone position and occlusion, as is possible with wire osteosynthesis.

Conceptually, MMF is not necessary after plate and screw osteosynthesis. However, when there is significant edema or joint damage, MMF may aid in patient comfort during the early postoperative period by providing occlusal equilibration. When the lower arch bar acts as a tension band splint, it should be left in place for three to four weeks. A liquid and then a soft diet is employed for the first two to three weeks. It may be necessary for a longer period, depending on the nature of the injury and the condition of the intraoral soft tissues.

Both titanium and Vitallium are quite compatible with tissue and theoretically can be left in indefinitely. Local irritation and cold intolerance are not infrequent indications for implant removal. The ASIF recommends that mandibular plates be removed when mandibular healing and remodeling are complete. Histologic analysis has shown healing to occur by six months in uncomplicated situations. Removal one year after fixation therefore should be safe.

Open Fractures

Open fractures are those that expose the fracture to the intraoral or external environment. Definitive plate and screw stabilization of open fractures should be performed within six to eight hours of the accident, if possible. If definitive surgical therapy is not possible within that time, internal and external wounds should be cleansed, the soft tissues should be closed, and the wound should be splinted by the placement of MMF until surgery can be performed.

Antibiotics

Antibiotics are administered when intraoral or extraoral open reductions are performed. They are administered preoperatively and for 48 to 72 hours postoperatively. As shown by the data of Luhr (1982), Spiessl (1976), and others, the rigid fixation of both open and closed mandibular fractures does not increase the incidence of infectious complications (and probably reduces it) when performed correctly. The incidence of infection is influenced by the severity of the fracture, the stability of fixation, and the condition of the soft tissues. Established infection should be drained, and purulent collections should be evacuated. Extraoral drainage may be necessary if a process is extensive or penetrates into the soft tissues of the neck. Devitalized bone fragments should be removed in this setting. However, if the fixation is rigid, it is not necessary to remove the internal hardware (see Chapter 19).

SUMMARY

The plate and screw fixation of mandibular fractures demands understanding of the biomechanical principles involved, precise anatomic reduction, and appropriate use of the implant systems. By fulfilling these requisites, restoration of the pre-injury anatomy with a minimum of postoperative morbidity is possible, even in the most difficult injury situations.

BIBLIOGRAPHY

Ardary WS: Plate and screw fixation in the management of mandible fractures. Clin Plast Surg 16:61, 1989.

Kahnberg KE: Extraction of teeth involved in the line of mandibular fractures. I. Indications for extraction based on a follow-up study of 185 mandibular fractures. Swed Dent J 3:27, 1979.

Klotch DW, Bilger JR: Plate fixation for open mandibular fractures. Laryngoscope 95: 1374, 1985.

Klotch D: Use of rigid internal fixation in the repair of complex and comminuted mandible fractures. Otolaryngol Clin 20:495, 1987.

Kruger E, Schilli W (eds): Oral and Maxillofacial Traumatology. Chicago, Quintessence Publishers, 1982.

Luhr HG: Compression plate osteosynthesis through the Luhr System. In Oral and Maxillofacial Traumatology, E Kruger, W Schilli (eds). Vol 1, p 319, Quintessence, Chicago, 1982.

Muller ME, Allgower M, Schneider R, Willenegger H: Manual of Internal Fixation. 1st and 2nd ed. Springer, Berlin, Heidelberg, New York, 1970, 1979.

Neiderdellman H, Schilli W, Duker J, Akuamoa-Boateng E: Osteosynthesis of mandibular fractures using lag screws. Int J Oral Surg 5:117, 1976.

Nishioka GJ, Van Sickels JE: Transoral plating of mandibular angle fractures: A technique. Oral Surg 66:531, 1988.

Prein J, Eschmann A, Spiessl B: Results of follow-up examinations in 81 patients with functionally stable mandibular osteosynthesis. Fortschr Kiefer Gesichtschir 21:304, 1976.

Rahn BA: Theoretical considerations in rigid fixation of facial bones. Clin Plast Surg 16:21, 1989.

Schneider SS, Stern M: Teeth in the line of mandibular fractures. J Oral Surg 29:107, 1971.

Schmoker R, Von Allen G, Tschopp HM: Application of functionally stable fixation in maxillofacial surgery according to the ASIF principles. J Oral Maxillofac Surg 40:457, 1982.

Schmoker R: Mandibular reconstruction using a special plate. J Maxillofacial Surg 11:99, 1983.

Spiessl B: New Concepts in Maxillofacial Bone Surgery. Springer, Berlin, 1976.

Spiessl B: Internal Fixation of the Mandible. Springer, Berlin, 1989.

CHAPTER 15

Lag Screws in Mandibular Fractures

Herbert Niederdellmann
Vivek Shetty

Of the various surgical options for the management of mandibular fractures, lag screw fixation is probably the most sensitive to technique and yet the most elegant method of achieving rigid internal fixation. This technique permits no latitude for operator error, so the surgeon performing lag screw osteosynthesis in the mandible must be conversant with the biomechanics of the mandible and the principles of lag screw osteosynthesis. Incorrect technique or failure to adhere to the sequential steps of the lag screw procedure tend to have a domino effect that manifests clinically as displacement of the fragments and concomitant malocclusion. This will adversely affect clinical outcome because restoration of premorbid occlusion is one of the hallmarks of accurate reduction and fixation of mandibular fractures. Used for the proper indications and correctly applied, lag screws ensure rigid immobilization of the fragments under functional loading of the mandible. They meet the major requirement of rigid internal fixation—namely, maximum stability achieved with a minimum of implant material. The high coefficient of fixation afforded by lag screws makes this technique a viable alternative to compression bone plates; and as such, the use of lag screws should be considered for every patient with facial fractures.

As enunciated in Chapter 4, the primary application for lag screws is in the management of mandibular fractures, where the anatomic conditions are more favorable than they are for midfacial fractures. However, even in the mandible, anatomic and biomechanic constraints restrict the sites available for the application of the lag screws. One of the basic biomechanical tenets of lag screw osteosynthesis is that a minimum of two, and preferably three, lag screws should be applied to overcome the forces of torsion and distraction acting across the fracture line. The absence of teeth renders oblique fractures in edentulous jaws particularly suitable for the application of lag screws. In the case of dentulous mandibles, the position of the roots of the teeth as well as of the mandibular nerve canal limit the area available for the application of the lag screws. This is especially true for fractures with minimal overlap of the fracture surfaces. Such limitations underscore the need for careful case selection for lag screw fixation and necessitate judicious placement of the lag screws across the fracture line. Indeed, a recognition of the biomechanical events taking place during functional loading of the mandible plays a significant role in the reduction of mandibular fractures with lag screws. This entails placing the lag screws at such sites and in a configuration that effectively neutralizes the tensile and torsional forces while creating dynamic compression between the fractured fragments; thereby resulting in a functionally stable mandible.

When one keeps in mind the potential for iatrogenic damage of poorly applied lag screws, the need to plan any lag screws reduction meticulously cannot be overemphasized. Careful study of preoperative radiographs will often allow the operator to determine whether lag screws can be used; this determination is substantiated by intraoperative assessment of the fracture site. Customarily, lag screw fixation of fractures in the anterior portion of the mandible can be carried out by a transoral approach, whereas fractures located more proximally are best approached transbuccally. For the transbuccal approach, a trocar is introduced through a stab incision, the detachable trocar point is removed, and a ring-shaped buccal retractor is mounted on the intraoral aspect of the trocar to fix it in place. This transbuccal channel facilitates the passage of instruments for lag screw insertion. A large extraoral incision is seldom necessary, thereby reducing the chances of injury to the facial nerve as well as facial scarring. Facial lacerations, if present, can be used to provide access to the fracture site. The screw holes should always be drilled at low speeds (up to 800 revolutions per minute), and drilling should be accompanied by copious irrigation. Because the holding power of the lag screw is dependent on the quality of bone it engages, any osteolysis at the screw interface induced by heat necrosis would compromise the lag effect.

Lag screws are versatile in their application and can be individualized to a variety of clinical situations. Some common applications of lag screw osteosynthesis in the mandible are described.

SAGITTAL FRACTURES

Lag screws are used primarily for the fixation of oblique fractures of the mandible caused by a shearing of the cortical plates. A more oblique fracture results in a greater area of interfragmentary contact; and, consequently, a superior lag effect is achieved with the cortical screws. Conversely, the minimal overlap of the fractured surfaces encountered in short sagittal fractures precludes placement of an adequate number of lag screws. In such cases the inadequate stability afforded by lag screw fixation, especially against the torsional component, is compensated for by stabilizing such fractures with the addition of a compression plate (see Figure 15.1). Such a plate serves to neutralize the rotational forces acting across the fracture line and increases the structural strength of the bone. The screw that passes through the plate hole overlying the fracture line is inserted in lag fashion, producing interfragmental compression. All remaining screws are inserted in a neutral position, alternating between the two sides of the fracture line. Placing the adjoining screws in an eccentric position would cause dynamic axial compression to develop between the fragments, and the resultant shear

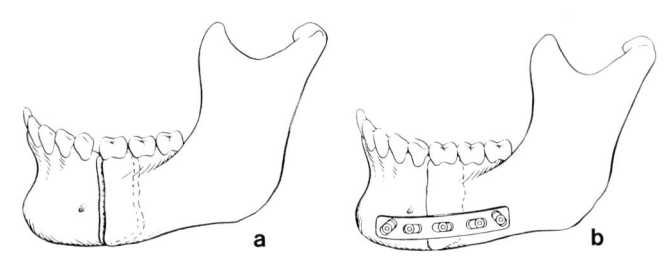

Figure 15.1 Short sagittal fracture reduced by a combination of lag screw and neutralization plate. The screw passing through the plate hole overlying the fracture surfaces is inserted in lag fashion.

stresses generated at the fracture site would dislodge the lag screw. In clinical situations that permit the application of only two lag screws, additional stabilization can be achieved by applying a tension band in the form of a dental splint or arch bar that connects the teeth on either side of the fracture line.

Occasionally, a single lag screw may be used to simplify a transverse fracture in order to facilitate subsequent reduction with a compression plate (see Figure 15.2a and b). Because the fixation afforded by the lag screw is biomechanically inadequate, it has to be buttressed against the torsion forces by a compression plate (see Figure 15.2c). Such neutralization plates are not necessary in the case of wide sagittal fractures because the large interdigitating fracture surfaces resist displacement following lag screw attachment of the fragments. Most wide sagittal fractures of the mandible attain functional rigidity as well as torsional stability following lag fixation with two or three 2.7-millimeters cortical screws (see Figure 15.3). As distraction forces are found predominantly in the tension zone, the initial lag screw is applied in this region in order to neutralize these forces. Basal reduction of the fracture surfaces is carried out around the first lag screw, and the surfaces are fixated by additional lag screws. In wide sagittal fractures, the static compression achieved by well placed lag screws is superior to that achieved by a dynamic compression plate (see Figure 15.4). When a large sagittal fracture is treated exclusively with screws, the bed

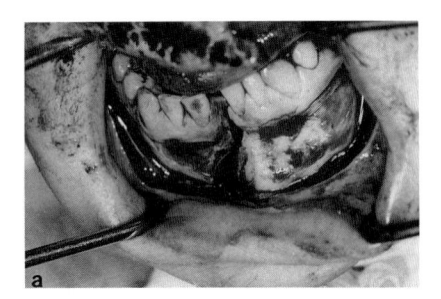

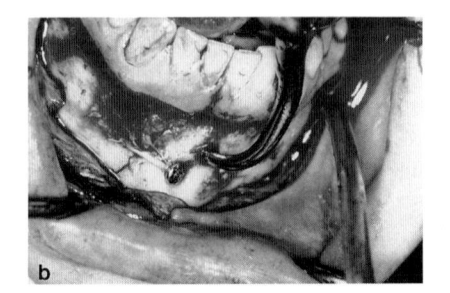

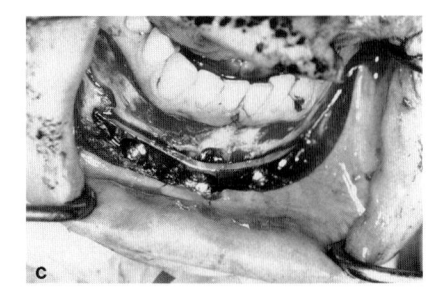

Figure 15.2 (a) Paramedian fracture of the mandible. (b) Fracture reduced with a lag screw. (c) The reduced fracture facilitates adaptation and application of a compression plate that stabilizes and protects the fracture against torsion forces.

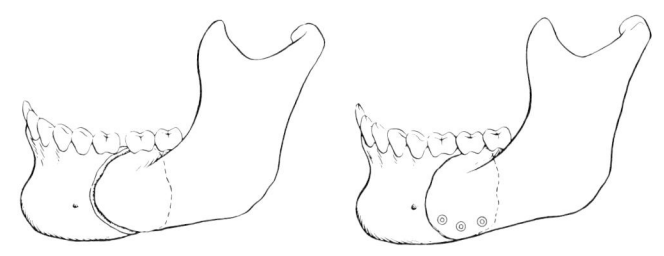

Figure 15.3 Lag screw fixation of a wide sagittal fracture. The functional rigidity and torsional stability are adequate for the biomechanical demands of the mandible.

in the outer cortical bone must be sufficient for the spherical screwhead. Thin portions of the cortical plate should be avoided to prevent fracture of the lateral cortical plate. If the anatomic conditions restrict the area available for application of a lag screw, small washers may be used to prevent the screwhead from sinking into cancellous bone or cracking the thin cortex.

MANDIBULAR ANGLE FRACTURES

The angle is one of the most frequent sites for mandibular fractures. A functionally stable osteosynthesis can be achieved in such fractures with a single lag screw. This is a significant departure from standard lag screw technique, in which two or more lag screws are inserted to prevent the rotational forces acting around a single lag screw. In order to appreciate this departure from the norm, it is necessary to consider the biomechanical factors that influence mandibular angle fractures.

Biomechanics of Angle Fractures

The mandible has a relatively wide lateral extension in the molar region because of the external oblique ridge, one of the buttresses of strength of the mandible. Inasmuch as the body is cantilevered off the ramus, functional loading of the mandible leads to tension forces at the upper border of the mandible and compression forces at the lower border (see Figure 15.5). A break in bone continuity causes the various muscle pulls to come into play; the displacement of bone fragments is influenced by the direction of the angle fracture. The elevator group of muscles—including the masseter, temporalis, medial pterygoids and lateral pterygoids—produces a superior, anterior, and medial displacement of the proximal fragment. Concurrent inferior and medial displacement of the distal fragment is caused by the depressor group, which includes the geniohyoid, genioglossus, mylohyoid, and digastric muscles. This results in distraction forces at the upper border and compression forces at the lower border of the angle fracture. Unlike in the other regions, torsional moments

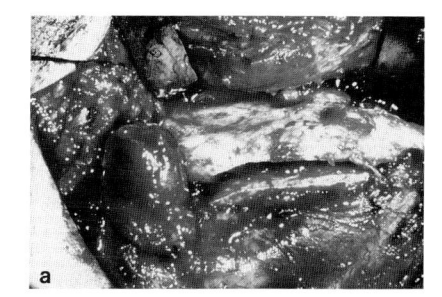

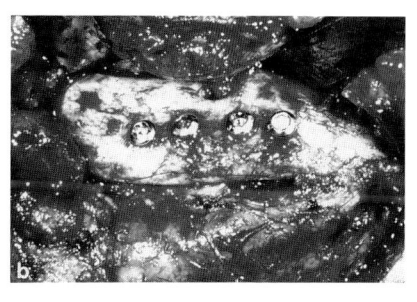

Figure 15.4 (a) A wide sagittal fracture caused by shearing of the cortical plates. (Courtesy of Professor J. Prein, Basel.) (b) Rigid internal fixation achieved by four lag screws. (Courtesy of Professor J. Prein, Basel.)

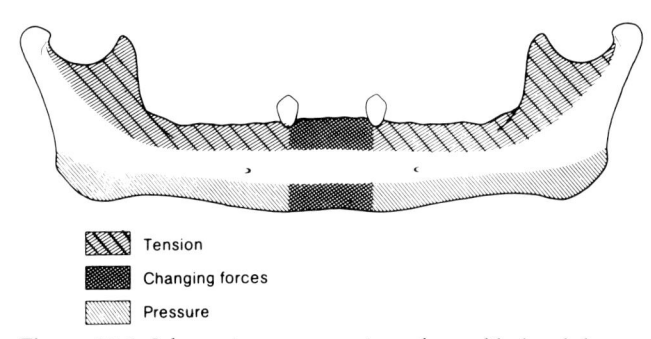

Figure 15.5 Schematic representation of mandibular deformation under functional loading.

are negligible because the angle of the mandible is well buttressed against rotational forces in the plane of the masticatory forces.

The anatomic and biomechanic conditions peculiar to the angle region make it suitable for the application of the tension band principle. Because the torsional component is minimal and the distracting forces are present only at the upper border, dynamic compression can be achieved by simply applying a tension band in this area. A single cortical screw passing through the external oblique ridge in lag fashion produces rigid internal fixation by acting as an internal device for force transfer. It absorbs the tensile forces occurring along the alveolar border and converts them into pressure forces. There is a concomitant reduction in the compressive forces at the lower border of the mandibular angle so that the forces of interfragmental compression are distributed equally across the fracture line. The intermeshing fracture surfaces help augment the stabilization achieved by lag screw fixation.

Operative Technique

The solitary lag screw technique is essentially an intraoral reduction, performed by way of a transbuccal channel (see Figure 15.6). After the fracture line is visualized with an intraoral incision, the premorbid occlusion is restored and the fracture is anatomically coapted. Any interposed soft tissue must be freed from the fracture line to avoid delayed healing or nonunion. Bone-holding clamps and maxillo-mandibular wiring help to immobilize the fragments throughout the procedure, especially in the case of unfavorably oriented fractures.

A cutaneous stab incision is made at the level of the lower border of the mandible in the premolar region. Gentle dissection with blunt scissors creates adequate access for insertion of the transbuccal trocar. Once the transbuccal channel has been established, a drill bit of 2.7-millimeter diameter protected by a drill guide is used to bore a gliding hole in the distal fragment (see Figure 15.7a). Drilling is initiated at the level of the external oblique ridge at sufficient distance from the fracture line. The drill bit is positioned at a very acute angle to the outer cortical bone and in a caudobuccal-craniolingual direction. Because the drill bit tends to slip when introduced at this acute angle, it is advisable to pit the bone surface initially with a small bur to provide purchase for the drill bit and to ensure precise orientation. On completion of the gliding hole, a special

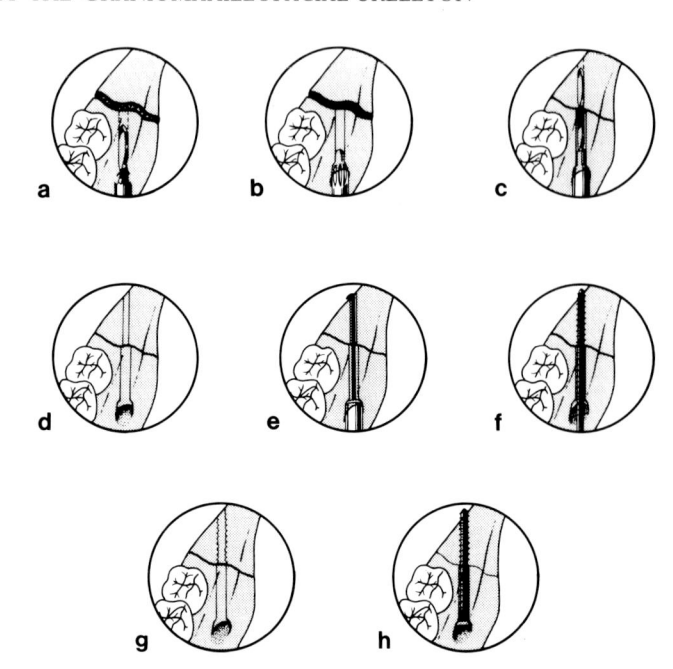

Figure 15.7 Lag screw fixation technique for mandibular angle fractures: (a) drilling the gliding hole (2.7 millimeter) in the distal fragment; (b) preparation of bed for screwhead with a countersink; (c) drilling the thread hole (2.0 millimeter) in the proximal fragment via an insert sleeve; (d) prepared bed, gliding hole, and thread hole; (e) determination of screw length with depth gauge; (f) tapping the thread hole with a 2.7-millimeter tap; (g) prepared fragments; (h) lag screw reduction of the fragments.

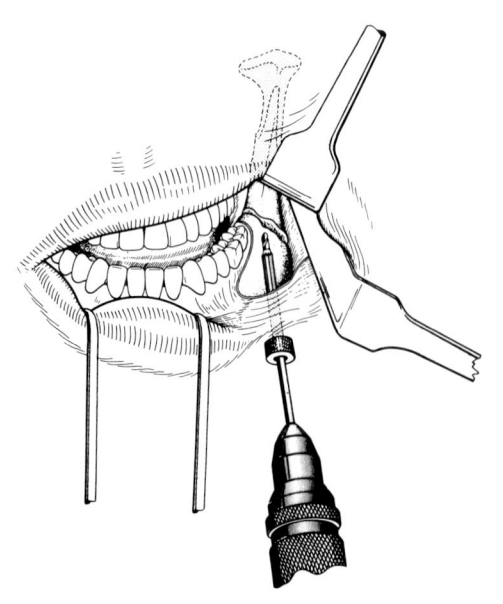

Figure 15.6 The combined intraoral/transbuccal approach. Intraoral use of the instrumentation is carried out via the transbuccal channel.

countersink drill with a centering guide pin is used to create a recess in the outer cortical bone over the gliding hole (see Figure 15.7b). This bony bed corresponds to the spherical undersurface of the screwhead, facilitating equitable distribution of pressure exerted by the screwhead and helping to sink the screwhead flush with the bone surface.

An insert sleeve with 2.7-millimeter outer diameter and 2.0-millimeter inner diameter is now placed in the gliding hole, and a thread hole is drilled into the proximal fragment along the predetermined axis with an extra-long 2.0-millimeter drill bit (see Figure 15.7c and d). The length of the hole for the screw is measured with a depth gauge (see Figure 15.7e); it usually ranges from 30 to 40 mm, depending on the clinical condition. Using the depth gauge before the tap is cut prevents damage to the threads in the proximal fragment. With a sharp 2.7-millimeter tap, the thread hole is tapped (see Figure 15.7f). The proximal and distal fragments must be coapted throughout the procedure to ensure that the gliding hole and the thread hole are coaxial (see Figure 15.7g). Lack of concentricity of the gliding hole and the thread hole would manifest as a disturbed occlusion

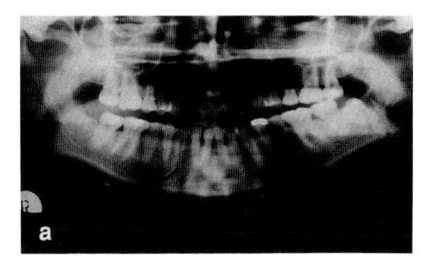

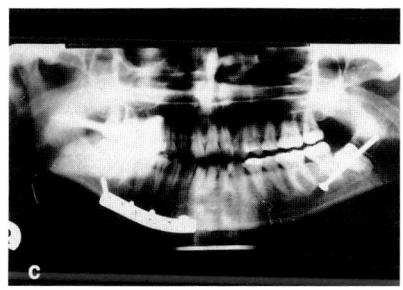

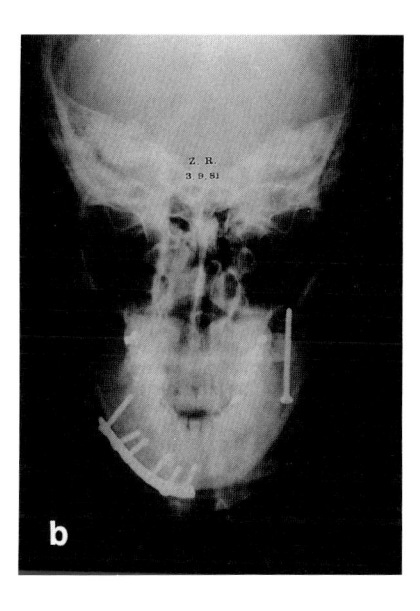

Figure 15.8 (a) Preoperative radiograph of a paramedian fracture associated with an angle fracture. (b) Status following lag screw fixation of the angle fracture and reduction of the concomitant paramedian fracture with a compression plate (PA view). (c) Panorex.

following lag screw reduction. A 2.7-millimeter cortical screw can now slide through the larger gliding hole in the distal fragment and obtain a firm hold in the thread of the proximal fragment. By firmly tightening the screw, the fracture surfaces are stabilized under pressure (see Figure 15.7h). Following insertion of the lag screw and removal of the trocar, the intraoral and the small cutaneous puncture incisions are closed with interrupted sutures. The occlusion is checked again, and MMF is removed.

When correctly placed, the lag screw runs obliquely through the body of the mandible in an anteroposterior direction. It enters the body of the mandible approximately in the region of the first molar at the level of the external oblique ridge and exits medially, anterior to the mandibular foramen. The inferior alveolar nerve always lies medial and inferior to the screw when the technique is carried out correctly, with the screw being inserted inferolateral to craniomedial. As lag effect of the screw depends partly on the length of the thread hole, drilling the screw hole at a very acute angle to the outer cortical plate ensures that the lag screw passes through a greater portion of the proximal fragment and engages a thread hole of adequate length. Concomitant fractures are reduced by lag screws or with an eccentric dynamic compression plate (see Figure 15.8a–c). Bilateral fractures of the mandibular angle can be reduced with one lag screw on either side (see Figure 15.9a–c); MMF is recommended for a week in such cases. Unerupted or impacted wisdom teeth constitute a structural weakness in the mandible and are often involved in the fracture line. If these teeth show no signs of severe loosening or inflammation, they should be left untouched in order to achieve as large a repositioning surface as possible and to maximize the tension band effect. Though the impacted molars are occasionally involved in the screw hole, this involvement does not affect healing. Most angle fractures are amenable to reduction with this technique; it is, however, not recommended for comminuted angle fractures or in children. Deceptively simple when performed by an experienced operator, this technique should be attempted only by a surgeon familiar with the biomechanics of the mandible and well experienced in the principles of rigid internal fixation using plates and screws.

CONDYLAR FRACTURES

The principle of lag screw osteosynthesis has been used to advantage in the management of certain condylar fractures. Rigid fixation permits an early return

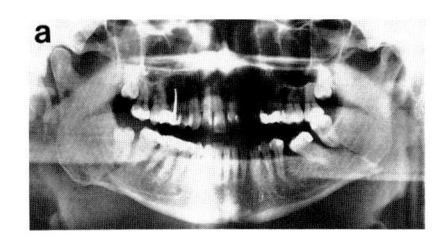

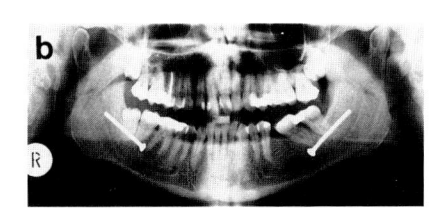

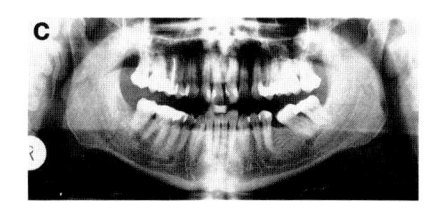

Figure 15.9 (a) Bilateral fractures of the mandibular angles. (b) Status following reduction with a solitary lag screw. (c) Status following removal of the lag screw after six months.

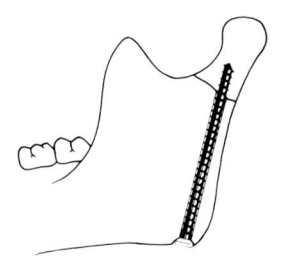

Figure 15.10 Lag screw fixation of high condylar fractures (Petzel technique).

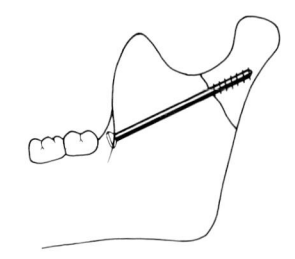

Figure 15.11 Reduction of low condylar fractures via an intraoral approach (Kitayama technique).

to function and precludes or minimizes adverse effects to the temporomandibular joint due to prolonged immobilization. The Petzel (1982) lag screw technique for the reduction of condylar fractures was originally designed to use a special screw pin that traverses the ascending ramus, but it can also be carried out with a long cortical screw. Using a percutaneous approach in the subangular region, a 2.7-millimeter gliding hole is created in the ramus with the help of a special drill guide. A special guide pin helps center the screw hole on the fracture surface. The gliding hole runs caudocranially and parallel to the posterior border of the ramus. The length of the screw is determined by measuring the guide hole and correlating it to the radiographs. A countersink is created over the gliding hole at the inferior border of the ramus. The ramus is retracted caudally; and the fracture reduced by an intraoral approach and held in place with a bone-holding forceps. A 2-millimeter thread hole is drilled along the predetermined axis into the aligned condylar fragment and then tapped. Inserting and tightening the lag screw stabilizes the fracture and compresses the fragments (see Figure 15.10).

A modification of this technique has been described by Kitayama (1989) for the treatment of basal condylar fractures. This procedure is carried out through an intraoral approach; the lag screw crosses the ramus diagonally to transfix the condyle (see Figure 15.11). The condylar region is exposed by using an intraoral incision similar to that used for a sagittal split ramus osteotomy. The mandible is retracted caudally with the assistance of a bone screw introduced percutaneously into the angle region, and the condylar fragment is repositioned with a condylar forceps. A gliding hole is drilled in the distal fragment with the help of a special drill guide, the tip of which positions on the fracture surface of the distal fragment and helps to orient the drilling axis. The condylar forceps helps to coapt the condylar fragment and hold it in position as a thread hole is drilled into it along the predetermined axis. A recess for the screwhead is prepared with a countersink, and the thread hole is tapped after the length of the screw is ascertained. The bone fragments are then fixated with a cortical screw of predetermined length.

Both of these procedures are technically demanding—even for the skilled surgeon—due to poor visibility and limited space. Kitayama recommends the use of fluoroscopy during the preparation of the gliding hole and for placing the screw. In addition to the difficult access to the surgical site, execution of these techniques is subject to clinical and anatomical restraints. They require special instruments and cannot be carried out if the thickness of the condylar neck is less than 5 millimeters or if the mandibular ramus is thin and curved. Accurate coaptation of the fractured segments throughout the procedure is critical to the success of these techniques.

COMMINUTED FRACTURES

Comminuted fractures, especially those caused by gunshot wounds, seriously impair the structural integrity of the mandible. In cases where the bony buttress is deficient or absent, the surgeon must seek to restore structural integrity with a minimum of implant material. Lag screws can be effectively used to simplify the fracture situation by combining the smaller fragments into larger ones. These larger fragments may then be reduced and stabilized with the help of additional lag screws or compression plates (see Figure 15.12). Lag screws can also be placed through a reconstruction plate when treating a severely comminuted mandible with small butterfly fragments. In such situations, all other screws must be placed neutrally to prevent overriding of the fragments. Otherwise, shear stresses generated at the site of lag screw fixation would loosen the lag screws, and interfragmentary compression would therefore be

Figure 15.12 (a) Lag screws used to simplify a comminuted angle fracture by combining the smaller fragments into larger ones. (b) This postoperative radiograph shows how the angle fracture has been reduced by the solitary lag screw technique.

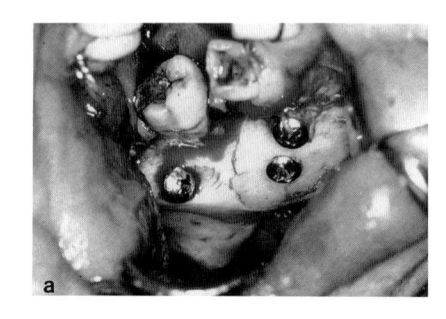

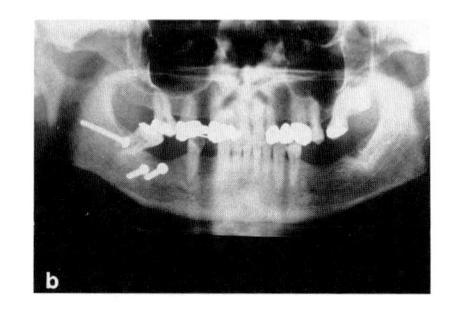

lost. In the case of segmental fractures, a lag screw can be used to attach a wedge-shaped fragment to the main body or transfix it to prevent displacement when the reconstruction plate is applied. Application of a lag screw entails minimal periosteal stripping, which is advantageous in comminuted fractures where extensive devascularization may jeopardize the viability of the free bone fragments.

GRAFT FIXATION

Small nonunion gaps can usually be treated by axial compression, but large gaps and defect fractures (such as those seen in gunshot wounds) must be restored with bone grafts. In such situations, screws placed through a reconstruction plate in lag fashion can help immobilize and compress the graft to the recipient bed, favoring revascularization.

Following MMF, an extraoral exposure is used to expose the recipient bed. The bony margins of the mandibular stumps are freshened until viable tissue is reached. The margins are decorticated, creating an overlap of 1.5 to 2 cm at the host recipient site so as to allow for mortising an appropriately shaped corticocancellous bone graft to the proximal and distal segments. The graft is secured and immobilized with a contoured bone plate; screws secure the graft to the mandible in lag fashion. A minimum of three screws should be used on each side of the graft; they should be inserted in a neutral fashion to avoid shear stresses on the lag screw

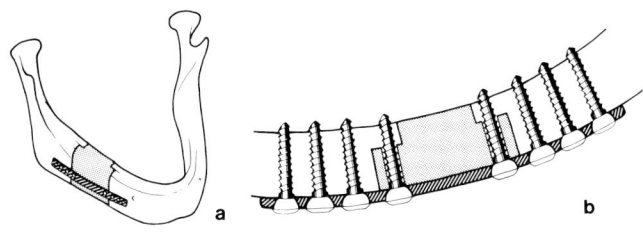

Figure 15.13 (a) Mortise inlay graft applied with the help of a reconstruction plate and lag screws. (b) Screws passing through the graft are inserted in lag fashion; the remaining screws are inserted in neutral fashion to avoid shear stresses on the lag screws.

(see Figure 15.13). Lag screws have a high coefficient of fixation, so they are more effective than wires for fixating a sliding bone graft to reconstruct a mandibular discontinuity defect.

SUMMARY

Applied in appropriate clinical situations, lag screw fixation is an appealing and effective alternative to the current systems of rigid internal fixation used for the management of mandibular fractures. The versatility of their application is defined by the ingenuity of the surgeon, as exemplified by the following case.

A 34-year-old patient was admitted to the hospital with multiple fractures of the mandible, including right paramedian, left angle, and condylar fractures (see Figure 15.14a). Following application of MMF, the para-

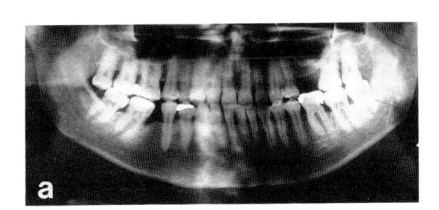

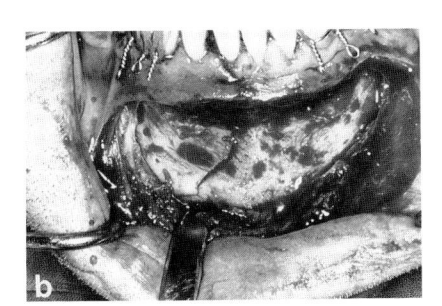

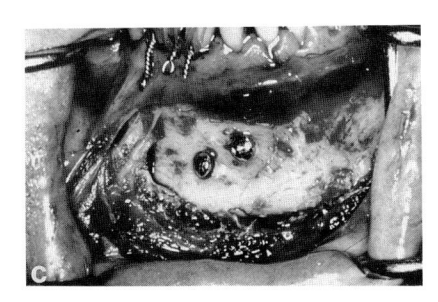

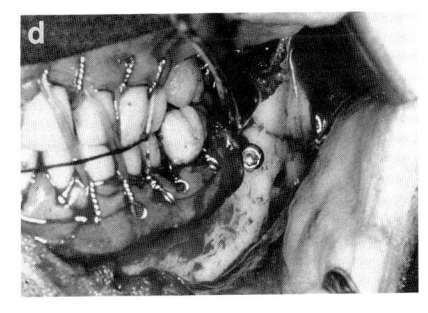

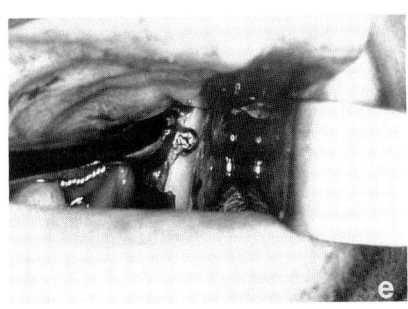

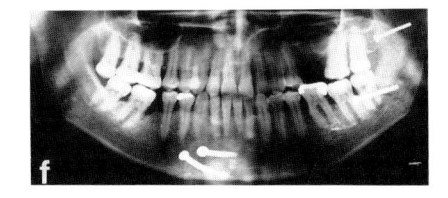

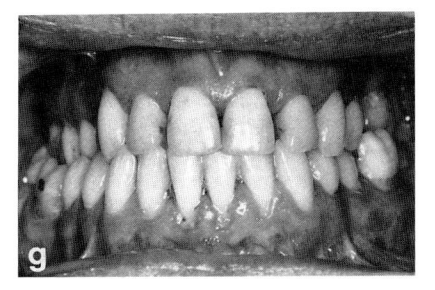

Figure 15.14 (a) Preoperative radiograph showing a right paramedian fracture and a left angle and condylar fracture. (b) Intraoperative view of the paramedian fracture. (c) Paramedian fracture reduced with lag screws. (d) Fixation of the left angle fracture with a lag screw. (e) Left condylar fracture reduced with a lag screw by way of an intraoral approach. (f) Postoperative radiograph showing reduction of the multiple fractures exclusively with lag screws. (g) Postoperative occlusion.

median fracture was first exposed and reduced with two lag screws (see Figure 15.14b and c) via an intraoral approach. The left angle fracture was then fixated by the solitary lag screw technique using a transbuccal approach (see Figure 15.14d), after which the left condylar fracture was reduced (see Figure 15.14e). Postoperative radiographs show the minimum use of implant material by judicious application of lag screws (see Figure 15.14f). Status at the time of removal of the lag screws evidences restoration of premorbid occlusion (see Figure 15.14g).

BIBLIOGRAPHY

Kitayama S: A new method of intra-oral reduction using a screw applied through the mandibular crest of condylar fractures. J Cranio Max Fac Surg 17: 16–23, 1989.

Niederdellmann H, Akuamoa-Boateng E: Internal fixation of fractures. Int J Oral Surg 7:152, 1978.

Niederdellmann H, Shetty V: Solitary lag screw osteosynthesis in the treatment of fractures of the angle of the mandible: A retrospective study. Plast Reconstr Surg 80; 1: 68–74, 1987.

Niederdellmann H, Shetty V, Collins JVC: Controlled osteosynthesis with the position screw. Int J Adult Orthodont Orthognat Surg 2: 159–162, 1987.

Petzel JR: Functionally stable traction-screw osteosynthesis of condylar fractures. J Oral Maxillofac Surg 40: 108–110, 1982.

CHAPTER 16

Rigid Fixation of Complex Mandibular Fractures

Joseph S. Gruss

Simple mandibular fractures may be adequately treated by conventional techniques or by rigid internal fixation according to the patient's choice, in the difficult patient, or in the patient for whom return for follow-up would be difficult. Alternatively, rigid internal fixation has become an absolute indication in certain clinical situations. The management of even simple mandibular fractures in the patient who is polytraumatized, is head injured, or has a cervical spine fracture has been revolutionized by the ability to fix the mandible rigidly, allowing immediate release of MMF and airway maintenance without tracheostomy in the majority of cases (see Figure 16.1). Similarly, the treatment of the fractured edentulous mandible and mandibular fractures associated with unstable midfacial fractures has been facilitated.

Treatment of the severely injured mandible with segmentation, comminution, or bone loss has traditionally been with an external fixation device. Interosseous wire and K-wire fixation, although used extensively, fail to provide three-dimensional stability to counteract the significant forces of function and mastication, even if prolonged MMF is used. It is in this group of patients, suffering complex fractures to the mandible, that rigid internal fixation with plates and screws has made a tremendous difference in treatment. A practical approach to the management of these difficult fractures with segmentation, comminution, and bone loss will be described.

BASIC PRINCIPLES

In the management of complex mandibular fractures, a thorough understanding of the basic principles will guide the surgeon in the stepwise, logical application of techniques, which can be applied and modified to the individual case as necessary. A carefully planned and progressively applied management strategy is essential in the difficult cases. Attempted shortcuts or omissions of technical steps invariably result in disastrous complications, which frequently condemn the patient to a prolonged and difficult phase of delayed reconstruction.

Diagnosis

In the polytrauma patient it may be very difficult to diagnose a mandibular fracture adequately with standard x rays. CT scanning of the mandible at the time of head and midfacial CT scan will often reveal, very accurately, the extent and pattern of mandibular injury (see Figure 16.2).

Exposure

In complex mandibular fractures, adequate exposure is essential in order to appreciate fully the extent and nature of the injury itself as well as its relationship to the stable areas of the mandible. In addition, wide exposure is critical to ensure adequate reduction and fixation of fracture segments. Intraoral exposure alone should be used only with fractures involving the anterior mandible. All other fractures should be exposed widely through an external incision. Pre-existing lacerations can be used separately, or they can be extended to provide adequate exposure. A combined intraoral and extraoral incision and approach may be needed in certain situations, but care must be taken to minimize the amount of periosteal stripping to lessen the chance of

Figure 16.1 (a) Polytrauma patient with panfacial fractures and cervical spine injury. Bilateral fracture of the mandible makes airway management difficult. (b) Reduction and rigid internal fixation with bilateral compression plates allows opening of the MMF immediately after surgery, ensuring an adequate airway and making nursing care much easier.

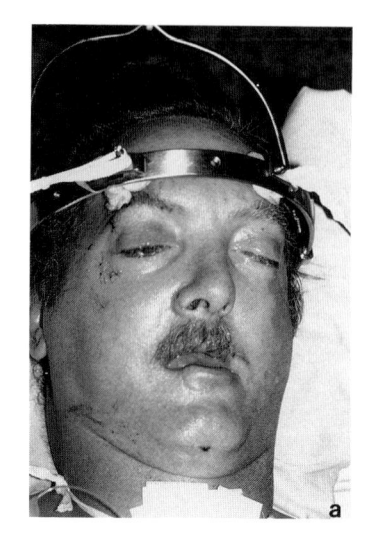

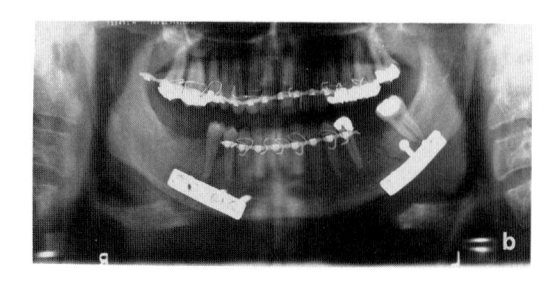

Figure 16.2 (a) CT scan reveals an oblique parasymphyseal fracture with comminution of the lingual cortex. In the repair of this fracture, it is essential to use a longer plate that goes beyond the sagittally split buccal cortex because screws placed in this area will be only monocortical. (b) CT scan illustrates bilateral condylar neck fractures. (c) CT scan illustrates bilateral condylar neck fractures. On the right side there is an intracapsular fracture. On the left side there is a markedly displaced condylar neck fracture. (d) Coronal CT scan gives excellent view of the condylar heads and necks and position of the ramus.

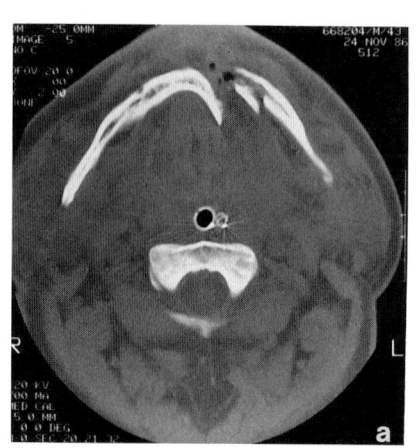

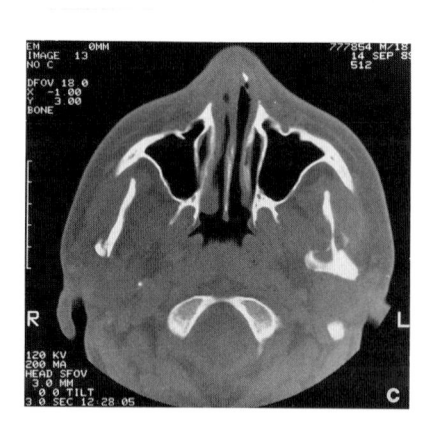

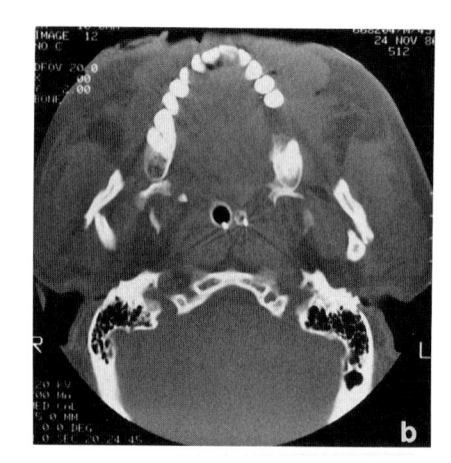

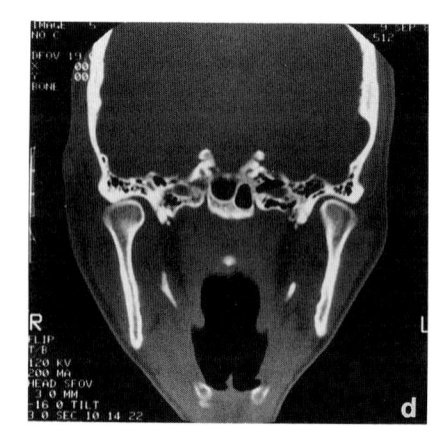

subsequent bone necrosis. The intraoral exposure will facilitate occlusal repositioning, and the extraoral approach will facilitate basal bone repair.

The edentulous mandible should always be exposed through an extraoral incision to minimize periosteal stripping. Only periosteum adjacent to the fracture needs to be elevated to allow adequate fracture reduction. The soft tissue adjacent to the fracture can be cleaned, without elevating the periosteum, and the plate is applied directly over the periosteum.

Maxillo-Mandibular Fixation (MMF)

The application of MMF is essential prior to plate application, to ensure the correct position of bony segments in segmental or comminuted fractures, or of the bone gap in fractures with bone loss. The mandibular arch bar may have to be applied in segments, to each bony segment containing teeth, to facilitate fracture reduction and correct occlusal repositioning. Once this is completed, continuity of the arch can be obtained by

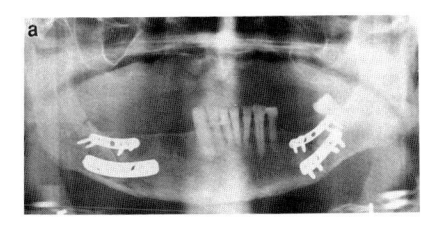

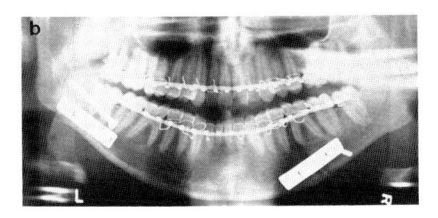

Figure 16.3 (a) Bilateral mandibular fracture with partially edentulous mandible. Repairs with bilateral Luhr compression plates at the inferior border and bilateral miniplates at the upper border acting as a tension band. Both repairs were done through an intraoral approach. (b) A tension band effect can be applied in the angle region by using a long lag screw placed through the thickest portion of the angle. A lag screw alone placed in the tension band area occasionally is sufficient to provide adequate stabilization. In many instances reinforcing the lag screw with a compression plate at the inferior border is preferable.

linking the arch bar across fracture gaps or by direct wiring around teeth adjacent to the fracture site. This is essential to produce the important tension banding effect of the arch bar on the mandibular upper border.

Tension Banding

Tension banding of the upper mandibular border can be provided most readily by an arch bar when there are teeth on both sides of the fracture, as previously described. When angle fractures are associated with segmentation or comminution anteriorly, controlling the tendency to medial and superior rotation of the proximal bone segment that does not contain teeth is difficult. A combination of miniplate and/or lag screw fixation at the upper border is frequently necessary to provide a tension band effect prior to final stabilization (see Figure 16.3).

Fracture Reduction and Stabilization

Following adequate exposure and occlusal repositioning using MMF, all fractures are reduced to reestablish the correct mandibular contour. Initial reduction, particularly in multiple segmented or comminuted fractures, may be by a combination of mandibular bone-holding clamps, interosseous wires, lag screws, and miniplates. Once contour is restored, final stabilization is by mandibular compression plates or reconstruction plates. In unstable or segmental fractures with good bone contact, a minimum of three screws in each lateral stable segment is necessary (three-hole principle of Spiessl). With severely comminuted fractures or fractures with bone loss, a minimum of four screws is necessary (four-hole principle).

Loose Bone Segments

In order to assess the fracture pattern adequately by direct inspection, to reduce, and to apply plate and screw fixation, sufficient periosteal stripping is required. Maintaining adequate periosteal and soft-tissue attachments to bone segments may be difficult or impossible, particularly if the fragments are severely displaced. Small cortical segments of bone, devoid of soft-tissue coverage, should be removed because they predispose to sequestrum formation and infection, even if internal fixation is adequate. Smaller corticocancellous segments can be discarded, if loose, particularly if adequate bony continuity can be established across the fracture site. Larger corticocancellous bone segments should be repositioned, whenever possible, particularly if they influence the provision of bony continuity. They can be repositioned with separate interosseous wires, lag screws, or miniplates; or they can be lagged directly to the overlying plate with screws.

Bone Grafting

The role, efficacy, and safety of primary bone grafting in the mandible is totally different from primary bone grafting in the upper face and midface. Primary bone grafting in the upper and midfacial region is a well proven, safe, and effective technique that has a high rate of success and low rate of complication. Because grafts in the upper face and midface are placed away from the salivary stream, a complete, watertight intraoral seal is not mandatory.

Primary bone grafts (nonvascularized) in the mandible are less predictable with significantly higher rates of resorption and infection. They are directly in contact with the salivary stream and therefore should not be used if there is any breach in the intraoral lining. Even without an obvious breach in intraoral lining, saliva can track down tooth sockets, particularly if the tooth has been loosened or injured. Primary bone grafting is occasionally used to bridge a small gap; to augment the thin, atrophic, edentulous mandible after the plate has been applied; or as a free vascularized bone graft. A strong mandibular reconstruction plate can adequately maintain the correct position of the lateral mandibular segments and bridge the bone gap, allowing safe, definitive secondary bone grafting once an intraoral seal is assured and soft tissue has healed.

Table 16.1 Classification of Segmental Fractures

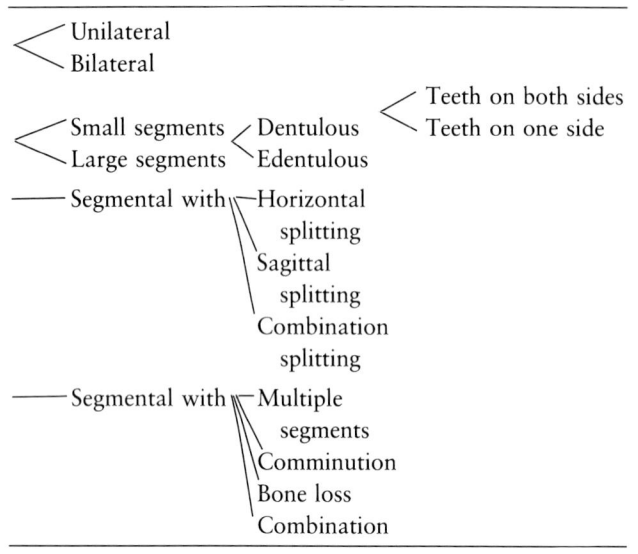

- Unilateral
- Bilateral
- Small segments / Large segments
  - Dentulous
    - Teeth on both sides
    - Teeth on one side
  - Edentulous
- Segmental with
  - Horizontal splitting
  - Sagittal splitting
  - Combination splitting
- Segmental with
  - Multiple segments
  - Comminution
  - Bone loss
  - Combination

Table 16.2 Management of Segmental Fractures

Adequate exposure
   intraoral
   extraoral
MMF
Reduce segments
Restore mandibular contour
   reduction forceps
   interosseous wires
   lag screws
   miniplates
Final stabilization
   compression plate
   reconstruction plate
Bone loss
   defect bridged with plate
   secondary bone grafting

SPECIFIC FRACTURES

Segmental Fractures

The sequential and correct principles of management of segmental fractures (see Table 16.1) have been outlined in the introduction and in Table 16.2. Their application to specific fractures will be described.

Large Segments

Segmental fractures with large intervening segments may be unilateral or bilateral. Common patterns of fracturing are as follows:

- *unilateral:* parasymphyseal and angle/ramus
  body and angle/ramus
- *bilateral:* parasymphyseal and opposite angle/ramus
  body and opposite angle
  bilateral body
  bilateral angle

The force needed to produce these fractures in a dentulous mandible is usually severe, and these fractures are frequently displaced and unstable. Because of the wide gap between the fractures, each fracture is usually treated with a separate plate (see Figures 16.4 and 16.5). Most important and difficult in the management of these fractures is ensuring optimal occlusal repositioning and reduction of both fractures prior to application of the plate. Because both fractures are usually exposed through separate incisions, visualizing and ensuring proper reduction of both fractures is essential. The reduction of one fracture can be maintained by a mandibular bone clamp, interosseous wire, lag screw, or tension band miniplate while the other plate is applied. Once this is completed, the final fixation is performed on the other fracture in isolation. If each fracture is exposed, reduced, and plated in turn, after seemingly perfect anatomical reduction on one side, an unrecog-

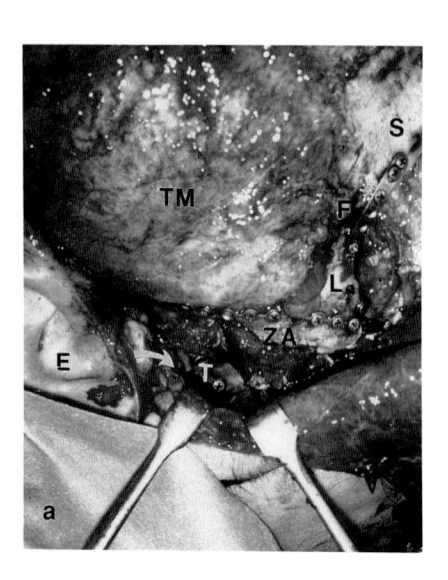

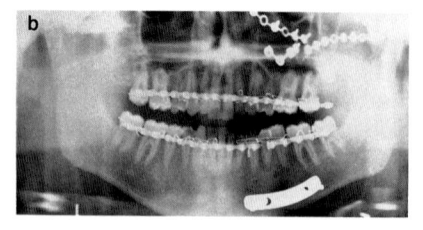

Figure 16.4 (a) When a unilateral, complex, segmental, displaced fracture of the body is associated with a displaced fracture of the condylar neck, reducing and fixing both the body fracture and the condylar neck fracture is often advisable. In this situation, the condylar neck fracture has been repaired through the coronal incision that has been used for orbitozygomatic repair. The body fracture has been repaired through an intraoral approach. The arrow points to the miniplate applied to the condylar neck. (T = temporomandibular joint, ZA = zygomatic arch, TM = temporalis muscle, E = ear, L = lateral orbital wall, F = fronto-zygomatic suture line, S = superior orbit.) (b) X-ray illustrates multiple miniplates repairing the orbitozygomatic complex, mini T-plate repairing the condylar neck fracture, and mandibular compression plate repairing the left body fracture.

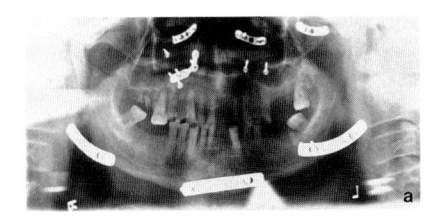

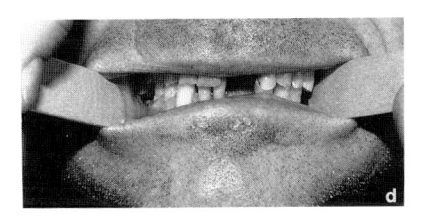

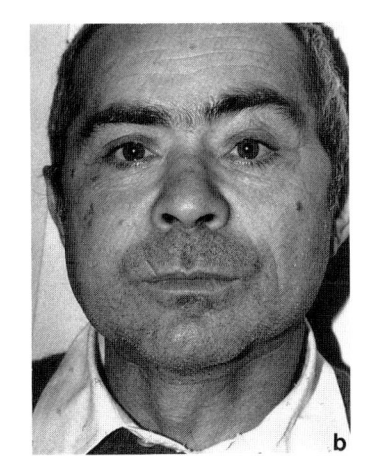

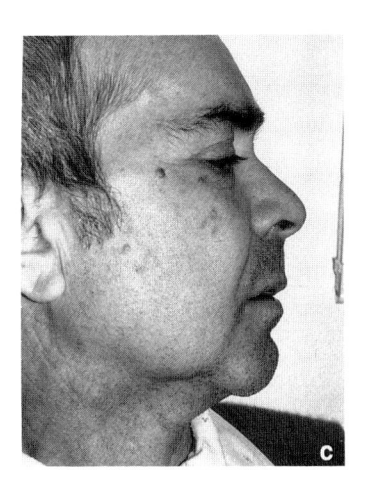

Figure 16.5 (a) Postoperative x-ray of patient with extensive panfacial injuries, including five fractures of the mandible. Displaced parasymphyseal and bilateral angle fractures are repaired with mandibular compression plates. Bilateral undisplaced condylar neck fractures are not repaired. All three mandibular plates have been inserted with an intraoral approach. (b) Facial appearance at two years shows good restoration of midfacial contour, height, and projection. (c) Lateral view illustrates good mandibular maxillary contour and projection. (d) In spite of mutilated occlusion and multiple tooth avulsions at the time of the injury, exact preoperative occlusion has been re-established by multiple plate fixation.

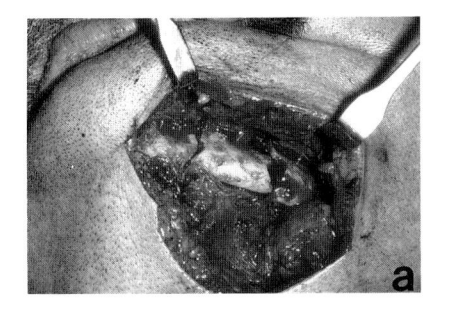

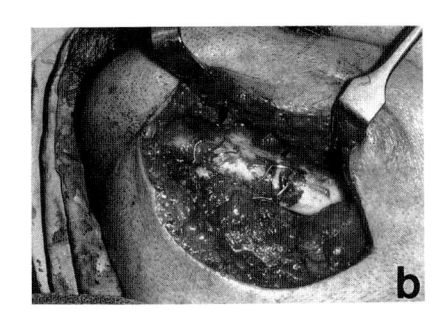

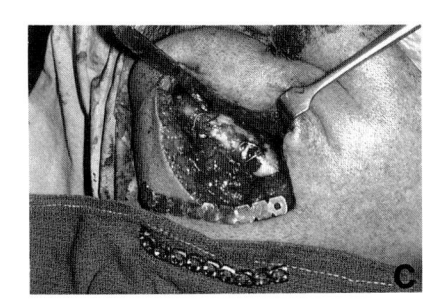

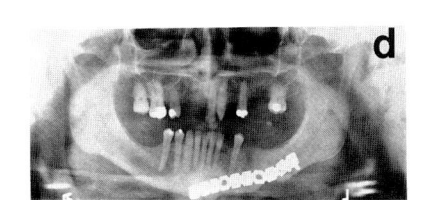

nized minor discrepancy may be translated into a major malalignment at the other fracture site, even with seemingly adequate MMF.

Once one plate has been applied, even minor discrepancies cannot be altered at the other fracture site, due to the rigid nature of the fixation. If such discrepancies are found, the initial plate must be removed and the integrated reduction and fixation must be recommenced.

Butterfly Segment

In the body of the mandible, the segmental fracture is often associated with a butterfly intervening segment (see Figure 16.6). This segment is repositioned and,

Figure 16.6 Segmental mandibular fracture with a butterfly fragment. In segmental fractures, comminuted fractures, or very difficult displaced fractures, an intraoral approach will often not give accurate assessment of the pattern of the fracture and allow accurate reduction and fixation. Whenever possible, complex fractures should be approached extraorally. (a) Extraoral approach to a complex segmental fracture of the body of the mandible. (b) The contour of the mandible is re-established by use of interosseous wires and figure-of-eight wires. (c) A template of the mandibular contour is taken and transferred to a reconstruction plate, which is bent exactly to the shape of the template. (d) The mandibular reconstruction plate now bridges the segmental segment, placing at least three screws in the proximal and distal segments. Two screws are placed in the intervening segment. This x ray, taken approximately six months after the repair, shows good healing across the fracture site.

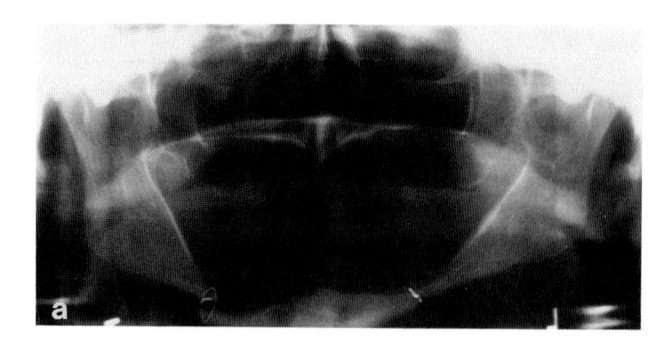

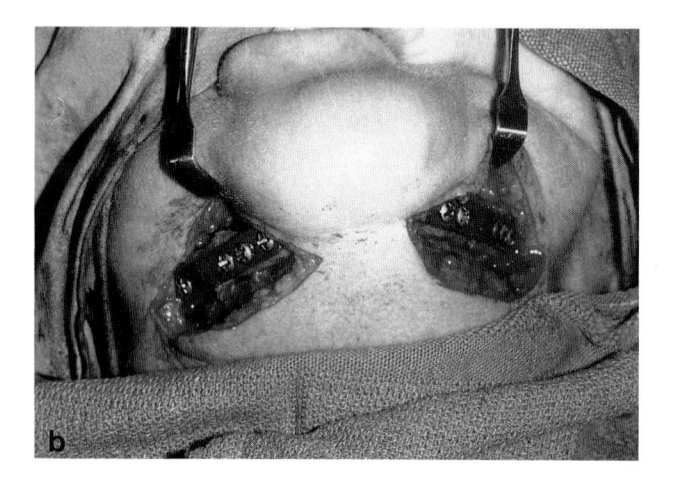

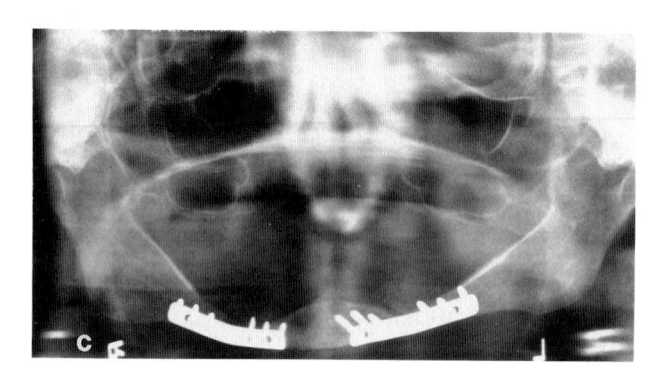

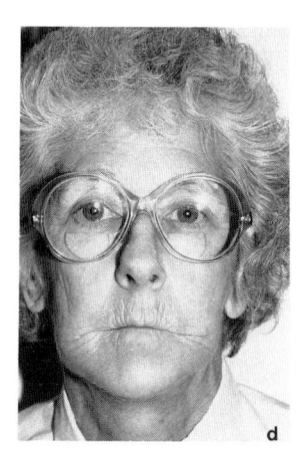

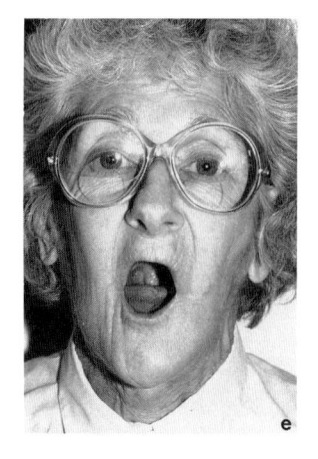

depending on the obliquity of the fracture on each end of the butterfly, either lag screws or lower-border interosseous wires will reestablish the proper mandibular contour. Final stabilization is provided by a reconstruction plate with a minimum of three screws in each outer segment. Whenever possible, separate screws are placed through the plate into the butterfly segment itself. Once fixation is completed, the interosseous wires can be removed.

Edentulous Segmental

Large Segments The force needed to fracture an atrophic, edentulous mandible is far less than that needed to fracture a fully dentulous mandible. Polytrauma in the elderly frequently results in a bilateral body fracture. The anterior, intervening mandibular segment becomes free-floating. The loss of anterior support of the tongue and laryngeal muscles allow their prolapse which may cause sudden and significant airway problems.

This situation is best treated by direct exposure of each fracture, minimal periosteal and soft-tissue stripping, and the application of a compression plate where possible (see Figure 16.7). Occasionally, the mandible is so thin that a miniplate may be required. Rigid fixation of this fracture facilitates management of the air-

Figure 16.7 The very thin, edentulous mandible may be difficult to repair with conventional techniques. (a) Attempted repair with two interosseous wires. (b) Edentulous mandible fractures should always be exposed through an extraoral incision because an intraoral incision requires too extensive stripping of the periosteum. Small incisions are made directly over the fracture, and only the periosteum at the fracture site is reflected. The remainder of the periosteum can be left intact on the bone, and the plate can be applied directly over the periosteum. Minimum stripping of the periosteum is important because the blood supply to thin, edentulous mandibles may arise almost entirely from the periosteum. (c) Postoperative x ray illustrates the fixation of the mandibular plates. Primary cancellous bone grafting from the iliac crest was inserted at the time of the plate repair to improve the chance of bony healing. The bone grafts can be seen at both fracture sites. Although it is sometimes possible to repair thin edentulous mandibles with miniplates, we feel, in the majority of cases, it is safer to use a bicortical mandibular plate. The mandibular plate can be placed into the thicker bone away from the fracture site. (d) Postoperative result with exact restoration of mandibular contour and projection. (e) Early restoration of mandibular function without the need for MMF.

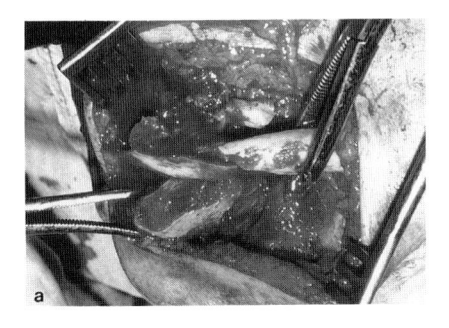

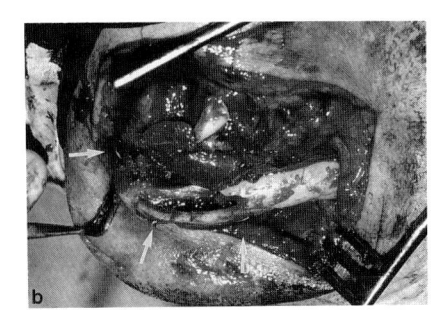

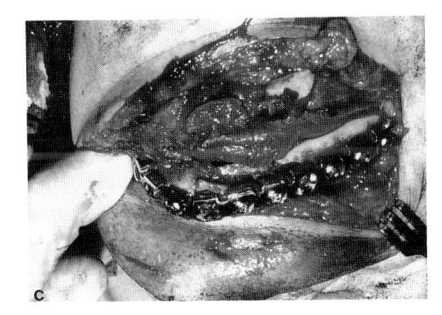

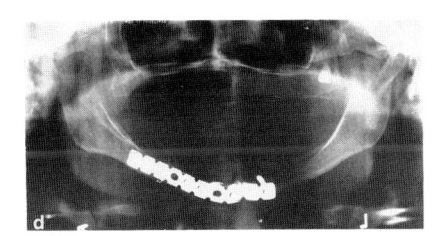

Figure 16.8 Complex comminuted fractures of the thin, edentulous mandible are also amenable to rigid internal fixation. (a) An extensive segmental fracture of a very thin, edentulous mandible exposed through an extraoral incision. Marked displacement of the multiple segments can be seen. (b) The mandibular contour is re-established using multiple interosseous wires and lag screws (arrows). (c) A long mandibular reconstruction plate is now used to provide the final form of stabilization. Even though this mandibular reconstruction plate is as large as the thin, edentulous mandible, it provides excellent and rigid stabilization of these complex and unstable fractures. (d) Postoperative panorex shows mandibular reconstruction plate bridging across the multiple segmental fractures. Once the bone has healed and the patient needs to be fitted with a denture, the mandibular reconstruction plate must be removed because it prevents prosthetic denture fitting.

way and postoperative care of the patient without the need for MMF with dentures wired to the upper and lower jaw.

Small Segments Multisegmented or comminuted fractures of the edentulous mandible are extremely difficult to treat (see Figure 16.8). Some surgeons think that the extensive periosteal stripping needed to expose these fractures will predispose to bone necrosis and that therefore external fixation should be used. In our experience, open reduction by an external incision facilitates optimal treatment. All fragments are reduced, and the mandibular contour is re-established by interosseous wires and lag screws. A long reconstruction plate then passes from each lateral stable segment across the area of comminution. Separate screws are placed from the plate to as many of the intervening segments as possible. The plate itself may be almost as large as the mandible itself, but this should not deter its use. The plate can be removed at a later stage to allow proper fitting of dentures. Additional bone grafts can be added primarily or, preferably, at the time of plate removal.

Horizontal Splitting

The mandible may split horizontally in all anatomic zones. Horizontal splitting in the tooth-bearing area poses a particular problem (see Figure 16.9). When the upper border, or alveolus, is split horizontally, a large tooth-bearing segment is displaced. This segment must be reattached to the main mandibular bone inferiorly. Because the teeth and tooth roots are contained within this segment, fixation is difficult; any form of fixation should not damage these structures. This tooth-bearing segment can be reattached to the main segment with interosseous wire or lag screws placed between the tooth roots. A reconstruction plate usually provides final stabilization.

Sagittal Splitting

Sagittal splitting of the inner and outer cortex commonly occurs in association with segmental fractures (see Figure 16.10). The obliquity of these fractures is ideally suited to multiple lag screw fixation alone or to lag screw fixation through a plate. In certain situations, sagittal splitting or comminution of the lingual cortex may occur with seemingly simple fracturing of the buccal cortex. This must be recognized, because standard management with a short compression plate may result in some screws having only monocortical purchase, leading to instability and eventual loss of fixation. This situation should be managed with a larger reconstruction plate with three or four screws on either side of the fracture site.

Multiple Segments or Comminution

When multiple segments or comminution are present, after adequate exposure and establishment of correct MMF, as many fragments as possible are reduced and linked together with a combination of inter-

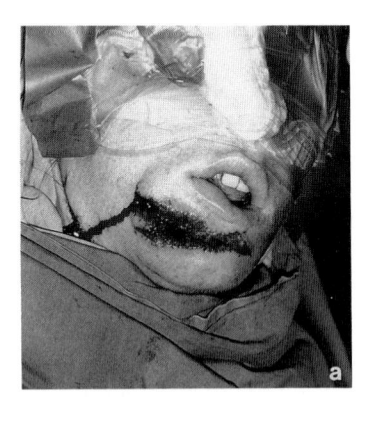

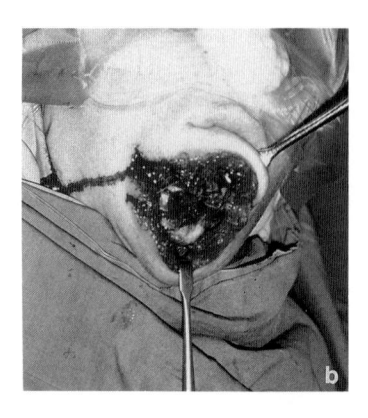

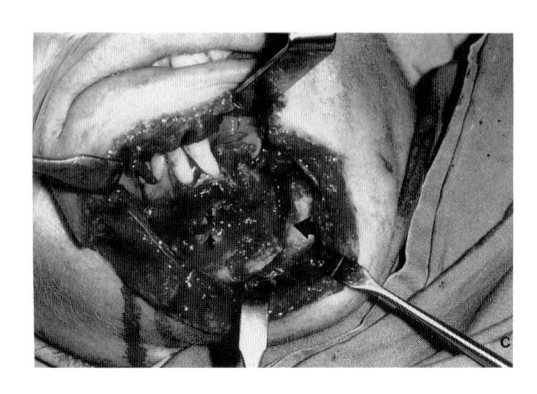

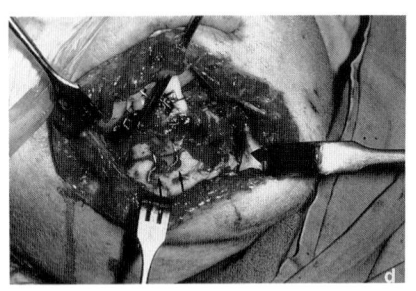

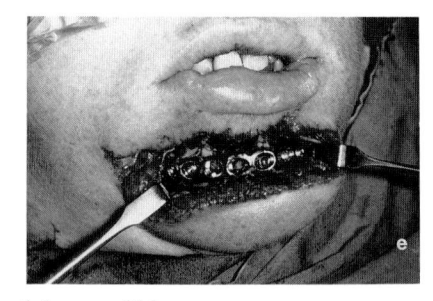

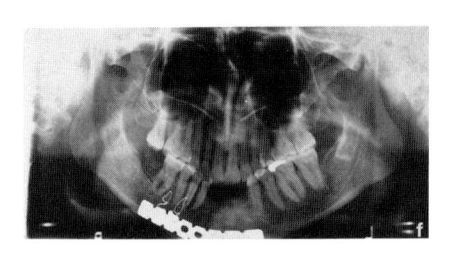

Figure 16.9 A complex segmental fracture of the mandible may be associated with horizontal and sagittal splitting of the mandible. In particular, the tooth-bearing segments may split horizontally. (a) A young female with complex open fractures of the mandible after being hit in the face with a motorized ski. (b) Severity of the degloving injury of the mandible and multiple comminuted fractures. (c) Small arrows indicate horizontal splitting of the tooth-bearing segment of the main inferior segment of the mandible. Large arrow illustrates anterior fracture through the parasymphyseal region. (d) Correct occlusion is applied by means of arch bars and interdental wiring. Multiple interosseous wires are placed between the tooth roots to reattach the tooth-bearing segment to the main inferior segment (arrows). (e) Final stabilization is now performed by bridging across the entire fractured segments with a long reconstruction plate. (f) Postoperative panorex indicates interosseous wires placed between the tooth roots and a long reconstruction plate with at least three screws on either side. (g) Appearance at two years illustrates healing of the severe soft-tissue injury with minimal shrinkage and contracture due to proper stabilization of the underlying bony injury. (h) Restoration of correct contour and occlusion.

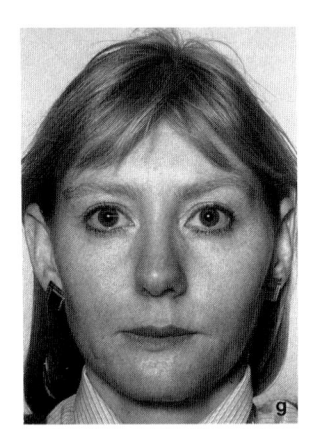

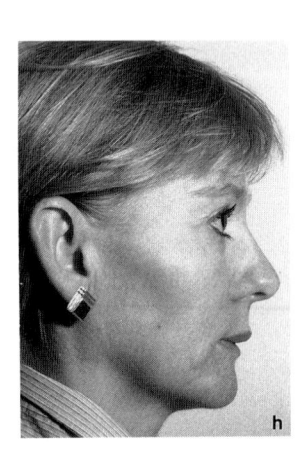

osseous wires, lag screws, and miniplates to restore the correct mandibular contour. A template is now taken of the mandible to allow exact contouring of a long reconstruction plate. Extending from the stable lateral mandible on each side, this plate provides final stabilization. Separate screws are placed through the plate into as many bony segments as possible. The plate bridges any bone gaps resulting from immediate bone loss or delayed resorption of bone segments, allowing safe delayed bone grafting (see Figures 16.11–16.15).

Fractures with Bone Defect

Mandibular fractures with a bone defect usually result following a blast to the facial region from a high-velocity rifle or shotgun (see Chapter 27). Occasionally, high-velocity blunt trauma will result in bone destruction or loss through large skin and mucosal lacerations. The stepwise, carefully planned progression of treat-

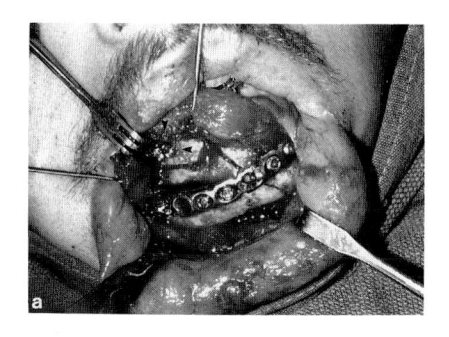

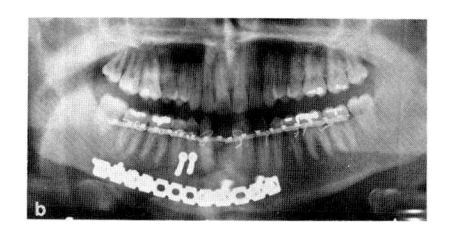

Rigid Fixation of Complex Mandibular Fractures 203

Figure 16.10 (a) Severe complex and comminuted injuries of the parasymphyseal region with splitting of the right tooth-bearing segments. These tooth-bearing segments may be repositioned by means of lag screws to the main inferior segment. Each lag screw must be placed between the tooth roots (arrows). A long reconstruction plate applies the final form of fixation to the parasymphyseal fractures. (b) This postoperative panorex illustrates the positions of the lag screws and the long reconstruction plate.

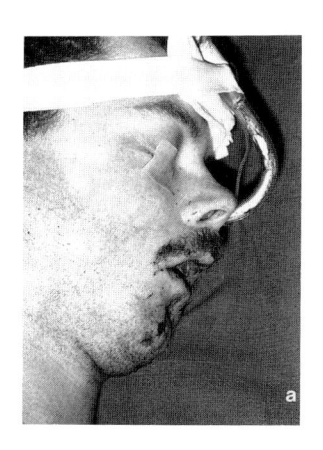

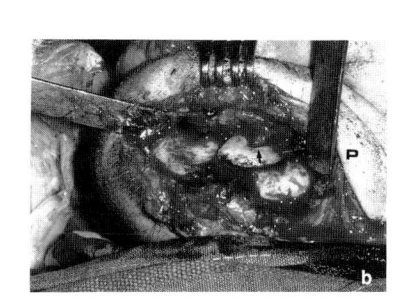

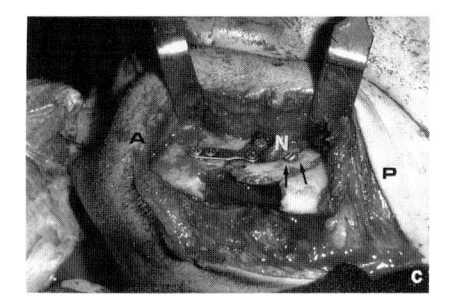

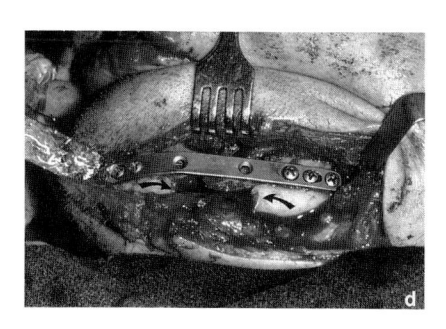

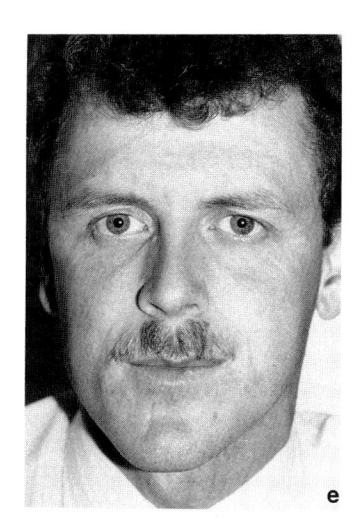

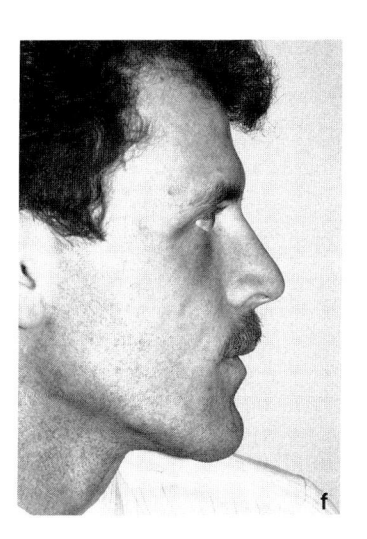

Figure 16.11 (a) A young man with severely displaced comminuted parasymphyseal and left body fractures. Marked backward depression of the entire mandibular complex can be seen. Such a patient may require intubation to preserve an adequate airway. (b) Multiple segmental fractures of the parasymphyseal and left body region can be seen. Arrow points to upper segment containing inferior alveolar nerve. (P = posterior.) (c) Initial mandibular contour is restored by lag screws (arrows); the central segment is placed back to the large posterior segment. The central segment is reattached to the anterior segment by means of a mini L-plate; the L portion ensures that the inferior alveolar nerve (N) is not damaged. (A = anterior, P = posterior.) (d) Final stabilization is now performed using a long mandibular plate, which bridges the area of comminution. At least three screws are used in both the anterior and posterior segments. Because bone-to-bone contact in the upper two thirds of the mandible is excellent, it is not necessary to bone graft the missing inferior segment of the mandible (arrows). (e) Postoperative appearance at two years illustrates restoration of facial contour and height. (f) Lateral view illustrates restoration of mandibular contour.

Figure 16.12 (a) A young male with a low-velocity gunshot wound of the left cheek and mandible. (b) At exploration, a fracture of the buccal cortex of the mandible looks simple and appears to require only a short compression plate. (c) Care must be taken not to misjudge the severity of these injuries. CT scan illustrates that although the outer cortex is not comminuted, the inner lingual cortex has multiple segmental fractures; therefore the use of a short plate in this patient will almost certainly result in all the screws being applied with only monocortical fixation. This fracture requires a long reconstruction plate with the screws placed away from the fracture site so that as much bicortical fixation can be obtained as possible. (d) Repair with a long reconstruction plate using at least four screws in either side. Accurate reduction of the fracture can be seen. (e) Postoperative panorex illustrates the positioning of the reconstruction plate along the inferior border of the mandible. (f) Following adequate repair of the fracture site, the reconstruction plate may be removed in certain cases. In this patient, the plate was removed because of persistent cold intolerance of the stainless steel plate.

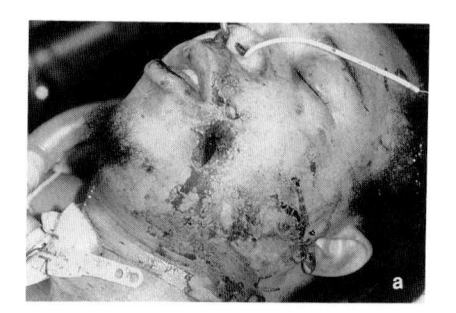

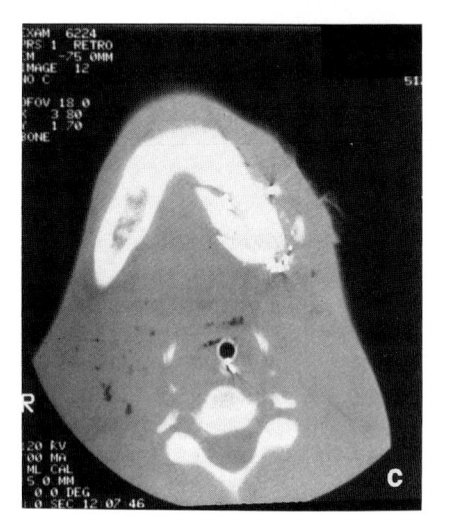

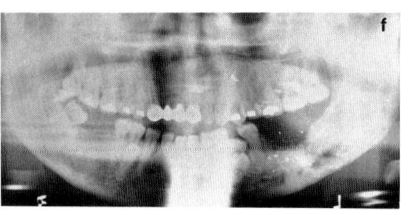

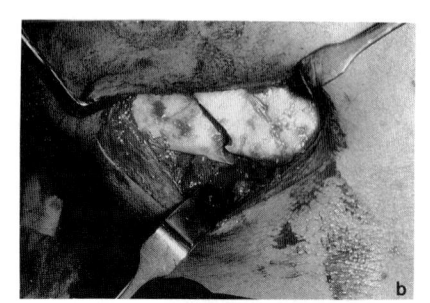

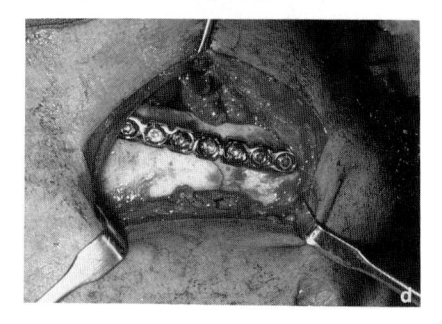

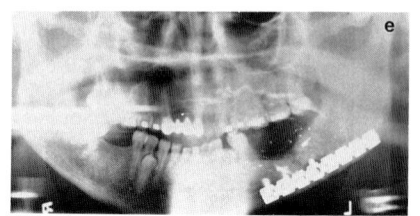

Table 16.3 Management of Mandibular Fractures with Bone Defect

Adequate exposure — intraoral / extraoral

MMF
  repositions remaining segments
  delineates bone gap

Template of gap and lateral segments

Reconstruction plate
  bridges gap
  stabilizes lateral segments

Soft tissue reconstruction
  intraoral
  external

Bone graft gap
  primary / secondary
  conventional / vascularized

ment principles has been outlined fully earlier in this chapter and in Table 16.3.

Adequate exposure is mandatory and can often be obtained directly through the soft-tissue injury. Careful, but thorough, debridement of all obviously damaged and devitalized soft tissue is necessary, as well as of small cortical bone segments devoid of soft-tissue coverage. If there is any doubt about the adequacy of debridement, the wound can be loosely sutured, covering as much exposed bone as possible, and covered with a moist dressing. The patient is then returned to be operated on at 48 to 72 hours for final, definitive reconstruction. The reconstruction plate bridges the gap and stabilizes the lateral segments. Primary bone grafting is rarely indicated. Soft-tissue reconstruction, both intraoral and external, can then be provided as needed.

The reconstruction plate provides alloplastic bridging of the bone gap. In the elderly edentulous patient, in whom dental rehabilitation is not planned, this bridging is permanent. If dentures are to be fitted or osteointegrated implants are to be inserted, then even-

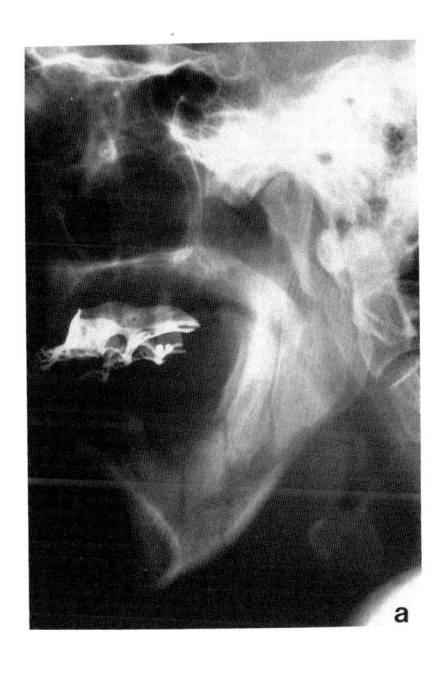

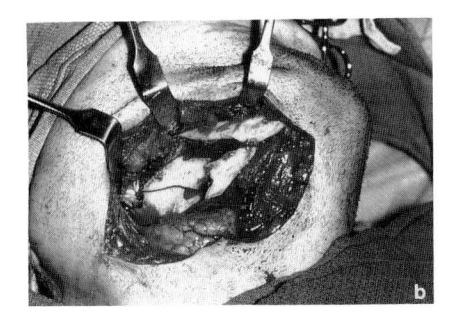

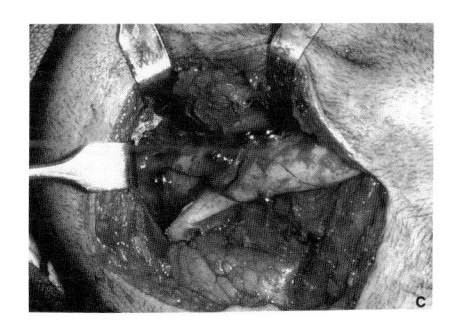

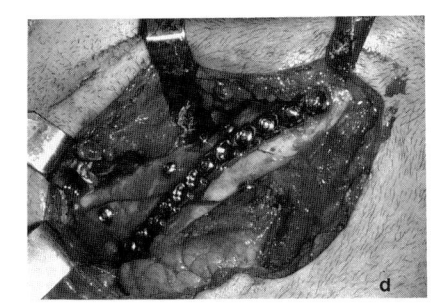

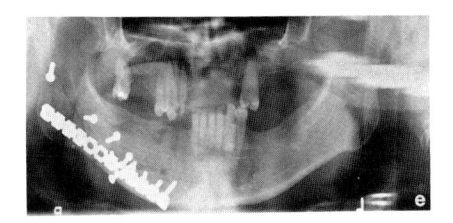

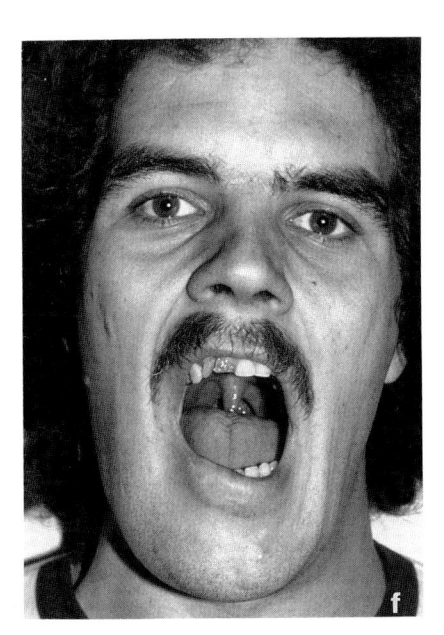

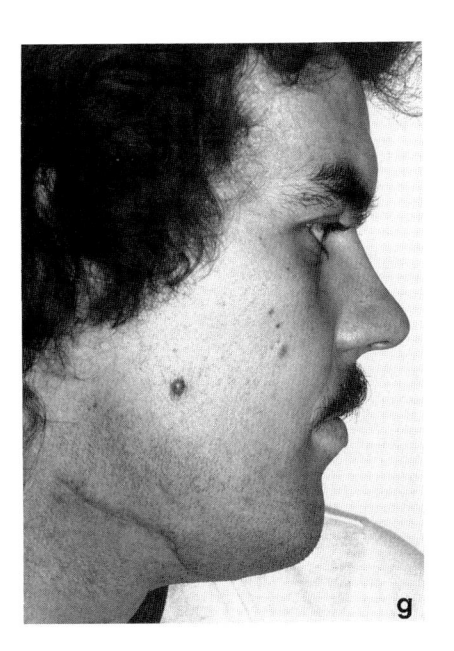

Rigid Fixation of Complex Mandibular Fractures 205

Figure 16.13 Multiple comminuted segmental fractures of the mandible are ideally repaired with multiple lag screws and plates. (a) Multiple comminuted segmental fractures of an edentulous mandible following an industrial accident. (b) Exposure through the pre-existing laceration extended anteriorly and posteriorly reveals multiple displaced segmental fractures of the mandible. (c) All the segmental fractures of the mandible are repositioned and initially fixed with multiple lag screws, reproducing the exact contour of the mandible. This fixation, although accurate, is not stable enough to provide a final form of fixation. (d) Final stabilization is performed by a long reconstruction plate, which bridges across all the segmental fractures, placing at least three screws in the anterior and posterior segments and multiple screws in the intervening segments. (e) Long reconstruction plate and multiple lag screws. (f) Rigid internal fixation results in rapid restoration of mandibular function. The patient, seen here two weeks after the repair, has excellent ability to open his mouth. (g) Lateral view showing restoration of mandibular contour. Laceration extended into incision can be seen.

Figure 16.14 A 16-year-old male with an accidental gunshot wound following a hunting accident with a high-velocity hunting rifle. (a) Massive injury to soft tissue and bone to the left side of the face. Note severe bursting type lacerations to the soft tissue extending right from the malar region down to the chin. (b) Multiple complex segmental and comminuted fractures of the mandible extend from the left ramus to the right body. The most important principle is first to apply arch bars and to place the patient in the proper occlusion. This assists in the reduction and alignment of the fractures. (c) The contour of the multiple segmental fractures is now re-established by the use of a long, miniadaptive plate on the left side. (d) Once the proper occlusion has been established and the correct contour of the mandible has been provided by the initial fixation with a miniplate, a long mandibular reconstruction plate is molded to the exact shape of the mandible to span across the multiple segmental areas from stable bone posteriorly to stable bone anteriorly. (e) On the right side, a mandibular compression plate repairs the fracture of the right body and angle region. Note the correct contour obtained by careful bending of the mandibular reconstruction plate. (f) Postoperative panorex reveals the method of fixation using miniplate, mandibular plate, and reconstruction plate, all in the one case. Note that the mandibular reconstruction plate has a minimun of four screws on either side of the fracture because this fracture is extremely unstable (the four-screw rule). (g) Six weeks after the injury, one notes good healing of the soft tissues, which have simply been repaired primarily. An obvious left facial palsy is present. (h) At six weeks, note excellent healing of the facial soft tissues without significant shrinkage or scar contracture due to the rigid fixation of the underlying bony skeletal support, which maintains expansion of the soft tissue in the phase of healing. (i) Appearance at seven months shows re-establishment of normal occlusion and regeneration of the facial nerve through the area of injury without any attempt at primary repair.

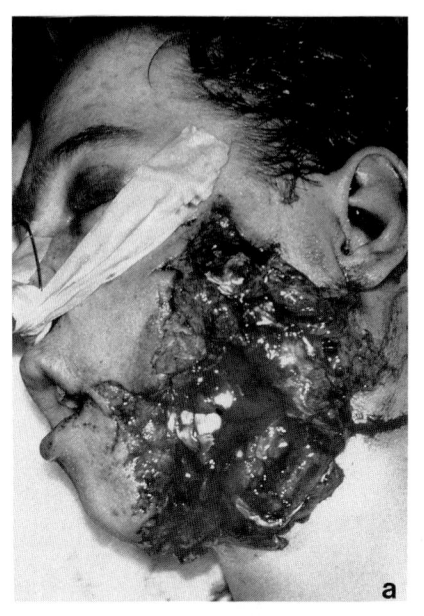

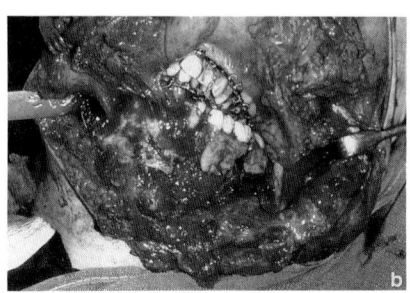

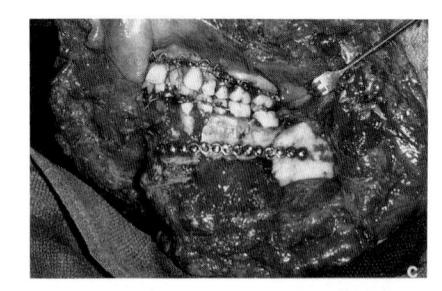

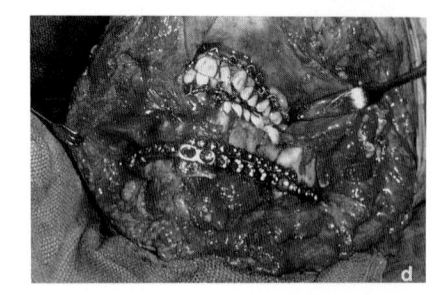

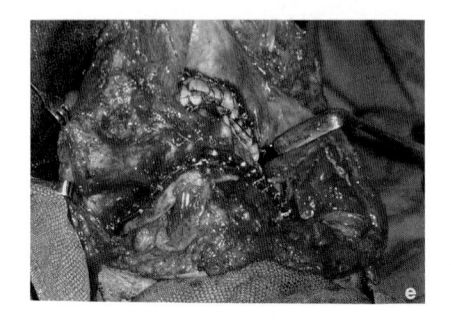

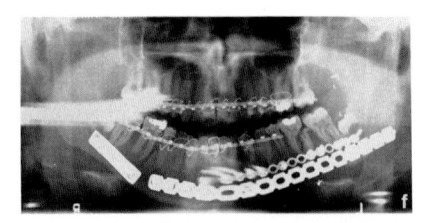

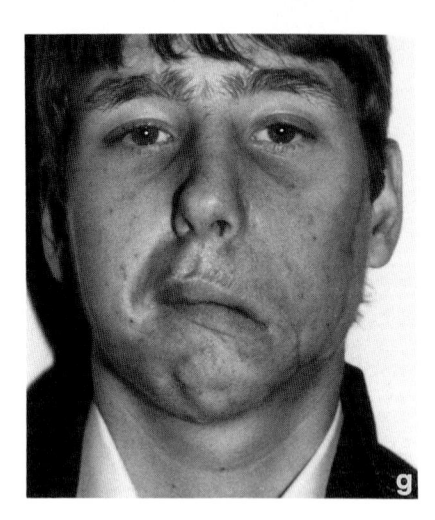

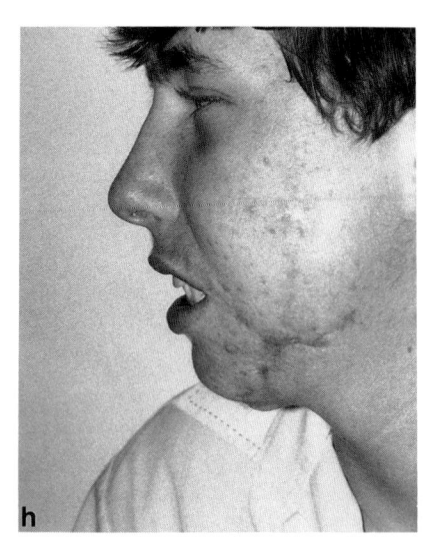

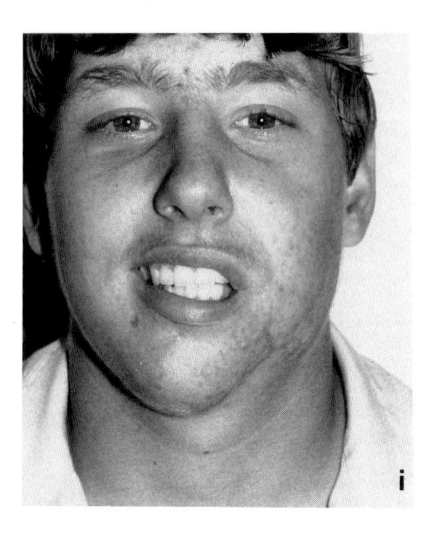

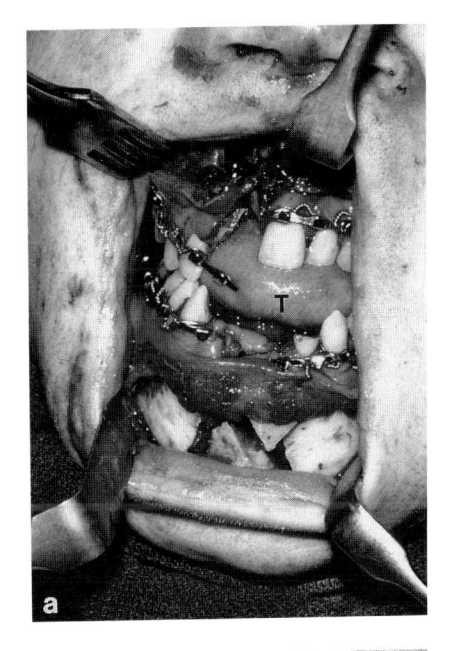

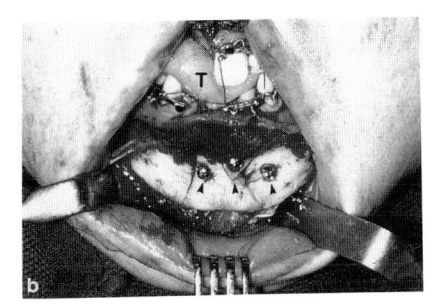

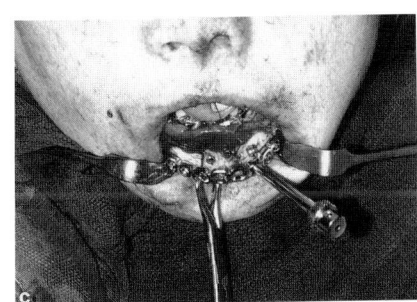

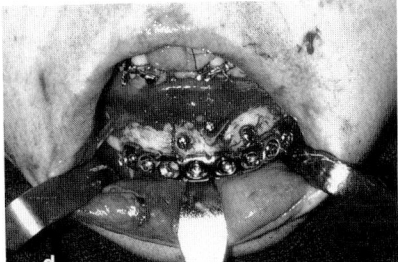

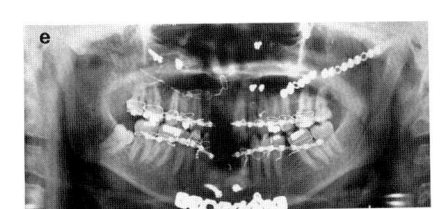

Figure 16.15 (a) A patient with massive panfacial and craniofacial injuries with multiple segmental fractures of the maxilla and mandible. Note that there are multiple areas of sagittal splitting of the palate as well as of the mandible and multiple areas of tooth loss. This makes the application of the correct occlusion difficult. Multiple segmental arch bars are applied, and the complex parasymphyseal fractures are exposed through an intraoral incision. (b) The occlusion is aligned and MMF is applied, taking into account the multiple missing teeth. The multiple segmental fractures of the mandible are now aligned and repaired with multiple lag screws (arrows). (T = tongue.) (c) A template is taken of the contour of the mandible. This is applied to a mandibular reconstruction plate, which is bent to the shape of the mandible and applied. Multiple lag screws are applied through the plate, lagging the individual fragments to the plate. (d) Completed repair with lag screws and long reconstruction plate, which maintains the shape of the symphyseal region. (e) Postoperative panorex illustrates the segmental arch bars as well as the mandibular plating, which maintains the gaps in the palate and mandible and prevents their collapse.

tual bone grafting is necessary. In the dentulous patient, the masticatory forces exerted on the remaining mandible and transmitted through the plate and screws will eventually loosen the screws, usually in the region of the angle or ramus where the bone is thinner and weaker. The masticatory forces may actually fracture the plate. In these patients, replacing the missing bone is essential to establish bony continuity across the mandible. Once the missing bone has been replaced, the plate is removed at 3 to 6 months to allow hypertrophy of the bone graft under the influence of functional stresses. If the plate is left in situ, its stress-shielding effect may cause atrophy of the bone graft.

The best source and type of bone graft to use is extremely controversial. Many surgeons have had excellent success with conventional bone grafting, even with large gaps. In our experience, bone gaps of less than 4 centimeters are ideally reconstructed with conventional iliac bone grafts. Gaps of 1 to 2 cm may be packed tightly with cancellous bone. Larger defects are reconstructed with block corticocancellous grafts. One cortex is removed, with manual instruments, leaving a block of cancellous bone with only one cortex. This bone graft is ideally made slightly larger than the defect and is wedged in place before the screws are tightened. As the screws are tightened, the graft is compressed and held between the bone ends. The cortical surface is applied adjacent to the plate, and additional screws can be inserted through the plate into the graft if necessary. These grafts are extremely resistant to infection and will often survive adequately even when significant infection occurs. Free rib and calvarial grafts are mainly cortical and have given much poorer results in our hands. Free calvarial grafts in particular have a very poor resistance to infection and usually have to be removed once infection occurs.

In bone gaps of greater than 4 centimeters, our results with conventional bone grafts have been variable and unpredictable. Therefore, we prefer to use free vascularized bone grafts for larger reconstructions. These grafts themselves are stabilized whenever possible with rigid internal fixation techniques.

BIBLIOGRAPHY

Ardary WC: Plate and screw fixation in the management of mandible fractures. Clin Plastic Surg 16:61, 1989.

Ellis E, Carlson DS: The effects of mandibular immobilization on the masticatory system. Clin Plast Surg 16:133, 1989.

Jeter TS, Van Sickels JE, Nishioka GJ: Intraoral open reduction with rigid internal fixation of mandibular subcondylar fractures. J Oral Maxillofac Surg 46:1113-1116, 1988.

Klotch D: Use of rigid internal fixation in the repair of complex and comminuted mandible fractures. Otolaryngol Clin North Am 20:495, 1987.

Luhr HG: Compression plate osteosynthesis through the Luhr System. In Oral and Maxillofacial Traumatology. E Kruger, W Schilli (eds). Vol 1, p 319, Chicago, Quintessence, 1982.

Niederdellmann H, Shetty V: Solitary lag screw osteosynthesis in the treatment of fractures of the angle of the mandible: A retrospective study. Plast Reconstr Surg 80:68, 1987.

Nishioka GJ, Van Sickels JE: Transoral plating of mandibular angle fractures: A technique. Oral Surg 66:531, 1988.

Perren SM, Huggler SM, Russenberger A: The reaction of cortical bone to compression. Acta Orthop Scand (Suppl) 125:3, 1969.

Rahn BA: Theoretical considerations in rigid fixation of facial bones. Clin Plast Surg 16:21, 1989.

Schmoker R: Mandibular reconstruction using a special plate. J Maxillofac Surg 11:99, 1983.

Schmoker R, von Allen G, Tschopp HM: Application of functionally stable fixation in maxillofacial surgery according to the ASIF principles. J Oral Maxillofac Surg 40:457, 1982.

Spiessl B: New Concepts in Maxillofacial Bone Surgery. Berlin, Springer, 1976.

Spiessl B: Internal Fixation of the Mandible. Berlin, Springer, 1989.

CHAPTER 17

Open Reduction and Rigid Fixation of Subcondylar Fractures

Thomas S. Jeter
Fred L. Hackney

Management of subcondylar fractures is controversial. Issues that complicate treatment are the degree of accompanying injury to soft tissue, age of the patient, location of the fracture, and subsequent position of the subcondylar fragment. Traditional management has been closed reduction with a few selected indications for open reduction. This approach has been predicated on studies in animals showing that closed reductions work well with the difficult access to this region of the mandible. However, problems with this therapy have been noted, such as limited opening, pain, occlusal shifts, late arthritic changes, dysfunction, and deformity such as asymmetry and open bite.

Concomitant injury to the soft tissues with bleeding into the joint space is an unknown factor, which may explain why some patients do well with closed reductions and others do not. The length of immobilization may play a role in preventing hypomobility in an injured joint. It has been suggested that one should explore the joint, in addition to doing an open reduction. Results of such an aggressive approach in large samples remain to be seen.

There are obvious differences between the child and the adult patient. In the young child, adaptive remodeling will often restore a functional condyle after a fracture; thus a conservative approach is usually indicated. Functional therapy is adequate if the resultant malocclusion is minimal, but a brief period of immobilization is necessary if a significant malocclusion is present. In either situation, long-term follow-up is necessary for observation of growth disturbances. This is in marked contrast to adults, in whom remodeling potential is less and the concern for growth disturbances is not important.

A variety of techniques have been available in the past to treat adult patients, but open reductions have gained popularity with the advent of rigid fixation. The plates may be placed using extraoral and intraoral approaches. Extraoral approaches include submandibular, preauricular, and postauricular techniques. These methods have been widely described in the use of wire osteosynthesis. However, an intraoral approach is possible with the use of rigid fixation. In this chapter, we present a brief review of pertinent anatomy, diagnosis, indications for open reduction, and selection of surgical approach. We then describe the treatment of subcondylar fractures with rigid fixation using an intraoral approach and a modification of the extraoral approach.

ANATOMY

The anatomy of the mandibular condyle and neck is relatively simple, but an understanding of important anatomical relationships and the functional aspects of the associated temporomandibular joint are important in diagnosis and treatment. The mandible consists of the tooth-bearing portion and the ramus, which extends upward from the mandibular angle. The mandibular angle and ramus provide attachment for the masseter muscle laterally and the medial pterygoid muscle medially. The ramus of the mandible extends superiorly to form two processes, the condylar and coronoid. The coronoid process is the superior extension of the anterior border of the ramus. Flattened in a medial lateral direction, it provides insertion along its medial, lateral, and anterior surfaces for the temporalis muscle. The superior extension of the posterior border of the ramus is the condylar process, which consists of the condylar neck and the condyle. The condyle is lengthened in a medial lateral direction; its longest dimension is approximately 1 to 2 cm. In contrast, the condyle is narrow in its anterior posterior dimension, but is curved slightly anterior in a spoonlike fashion. The long axis of the condyle is directed posteriorly and medially, such that a line drawn through its long axis would intersect a similar line from the opposite condyle at the anterior border of the foramen magnum. The condylar neck, which supports the condyle, contains a depression on its anterior aspect for the insertion of the lateral pterygoid muscle. This depression is often referred to as the pterygoid fovea. Unilateral contraction of the lateral pterygoid muscle moves the mandibular condyle inferiorly and anteriorly along the articular eminence, resulting in the mandible deviating to the opposite side. Bilateral contraction of the lateral pterygoid muscles, in conjunction with contraction of the suprahyoid muscles, causes the mouth to open (see Figure 17.1). The notch between the condylar and coronoid processes is most commonly referred to as the sigmoid notch, but may also be called the mandibular notch.

Several vascular relationships to the condylar process are important if hemorrhage is to be avoided. The nerves and blood supply to the masseter muscle pass through the sigmoid notch to enter the muscle on its posterior aspect, a relationship that may result in hemorrhage if the dissection of this area does not remain subperiosteal. Additionally, posterior to the ramus is the upper portion of the external carotid artery, which gives off the maxillary artery that courses medial to the condylar neck. The maxillary artery gives off the middle meningeal artery, which courses superiorly on the medial aspect of the condylar neck and condyle (see Figure 17.2). Thus control of the depth of medial penetration with drilling instruments is important when screw holes are placed in the condylar neck.

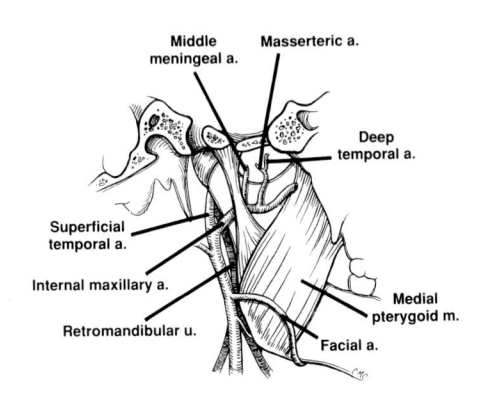

Figure 17.2 The important vascular relationships to the condylar neck are illustrated in this medial view. Note the positions of the maxillary, masseteric, and middle meningeal arteries.

The condyle is enclosed in a capsule, usually referred to as the capsule of the temporomandibular joint. The capsule attaches superiorly to the circumference of the articular fossa and eminence of the temporomandibular joint and inferiorly blends with the periosteum of the condylar neck. The capsule is thin and loose, except along its lateral side, where it is thickened to form the temporomandibular ligament. The capsule is more likely to rupture on the weaker medial aspect, thus resulting in medial displacement of the condyle when the condylar neck is fractured.

The temporomandibular joint also contains an articular disc composed of dense fibrous connective tissue. This disc is thicker at its periphery, where it is attached to the joint capsule; but it also is firmly and independently attached to the condyle at the condyle's medial and lateral poles. This allows the disc to move with the condyle during function but may also result in injury the disc from condylar displacement associated with fractures.

DIAGNOSIS

Diagnosis of mandibular subcondylar fractures depends on adequate history, physical findings, and radiographic confirmation. The mechanism of injury should alert one to the possibility of this type of fracture. A history of a blow to the side of the mandible should lead one to suspect a subcondylar fracture on the contralateral side. This type of injury often is associated with a concomitant parasymphysis fracture on the side of the blow (see Figure 17.3). Another common pattern occurs when a direct blow to the chin is sustained, resulting in bilateral subcondylar fractures (see Figure 17.4). Additionally, when massive facial trauma is sustained, a subcondylar fracture should always be suspected and must be ruled out with appropriate examination and radiographic studies.

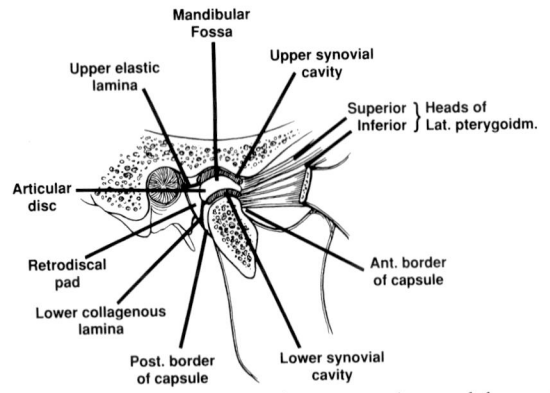

Figure 17.1 The muscular attachments to the condylar neck and mandibular ramus. The lateral pterygoid muscles attach to the condylar neck. Bilateral contraction of these muscles, in conjunction with contraction of the suprahyoid muscles, moves the condyle inferiorly and anteriorly, opening the mouth.

Open Reduction and Rigid Fixation of Subcondylar Fractures

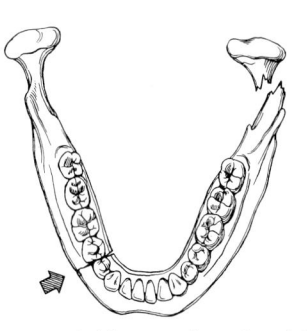

Figure 17.3 A blow to the side of the mandible often results in a contralateral subcondylar fracture and an ipsilateral parasymphysis fracture.

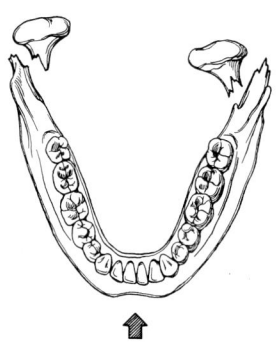

Figure 17.4 A direct blow to the chin often results in bilateral subcondylar fractures.

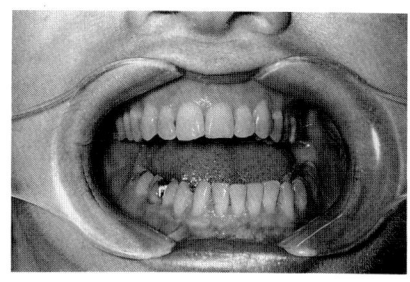

Figure 17.5 The mandible deviates to the side of the fracture when the mouth is opened.

Physical examination should concentrate on evaluation of the range of mandibular motion because the position of the condylar neck makes direct palpation of a fracture difficult. When a subcondylar fracture is present, the mandible will deviate to the side of the fracture when the mouth is opened (see Figure 17.5). The fracture prevents effective function of the lateral pterygoid muscle, and the condyle is not advanced along the articular eminence (see Figure 17.6). The unopposed action of the contralateral lateral pterygoid muscle causes the mandible to deviate to the injured side. However the patient must be able to open the mouth enough usually more than about 15 millimeters, to demonstrate that a deviation is present. If the patient is unable to open the mouth because of pain or trismus, the loss of lateral pterygoid function will result in the inability to shift the mandible to the opposite side of the fracture with the mouth in a closed position. The patient will be able to shift the mandible to the affected side because the unfractured side will be advanced normally by the functioning lateral pterygoid muscle (see Figure 17.7).

Bilateral subcondylar fractures may cause a complex of symptoms from the telescoping of the fractured segments. The contraction of the masseter and medial pterygoid muscles pulls the ramus superiorly, shortening the ramus at the fracture site; and contraction of the suprahyoid muscles pulls the distal mandibular segment inferiorly and posteriorly. This causes lengthening of the anterior face, anterior open bite, and a receded chin. The patient will be unable to produce normal occlusion of the dentition because of the lose of structural integrity of the mandible. With unilateral fractures, the same mechanism—telescoping of the fracture segments—may result in premature contact of the dentition on the affected side, with the appearance of an open bite anteriorly on the opposite side.

Other possible findings when a subcondylar fracture is present include edema and tenderness over the temporomandibular joint. However, this is a nospecific finding and may occur with concomitant contusion of the temporomandibular joint soft tissues. Additionally, the external auditory canal should be inspected for ecchymosis or laceration, which may have resulted from posterior displacement of the condyle.

Radiographic evaluation should include a modified Towne's projection, right and left lateral oblique views, lateral and anterior-posterior views of the mandible (see Figures 17.8–17.10). A panoramic radiograph may be more useful than the lateral and oblique mandibular projections. Fracture lines, fracture dis-

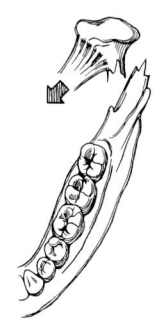

Figure 17.6 The subcondylar fracture occurs below the attachment of the lateral pterygoid muscle, thus preventing movement of the mandible.

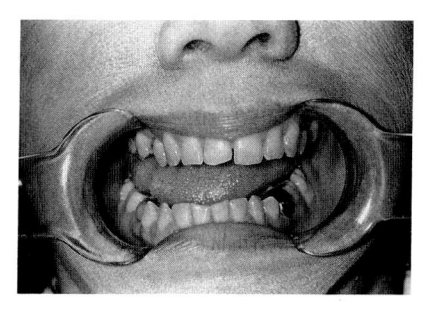

Figure 17.7 The patient will be able to shift the mandible only to the side of the fracture.

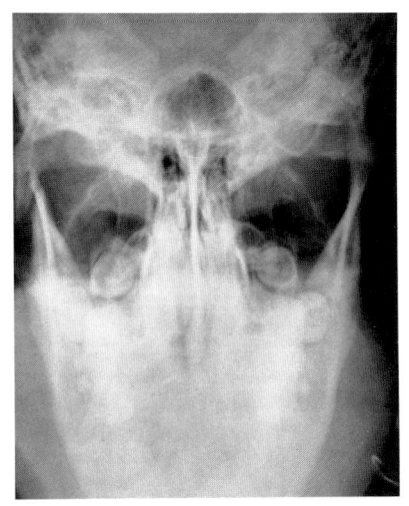

Figure 17.8 A Towne's projection showing a subcondylar fracture.

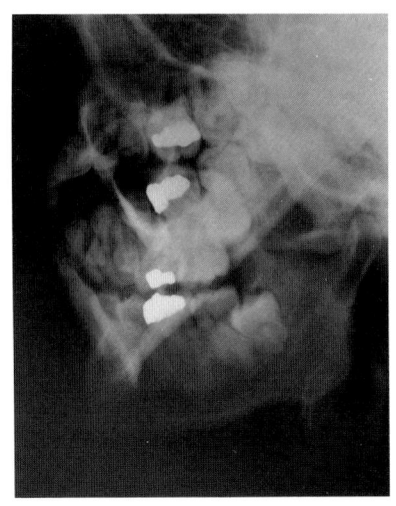

Figure 17.9 A lateral oblique radiograph showing a subcondylar fracture.

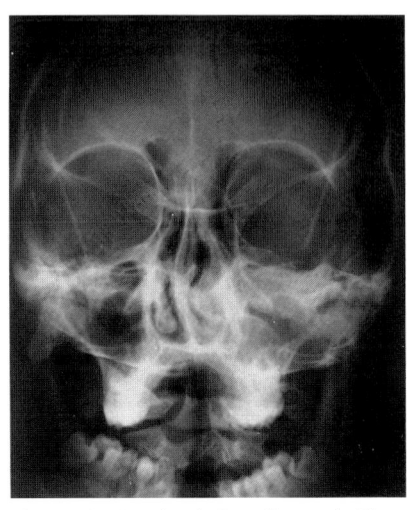

Figure 17.10 An A-P radiograph illustrating a subcondylar fracture.

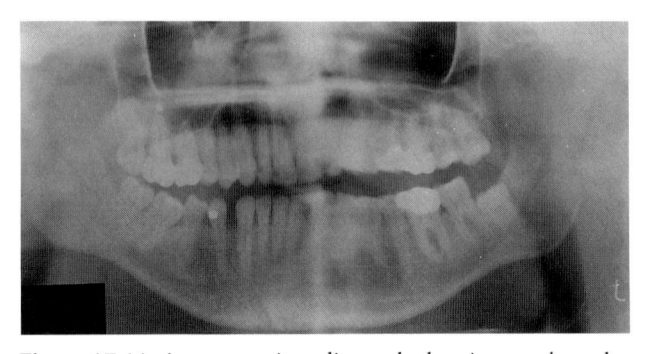

Figure 17.11 A panoramic radiograph showing a subcondylar fracture. This fracture is evidenced by the anterior angulation of the condylar neck, as compared with the opposite side.

placement, and overlapping of the fracture segments should be searched for on each radiograph. The only indication of a subcondylar fracture may be an anterior angulation of the condylar neck evident on the oblique, lateral, or panoramic radiograph (see Figure 17.11). This is due to the overlapping and anterior displacement at the fracture line. The modified Towne's view will frequently demonstrate medial angulation of the condyle. CT scans can precisely define the status of the condyle and its relation to the fossa.

TREATMENT

Indications

The indications for open reduction of subcondylar fractures are the same for both intraoral and extraoral approaches. Some authors have listed absolute and relative indications for open reduction of subcondylar fractures; however, the decision to perform an open reduction should be made for each patient individually.

Findings where an open reduction should be considered include the following:

1. the inability to obtain an adequate dental occlusion by closed reduction;
2. interference of mandibular movement by a displaced segment;
3. open facial wounds with exposure of the condyle or a foreign body in the temporomandibular joint;
4. subcondylar fractures associated with panfacial fractures requiring reestablishment of posterior vertical facial height;
5. subcondylar fractures in an edentulous patient where a splint is unavailable or impossible to use secondary to atrophic bone loss;
6. patients with medical conditions such as seizure disorders, substance abuse, neurologic injury, mental retardation, or psychiatric illness, where MMF may complicate the underlying condition;
7. fractures with unstable occlusions secondary to dentofacial deformities, periodontal disease, loss of teeth, and active orthodontics; and
8. any other patient in whom early function is indicated for medical-dental reasons or is desired by the patient.

Selection of Surgical Approach

When an open reduction is indicated, selection of an appropriate surgical approach is based on the ease of surgical access. One should radiographically evaluate the position of the fracture. A fracture that exits the posterior border of the ramus inferior to the sigmoid notch is amenable to rigid fixation with an intraoral approach (see Figure 17.12). The more inferior the po-

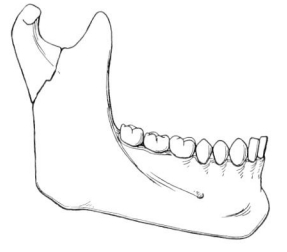

Figure 17.12 A fracture exiting the posterior border of the ramus at a level inferior to the level of the sigmoid notch may be amenable to the intraoral approach.

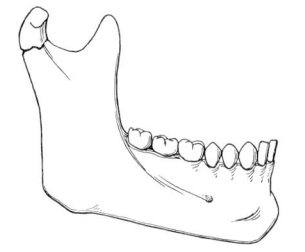

Figure 17.13 A fracture exiting the posterior border superior to the level of the sigmoid notch is best approached extraorally.

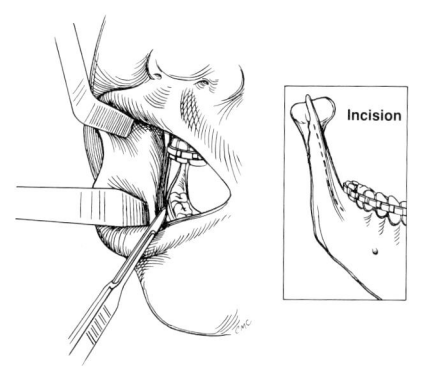

Figure 17.14 The intraoral incision and exposure for approaching the condylar neck.

sition of the fracture, the easier access will be for application of the fixation with this approach. The intraoral approach has the advantages of virtually eliminating a facial scar, minimizing injury to the facial nerve, and allowing the operator to observe the dental occlusion while placing the fixation. Direct observation of the occlusion may help prevent malocclusions that are produced during application of the fixation; however, the intraoral approach is more technically demanding than the extraoral approach. A fracture requiring an open reduction that exits the posterior border superior to the sigmoid notch may best be treated with an extraoral approach (see Figure 17.13), because access via an intraoral approach may be poor. The extraoral approach has the disadvantages of producing a facial scar and possible injury to the facial nerve.

Intraoral Approach

We describe the intraoral approach first and in detail. Utilizing general anesthesia, the procedure is begun with injection of local anesthetic with a vasoconstrictor into the medial and lateral regions of the mandibular ramus. While vasoconstriction is taking place, maxillary and mandibular arch bars are placed. It is recommended that all the teeth be incorporated by the arch bars, including the incisors. An incision is made through the soft tissue and the periosteum overlying the external oblique ridge (see Figure 17.14). The lateral aspect of the ramus is then exposed so that the entire lateral surface from the sigmoid notch to the angle is visualized. It is important to release the periosteum overlying the posterior and inferior borders of the ramus and the angle region to allow good access. This can be accomplished by stripping the attachments of the masseter with a J stripper. A fiberoptic retractor* is inserted to expose the fracture site. If the coronoid

process flares laterally, obscuring vision, an osteotomy is made that allows the coronoid process to be retracted medially. This is rarely necessary. If the condyle is displaced medially, a Kocher clamp or a periosteal elevator is used to manipulate the condyle laterally. Condyles that are displaced laterally can be similarly manipulated, usually without much difficulty.

Once the condyle is in a reduced position, the patient is placed into MMF. Occasionally, medially displaced fractures will not maintain a reduced position secondary to muscle pull. In this situation the condyle can be held in a reduced position by placing the patient tightly into MMF on the contralateral side and loosely on the ipsilateral side of the fracture. A towel clamp is then placed percutaneously at the mandibular angle on the fractured side to provide inferior traction of the mandible. With traction, the medially displaced condylar process can be manipulated laterally until it is seated in the articular fossa. After the condyle is seated in the articular fossa, it can be maintained in the reduced position by tightening the MMF on the side of the fracture.

Adequate MMF is important while using rigid fixation. Placement of the bone plate may produce shifts of the bony fragments when the bone is pulled to the bone plate during placement of the screws. This can occur if the tooth-bearing fragment of bone is not adequately stabilized with MMF. Minor shifts during screw placement may produce major malocclusions postoperatively, but this can be minimized by tight MMF as well as direct observation of the dental occlusion during plate and screw application.

Once the condyle is in the articular fossa, the modified LeVasseur-Merrill retractor can be used to engage the posterior border of the condylar neck (see Figure 17.15). Next, a small trocar* is inserted percutaneously through the preauricular region over the fracture. Using a 0.062-inch threaded Kirschner wire or a 1.5-millimeter drill through the trocar and copious saline irrigation, a screw hole is placed through the

---
*Available from Walter Lorenz Surgical Instrument Company, Jacksonville, Fl.

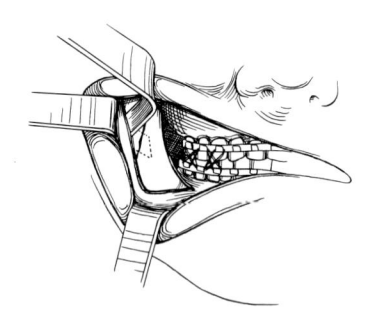

Figure 17.15 The condylar fracture is reduced in the articular fossa, and its position is maintained with the modified LeVasseur-Merrill retractor. (Jeter et al. 1988.)

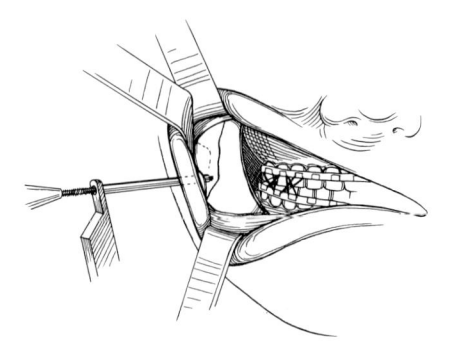

Figure 17.16 The screw holes are drilled percutaneously. The first screw hole is placed in the proximal fragment 3 to 4 mm superior to the fracture. (Jeter et al. 1988.)

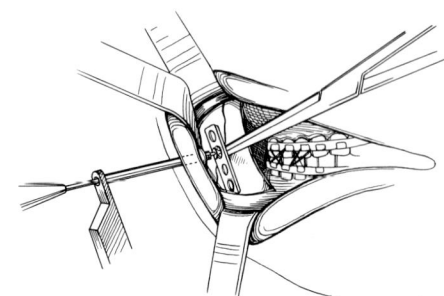

Figure 17.17 The bone plate and screw are held with a clamp as a single unit; the screw is placed and tightened percutaneously. (Jeter et al. 1988.)

proximal fragment 3 to 4 mm superior to the fracture, just anterior to the posterior border of the condylar neck and ramus, where the bone is thickest (see Figure 17.16). The modified LeVasseur-Merrill retractor may be used to provide stabilization of the condylar fragment during placement of the screw. The depth of the screw hole is measured and recorded with a depth gauge* inserted through the trocar and bone. A minifragment 2-millimeter dynamic compression bone plate is then adapted across the fracture parallel with the posterior border of the ramus and neck of the condylar process. A plate that will provide holes for at least two screws, and preferably three, in each segment should be selected. Care should be taken not to place the bone plate too far anteriorly because the bone is thin beneath the sigmoid notch. One must also be cognizant of the pathway of the inferior alveolar nerve, which can be located on the radiographs. Occasionally, the condylar process will not stay passively in an upright position, but will remain in a slightly medial position. When this occurs, the bone plate can be contoured so that the fractured segment will be in a reduced anatomic position when the plate is screwed into place.

After the bone plate has been contoured, a modified right-angle clamp* is used to grasp the plate, insert it, and check its adaptation. Next, a 2-millimeter-diameter screw of appropriate length is inserted in one of the central holes in the bone plate, and the screw-holding clamp* is applied to the screw on the internal surface of the plate (see Figure 17.17). Then the plate and screw are taken intraorally and positioned over the screw hole in the proximal fragment close to the fracture. A small screwdriver is inserted through the trocar, and the screw is placed in the screw hole and tightened slightly. The plate should still be loose enough that it can be rotated into proper alignment.

A second screw hole is then offset drilled in the distal fragment through one of the holes in the bone plate, and a screw is placed securely but not tightly. The other holes in the bone plate are now offset drilled with a 0.062-inch threaded Kirschner wire or a 1.5-millimeter drill. Offset holes are drilled in the plate away from the fracture so that when the screws are tightened some compression can take place. When the superior holes are drilled in the proximal fragment, there is a tendency to drill them with a slightly superior angulation because the tissue cannot be retracted laterally near the condyle. If a long screw is placed in the most superior hole, it can perforate the articular surface. To avoid this, a short, 6- or 8-millimeter, screw may be used. When the bone plate is placed and the superior holes are drilled, an additional retractor often can help to retract the tissue that is in close proximity to the condyle superiorly. The remaining screws are now inserted (as previously described) and tightened. The two previously placed screws are also tightened. The final position of the plate should be parallel to the posterior border of the condylar neck and ramus (see Figure 17.18).

MMF is removed, and the dental occlusion is checked to make certain that there are no discrepancies. If a coronoidectomy has been done for access, the co-

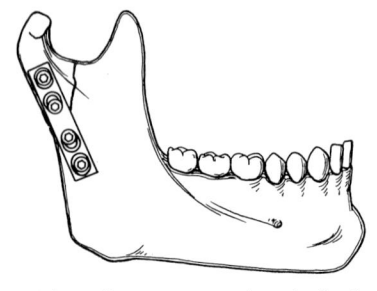

Figure 17.18 After all screws are placed, the bone plate should be parallel to the posterior border of the condylar neck and ramus.

---

*Available from Walter Lorenz Surgical Instrument Company, Jacksonville, Fl.

Open Reduction and Rigid Fixation of Subcondylar Fractures 215

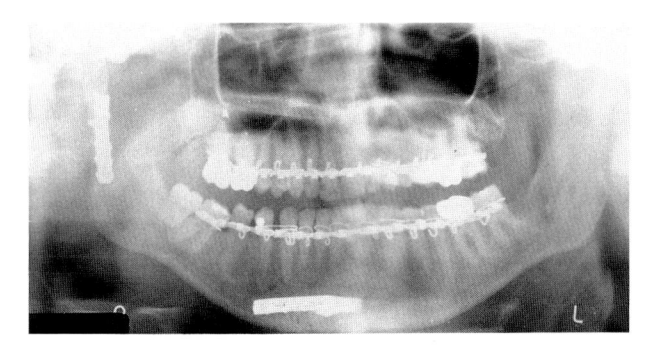

Figure 17.19 Postoperative radiograph.

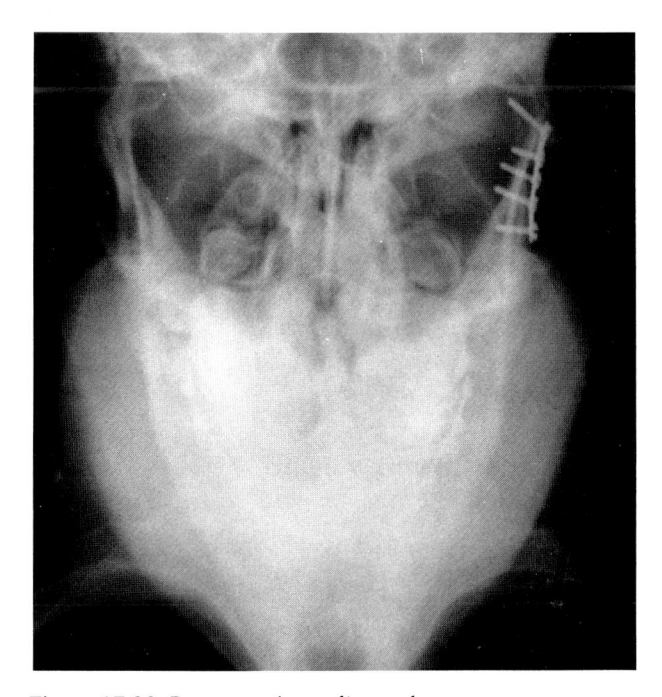

Figure 17.20 Postoperative radiograph.

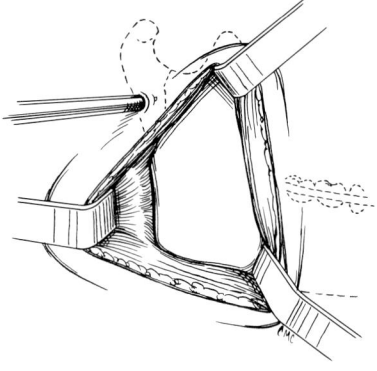

Figure 17.21 The extraoral approach via a submandibular incision is illustrated. The holes are drilled and the screwdriver is used through the trocar, as in the intraoral approach. The plate and screws are manipulated into position via submandibular incision.

ronoid process may remain medially displaced. It can be repositioned laterally into alignment and plated in a similar fashion, but this usually is not necessary.

After the operation is completed, the wound is irrigated with sterile saline solution and closed in two layers (periosteum and mucosa) with 3-0 chromic continuous sutures. Two training elastics are placed bilaterally to guide the patient's occlusion while functioning during the early postoperative period. During this period a transient slight opening of the posterior occlusion of the ipsilateral side can be expected due to edema in the joint. A pressure dressing is placed over the mandibular ramus. A drain is not necessary. Postoperative radiographs are obtained to evaluate the reduction, alignment, and placement of the bone plate and screws (see Figures 17.19 and 17.20). The patient is started on a liquid diet immediately, but allowed to progress to a soft mechanical diet within a few days after surgery. Within the first few days after surgery, the patient is encouraged to use passive range-of-motion exercises.

Extraoral Approaches

If open reduction is required and the transoral approach would be difficult due to the superior location of the fracture (see Figure 17.13), the fracture can be approached by a posteriorly placed submandibular incision. MMF is applied before the incision is made. The fracture is reduced and the plate is adapted through the submandibular incision, but a trocar is inserted percutaneously in the preauricular region over the fracture. The holes are drilled and the screw driver is used through the trocar as in the intraoral approach; the plate and screws are manipulated into position via submandibular incision (see Figure 17.21). It may be necessary to re-enter the oral cavity to loosen the MMF on the side of the fracture to assist in maintaining reduction of the fracture, as described in the intraoral approach. Also, it may be necessary to place an instrument or finger on the medial side of the ramus to manipulate a medially displaced fracture into the operative site for reduction. After the bone plate is secure, the MMF is removed and the occlusion is evaluated before the incision is closed. Postoperative diet and physiotherapy are the same as with the intraoral approach. Other extraoral approaches are the preauricular and postauricular, in which the bone plate can be applied directly without use of the trocar. These approaches often must be combined with the submandibular approach for adequate access. In this situation the use of the trocar obviates the need for a second incision in addition to the submandibular incision.

COMPLICATIONS

Complications with open reduction of subcondylar fractures by an intraoral approach have been limited. Postoperative occlusal discrepancies have occasionally been noted. These can be minimized by application of tight MMF during placement of the bone plates and by

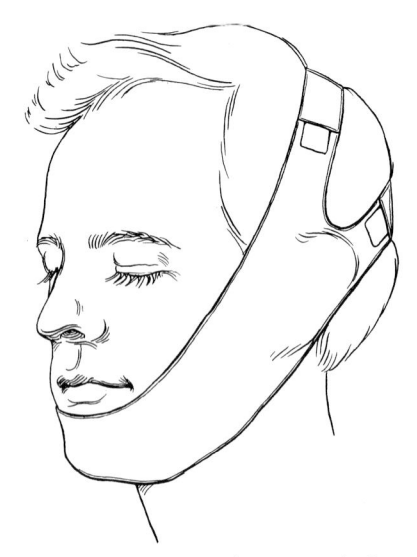

Figure 17.22 The postoperative dressing, which applies pressure over the mandibular ramus, should be left in place for 24 to 48 hours.

anatomic adaptation of the plates. Minor occlusal abnormalities can be corrected with judicial use of light elastics, but more severe discrepancies may require occlusal adjustment or reoperation. Dehiscence of the intraoral incision may also occur. This usually does not require removal of the bone plates and can be managed with frequent wound irrigation until the incision heals. One episode of postoperative wound hematoma has been noted. The hematoma, in the area of the masseter muscle, was managed with antibiotics, aspiration, and application of a pressure dressing. This underscores the importance of keeping the dissection subperiosteal to avoid hemorrhage, of maintaining adequate hemostasis before closure, and of using a postoperative pressure dressing, which is left in place for 24 to 48 hours (see Figure 17.22). One patient sustained a transient facial nerve injury that resolved in a few weeks. Significant injuries to the parotid gland, auriculotemporal nerve, superficial temporal artery, transverse facial artery, middle meningeal artery, or masseteric artery have not been noted.

LONG-TERM RESULTS

Results with this method of treatment of subcondylar fractures, for as long as five years, have revealed few problems. Problems such as limited opening interfering with function, occlusal shifts, late arthritic changes, dysfunction, and deformity such as asymmetry and open bite have been previously noted. Even though such problems have been noted with closed reductions, only continued assessment of rigid fixation will reveal if these problems occur less with open reductions.

BIBLIOGRAPHY

Bradley PF: Injuries of the condylar and coronoid process. In Maxillofacial Injuries, Vol 1. Rowe NL, Williams JL (eds). New York, Churchill Livingstone, 1985, pp 337–362.

Brown AE, Obeid G: A simplified method for the internal fixation of fractures of the mandibular condyle. Br J Oral Maxillofac Surg 22:145–150, 1978.

Chuong R, Piper MA: Open reduction of condylar fractures of the mandible in conjunction with repair of discal injury: A preliminary report. J Oral Maxillofac Surg 46:257–263, 1988.

Gerlock AJ, McBride KL, Sinn DP: Clinical and Radiographic Interpretation of Facial Fractures. Boston, Little, Brown 1981.

Hollinshead WH: Anatomy for Surgeons. Vol 1: The Head and Neck. Philadelphia, Harper and Row, 1982.

Hoopes JE, Wolfort FG, Jabaley ME: Operative treatment of fractures of the mandibular condyle in children using the post-auricular approach. Plast Reconstr Surg 46:357–362, 1970.

Jeter TS, Van Sickels JE, Nishioka GJ: Intraoral open reduction with rigid internal fixation of mandibular subcondylar fractures. J Oral Maxillofac Surg 46:1113–1116, 1988.

Koberg WR, Momma W-G: Treatment of fractures of the articular process by functional stable osteosynthesis using miniaturized dynamic compression plates. Int J Oral Surg 7:256–262, 1978.

Peters RA, Caldwell JB, Olsen TW: A technique for open reduction of subcondylar fractures. Oral Surg Oral Med Oral Path 41:273–280, 1976.

Robinson R, Yoon C: New onlay-inlay metal splint for immobilization of mandibular subcondylar fractures. Am J Surg 100:845–849, 1960.

Schule H: Injuries of the temporomandibular joint. In Oral and Maxillofacial Traumatology, Vol. 2. Kruger E, Schilli W (eds). Chicago, Quintessence, 1986, pp 45–101.

Walker RV: Traumatic mandibular condylar fracture dislocations: Effect on growth in the Macaca rhesus monkey. Am J Surg 100:850–863, 1960.

Zide MF, Kent JN: Indications for open reduction of mandibular condyle fractures. J Oral Maxillofac Surg 41:89–98, 1983.

CHAPTER 18

Complications of Rigid Internal Fixation of the Mandible

Joseph S. Gruss

Many simple mandibular fractures can be managed by conventional techniques with maxillomandibular fixation (MMF). Rigid internal fixation of the mandible using plates and screws has brought a new dimension to the treatment of more complex mandibular fractures. The indications, both relative and absolute, have been well defined: Their use in the polytrauma patient, with associated midfacial fractures and when the mandible is edentulous or comminuted, or has segmental fractures and bone loss, have revolutionized the care of these patients, who were previously very difficult to manage. The advantages of the immediate or early release of MMF following completion of fixation—for patient management and temporomandibular joint function—have been extensively delineated. However, as with any new surgical procedure, this procedure offers many potential disadvantages.

The surgeon beginning to use internal fixation must understand that complications occurring with internal fixation will invariably be much worse than with conventional techniques. All the systems currently on the market are so well designed and engineered that rarely, if ever, does a failure of the system cause complications. Poor or inadequate results and complications invariably are due to operator error. As with any new technique, the operator must be fully versed in both the theoretical and the practical aspects of internal fixation. The surgeon must recognize the difficulty inherent in these techniques and the fact that proper internal fixation of a complex mandibular fracture is one of the most challenging procedures in maxillofacial surgery. The correct incisions and surgical approaches must be used in combination with a thorough understanding of the basic and applied principles of internal fixation, together with the ability and training to use the sophisticated equipment properly.

Notwithstanding, complications, failures and errors may still occur due to poor patient selection, poor selection of the correct technique, or improper application of techniques. In this chapter we define in a practical manner the reasons mistakes are made and how they can be avoided, based on long-term combined experience with many cases of both use and abuse of internal fixation.

COMPLICATIONS AND TECHNICAL PROBLEMS

Complications are invariably due to technical errors. A proper and thorough understanding of the information in this chapter will reduce the likelihood of failures and complications.

Incisions/Exposure

Intraoral placement of most mandibular plates is the standard for which most surgeons should aim in the evolution and refinement of their technical expertise in care of mandibular fractures. Intraoral exposure and placement of plates on the anterior mandible is relatively simple as long as the inferior alveolar nerve and tooth roots are avoided. Although intraoral placement for the ramus, angle, and posterior body can be performed without an external scar and without risk of damage to the marginal mandibular branch of the facial nerve, the inherent technical difficulties in performing these techniques may result in disastrous complications. The surgeon may have difficulty in appreciating the exact configuration of the fracture, and it may be extremely difficult to reduce and maintain reduction of the fracture while the plate is contoured, because of lack of access and the inability to use the standard bone-reduction appliances currently available. Drilling and screw placement, usually done through a trocar placed through an external stab incision, may be difficult, and it is easy to place the plate in the wrong position in relation to the lower border of the mandible, the inferior alveolar nerve, or the fracture itself. Intraoral placement of plates in the posterior mandible should be used only when the surgeon has become fully experienced with the extraoral placement of plates. Only then will the inherent difficulties and potential errors of intraoral plating be appreciated.

Intraoral plating of posterior fractures should be reserved—even in experienced hands—for the relatively simple fracture (commonly angle or posterior body fracture). Comminuted or segmental fractures or fractures with bone loss should be exposed through the external incisions to facilitate adequate exposure, reduction, and fixation. In addition, fractures in the edentulous mandible should be exposed through a small external incision to minimize the degree of periosteal dissection. Intraoral exposure always requires more extensive subperiosteal dissection of bone, and this may be extremely detrimental to the healing of the fracture in the thin edentulous mandible.

Maxillo-Mandibular Fixation

The application of MMF with the patient in the correct premorbid dental occlusion, *prior* to bending and applying the plate, is essential in *all* cases except in the treatment of the edentulous maxilla or mandible. There is a great tendency, particularly with the inexperienced surgeon, to assume that if seemingly perfect anatomical reduction is obtained at the fracture site, the occlusion must be correct. However, at surgery, only the reduction of the buccal cortex is visualized in one plane, and potential distraction of the fracture on the lingual side as well as minor degrees of rotation may exist. Once the plate has been applied, it is impossible to adjust the occlusion. Postoperative orthodontics can compensate only with dental movement and cannot alter the position of bone segments held rigidly in the wrong position by plates and screws. The MMF is released only when the plates and screws have been applied.

Positioning the Condyles

Proper positioning of the mandibular condyles in the glenoid fossa has become an important consideration with the use of rigid internal fixation in orthognathic surgery. Failure to seat the condyles properly will often result in malocclusion, usually with an anterior open bite deformity, once the MMF is removed after internal fixation is completed. Similar problems can arise with the treatment of mandibular fractures, particularly when associated with midfacial fractures of the Le Fort type. Seemingly correct occlusion can be established with the condyles usually pulled in an inferior and anterior direction, due to rotation of the mandible forward and upward to meet the fractured maxilla. If the maxillary buttresses and mandibular fractures are then rigidly plated, this position of the mandible is maintained until the MMF is released at the end of the procedure. As soon as this is done, the muscles of mastication pull the condyles back into their proper position in the fossa, causing malocclusion and an anterior open-bite deformity. This can be avoided by repositioning the condyles in the glenoid fossa with gentle upward and forward traction before and during the application of the maxillary and mandibular plates.

Plate Contouring

Once the fracture has been exposed, MMF has been applied, and the fracture has been reduced, the correct plate is chosen and adapted to fit *passively* to the contours of the mandible, using specially designed bending instruments. This is one of the most critical steps in ensuring success; the plate must be accurately and meticulously bent. If the plate is not bent accurately, the underlying bone will be pulled toward the plate, causing a corresponding shift at the occlusal level.

One of the problems in obtaining accurate fixation at the fracture site is that only the reduction at the anterior or buccal cortex is visualized. Seemingly adequate reduction of the buccal cortex may be accompanied by distraction of the posterior or lingual cortex; this distraction will not be appreciated until the patient presents later with an occlusal disharmony. If compression osteosynthesis is used as the buccal cortex is compressed the distraction of the lingual cortex may be increased. This complication is prevented by *controlled overbending* of the plate. After the plate is perfectly and passively adapted, it is slightly overbent; and as the plate is compressed against the underlying bone surface as screws are inserted, the slight overbending causes closure and compression of the lingual fracture gap (see Figure 18.1). Failure to take the time and trouble to bend the thicker and stronger mandibular plates accurately is one of the most common causes of complications in rigid fixation of the mandible.

Plate Length

The success of rigid internal fixation of the mandible depends on the strength of the fixation being greater than the functional forces acting on the mandible. Increased strength is produced by a stronger plate, a longer plate with more screws, compression across the

Complications of Internal Fixation of the Mandible 219

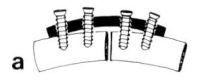

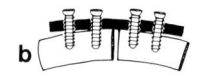

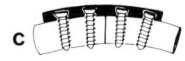

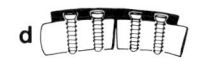

Figure 18.1 On the right, the plate has been inadequately adapted to the contour of the bone. As the screws are driven into the bone, the bone is pulled towards the plate thus causing a distraction at the distal cortex. On the left side, with controlled overbending as the screws are inserted into the bone, there is compression across both the proximal and the distal cortices as the plate is compressed against the bone itself.

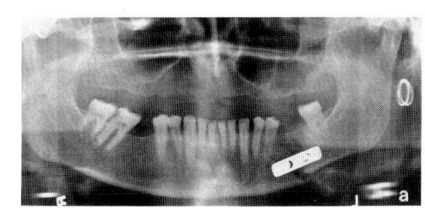

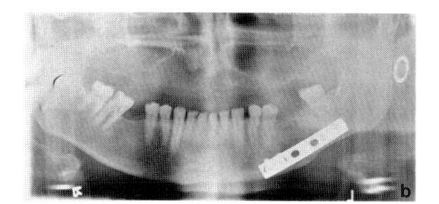

Figure 18.2 (a) Oblique unstable left-body fracture with inadequate dentition. Too short a plate has been used, and the inner two screws have been placed too close to the fracture site. This provides inadequate stability for this unstable fracture, and eventually the inner two screws will loosen, causing an unstable situation and a nonunion. (b) Removing the short plate, applying a longer plate, and placing the screws away from the fracture site results in mechanical stability. This stability overcomes the forces of mastication, and so the bone can heal normally.

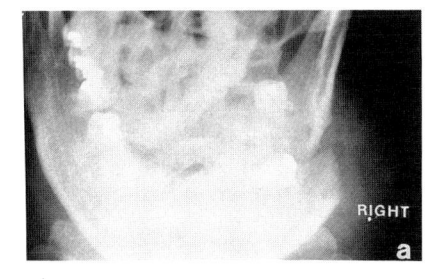

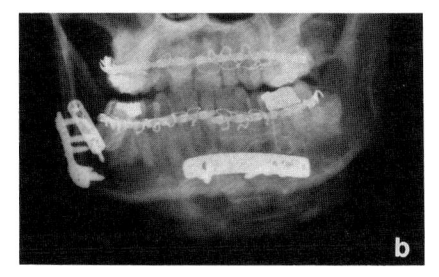

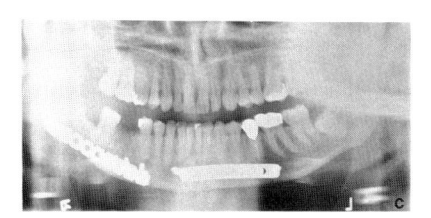

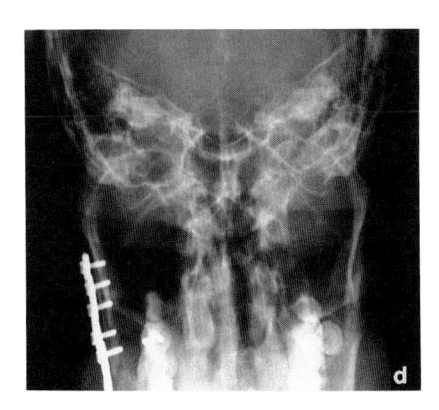

Figure 18.3 (a) A very unstable displaced right-angle fracture with some comminution in combination with a displaced and unstable parasymphyseal fracture. (b) This unstable fracture has been repaired with a short four-hole compression plate at the inferior border of the mandible and a miniplate at the upper border, acting as a tension band. Inadequate fixation and stability of the right angle caused the plate to loosen, necessitating the removal of these plates. (c) Restabilization with a long, curved reconstruction plate placing at least 3 screws in each side of the fracture site. In displaced and unstable angle fractures, use of at least three screws on either side of the fracture site is important. The loss of fixation of just one screw on either side will result in an unstable situation. (d) Fixation at the upper aspect of the plate through the ramus with five screws. Note that all five of these screws are placed through both cortices.

fracture site, and the use of multiple plates. Care must be taken to choose a plate of correct length. A minimum of two screws on each side of the fracture is necessary to control rotation and to ensure adequate stability. In addition, if a short plate with only two screws is used, compression across the fracture site is necessary to counteract functional forces. A short four-hole plate should be used only in a relatively simple, uncomminuted transverse fracture with good apposition of the bone ends. When the fracture is less stable and has obliquity or sagittal splitting of the inner and outer bone cortices at the fracture site, a longer plate is needed. The screws should be placed away from the fracture site to produce a longer lever arm and to increase the mechanical advantage across the fracture site. In addition, with obliquity or sagittal splitting at the fracture site, the screws closest to the fracture site in a short plate may purchase only one cortex. Loosening of this screw will result in inadequate fixation, plate loosening, and failure of repair. In a more unstable oblique fracture, especially if there is any comminution or segmentation at the fracture site, it is always safer to use a longer plate with at least three screws on either side of the fracture site. If one screw loosens, the remaining two screws will usually be adequate to maintain sufficient stability across the fracture site to allow uncomplicated healing. The use of a plate that is too short with screws placed too close to the fracture site is one of the most common causes of failure of internal fixation (see Figures 18.2–18.5).

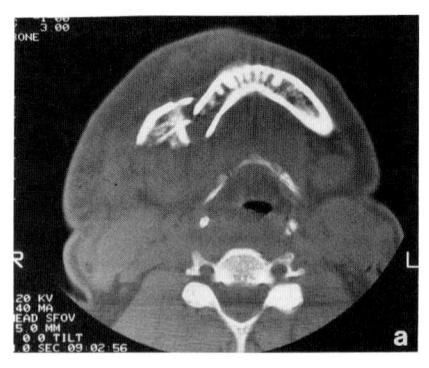

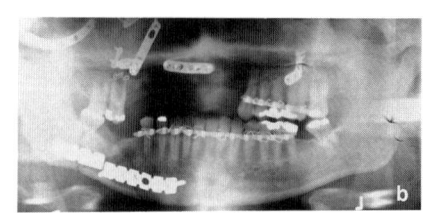

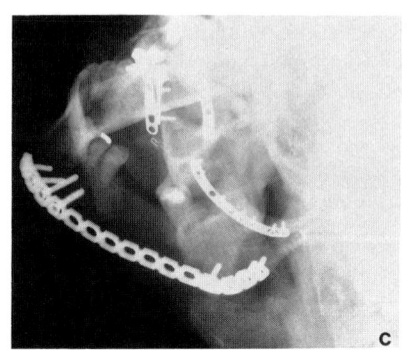

Figure 18.4 (a) This axial CT scan through the mandible shows markedly comminuted segmental and displaced fractures of the right body and angle of the mandible associated with comminuted midfacial fractures. (b) The two separate areas of fracturing of the right body were repaired with two separate short reconstruction plates. An insufficient number of screws are placed on either side of each fracture site, and a weak area will form at the junction between the two plates. The bone between the two plates will eventually refracture, and both plates will become loose. (c) The two plates have been removed, and a long reconstruction plate has been applied. Fixation is performed at the stable bone outside the area of fracturing on either side with a minimum of four screws on either side. In a situation with multiple segmental fractures, bridging across the area of segmentation and comminution and using at least four screws on either end (the four-screw rule) are essential.

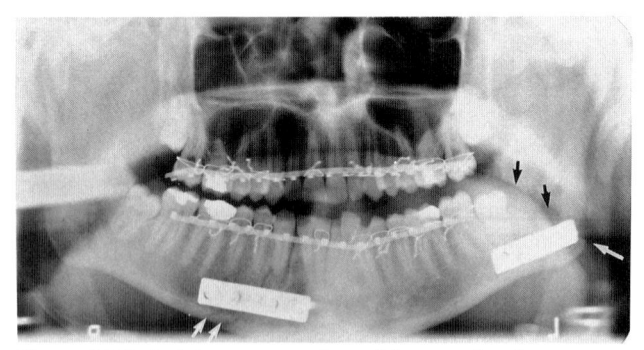

Figure 18.5 A right parasymphyseal fracture has been repaired with a short four-hole compression plate. Note the area of segmentation at the inferior border of the mandible; this indicates marked instability of this fracture. On the left angle, a short plate has been placed in the wrong position—the most posterior screw was placed right through the fracture site. This fracture was inadequately fixed and therefore mobile. Thus the fixation of the right parasymphyseal fracture will loosen, due to the fact that only two screws were placed on either side of an unstable fracture. Both plates in this instance were too short. The parasymphyseal fracture should have been repaired with a six-hole plate, and the angle fracture should have been repaired with a curved six-hole plate or a curved reconstruction plate; at least three holes should have been placed on either side of the fracture.

Incorrect Plate

It is important not only to choose the correct length of plate and number of screws but also to use the correct plates—that is, those designed for *mandibular* rigid fixation. Specific, strong mandibular compression and reconstruction plates have been specially designed to counteract the considerable forces acting on the mandible. Their use is particularly important when one considers that the common mandibular plate is placed on the pressure area at the inferior mandibular border. Thus it has to withstand far greater forces than it would if it were placed on the tension area at the upper border (tooth roots) or on the midline of the ramus or body (inferior alveolar nerve). The use of thinner and weaker metacarpal or forearm plates will invariably result in inadequate stability and loosening of screws and plates. Use of the wrong type of plate has led many centers to condemn internal fixation of the mandible.

The use of miniplates for mandibular fracture fixation has been popularized by Champy. These miniplates are placed on the tension areas of the mandible with monocortical fixation to prevent damage to the underlying tooth roots. Multiple plates may be needed to obtain adequate stability. Miniplates used in other areas of the mandible, in place of proper mandibular plates, are much too weak to counteract the functional forces across the fracture site. Their use usually must be accompanied by prolonged MMF, which negates the advantages of proper internal fixation (see Figures 18.6–18.9).

Complications of Internal Fixation of the Mandible 221

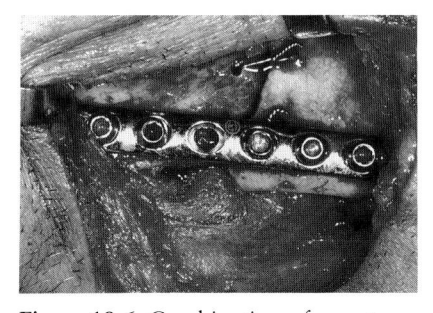

Figure 18.6 Combination of a metacarpal semitubular compression plate and multiple interosseous wires to repair a mandibular fracture. These plates are not designed for mandibular fractures and will not withstand the significant functional stresses of mastication. Only the specially designed mandibular plates should be used in this situation.

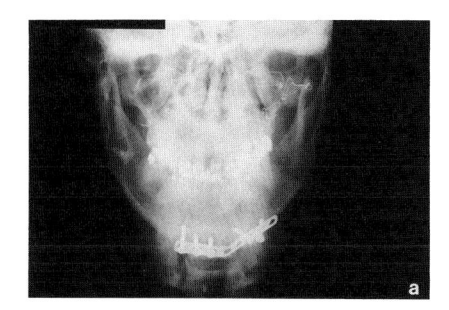

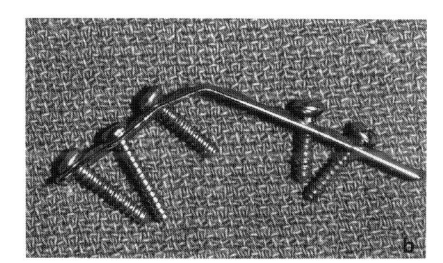

Figure 18.7 (a) An unstable parasymphyseal fracture repaired with a finger plate. The plate, of inadequate strength, will bend with masticatory forces, and all screws will loosen. (b) After the plate is removed, one can see the distortion produced by the masticatory forces.

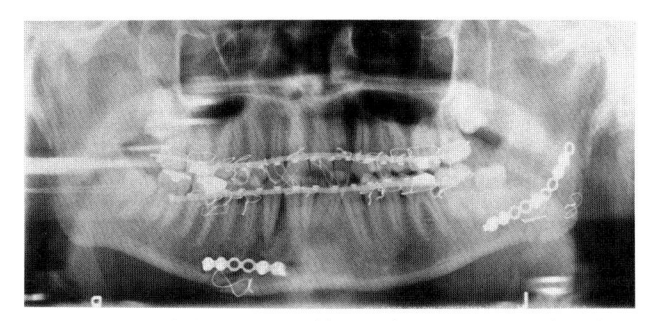

Figure 18.8 A bilateral mandibular fracture repaired with a combination of interosseous wires and miniplates. The miniplate at the left end is placed too high over the region of the inferior alveolar nerve. Because of insufficient stabilization this patient had to be kept in MMF for six weeks.

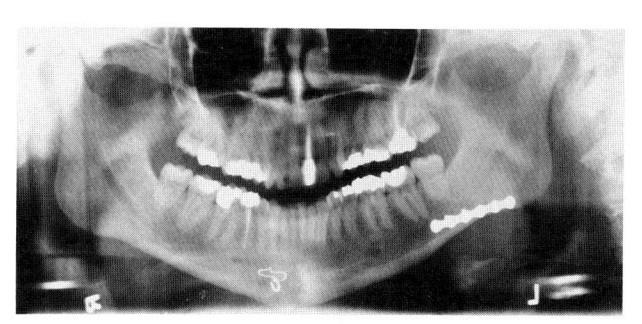

Figure 18.9 This bilateral mandibular fracture in a professional singer was repaired with an interosseous wire at the parasymphyseal region and a miniplate at the left body region. The anterior two screws of the miniplate are placed through the nerve canal, causing permanent anesthesia of the left side of the lip. This resulted in prolonged disability and difficulty for the patient as a professional singer. Internal fixation with miniplates, when used as in this situation, results in much worse complications than if an interosseous wire were used.

Improper Plate Placement

The common mandibular plate is fixed along the inferior border of the mandible with bicortical screws. The plate must be carefully bent and applied. If the plate protrudes beyond the mandibular border, it will be palpable and the overlying skin tender, necessitating plate removal. If the plate is placed too close to the mandibular border, the screw may gain inadequate purchase and may loosen. The most difficult area for plate placement is in angle fractures, where there is a tendency for straight plates to be placed directly across the angle. The plate may be placed too low, or the edges may protrude too high, damaging the inferior alveolar nerve. To facilitate placement of plates in angle fractures, a curved compression plate or prebent reconstruction plate is preferable. In ramus and body fractures, the inferior alveolar nerve must be avoided and, in the body and symphyseal regions, the tooth roots must be protected. In the symphyseal/parasymphyseal region anterior to the inferior alveolar canal, the plates can be placed higher on the mandible to facilitate ease of plate placement and stability without risk of nerve injury (see Figures 18.10–18.18).

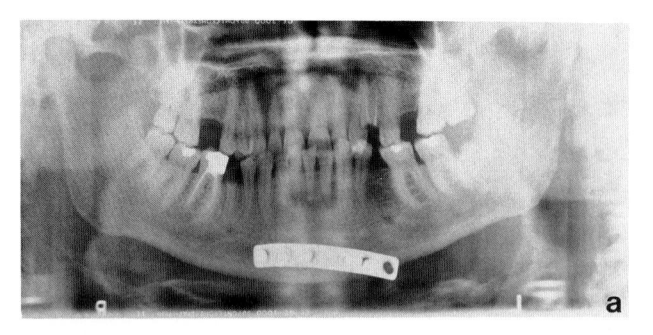

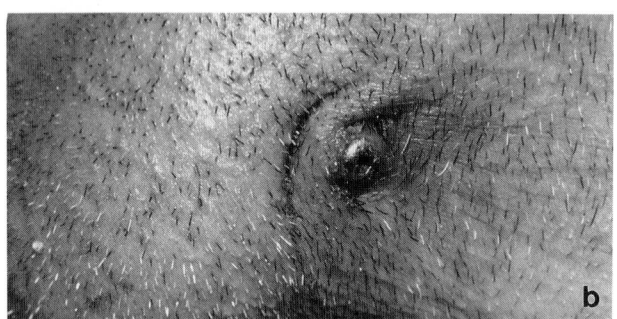

Figure 18.10 (a) Six-hole compression plate used to repair an unstable symphyseal fracture. The plate was inadequately contoured to the bone, so that the edge of the plate extended over the edge of the mandible bone. This caused the final screw, which had inadequate purchase in the bone, to become loose. This plate was palpable by the patient. (b) The extrusion of the loose screw through a sinus tract is shown. The entire plate had to be removed.

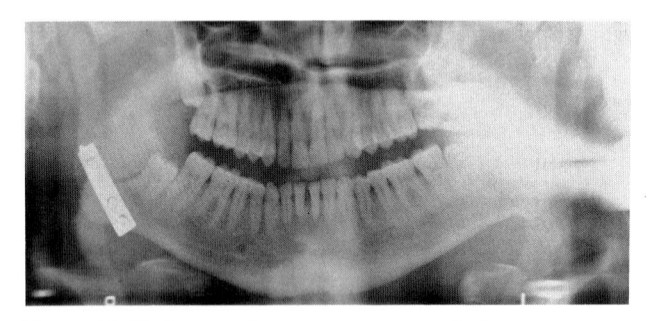

Figure 18.11 In most instances, a true angle fracture cannot be adequately repaired with a straight compression plate, as seen in this case. The compression plate has been inadequately shaped and extends beyond the border of the mandible. In this situation, it is preferable to use a curved compression plate or a curved reconstruction plate so that the plate can be placed adequately along the inferior border of the mandible without risk of plate protrusion or damage to the inferior alveolar nerve.

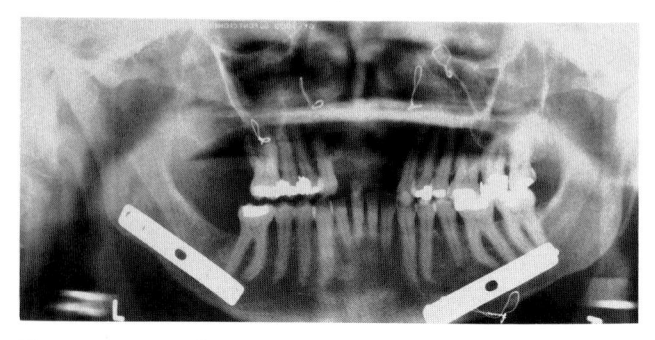

Figure 18.12 In this situation, both compression plates have been placed too high on the mandible, resulting in damage to both inferior alveolar nerves. Plates used in mandibular repair must be placed on the inferior border of the mandible, away from the inferior alveolar nerve.

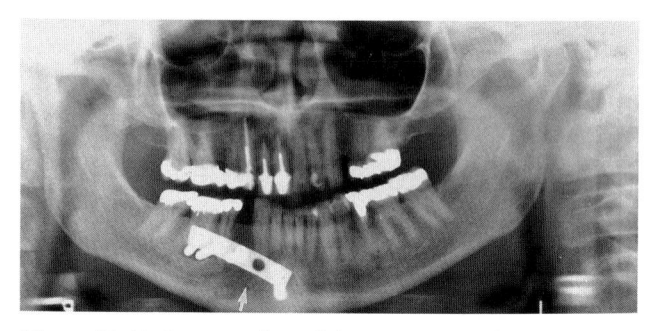

Figure 18.13 Parasymphyseal fracture repaired with a compression plate placed through an intraoral incision. The plate was placed above the nerve, and thus the upper two screws were placed through the apices of the tooth roots. In addition, the plate was placed in the wrong position: Three screws were placed on one side of the fracture, and only one screw was placed on the opposite of the fracture. This is inadequate fixation, as well as the wrong place for this plate, which should be placed below the nerve.

Incorrect Screw Placement

Acute Fracture

The importance of using an adequate number of screws on each side of the fracture and avoiding screw placement too close to the fracture site and mandibular border has been described. Atraumatic surgical drilling of the screw hole is essential to prevent bone necrosis and eventual loosening of screws. The pilot hole should be drilled at less than 1000 revolutions per minute with copious cooling and irrigation. All bone debris should be carefully flushed from the hole. A depth gauge indicates the correct length of screw to ensure bicortical fixation. If there is any doubt about screw purchase, the

Complications of Internal Fixation of the Mandible 223

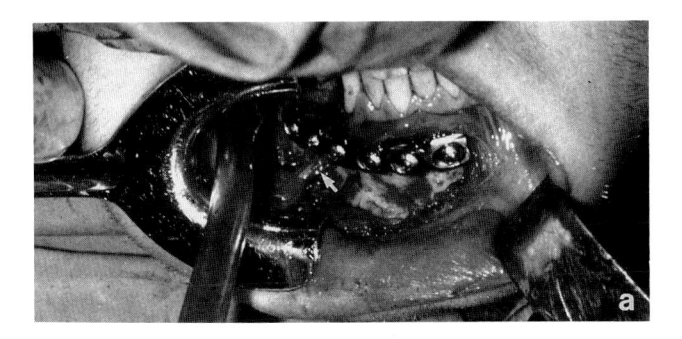

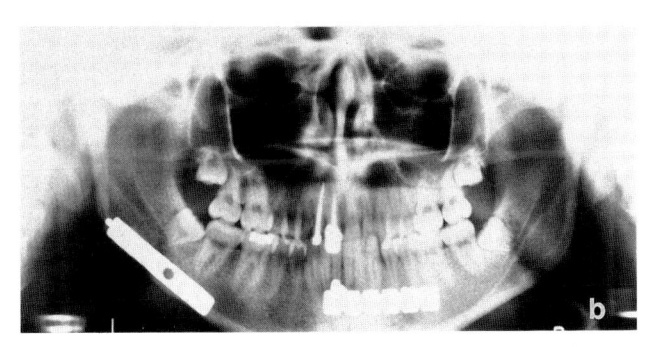

Figure 18.14 (a) Parasymphyseal fracture repaired with a small reconstruction plate, which was placed too high on the mandible above the inferior alveolar nerve (arrows) resulting in injury to the tooth roots. (b) X ray shows placement of the reconstruction plate too high on the mandible. This plate should have been placed below the nerve.

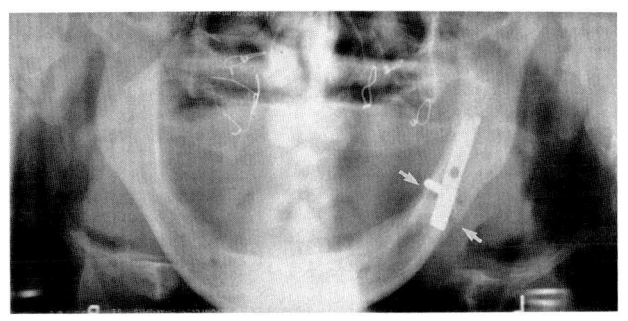

Figure 18.15 An edentulous body fracture repaired with a compression plate. Note that the plate, which has been placed in the wrong position, crosses the inferior alveolar nerve. In addition, the lower screw has been placed through the fracture; only one screw is therefore below the fracture. The plate will eventually loosen and there will be a nonunion. This plate had to be removed and replaced with a reconstruction plate.

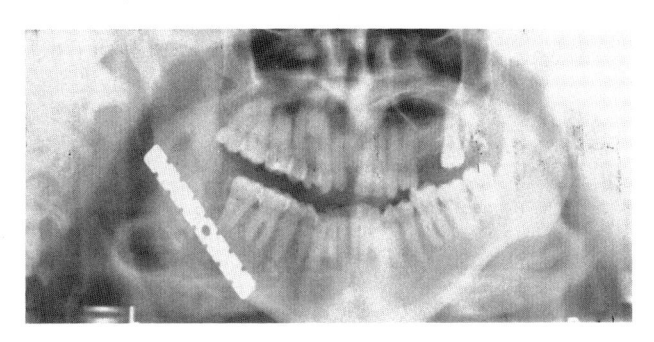

Figure 18.16 Incorrect placement of a reconstruction plate at the angle region. Note that the plate has not been contoured to the shape of the mandible in this region and has been placed perfectly straight across the angle. The reconstruction plate should be bent to follow the contours of the mandible and should be angled across the angle.

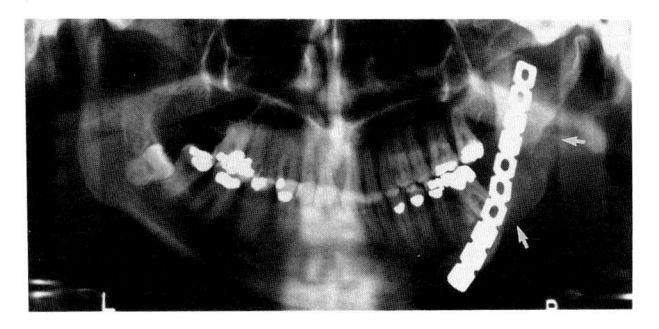

Figure 18.17 A reconstruction plate used for fixation of a very complex angle fracture. Note that the plate has been placed in the wrong direction. The plate itself is too long; note that the upper screws are unusable. In addition, there is inadequate reduction of the fracture site, and a marked step deformity can be seen (arrows).

screw should be removed and replaced by an emergency screw to prevent the inevitable screw loosening, which leads to bony infection, sequestration, and sinus formation (see Figures 18.19–18.21).

Nonunion

After any infection is controlled by antibiotics and debridement, adequate bony stabilization is necessary to ensure subsequent union with or without bone grafting. With a fibrous union, compression plating usually ensures healing. When a bony gap is present, a reconstruction plate is necessary to bridge the bony gap and ensure enough stability for subsequent bony healing. At the time of plate placement, the bone adjacent to the nonunion site may look entirely normal on x ray and to direct inspection. However, this bone, in the great majority of cases, is abnormal and inadequate to withstand screw placement. Screws placed too close to the nonunion site will invariably loosen and the fixation may fail. Screws should be placed at least 1 centimeter from the edge of the nonunion site to ensure adequate bony purchase (see Figure 18.22).

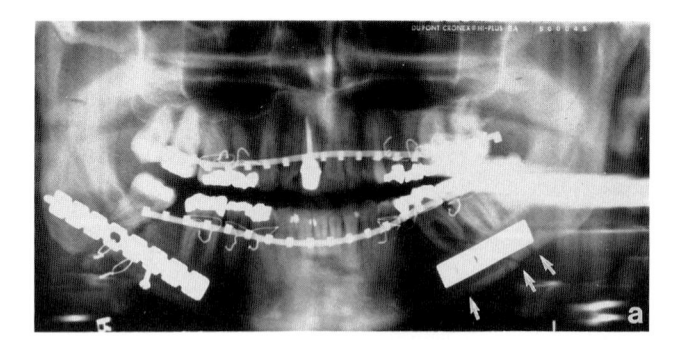

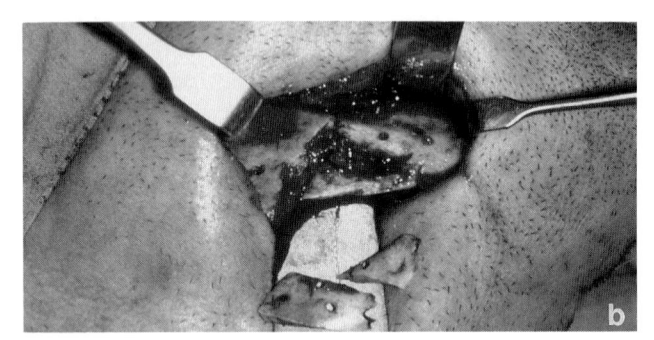

Figure 18.18 (a) A complex bilateral mandibular fracture. On the left side, a complex body fracture has been repaired with too short a plate. One can see the segmental nature of the fracture, and the screws are placed too close to the fracture site, resulting in inadequate fixation. On the right side, a very complex unstable angle fracture with some bone loss at the inferior border is repaired with a straight reconstruction plate that goes across the midline of the mandible in the region of the inferior alveolar nerve. In addition, the position of the right molar tooth has not been controlled. The tooth is displaced upward and inward, acting as a block, resulting in an open bite deformity. (b) At operation, multiple small cortical segments were found anchored to the plate and underlying bone with multiple interosseous wires. When there are small cortical fragments completely devoid of their periosteal attachments, it is not necessary to reattach these or replace them if there is good bone-to-bone contact superiorly, as in this case. (c) The right posterior molar tooth was controlled by use of the arch bar, and a miniadaptive plate at the upper border was used as a tension band. The posterior miniscrew is placed only monocortically so as not to injure the roots of the molar tooth. (d) A properly contoured reconstruction plate is now used to rigidly stabilize the remainder of the angle fracture. At least three screws are placed on either side of the fracture site. In addition, the opposite compression plate, which is too short, is replaced with a longer reconstruction plate. Here, at least three screws are placed on either side of the fracture site (the three-screw rule).

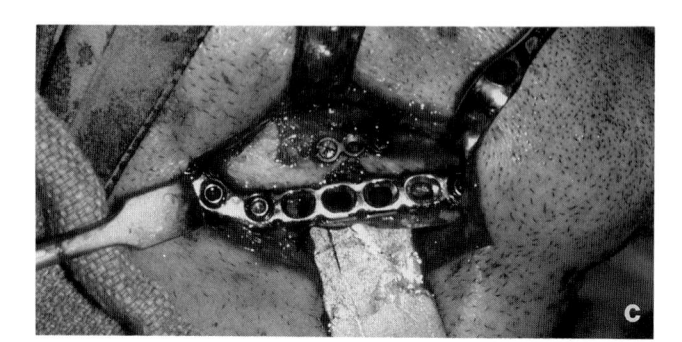

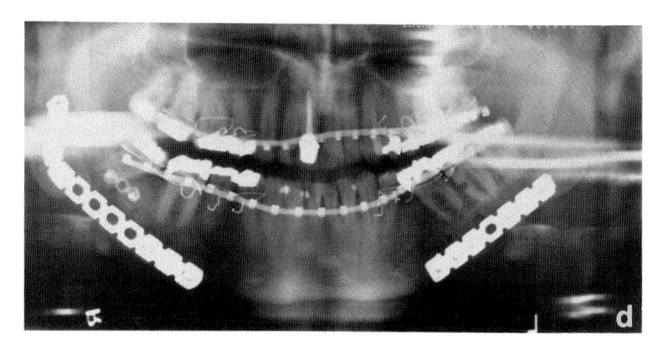

Pathological Bone

Rarely, the mandibular bone may be involved in an extensive or generalized disease process, such as infection. Pathologically abnormal bone will not give adequate purchase for insertion of more than one screw. The physical trauma of drilling for and inserting many screws may cause rapid degeneration of bone stock, loosening of screws and plates, and multiple pathological fractures. Plates and screws should not be placed in pathologically abnormal bone. Stabilization in this instance should be with external fixation with the pins placed well away from the involved area (see Figure 18.23).

Tension Banding

Due to the position of the tooth roots and inferior alveolar nerve, the majority of mandibular compression and reconstruction plates have to be placed on the inferior border of the mandible in the zone of pressure forces. As the plate and screws are applied, particularly if compression is used, gaps tend to form at the upper border of the mandible due to the inability of the inferiorly placed plate to neutralize the tension forces in this area. Failure to recognize this will frequently result in a shift of the previously established occlusion as the screws are tightened (see Figure 18.24). This malocclusion, occurring after seemingly perfect occlusal repositioning and

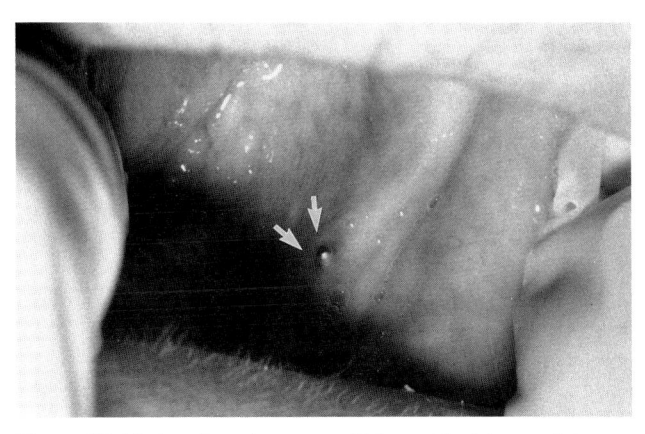

Figure 18.19 In edentulous mandibles with thin overlying mucosa, the screws must not be placed too long because they may erode through the mucosal surface and interfere with fitting of the dentures.

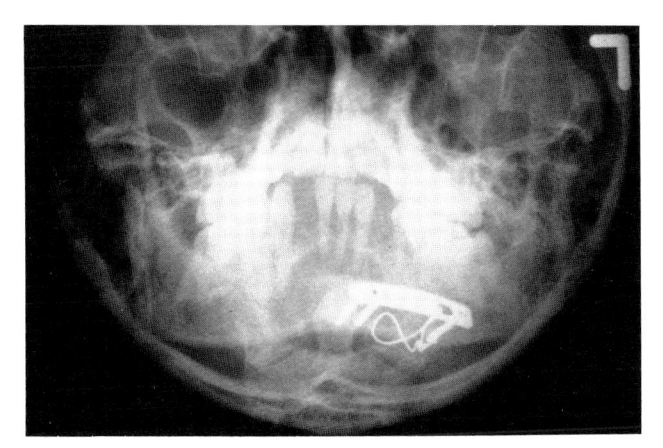

Figure 18.20 A parasymphyseal fracture repaired with a mandibular compression plate. On one side, there has been loss of screw fixation, and the surgeon has applied an interosseous wire through the screw hole to replace the loose screw. In this situation, the loose screw should be replaced with a rescue screw. The situation is unstable because there is only one screw on one side of the fracture and two screws on the other side. This resulted in a significant infection and nonunion. If a rescue screw is not available, this short plate should be removed, and a longer plate should be placed with the screws away from the fracture site. At least three screws should be placed on either side of the fracture site.

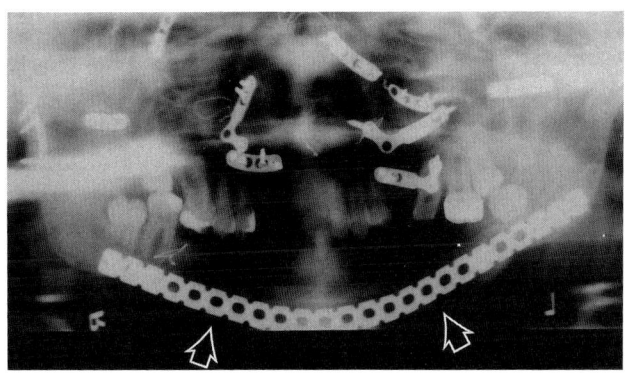

Figure 18.21 A long reconstruction plate used to bridge two traumatic gaps. Note that only three screws have been placed on either side. This caused the plate eventually to loosen. When plates are placed across large gaps such as this, a minimum of four (and preferably more) screws should be placed on either side because the masticatory forces acting on the plate are significant. With placement of insufficient screws the plate will become loose.

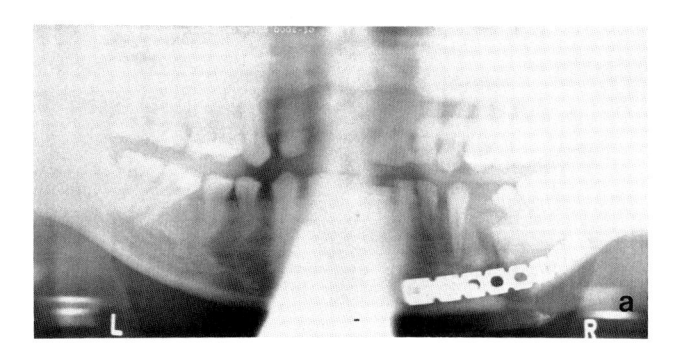

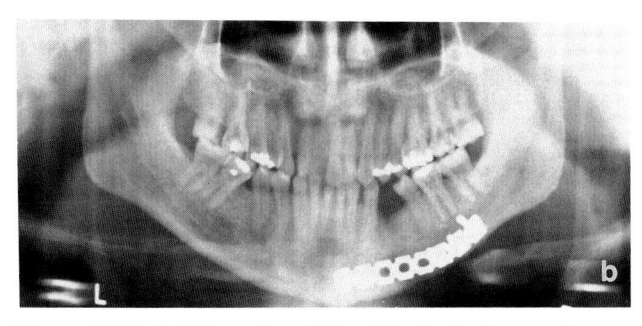

Figure 18.22 (a) Nonunion of the right body fracture is stabilized with a reconstruction plate. Note that the inner screws have been placed too close to the fracture site, resulting in loosening of these screws and continued drainage. This is not an indication to remove the plate; only the loose screws have to be removed. (b) Six months later, after only the loose screws adjacent to the nonunion site have been removed (the other screws have been left in situ) the fracture with nonunion has healed completely.

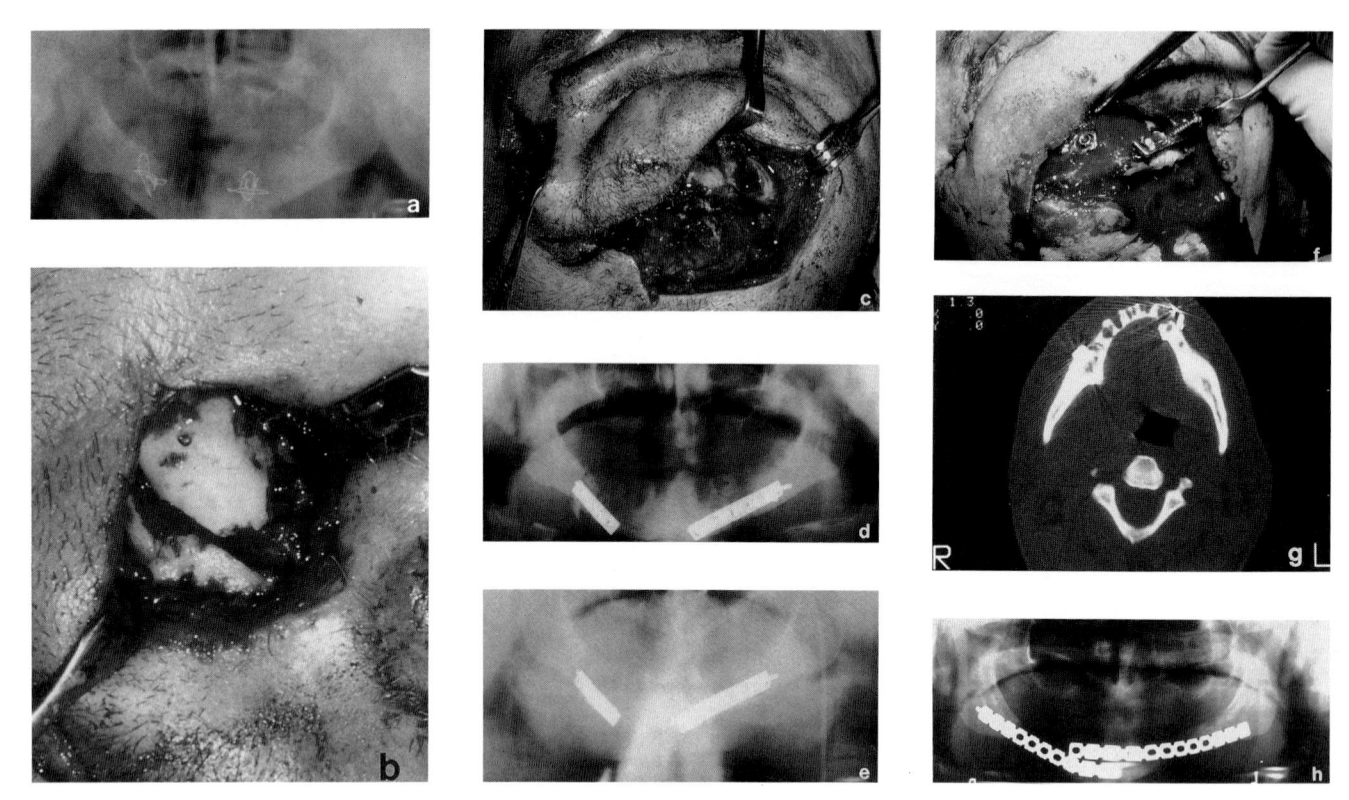

Figure 18.23 (a) A 25-year-old man with bilateral body fractures of a recently edentulous mandible. This patient had all his teeth removed two weeks prior to the accident and had a severe periodontal infection after the tooth removal. An attempt was made to repair this using heavy interosseous wires, but this has failed. (b) At the time of exploration, the mandibular bone looks normal. (c) Both fractures were explored using the pre-existing laceration and previous incisions. Again, the bone on the left side looks normal macroscopically. (d) Two compression plates were placed, one in each fracture site. Ten days after the repair, there is significant draining from both incisions. Panorex x-ray revealed a loosening of both plates and disintegration of both fracture sites. (e) Panorex taken four days later shows total loosening of both plates and rapid disintegration of the bone under the plates. (f) At exploration, virtually all screws were loose, and so the plates were removed. (g) Retrospective analysis of the CT scan of the mandible taken at the time of admission shows that the mandibular bone was abnormal from the recent tooth removal and infection. Pathologically abnormal bone such as this is an absolute contraindication to the insertion of plates and screws as this will frequently exacerbate the pathological process, resulting in rapid degeneration and loosening of the plates and screws. In this situation, it is preferable either to bridge the area of pathologically abnormal bone with a long reconstruction plate or to place an external fixation device well away from the area of pathological bone. (h) The application of two long reconstruction plates after removal of the two compression plates. This resulted in rapid resolution of the infection. Subsequent bone grafts had to be inserted into the bone gaps on either side. It would have been preferable in this case to use one long reconstruction plate going from one angle to the other.

anatomical internal fixation at the time of surgery, may manifest only in the postoperative period after the MMF is released.

Thus, whenever possible, *tension banding* at the upper border of the mandible should be used to counteract the tension forces in this area. Tension banding can be accomplished by the use of either an arch bar, an eccentric dynamic compression plate (EDCP), or an upper border plate with either a two-hole dynamic compression plate (DCP) or a miniplate.

Arch Bar

The arch bar, the simplest method of tension banding, is used with fractures occurring between tooth-bearing segments.

Eccentric Dynamic Compression Plate

The eccentric dynamic compression plate (standard AO set, special-order Luhr set) produces compression in two directions; the inner, straight holes along the inferior border of the mandible and the outer, oblique holes toward the superior border produce a tension banding effect. Because of the necessity to produce compression and bony movement in two directions, the injudicious use of this plate may cause uncontrollable bony shifts, leading to malocclusion in the dentulous patient. The inexperienced surgeon should use it with extreme caution in the dentulous mandible, whereas in the edentulous or partially dentulous mandible the eccentric compression is easier to control and its use is facilitated.

Upper Border Plate

With insufficient teeth, or teeth only on one side of the fracture (for example, an angle fracture), the simplest and safest means of providing tension banding is with an upper border miniplate. When angle fractures are exposed via an intraoral approach, a miniplate applied first to the upper border of the posterior edentulous segment with bicortical screws can be used as a handle to control this segment and aid in fracture reduction. The anterior screw or screws may have to be placed with monocortical fixation to prevent damage to the tooth roots. Once the upper border miniplate has been applied, it is much easier to bend and apply the lower border compression plate accurately.

Compression Osteosynthesis

One of the most important areas of misunderstanding and potential causes of complications is a lack of appreciation of compression osteosynthesis and its underlying role in the provision of rigid internal fixation of the mandible. Compression of the bone ends at a fracture or osteotomy site has been shown to produce primary or direct bone healing. Primary bone healing is more rapid than secondary or indirect bone healing because of the initial formation of cartilage bone. Mandibular bone will heal just as adequately without compression, however, although at a slower pace. Therefore compression is not necessary to ensure adequate bone healing of mandibular fractures.

Dynamic compression of the bone ends at the fracture or osteotomy site by the proper use of the compression holes in the standard mandibular compression plate will lead to increased stability of fixation and ultimately to primary bone healing. Compression therefore increases stability and is the easiest method to ensure the rigidity of internal fixation.

Dynamic compression at the fracture site has to produce a shift of bone segments. This shift, if not controlled, can be easily transmitted to the occlusal plane and condylar head, causing occlusal shifts and condylar torque. Failure to appreciate this is a common cause of postoperative malocclusion after seemingly accurate occlusal and fracture reduction at the time of surgery.

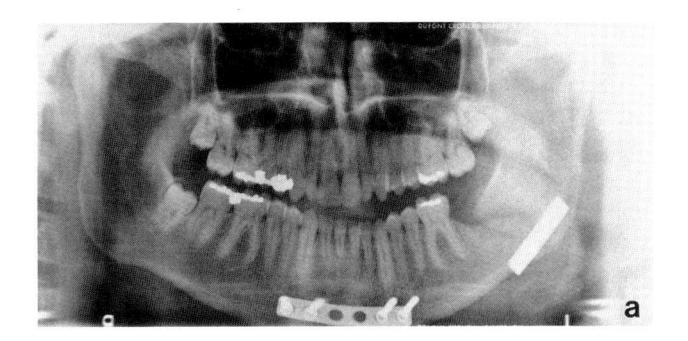

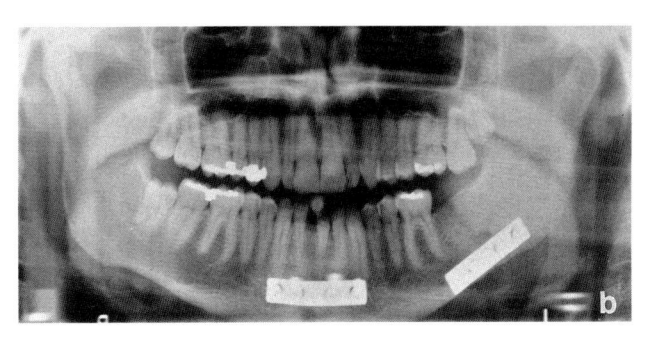

Figure 18.24 (a) A left angle fracture has been repaired with a short compression plate. No attempt at tension banding has been made, and so the fracture site has opened at the upper border of the mandible, resulting in a significant malocclusion. (b) Secondary osteotomy had to be performed at both fracture sites. The fracture sites are now repaired with two eccentric dynamic compression plates. There is now a proper tension banding effect, and the fracture at both sides has healed rapidly.

In order to use compression safely, surgeons, particularly less experienced ones, must ensure good bone-to-bone contact of the fracture ends. This will enable the fracture ends to "lock together" during compression without sliding or oblique torquing. Compression osteosynthesis is contraindicated, or should be used with extreme caution, when there are oblique fractures, sagittal splitting of inner and outer cortex, segmental fractures, comminuted fractures, or fractures with bone loss.

Instead of compression osteosynthesis with a plate, the following techniques can be used to produce adequate stability at the fracture site.

Longer Plate (Neutralization or Stabilization Plate)

Compression osteosynthesis allows the use of a shorter plate with less screws. Use of a longer plate with more screws, placed in the neutral, or noncompressive, mode, will allow equal stability to neutralize the forces acting across the fracture site and ensure adequate bone healing (see Figure 18.25).

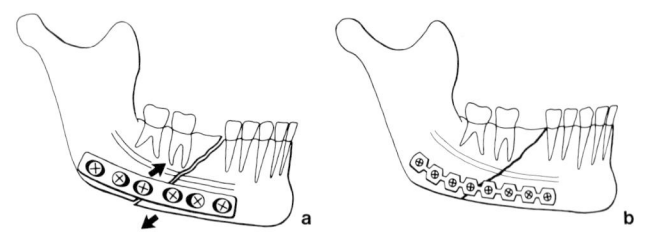

Figure 18.25 (a) A displaced and unstable oblique fracture. Any attempt at compression of this fracture may cause the fracture segment to slide on each other, resulting in a severe malocclusion. (b) In fractures with marked obliquity, it is safer to use a long reconstruction plate, placing more screws in either side of the fracture without compression, thus neutralizing the forces.

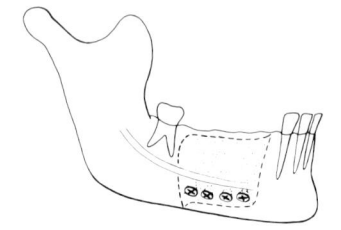

Figure 18.26 In markedly oblique fractures with sagittal splitting of the inner and outer table, multiple lag screws can be used to provide fixation instead of a plate.

Lag Screws

With oblique, segmental, or comminuted fractures, lag screw fixation provides direct interfragmentary compression under each screwhead. A long stabilization plate provides the final fixation, and all subsequent screws are placed in the neutral mode (see Figures 18.26 and 18.27).

Lag Screw Through Plate

In oblique or sagittal fractures, a lag screw can be applied directly through the plate, providing direct compression across the fracture site between the plate and screwhead proximally and between the screw threads distally. This direct compression with a screw across the fracture site prevents sliding of bone ends and is different from the indirect compression produced by a dynamic compression plate. Once compression has been achieved with a lag screw through the plate, all other screws are placed in the neutral mode; any further attempt to provide compression via the plate will loosen the lag screws (see Figure 18.28).

A common misconception in osteosynthesis is that the greatest degree of compression possible should be applied to increase rigidity of fixation and bone healing. Various technical maneuvers can be used to increase the degree of compression. After the first compression screw is partially inserted, the plate is pulled toward the fracture so that the edge of the plate is in direct contact with the screw. The opposite screw hole is now drilled as close as possible to the outer portion of the compression hole, and the screw is inserted. As both screws are tightened, theoretically maximal compression is produced. In practice, this maneuver, because the screw actively contacts the plate edge during insertion, will frequently cause the screw to fail; the screwhead will shear off from the shaft. In addition, excess compression applied to the fracture or osteotomy site may cause

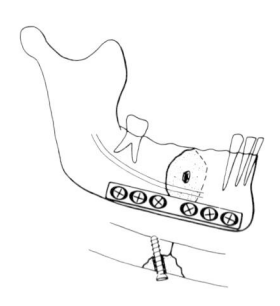

Figure 18.27 In certain situations, lag screw fixation can be combined with plate fixation. Once the lag screw has been applied, compression must be applied very carefully, or not at all; injudicious use of compression may result in loosening of the lag screw fixation. In this situation, use of a long neutralization plate without compression is safer.

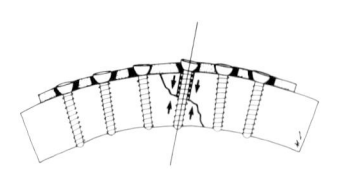

Figure 18.28 In certain situations, a lag screw can be used through the plate. This will provide direct interfragmentary compression underneath the lag screw. Once the lag screw has been inserted, all other screws must be inserted in the neutral position because attempts to compress these screws will loosen the lag screw.

detrimental bone changes or necrosis, resulting in delay of bone healing. Compression should always be gently and accurately applied, without undue force, to facilitate direct or primary bone healing. There is no advantage at all in applying extra compression.

Soft-Tissue Cover

The provision of adequate soft-tissue cover over all nonautogenous implants, including plates and screws, is essential to ensure adequate healing and lessen the risk of infection. A mandibular plate is occasionally ex-

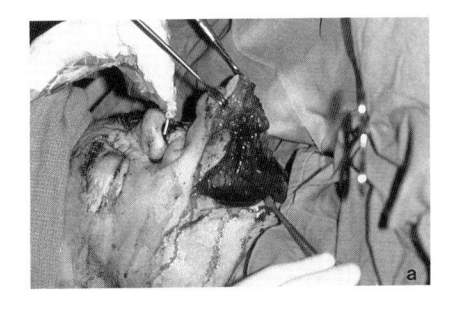

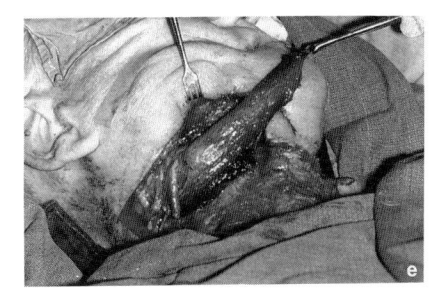

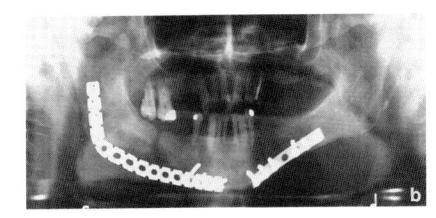

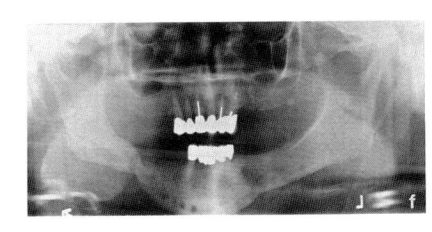

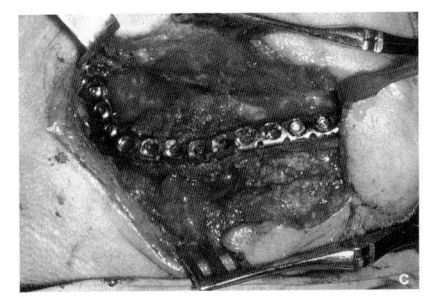

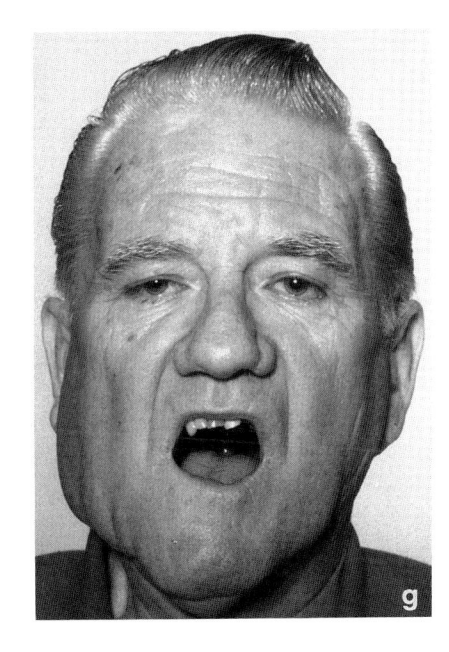

Figure 18.29 (a) Very complex multiple mandibular fractures with severe injury to soft tissue. (b) Fractures repaired with a six-hole compression plate at the left body and a long reconstruction plate bridging the bony gap at the right body. Due to the significant soft-tissue injury, both externally and of the intraoral lining, no immediate bone grafting was performed. (c) At three months, the incision is reopened, and cancellous bone is packed into the bone gap underneath the reconstruction plate. (d) At six months, the overlying skin is adhering to the underlying plate, resulting in eventual plate erosion. (e) Because there was still concern that the bone had not healed completely, the incision was reopened, soft tissue was freed from the plate, and the sternomastoid muscle was mobilized and used to cover the plate completely. (f) Osteointegrated implants were placed in the region of the bone grafts. (g) Restoration of contour and function.

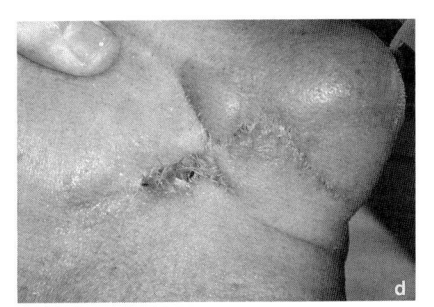

posed through an intraoral incision. As long as the plate and screws are rigidly fixed to the bone and the patient has not received previous radiotherapy, routine and frequent mouth and wound care will invariably help the wound to close over the plate.

Occasionally, when severe soft-tissue injury occurs external to the plate, the scarred soft tissues may eventually adhere to the plate and undergo subsequent necrosis, thus exposing the plate. If bone has already healed, then the plate is simply removed. If the plate is still necessary to ensure adequate bone healing, then as long as it is adequately fixed in place, it does not have to be removed but can be covered with local soft tissue or muscle flaps (see Figure 18.29). Plates that are exposed intraorally or externally need to be removed only if they become loosened, because if they are loose the metal will act as a foreign body and predispose to infection.

Bone Continuity

When fractures of the dentulous mandible with bone loss are bridged by reconstruction plates, failure to produce bone continuity across the fracture gap with bone grafts will invariably produce late loosening or fracture of the plate. The plate itself, in this situation, provides only a temporary alloplastic bridging of the bone gap. It cannot withstand the continuous masticatory forces applied across the gap, particularly in a younger person with adequate dentition. Delayed bone grafting with conventional or free vascularized techniques should always be performed, except in the elderly patient with an edentulous mandible, where the masticatory forces are considerably less. Primary bone grafting of mandibular defects, particularly with associated mucosal injury or loss, has proven unreliable in our hands and has a significant incidence of acute infection (see Figures 18.30–18.32).

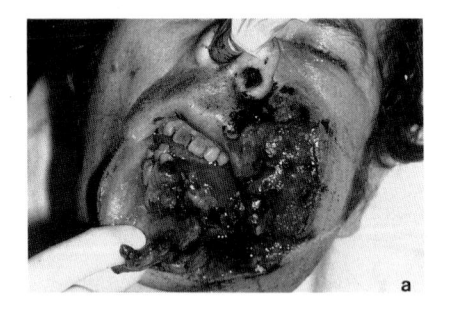

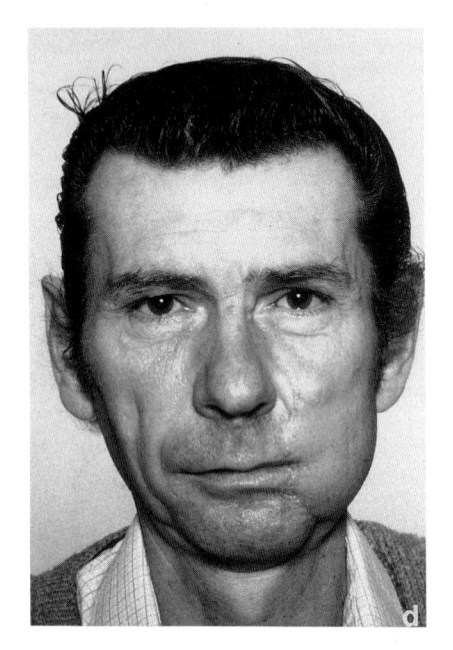

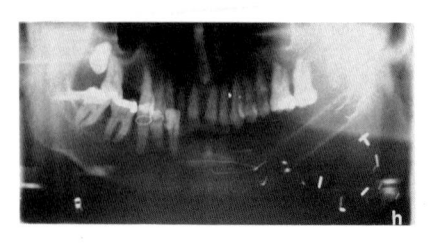

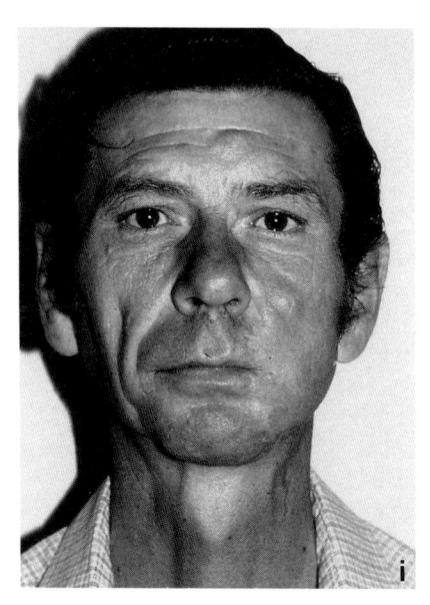

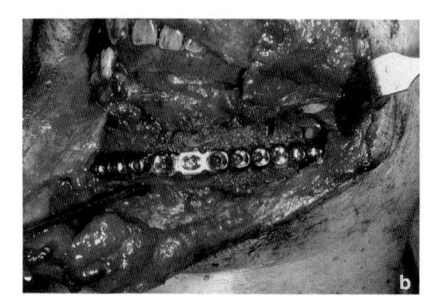

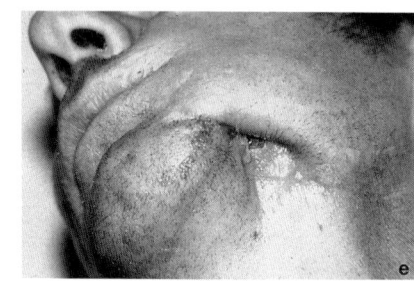

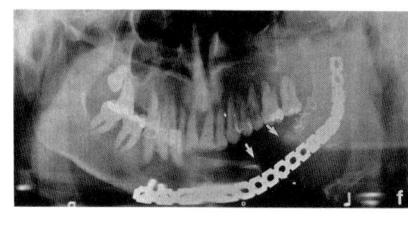

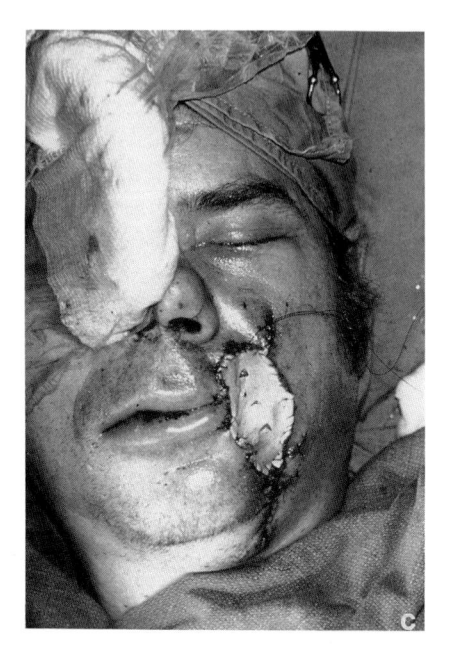

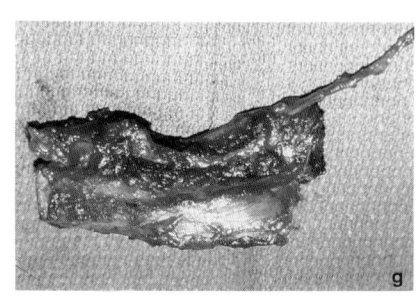

Figure 18.30 (a) A massive gunshot wound of the left cheek and mandible with severe destruction of intraoral lining and bone. (b) Bridging of the mandibular gap with a reconstruction plate and application of primary bone grafting using iliac cancellous bone. (c) Primary reconstruction of facial soft tissue with application of a split skin graft. (d) Facial appearance at two years following eventual excision of the skin graft and cheek rotation flaps. Note excellent contour and esthetic reconstruction. (e) After 2½ years, the patient presents with a draining sinus in the left upper neck. (f) Panorex reveals residual bone gap (arrows). Primary bone grafting has failed to obtain bony healing, and continued masticatory forces resulted in eventual loosening of the plate. (g) Free vascularized iliac crest graft is harvested. (h) Iliac crest graft is placed in the gap. (i) Eventual healing of the mandibular bone gap.

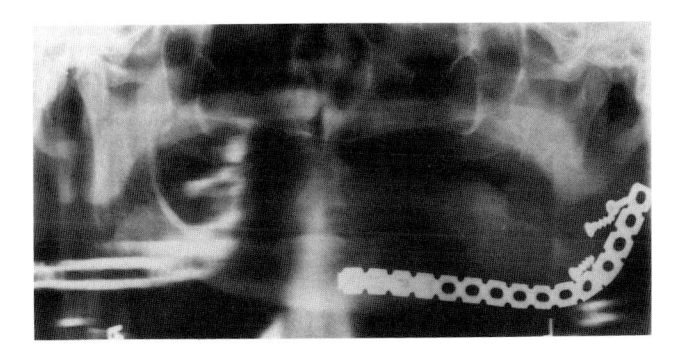

Figure 18.31 In the thin, edentulous mandible fixing a plate to the thin bone of the ramus is difficult. Particularly when bony gaps are being bridged, it is not uncommon for the screws placed into the ramus to pull out eventually. Care must be taken to place at least three screws, and preferably more, into the ramus with careful bicortical fixation.

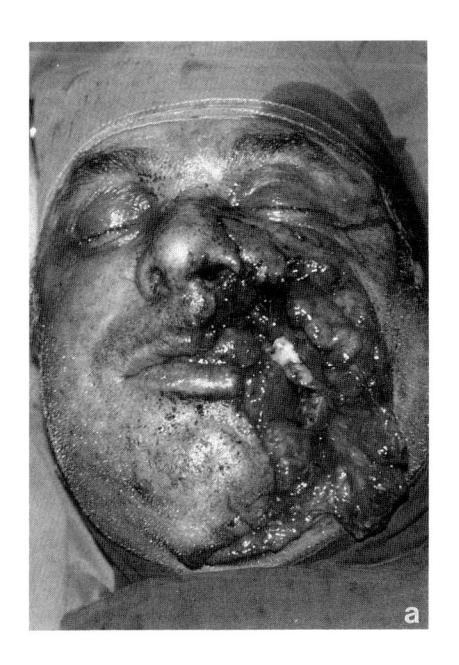

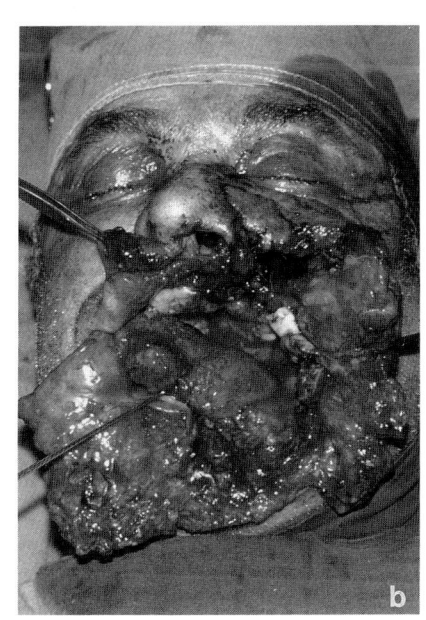

Figure 18.32 (a) A male patient with massive gunshot wound of the face. (b) Extensive bone loss in the maxilla and mandible. (c) Panorex x ray reveals multiple segmental fractures and bone loss. (d) Fixation of the multiple fractures using compression, reconstruction, and miniplates. Note several mistakes. The compression plate placed on the right body fracture has not resulted in good anatomical alignment of the fracture. Primary bone grafts have been inserted into the gap in the left body fracture. (e) Patient 1 week after the repair shows massive swelling to the left side of the chin. Eventual abscess formation necessitated removal of all bone grafts.

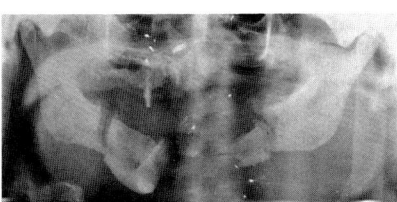

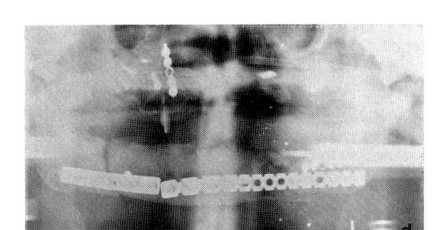

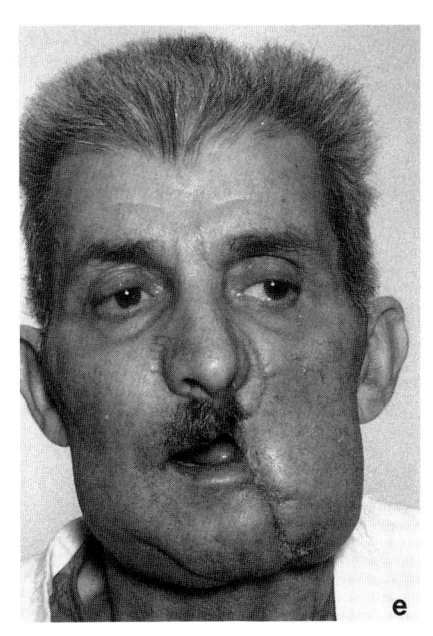

BIBLIOGRAPHY

Beckers HL: Treatment of initially infected mandibular fractures with bone plates. J Oral Surg 37:310, 1979.

Davidson TM, Bone RC, Nahum AM: Mandibular fracture complications. Arch Otolaryngol, 102 (10):627–30, 1976.

Fischer-Brandies E, Dielart E: The infected mandibular fracture. Arch Orthop Trauma Surg 103:337, 1984.

Girdano AM, Foster CA, Boies LR, Maisel RH: Chronic osteomyelitis following mandibular fractures and its treatment. Arch Otolaryngol 108:30, 1982.

Kappel DA, Craft PD, Robinson DW, Masters FW: The significance of persistent radiolucency of mandibular fractures. Plast Reconstr Surg 53:38, 1974.

Levine PA: AO compression plating technique for treating fractures of the edentulous mandible. Otolaryngol Clin North Am 21:457–477, 1987.

Mathog RH: Non union of the mandible. Otolaryngol Clin North Am 16:533, 1983.

Prein J, Kellam RM: Rigid internal fixation of mandibular fractures: Basics of AO technique. Otolaryngol Clin North Am 20:441–456, 1987.

Rahn BA: Direct and indirect bone healing after operating fracture treatment. Otolaryngol Clin North Am 20:425, 1987.

Schneider SS, Stern M: Teeth in the line of mandibular fractures. J Oral Surg 29:107, 1971.

Souyris F, Lamarch JP, Mirfakhra I: Treatment of mandibular fractures by intraoral placement of bone plates. J Oral Surg 38:33, 1980.

Worthington P, Champy M: Monocortical miniplate osteosynthesis. Otolaryngol Clin North Am 20:607, 1987.

CHAPTER 19

Management of Infected Fractures and Nonunions of the Mandible

Roland R. Schmoker

The classic concept of the pathogenesis of nonunion was presented by Lexer (1922), who theorized that the connective tissue at the fracture site no longer had sufficient biologic potential to bring about fracture healing. He believed that the key to treatment was to reactivate the healing process by providing an adequate biologic stimulus. To effect this, Lexer advocated resection of the scarred tissue at the nonunion site, opening the first medullary cavity, and stimulation by placing a cortical bone graft between the fracture ends.

This concept led to the development of the classic conventional treatment principle, which holds that the primary therapeutic goal is to convert an infected nonunion to an aseptic nonunion. This is accomplished by sequestrectomy, the removal of any internal fixation material, MMF, and antibiotic therapy. After the infection has cleared, fistulous tracts are excised, and soft-tissue integrity is restored using flap techniques. Six to 12 months are allowed for soft-tissue healing, whereupon osseous continuity is reestablished secondarily by resecting the nonunion and restoring osteogenic potential by an interposed or onlay bone graft. The main problem of this classic treatment concept, pointed out by Weber and Cech (1976), is that fracture consolidation cannot take place in the presence of infection, and an infection cannot resolve in the presence of a fracture.

In this chapter, we describe techniques based on principles of rigid internal fixation. These techniques reconcile the contradiction of the conventional approach, thereby allowing successful management of infected fractures and nonunions of the mandible.

DEFINITIONS

In contrast to classic *osteomyelitis*, which involves the bone marrow, typically progresses from a primary acute to secondary chronic stage, and can occur independent of fractures, the localized infection of a fracture line tends to involve the cortex, periosteum, and adjacent soft tissues. Because necrotic post-traumatic cortical fragments generally form the true focus of infection, the term *fracture-line osteitis* describes this condition most accurately and should replace the older term "fracture-line osteomyelitis."

Differentiation between a delayed union and a nonunion may be difficult in the mandible. The typical radiographic criteria of nonunion in long bones—such as sealing of the medullary cavity and a failure of periosteal callus formation across the fracture site—are appreciated infrequently in situations other than the edentulous jaw. Most nonunions in the dentulous mandible are manifested only by a rounding of the basal cortex and, occasionally, by the appearance of a faint border that resembles lamina dura around the ends of the fragments. With conservative treatment it is unlikely that a radiographically visible callus will form even when fracture healing is undisturbed.

Various authors have proposed a time factor as the basis for establishing a workable clinical definition of nonunion. In long bones, many experts state that nonunion may be diagnosed in a fracture that has failed to unite within five months; Muller et al. (1970, 1979) extend that period to eight months. For mandibular fractures, Spiessl (1988) states a period of eight months or in some cases four months, Luhr (1973) states three months, and Schmoker and Spiessl (1976) four months.

PATHOGENESIS

The mandible is especially susceptible to infection and nonunion because of its unique location and functional role. Because of their close relation to teeth, periodontium, and gingiva, all fractures in the edentulous portion of the mandible and most fractures in areas covered by the gingiva should be considered open, contaminated fractures. The potential for complications is compounded by the fact that even after operative treatment, the fracture line openly communicates with the contaminated oral cavity via the periodontium of the involved tooth throughout the healing period. It should be noted, however, that the process that actually sustains the osteitis is the secondary infection of necrotic portions of the cortex and not the exposure and contamination per se.

Disputing the notion that nonunion represents a closed process based on inferior interstitial tissue that lacks healing potential, Pauwels (1965) attributed the development of nonunion to unfavorable mechanical loading of the fracture. Pauwels (1965) taught that mechanical immobilization of the fragments by compression promotes healing and consolidation, whereas bending and shear have the opposite effect of promoting nonunion.

Segmuller et al. (1969, in Weber 1976) used isotope scanning to show that, in the great majority of cases, the expanded, sclerotic bone ends are not dead bone but actually represent reactive bone deposition with an excellent blood supply and the interposition of connective tissue and cartilage. The resorptive breakdown and reactive widening of the bone ends may be interpreted as a biologic response to mechanical unrest at the fracture site. This response represents an attempt to reduce stresses on new blood vessels permeating the nonunion by increasing the distance between the bone ends and widening the cross section of the interposed connective tissue. This process, together with the increasing stability provided by callus formation, is aimed at promoting eventual consolidation of the nonunion.

CLASSIFICATION, SYMPTOMS, AND DIAGNOSIS

A classification of fracture-line osteitis and nonunions is presented in Table 19.1 and discussed below. A delayed or nonunion often results from, or is compounded by, acute or late osteitis.

Osteitis

Early Osteitis

Patients with early osteitis present within a month after trauma with symptoms of an abscess or soft-tissue infiltration not wholly attributable to a superficial soft-tissue infection.

Late Osteitis

Following a symptom-free interval of at least one month, the patient with late osteitis presents with soft-tissue symptoms (often mild) of redness, heat, tenderness to pressure, and incipient fistulization. Toward the end of the second month, radiographic evidence shows poor bone healing. Devitalized bone fragments show increasing sclerosis as a sign of impending sequestration. The fracture line appears less sharp but is very conspicuous as a result of osteolysis.

If internal fixation has been performed, instability is manifested by incipient periosteal callus formation. A careful comparison of radiographic findings with initial postoperative x-rays will often reveal early signs of screw loosening.

Delayed Union

Aseptic

Delayed union is signified by radiographic evidence of impaired healing noted between two and four months after the injury.

An aseptic union may produce symptoms consistent with instability but, in some cases, produces no clinical symptoms and is appreciated only on x-ray films.

Infected Delayed Union

Infected delayed union is characterized by fistulization and signs of chronic osteitis. These conditions are due to either the development of sequestra or infected, devitalized bone areas, or they are due to loose implant material with mechanical instability at the fracture site.

Nonunion

Nonunion is defined a failure of consolidation after four months, with clinical and radiographic evidence of impaired healing. Contact nonunion, where the bone ends are apposed in good alignment, is distinguished from nonunions with a bone defect or deformity.

Aseptic

With aseptic nonunion no clinically overt infection is found, and radiographs show no osseous defect or deformity. The reactive, vascular nonunion is the most

Table 19.1 Classification of Disturbances of Bone Healing

Osteitis
Early
Late

Delayed Union
Aseptic
Infected

Nonunion

Contact Nonunion
Aseptic
    Reactive, vascular
    Nonreactive, avascular
Infected
    Previously infected nonunion
    Actively infected nonunion

Bone Defect or Deformity Nonunion
Aseptic
    Reactive, vascular
    Nonreactive, avascular
Infected
    Previously infected
    Actively infected

---

common disturbance of fracture healing, developing in response to mechanical unrest at the fracture site. It is accompanied by increased perfusion, resorption, and rounding of the bone ends. Occasionally the bone ends hypertrophy, resembling an "elephant foot" on x-ray films, especially in edentulous patients. As an expression of the reactive component, the vascular nonunion will consolidate without resection of the bone ends when it is rigidly immobilized by interfragmental compression.

The nonreactive, avascular nonunion is a rare disturbance of bone healing that predominantly affects the severely atrophic, osteoporotic, edentulous mandible. It is especially common in cases where masticatory stimuli have been abolished by MMF performed alone or as an adjunct to internal fixation with interosseous wires or miniplates. It may also occur in the dentulous mandible affected by a comminuted fracture with devitalized bone fragments. The bone ends show no reactive expansion due to lack of blood supply.

Infected Nonunion

The previously infected nonunion is marked by radiographic signs of previous fracture-line osteitis and subsequent osteitis-free nonunion. There are no reactive or nonreactive bone changes.

In an actively infected nonunion, there is persistent chronic osteitis and fistulous drainage arising from sequestered or infected, devitalized bone, a loose screw, or other unstable internal fixation material.

Nonunions with a Bone Defect or Deformity

Nonunions with a bone defect or deformity differ from contact nonunions with correctly aligned fragments in that there is a defect between the bone ends caused by primary traumatic bone loss, secondary bone resorption, the sequestration of devitalized bone, or inadequate fixation measures. In other cases there may be malalignment of the fragments with associated deformity.

Aseptic Nonunion with a Bone Defect or Deformity

The reactive vascular form of the aseptic nonunion with a bone defect or deformity is characterized radiographically by viable, rounded or widened bone ends either separated by a defect or showing gross malalignment.

In the nonreactive avascular form there is no clinically overt infection, but radiographs show foci of devitalization in the mandibular stumps or intervening fragments.

Infected Nonunion with a Bone Defect or Deformity

The previously infected nonunion with a bone defect or deformity shows radiographic signs of prior osteitis and associated bone resorption with no clinical evidence of infection. In the actively infected nonunion there is persistent chronic osteitis and drainage. In some cases an accurate classification must rely not only on the clinical picture and x-ray findings but also on the clinical history, as for example in a previously infected nonunion with a bone defect (see Figure 19.1).

THERAPEUTIC CONCEPTS

The instability inherent in the attempted immobilization by MMF or MMF and interosseous wiring is the major cause of poor fracture healing. In an effort to compensate, the period of MMF was often prolonged. Despite, or perhaps because of, this prolonged immobilization, difficult avascular nonunions were a relatively frequent complication, especially in the atrophic and edentulous mandible.

This situation improved greatly with the introduction of functionally stable internal fixation with the dynamic compression plate (Spiessl and Schroll 1972). The early design, which used thin titanium plates, were not strong enough to withstand the high masticatory loads produced by certain patients. The incidence of postoperative complications declined dramatically with the introduction of thicker, more stable plates, and especially with the use of the eccentric dynamic compression plate

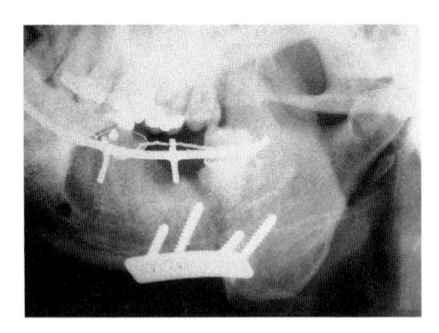

Figure 19.1 X-ray film of a 30-year-old patient four months after osteosynthesis of a preangular mandibular fracture with a four-hole DCP. The plate of choice at the base of the mandible would be an EDCP—if possible, a six-hole EDCP. The DCP used without a buttress far from the plate in the alveolar region provides insufficient stability. As a consequence of this instability, the following findings can be seen on the x-ray film: resorption, rounding, and a slight hypertrophic expansion of the bone ends; loosening of both screws in the anterior fragment with loss of anchorage of the screwheads in their plate holes; beginning osteolysis around the thread of these screws; fistulization and signs of chronic osteitis; secondary bone resorption and the beginning of sequestration of devitalized bone; and a slight deviation of the fragments. An accurate classification of a changeover from an aseptic delayed union in a nonunion and in an infected nonunion with defect and deformity must rely not only on all these x-ray findings but also on the clinical history and the clinical picture.

(EDCP) (Schmoker 1973, 1976), which exerts an eccentric compressive force better adapted to the mechanical loads on the mandible. Similar improvements have come with systematic application of the reconstruction plate to mandibular comminuted fractures and fractures with bone loss (Schmoker 1983, 1987).

With the refined implants presently available, disturbances of bone healing can no longer be attributed to deficiencies of the fixation material but rather to faulty application. The most common sources of error were analyzed in an earlier publication (Schmoker and Spiessl 1978). They are provided in Table 19.2. This review of case material, based on 20 years of experience with functionally stable internal fixations, shows that the fundamental causes of osteitis and nonunion are deficient blood supply and mechanical instability.

CLINICAL ASPECTS AND TREATMENT

The fundamental objectives in the treatment of infected fractures and nonunions of the mandible include the elimination of acute and chronic infection; bony consolidation, which may require the bridging of segmental defects; and the correction of any deformity. These objectives are accomplished by the use of long-standing fundamental principles of surgery and by use

Table 19.2 Causes of Osteitis, Delayed Union, and Nonunion

Faulty asepsis
Inadequate debridement
Inadequate hemostasis
Absence of closed drainage
Absence of antibiotic prophylaxis for a fracture in a dentulous area (that is, a fracture communicating with the oral cavity)
Trauma-related or surgery-related disruption of blood flow to bone and surrounding soft tissues, including obstruction of revascularization by implant material
Devitalized bone fragments (sequestra)
Avascular areas in the bone ends
Tooth in the fracture line with conservative fracture treatment
Devascularized tooth in a comminuted fracture line
Partially impacted wisdom tooth in the fracture line
Inappropriate conservative fracture treatment
Internal fixation by interosseous wiring
Functionally unstable internal fixation with miniplates
Screw in the fracture line
Screw transfixing the fracture line (other than a lag screw)
Central compression at the basal margin of the mandible with a DCP, resulting in a deficient alveolar buttress, instead of eccentric compression with an EDCP
Deficient lingual buttress due to inadequate overbending of the plate
Compression plating of a comminuted fracture or fracture with bone loss, resulting in a deficient bony buttress, instead of reconstruction plating
Insufficient plate length, that is, compression plate too short to allow at least two bicortical screws in each fragment, or reconstruction plate too short to allow three bicortical screws in each fragment

of proper rigid fixation techniques. Depending on the clinical situation, the methods used are incisions and drainage, fistulectomy and suction irrigation, compression plating, reconstruction plating, corrective osteotomy, and combination therapy. In some respects these techniques represent a radical departure from the classic approach based on converting an infected nonunion to an aseptic nonunion and eventually resecting the nonunion after a prolonged waiting period. The proven capabilities of internal fixation in various areas of mandibular surgery have led to this fundamental change in the management of nonunions. The application of these new therapeutic principles can significantly shorten treatment time and alleviate patient discomfort (Burri 1974, Rittman 1974, Schmoker 1978, Spiessl 1972, 1982, 1988) (see Table 19.3). Effective treatment of difficult complications is of prime importance in the traumatology of the mandible. Furthermore, experience gained in this area has yielded valuable insights that can be applied to the primary treatment of mandibular fractures.

Table 19.3 Treatment of Bone Healing Disturbances

Diagnosis	Treatment
Osteitis	
Early osteitis	Incision and drainage
Late osteitis	Fistulectomy and suction irrigation
Delayed Union	
Aseptic	Compression plating
Infected	Combination therapy
Nonunion	
Contact Nonunion	
Noninfected	
Reactive, vascular	Compression plating
Nonreactive, avascular	Reconstruction plating
Infected	
Previously infected	
edentulous	Reconstruction plating
dentulous	Corrective osteotomy
Actively infected	Combination therapy
Nonunion with a Bone Defect or Deformity	
Noninfected	
Reactive, vascular	
edentulous	Reconstruction plating
dentulous	Corrective osteotomy
Infected	
Previously infected	
edentulous	Reconstruction plating
dentulous	Corrective osteotomy
Actively infected	Combination therapy

The following section describes the individual therapeutic techniques as they are applied in practice (Texhammer 1984).

Incision and Drainage

Acute osteitis produces the typical manifestations of a perimandibular abscess. The osteitis usually necessitates immediate incision, wound culturing to determine antibiotic sensitivities, and appropriate drainage. In addition, the wound must be explored to identify and eliminate infectious foci, especially devitalized bone fragments that may form sequestra.

Internal fixation material, if solidly attached, should be left alone. A loose screw can be replaced by an emergency screw of slightly larger diameter (3.2 millimeter instead of 2.7 millimeter). If the internal fixation is no longer stable, however, all implants should be removed. Additional operative measures, such as revisionary fixation or cancellous bone grafting, are withheld in the acute stage of infection. Such measures may be undertaken three to four weeks later, after the infection has cleared under a regimen of daily irrigations through the drains and specific antibiotic treatment.

Fistulectomy

Signs of chronic infection such as local heat, redness, tenderness, and fistulization can arise in association with late osteitis, an infected delayed union, or an infected nonunion. These symptoms are an indication for operative exposure with fistulectomy, wound culturing for antibiotic sensitivity, and debridement (Burri 1975, Rittmann 1974). Meanwhile a systematic search is made for potential infectious foci. Sequestra, devitalized bone fragments, or a partially impacted wisdom tooth in the fracture line must be removed. In cases where the infection arises from a tooth in the fracture line, the offending tooth will necessitate root treatment, especially when there is a comminuted fracture with impairment of revascularization (Schmoker and Spiessl 1976).

The anchorage of the implant material is checked, and the stability of the fracture is assessed. A single loose screw can be replaced by an emergency screw with a slightly larger diameter. If multiple screws are loose but the fracture has already consolidated, removal of the implants is all that is required.

Loose internal fixation in an unconsolidated fracture is managed by removing the old fixation material and instituting appropriate combination therapy (see below) that includes revisionary fixation of the fracture (Schmoker and Spiessl 1976, Speissl 1988).

The soft tissues are closed over adequate drainage, and specific antibiotic therapy and daily suction irrigation are maintained until the infection clears. With the fracture stabilized, the infection should resolve within a short time. The drains are left in place for several days after antibiotic treatment is discontinued.

Compression Plating

The reactive, vascular contact nonunion is the most common late sequela to neglected fracture treatment, conservative fracture treatment, or inadequate internal fixation with miniplates or interosseous wires. Schenk et al. (1968, in Weber 1973) were able to show that a nonunion will undergo revascularization, and the well-perfused bone ends will proceed to osseous union, under the mechanical rest provided by a stable internal fixation. Accordingly, the treatment of a vascular, reactive contact nonunion should follow the very same principles that apply to the internal fixation of fractures. This includes avoiding the major errors responsible for loss of implant stability:

- a screw in or crossing the fracture line,
- deficient lingual or alveolar buttress opposite the plate,
- insufficient length of the implant, and
- use of a dynamic compression plate (DCP) (Spiessl 1972) instead of an eccentric dynamic compression plate (EDCP) (Schmoker 1973,

1976) or a three-dimensionally bendable reconstruction plate (3-DBRP) (Schmoker 1983, 1987).

Effective treatment requires the noncompromising stabilization effected by compression fixation. Proceeding from the chin toward the mandibular angle, compression plating of the contact nonunion is performed with the implants listed in Table 19.4 and presented in Figures 19.2–19.5. The correct indications for the individual implants are of primary concern for obtaining optimum compression across the nonunion.

The Dynamic Compression Plate

A median or paramedian nonunion in the *interforaminal* mandible can be adequately stabilized by a six-hole DCP applied infra-apically, that is, over the center of the nonunion (see Figure 19.2b). The stability of the fixation depends critically on having a competent bony buttress opposite the plate. This can be achieved by overbending the plate to compress the fragments on the lingual side. A dental splint encompassing three teeth on each side of the nonunion reduces the potentially harmful, short-acting dynamic masticatory forces acting on the nonunion. However, the splint has no tension-band effect on the long-acting static compressive forces because of its mobile dental anchorage in the periodontium.

Following the plate and tension band principle of Spiessl and Schroll (1972), a two-hole DCP applied as a tension band on the tension side of the alveolar process combined with a four-hole DCP applied as a stabilization plate on the pressure side of the basal margin of the mandible (see Figure 19.4b) is the configuration of choice for stabilizing a preangular nonunion in patients with a missing third molar or a shortened dental arch.

Table 19.4 Plate Selection for Contact Nonunion

Area	Plate
Interforaminal region (Figure 19.1)	EDCP basal (Figure 19.2a) DCP infra-apical (Figure 19.2b)
Body of mandible (Figure 19.2)	EDCP basal EDCP (Figure 19.3a) infra-apical (Figure 19.3b)
Preangular region (Figure 19.3)	EDCP basal (Figure 19.4a) DCP and tension-band plate (Figure 19.4b)
Angle region (Figure 19.4)	3-DBRP (Figure 19.5a) 2-DBRP and tension-band plate (Figure 19.5b)

The Eccentric Dynamic Compression Plate

The EDCP, which exerts an eccentric compressive force, is the plate of choice for producing interfragmental compression at the base of the mandible (Schmoker 1973, 1976). The four-hole or six-hole EDCP is considered the universal plate for the stabilization and compression of nonunions located anywhere in the body of the dentulous or edentulous mandible (see Figures 19.2a, 19.3, and 19.4). The stability necessary for immobilizing the nonunion is derived from the buttress that the EDCP produces through its compressive action on the alveolar process.

The dental splint, with its mobile periodontal anchorage, does not contribute to stabilization by compression. It does, however, reduce the dynamic masticatory forces that perpetuate the nonunion and thus minimizes their impact on the fracture site.

Lag Screw

In all sagittal nonunions with an oblique fracture line, optimum localized compression can be produced by passing a lag screw across the fracture site close to the center of the fracture surface. The screw may be used alone, or it may be inserted through a plate hole.

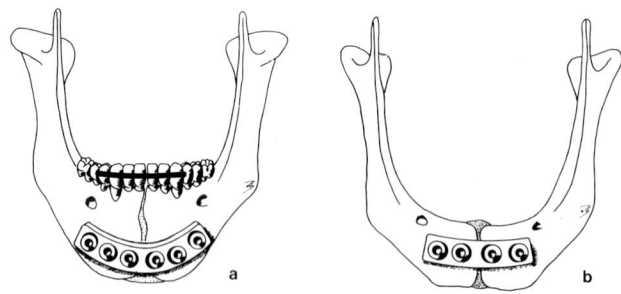

Figure 19.2 Contact nonunion in the interforaminal region. (a) For a basal (eccentric) plate position, compression plating with the EDCP can be applied anywhere on the mandibular body. In the symphyseal area applying an EDCP to the basal, rounded portion of the chin with no bending is easier than to apply a DCP to the infra-apical area, where an anatomic midline bulge with lateral indentations extending from the chin to the alveolar process complicates adaptation and overbending of the plate. The eccentric compressive action of the EDCP neutralizes the alternation of tension and pressure on the nonunion that typically occurs in the chin area. (b) For an infra-apical (central) plate position: compression plating with the DCP. A four-hole plate is satisfactory in the edentulous mandible, whereas the dentulous mandible requires a six-hole plate due to the alternative tensile and compressive loading of an infra-apical plate in the chin area. The DCP can be applied only centrally; if the nonunion is farther from the midline, a six-hole plate cannot be applied infra-apically without impinging on the emerging mental nerve.

Reconstruction Plating

The nonreactive avascular nonunion, characterized by devitalized bone fragments or avascular bone ends and occurring chiefly in the atrophic, osteoporotic, edentulous jaw, is difficult to manage by compression plating alone, which may bring about consolidation only through a protracted course of healing. If a functionally stable compression plate is already in place, an expectant approach may be taken because the prolonged healing process itself does not constitute an ordeal for the patient.

The Three-Dimensionally Bendable Reconstruction Plate

The three-dimensionally bendable reconstruction plate (3-DBRP) (Schmoker 1983, 1987) was designed basically for the bridging of defects, but the pre-bent four- or six-hole plate is excellent for stabilizing nonunions in the angle region. In this region, the 3-DBRP can be combined with a two-hole tension-band plate in patients with a shortened dental arch (see Figure 19.5).

If functionally stable internal fixation is not in place, as in the case of miniplate fixation where there is little prospect for healing of the nonunion despite (or because of) the need for MMF, the devitalized portion of the nonunion should be resected to accelerate healing (see Figure 19.6). This creates a defect like that seen in a nonunion with a bone defect or following the realignment of a nonunion with angular deformity. The same applies to a previously infected nonunion that has progressed to a nonunion with a bone defect or deformity.

In an avascular nonunion, correct positioning of the fragments is easily accomplished even in the dentulous patient by adapting the reconstruction plate before the resection is performed (see Figure 19.6a). In a nonunion with a bone defect or deformity, on the other hand, reduction without measures like those required in a corrective osteotomy can be recommended only in the edentulous jaw.

Reconstruction is accomplished with the 3-DBRP and an interposed corticocancellous bone graft tailored to the size of the defect (see Figure 19.6b). With the screws placed through the center of the plate holes but not tightened, the graft is wedged in between the mandibular stumps to push them apart slightly and to move the screws to an eccentric position in the plate holes. When the screws are then driven home, the graft will be tightly compressed between the mandibular stumps and will act as a solid buttress to augment the stability of the fixation.

Corrective Osteotomy

In the dentulous portion of the mandible, the stumps of a nonunion with a bone defect or deformity (see Figure 19.7) or of a previously infected nonunion

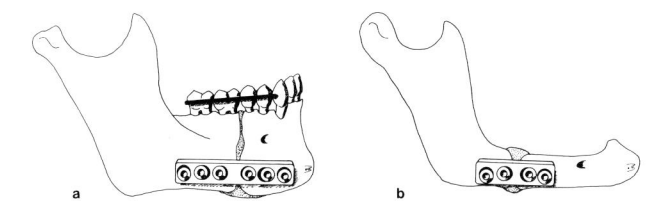

Figure 19.3 Contact nonunion in the mandibular body located distal to the mandibular angle. The plate must be applied basally, so use of the EDCP is indicated. (a) In the dentulous mandible: compression plating with a six-hole EDCP on the lower mandibular border. The static compressive force of the EDCP is not affected by the splint with its mobile periodontal anchorage. However, the splint does reduce dynamic masticatory forces acting on the nonunion. (b) In the edentulous mandible: compression plating with a four-hole EDCP on the lower mandibular border.

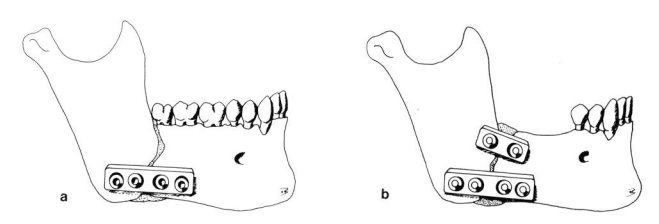

Figure 19.4 Contact nonunion in the preangular region. (a) With an unshortened dental arch: compression plating with a four- or six-hole EDCP. (b) With a shortened dental arch: compression by a plate and tension-band system. A two-hole DCP is applied as a tension band on the tension side of the alveolar process, and a four-hole DCP is applied as a stabilization plate on the pressure side of the mandibular base.

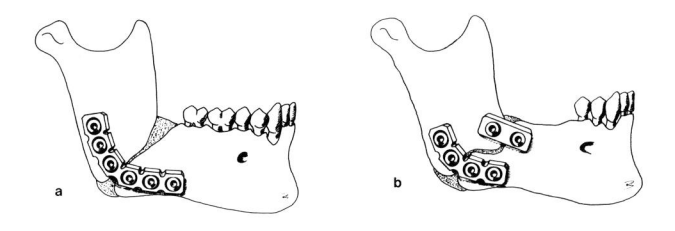

Figure 19.5 Contact nonunion in the angle region. (a) With an unshortened dental arch: compression plating with a pre-bent six-hole 3-DBRP. Interfragmental compression is produced entirely by the reduction-compression forceps, so the screws are centered in the plate holes. (b) With a shortened dental arch: compression by a plate and tension-band system. A two-hole DCP is applied as a tension band on the tension side of the alveolar process, and a four-hole 3-DBRP is applied as a stabilization plate on the pressure side of the lower mandibular border.

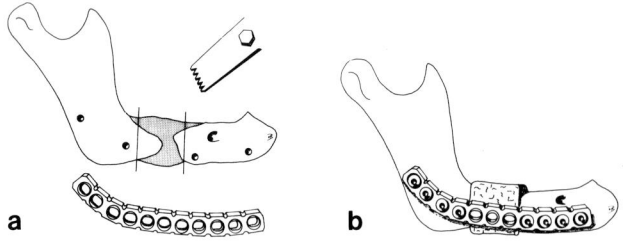

Figure 19.6 Nonunion with a bone defect or deformity in the edentulous mandible and a resected, nonreactive, avascular contact nonunion: reconstruction plating. The lack of a bony buttress means that the nonunion cannot be stabilized by interfragmental compression, so reconstruction plating is indicated. Stability is produced by a heavy-duty implant (that is, a 3-DBRP) bridging the defect. (a) Adaptation of the reconstruction plate: With the jaw correctly reduced, a 3-DBRP is adapted to the bone, and its position is marked by two drill holes at each end. Resection of the nonunion is then carried out. (b) Bone grafting: The plate is applied without tightening the screws. A cancellous bone graft is fitted into the defect so that it moves the screws in both mandibular stumps into an eccentric position relative to the plate holes. Alternative tightening of the screws compresses the bone graft between the bone ends and holds it in place. The stability-enhancing effect of the bony buttress lasts only until remodeling of the bone graft begins. During remodeling, stability is provided solely by the bridging action of the reconstruction plate.

that has been resected cannot easily be placed into a proper occlusal relation with the maxilla at operation, as can be done in a displaced comminuted fracture or a fracture with bone loss. This is due to the compensatory shifting of one or more teeth that occurs in response to a prolonged deformity of the jaw. It is necessary in such cases to simulate the operation on models of the dental arches (see Figure 19.7a) like those used for the planning of corrective osteotomies in orthognathic surgery. A saw cut is made through the model in the area of the nonunion, and it is determined whether the original occlusion can be reestablished (see Figure 19.7b).

In many cases this can be accomplished by simple grinding in the expectation that some spontaneous repositioning of shifted teeth will occur following operative repositioning of the mandibular stumps. In other cases it will be necessary to incorporate preoperative or postoperative orthodontic measures into the treatment plan in order to restore the original occlusion.

The simulation model is used to prepare a lingual "key plate" made of methylmethacrylate, and a dental splint or orthodontic arch bar (if there has been preliminary orthodontic treatment) is prepared and placed on the vestibular side (see Figure 19.7b). Following resection of the nonunion, these appliances are ligated to the teeth to establish the desired occlusion (see Figure 19.7c) and are left in place for six weeks. MMF is maintained only during the operation itself.

When the mandible is reconstructed using the 3-DBRP (see Figure 19.7d), the screws are inserted through the plate in the neutral position and left somewhat loose. Then a corticocancellous bone graft is interposed so that it moves the screws in both mandibular stumps from the neutral to the eccentric position in the plate holes. Tightening the screws will compress the graft between the fragments and create a bony buttress to stabilize the fixation.

Combination Therapy

Infection cannot resolve in the presence of a fracture, and bony consolidation of a fracture cannot occur in the presence of infection. This is the essential flaw in the classic, conventional treatment concept, with its staged approach to curing the infection and resecting the nonunion.

The techniques of functionally stable internal fixation that have proved effective in various areas of mandibular bone surgery have led to a reordering of priorities in favor of a combined treatment principle centering on the forced restoration of bony continuity. With this modern combination therapy, even complex problem cases involving an infected nonunion with a bone defect or deformity can be successfully managed by a single-stage procedure with little risk of complications. The only exception is the acute infection, which must be treated before combination therapy is initiated. Consequently a two-stage procedure is required.

The process of combination therapy first requires culturing the site to determine antibiotic sensitivities. Later, fistulectomy and debridement are performed and specific antibiotic treatment is administered. The wound is systematically explored for potential infectious foci. Sequestra, devitalized bone, and a partially impacted wisdom tooth in the fracture line, if present, must be removed. The tooth in the fracture line is examined for vitality and periapical osteolysis, which may necessitate corresponding treatment.

Internal fixation material on an infected nonunion is invariably loose or incorrectly applied and therefore must be removed. A delayed union or contact nonunion requires compression plating with a six-hole EDCP (see Figures 19.2, 19.2a, and 19.3). Alternatively, a median or paramedian nonunion may be fixed with a six-hole DCP applied infra-apically (see Figure 19.2b). For a nonunion in the angle region, it is preferable to combine a two-hole tension-band plate on the alveolar process (if there is room for it) with a basally applied four-hole DCP (see Figure 19.3b) or a pre-bent four-hole 3-DBRP (see Figure 19.5b).

The resected, avascular nonreactive nonunion or the more common nonunion with a bone defect or de-

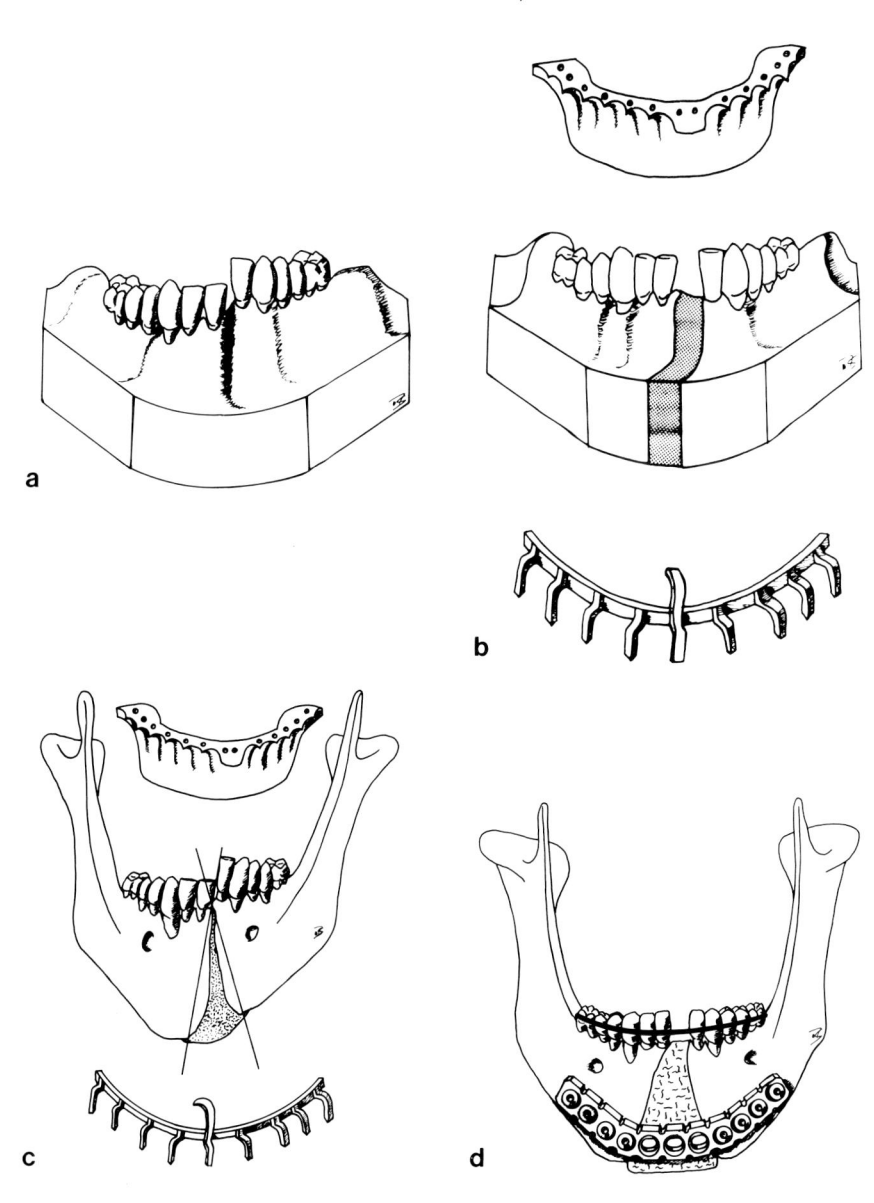

Figure 19.7 Nonunion with a bone defect or deformity in the dentulous mandible: corrective osteotomy. A long-standing jaw deformity results in compensatory shifting of the dentition. Thus the occlusion cannot be restored intraoperatively as it can with a displaced fracture, and a procedure like that for a corrective osteotomy is indicated. (a) Model simulation: A model of the dental arch shows the deformity at the site of the nonunion. The model is sectioned at that location, and an attempt is made to restore the original occlusion. (b) Key plate and dental splint: Simulation model with dental segments correctly occluded to the maxilla. A lingual key plate is prepared from methylmethacrylate, and a dental splint is adapted to the arch. The key plate makes it easier to position the mandibular stumps in correct occlusion by interlocking with the lingual tooth surfaces by a key-in-lock mechanism. (c) Resection and retention: Resection of the nonunion. The dental segments are held in position by wiring the lingual key plate and dental splint in place; they stabilize the dental arch for six weeks. Additional retention is provided by intraoperative MMF. (d) Fixation and bone grafting: The 3-DBRP is adapted and attached without tightening the screws completely. A bone graft is fitted into the defect so that it moves the screws in both mandibular stumps from the neutral to the eccentric position in the plate holes. Final tightening of the screws compresses the graft between the bone ends.

formity occurring in the edentulous mandible is managed with a 3-DBRP and an interposed bone graft as described in the section on reconstruction plating (see Figure 19.6). A nonunion with a bone defect or deformity in the dentulous mandible calls for the preparations and operative measures outlined in the section on corrective osteotomy (see Figure 19.7).

Combination therapy is concluded by establishing adequate drainage. The wound is irrigated daily through the drains until the infection resolves completely. Several days after antibiotics are discontinued, the drains may be removed. Case reports illustrating the clinical aspects and therapy of infected fractures and nonunions of the mandible are presented in Figures 19.8–19.11.

Figure 19.8 Infected delayed union: combination therapy. A 48-year-old man sustained a spontaneous fracture of the left mandibular angle while chewing food several days after surgical removal of the wisdom tooth. A dentist treated the fracture with MMF for six weeks. A chronic late osteitis ensued, with swelling and intraoral fistulization. (a) X ray at 12 weeks shows signs of an infected delayed union with sequestration of a bone fragment in the region of a fragment fracture. (b) Specific antibiotic treatment was administered concurrently with combination therapy involving fistulectomy, reconstruction with a six-hole 3-DBRP, and cancellous bone grafting.

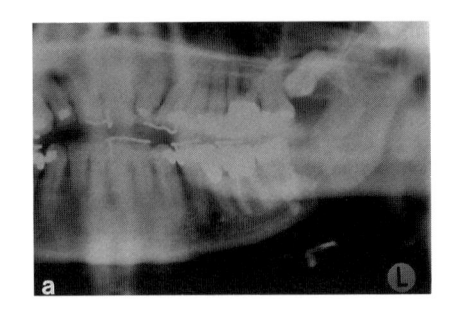

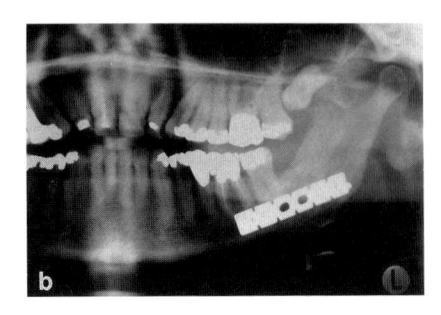

Figure 19.9 Infected contact nonunion: combination therapy. A 28-year-old man presented with signs of acute early osteitis (swelling, redness, fracture-line abscess) one week after sustaining a low subcondylar fracture and an undisplaced mandibular fracture in the left cuspid area treated conservatively by MMF. Following incision, suction irrigation, and specific antibiotic therapy, the infection cleared within a week. (a) Because of the infection, the period of MMF was extended from four to six weeks. After that time there was slight resorption of the bone ends with minimal consolidation of the fracture, so the MMF was extended another two weeks (eight weeks in all). (b) After 12 weeks the patient presented with signs of a chronic late osteitis, and at 17 weeks a springy mobility was noted at the fracture site. An infected contact nonunion was diagnosed, and combination therapy was instituted with fistulectomy and compression plating with an infra-apical six-hole DCP. Specific antibiotic therapy was reinitiated, and uncomplicated healing ensued.

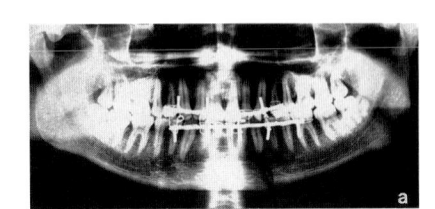

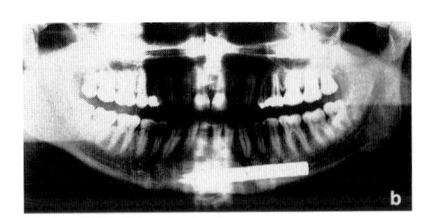

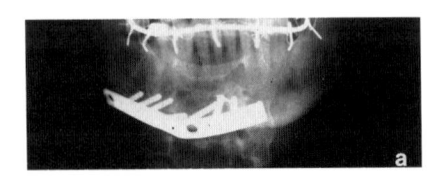

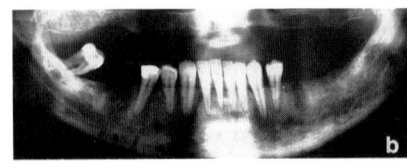

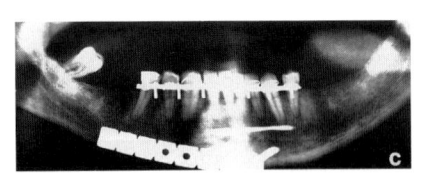

Figure 19.10 Infected nonunion with a bone defect: combination therapy. In a job-related injury, a 40-year-old man sustained a comminuted fracture of the right mandible with bone loss, a left subcondylar fracture, and a Le Fort III fracture. The comminuted fracture was fixed with a 10-hole DCP. (The following errors were made: no antibiotic coverage, failure to canalize a subluxated canine tooth in the area of comminution and bone loss, DCP applied basally, plate too weak for bridging.) (a) At 14 weeks a chronic, late osteitis developed, with radiographic signs of a loose screw. At reoperation in week 16 the internal fixation was removed along with several sequestra. The fracture appeared stable, so revisionary fixation was considered unnecessary. (b) At 24 weeks the patient presented again with an infection. An infected nonunion with a bone defect was diagnosed on examination. (c) Specific antibiotic treatment was given concurrently with combination therapy involving fistulectomy, canalization of the canine tooth in the area of the defect, reconstruction with an eight-hole 3-DBRP, and bone grafting. The fracture went on to uncomplicated union.

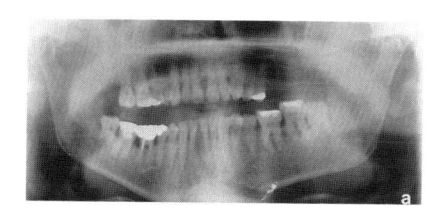

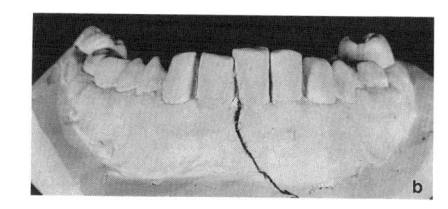

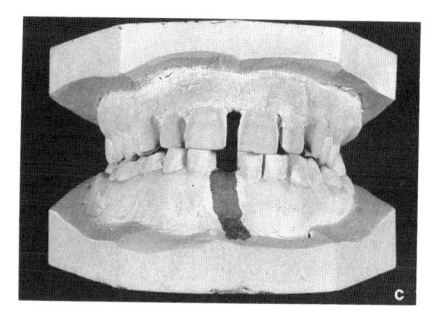

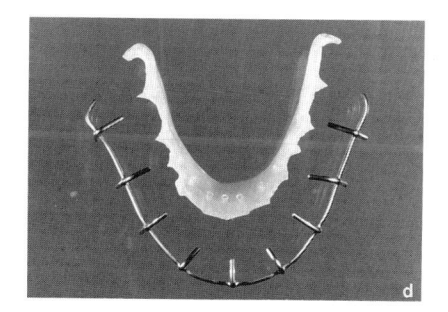

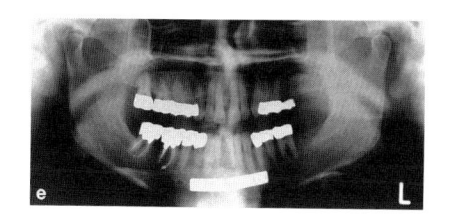

Figure 19.11 Previously infected nonunion with deformity. A 44-year-old man sustained a fracture of the chin area in an automobile accident. A general surgeon treated the fracture by interosseous wiring. (The following errors were made: occlusion was not established, MMF was not applied.) (a) At 19 weeks, after recurrent bouts of swelling, the patient presented with a previously infected nonunion with bony deformity. (b) The jaw model shows a conspicuous step-off deformity with loss of space for the luxated incisor. The deformity is manifested by pronounced malocclusion. (c) The correct position of the fragments is simulated by sectioning the jaw model at the site of the nonunion and restoring the dental arches to the original occlusion. (d) The model is used to prepare a methylmethacrylate lingual key plate and a buccal dental splint. (e) Following the procedure for a corrective osteotomy, the nonunion was resected under antibiotic coverage, the fragments were positioned with the aid of the lingual key plate, the dental arch was stabilized with the dental splint, the occlusion was retained intraoperatively by MMF, and the osteotomy site was fixed with a six-hole DCP and a bone graft. Uncomplicated healing ensued.

SUMMARY

The main problem with the conventional, classic treatment of fracture line osteitis, delayed union, and nonunion lies in the interdependency of fracture healing and infection. This has prompted the development of a specific combination therapy aimed at curing the infection and eliminating the disturbance of bone healing in a one-stage procedure. The internal fixation techniques that have proven their efficacy in the management of nonunions are also optimum for the primary treatment of fractures and are associated with the lowest rate of complications.

BIBLIOGRAPHY

Burri C: Post-Traumatic Osteomyelitis. Bern, Stuttgart, Vienna Huber, 1975, p. 169.

Lexer E: Über die Entstehung von Pseudarthrosen nach Frakturen und nach Knochentransplantationen. Langenbecks Arch Klin Chir eitis 119:520, 1922.

Luhr HG: Moderne Verfahren bei der Behandlung der Unterkieferpseudarthrose. Akt Traumatologie 3: 165, 1973.

Müller ME, Allgöwer M, Schneider R, Willenegger H: Manual of Internal Fixation. 1st and 2nd editions. Berlin, Heidelberg, New York, Springer, 1970 and 1979.

Pauwels F: Gesammelte Abhandlungen zur funktionellen Anatomie des Bewegungsapparates. Berlin, Heidelberg, New York, Springer, 1965.

Rittmann WW, Perren SM: Cortical Bone Healing after Internal Fixation and Infection. Berlin, Heidelberg, New York, Springer, 1974.

Schmoker R: Internal fixation of mandibular fractures using an eccentric dynamic compression plate (EDCP). (Universität Basel: medical dissertation, 1973). In New Concepts in Maxillofacial Bone Surgery. Spiessl B (ed). Berlin, Heidelberg, New York, Springer, 1976.

Schmoker R: Mandibular reconstruction using a special plate. J Maxillofac Surg 11:99, 1983.

Schmoker R: Functional Reconstruction of the Mandible. Berlin, Heidelberg, New York, London, Paris, Tokyo, Springer, 1987.

Schmoker R, Spiessl B: Infektion nach Osteosynthese von Unterkieferfrakturen. Kasuistik, Ursache,

Verhütung, Behandlung. Akt Traumatologie, 6:297, 1976.

Schmoker R, Spiessl B: Fehlermöglichkeiten bei der Osteosynthese von Unterkieferfrakturen. Dtsch Z Mund-Kiefer-Gesichtschir 2:129, 1978.

Spiessl B: Rigid Internal Fixation of the Mandible. Berlin, Heidelberg, New York, London, Paris, Tokyo, Springer, 1988.

Spiessl B, Hochstetter A: Unspezifische pyogene Infektionen im Kiefer-Gesichts-Bereich. In Allgemeine und spezielle Chirurgie, 4. Aufl. Allgöwer M (ed). Berlin, Heidelberg, New York, Springer, 1982.

Spiessl B, Schroll K: Gesichtsschädel. In Spezielle Frakturen- und Luxationslehre. Nigst H (ed). Stuttgart, Thieme, 1972.

Texhammar R, Schmoker R: Stable Internal Fixation in Maxillofacial Bone Surgery. Berlin, Heidelberg, New York, Tokyo, Springer, 1984.

Weber BG, Cech O: Pseudarthrosis: Pathophysiology, biomechanics, therapy, results. Bern: Huber, 1976.

CHAPTER 20

Rigid Fixation of Le Fort Maxillary Fractures

Joseph S. Gruss

John H. Phillips

The classic patterns of midfacial fractures occurring in the lines of weakness of the face, as originally described by Le Fort, are rarely encountered in clinical practice. The great majority of maxillary fractures consist of combinations and permutations of Le Fort type fractures. To add a further dimension of complexity to these fractures, injury patterns following high-speed motor vehicle accidents are often associated with a significant component of comminution of the maxilla. The aim of treatment of Le Fort fractures is the correct anatomical restoration of the maxilla in relation to the cranial base above and the mandible below and the reconstruction of any associated craniofacial, nasoethmoid-orbital, and zygomatic fractures. The plethora of techniques described for the management of these injuries attests to the fact that controversy and confusion still surround the management of these patients.

A variety of techniques for the treatment of both the acute maxillary injury and the post treatment complications have been described. Some authors have stressed that multiple small bone fragments in the maxilla can be left to heal by bony apposition, and no form of open reduction, which might disrupt the relationship of these small fragments and the overlying periosteum, is recommended. These authors feel that compression of the maxilla to the cranial base will assist apposition of fragments and facilitate healing.

Numerous methods of internal craniofacial suspension have been described suspending the maxilla or maxillo-mandibular complex to a stable portion of the skull, zygoma, or orbit (see Figure 20.1). Secondary deformity following this type of management is common. Midface elongation, common to the untreated Le Fort fractures, is replaced with problems of midfacial compression and retrusion following the surgically treated Le Fort fracture. A study by Ferraro and Berggren (1973) noted that 62% of Le Fort fractures treated with craniofacial suspension had late posterosuperior maxillary displacement. The midfacial collapse in these patients is most likely due to excessive tightening and compression of the comminuted maxillary buttresses by the craniofacial suspension wires. The loss of anterior projection is related to the fact that the vector force of

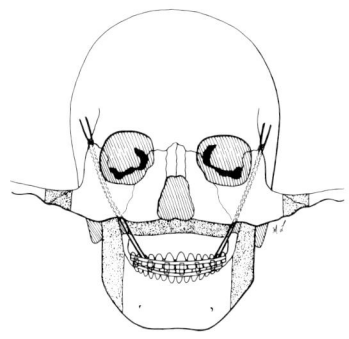

Figure 20.1 A complex midfacial fracture is stabilized with internal craniofacial suspension wires. Certain areas of the craniofacial skeleton tend to collapse, and this causes inadequate projection, increased facial width, and decreased facial height. The unstable areas are marked with stippling. Collapse through the zygomatic arch increases facial width. Telescoping of the maxilla through the unstable areas of the buttresses decreases the height of the mandibular ramus, particularly with condylar neck fractures, and leads to a decrease in facial height.

Figure 20.2 (a) Typical appearance of a young patient with severe midfacial fractures, treated with Adams suspension and MMF for nine months. Note the marked facial retrusion and shortening and widening through the arches. (b) Lateral view demonstrates severe dish face deformity.

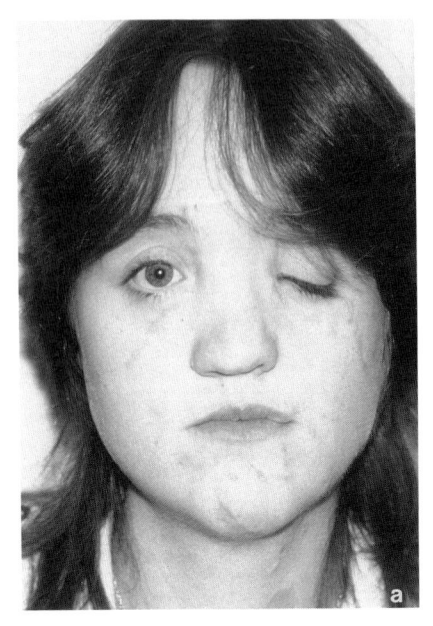

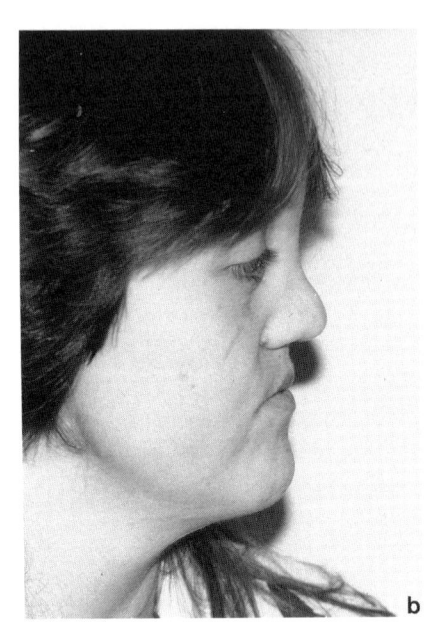

the pull of these wires is in a superior direction and thus will have no effect in maintaining adequate anterior maxillary projection (see Figure 20.2).

External craniofacial suspension devices have been recommended to correct this problem of compression and retrusion, particularly when a Le Fort fracture of the midface occurs in combination with bilateral condylar neck fractures of the mandible (see Figure 20.3). These devices, however, are difficult to apply, uncomfortable for the patient to wear for a prolonged period, and require constant adjustment. Manson et al. (1980) recognized the difficulties associated with the use of both internal craniofacial suspension wires and external craniofacial fixation in the management of these complex maxillary fractures. He recommended that the midface be divided into upper and lower regions and suggested the upper midface (including the orbital and naso-ethmoidal regions) be stabilized by interfragmentary wiring and then related to an intact frontal cranium. The lower midface was related, through proper occlusion, to a stabilized mandible, which had been correctly oriented to the cranial base. The comminuted areas of the maxillary buttresses were then left free. Although these techniques would decrease the incidence of midfacial retrusion and collapse, they would not prevent midfacial elongation, and, in the presence of condylar neck fractures, external fixation was still recommended. Concomitant sagittal fractures of the maxilla would be difficult to control with this method. Immobilization with interdental fixation was recommended for a minimum of 6 to 8 weeks. Later Manson et al. (1985) recognized that these comminuted buttresses cannot be left free, but must be wired directly and bone grafted when necessary.

Bonnano and Converse (1975) described the insertion of a block of iliac bone graft at the site of the comminuted posterior buttress in an attempt to hold the maxilla forward and prevent late maxillary collapse and retrusion. The results of their work were not presented and thus evaluation of this technique is difficult.

The surgical treatment utilized in our patient population is based directly on several basic principles. Our aim of treatment in complex Le Fort fractures of the maxilla is the exact and systematic evaluation of the extent and pattern of injury of the maxilla and associated injuries of the cranium, orbits, nose, zygoma, and mandible. Once the entire injury pattern has been defined, the normal position of the midface in relation to the skull and orbits above and the mandible below is re-established. This involves (1) fixation of the maxilla

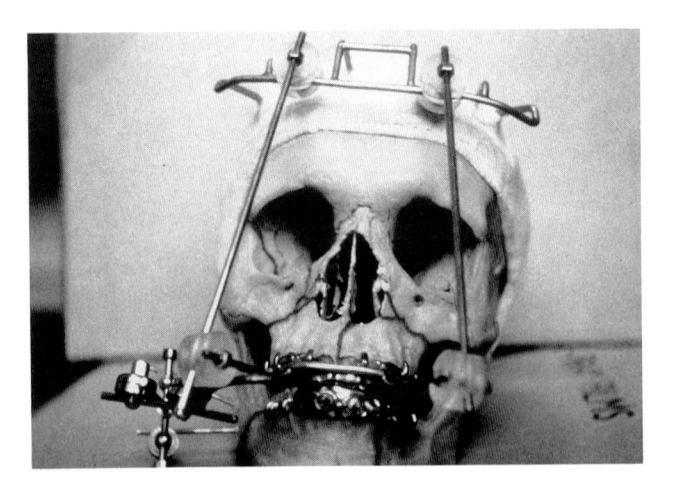

Figure 20.3 Craniofacial external suspension devices have been designed to maintain the facial projection and height. Even though the relationship of the occlusal segments to the skull base can be maintained with an external fixation device, maintaining correct midfacial contour and projection with these devices is impossible.

to the stable skull and orbits above, (2) re-establishment of normal maxillo-mandibular occlusal relationships below, and (3) evaluation and re-establishment of normal maxillary height and projection. Comminution of one or more of the anterior maxillary buttresses in combination with displacement, dislocation, or actual destruction of bony segments is common and will magnify the difficulty of determining both maxillary height and projection and of achieving maxillary stabilization and correct anatomical restoration.

The key, however, to reconstruction of complex Le Fort fractures, no matter how severe, is by direct exposure of all involved fractures, followed by reduction and anatomical reconstruction of the medial and lateral maxillary buttresses. Stabilization of the buttresses can be affected by interosseous wiring or miniplates. Unstable, comminuted, or missing buttresses can be reinforced or replaced with primary bone grafts using split rib or split skull grafts. This will facilitate the restoration of normal horizontal and vertical height and projection of the maxilla and midface and ensure that no relapse occurs during the period of soft-tissue healing and scar contracture. All fracture sites must be exposed directly in order to assess the degree of comminution, displacement, and dislocation of the fracture fragments and bone segments. This will allow the fractures to be reduced and stabilized in a normal relationship to the neighboring bony segments. The use of selected exposure and wiring not infrequently results in fractures being wired together in an unreduced position.

Sagittal fractures of the maxilla and palate increase the instability of the associated Le Fort fractures. Extension of the exposure and accurate reduction and fixation of all fractures, in combination with exact restoration of maxillary height and mandibular occlusion, will correct this injury pattern without the need for a palatal splint.

ANATOMICAL CONSIDERATIONS

The midface consists of pneumatic cavities, or sinuses, which are reinforced by vertically or horizontally oriented struts of bone. The importance of these pillars, or buttresses, has been described by Sicher and DeBrul (1970) and re-emphasized recently by Manson et al. (1980). The three principal maxillary buttresses are (1) the medial buttress (the nasomaxillary buttress, extending from the anterior maxillary alveolus, along the pyriform aperture and the nasal process of the maxilla to the frontal cranial attachment), (2) the lateral buttress (the zygomaticomaxillary buttress extending from the lateral maxillary alveolus to the zygomatic process of the frontal bone and laterally to the zygomatic arch), and (3) the posterior buttress (the pterygomaxillary buttress, which attaches the maxilla posteriorly to the pterygoid plate of the sphenoid bone) (see Figure 20.4). The two anterior buttresses (the medial and lateral but-

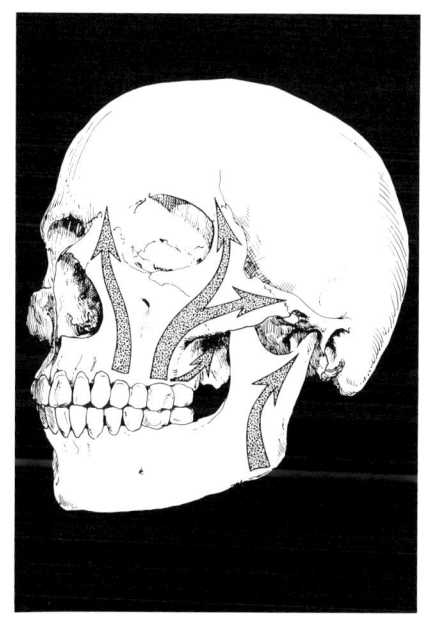

Figure 20.4 Diagram of the maxillary buttresses showing the two anterior buttresses (medial and nasomaxillary and lateral or zygomaticomaxillary) and the posterior buttress (pterygomaxillary). The relationship of these buttresses to the cranial base above, the mandible below, and the correct occlusion is seen.

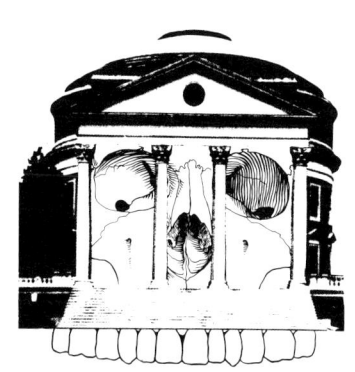

Figure 20.5 Diagram of the four anterior maxillary buttresses maintaining the position of the maxilla in relation to the cranium and carnial base above and the occlusal surface below. These buttresses are analogous to the supporting pillars of the roof of a building; the position and stability of each is interrelated. Exact anatomic reconstruction of the four anterior buttresses will allow exact repositioning of the maxilla in relation to the cranial base and will allow reconstruction of the exact vertical and horizontal projection and height of the maxilla. No reconstruction is needed at the posterior buttress.

tresses) and the posterior buttress provide a system of buttresses enclosing the functional units of the oral, nasal, and orbital regions.

These buttresses maintain the position of the maxilla in relation to the cranial base above and the mandible below. Exact anatomical reconstruction of the four anterior buttresses (see Figure 20.5) (medial and lateral

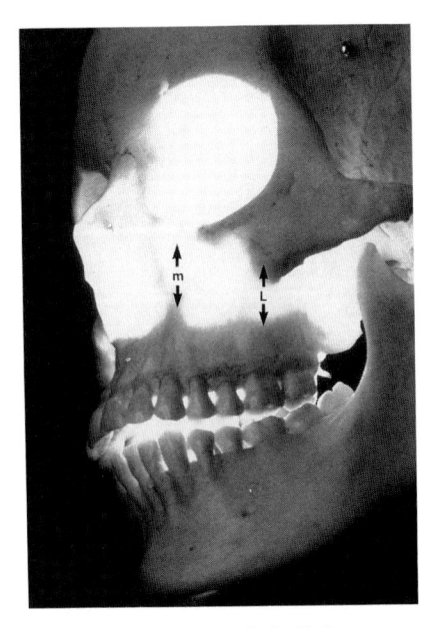

Figure 20.6 This transilluminated skull demonstrates the actual bony anatomy of the buttress system. Thinness of the anterior maxillary buttresses in relation to the other facial bones is evident; this predisposes to comminution of these buttresses in severe maxillary injuries (M = medial, L = lateral).

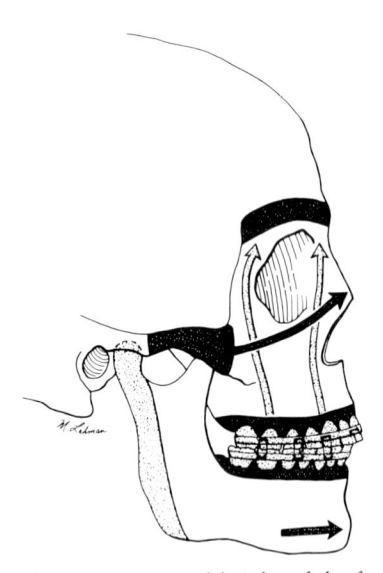

Figure 20.7 The correct vertical height of the face is restored by reconstruction of the vertical height of the ramus. The correct facial width and projection and anteroposterior projection are restored by reconstruction of the frontal bar, the zygomatic arches, and the occlusion, as well as of the anterior mandible.

on both sides) will allow exact repositioning of the maxilla in its correct anteroposterior position in relation to the cranial base and allow reconstruction of the exact vertical height and horizontal projection of the maxilla. No reconstruction is needed of the posterior buttress because the four anterior buttresses will maintain correct position of the maxilla. The intact mandible provides an additional buttress in relation to the cranial base, and the re-establishment of normal maxillomandibular occlusion will provide additional support to the reconstructed maxilla (see Figures 20.6 and 20.7).

PRINCIPLES OF SURGICAL REPAIR

The surgical technique has developed directly from reconstructive craniofacial surgery utilizing direct fixation and immediate bone grafting. The principles of repair involve four important concepts. First, reconstruction of the anterior maxillary buttresses is the key to maxillary repair. Second, direct exposure and fixation of these buttresses provides exact anatomical reconstruction. Third, reinforcement of unstable buttresses with bone grafts or miniplates or replacement of comminuted or damaged buttresses with immediate bone grafting will allow reconstruction and stabilization of even the most severe injuries without the need for any internal cranial suspension or external fixation devices. Finally, buttress reconstruction will prevent late midfacial collapse or elongation and secondary deformity.

SURGICAL PROCEDURE

The maxillary fractures are exposed through an upper gingivobuccal sulcus incision. Both maxillae are exposed subperiosteally to facilitate complete identification of all four anterior buttresses. The upper buccal sulcus incision communicates with the eyelid (blepharoplasty type) and upper facial incisions to provide complete periosteal stripping of the entire craniofacial skeleton where needed. Only then can the exact amount of comminution, displacement, and actual dislocation of bony segments be identified; and only then can the exact position of the maxillary buttresses, in relationship to each other and to other facial fractures, be assessed. All fractures are then reduced and internally fixed with miniplates. No attempt is made to retain periosteal attachments to small fragments of bone because this hinders adequate exposure of the maxillary buttresses. All small, loose fragments of bone and torn maxillary sinus mucosa are carefully removed; no drainage of the sinus is performed.

In Le Fort fractures in which an intact mandible and normal dentition are present, correct occlusion is re-established first using MMF. In Le Fort I fractures, both lateral and medial buttresses are repaired. In Le Fort II type fractures, additional fixation may be performed at the nasofrontal region and medial portions of the orbital rims. In Le Fort III fractures, buttress stabilization is combined with more extensive fixation at the nasoethmoid-orbital and fronto-zygomatic regions, the orbital rims, and zygomas as required.

When the Le Fort fractures are associated with fractures of the mandibular angle, body, or parasymphyseal region, and there are no sagittal fractures of the palate or fractures of the condylar neck, the correct occlusion is established first. The mandibular fractures are then repaired using compression plates, allowing rigid internal fixation. Maxillary buttress and upper facial repairs are then completed.

In the edentulous patient, careful anatomical reduction and fixation of the anterior maxillary buttresses is performed. No form of MMF is needed, and minor occlusal discrepancies are corrected by denture adjustments. Associated mandibular fractures are stabilized using internal fixation technique.

Le Fort type fractures associated with sagittal fractures of the palate require the re-establishment of normal occlusion in combination with direct fixation across the anterior buttresses and the palatal fractures anteriorly or posteriorly through an incision made in the palatal mucosa. Bone grafts or miniplates placed transversely across the sagittal fractures facilitate reinforcement of the unstable segments.

Bilateral condylar neck fractures of the dentulous mandible result in a loss of vertical mandibular height. In the repair of associated Le Fort type fractures of the maxilla, the position of the mandible in relation to the cranial base cannot be used as a guide and aid in maxillary stabilization. In this situation, a reverse order of fixation is used. The upper face and anterior maxillary buttresses are repaired, thus re-establishing the correct relationship of the maxilla to the cranium and cranial base. Once the maxilla has been stabilized, any fractures of the mandibular angle, body, or symphysis are repaired using rigid fixation techniques and correct maxillary-mandibular occlusion is re-established by MMF. The correct re-establishment of maxillary height and projection maintains the correct mandibular height in relation to the cranial base without the need for external fixation devices or open reduction of the condylar neck fractures. This will necessitate the maintenance of MMF for four to six weeks. If the condylar neck fractures are complex, with displacement of the head out of the fossa, or if the MMF needs to be released to maintain a patent airway or to ease nursing care, then open reduction and internal fixation with miniplates of the condylar neck fractures can be performed.

Le Fort type fractures associated with bilateral condylar neck fractures in an edentulous mandible provide a unique problem. The maxillary fractures are stabilized to the cranium as outlined, and any mandibular body fracture is repaired with rigid fixation techniques. Mandibular and maxillary splints are then used to facilitate MMF and maintenance of correct mandibular height. Open reduction and internal fixation of the mandibular condyles or the use of an external fixation device is necessary if it is not possible to fashion splints.

Special note must be taken concerning Le Fort fractures with impaction. These fractures may appear to be relatively stable and show minimal external deformity or movement on palpation. However, when these fractures are disimpacted and reduced, they may become extremely unstable and require extensive internal fixation and bone grafting.

HISTORICAL CONCEPTS

The limitations and potential complications associated with the use of internal craniofacial suspension and external fixation devices have been previously described. Before the development of miniplating systems for upper and midfacial reconstruction, interosseous wiring was used extensively to establish bony continuity (see Figures 20.8 and 20.9). Comminuted areas were reinforced with primary bone grafts (see Figures 20.10, 20.11, and 20.12). Associated mandibular fractures were repaired with rigid compression plating.

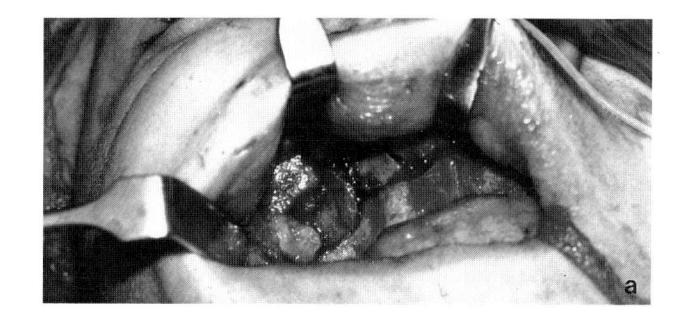

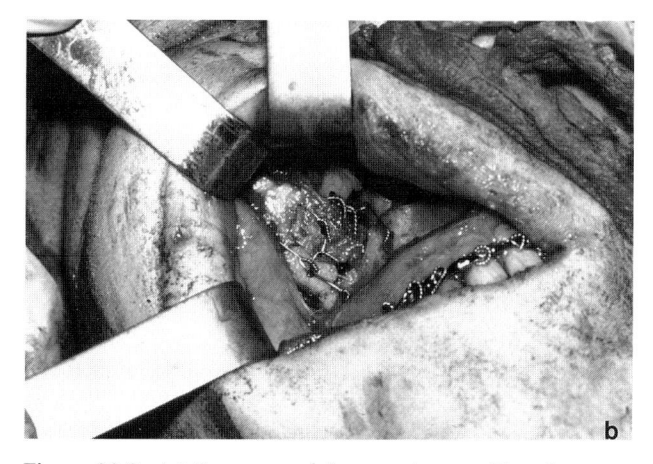

Figure 20.8 (a) Exposure of the anterior maxillary buttresses is performed through an upper gingivobuccal sulcus incision. Note multiple comminuted fractures of both anterior maxillary buttresses. (b) Prior to the advent of miniplates, fractures had to be repaired with multiple interosseous wires; chain link had to be used when necessary. The difficulties associated with adequate restoration of the height of the buttresses can be seen.

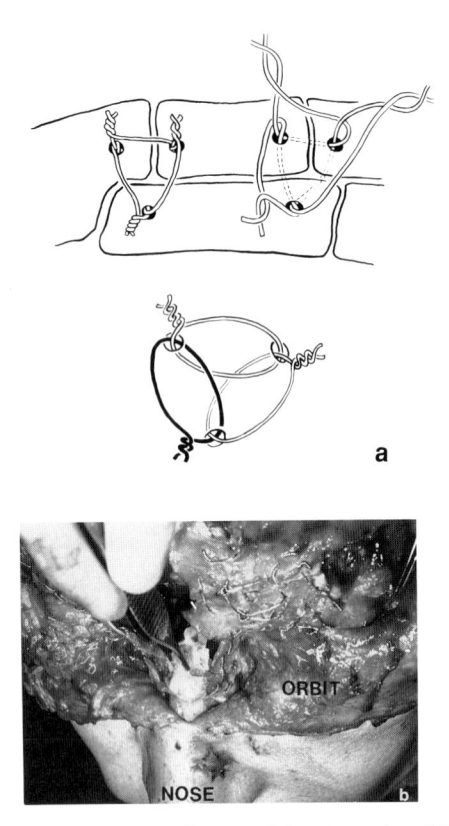

Figure 20.9 (a) Method of internal fixation of multiple small fragments to provide structural stability. Each fragment is wired to as many adjacent fragments as possible, utilizing the same drill holes. The wires themselves can be linked together to provide relatively stable fixation without the danger of wires pulling through bone. (b) Extensive areas of the craniofacial skeleton were originally fixed with extensive chain-link wiring prior to the development of miniplates. Even though extensive and multiple wiring was used, fixation was never rigid, and accurate bony healing in the reduced position was compromised by soft-tissue scarring and contracture in the healing phase.

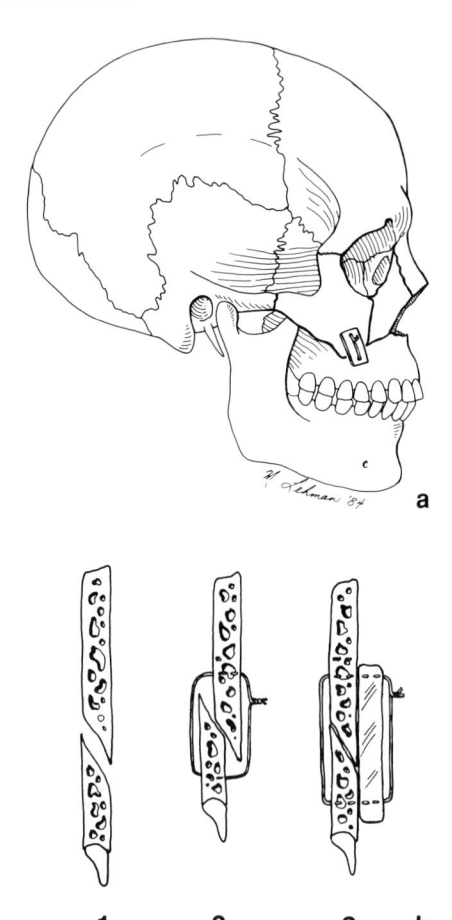

Figure 20.10 (a) Buttress stabilization prior to the advent of miniplates. Unstable oblique fracture of the anterior maxillary buttress are stabilized by the incorporation of a small bone graft at the wiring site. Similar stabilization can now be accomplished by the use of a miniplate. (b) Close-up view shows the inability of an interosseous wire to maintain reduction. The buttressing effect of the bone graft, exactly the same as a miniplate, is seen.

Even with extensive interosseous wiring combined with bone grafting, maintaining the intraoperative reduction was often difficult because the interosseous wires do not maintain three-dimensional stability. Particularly with comminuted fractures of the zygomatic arches, there was a tendency for the midface to retrude in an anteroposterior dimension with widening through the zygomatic arches. In addition, vertical shortening would occur due to failure to maintain adequate buttress height (see Figure 20.13).

With the development of newer, more sophisticated miniplate systems, miniplate fixation of the midface has almost totally replaced interosseous wires as our primary method of fixation and has solved the problems of arch and buttress collapse. Has the more extensive use of miniplates reduced the need for immediate bone grafting?

A careful analysis of cases treated over the past 11½ years led to the following conclusions: (1) miniplate fixation has reduced the need for primary bone grafts in the repair of the anterior maxillary buttresses and orbital rims; (2) the need for bone grafting in the craniofrontal region is slightly reduced when miniplates are used; (3) the need for immediate bone grafts has remained the same for repair of orbital wall defects and to reconstruct nasal support.

SPECIFIC FACTORS IN MINIPLATE FIXATION

Buttress Plating

Whenever possible, separate plates are used to repair both medial and lateral anterior maxillary buttresses. The lateral buttress plate should extend from

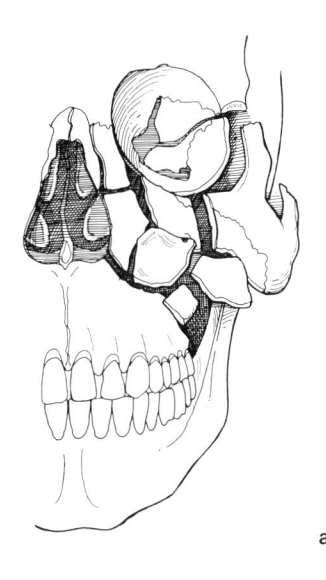

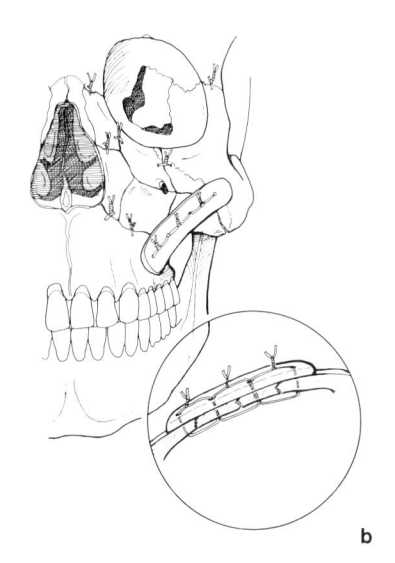

Figure 20.11 (a) Reinforcement in comminuted fractures of the anterior buttresses. (b) Incorporation of a carefully contoured and measured bone graft into the site of a comminuted or segmental fracture of the anterior buttress produces buttress reinforcement, stabilization, and re-establishment of the correct maxillary height. This can now be performed much more readily with a miniplate.

the strong, thick bone of the zygomatic body above to the thinner lateral buttress below. At least two screws are needed on both sides of the fracture. Care must be taken to avoid the tooth roots when inserting the lower screws (see Figures 20.14 and 20.15).

A fracture through the lateral buttress may be low, directly adjacent to the tooth roots. In this situation, the lateral buttress can be bypassed by extending the plate from the zygomatic body above to the medial buttress, or the region of the anterior nasal spine, below.

Care must be taken to align the plates along the lateral and medial buttresses. Screw placement through the thin bone of the anterior wall of the antrum should be avoided.

In the edentulous maxilla, placing the plates too low on the buttress will prevent adequate denture fitting. After the fracture has healed adequately, these plates must be removed.

Miniplates used for buttress fixation occasionally will become exposed through the upper buccal sulcus incision. As long as these plates remain rigidly fixed to bone, they will rarely become infected. The mouth is kept clean by frequent irrigation until the fracture heals adequately. Then the exposed plate can be safely removed.

Buttress Reconstruction

In high-velocity trauma, severe buttress comminution or bone loss is not uncommon. In addition, the thickness and strength of the buttresses vary greatly, and comminution and bone loss may occur with trauma of relatively low velocity. It is commonly asked whether a miniplate can safely bridge a bone gap and, if so, what the maximal bridging distance is before a bone graft is needed. The ability of plates to bridge bone gaps has not been studied experimentally; the following principles are based on our clinical experience and impression.

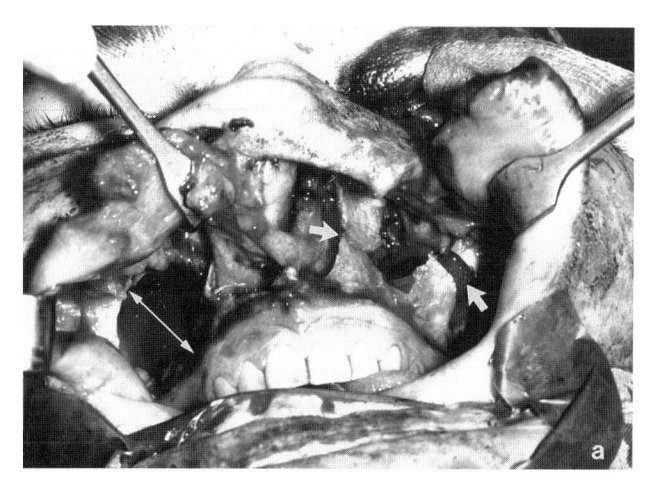

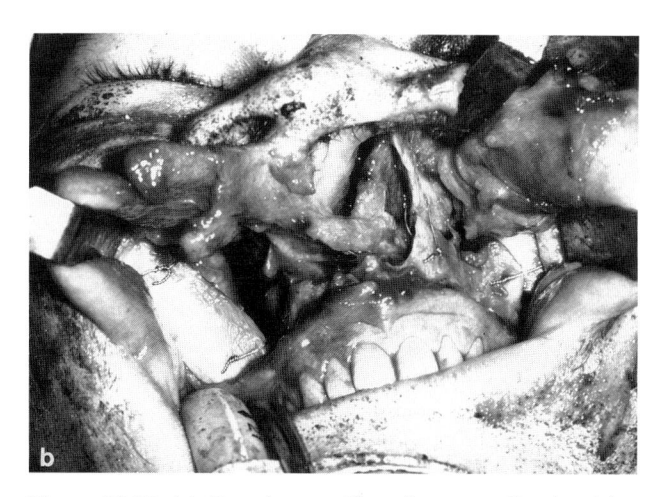

Figure 20.12 (a) Complex maxillary fractures. On the right side both anterior maxillary buttresses are lost. On the left side, oblique fractures are present through both maxillary buttresses. (b) The right maxillary buttress has been replaced with a split rib graft held in place with interosseous wires. On the left side, the two buttress fractures have been repaired with interosseous wire fixation. Note how the interosseous wires allow sliding and overlap of fracture sites, with loss of vertical maxillary height.

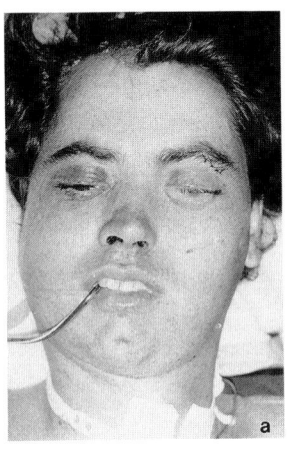

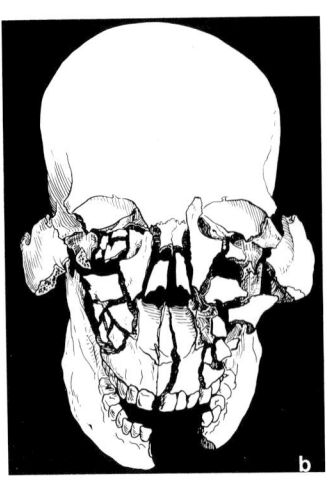

Figure 20.13 (a) A young male with massive panfacial injury. Note marked facial longation and collapse and marked increase in facial width through the zygomatic arches. (b) Artist's depiction of complex midfacial and mandibular fractures. (c) Extensive repair with multiple interosseous wires. Note extensive interosseous wires at both zygomatic arches. Even with this, an onlay rib graft must be placed at the right zygomatic body because of the perceived lack of projection in this area. The mandible has been repaired with a compression plate, and extensive bone grafting has been performed to the maxillary buttresses. (d) Anteroposterior appearance on the operating table shows restoration of facial height and midfacial projection. (e) Preoperative lateral view shows market facial elongation and midfacial and mandibular collapse. (f) Result on the operating table shows restoration of midfacial and mandibular projection and height. (g) At two years, the occlusion has been perfectly restored. (h) Anteroposterior examination at two years demonstrates progressive widening of the midface through the zygomatic arches with depression of the zygomatic bodies and sagging of the midfacial soft tissue, resulting in increase in scleral show. This has come about due to inadequate ability of extensive interosseous wiring and bone grafting to maintain the reduction obtained in the operating room. Particularly, inadequate stabilization of the zygomatic arches has resulted in widening of the midface and midfacial collapse, even though the normal occlusion has been maintained. (i) Lateral view at two years demonstrates midfacial collapse with loss of projection.

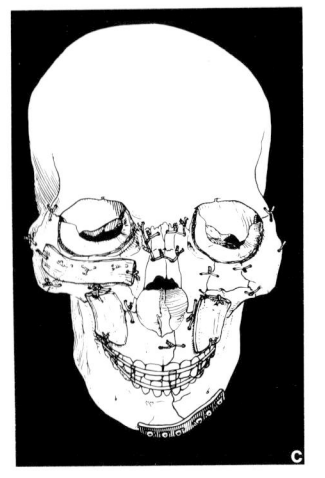

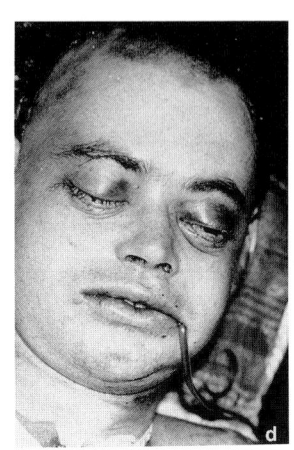

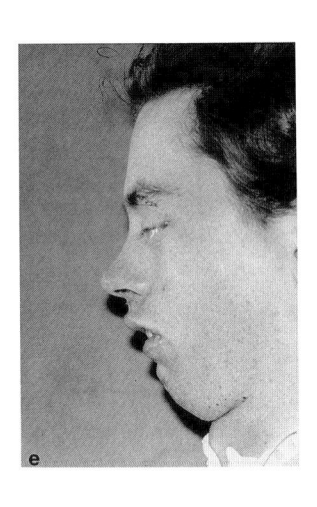

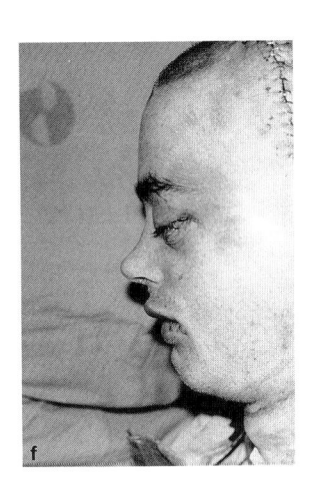

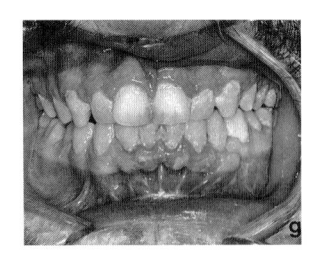

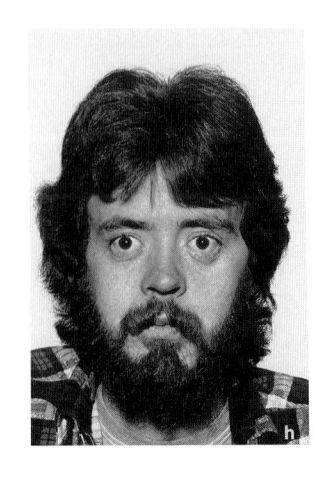

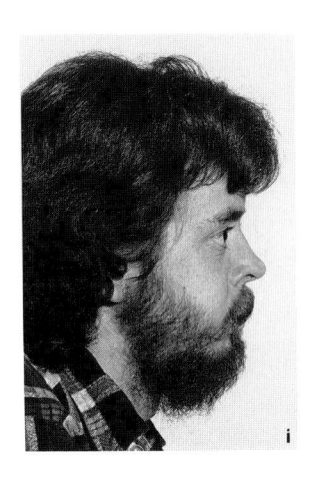

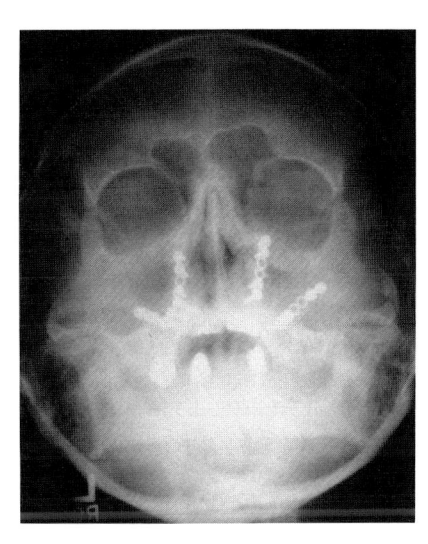

Figure 20.14 A partially edentulous patient with a simple Le Fort I fracture is repaired with four miniplates place on each of the anterior maxillary buttresses. There is no need to maintain any form of MMF.

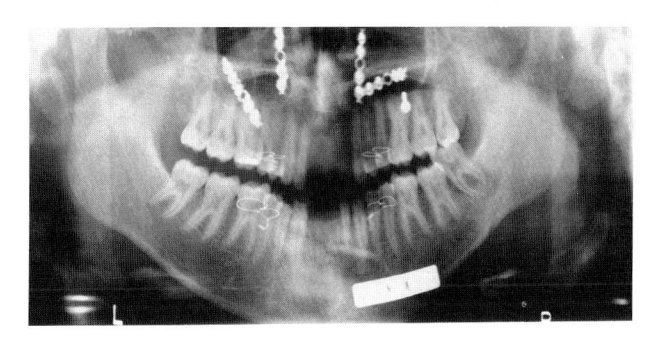

Figure 20.15 When the Le Fort I fracture is combined with a mandibular fracture, the patient is placed in the correct occlusion. The four anterior buttresses are repaired with miniplates. The mandible is repaired with a compression plate. The MMF can then be released.

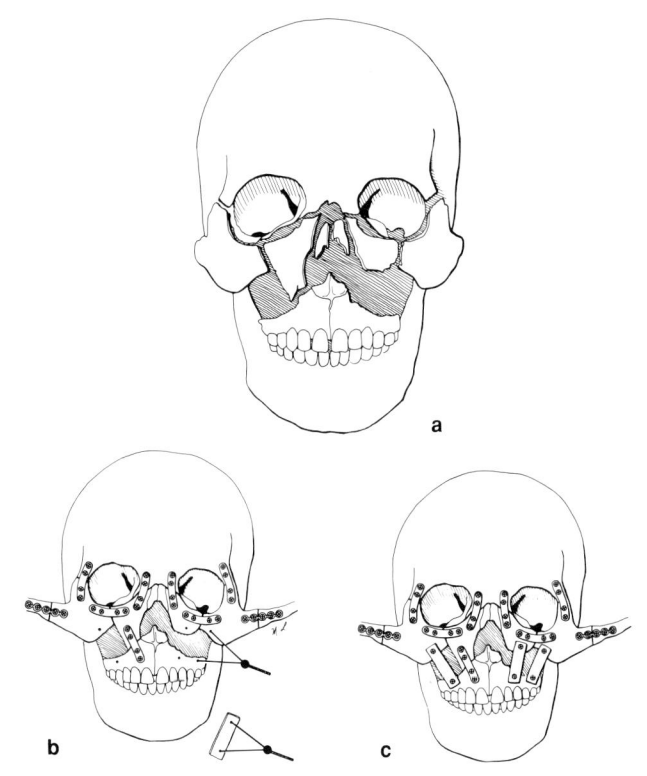

Figure 20.16 (a) Diagram of severe maxillary injury showing destruction of three of the four anterior maxillary buttresses. (b) Upper craniofacial repair is completed with fixation of the zygomatic arches, zygoma, orbits, and nasoethmoid region, establishing the correct upper, outer facial frame. The remaining medial buttress is now stabilized in the correct relationship to the cranial base above and the mandible below, thus re-establishing the normal maxillary height and projection. Exact measurements are now taken of each missing anterior maxillary buttress; these measurements are then transferred to a bone graft. (c) Each missing buttress is replaced with a carefully contoured and measured bone graft, resulting in re-establishment of the normal maxillary height and projection.

1. Miniplates can bridge gaps of up to approximately 0.5 centimeters in most areas of the craniofacial skeleton.
2. The ability to bridge gaps depends on the specific area of the craniofacial skeleton. Minimal muscular forces act on the craniofrontal and orbital region, and gaps in this region can be more readily bridged. The zygoma and maxilla are under the influence of greater muscular and masticatory forces, and therefore bridging is less successful.
3. Gaps of greater than 0.5 centimeters should be replaced with bone grafts, particularly in the lower midface, because plates and screws tend to loosen before bony continuity is restored.
4. Bone grafts can completely bridge the gap, being held in place at either end with lag screws; or a miniplate can bridge the gap, and the exact amount of bone graft can be wedged underneath the plate into the gap and held in place with screws placed from the plate directly into the bone graft (see Figures 20.16, 20.17, and 20.18).
5. In comminuted fractures, extensive bone may be lost or the anterior wall of the antrum may be destroyed. Although bone loss in this area does not affect the provision of stability with buttress fixation, it predisposes to the prolapse of overlying soft tissue or the buccal fat pad into the open antral cavity. Significant loss of the anterior wall of the antrum

Figure 20.17 A bone graft replacing the right lateral buttress held in place with four lag screws. The inferior orbital nerve can be seen above the bone graft.

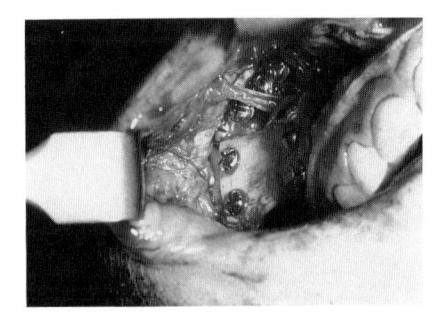

Figure 20.18 (a) Alternative method of buttress replacement. A miniplate bridges the bone gap in the buttress and is fixed rigidly in place at either end. (b) A carefully measured and contoured bone graft is now wedged into the gap and fixed to the overlying plate with two screws (B = bone graft). (c) On the opposite side, a larger bone gap is bridged by a long miniadaptive plate, which is anchored to the region of the anterionasal spine anteriorly and to the zygomatic body posteriorly. The width of the gap can be seen (arrows). (d) A long, carefully measured and contoured split calvarial bone graft (B) now replaces the bone gap and is fixed to the overlying plate with four screws.

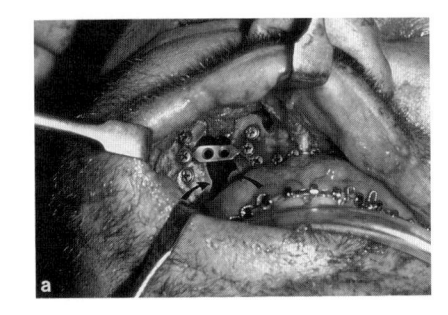

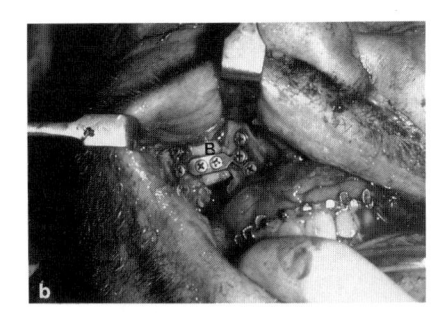

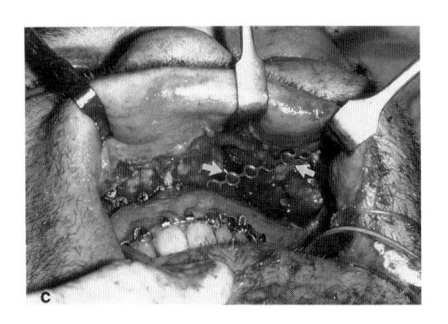

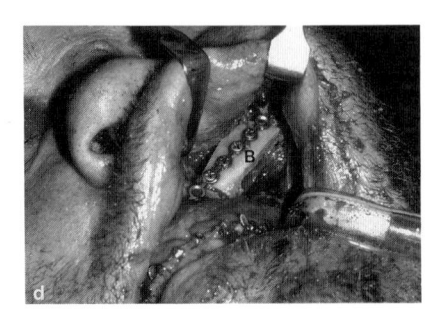

should be replaced by bone grafts to prevent soft-tissue prolapse and to maintain midfacial contour (see Figure 20.19).

Mandible Plating

Compression or reconstruction plate fixation of mandibular fractures resulting in rigid internal fixation, and miniplate and bone graft fixation of the maxillary buttresses combined with mandibular fixation have significantly improved both the intraoperative and postoperative management of these patients. Intraoperatively, the oral reinforced armor endotracheal tube can be pushed to the side, lateral to the posterior molar teeth, and interdental fixation can be applied. Once the maxillary and mandibular stabilization has been completed, the interdental wires can be released, and the endotracheal tube can be left in place until the patient no longer requires airway management. The interdental wires or elastics can be replaced, if necessary. In the great majority of patients, however, following rigid maxillary and mandibular repair, subsequent interdental fixation is not required and the need for tracheostomy is thus obviated. Airway management in this way facilitates the care of the polytrauma patient and the patient with a head injury or cervical spine fracture (see Figure 20.15). Only if Le Fort fractures are associated with bilateral condylar neck fractures, is maintenance of interdental fixation following completion of repair essential; a tracheostomy is usually needed in these patients. Rigid internal fixation of both the maxilla and the mandible will allow early removal of interdental fixation, if used, often at a maximum of three to four weeks following repair. In the edentulous patient, no form of interdental fixation is needed, resulting in early resumption of diet.

Mandibular Condylar Positioning

In the rigid fixation of elective midfacial and mandibular osteotomies for the correction of dentofacial deformities, the need for correct positioning of the mandibular condyle within the glenoid fossa has been well recognized. With rigid fixation of midfacial and mandibular fractures, the need for correct condylar positioning is just as important.

It is essential to understand that even with an intact mandible, the position of the occlusion is not stable when midfacial fractures are present. The position of the occlusal segments in relation to the cranial base may vary in an anteroposterior or vertical dimension, with changes in condylar position in relation to the glenoid

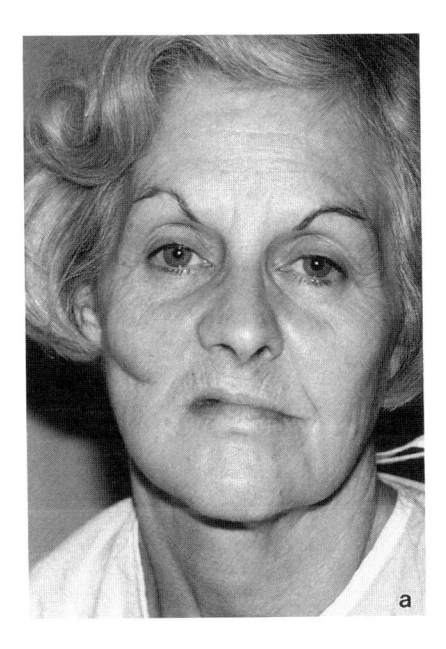

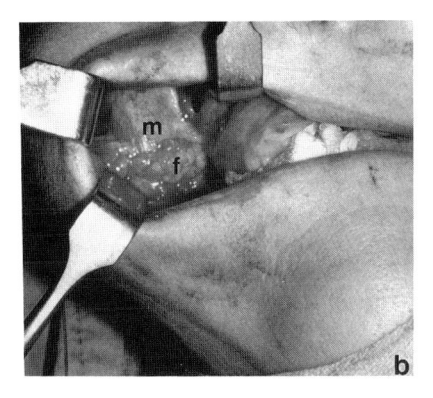

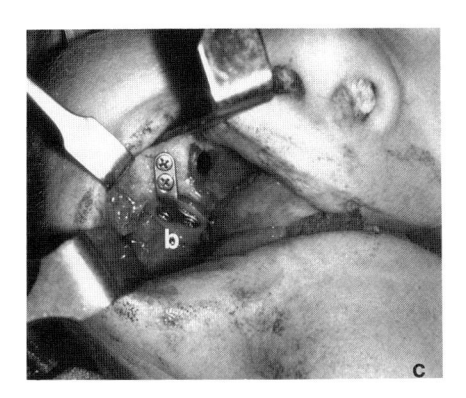

Figure 20.19 (a) A patient following a maxillary fracture with loss of the anterior wall of the maxilla and severe soft-tissue ptosis and prolapse into the maxillary antrum through the area of bone loss. (b) At exploration, the buccal fat pad (F) can be seen protruding through the open anterior maxillary wall (M = maxilla). (c) The defect in the anterior maxillary wall must be replaced with a split calvarial bone graft (B), held in place with a miniplate.

fossa. Thus, relating the entire repair of the upper face and midface to the occlusion alone may frequently result in post treatment deformities and malalignments that are difficult to explain. This is particularly liable to occur in the presence of coexisting condylar neck fractures and displaced fractures of the zygomatic arches.

In the reduction of a Le Fort midfacial fracture with an intact mandible, after the correct occlusion is established, there is a tendency to pull the mandible and occluded inferior maxilla forward and upward to meet the maxillary fractures above. This results in autorotation of the mandible due to a change in condylar positioning within the glenoid fossa. Miniplates are applied at the anterior maxillary buttresses, producing seemingly perfect reduction and internal fixation. When the interdental fixation is now released, the mandibular condyle rotates back into its correct position in the glenoid fossa and an unexplained open bite results.

Thus, the correct position of the condyle within the glenoid fossa must be ensured before the application of mandibular or buttress plates. This can be accomplished by gentle forward and upward pressure on the mandible to seat the condyle into the anterior aspect of the glenoid fossa.

Displaced Zygomatic Arch

The status of the zygomatic arch is the key to the repair of complex midfacial injuries. The position of the zygomatic arch, between its temporal attachment posteriorly and the zygomatic body and lateral orbit anteriorly, predetermines the position of the lateral and midfacial bones. A careful review of our early patients treated with extensive midfacial fixation and immediate bone grafting without zygomatic arch fixation has shown, in a significant number, late flatness of the zygomatic bodies and midface and an obvious shortening of the zygomatic arch, both clinically and on x ray. In all complex orbitozygomatic and midfacial fractures that show a shortening or loss of projection of the zygomatic arch on axial computer tomographic (CT) scanning (see Figure 20.20), stabilization of the zygomatic arch first is essential. Careful stabilization of the zygomatic arch itself, using miniplates and lag screws in combination with miniplate fixation at the fronto-zygomatic suture line, will produce exact restoration of correct projection of the zygomatic body and the lateral orbital wall in relation to the cranial base. This produces an intact outer facial frame. The upper inner facial frame, composed of the orbital rims and nasoethmoid-orbital bones, can now be exactly repositioned within this outer facial frame. As long as fractures are present at the Le Fort I level, this upper and outer fixation can be performed independent of the occlusion. The patient can now be placed in the correct occlusion, and the final step is the repair at the anterior maxillary buttresses. This should produce an exact three-dimensional anatomical reconstruction with normal midfacial projection.

Extensive bone loss and comminution may occur at more than one anterior maxillary buttress. It is rare for more than three out of the four buttresses to be lost, and the remaining buttress can be used to obtain the correct vertical height of the maxilla. The outer and upper, inner facial frames are first reconstituted. The correct occlusion is produced, and the condyles are seated correctly in the glenoid fossa. The remaining buttress is now accurately reduced and internally fixed with a miniplate, re-establishing the correct maxillary position in a vertical and anteroposterior dimension. The

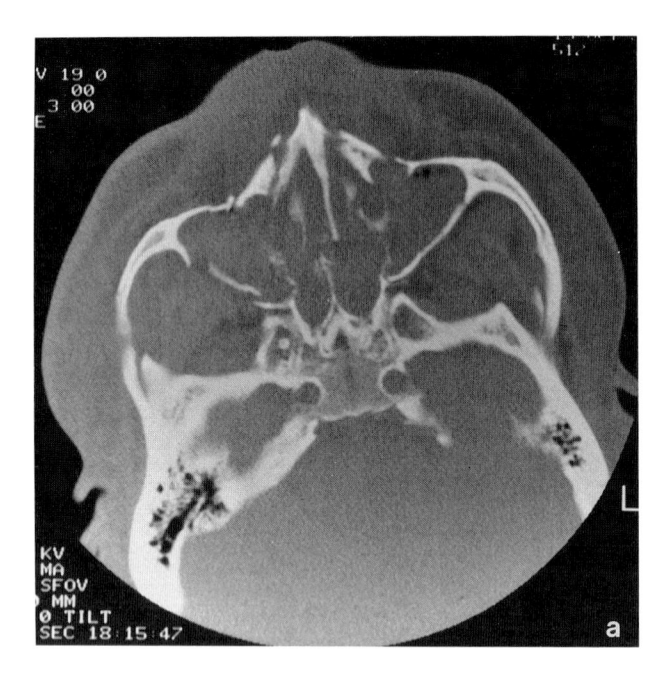

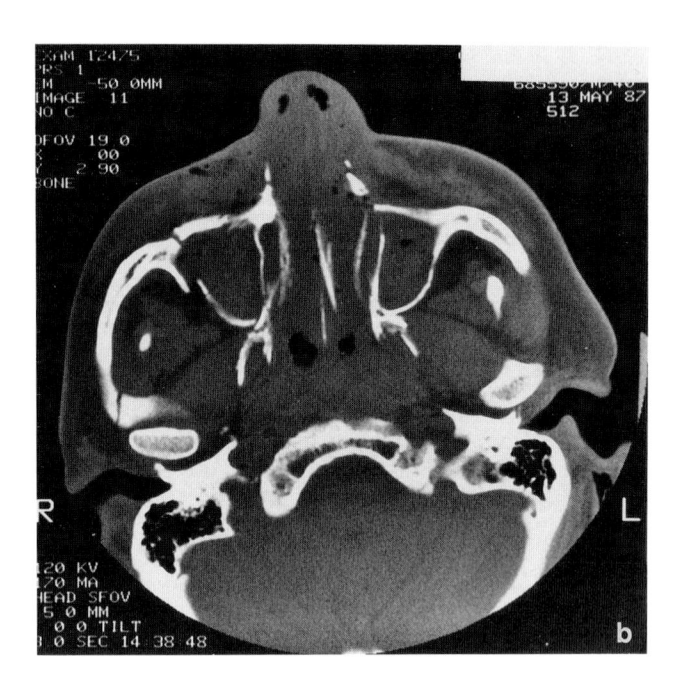

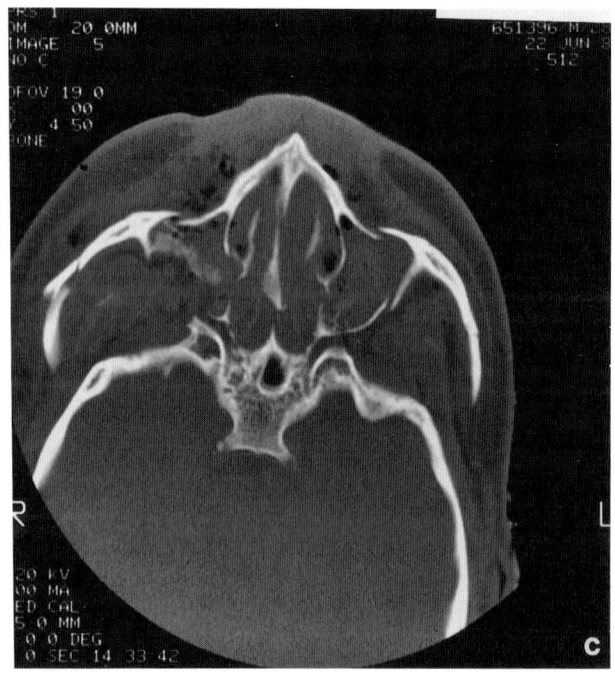

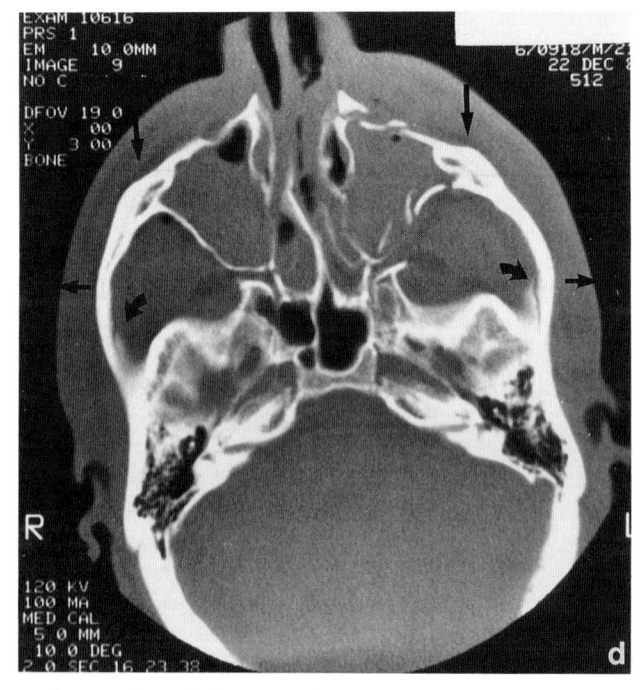

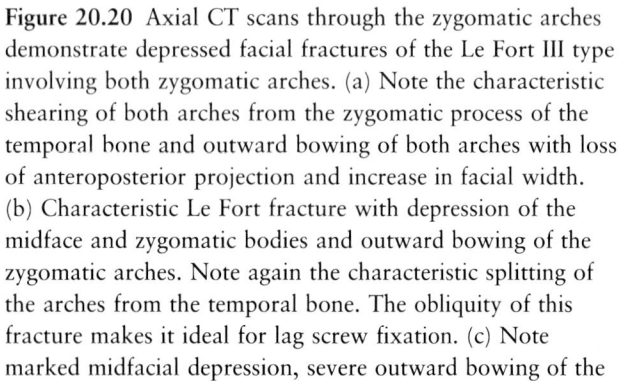

Figure 20.20 Axial CT scans through the zygomatic arches demonstrate depressed facial fractures of the Le Fort III type involving both zygomatic arches. (a) Note the characteristic shearing of both arches from the zygomatic process of the temporal bone and outward bowing of both arches with loss of anteroposterior projection and increase in facial width. (b) Characteristic Le Fort fracture with depression of the midface and zygomatic bodies and outward bowing of the zygomatic arches. Note again the characteristic splitting of the arches from the temporal bone. The obliquity of this fracture makes it ideal for lag screw fixation. (c) Note marked midfacial depression, severe outward bowing of the arches, and marked increased in facial width. Note again the characteristic shearing of the posterior aspect of the right arch from the zygomatic process of the temporal bone. Note how close this fracture is to the temporomandibular joint. The placement of lag screws in this area must be done with care so as not to place the screws into the temporomandibular joint. (d) Marked midfacial depression with multiple segmental fractures of both arches and severe outward bowing of the zygomatic arches. Note the characteristic splitting of the arches from the temporal bone. The obliquity of this fracture make it ideal for lag screw fixation.

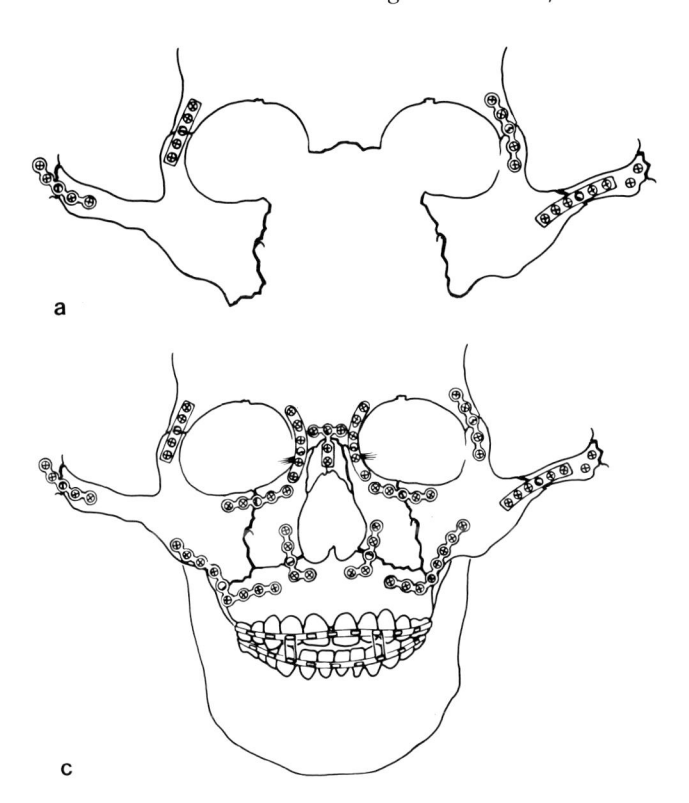

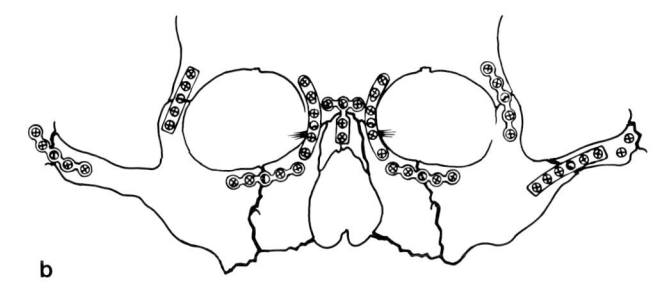

Figure 20.21 (a) Initial restoration of the zygomatic arch and fronto-zygomatic suture line produces an outer facial frame with the exact anteroposterior projection and transverse facial width. (b) The upper, inner facial frame, composed of the infraorbital rim and nasoethmoid region, is now repaired within this outer facial frame. As long as there are fractures at the Le Fort I level, this repair can be performed entirely independent of the occlusion. (c) Lower facial repair is now completed by re-establishing the correct occlusion and completing the repair at the four anterior maxillary buttresses. At the completion of the repair, the MMF can be released in most cases, ensuring an adequate airway in the immediate postoperative period.

gaps in the other three buttresses are now replaced with carefully measured bone grafts or bridged by miniplates with bone grafts placed beneath the plates in the buttress gap (see Figures 20.21 and 20.22).

Sagittal Maxillary Fractures

When sagittal fractures of the maxilla occur, with splitting of the palate, reconstructing the correct maxillary arch and restoring the correct width and projection may be difficult. Prior stabilization of the zygomatic arches produces an outer facial frame and sets the correct position of the upper portion of the lateral and medial maxillary buttresses. Establishing the correct occlusion with the intact mandible, in combination with accurate reduction and fixation at the anterior maxillary buttresses, should ensure correct positioning of the sagittally split segments. Additional miniplates can be applied horizontally across the sagittal fracture at the anterior maxilla, or the palatal fracture itself can be exposed and plated directly through a small incision in the palatal mucosa (see Chapter 26).

Panfacial Fractures

When a complex Le Fort fracture is associated with displaced zygomatic arches, sagittal palatal splitting, mandibular body or parasymphyseal and bilateral condylar neck fractures, all reference points in relation to the cranial base are lost. The difficulty here is setting the correct facial width. If the correct width is not set, the facial projection will be deficient.

With sagittal palatal fractures, combined with mandibular body or parasymphyseal and bilateral condylar neck fractures, the midface and mandible tend to be splayed open. The seemingly correct occlusion can be established at this time, and the mandibular body or parasymphyseal fracture can be rigidly plated. If the midfacial repair is then related to the seemingly correct and stable occlusion, the whole midface will be fixed in the wrong position, producing an increase in facial width and a decrease in facial projection (see Figures 20.23, and 20.24).

The key in this situation is to reduce and repair the zygomatic arches first to produce an outer facial frame with the correct width. The upper, inner facial frame is repaired within this outer frame. The position of the upper portions of the lateral and medial maxillary buttresses are next established with the correct midfacial width and projection. The maxilla is then reduced to these buttresses, and the correct maxillary width and arch contour are obtained by repair across the four anterior buttresses. Additional plating across the sagittal fractures anteriorly or at the hard palate can be added at this time.

The mandible is then placed into the correct occlusal relationship with the reconstructed maxillary arch. The anterior mandibular fracture is rigidly fixed with a

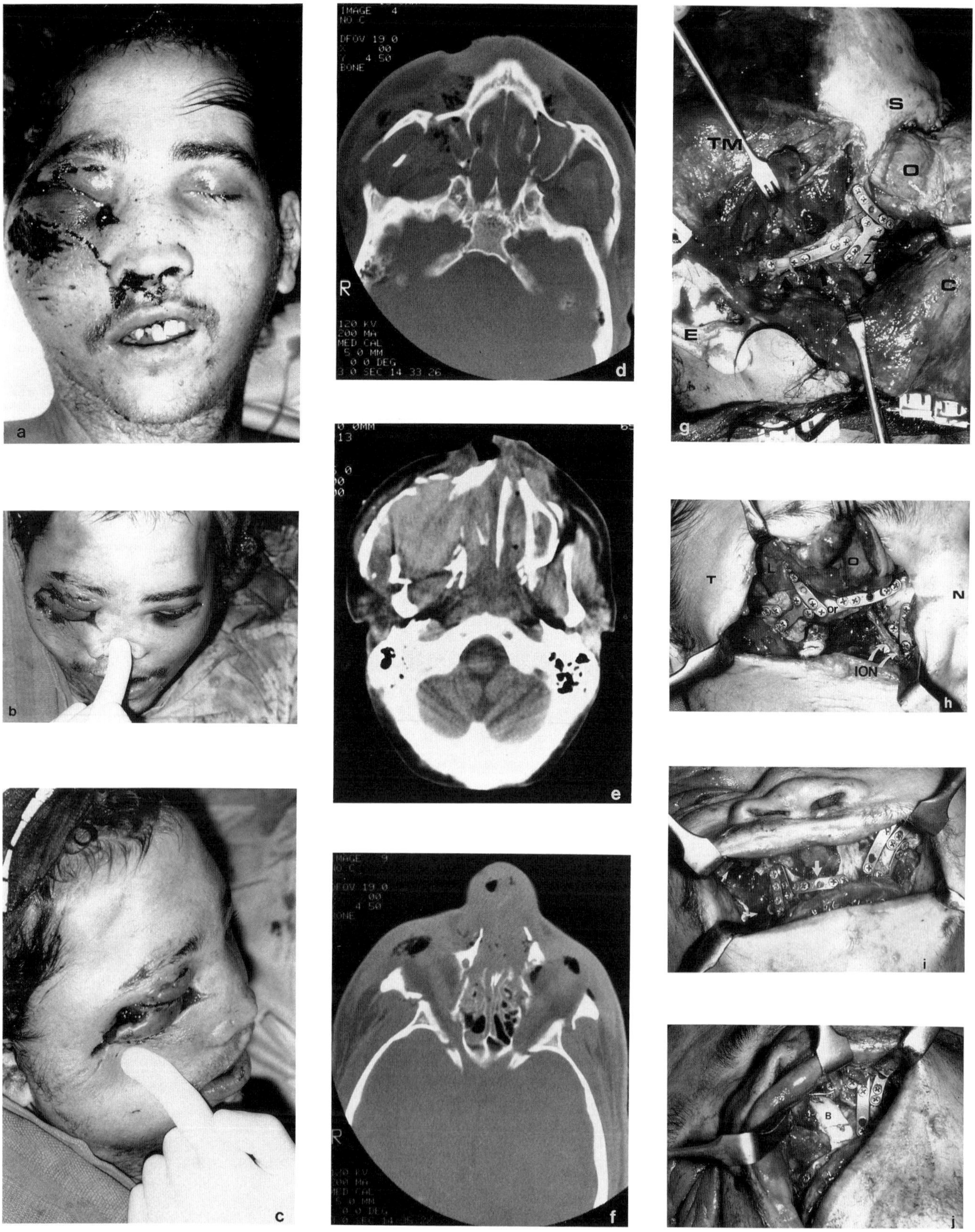
a
b
c
d
e
f
TM
S
O
Z
C
E
g
T
L
O
N
or
ION
h
i
B
j

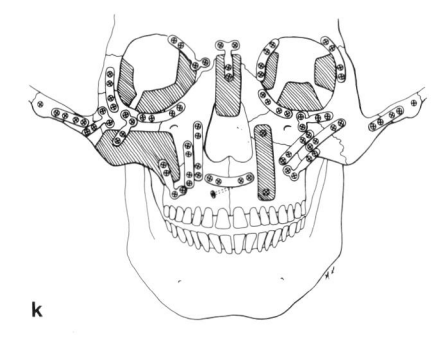

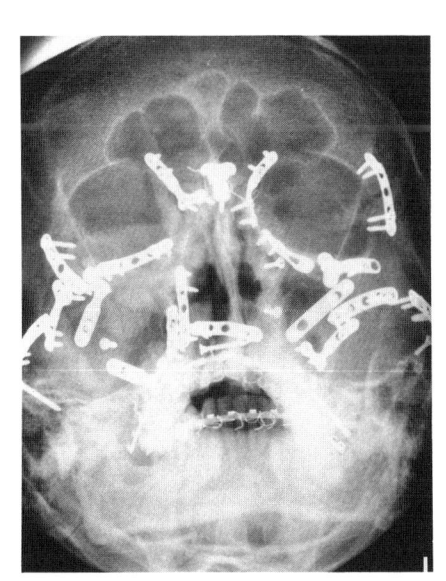

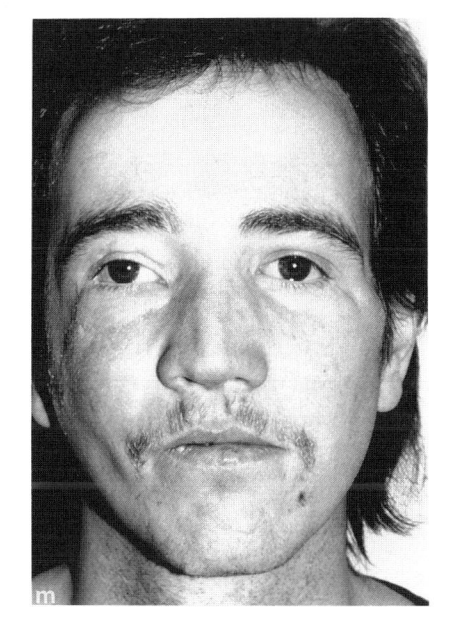

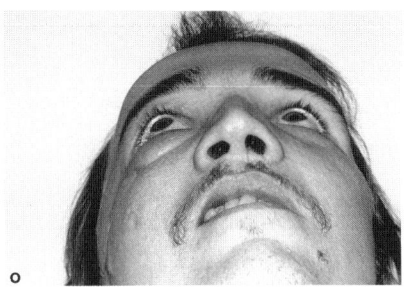

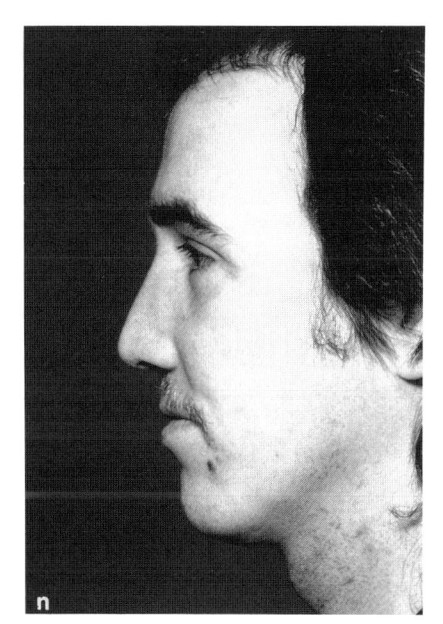

Figure 20.22 (a) Patient with extensive comminuted midfacial fractures involving both zygomatic arches, orbits, naso-ethmoid, and maxilla in association with a life-threatening epistaxis. Severe flattening of the midface in association with increase in transverse facial width is seen. (b) Loss of central midfacial support with central maxillary crush. (c) Collapse and loss of projection of the right orbitozygomaticomaxillary complex is seen. (d) Axial CT scan through the arches shows marked collapse of the midface and multiple segmental fractures of the arches, with loss of projection and outward bowing. (e) Axial CT scan shows extensive destruction of the right maxilla and increase in facial width. (f) Axial CT scan shows marked posterior and lateral displacement of the naso-ethmoid complex and marked lateral and posterior displacement of both zygomatic complexes. Note the comminution and bone loss of both lateral orbital walls. (g) Repair of right zygomatic arch and zygomatic body. Note the lag screw used at the posterior oblique fracture at the zygomatic process of the temporal bone. Note the necessity to use multiple miniplates going in different directions prior to the development of the miniadaptive plate, which is able to be contoured in a 3-dimensional fashion, allowing the plate to repair multiple fractures in different directions. (h) Repair along the orbital rim (OR) and inferior orbital margin with multiple miniplates. Plates can also be seen along the medial maxillary buttress. A miniadaptive plate would have been ideal to repair most of these fractures, because it could have been bent exactly to the shape of the orbital rim. The infraorbital nerve (ION) can be seen. (i) Extensive miniplate fixation of the maxillary buttresses. Note the bone gap in the right lateral buttress and transverse miniplate (arrow) across the region of the anterior spine to fix the sagittal palatal fracture rigidly in the midline. (j) The comminuted left medial buttress is now replaced with a split calvarial bone graft held in place with lag screws. Similar bone grafts were used to repair the right maxillary buttresses. (k) This artist's drawing depicts extensive miniplate fixation and immediate bone grafting. Prior repair of both zygomatic arches restores an outer facial frame and allows exact reconstruction of the remainder of the midface, notwithstanding the severity of the injury. Extensive split calvarial bone grafting has been utilized in both orbits, nose, right zygoma, and both maxillae. (l) Postoperative x ray demonstrates three-dimensional reconstruction with extensive miniplate and screw fixation. (m) Appearance at two years following one-stage correction. Note the restoration of transverse facial width. (n) This lateral view shows restoration of anteroposterior projection of the midface and nasal contour with primary nasal bone grafting. (o) This inferior view shows the restoration of anteroposterior projection of the midface and nasal contour with primary nasal bone grafting.

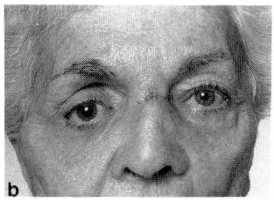

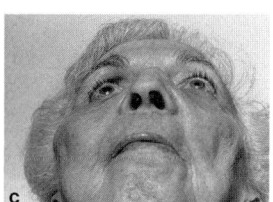

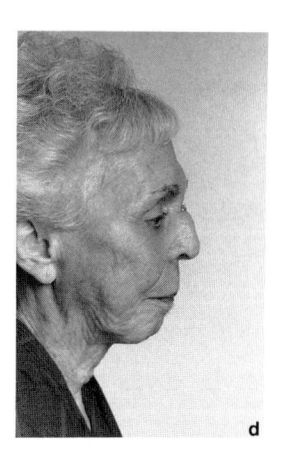

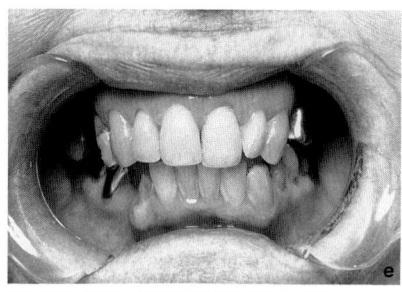

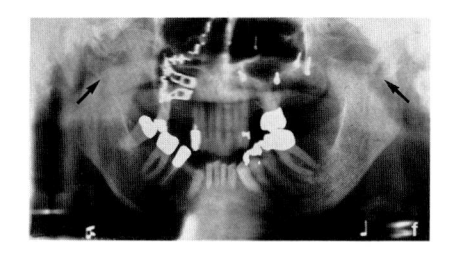

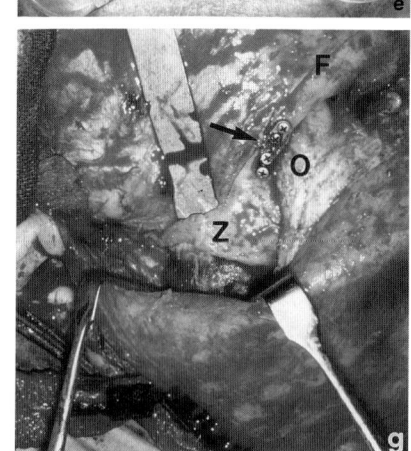

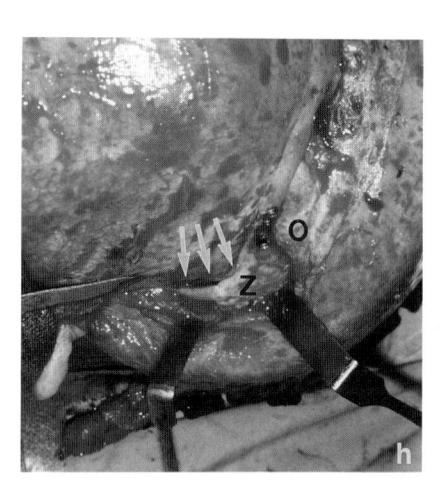

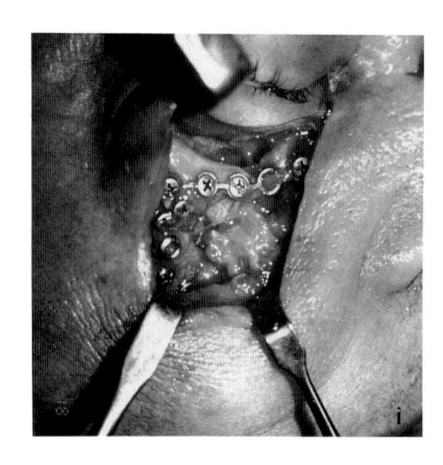

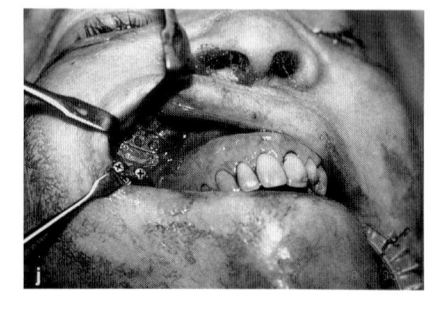

Figure 20.23 (a) A patient with severe maxillary fractures, right orbitozygomatic fractures, and bilateral condylar neck fractures, which were repaired with extensive miniplates and bone grafts. Note that the entire lower facial midline is shifted 2 centimeters to the right and there is a severe widening of the right midface through the zygomatic complex. In addition, there is a residual right enophthalmos and vertical ocular dystopia. (b) Severity of the increased width of the right side of the midface and the vertical dystopia of the right orbit and enophthalmos can be seen. (c) This inferior view demonstrates severe widening through the zygomatic arch of the right side of the face, combined with the enophthalmos. (d) This lateral view demonstrates marked lower facial retrusion due to shortening of the ramus height through the condylar neck fractures. (e) The occlusal midline is restored, but the entire midline of the occlusion is shifted 2 centimeters to the right. (f) Marked shortening of the vertical height of both mandibular rami. Note also the extensive miniplate and screw fixation in the midface. (g) At secondary exploration, note the miniplate fixation of the fronto-zygomatic suture line and the marked outward bowing and shortening in the anteroposterior direction of the zygomatic arch. (h) This view from above demonstrates the rigid fixation of the orbitozygomatic complex in its laterally displaced position with marked bowing and shortening of the zygomatic arch. (i) Extensive miniplate fixation of the midfacial fractures. (j) Extensive miniplate fixation of the right maxillary buttresses. In this situation, the patient was first placed in occlusion and then maxillary buttresses were stabilized, so that the entire occlusal segments were stabilized to the right of the midline. Then the zygomatic complex was stabilized, also in the wrong position, with marked widening of the right side of the midface. Even though the patient's occlusal midline was re-established, the whole facial skeleton was ridigly fixed 2 centimeters to the right of the midline. This resulted in a marked increase in the orbital volume on the right side, with enophthalmos and vertical dystopia. In these cases, it is essential to start with the upper facial skeleton, repairing the zygomatic arch and zygomatic complex first. This establishes the outer facial frame, and the rest of the repair can then be completed.

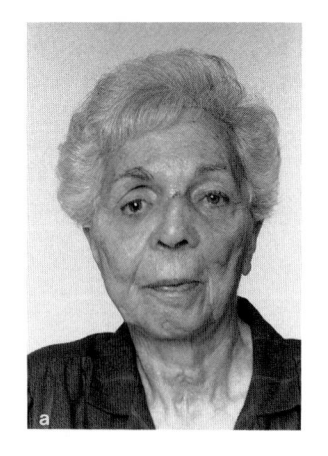

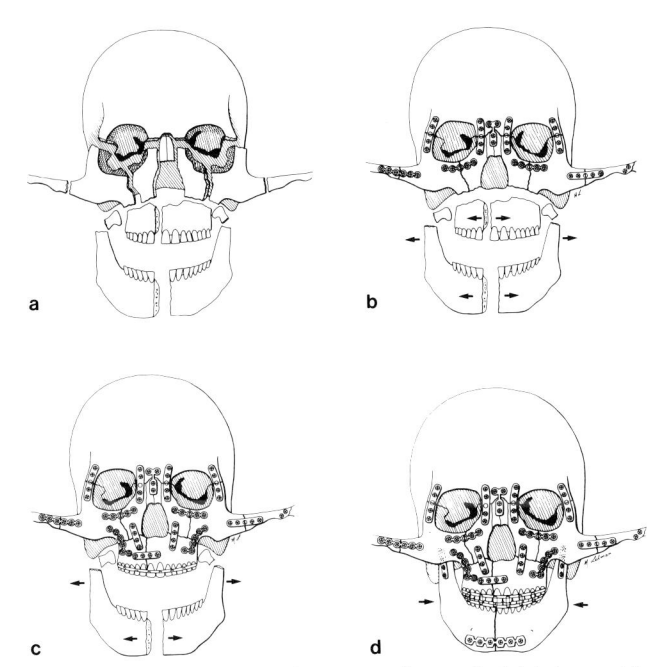

Figure 20.24 (a) Artist's depiction of a panfacial injury with Le Fort III fracture of the midface, bilateral displaced zygomatic arch fractures, and midline splitting of the sagittal splitting of the hard palate, parasymphyseal fracture, and bilateral condylar neck fractures. This demonstrates the most difficult and unstable situation in repair of facial fractures. (b) The correct repair must commence with upper facial repair, fixing the zygomatic arches in the upper midface. If this is not done, it is virtually impossible to set the correct width of the maxillary arch and mandibular arch because these arches tend to splay outward. Without the anatomically reduced zygomatic arches as a guide, it is extremely difficult to properly reduce the splayed maxillary and mandibular arches. (c) Once the upper facial repair has been established, the position of the anterior maxillary buttresses can be established, thus exactly determining the width of the maxillary arch. The repair is now completed at the Le Fort I level, and further rigid fixation is used across the sagittal fracture of the palate. If necessary, separate miniplates can be applied to the palatal fracture through incisions in the palatal mucosa. (d) Now that the maxillary width has been established in relation to the upper facial width, the lower facial width can be exactly restabilized with use of a mandibular plate at the parasymphyseal fracture and a miniplate at the condylar neck fractures if needed. Care must be taken to push inward at both angle regions to obtain the correct width of the mandibular arch.

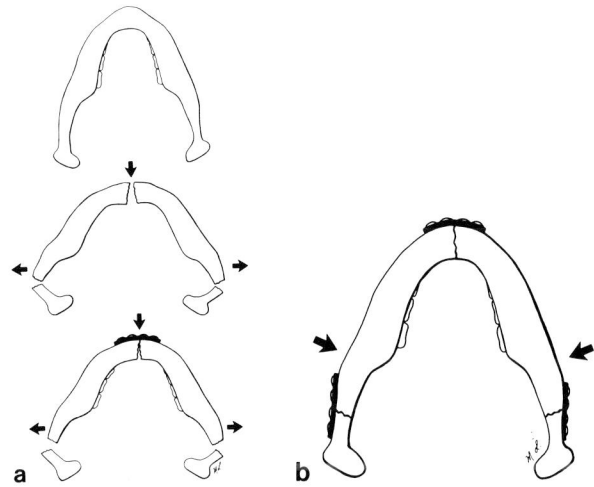

Figure 20.25 (a) When a parasymphyseal fracture is associated with bilateral condylar neck fractures, the width of the mandible increases markedly. If the fracture is repaired by simply reducing the anterior cortex of the mandible so that it looks anatomical and placing a plate on this fracture, it is not uncommon for the mandible to be rigidly stabilized with its arch much too wide because the lingual cortex of the parasymphyseal fracture, as well as the condylar neck fractures, can open. (b) By relating the width of the mandibular arch to the previously stabilized upper facial arch, and by fixing both condylar neck fractures and pushing inward to reduce the lingual cortex of the parasymphyseal fracture, rigid stabilization can be performed at these three sites, thus exactly recreating the natural mandibular arch without increasing the width of the arch.

compression or reconstruction plate. Care is taken to apply medial pressure at both mandibular angles during contour and application of the plate. Open reduction of the condylar neck fractures is performed whenever possible. This ensures establishment of the correct mandibular contour, width, and projection (see Figure 20.25).

In Chapter 26 Markowitz and Manson present a different sequence but abide by the same principles for treating the panfacial fracture.

Maxillary Sinus Drainage

The need for drainage of the maxillary sinus by means of either nasal antrostomy or a drain in the gingivobuccal sulcus at the time of fracture repair is controversial. In our experience, sinus infection after repair is rare and is almost always due to loosening of a screw, plate, or bone graft. Once the loose screw, plate, or bone graft is removed, the infection rapidly subsides. Careful debridement of small bone fragments and torn sinus mucosa, in combination with rigid fixation of the maxillary buttress, seems to prevent maxillary sinus infections.

BIBLIOGRAPHY

Adams WM: Internal wiring fixation of facial fractures. Surg 12:523, 1942.

Alling CC, Davis BP: Compound, comminuted, complex maxillofacial fractures. J Oral Surg 32:415, 1974.

Bonanno PC, Converse JM: Primary bone grafting in management of facial fractures. NY State J Med 75:710, 1975.

Dingman RO, Alling CC: Open reduction and internal wire fixation of maxillofacial fractures. J Oral Surg 12:140, 1954.

Dingman RO, Natvig P: Surgery of Facial Fractures. Philadelphia, Saunders, 1964.

Ferraro JW, Berggren RB: Treatment of complex facial fractures. J Trauma 13:783, 1973.

Georgiade N, Nash T: An external cranial fixation apparatus for severe maxillofacial injuries. Plast Reconstr Surg 38:142, 1966.

Gruss JS: Fronto-naso-orbital trauma. Clin Plast Surg 9:577, 1982.

Gruss JS, Mackinnon SE: Complex maxillary fractures: Role of buttress reconstruction and immediate bone grafts. Plast Reconstr Surg 78:9, 1986.

Gruss JS, Mackinnon SE, Kassel EE, et al: The role of primary bone grafting in complex craniomaxillofacial trauma. Plast Reconstr Surg 75:17, 1985.

Gruss JS, Phillips JH: Complex facial trauma: The evolving role of rigid fixation and immediate bone graft reconstruction. Clin Plast Surg 16:93, 1989.

Gruss JS, Van Wyck L, Phillips JH, Antonyshyn O: The importance of the zygomatic arch in complex midfacial fracture repair and correction of posttraumatic orbitozygomatic deformities. Plast Reconstr Surg 85:878, 1990.

Irby WB: Facial Trauma and Concomitant Problems. 2nd ed. St Louis, Mosby, 1979.

Kazanjian VH, Converse JM: Surgical Treatment of Facial Injuries. 3rd ed. Baltimore, Williams and Wilkins, 1974.

Kruger GO: Textbook of Oral and Maxillofacial Surgery. St. Louis, Mosby, 1979.

Kuepper RC, Harrigan WF: Treatment of midfacial fractures at Bellevue Hospital Centre 1955–1976. J Oral Surg 35:420, 1977.

Le Fort R: Etude experimental sur les fractures de la machoire superieure, Parts I, II, III. Rev Chir Paris 23:201, 360, 479, 1901.

Manson PN, et al: Rigid stabilization of sagittal fractures of the maxilla and palate. Plast Reconstr Surg 85:711, 1990.

Manson PN, Crawley WA, Yaremchuk MJ, et al: Midface fractures: Advantages of immediate extended open reduction and bone grafting. Plast Reconstr Surg 76:1, 1985.

Manson PN, Hoopes JE, Su CT: Structural pillars of the facial skeleton: An approach to the management of Le Fort fractures. Plast Reconstr Surg 66:54, 1980.

Manson PN, Glassman D, Vanderkolf C, Petty P, Crawley WA: Rigid stabilization of sagittal fractures of the maxilla and palate. Plast Reconstr Surg 85:711, 1990.

Manson PN, Shack RB, Leonard LG, et al: Sagittal fractures of the maxilla and palate. Plast Reconstr Surg 72:484, 1983.

Markowitz BL, Manson PN: Panfacial fractures: Organization of treatment. Clin Plast Surg 16:105, 1989.

Merville LC: Multiple dislocations of the facial skeleton. J Maxillofac Surg 2:187, 1974.

Rowe NL, Killey HC: Fractures of the Facial Skeleton. 2nd ed. Edinburgh, Churchill Livingstone, 1968.

Schilli W, Ewers R, Niederellmann H: Bone fixation with screws and plates in the maxillo-facial region. Int J Oral Surg 10:329, 1981.

Schilli W: Midface fractures: Advantages of immediate extended open reduction and bone grafting (discussion). Plast Reconstr Surg 76:11, 1985.

Schultz RC: Facial Injuries. 2nd ed. Chicago, Year Book, 1977.

Sicher H, DeBrul EL: Oral Anatomy. 5th ed. St. Louis, Mosby, 1970, p. 78.

Spiessl B: New Concepts in Maxillofacial Bone Surgery. Berlin, Springer-Verlag, 1976.

CHAPTER 21

Rigid Fixation of Zygomatic Fractures

Joseph S. Gruss
John H. Phillips

Zygomatic fractures are one of the most common injuries of the facial skeleton. They are usually regarded as simple injuries requiring simple treatment. Failure of surgeons to appreciate the complexity of these fractures, their pathological anatomy, and the deforming forces acting on them, have combined to result in zygomatic complex fractures being the most common cause of posttreatment morbidity and deformity of all facial fractures. Posttreatment depression of the orbitozygomatic complex, often associated with enophthalmos, is one of the most difficult deformities to treat secondarily. Enophthalmos and ocular dystopia with coexistent diplopia, once established, may be impossible to correct adequately (see Figures 21.1 and 21.2).

The zygomatic bone itself is a complex, three-dimensional structure that is intimately associated with the adjacent facial bones. Zygomatic fractures, rarely truly isolated (except arch fractures), are associated with fracture of the maxilla and orbit. Depending on the force and direction of the impact, zygomatic fractures may be associated with fracture of the maxillary complex or frontal bone. The relationship of the zygomatic bone to these complexes, in addition to coexisting injury of these areas, is a key feature in the correct treatment of zygomatic fractures and the resultant secondary deformity after inadequate treatment.

Fractures of the zygomatic complex have been regarded by some surgeons as "tripod" fractures, the seat of the stool being the zygomatic bone and the legs the frontal process, the inferior orbital margin, and the zygomaticomaxillary buttress. The zygomatic arch is ignored (see Figure 21.3a).

Zygomatic complex fractures should never be considered as a "tripod," they are always a "quadrapod," because the fracture of the zygomatic arch is critical to their understanding and treatment. Accurate assessment of the position of the zygomatic arch in relation to the cranial base posteriorly and the midface anteriorly is the key to the acute repair of complex zygomatic and midface fractures and the secondary re-

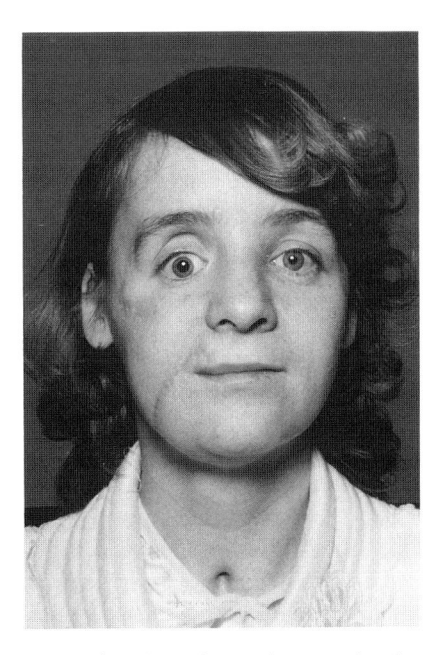

Figure 21.1 This female with poorly treated right zygomatic injuries illustrates all the typical features. She demonstrates severe enophthalmos, vertical ocular dystopia, severe flattening of the malar process, deformity and malposition of the lateral canthus, and severe ptosis of the soft tissues of the right cheek and eyelid.

Figure 21.2 This young male patient shows typical features of an inadequately reduced orbitozygomatic injury. (a) Inferior view demonstrates enophthalmos and flattening of the entire zygomatic complex. Note the characteristic widening of the facial width on the left side with outward bowing of the zygomatic arch. (b) Axial CT scan through the zygomatic arches demonstrates the characteristic depression of the zygomatic body and outward collapse and bowing of the zygomatic arch (note that the zygoma is aligned at the intraorbital rim).

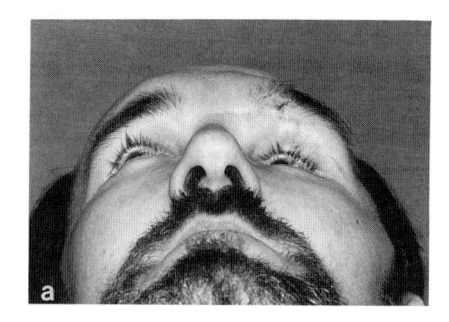

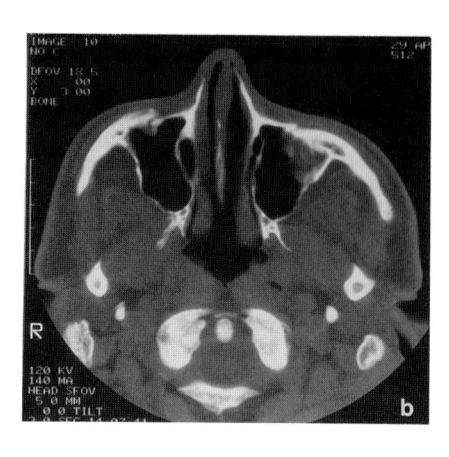

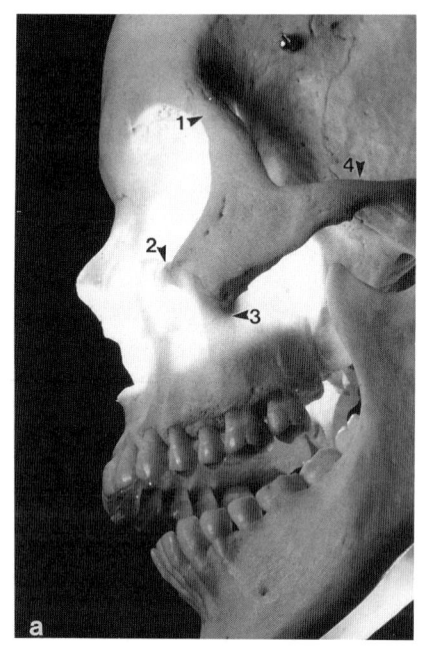

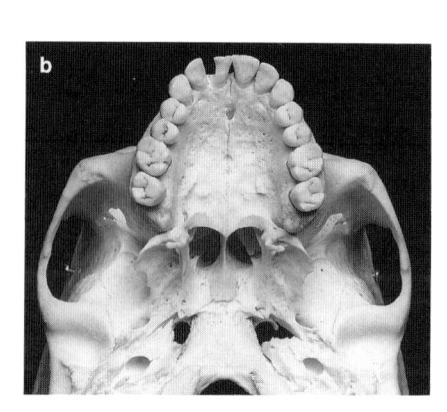

Figure 21.3 (a) This transilluminated skull demonstrates the quadrapod nature of the zygomatic complex. In complex injuries, fracturing and displacement usually occur at all four sites of fracturing and not as a tripod, as is commonly held. Note the relative thinness of the bone at the zygomaticomaxillary buttress (3) as well as at the inferior orbital rim. This predisposes to a higher degree of comminution at the buttress and at the orbital rim in high-velocity injuries. Thus in severely displaced high-velocity injuries with comminution, visualization of at least three, and sometimes all four, sites of fracturing is essential to obtain the correct three-dimensional reduction and fixation of these fractures. (b) This basal view of the skull illustrates the extreme importance of the zygomatic arches in the reduction and stabilization of complex injuries. The zygomatic arch is the structure that links the base of the skull with the zygomatic body. The zygomatic arches, by their position, determine the facial width and projection. The zygomatic arch is not a true arch but is curved in its posterior and anterior portions and is relatively flat in its central portion. Thus reconstruction of the arch must conform to this configuration. In the central portion, the arch should always be reconstructed in a flattened dimension.

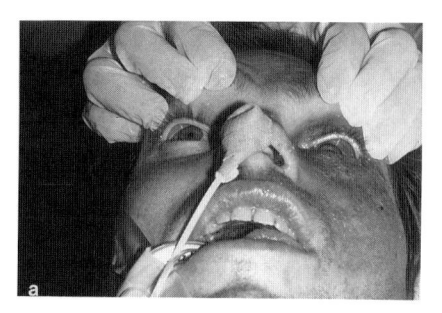

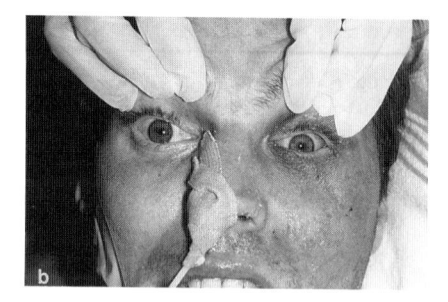

Figure 21.4 (a) Inferior view of young patient with very complex, comminuted, high-velocity orbitozygomatic injuries and severe, acute enophthalmos due to massive orbital enlargement. Acute enophthalmos such as this should warn the surgeon of the severity of the injury. These injuries usually require a three-dimensional reconstruction of the entire complex through the coronal incision. Exact reconstruction of the orbital volume with deep orbital bone grafting is required. (b) Anterior view of same patient shows severe enophthalmos, vertical ocular dystopia, and flattening of the orbitozygomatic arch resulting in increase in facial width on the left side.

construction of post-traumatic deformities of the orbitozygomaticomaxillary complex (see Figure 21.3b).

The zygomatic arch may be fractured in isolation, but it is more commonly fractured in association with complex orbitozygomatic and midfacial injuries. The principles of exposure and repair of facial bone in complex facial injuries utilizing craniofacial surgical techniques, extended exposure, rigid internal fixation, and primary bone grafting have become standard. Following our initial experience with these techniques, we still noted some patients with residual depression in the orbitozygomatic area and the midface and increase in facial width. A careful analysis of these patients and other patients referred for correction of late post-traumatic deformities, with clinical, cephalometric and radiological examinations, consistently demonstrated deformity of the zygomatic arch or arches in bilateral injuries. This collapse, or outward bowing, of the zygomatic arch was indicative of inadequate restoration of midfacial projection and contour.

SURGICAL ANATOMY

The zygomatic complex is bounded by the zygomaticofrontal, maxillary, temporal, and sphenoidal suture lines. The arch furnishes attachments for the masseter muscle and temporalis fascia. The broad attachment of the masseter muscle produces the major deforming force on the zygomatic body and arch. The superficial temporal vessels and frontal branch of the facial nerve lie superficial; and the internal maxillary vessels, temporomandibular joint (TMJ), coronoid process, and temporalis muscle are located deep to the zygomatic arch.

The arch maintains the forward projection of the malar prominence. Its situation between the zygomatic process of the temporal bone posteriorly and the zygomatic body anteriorly predetermines the position of the zygomatic bone in relation to the skull base in the anteroposterior, vertical, and transverse dimensions, forming an outer facial frame (see Figure 21.3). The inner facial frame, composed of frontal, orbital, and naso-ethmoid bones and the anterior maxillary buttresses are intimately related to the position of the zygoma. Disruption of the outer facial frame influences the ultimate positioning of the inner facial frame to which it is linked by the zygomatic arch. Improper reconstruction of the arch will therefore lead to malposition of facial bones and asymmetry and/or associated masticatory problems due to impingement of the underlying coronoid process and TMJ.

DIAGNOSIS

Disruption of the zygomatic arch should be suspected following all complex orbitozygomatic, maxillary, and midfacial fractures. The well known signs and symptoms of malar fracture are (1) subconjunctival and circumorbital ecchymosis, (2) anesthesia in the distribution of the infraorbital nerve, (3) a palpable step and associated tenderness of the orbital rim, (4) emphysema of the overlying tissues, (5) diplopia and enophthalmos (see Figure 21.4), and (6) trismus and ecchymosis and/or palpable fractures in the upper buccal sulcus. These signs may all be present to varying degrees. Significant depression of the zygomatic body is often associated with acute enophthalmos and depression or bulging of the temporal region, depending on the angulation of the arch fracture. These signs are more certain evidence of arch disruption. Le Fort III fractures with loss of anteroposterior midface projection and increase in transverse facial width are usually indicative of bilateral arch disruption.

Severe panfacial edema may mask these signs, however, and so radiologic assessment of the arches is essential for accurate diagnosis. Plain radiologic films consisting of the Water's and reverse Water's views identify displacement of the frontozygomatic area, orbital rim, maxillary buttress, and zygomatic body. The Caldwell and submental vertex views identify involvement of the zygomatic arch.

Axial computer tomographic (CT) scans have greatly facilitated the assessment of arch injury, and the position and degree of pattern of injury (see Figures 21.5–21.8). In unilateral injuries, the injured arch can be compared to the uninjured side. In bilateral injuries (Le Fort III fracture), the deformed arches are compared to normal scans or to the normal anatomic configuration and projection of a dry skull model. Three-dimensional CT scans demonstrate the positions of both arch and body but, in our experience, have not always been as accurate or useful as the standard axial CT.

CLASSIFICATION

Zygomatic fractures have been extensively classified by Knight and North (1961) according to their displacement, and by Rowe and Killey (1955).

Many authors have recognized that the degree of displacement and the complexity of the injury is often related to the velocity of the injury. Low-velocity injuries tend to have less displacement and greenstick of linear fractures, whereas high-velocity injuries predispose to segmentation, comminution, and significant displacement and involvement of contiguous areas of the facial skeleton. Jackson (1989) proposed a simplified classification based on this:

Group I: Undisplaced fractures, which require no treatment but need careful follow-up

Group II: Localized segmental fractures, which require exposure, direct fixation, and follow-up

Group III: Displaced tripod fractures, which usually are low velocity and require either simple

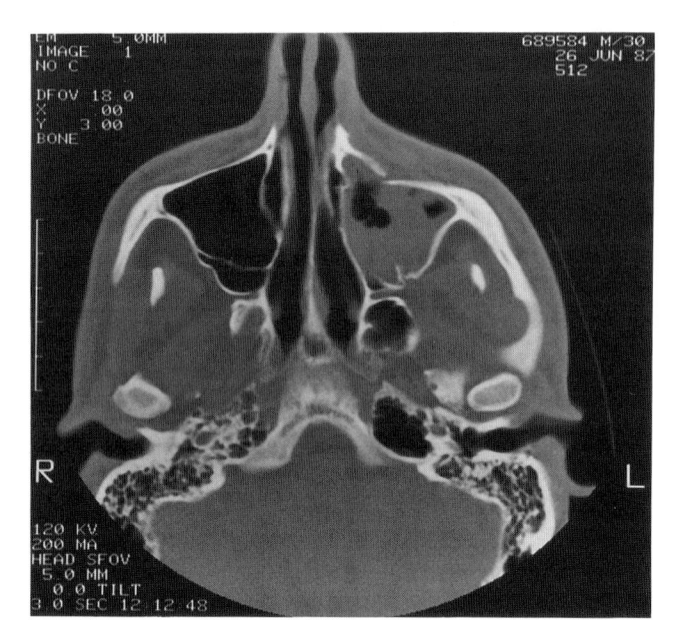

Figure 21.5 This axial CT scan through depressed orbitozygomatic complex injury shows depression of the zygomatic body. There is no severe bowing of the zygomatic arch or telescoping and loss of length of the arch, so this fracture can be repaired with an anterior approach. Exploration and repair of the zygomatic arch are not necessary.

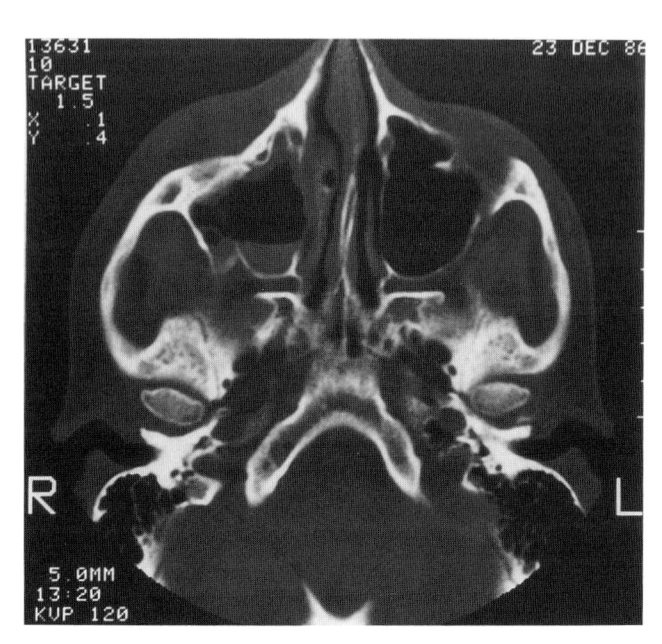

Figure 21.6 This orbitozygomatic axial CT scan demonstrates orbitozyomatic injury with depression of the right zygomatic body. Note the characteristic bowing of the zygomatic arch. This injury can usually be repaired without direct exploration of the arch. However, during the repair, it is important to apply external pressure to the arch to force the zygomatic body forward.

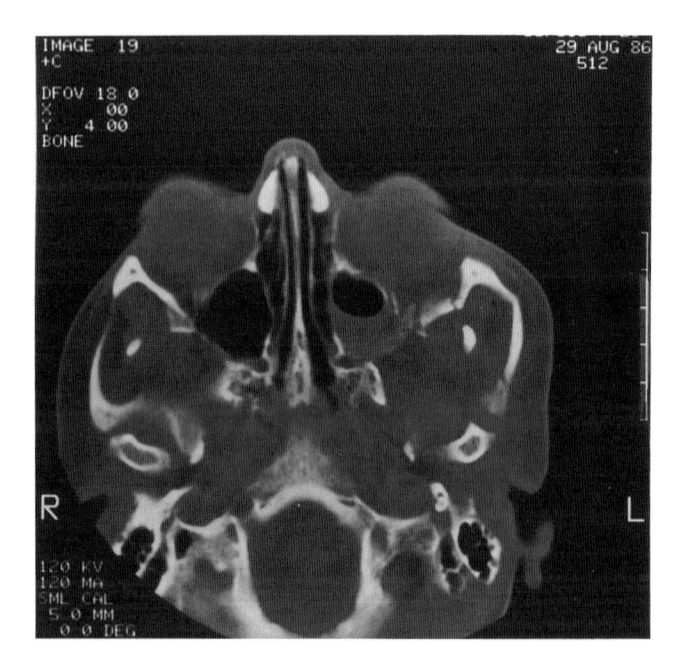

Figure 21.7 Marked fracturing of the lateral wall of the orbit and zygomatic arch with multiple segmental fractures of the arch and outward collapse and bowing. In order to reposition this orbitozygomatic complex accurately in three dimensions, it is essential to explore the arch to obtain adequate reduction and fixation.

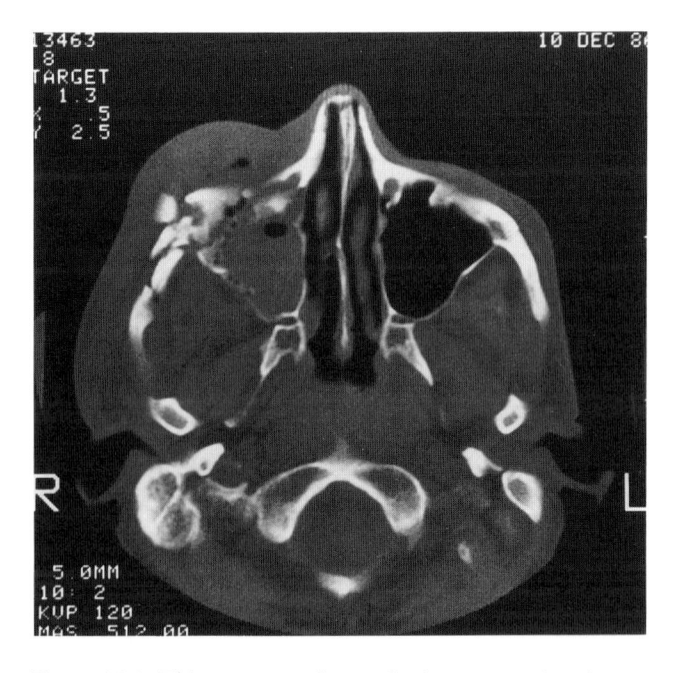

Figure 21.8 This very complex multiple segmental and comminuted fracture of the right orbitozygomatic complex and arch requires a three-dimensional repair with four-point stabilization and fixation.

elevation or elevation, direct exposure, and fixation with careful follow-up

Group IV: Badly displaced, sometimes comminuted, fractures, which usually are high velocity and usually require more careful analysis, wide surgical exposure, and more rigid fixation.

On the basis of extensive radiologic review, combined with direct observation of the fracture pattern at the time of exposure and fixation, it is evident that both the zygomatic body and the arch can be fractured and displaced in various patterns. The zygomatic body or arch can occasionally be fractured in isolation, but more commonly such fractures are associated with injury patterns involving the orbitozygomaticomaxillary complex alone or in association with complex midfacial fractures of the Le Fort III pattern.

Because the type and pattern of zygomatic arch fracture is the key to stabilization of these injuries, the arch fractures should be further subdivided within these proposed classification systems to reflect the possible combinations and permutations of both coexisting and isolated injuries of body and arch.

Classification of Zygomatic Fractures

1. Zygomatic body
   (a) Intact
   (b) Undisplaced
   (c) Segmental
   (d) Displaced
   (e) Comminuted
2. Zygomatic arch
   (a) Intact
   (b) Undisplaced
   (c) Segmental
   (d) Displaced
      (i) Inferiorly with depression and/or telescoping
      (ii) Laterally with outward bowing and/or telescoping
   (e) Comminuted

PRINCIPLES OF SURGICAL REPAIR

On the basis of careful clinical and radiologic examination, combined with direct inspection at the time of surgery, a pattern of injury is ascertained and the status of the arch is identified. The classification now aids in making the correct choice of treatment.

Undisplaced fractures require no treatment but should be followed up carefully.

Isolated arch fractures can be managed with closed reduction techniques, as can minimally displaced zygomatic fractures manifesting no separation at the fronto-zygomatic suture, no disruption of the orbital floor or medial wall and zygomatic arch on radiologic examination, minimal step deformity at the infraorbital rim, and no enophthalmos.

Displaced zygomatic fractures require careful assessment and meticulous open reduction and fixation. The extent of zygomatic exposure depends on the status of the zygomatic arch. Undisplaced or minimally displaced arch fractures with maintenance of adequate arch projection are exposed through a lateral upper blepharoplasty, subciliary and upper buccal sulcus incisions. Three-point fixation is then performed at the fronto-zygomatic suture, inferior orbital rim, and zygomaticomaxillary buttress (Figures 21.9 and 21.10).

The subciliary incision splits the muscle. Careful inferior dissection superficial to the orbital septum should be down to bone. No attempt is made to close the deeper layers in the eyelid itself, because this may inadvertently shorten the orbital septum. One-layer closure of the skin is performed. Heavy anchoring sutures, placed from the musculofascial layers of the cheek below to the malar bone and orbital rim or deep temporal fascia, help support the soft tissues of the cheek in the immediate postoperative period, preventing inferior tension on the eyelid and sagging of soft tissue in the cheek. Careful reattachment of the lateral canthal ligament to the inner surface of the lateral orbital rim, with a separate wire suture, provides additional support to the lower eyelid and prevents residual lateral canthal deformity, which was frequently noted in our initial cases (see Figure 21.11).

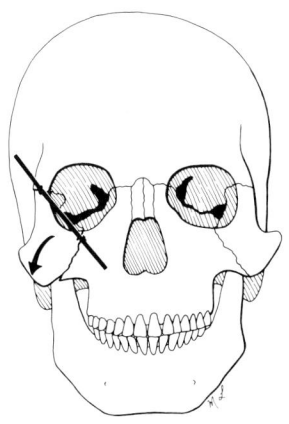

Figure 21.9 In displaced, unstable fractures of the orbitozygomatic complex, two-point stabilization with interosseous wires at the fronto-zygomatic suture line and the infraorbital rim, as is commonly practiced, will still allow rotation around these two points in the axis shown. As the masseter muscle contracts, it tends to pull the whole complex in a downward direction, causing residual depression of the orbitozygomatic complex. The possibility of this occurring is increased by any degree of comminution or bone loss at the zygomaticomaxilllary buttress.

Figure 21.10 (a) Patient with severely displaced orbitozygomatic complex but no collapse or loss of projection of the zygomatic arch. Here, exposure and repair of three points is satisfactory. Fixation at the fronto-zygomatic suture line, the infraorbital rim, and the zygomaticomaxillary buttress can be seen. (b) Accurate reduction at three points allows identification of a small degree of bone loss at the infraorbital rim. If the three points were not accurately visualized and repaired, this gap would tend to collapse, resulting in residual depression of the orbitozygomatic complex, even with rigid fixation. Once plates have been applied to the fronto-zygomatic suture line and buttress, this gap is visualized. (c) Because this gap is less than ½ centimeter, it can be bridged by a miniplate. Bone graft (B) to repair small defect of the orbital floor can be seen. This bone graft was harvested from the anterior wall of the antrum. Although in the occasional patient a bone graft of satisfactory size can be found in this region, it is not advisable to use this bone because a large gap in the anterior wall of the antrum will be left. Thus soft tissue or the buccal fat pad may prolapse into the antrum, causing a significant soft tissue abnormality. (d) In some patients, the fracture of the lateral zygomaticomaxillary buttress is low, adjacent to the tooth roots (L). In this situation, attempts at placing the palate from the zygomatic body above (Z) to the lateral buttress below (L) will cause the lower screws to be applied through the tooth roots. In this situation, it is preferable to place the plate from the zygomatic body above to the medial buttress below (M), thus bypassing the lateral buttress. Particularly in displaced orbitozygomatic fractures with comminution and bone loss at the lateral buttress, it is important always to provide this point of fixation because this buttress repair is the direct antagonist to the pull of the masseter muscle. (e) Patient at two years after one-stage repair. (f) Exact restoration of orbitozygomatic complex and position of the ocular globe.

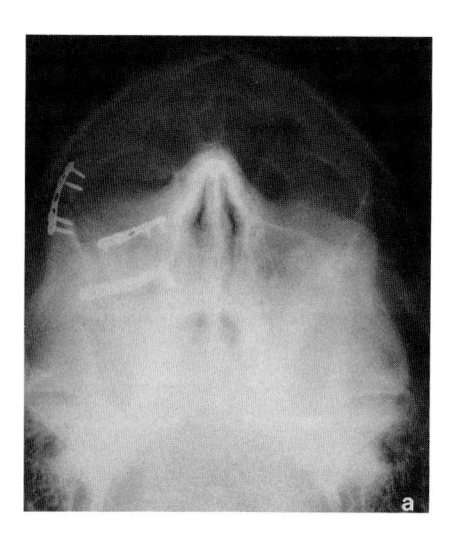

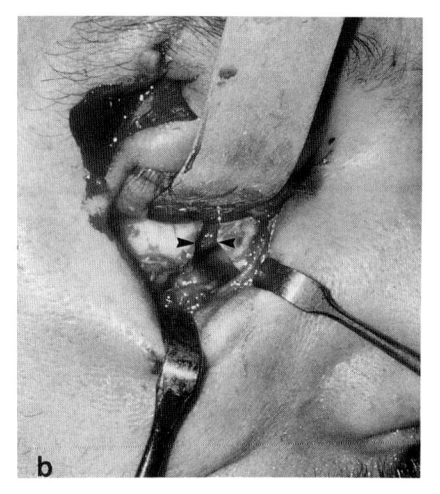

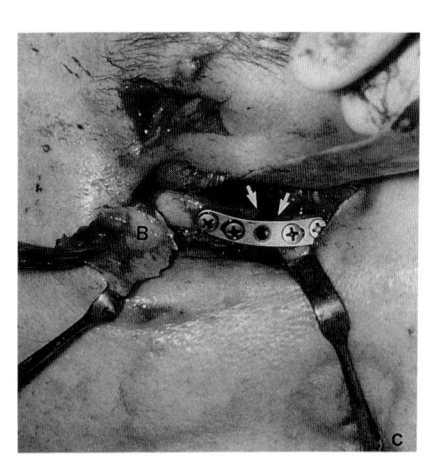

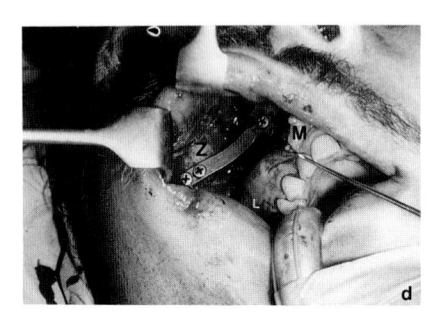

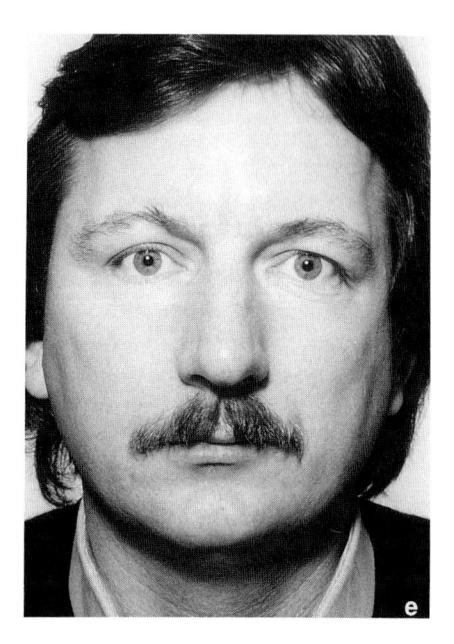

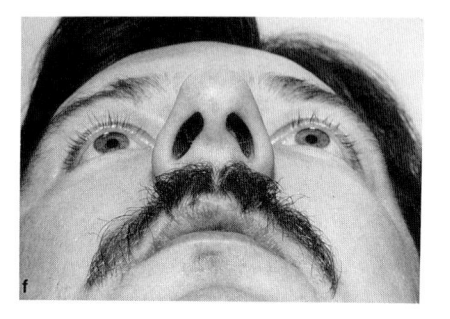

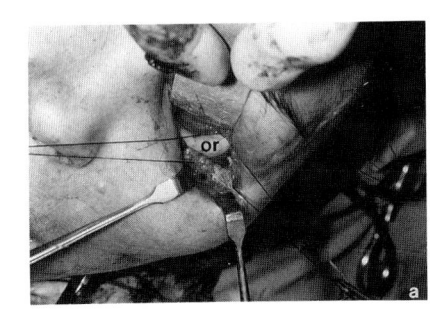

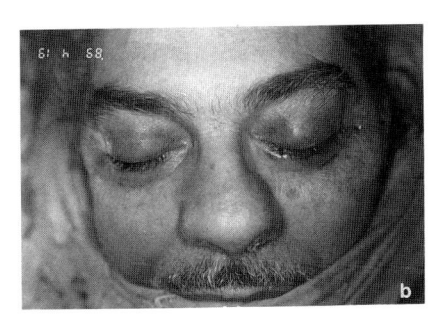

Figure 21.11 (a) Typical resuspension of the midfacial soft tissues and periosteum through multiple drill holes in the inferior orbital rim (OR). (b) After resuspension of soft tissue to the bone. Note the characteristic suspension and repositioning of the left soft tissues of the cheek and the support this provides to the lower eyelid. Resuspension of the facial soft tissues has resulted in marked decrease in the incidence of postoperative ectropion following subciliary incisions.

Displaced arch fractures with loss of anteroposterior projection require substitution of the upper blepharoplasty incision with a bicoronal incision. Following exposure and repositioning of bony fragments, a temporary interosseous wire is inserted at the fronto-zygomatic fracture site. The correct rotation and anteroposterior projection of the arch and body are carefully checked by ensuring proper alignment of the lateral orbital wall, inferior orbital rim, and zygomaticomaxillary buttress. Rigid fixation of the arch is performed using miniplates and screws, and miniplate fixation then replaces the temporary interosseous wire at the fronto-zygomatic fracture. The zygomaticomaxillary buttress is reinforced with a miniplate, and the infraorbital rim is repaired with a miniplate, a microplate, or interosseous wire. Immediate bone grafts reconstruct any gaps in the orbital rim, arch, or buttress and repair deficits in the orbital walls (see Figure 21.12).

Exposure of the Zygomatic Arch

Safe exposure of the entire zygomatic arch and assessment of its exact relationship to the remaining craniofacial skeleton can be accomplished only through an extended coronal incision. The scalp flap must be dissected meticulously in order to prevent postoperative morbidity relating to

1. weakness or permanent paralysis of the frontal branch of the facial nerve,
2. atrophy of the temporalis muscle resulting in clinically apparent temporal depression, and
3. displacement of the lateral canthal ligament resulting in downward inclination of the lateral canthus (see Figure 21.13).

The key to prevention of damage to the frontal branch of the facial nerve is an understanding of its intimate anatomic relationship with the temporoparietal fascia (superficial temporal fascia) and the superficial musculoaponeurotic system (SMAS) in the cheek (see Figures 21.14 and 21.15).

Dissections of cadavers, combined with careful delineation of the frontal nerve during extended parotid dissections, have confirmed the exact anatomic relationship in this region. The SMAS fascia in the cheek is continuous above the zygomatic arch with the temporoparietal fascia, which, in turn, is continuous with the galea above. This layer is separate from the deep temporal fascia covering the temporalis muscle itself, which is continuous above with the pericranium and below attaches to the periosteum overlying the zygomatic arch. The temporalis muscle itself passes below the zygomatic arch to attach to the mandible.

In the cheek, the frontal branch of the facial nerve runs anterosuperiorly, deep to the SMAS fascia. It consistently pierces the SMAS fascia at the lower border of the zygomatic arch and then runs superficial to the contiguous temporoparietal fascia in the temporal region. Thus, the key to preservation of the frontal nerve is careful dissection between the deep temporal fascia and superficial temporoparietal fascia and the elevation with the scalp flap of the temporoparietal fascia and nerve.

The coronal flap is elevated in a plane that is deep to the galea, leaving the pericranium intact. At the upper border of the temporalis muscle, care is taken to raise the temporoparietal fascia with the coronal flap. Dissection proceeds inferiorly between the temporoparietal fascia and deep temporal fascia. Above the zygomatic arch, the temporal fat pad is encountered. Its consistent position on the deep temporal fascia and beneath the temporoparietal fascia indicates the correct plane of dissection. Approximately 1/2 centimeter above the arch, an incision is made through the temporal fat pad and the deep temporal fascia, and the upper border of the arch is identified subperiosteally. The frontal branch lying above the temporoparietal fascia and periosteum is thus protected.

The pericranium is incised approximately 1 to 2 cm above the superior orbital rim, and subperiosteal dissection of the superior orbital rim proceeds inferolaterally along the fronto-zygomatic process; thus the fracture or deformity at the fronto-zygomatic suture is identified. Dissection continues along the lateral orbital rim until the anterior aspect of the zygomatic arch is encountered. The posterior dissection under the temporoparietal fascia and the anterior dissection along the

Figure 21.12 (a) Female with complex displaced right orbitozygomatic complex. Note the characteristic sagging of her facial soft tissues, depression of the lateral canthus, and acute enophthalmos. (b) This axial CT scan demonstrates the multiple segmental nature of the orbital rim fractures and marked depression of the entire orbitozygomatic complex. (c) This axial CT scan demonstrates marked displacement and backward telescoping of the lateral orbital wall and zygomatic arch. In addition, the characteristic bulge of the maxillary sinus into the posterior orbit is lost. This indicates the need for extensive three-dimensional reconstruction through a four-point reduction and stabilization, as well as deep orbital bone grafting. (d) Three-dimensional reconstruction with older, stainless steel, miniplates. The comminuted segmental fracture of the infraorbital rim has been repaired with multiple interosseous wires in combination with extensive deep orbital bone grafting. (e) This repair, performed eight years ago, demonstrates excellent restoration of the bony orbitozygomatic architecture and globe position, but manifests soft-tissue problems that were previously not recognized. Note the characteristic displacement of the lateral canthus because it was not reattached after a coronal exposure. Also note the characteristic ptosis of the medial portion of the soft tissues of the cheek due to failure to resuspend these tissues to the reconstructed bony skeleton at the end of the procedure. (f) Perfect three-dimensional restoration of the bony orbitozygomatic complex and eye position from an inferior view.

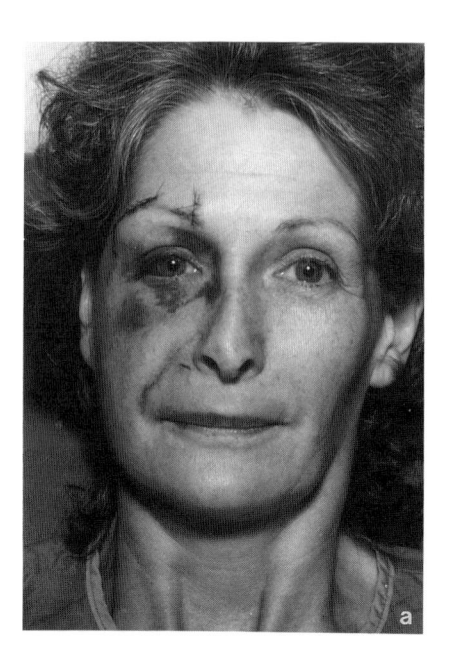

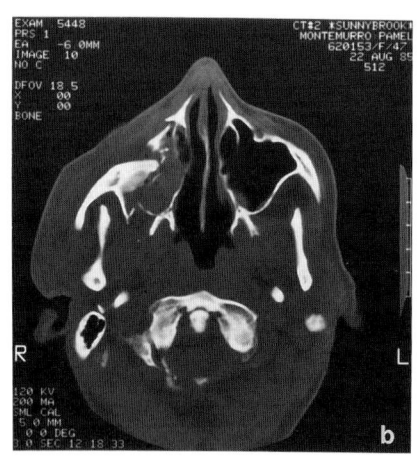

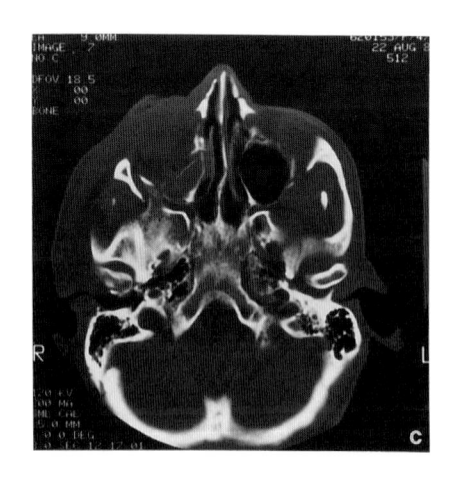

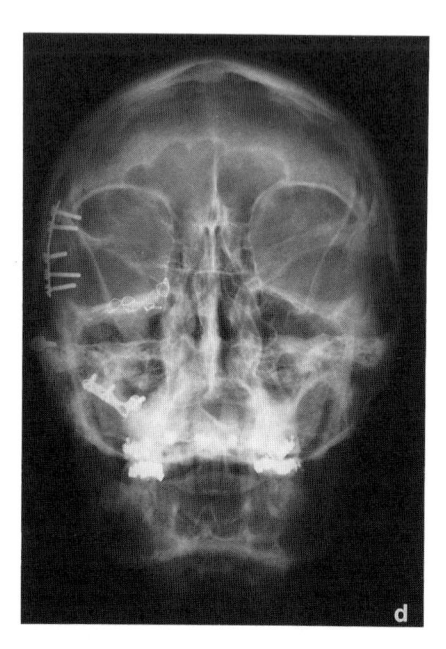

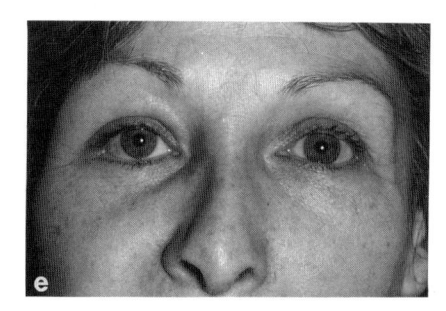

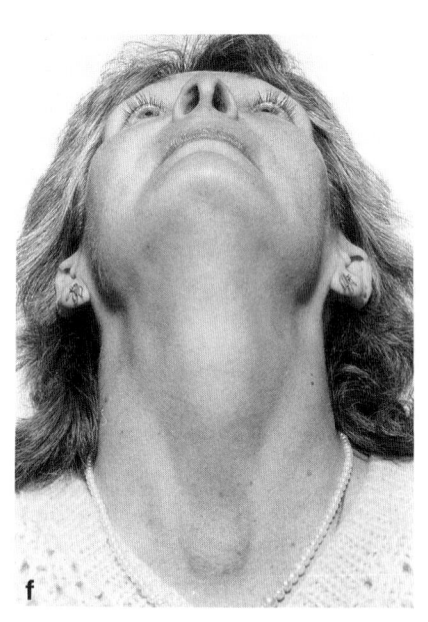

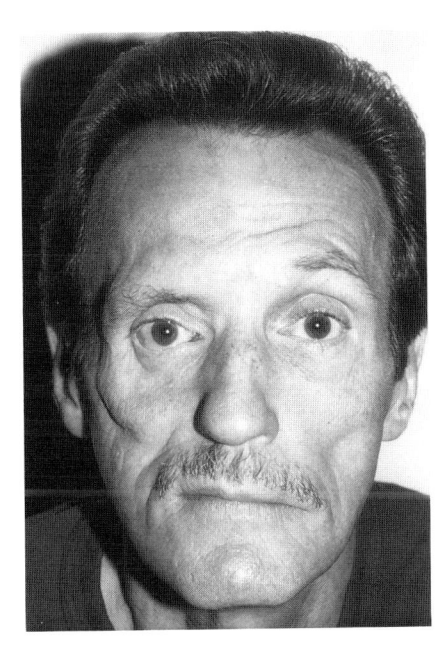

Figure 21.13 Multiple attempts have been made to repair this patient's complex right orbitozygomatic fracture. Many typical mistakes are illustrated here. Exposure of the zygomatic arch through a coronal incision has left him with severe right temporal hollow due to atrophy of the temporalis muscle. The right side of the forehead is paralyzed following injury to the frontal branch of the facial nerve. He has severe ptosis of the right lower eyelid and soft tissues of the right cheek, which were not suspended after the operative procedures. There is asymmetry and deformity of the orbitozygomatic complex.

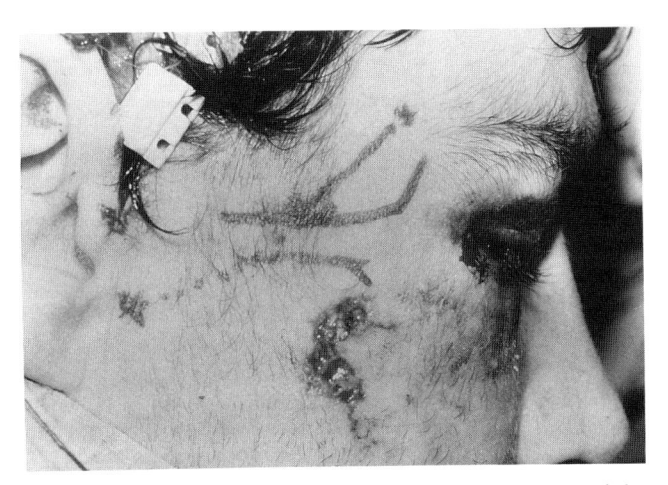

Figure 21.14 The skin markings of the frontal branch of the facial nerve in relation to the zygomatic arch are illustrated. It is essential to understand the anatomy of the frontal branch of the facial nerve in relation to the coronal approach to the zygomatic arch. Below the arch the nerve is under the SMAS fascia, and above the arch it is above the temporoparietal fascia, which is continuous with the SMAS.

lateral rim are now linked subperiosteally, and the entire zygomatic arch is identified. Complete release of the insertion of the masseter muscle onto the arch and body is essential to allow mobilization of the zygoma from its displaced position.

The craniofacial exposure is increased by extending the preauricular skin incision down to the earlobe and continuing the subperiosteal dissection inferiorly. Adequate exposure of the TMJ, coronoid process, mandibular ramus, upper two thirds of the maxilla, and inferior orbital rim is obtained. In order to obtain adequate inferior exposure, the superficial temporal vessels may have to be divided at their entrance into the coronal flap.

The postoperative temporal depression due to atrophy of the temporalis muscle can be minimized by preventing incisions into the muscle itself or by lifting it out of its bed. Exposure of the lateral orbital wall and rim should be obtained with as little elevation of the temporalis muscle as possible. Following completion of repair, the incised deep temporal fascia is reapproximated to the periosteum overlying the zygomatic arch to prevent postoperative prominence of the arch due to malposition and atrophy of the surrounding soft-tissue structures.

APPLIED ANATOMIC PRINCIPLES

It is essential to understand certain important anatomic and pathologic features of zygomatic complex fractures and their relation to proper reduction and rigid internal fixation.

Fronto-zygomatic Suture Line

Fractures at the fronto-zygomatic suture line give the poorest index of degree of rotation and displacement of the rest of the zygomatic complex. Severe degrees of injury, displacement, and comminution of the zygoma may be accompanied by minimal separation or displacement at the fronto-zygomatic fracture site. Fixation with interosseous wires, particularly at the fronto-zygomatic suture, allows rotation of the zygomatic body and arch, due to the deforming pull of the masseter muscle. Miniplates are ideally suited to repair the fronto-zygomatic region, zygomaticomaxillary buttress, and arch.

Stabilization of displaced zygomatic fractures using one miniplate at the fronto-zygomatic suture has recently been advocated. This method, although technically feasible, has certain important drawbacks. In our experience, the fronto-zygomatic fracture is the least helpful site in determining degrees of zygomatic displacement and rotation. Many severely displaced fractures of the zygomatic body and arch will have minimal deformation at the fronto-zygomatic suture (see Figure 21.16). In addition, the key aim of zygomatic fracture

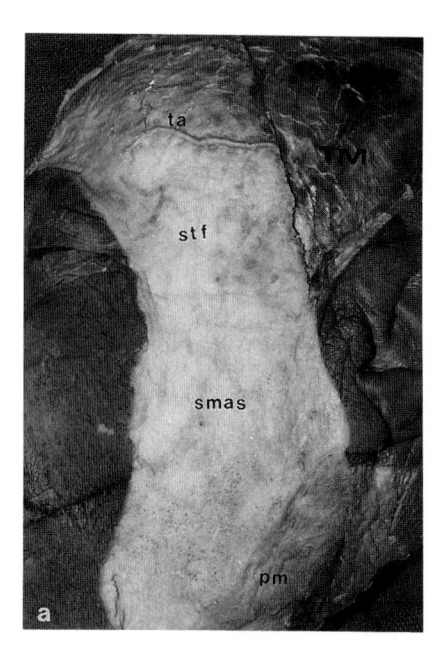

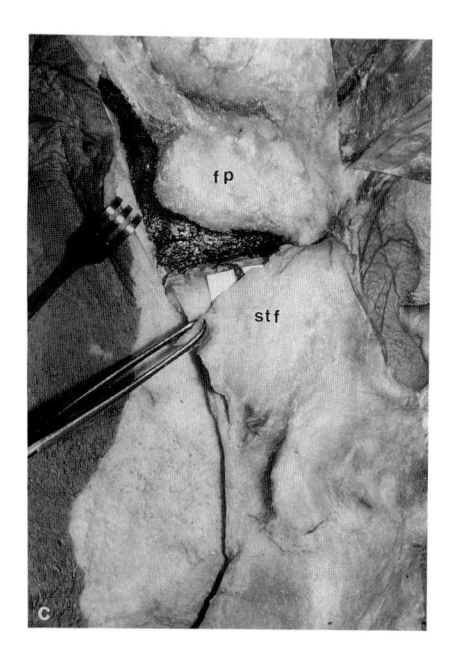

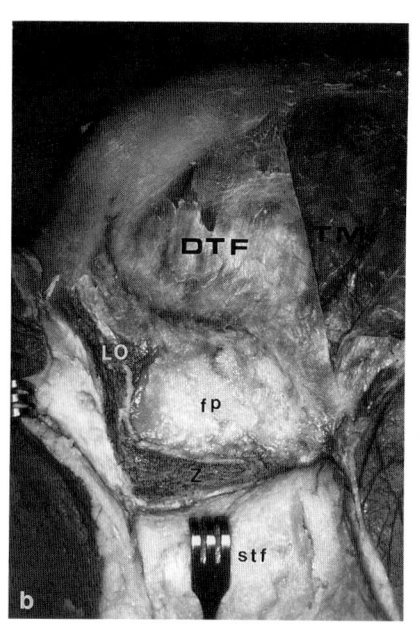

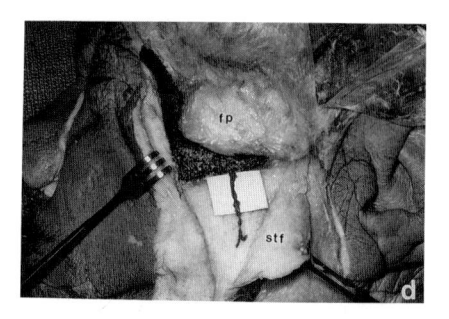

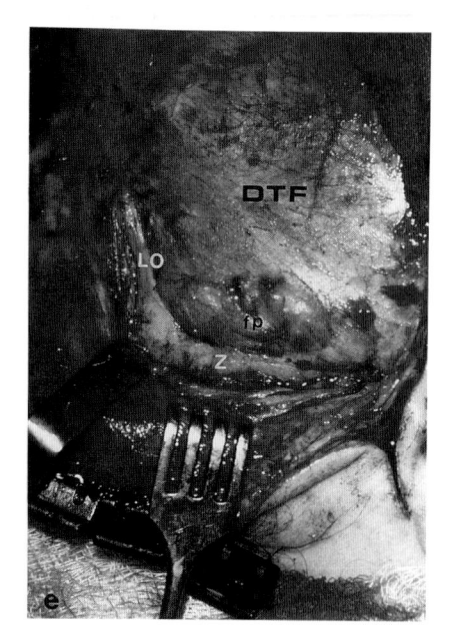

Figure 21.15 (a) A cadaver dissection illustrates the important anatomy in the temporal region in relation to the frontal branch of the facial nerve. The superfical temporoparietal fascia (STF) contains the superficial temporal artery (TA). This superficial temporoparietal fascia is separate from the deep temporal fascia that covers the temporalis muscle itself (TM). The superficial temporoparietal fascia extends downward, crosses the zygomatic arch, and is continuous in the cheek with the SMAS fascia. The SMAS fascia then continues downward into the neck as the platysma muscle (PM). (b) In order to identify the zygomatic arch and lateral orbital wall superiosteally, dissection is carried out between the superficial temporoparietal fascia and the deep temporal fascia (DTF) covering the temporalis muscle (TM) itself. The superficial temporoparietal fascia must be raised with the coronal flap. The correct level of dissection is ensured by the visualization of the characteristic temporal fat pad (FP), which lies between the superficial temporoparietal fascia and the deep temporal fascia. Approximately ½ centimeter above the zygomatic arch an incision is made through the bottom portion of the temporal fat pad and onto the top of the arch, where the periosteum is incised. The periosteum overlying the arch is then reflected forward in continuity with the superficial temporoparietal fascia. Dissection then continues down the lateral orbital margin and communicates with the dissection of the zygomatic arch to allow exposure of the entire lateral orbitozygomatic complex. (c) The frontal branch of the facial nerve pierces the superficial temporoparietal fascia just below the arch where it comes from a deep to a more superficial level. Thus, staying beneath the superficial temporal fascia and the periosteum allows the protection of the nerve. (d) Dissection of the frontal branch of the facial nerve shows its typical position at the inferior border of the zygomatic arch, lying above the superficial temporoparietal fascia, which has been reflected forward. Thus raising the coronal flap with the superficial temporoparietal fascia on the flap and, in addition, raising the periosteum over the zygomatic arch, will always protect the frontal branch of the facial nerve. In complex cases requiring extensive retraction of the skin flaps, temporary paresis of the frontal branch of the facial nerve is not uncommon. Full recovery of this nerve may take months if the traction injury is severe. (e) Dissection of the zygomatic arch (Z) and lateral orbital wall (LO) in a clinical situation shows the characteristic appearance and position of the temporal fat pad lying between the deep temporal fascia and the superficial temporoparietal fascia, which is attached to the coronal flap.

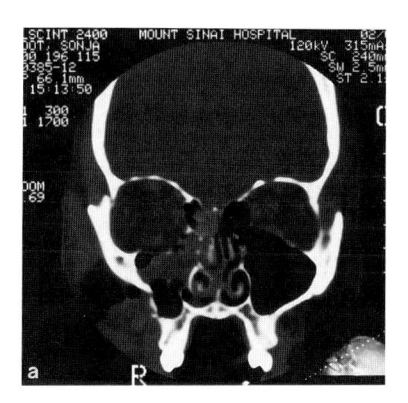

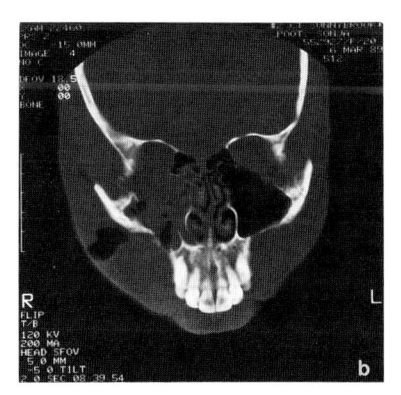

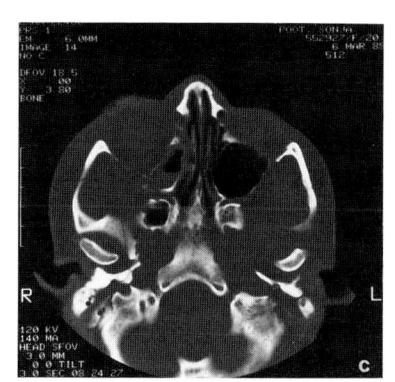

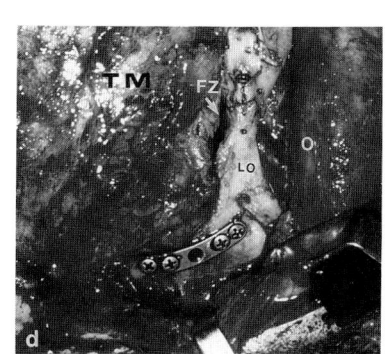

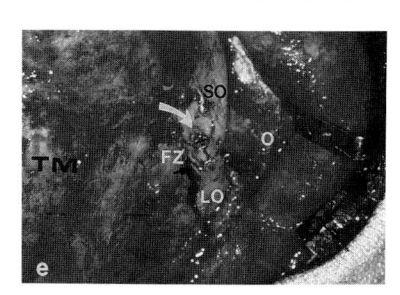

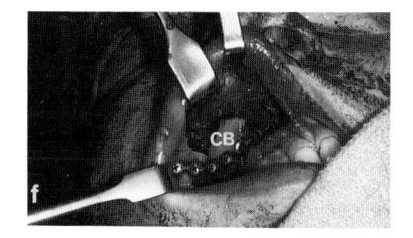

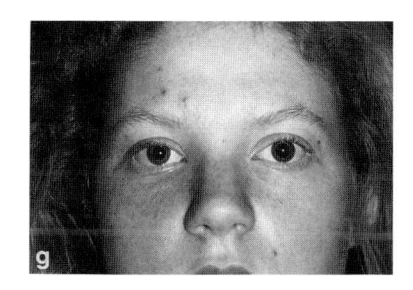

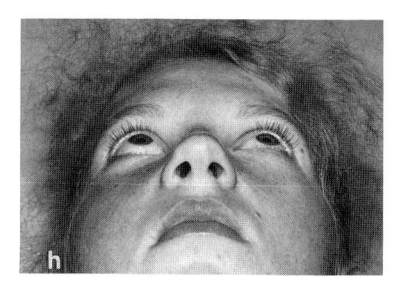

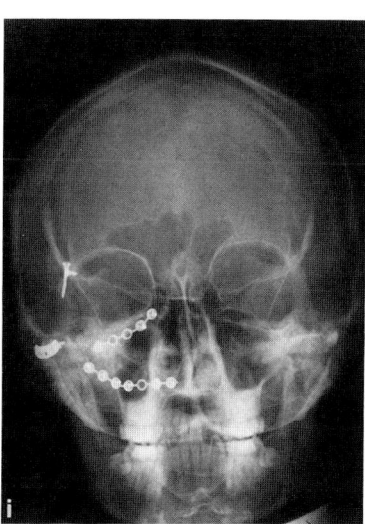

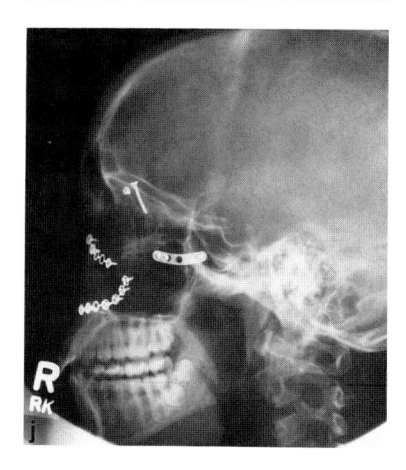

Figure 21.16 (a) Female with very severe complex right orbitozygomatic injury. Note the small displacement at the ZF suture. Note the severe blowout fracture of the medial wall and floor of the orbit with loss of the maxillary sinus bulge that is evident on the normal left side. (b) This coronal CT scan shows deep orbital loss extending back into the apex of the orbit. (c) This axial scan through the deep orbit shows characteristic loss of the deep orbital bulge. This indicates the necessity for deep orbital exploration and bone grafting. (d) In some patients, once the fronto-zygomatic suture line has been temporarily stabilized with interosseous wire and the zygomatic arch has been repaired with adequate transverse and forward projection, the fronto-zygomatic suture line can be stabilized with a long lag screw which will provide compression across this fracture line. A small amount of bone is burred out above the fronto-zygomatic suture line, to countersink the head of the lag screw. (FZ = fronto-zygomatic.) (e) This superior view shows the lag screw that is countersunk into the bone (large arrow). (f) This severely comminuted fracture of the zygomatic maxillary buttress is bridged with a long mini-adaptive plate. A large cranial bone graft (CB) is used to fill in the gap; it is anchored to the underlying plate with two screws. Note that the cranial bone graft is placed in such a way that a large extension of the bone graft extends over the comminuted anterior wall of the maxillary antrum. This will prevent soft tissue and buccal fat pads sinking into the antrum. (g) Results of extensive open reduction and internal fixation with multiple miniplates and lag screws through coronal, subciliary muscle splitting and upper buccal sulcus incisions. (h) Exact restoration of the orbitozygomatic complex and globe position. There is a slight tethering and shortening of the right lower eyelid when the patient looks upward, resulting in a slight ectropion. (i) Three-dimensional reconstruction with multiple miniplates and a lag screw to the fronto-zygomatic suture line is seen. (j) This lateral x ray illustrates the fixation of the fronto-zygomatic suture line using lag screws.

treatment—restoring normal zygomatic position and orbital volume to prevent the occurrence of enophthalmos and oculo-orbital dystopia—cannot be accomplished without orbital exploration to delineate and repair injury to the orbital floor, and the medial and lateral walls. Displaced orbitozygomatic fractures, with impaction of the lateral and inferior orbital rims, not uncommonly show little evidence of bony disruption and displacement of the orbital walls on initial radiologic examination. Bony displacement or loss may become apparent only following adequate reduction and stabilization of the orbitozygomatic complex (see Figure 21.17). Thus orbital exploration is essential following the repair of a displaced zygomatic fracture to prevent the occurrence of enophthalmos and oculo-orbital dystopia, which may be extremely difficult to repair by secondary surgery.

In zygomatic fractures without significant displacement and no comminution or orbital wall injury, a single minicompression plate may be used at the fronto-zygomatic suture line but only if the orbital rim, lateral orbital wall, and zygomaticomaxillary buttress are exposed as well, to ensure accurate three-dimensional reduction.

Palpability and even visibility of the miniplate may be a problem in thin-skinned individuals in the periorbital area. In complex injuries, this can be avoided by placing the plate posteriorly (see Figure 21.18) or, sometimes, by using large lag screws at the zygomatic frontal area (see Figure 21.16). In less severe injuries interosseous wire or microplate fixation (see Figure 21.19) may be used when coupled with sufficient stabilization elsewhere.

Zygomatic Arch

The importance of accurate reduction and fixation of the zygomatic arch has been stressed (see Figure 21.20). The most common mistake made is to reconstruct the arch as an "arch," thus failing to establish the correct facial width and projection (see Figures 21.21, 21.22 and 21.23). The arch is not a true arch. It is curved at its origin from the temporal bone and at its junction with the zygomatic body, but the central two thirds is flat (see Figure 21.3b). When the arch is plated, care must be taken to flatten the middle portion of the arch to ensure reconstruction of the correct anatomic configuration.

PATTERN OF ARCH FRACTURES

Accurate assessment of radiographs and direct inspection at operation of over 500 displaced zygomatic arch fractures have uncovered a consistent fracture pattern (see Figure 21.24). The posterior and anterior suture lines are the sites most commonly involved. An oblique fracture of the posterior arch as it joins the zygomatic process of the temporal bone is the most common finding. Mid arch fractures, in association with a segmental displacement, are also frequent findings. Segmental and comminuted fractures of the arch are frequently associated with a transverse or oblique fracture through the thickest and most anterior portion of the zygomatic body, indicating the severity of the force applied directly to the zygomatic body.

Inferior Orbital Rim

The inferior orbital rim is important in the assessment of accurate reduction of the whole complex; but it is the least important site for rigid internal fixation, and it is at this site where plates are most easily palpated. Following accurate and stable reduction and fixation of the other two or three sites of fracturing, if the inferior orbital rim is uncomminuted, it can be repaired with an interosseous wire or microplate (see Figure 21.19 and 21.25). When it is comminuted, a standard mini adaption plate or microplate is used to bridge the comminuted segments, which are individually lagged to the overlying plate with screws (see Figures 21.20h and i and Figure 21.26).

Zygomaticomaxillary Buttress

Fractures at the zygomaticomaxillary buttress site are an important index of the degree of rotation of the whole complex. Accurate reduction and stable fixation is important because this buttress acts as the direct antagonist to the pull of the masseter muscle. Comminution of this buttress or actual bone loss is not uncommon. Comminuted fractures are buttressed by miniplates, and areas of bone loss are similarly bridged (see Figure 21.16f). It is important to bridge the bone gap with a bone graft that can be fixed to the overlying plate; failure to ensure bony continuity across the gap may allow masticatory forces to loosen the plate.

Occasionally, this fracture may be low, directly at the level of the apices of the tooth roots. If the inferior screws cannot be safely inserted without damage to the tooth roots, then the plate is placed from the upper portion of the buttress laterally to the stable medial nasomaxillary buttress, thus bypassing the inferior portion of the zygomaticomaxillary buttress (see Figure 21.10d).

Lateral Orbital Wall

The lateral orbital wall, the thickest wall of the orbit, is rarely comminuted (approximately 10% of displaced orbital fractures are comminuted). This wall provides the final and most accurate point of adjustment and assessment of fracture reduction, particularly if there is comminution at any of the three or four sites of exposure (see Figure 21.27). If this wall is comminuted, primary bone graft reconstruction of the defect is essential to restore normal orbital volume and to pre-

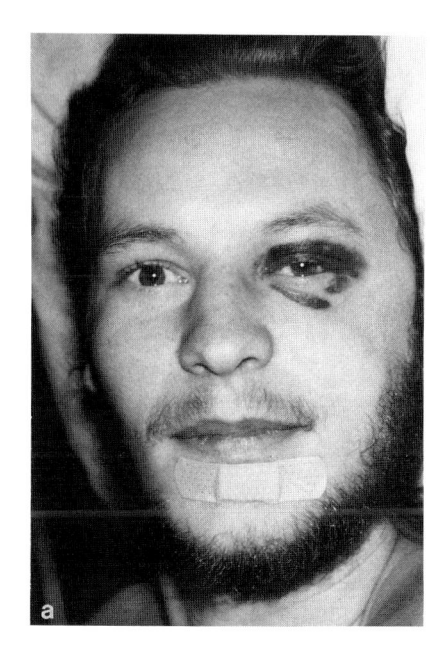

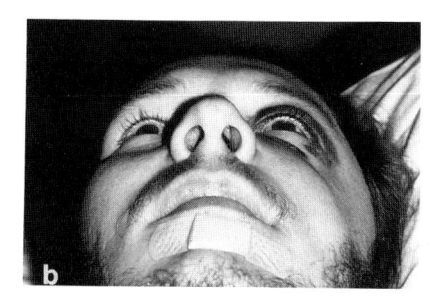

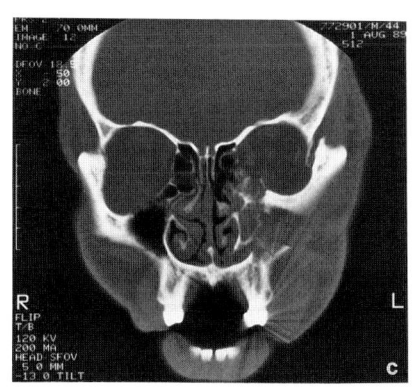

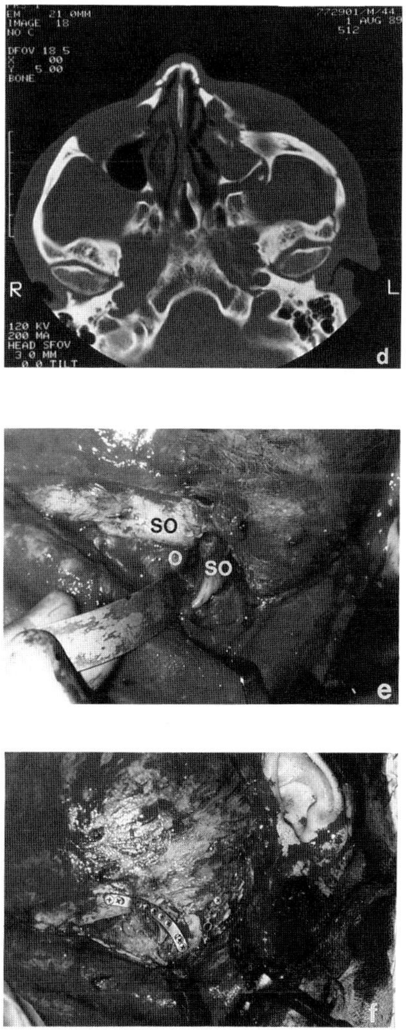

Rigid Fixation of Zygomatic Fractures 275

Figure 21.17 (a) Patient with severe inward displacement of complex orbitozygomatic fractures resulting in characteristic blow-in fracture of the orbit with upward and outward displacement of the ocular globe. (b) Characteristic loss of zygomatic projection is seen with concomitant proptosis of the left ocular globe. (c) This coronal CT scan demonstrates marked inward rotation of the entire orbitozygomatic complex, resulting in a diminution of the left orbital volume. (d) This axial CT scan shows marked blow-in of the left orbitozygomatic complex with loss of anteroposterior projection and multiple segmental fractures of the arch. (e) Accurate restoration requires the use of a coronal incision. Multiple segmental fractures of the arch and lateral orbital wall (LO) can be seen with marked inward displacement of the lateral orbital wall. (f) Accurate three-dimensional reconstruction of the lateral orbital wall and zygomatic arch with multiple miniplates can be seen. Reduction of the blow-in segments which usually reveal large deficits in the orbital walls. Re-exploration of the orbit at the end of the reduction of the rims is essential to assess the size of the deficits which require reconstruction with split calvarial bone grafts to prevent the occurrence of enophthalmos.

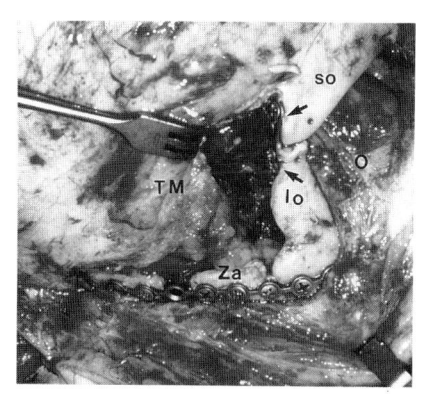

Figure 21.18 In female patients, the plate applied at the fronto-zygomatic suture line may often be palpable. The plate may be applied on the posterior aspect of the fronto-zygomatic suture line (arrows). It is essential not to raise the temporalis muscle significantly because this predisposes to atrophy and postoperative hollowing in the temporal region. The previously stabilized zygomatic arch can be seen. (LO = lateral orbit, SO = superior orbit, O = orbit, T = temporalis muscle.)

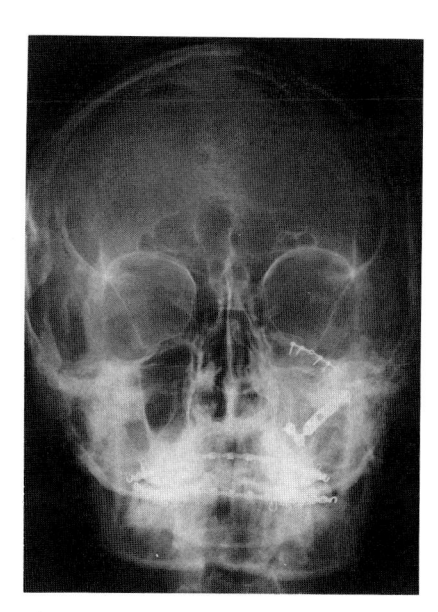

Figure 21.19 Post-op x-ray after fixation of noncomminuted low energy zygomatic fracture in 20-year-old female. Microplate fixation was applied at the infraorbital area. A miniplate was used for stabilization at the zygomaticomaxillary buttress. The patient had a left subcondylar fracture treated with MMF.

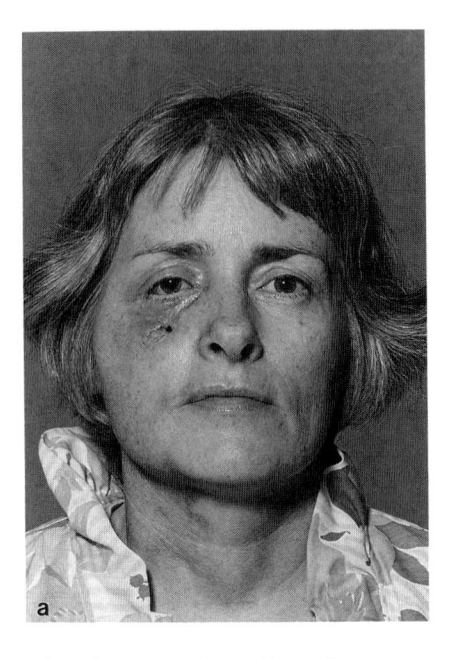

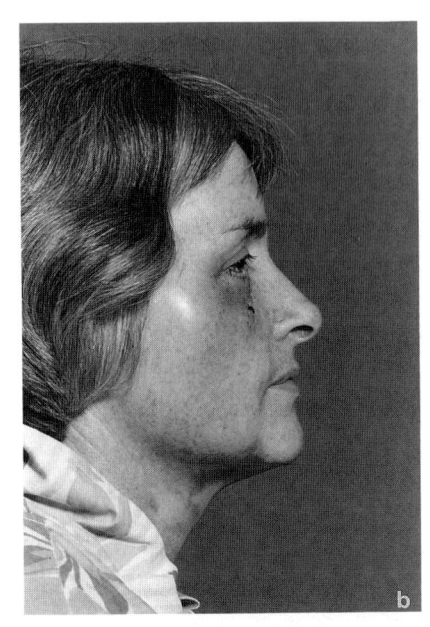

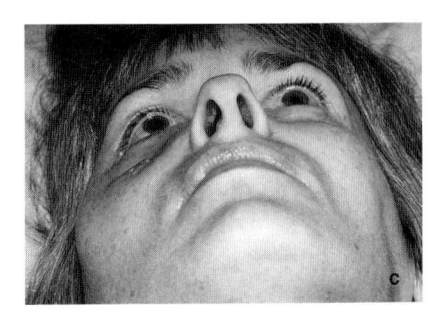

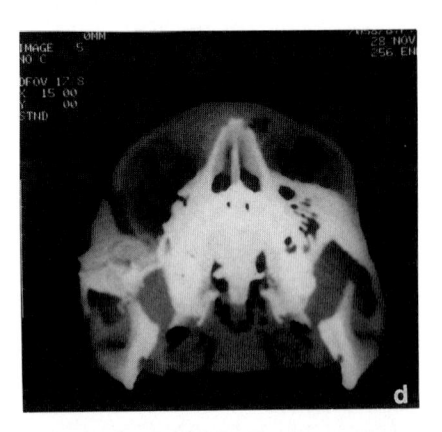

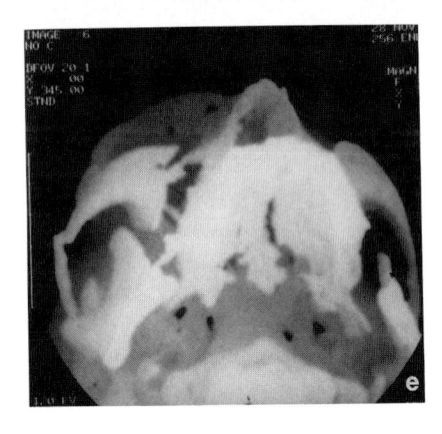

Figure 21.20 Female patient with very complex displaced right orbitozygomatic injury. (a) Marked depression of the right orbitozygomatic complex and marked increase in facial width on the right side due to outward bowing of the zygomatic arch. Acute enophthalmos can be seen. (b) This lateral view illustrates marked depression of the anterior projection of the zygomatic complex and marked outward bowing of the arch, which is protruding through the lateral cheek skin. (c) Marked flattening of the orbitozygomatic complex and marked increase in facial width. Enophthalmos can be seen. (d) This three-dimensional CT scan shows characteristic telescoping of the zygomatic arch and marked downward and outward displacement of the entire orbitozygomatic complex. A large gap in the lateral orbital wall can be seen. In addition, impingement of the depressed zygomatic body on the coronoid process of the mandible can be seen. (e) This three-dimensional CT scan demonstrates characteristic telescoping of the zygomatic arch. (f) This axial CT scan demonstrates marked depression of the zygomatic body and multiple segmental fractures of the zygomatic arch with collapse and outward bowing. (g) This view from above shows coronal flap (C) reflected downward. Multiple segmental fractures of the arch have been initially wired using interosseous wires. Accurate stabilization of the lateral portion of the orbitozygomatic complex at the fronto-zygomatic suture line and the zygomatic arch has resulted in the production of a stable outer frame with the correct anteroposterior projection and facial width. (E = ear, S = superior orbit, O = orbit, ZA = zygomatic arch.) (h) Following exact stabilization of the lateral zygomatic frame, the exact amount of missing inferior orbital margin can be identified; and the gap in the inferior orbital margin is bridged with a long miniplate. Failure first to stabilize the zygomatic complex at the arch and fronto-zygomatic suture line would almost certainly result in a tendency to collapse the defect at the infraorbital margin and lateral zygomaticomaxillary buttress, resulting in residual post-treatment depression. (i) A large deficit in the infraorbital rim is bridged with a carefully contoured split calvarial bone graft (B). The bone graft is fixed to the overlying plate with three screws. (j) With prior lateral stabilization, the deficit at the zygomaticomaxillary buttress is accurately reproduced (arrows). (k) This deficit is bridged by a miniplate, and the deficit itself is filled in with a split calvarial bone graft (B) that is fixed to the overlying plate. Particularly in the tooth bearing segments that are under masticatory forces, it is essential to bridge bony gaps with bone and not to rely on the plate fixation alone. (l) Postoperative x ray. (m) Postoperative result at two years. Note exact restoration of bony orbitozygomatic complex. Slight depression of the soft tissue in the anterior upper cheek is evident; direct injury in this area caused atrophy of the soft tissues. (n) This inferior view demonstrates exact reconstruction of the orbitozygomatic skeletal complex. Slight right exophthalmos has resulted from overcorrection of the deep orbital bone grafting on the right side, but there is no diplopia or visual disturbances. (o) This lateral view demonstrates restoration of projection and contour of the orbitozygomatic complex.

Rigid Fixation of Zygomatic Fractures 277

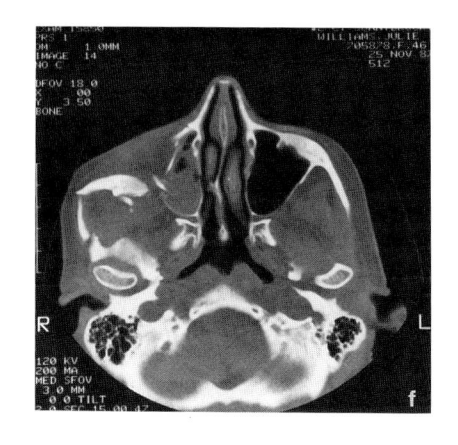

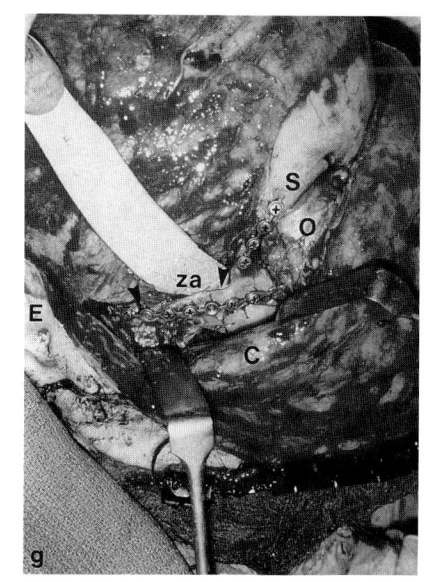

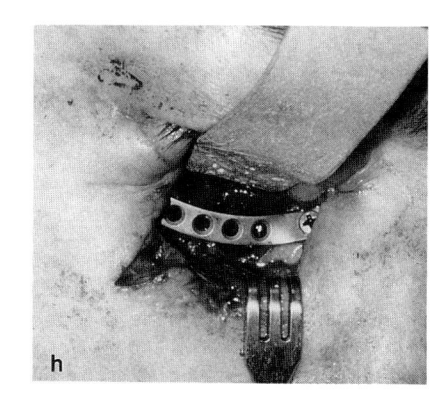

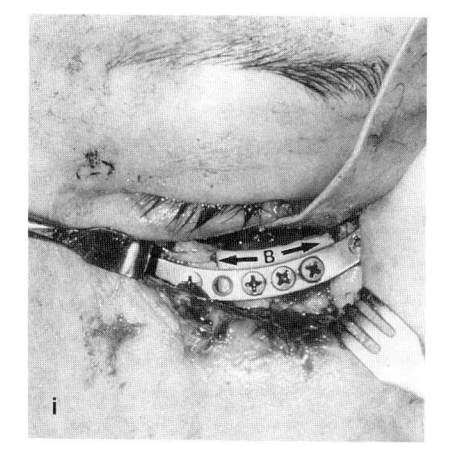

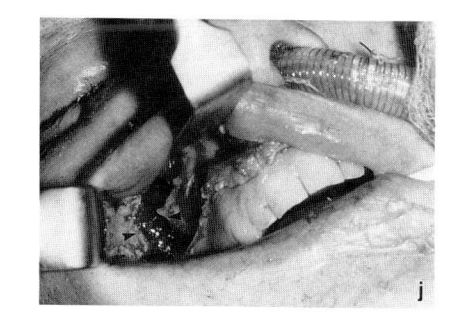

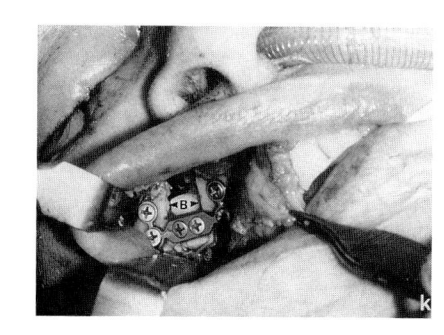

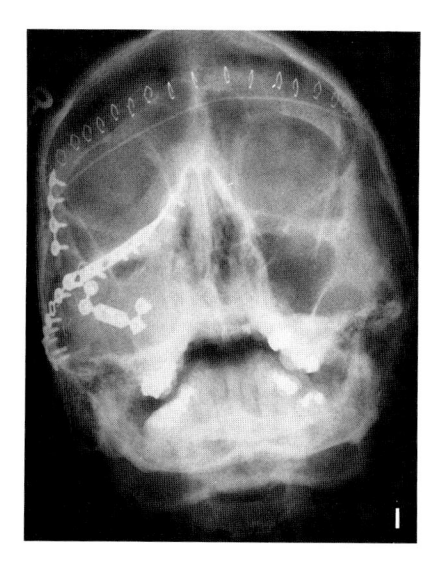

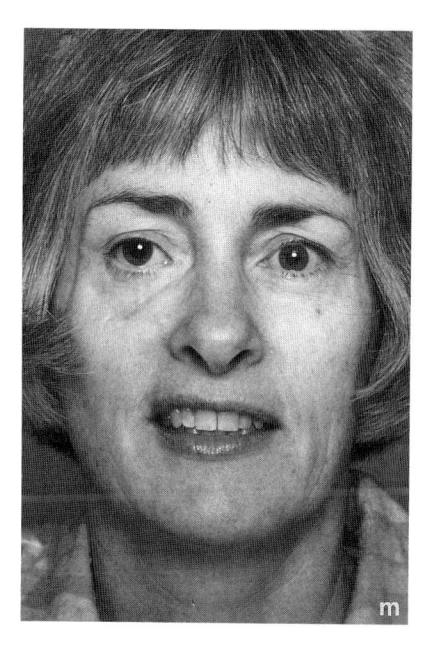

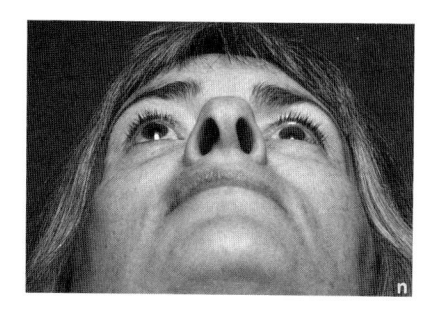

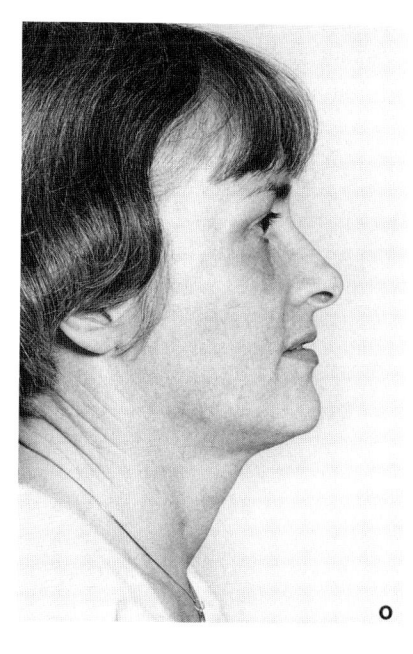

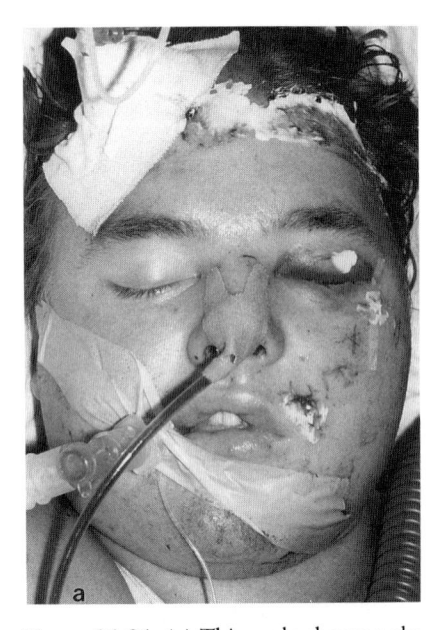

Figure 21.21 (a) This male shows polytrauma, severe head injury needing a Richmond screw, and very complex left orbitozygomatic injuries. Note the severe panfacial edema that very often masks the severity of these injuries. (b) This axial CT scan shows multiple segmental displaced fractures of the left zygomatic arch. (c) Very significantly displaced left orbitozygomatic injury with outward bowing of the zygomatic arch and marked downward depression of the zygomatic body. (d) Three-dimensional repair with extensive use of the old stainless steel miniplates. (e) Accurate restoration of orbital volume and globe position. However, there is a slight residual depression of the zygomatic body and a slight increase in facial width on the left side. (f) This anterior view demonstrates slight flattening of the zygomatic body region, characteristic sagging of the facial soft tissues, and inferior displacement of the lateral canthus which was not replaced by lateral canthopexy. (g) Characteristic and common mistake of reconstructing the zygomatic arch as an arch and failure to flatten the reconstruction of the mid portion of the arch.

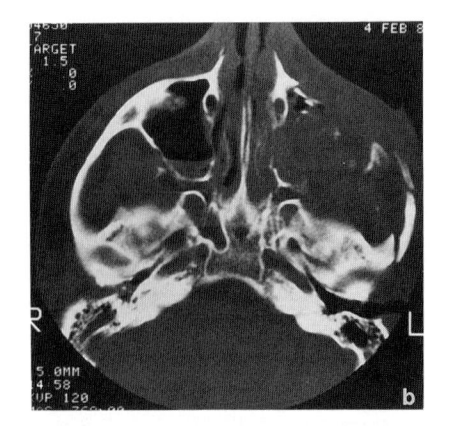

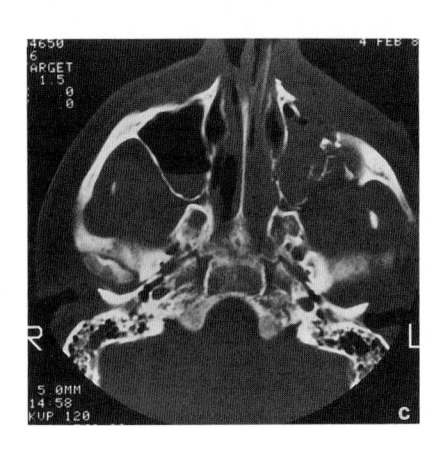

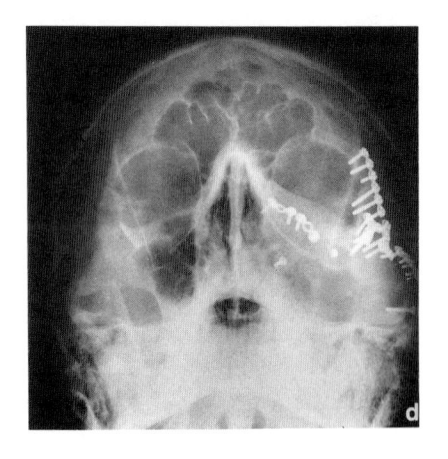

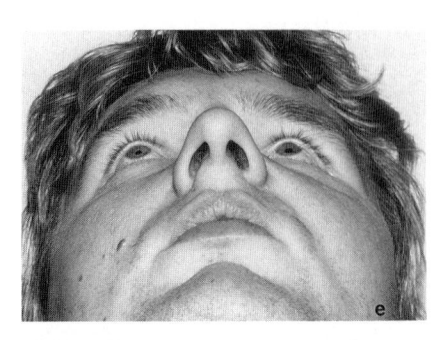

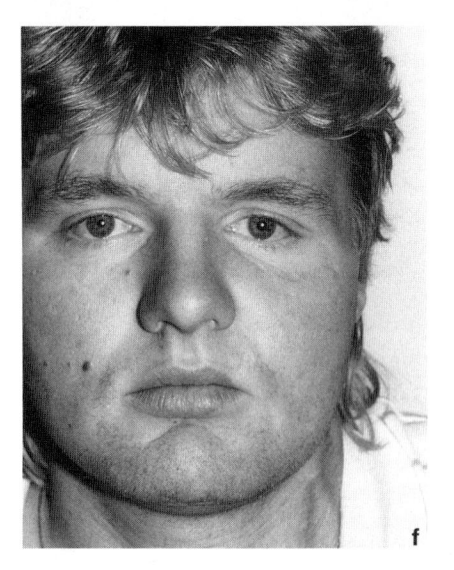

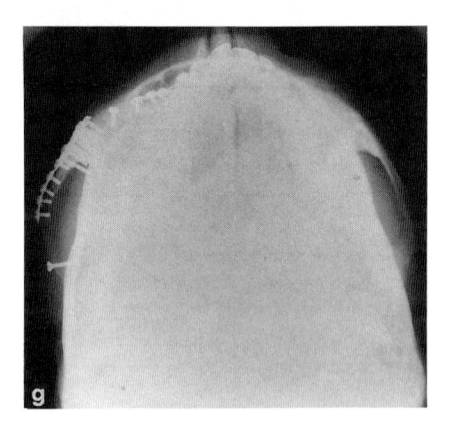

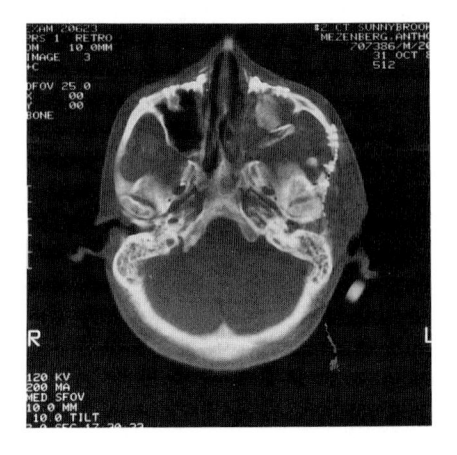

Figure 21.22 Extensive open reduction and internal fixation of left orbitozygomatic complex injury with reconstruction of the zygomatic arch as a true arch, resulting in residual depression of the zygomatic body.

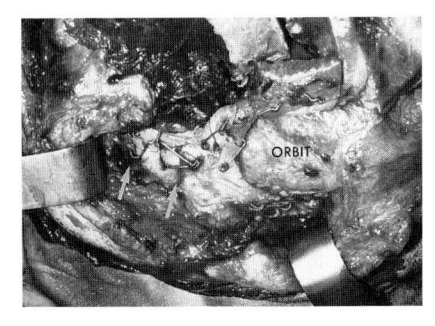

Figure 21.23 Before the advent of miniplates for midfacial repair, we attempted to repair complex fractures of the zygomatic arch with multiple interosseous wires, using chain-link wiring where necessary (arrows). Even though this form of fixation seemed to provide adequate stabilization on the operating table, interosseous wires, even when used in a multiple fashion or with chain-link wiring, failed in many cases to maintain the position of the stabilized zygomatic arch on a long-term basis.

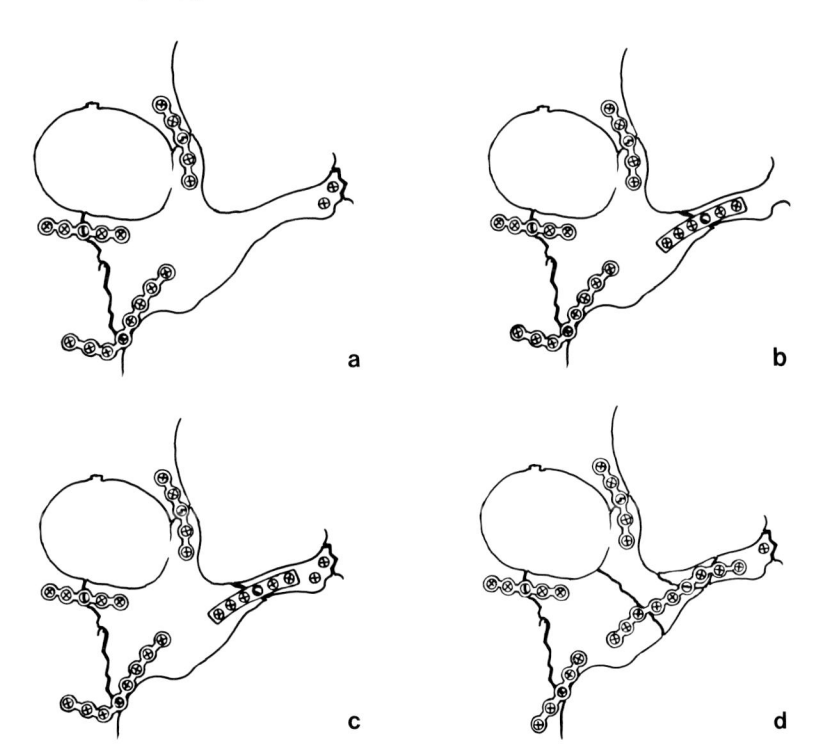

Figure 21.24 Fractures of the zygomatic arch in relation to fractures of the entire complex tend to follow a well defined pattern. (a) The zygomatic arch is commonly split from its attachment to the zygomatic process of the temporal bone. This fracture is usually oblique and is ideally amenable to lag screw fixation. (b) The arch may be fractured in its middle portion, and this fracture is repaired using a miniplate. Compression may be used if needed. (c) In some situations the arch is fractured in its middle portion as well as split away from its junction to the zygomatic process of the temporal bone. Here, a combination of posterior lag screws and miniplate at the middle of the arch is utilized in association with fixation at the other three points of fixation. (d) In comminuted or segmental fractures of the arch, posterior lag screws may have to be combined with long miniadaptive plates to cross all the different segments. They are positioned from stable bone anteriorly to stable bone posteriorly. Separate screws are placed into intervening segments wherever possible.

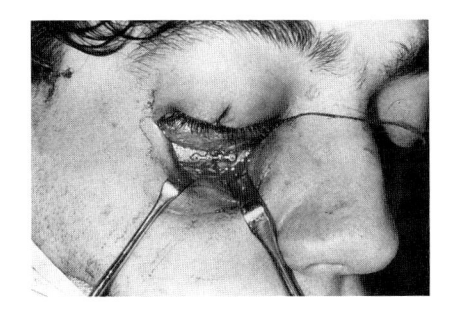

Figure 21.25 If adequate fixation is applied at the fronto-zygomatic suture line and the other two points, the infraorbital margin is the least important point of fixation. It can be repaired with an interosseous wire or a microplate, as illustrated here, because this is less likely to be felt, particularly by young females.

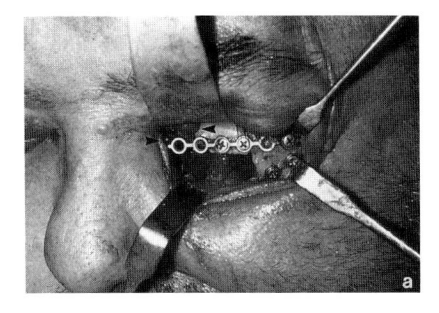

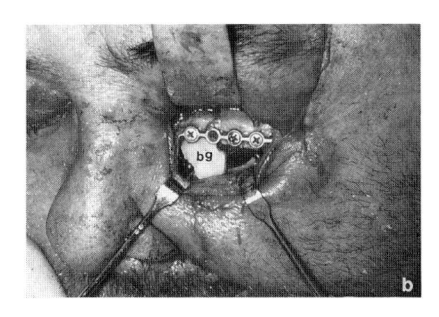

Figure 21.26 (a) In this case, after stabilization of the residual orbital rim inferiorly with a long miniadaptive plate, it is evident that there is a large bony gap on the medial aspect of the orbital rim (arrows). Extensive bone loss in the anterior maxilla around the inferior orbital nerve can be seen. (b) This bony gap in the infraorbital margin is replaced with a split calvarial bone graft using an extension of the bone graft downward to replace the anterior wall of the maxilla and to maintain soft-tissue expansion in this area. (BG = bone graft.)

280 RIGID FIXATION OF THE CRANIOMAXILLOFACIAL SKELETON

Figure 21.27 In addition to the four characteristic points of reduction and stabilization, the lateral orbital wall is the final key point to assess accurate reduction of the complex in a three-dimensional fashion. (a) Characteristic step deformity at the lateral orbital wall. It is rare for the lateral orbital wall to be comminuted, even with comminuted fractures at the other four points. Accurate reduction at this point is the final and most accurate determination of the exact repositioning of the orbitozygomatic complex. (b) In approximately 10% of complex displaced orbitozygomatic fractures, there is comminution or bone loss in the lateral orbital wall. In this situation, the lateral orbital wall cannot aid in the reduction of the fracture; therefore, accurate reduction must be predetermined by an inspection of the other four points of fracturing. (c) Actual bone loss in the lateral orbital wall in association with a severe fracture of the medial wall. After the entire orbitozygomatic complex has been restabilized, the lateral orbital wall needs to be inspected for any deficits. Failure to repair the lateral orbital wall will invariably result in an increase in orbital volume and enophthalmos. (d) In most situations, the lateral orbital wall deficit can be repaired by means of a bone graft placed on the inside of the orbital rim. This bone graft can almost always be wedged into place along the remaining ledges. However, in certain situations with massive loss of the lateral orbital wall, the defect must be repaired by external bone graft. This picture illustrates a massive deficit of the lateral orbital wall with herniation of periorbital contents through the lateral orbital wall (arrow). (TM = temporalis muscle, SO = superior orbit, O = orbit, Z = zygoma.) (e) After careful three-dimensional stabilization of the orbitozygomatic complex, the hole in the lateral orbit is repaired using an external bone graft in the temporal fossa (B). This bone is stabilized with a miniplate, which is anchored either to the fronto-zygomatic region or to the temporal bone itself. Care must be taken to reposition the reflected temporalis muscle (TM) to prevent the characteristic hollow that occurs after this approach.

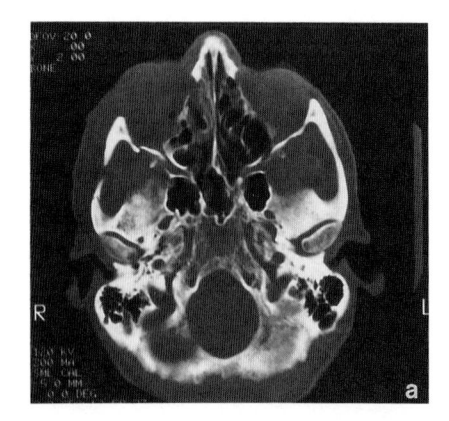

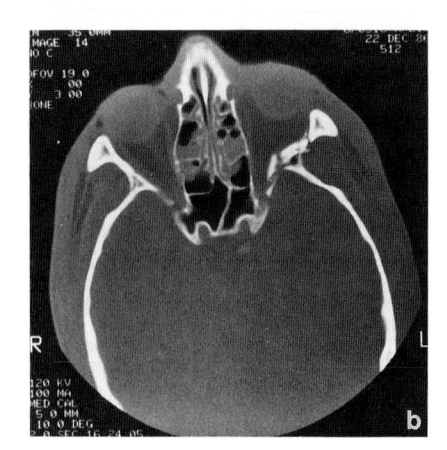

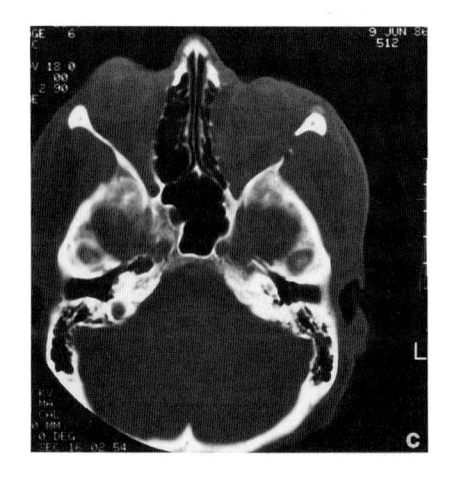

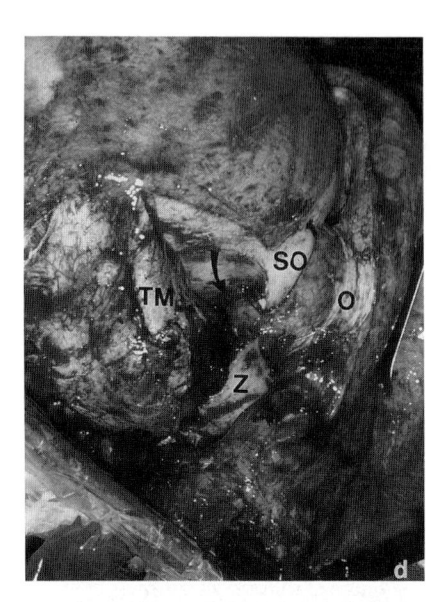

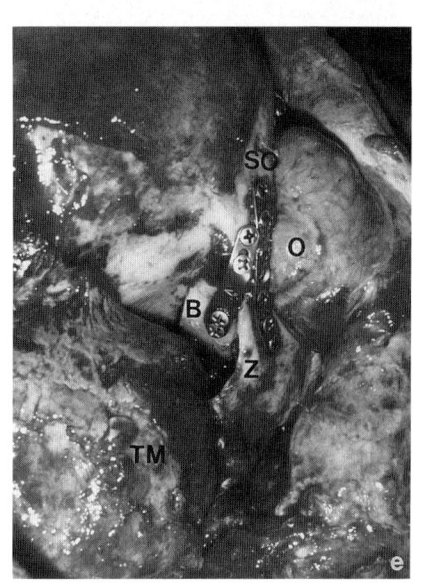

vent herniation of orbital fat into the temporal fossa. In most defects, split calvarial bone grafts are placed inside the orbit after completion of three- or four-point fixation. In certain extensive defects, the bone graft is placed externally and fixed with a miniplate to the bone in the region of the temporal fossa; 3- or 4-millimeter screws are used to prevent inadvertent intracranial penetration.

Unilateral Nasoethmoid-orbital Fractures

Occasionally a zygomatic complex fracture is associated with a unilateral nasoethmoid-orbital fracture. The frontonasal buttress is displaced laterally and in-

Figure 21.28 Patient with left orbitozygomatic injuries undergoing extensive open reduction and miniplate fixation without adequate reduction of the displaced bone segments prior to miniplate application. (a) Post-treatment deformity with inward collapse of the orbitozygomatic complex, loss of zygomatic projection, and left ocular orbital dystopia and enophthalmos. (b) This inferior view shows typical depression and inward displacement of the orbitozygomatic complex and enophthalmos. (c) Extensive use of miniplate stabilization is shown. Miniplates have been applied without adequate reduction of the underlying bony segments. (d) This inferior view shows incorrect placement of the miniplates without adequate contouring to reproduce the exact contours of the anterior maxilla and orbitozygomatic complex. (e) This axial CT scan illustrates residual outward bowing of the zygomatic arch and downward depression of the zygomatic complex. (f) Inadequate reduction of the lateral orbital wall and inferior orbital rim. Note that inadequate restoration of the normal orbital walls, particularly medial and inferior, has resulted in marked increase in orbital volume. (g) Multilayered Silastic prosthesis can be seen prolapsed into the maxillary antrum. This is the cause of residual bony deficit in the deep orbit. It is essential first to accurately reduce all bony segments prior to the application of miniplate fixation. The use of rigid internal fixation will not guarantee accurate repair of a complex injury. Miniplate fixation will do no more than provide the most sophisticated form of fixation once the bony segments have been accurately reduced.

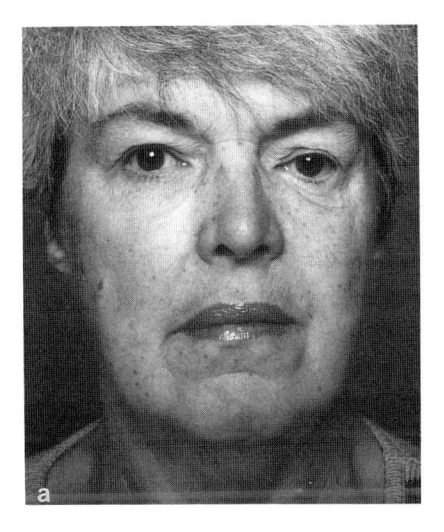

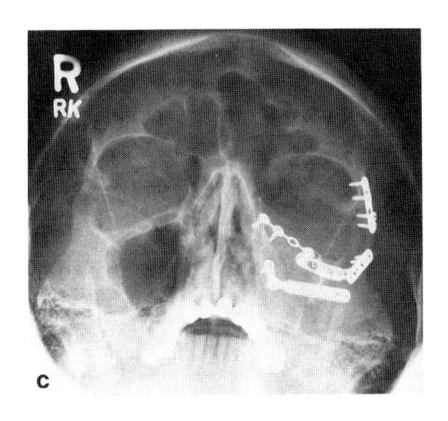

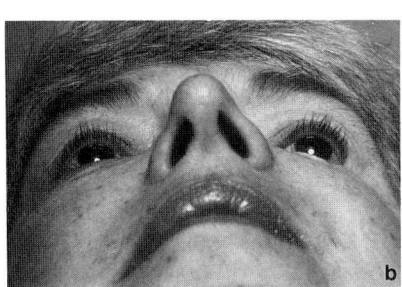

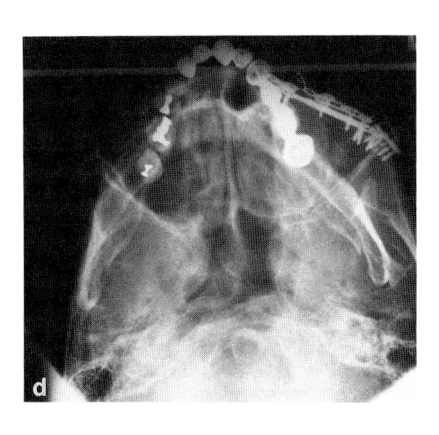

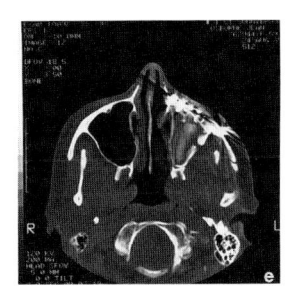

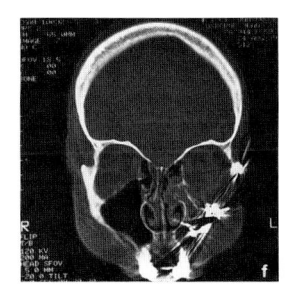

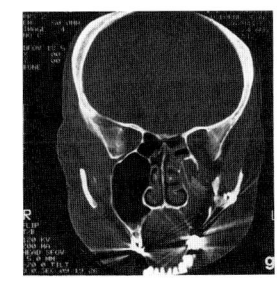

feriorly, resulting in displacement of the medial portion of the inferior orbital rim. If this is not recognized, reduction and fixation of the zygomatic complex to this unreduced segment will result in residual post-treatment deformity and displacement. Inability to obtain accurate reduction at the lateral orbital wall with seemingly accurate reduction at the other three or four sites may be indicative of an unrecognized displaced nasoethmoid-orbital fracture.

SUMMARY

Appreciation of the anatomic complexity of the zygomatic region and the ability to provide exposure without morbidity now allows anatomic reconstruction of the most complex zygomatic injuries. Key is anatomic repositioning the orientation provided by the zygomatic arch. The arch not only determines the proper projection of the malar complex but also determines facial width. A thorough understanding, assessment, exposure, and repair of the zygomatic arch will facilitate management of acute and established orbitozygomatic and midfacial injuries. It is critical to remember that the precise anatomic realignment permitted by extended exposure techniques and maintained by rigid fixation techniques allows stable restoration of the preinjury appearance and not the rigid fixation per se. The morbidity associated with improper extended exposure techniques and misapplied rigid fixation can cause deformities that may be extremely difficult, if not impossible, to correct (see Figures 21.13 and 21.28).

BIBLIOGRAPHY

Antonyshyn O, Gruss JS: Complex orbital trauma: The role of rigid fixation and primary bone grafting. Adv Ophth Plast Reconstr Surg 7:61, 1988.

Davidson J, Nickerson D, Nickerson B: Zygomatic fracture: Comparison of methods of internal fixation. Plast Reconstr Surg 86:25, 1990.

Eisele DW, Ducket LG: Single point stabilization of zygomatic fractures with the minicompression plate. Arch Otolaryngol Head and Neck Surg 113:267, 1987.

Ellis E, Elatter A, Moos KF: An analysis of 2067 cases of zygomatico-orbital fractures. J Oral Maxillofac Surg 43:417, 1985.

Glassman RD, Manson PN, Vanderkolk CA et al.: Rigid fixation of internal orbital fractures. Plast Reconstr Surg 86:1103, 1990.

Gruss JS, Van Wyck L, Phillips JH, Antonyshyn O: The importance of the zygomatic arch in complex midfacial fracture repair and correction of post traumatic orbitozygomatic deformities. Plast Reconstr Surg 85:878, 1990.

Jackson IT: Classification and treatment of orbitozygomatic and orbitoethmoid fractures: The place of bone grafting and rigid fixation. Clin Plast Surg 16:77, 1989.

Jackson IT: Classification and treatment of orbitozygomatic and orbitoethmoid fractures: The place of bone grafting and rigid fixation. Clin Plast Surg 16:77, 1989.

Karlan MS, Cassisi NJ: Fractures of the zygoma. Arch Otolaryngol 105:320, 1979.

Knight JS, North JF: The classification of malar fractures: An analysis of displacement as a guide to treatment. Br J Plast Surg 13:325, 1961.

Lasargil MG, Reichman MV, Kubik S: Preservation of the frontotemporal branch of the facial nerve using the interfascial temporalis flap for pterional craniotomy. J Neurosurg 67:463, 1987.

Manson PN: Internal fixation of malar fractures. (Letter) Plast Reconstr Surg 85:481, 1990.

Manson PN, Crawley WA, Yaremchuk MJ, et al: Midface fractures: Advantages of immediate extended open reduction and bone grafting. Plast Reconstr Surg 76:1, 1985.

Rinehart GC, Marshall JL, Hemmer KM, Bresina S: Internal fixation of malar fractures: An experimental biophysical study. Plast Reconstr Surg 84:21, 1989.

Rowe NL, Killey HC: Fractures of the facial skeleton. Baltimore, Williams and Wilkins, 1955.

CHAPTER 22

Rigid Fixation of Nasoethmoid-orbital Fractures

Joseph S. Gruss

A direct blow to the midface may result in fractures of the bony nasoethmoid-orbital complex and injury to the adjacent soft tissues. These injuries may be confined to the nasoethmoid-orbital complex, but are more frequently associated with other facial fractures and are often complicated by multisystem trauma.

Nasoethmoid-orbital injuries are the most difficult and challenging of all facial injuries to treat. Their complexity is enhanced by the predisposition to comminution of the nasal bones, medial wall, and floor of the orbit and by the intricate anatomy of the region. Concomitant injury of the anterior cranial fossa, frontal sinus, ocular globe and optic nerve, medial canthal ligaments, and nasolacrimal apparatus adds to this complexity.

Closed reduction and external splint fixation has been recommended by many authors (see Figure 22.1). This usually involves external nasal compression with lead plates held together with transnasal wires. These may produce an acceptable result in only the less severe cases. With severe comminution and posterior, lateral, and inferior displacement and dislocation of the medial orbital rim and wall, the axis of these bony segments lies below and posterior to the axis of the stable inferior orbital rim. Without direct exploration and inspection of the fracture pattern and fragment situation, including these fragments adequately in the transnasal wiring and holding them in their "elevated" position for any length of time is virtually impossible. The use of lead plates often results in an unnatural appearance of the nose, with characteristic flattening, collapse, and inward telescoping of the nasal bones (see Figure 22.2). This is particularly evident in the markedly comminuted nasoethmoid-orbital fractures in which external compression causes further collapse and inward compression of the multiple unstable fragments. This can be readily demonstrated by the application of lead plates to these fractures at the time of open reduction. In addition, lead plates and transnasal wires will usually not correct the medial canthal displacement or disinsertion. Inadequate initial treatment will often result in severe deformity; such a deformity may be extremely

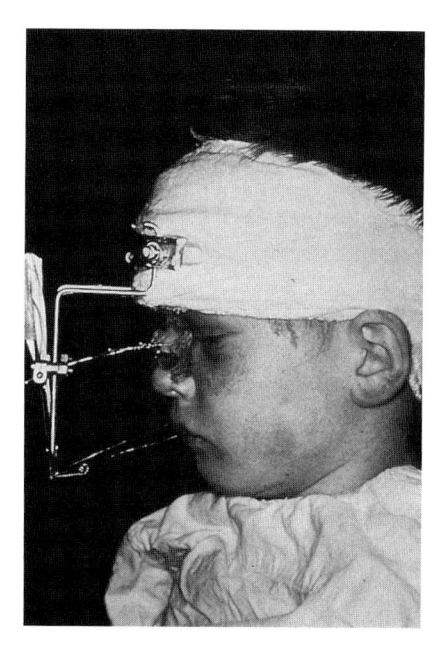

Figure 22.1 This young patient's midfacial and nasoethmoid-orbital fractures are treated with external fixation. Note the lead plate compression for the nasoethmoid region, which is anchored additionally to the external fixation device to try to pull this region forward.

Figure 22.2 (a) This female patient's nasoethmoid-orbital injury was treated with lead plate compression. Note the typical post-treatment deformity, with collapse of the nasal bones and severe blunting and scarring of both medial canthal regions. This is extremely difficult or impossible to correct on a secondary basis. (Photo courtesy of Dr. M. Vincent.) (b) This lateral view shows typical collapse of the nasal bridge and telescoping of the nasal bones with shortening of the entire nasal complex.

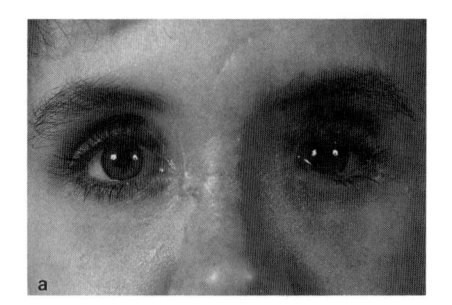

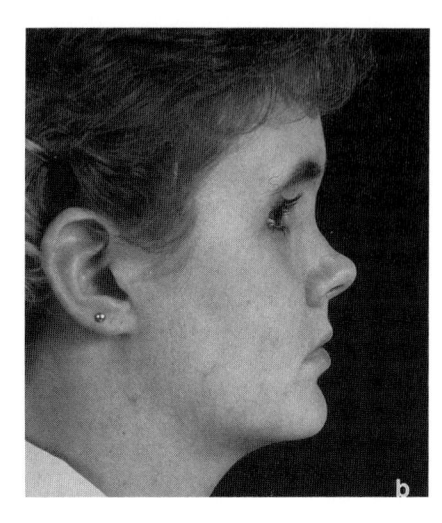

difficult or impossible to correct secondarily. Optimal management involves early surgical exploration and meticulous repair of bone and soft tissue utilizing the principles learned from reconstructive craniofacial surgery.

Nasoethmoid-orbital injuries have been described in detail by numerous authors, but no adequate classification of these injuries has existed. The patterns of injury, often complex, do not fit the classic patterns described by Le Fort. The recognition of several distinct injury patterns has led to formulation of a comprehensive classification of nasoethmoid-orbital injuries. An understanding of this classification will facilitate the recognition and diagnosis of these injuries and aid in the correct choice of treatment for each specific pattern of injury.

PATHOLOGICAL ANATOMY

The nasoethmoid-orbital region represents the anatomic crossroad of the nasal, orbital, and cranial cavities. The interorbital space is the area behind the nasal bones, between the medial walls of the orbits, and beneath the floor of the anterior cranial fossa. It contains the two ethmoid labyrinths, the upper portion of the nasal cavity, the nasal septum, and a portion of the superior and medial turbinates. The roof is formed by the cribriform plate medially and the roof of the ethmoid sinus laterally. The cribriform plate is traversed by numerous olfactory canals. The junction of the ethmoid roof and the cribriform plate is the weakest portion of the roof of the interorbital space, and the dura is tightly adherent in this area. Fractures extending into this area and through the posterior wall of the frontal sinus may produce dural lacerations and cerebral injury. Injuries in the region of the cribriform plate may damage the olfactory nerves. The nasal bones, vomerine bone, perpendicular plate of the ethmoid, and ethmoid labyrinths are thin and predisposed to comminuted fractures, possibly restricting the nasal airway. Conversely, the nasal process of the frontal bone and the frontal process of the maxilla are strong and comminution is rare.

The medial wall of the orbit is composed of the lacrimal bone anteriorly and the lamina papyracea of the ethmoid bone posteriorly. These bones are extremely thin and fragile and invariably comminute. The continuity of the lamina papyracea with the thin portion of the orbital floor facilitates a concomitant blowout fracture in this area. The optic foramen is situated in the posteromedial aspect of the orbit at the posterior limit of the lamina papyraceá. Severe fractures of the medial orbital wall may injure the optic nerve, and direct injury to the globe may occur from displaced bone fragments. The lacrimal bone contains the lacrimal sac. The nasolacrimal duct lies within the bone of the lateral wall and enters the nasal cavity in the inferior meatus under the inferior turbinate. Fractures with displaced bone segments may cause injury or external compression of the nasolacrimal duct in its bony canal.

MEDIAL CANTHAL LIGAMENT

The critical principle in the management of injury to the medial canthal ligament is the accurate and comprehensive reconstruction of the medial canthal region, including repositioning of the medial canthal tendon to correct the traumatic telecanthus. Traumatic telecanthus may be due to (1) lateral displacement of the medial canthal ligament still attached to the frontonasal buttress (see Figure 22.3), (2) lateral displacement of the canthal ligament attached to a small fragment of bone, or (3) direct laceration of the ligament itself (see Figure 22.4).

In the great majority of cases, the medial canthal ligament is displaced laterally but still attached to the large frontonasal buttress, which rarely comminutes. Our experience agrees with that of Manson (1983), who

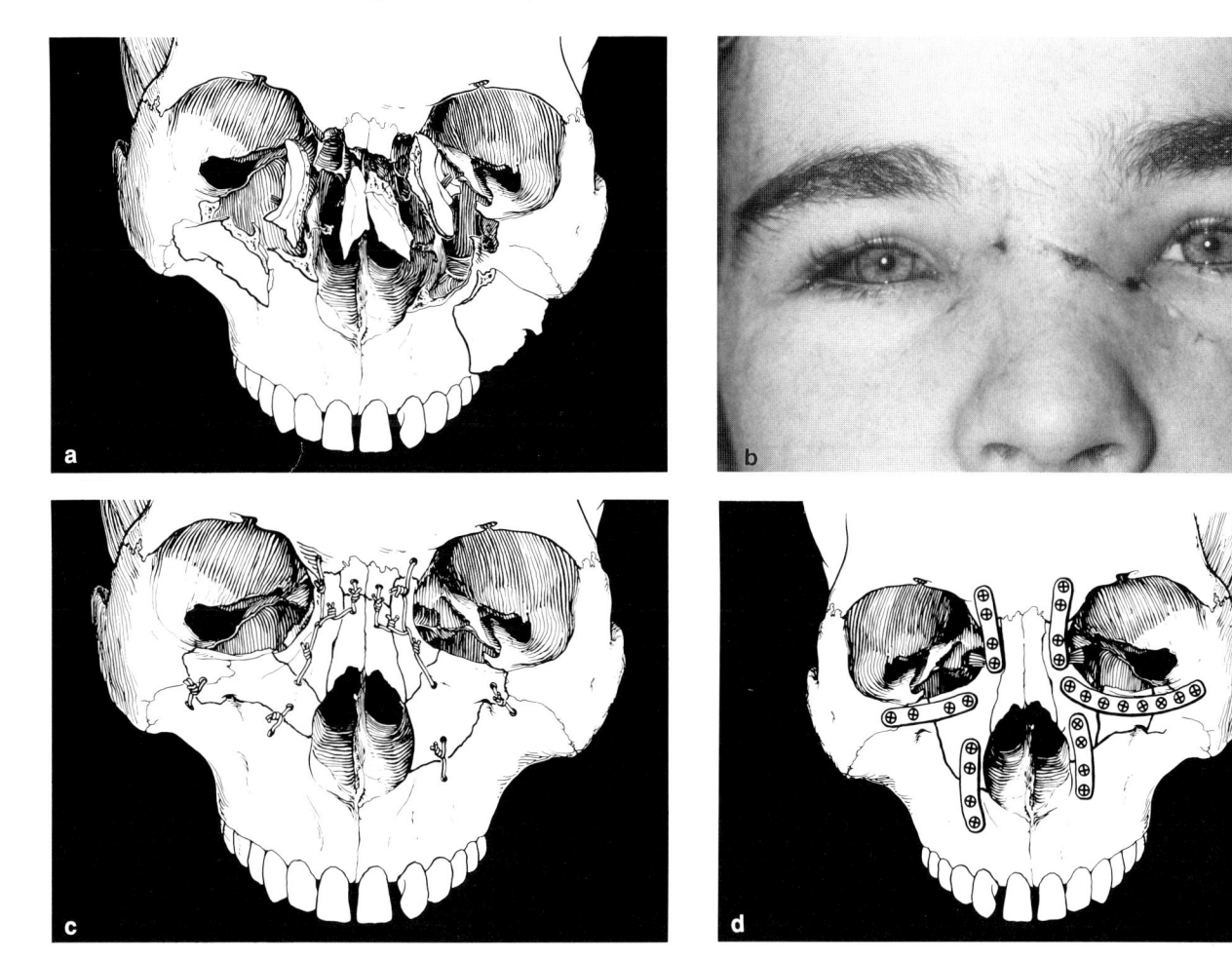

Figure 22.3 (a) Artist's depiction of the typical pattern of bony injury in the bony nasoethmoid fracture. Note that the strong frontonasal buttress is detached superiorly and inferiorly and displaced inferiorly and posteriorly, taking the medial canthal ligament with it. The most important principle of repair is the repositioning of this bone segment and the careful dissection of the segment prior to fixation to maintain the attachment of the ligament. (b) The typical clinical appearance of a patient with bony nasoethmoid injury. Telecanthus can be seen with flattening of the nasal bridge. The distal cartilaginous nasal support is maintained. (c) Prior to the advent of miniplates, these fractures were repaired with extensive interosseous wiring using chain-link wiring. This provided good fixation in many cases, maintaining the position of these segments was difficult when these fractures were severely comminuted. In addition, it was often necessary to strip the ligament off the bone to allow proper placement of the wires. (d) Common positioning of miniplates in the typical nasoethmoid injury. The upper plates are placed across the upper portion of the fracture at the frontonasal region and below the ridge of the bone so that they are rarely palpable. The lower portion of a miniplate is placed in such a way that it is adjacent to the canthal ligament. In this way, the canthal ligament is exactly repositioned. In relatively stable and uncomminuted fractures, the plate at the frontonasal, as well as the plate at the infraorbital rim, can be a microplate rather than a miniplate. However, in more unstable fractures and those with comminution, it is easier to use miniplates because the microplates are more difficult to apply and, in certain situations, will not give adequate stability.

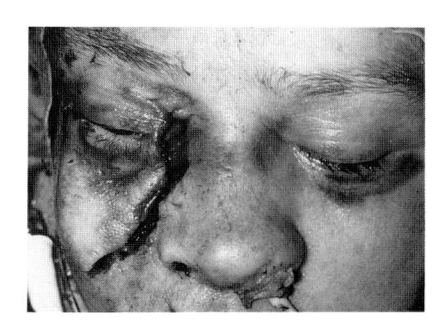

Figure 22.4 This patient has direct laceration across the nasoethmoid region, resulting in direct laceration of the medial canthal tendon. Detachment of the medial canthal tendon from bone is rare and requires direct transnasal wiring of the canthal ligament.

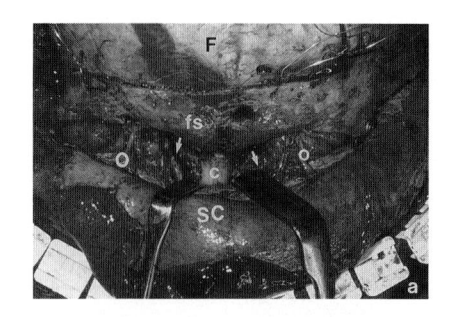

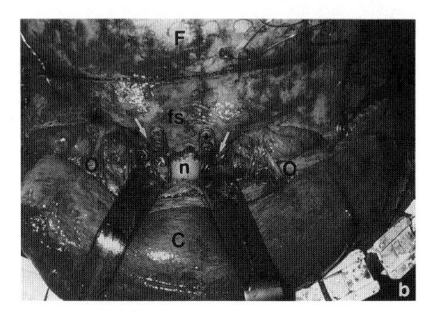

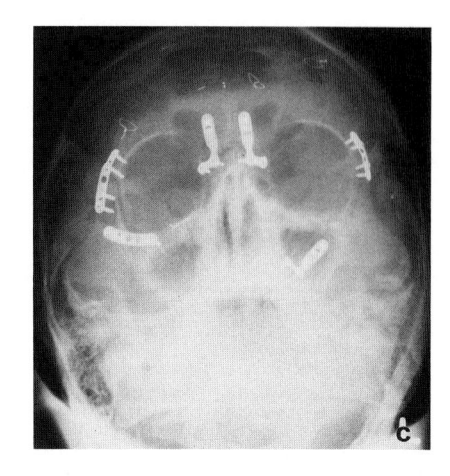

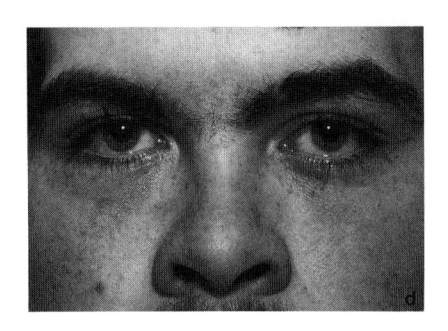

Figure 22.5 (a) In this young patient who had suffered massive panfacial injuries and a severe nasoethmoid-orbital crush, exposure through the coronal incision after the neurosurgical repair reveals the dissection of the displaced frontonasal segments (white arrows). The nasal bone (N) can be seen. Care was taken not to strip the canthal ligaments from these segments. (O = orbits, F = frontal bone, C = coronal flap.) (b) The displaced frontonasal segments are reduced perfectly and repositioned with a miniplate on each side (white arrows). The lower two screws are placed close to the canthal ligament. (c) This postoperative x ray shows the positioning of the miniplates in the frontonasal region in combination with miniplate and interosseous wire fixation in other areas of the craniofacial skeleton. (d) This close-up view of the nasoethmoid region shows normal restoration of intercanthal distance and position and intercanthal anatomy. Note the characteristic anatomic appearance of the medial canthal region with slight downward tilt, which is not changed because the canthal ligaments were not wired in a transnasal fashion.

found that in 92% of cases with a closed injury the canthus was attached to a large bone segment.

The previous misconception in the treatment of injuries to the medial canthal ligament—that these injuries were always comminuted and were not amenable to open reduction—led to their invariable treatment with external compression plates. Accurate delineation of the exact fracture pattern has demonstrated that the strong frontonasal buttress containing the medial canthal ligament rarely comminutes. Comminution commonly occurs in the more delicate nasal bones anteriorly and in the medial and inferior orbital walls posteriorly. Thus careful delineation of the frontonasal buttress, which contains the medial canthal ligament, and its accurate repositioning and fixation, will result in accurate reconstruction of the medial canthal region and the correction of traumatic telecanthus (see Figures 22.3 and 22.5). It is necessary to wire the ligament transnasally only if it is avulsed with a small fragment of bone or directly lacerated.

CLASSIFICATION AND MANAGEMENT

One third of nasoethmoid-orbital fractures are unilateral, and two thirds are bilateral. They are associated with other facial fractures in greater than 90% of cases. Five clinical types of fractures have been recognized, each of which may occasionally have a combination of features (see Table 22.1). Based on the recognition of each fracture type and pattern, a specific reconstructive protocol has been developed to ensure optimal repair.

Type 1: Fractures Isolated to the Bony Nasoethmoid-orbital Region

This injury occurs following a direct blow to the nasal bony dorsum. In the rarer, less severe injury, the nasal bones and a portion of the medial orbital wall are telescoped backward into the interorbital space, either in one segment or with minimal comminution of bone. These fractures may be impacted and difficult to reduce.

Table 22.1 Classification of Nasoethmoid-Orbital Injuries

Type 1: Isolated bony nasoethmoid-orbital injury

Type 2: Bony nasoethmoid-orbital and central maxilla
   2A: Central maxilla only
   2B: Central and one lateral maxilla
   2C: Central and bilateral lateral maxillae

Type 3: Extended nasoethmoid-orbital injury
   3A: With craniofacial injuries
   3B: With Le Fort II and III fractures

Type 4: Nasoethmoid-orbital with orbital displacement
   4A: With oculo-orbital displacement
   4B: With orbital dystopia

Type 5: Nasoethmoid-orbital with bone loss

Open reduction is achieved through pre-existing lacerations, an "open sky" approach (or preferably a coronal incision) and direct fixation at the frontonasal and medial orbital region is performed.

In the more common injury (see Figure 22.3), the nasal bones are telescoped backward into the interorbital space in one segment, two separate segments, or multiple comminuted fragments. The nasal process of the frontal bone is usually preserved. The frontal process of the maxilla detaches at the frontonasal region and at the medial aspect of the inferior orbital rim and shifts in a posterior and lateral direction—usually in one or two segments. Severe comminution is rare. Cartilaginous or distal nasal support is always maintained. The medial canthal ligament and its attachment to the anterior lacrimal crest becomes laterally displaced, producing a traumatic telecanthus.

All fractures are identified, reduced, and stabilized with interosseous fixation. The need for immediate bone grafts is now assessed.

Type 2: Nasoethmoid-orbital Injury Associated With Fractures of the Central Maxilla

A nasoethmoid-orbital injury associated with fractures of the central maxilla is produced by a direct blow over the nasal bony and cartilaginous dorsum, nasal tip, and central maxilla. In addition to the fractures of the bony nasoethmoid-orbital region previously described, there is extensive comminution of the perpendicular plate of the ethmoid, maxillary crest, vomerine bone, and central maxilla (nasomaxillary buttresses). The cartilaginous and bony nasal support may be crushed. Pressure exerted on the nasal tip causes prolapse of the distal nose into the pyriform aperture and is pathognomonic of this injury. Three injury patterns have been recognized; they are related to the severity of the maxillary injury (see Figure 22.6).

Type 2A

A Type 2A injury is produced by a direct central blow to the midface. In this injury, the maxillary fractures are confined to the central maxilla (nasomaxillary buttresses). The fracture pattern extends from the previously described fracture of the medial portion of the inferior orbital rim, downward to completely encircle the pyriform aperture. The entire bony nasoethmoid-orbital and central maxilla is crushed backward. Both lateral orbitozygomaticomaxillary regions are stable.

Type 2B

An oblique force to the central midface causes a Type 2B injury (see Figure 22.7). In addition to the Type 2A fracture pattern, the maxillary fractures extend laterally on the side of the injury to involve the maxillary body and lateral zygomaticomaxillary buttress. This area is crushed inward in combination with a central maxillary injury. The maxilla itself is usually stable to palpation.

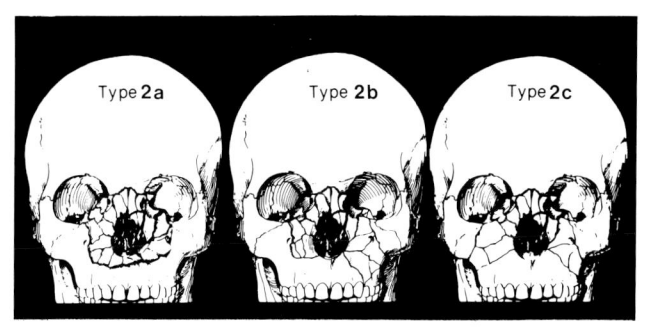

Figure 22.6 Patterns of Type 2 injury with central maxillary crush. All injuries have loss of distal nasal support and require primary nasal bone graft reconstruction.

Type 2C

In the Type 2C injury, the force to the central midface is so severe that the inward buckling and crushing of the central maxilla extends laterally on both sides and may involve both zygomaticomaxillary buttresses. The entire central midface and anterior maxilla is crushed inwards, often producing the most severe of all deformities in nasoethmoid-orbital injuries (see Figures 22.8 and 22.9). The crushing may be confined to the anterior maxilla, and the posterior pterygomaxillary buttress may be either intact or fractured, producing mobility of the maxilla.

The bony nasoethmoid-orbital and maxillary fractures are reduced and repaired as described previously. Re-establishment of bony continuity and stability of the frontal process of the maxilla and bony nasal dorsum is almost always possible with interfragmentary fixation. However, the loss of distal cartilaginous nasal support can be repaired only by the use of immediate bone grafts to the nose.

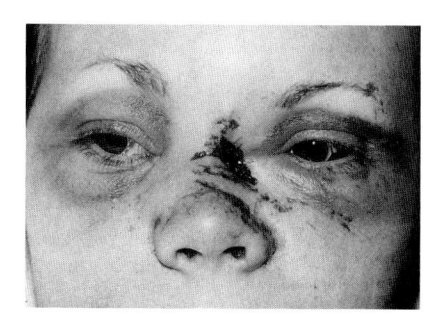

Figure 22.7 Severe Type 2B injury with oblique crush to the central midface and loss of distal nasal support. The injury extends into the left lateral maxilla.

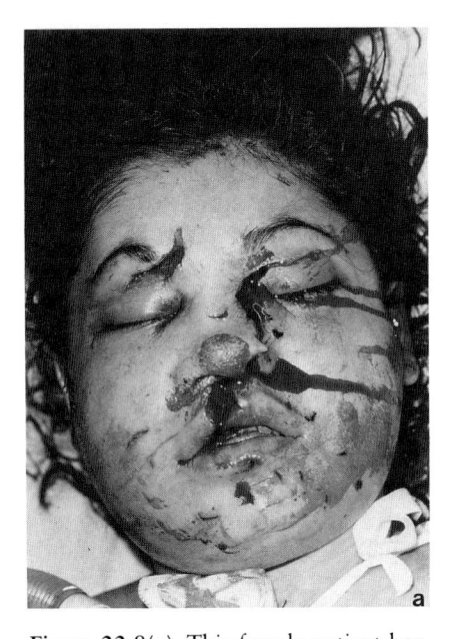

Figure 22.8(a) This female patient has severe panfacial injuries. Note the severe central maxillary crush and nasoethmoid injury. **(b)** Pressure on the distal portion of the nose reveals the pathognomonic feature of a central maxillary crush with loss of distal nasal support. **(c)** This lateral view shows the loss of distal nasal support. This injury requires immediate bone grafting to the nose. **(d)** This lateral view of the patient at five years shows good restoration of the nasal contour with a primary nasal bone graft. **(e)** This anteroposterior view demonstrates fairly good restoration of midfacial anatomy. There is a slight enophthalmos of the left eye and a ptosis of the left upper eyelid due to a superior orbital fissure syndrome. However, the medial canthal region, although having a correct intercanthal distance, is abnormal because the canthi have a pulled appearance due to the necessity of wiring the canthal ligaments in a transnasal fashion. When the canthal ligaments are wired transnasally, this unnatural appearance of the medial canthal region will not infrequently result. This patient, treated more than 10 years ago, reveals the problem that frequently occurs when the canthal ligaments are dissected off the bone in the exposure of the medial canthal region.

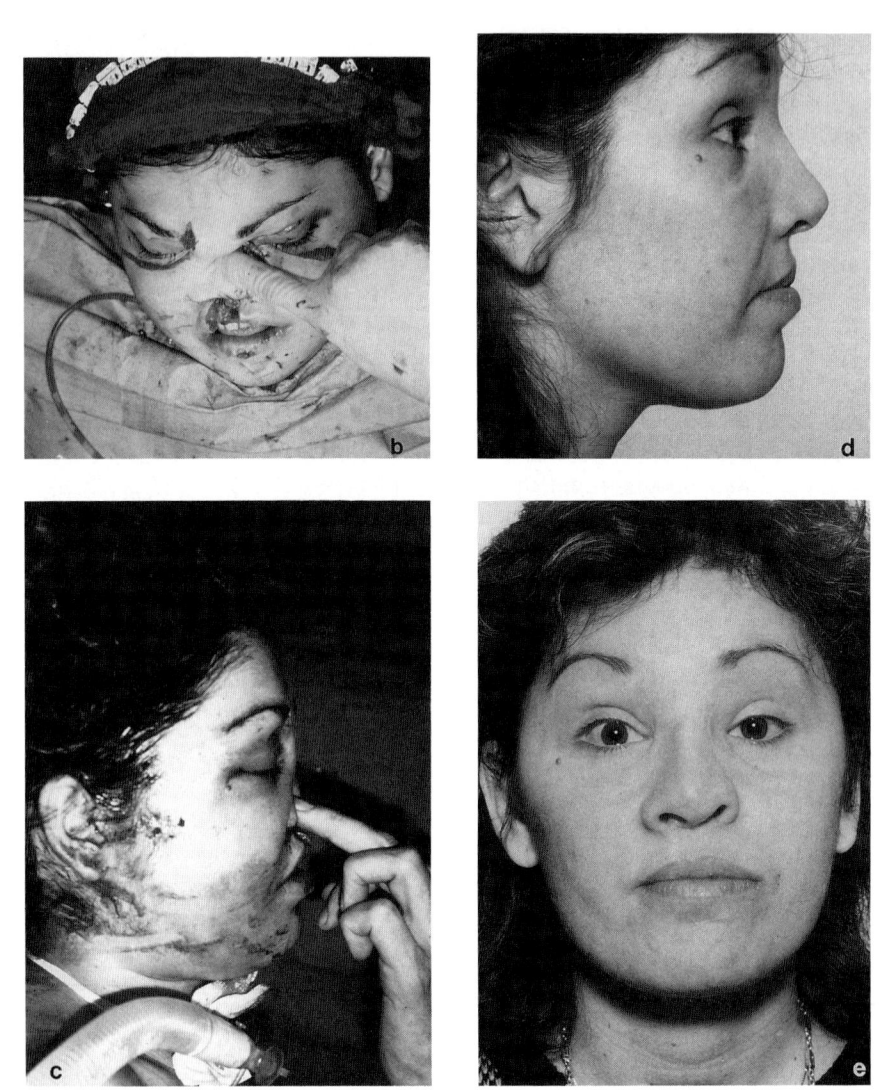

Type 3: Extended Nasoethmoid-orbital Injuries

Injuries of the nasoethmoid-orbital region may occur as an extension of injuries to other sites in the craniofacial skeleton.

Type 3A: With Craniofacial Injuries (Frontobasilar Injuries)

A severe force applied to the frontal bone, frontal sinuses, central portion of the superior orbits, or glabellar region may cause concomitant injury of the nasoethmoid-orbital region. Injuries may involve the anterior wall of the frontal sinus without intracranial penetration, or they may extend through the posterior wall of the sinus and the cribriform plate and ethmoid roof, causing dural laceration, cerebrospinal fluid rhinorrhea, and even cerebral injury. A combined approach is used, consisting of initial neurosurgical repair followed by facial bone repair.

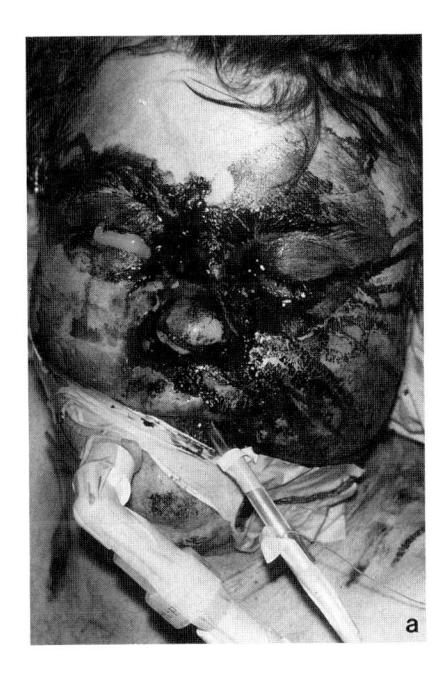

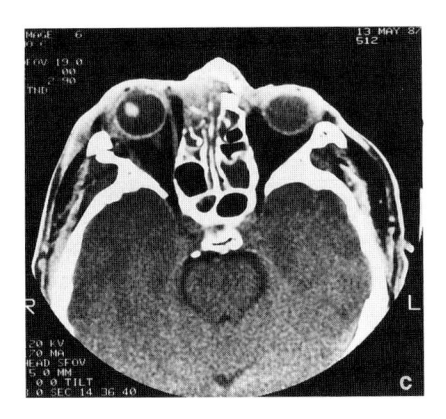

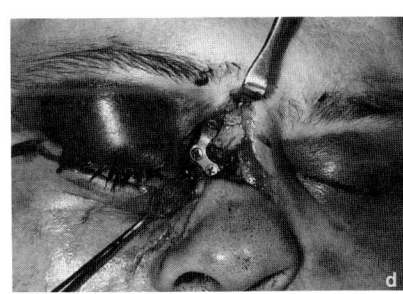

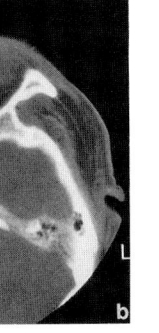

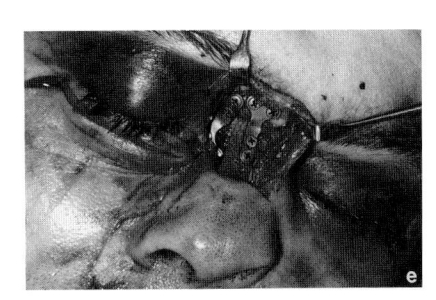

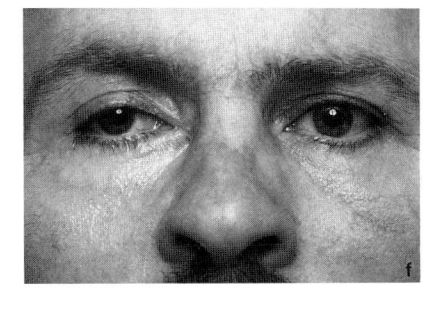

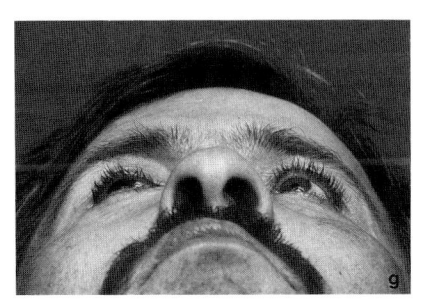

Figure 22.9 (a) This male patient, involved in an industrial accident, was hit across the central midface with a 1,000-pound metal beam. (b) This axial CT scan shows comminuted nasoethmoid fractures. Note the marked lateral displacement of the right frontonasal buttress, which is impinging on the ocular globe. (c) This injury has resulted in a true dislocation of the lens of the globe. (d) Midfacial and orbital fractures are exposed through the preexisting lacerations, in combination with a coronal incision. The large laterally displaced frontonasal segment still containing the canthal ligament is carefully identified and repositioned; it is held in place with a miniplate. (e) A primary split calvarial nasal bone graft is inserted into the nasal tip and anchored to the nasoglabellar region with a miniplate. The remainder of the orbital and maxillary fractures are repaired with miniplates. (f) Appearance at 1½ years shows exact repositioning of the right medial canthal ligament without the need for transnasal wiring. (g) Restoration of midfacial projection and height and globe position.

Type 3B: Le Fort II and III Fractures

Le Fort II and III fractures are produced by a direct blow to the maxilla or maxillo-mandibular complex. The fractures pass through the medial orbital region and bridge of the nose, thus involving the bony nasoethmoid-orbital region. Even in severe comminuted fractures, distal nasal support is usually maintained. Occasionally, concomitant injury to the distal nose may result in loss of cartilaginous nasal support. Primary nasal bone grafting is required here, in combination with reduction and internal fixation of the Le Fort fractures. When a displaced nasoethmoid-orbital fracture is associated with a Le Fort III fracture that involves posterior or lateral displacement of the zygomatic arch or arches, then all reference points for accurate fixation of the nasoethmoid-orbital fractures are lost. The zygomatic arch is exposed, accurately reduced, and rigidly fixed with miniplates and lag screws, establishing an outer facial frame with the exact facial width and projection. This will accurately reposition the lateral segment of the inferior orbital rim in relation to the skull base. The upper facial repair is completed by reducing the frontonasal buttress between the stabilized inferior orbital rim below and the frontonasal fracture site above and rigidly fixing this key segment in place using miniplates. Once this is done, the traumatic telecanthus is corrected and the possible need for nasal and deep orbital bone grafting is assessed.

Type 4: Nasoethmoid-orbital Fractures With Oculo-orbital Displacement or Dystopia

The Type 4 injury is characterized by injury in the nasoethmoid-orbital region associated with lateral and downward displacement of the ocular globe and orbit (see Figure 22.10). A number of different patterns of this injury have been recognized. Two distinct patterns are common.

Type 4A

In the Type 4A injury, the orbit is detached medially by the nasoethmoid-orbital fractures; laterally at the fronto-zygomatic suture line; and inferiorly by concomitant fractures of the zygomatic, maxillary, and nasomaxillary buttresses of the maxilla. The inferior two thirds of the orbit and its contents shift downward and outward, giving a picture of a typical nasoethmoid-orbital injury associated with an oculo-orbital displacement.

Type 4B

In addition to the pattern of a Type 4A injury, the orbit may be detached superiorly from the frontal bone with associated supraorbital fractures on that side, producing a Type 4B injury (see Figure 22.11). The orbital shift is accentuated in this type of injury; the entire bony orbit is displaced downward and outward, producing a true orbital dystopia. Intracranial extension of fractures may occur with this injury. Reconstruction involves repositioning and fixing the displaced orbit and repairing the other coexisting fractures.

Type 5: Nasoethmoid-orbital Fractures with Loss of Bone

Certain severe injuries to the nasoethmoid-orbital region may result in areas of bony destruction or loss of small or large segments of bone through large skin or mucosal lacerations. All this is in addition to the pattern of nasoethmoid-orbital injury described previously. In this situation a reverse order of fixation is employed. The remaining fracture segments are stabilized to one another and to the residual facial skeleton, after which the exact amount of missing bone can be ascertained. All the missing or severely damaged bone is replaced with primary bone grafting, usually using split calvarial bone grafts and occasionally using split rib grafts.

EXPOSURE

The extent of the exposure depends on the type of fracture. Displaced fractures invariably need a coronal incision for adequate visualization of the exact fracture pattern and to allow accurate fixation with miniplates. The use of pre-existing lacerations or an "open sky" approach will frequently not give adequate exposure. The coronal incision is combined with subciliary and upper buccal sulcus incisions as needed. The zygomatic arch is exposed through the coronal incision when necessary.

SPECIFIC ROLE OF PLATE AND SCREW FIXATION

Frontonasal Buttress Fixation

The frontonasal buttress, with its attached medial canthal ligament, may be markedly displaced or dislocated, usually in an inferior and posterior direction. This bony segment must be carefully identified and reduced. Interosseous wire fixation frequently failed to maintain reduction completely, resulting in post-treatment lateral displacement with mild to significant recurrence of the telecanthus and canthal asymmetries. Once this buttress has been accurately reduced, miniplate fixation across

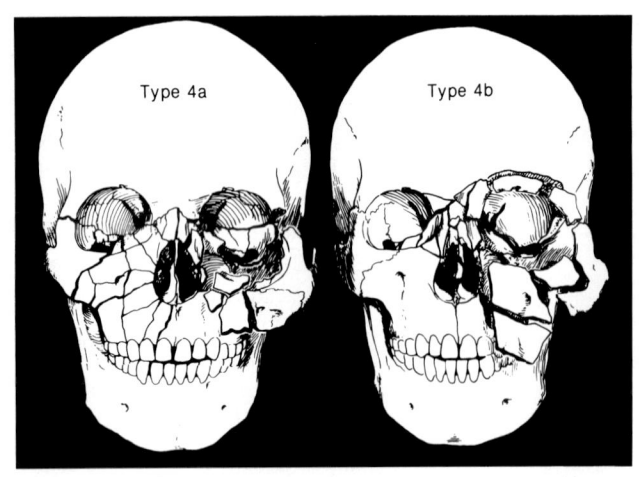

Figure 22.10 Common patterns of Type 4 injuries show bony nasoethmoid-orbital injury, in combination with orbital detachment and displacement. Type 4A injury shows a typical ocular orbital displacement. In a Type 4B injury, with extension up into the cranial region, this produces a true orbital dystopia with displacement of all four walls and rims of the orbit.

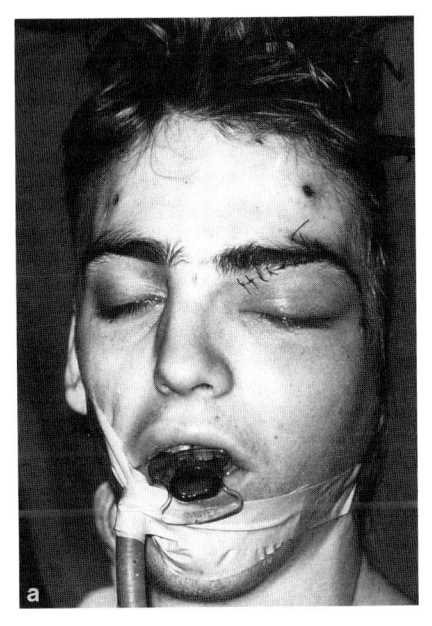

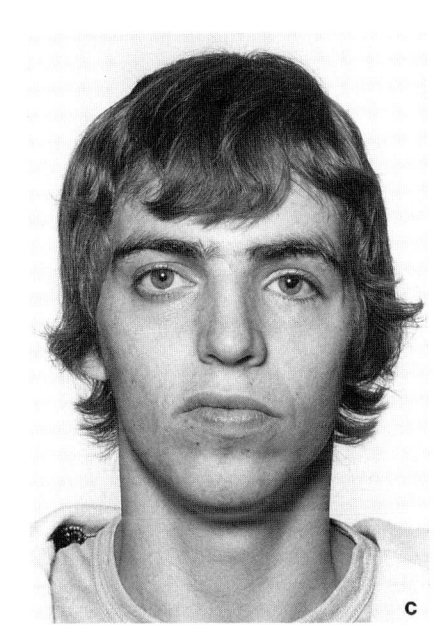

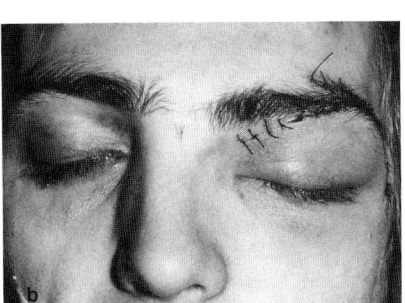

Figure 22.11 (a) This man has Type 4B injury and left orbital dystopia. Downward and lateral shift of the orbit is accentuated by total orbital detachment. Telecanthus on the side of the dystopia is increased. (b) This close-up view shows the true orbital dystopia and telecanthus on the left side. (c) Appearance at four years shows good restoration of the positions of the globe and orbital and correction of telecanthus. This patient was treated approximately ten years ago, prior to the institution of soft-tissue suspension and lateral canthopexy. Note that the lateral canthal tendon remains disinserted and depressed and the soft tissues of the left cheek and malar region are ptotic, giving the appearance of a slight depression in this area.

Comminuted Fracture

When the frontonasal buttress comminutes, fixation may be extremely difficult (see Figures 22.13 and 22.14). A long mini-adaptive plate is placed from the stable frontal region above, down to the stable lateral portion of the inferior orbital rim below, through a subperiosteal tunnel over the comminuted segments of the frontonasal buttress. The plate is carefully bent and adapted to the correct contour. If contouring is difficult, the mini-adaptive plate can be carefully contoured on a skull model to obtain the exact contour of the frontonasal buttress region. The plate is then sterilized.

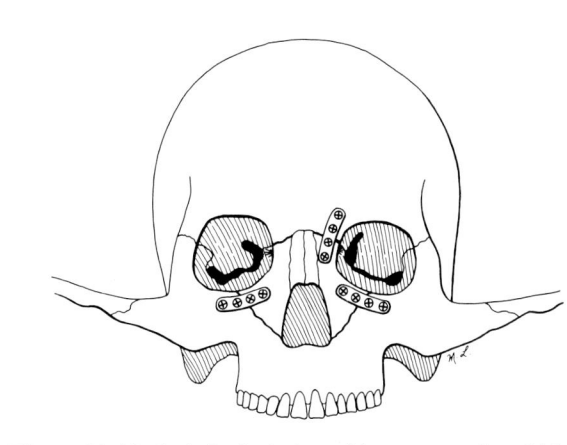

the upper and lower fracture sites provides rigid fixation without the risk of post-treatment relapse.

In displaced fractures, miniplates are applied across the frontonasal fracture and at the inferior orbital rim. The upper plate is placed from the inferior aspect of the stable frontal bone and, whenever possible, posterior to the medial portion of the supraorbital margin. The miniplate crosses the fracture site and the two inferior screws are placed as close as possible to the medial canthal tendon attachment. Whenever possible, the plate itself is placed behind the ridge of the medial orbital rim. The patient rarely complains of the plate being palpable, and it rarely needs removal. In less displaced fractures, a microplate may be used. The inferior fracture site is stabilized with a miniplate along the inferior orbital rim. Commonly, a mini-adaptive plate is used because it is easier to contour and is less palpable. In less severely displaced fractures, a microplate may be used.

In certain situations, the major displacement of the nasofrontal buttress may occur inferiorly at the inferior orbital margin with a greenstick type fracture superiorly. In this situation, the segment can be reduced from below, and an inferior junctional plate is applied alone (see Figure 22.12).

Figure 22.12 Artist's depiction of bony nasoethmoid injuries with little displacement. The left side shows the characteristic repair across the frontonasal suture line and the infraorbital margin at the junctions of the fracture. The right side shows the frontonasal segment displaced, and there is a greenstick fracture at the frontonasal region. This fracture can be reduced from below, and one plate can be placed across the infraorbital margin.

Figure 22.13 (a) The right naso-orbital region shows a multiple segmental comminuted fracture. The left side shows a significant comminuted fracture with bone destruction and loss. (b) The fractures of part (a) are ideally repaired with three-dimensionally bendable mini-adaption plates. On the right side, with multiple segmental fractures, the mini-adaptor plate is carefully bent to the shape of the affected orbital rim. This can be done in situ, or the plate can be carefully contoured on a skull model. The plate can then be sterilized and anchored superiorly to the intact frontal bone and inferiorly to the lateral portion of the orbital rim with at least two screws on either side. The intervening comminuted segments are now brought up to the plate and lagged with screws, which are placed in each segment, thus re-establishing the correct contour. In comminuted fractures such as this, the ligament is either avulsed or has to be stripped in order to allow adequate exposure and fixation. The ligament therefore must be rewired transnasally. On the left side, where the nasoethmoid segment is lost, the plate is bent in a similar fashion and attached both superiorly and inferiorly to at least two screws. A bone graft is now taken, carefully contoured to the shape of the missing nasoethmoid complex, and fixed to the overlying plate with multiple screws. Deep orbital and nasal bone grafting is then performed as needed.

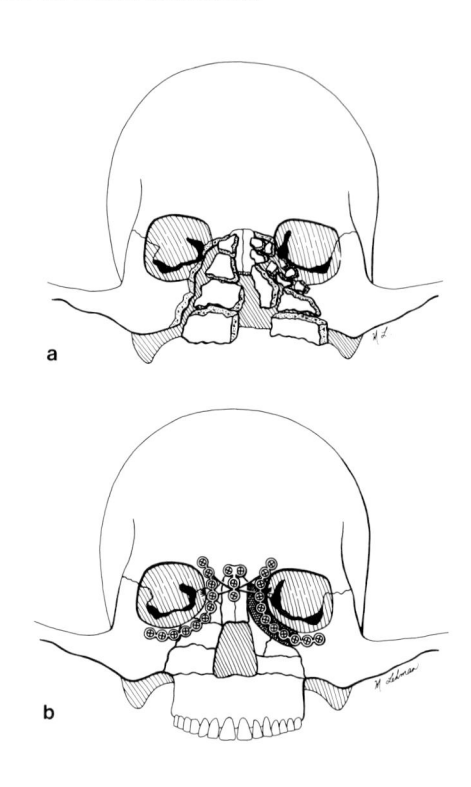

The correctly contoured plate is now inserted through the subperiosteal tunnel and fixed superiorly to the frontal region and inferiorly to the lateral portion of the inferior orbital rim, using a minimum of two screws at each site. Each intervening bone segment is now lagged to the plate with one or more screws until all the contiguous fractures are reduced and rigidly fixed. The canthal ligament can now be wired transnasally through the stabilized segment.

Bone Loss

When there is actual bone loss involving a portion of the entire frontonasal buttress, a mini-adaptive plate is similarly bent, either in situ or on a skull model, to conform to the correct frontonasal buttress contour. The plate is inserted and fixed superiorly to the frontal bone and inferiorly to the inferior orbital rim. The bone gap is now replaced with a carefully contoured split calvarial or split rib graft which is lagged to the overlying

Figure 22.14 (a) This male has complex frontonasal ethmoid injury after a motor vehicle accident. Note the severe telescoping of the entire nasoethmoid complex. (b) This close-up view shows the complex telescoped nasoethmoid-orbital injury. (c) This lateral view shows marked telescoping of the entire nasoethmoid complex. (d) This axial CT scan shows the comminution and degree of posterior displacement of the entire frontonaso-ethmoid complex. (e) After neurosurgical and dural repair, the frontal sinus is exenterated and the base of the frontal sinus is packed with bone grafts. A galeal frontalis flap (GF) has been raised with a base adjacent to the frontal sinus. Two long mini-adaptive plates have been carefully contoured to each naso-ethmoid region and have been anchored superiorly and inferiorly with multiple screws (arrows). The transnasal wire that has been anchored to the right medial canthus and passed transnasally is evident (large arrow). (f) The frontal bone (F) has been replaced and fixed with miniplates. The anterior wall of the frontal sinus (FS) has been reconstructed with a split calvarial bone graft, which is anchored with a long transverse miniplate. The galeal frontalis flap (GF) has been tunnelled through an opening in the left orbital roof into the frontal sinus and anchored across the bone grafts that were placed in the frontal sinus floor. A further mini T-plate now jumps across the transverse mini-adaptive plate to anchor the nasal bone graft (N). The transnasal canthopexy wire is now anchored to one of the screws in the left supraorbital region (large arrow). (g) This x ray shows three-dimensional reconstruction with multiple miniplates. The long mini-adaptive plate across the frontal sinus and across the right nasoethmoid region can be seen lagging the multiple comminuted segments to the plate. Two long mini-adaptive plates have been used as junctional plates in the left nasoethmoid region. The transnasal canthopexy wire can be seen. (h) Appearance at one year shows restoration of midfacial projection and contour. (i) This close-up view shows restoration of the intercanthal distance. There is a slight thickening of the soft tissue over the bridge of the nose. The soft tissues in the right medial orbital region reveal that a recent dacryocystorhinostomy has been performed. (j) This lateral view shows exact restoration of midfacial and nasal projection and contour.

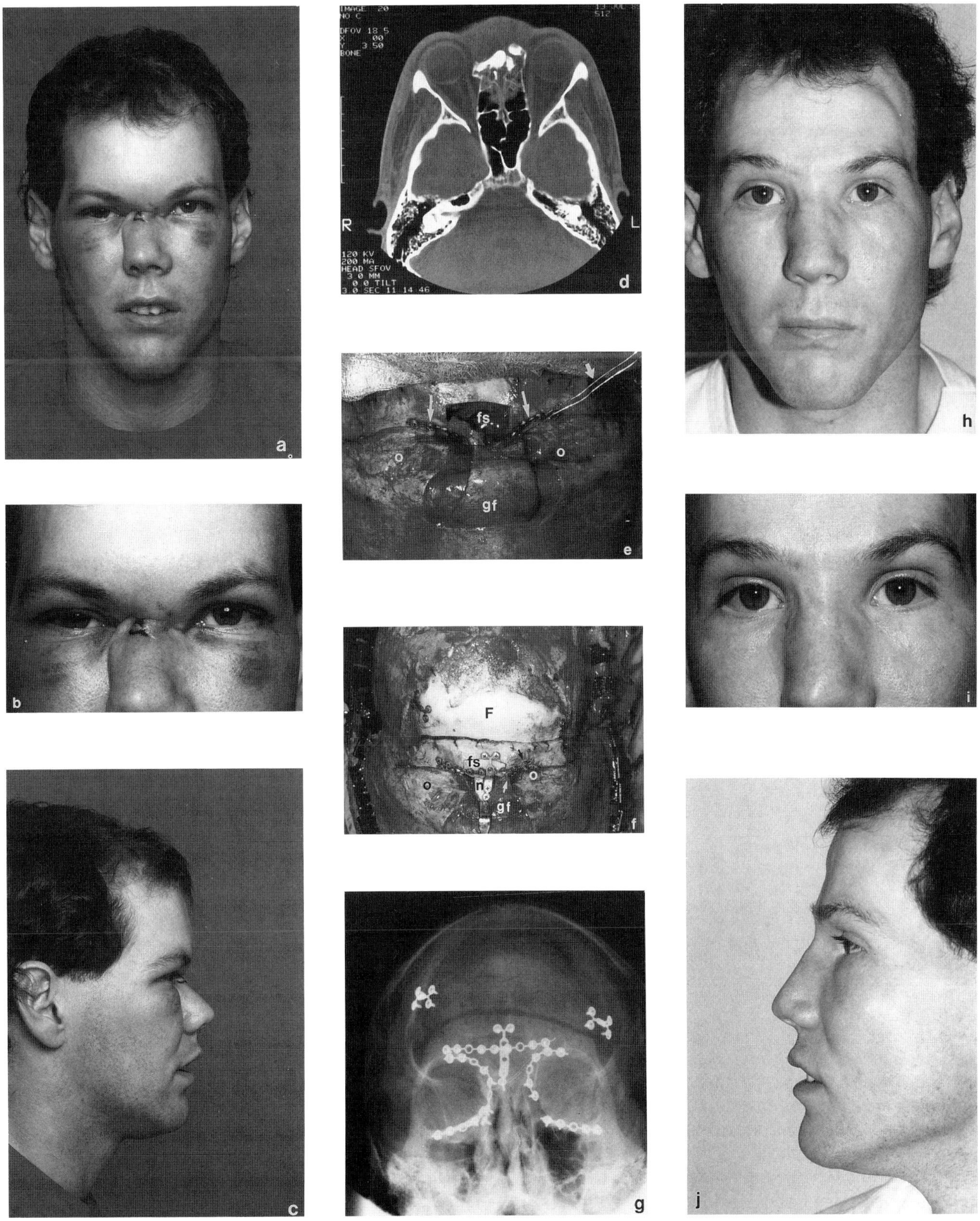
IMAGE 20
NO C
DFOV 18.5
X 00
Y 3.50
BONE
R
L
120 KV
200 MA
HEAD SFOV
3.0 MM
0.0 TILT
3.0 SEC 11 14 46
a
b
c
d
fs
o
o
gf
e
F
fs
o
n
o
gf
f
g
h
i
j

plate with multiple screws. The medial canthal ligament is now wired transnasally through the reconstructed medial orbital rim.

Small Bone Fragment

Rarely, massive bone destruction or loss through open skin and mucosal lacerations may occur. The medial canthal ligament may be found still attached to a small fragment of bone. If this fragment of bone is sufficiently large to allow the placement of at least two screws, then a small double T-plate can be carefully contoured and two screws inserted into each bone segment containing the canthal ligament. This will allow the canthal ligaments to be repositioned accurately without the need for transnasal wiring. The frontonasal buttress can now be reconstructed (see Figure 22.15).

Nasal Bone Graft Fixation

Initially, costochondral grafts were used for primary nasal bone grafting. These grafts often gave excellent results, but the resorption of the bone at the base of the graft was variable and unpredictable. Internal fixation of rib is difficult because the cortex tends to crack when a screw is inserted, making countersinking of the screwhead risky.

Thin split calvarial bone grafts have been the principal source for nasal bone grafts over the past eight years. The thick cortical bone can be exactly contoured to provide a thin nasal dorsum. The graft tip is inserted underneath the lower lateral cartilages, whenever possible, to provide a natural tip contour and projection. These grafts rarely resorb when fixed at their base, although minor degrees of tip resorption occasionally occur.

When there is comminution of the underlying nasal bones, a flat ledge is burred into the residual nasal bones superiorly and a small pocket is created superiorly in the frontal bone at the nasal root. The correctly sized and sloped graft is wedged into the superior bony pocket and allowed to rest on the created ledge. A mini T-plate is now carefully bent, and the T portion is applied to the frontal bone with a minimum of two screws. A minimum of two screws are now applied through the plate and then through the bone graft itself to produce a cantilever effect. The angle of the cantilever can be adjusted by adjusting the angle of the bend in the mini-plate (see Figures 22.14, 22.15, and 22.16).

If the underlying nasal bone is stable, and distal cartilaginous nasal support is lost, the bone graft can be rigidly fixed to the underlying nasal bone with two or three lag screws. Care must be taken not to burr down the cortex of the nasal bone; this will weaken the lag screw fixation. Calvarial bone provides an ideal situation for lag screw fixation. The thick cortical bone

Figure 22.15 (a) This 60-year-old male has massive panfacial injury and severe nasoethmoid-orbital crush after having impacted his midface on the dashboard of a car. Note the marked telecanthus and the large open laceration of the nasoethmoid region with loss of midfacial projection. (b) This lateral view shows the severe telescoping of the nasoethmoid-orbital complex posteriorly and loss of midfacial projection. (c) Exposure through the pre-existing laceration and coronal incision shows that virtually all the bone in the nasoethmoid-orbital region is missing. However, two small fragments of bone (white arrows) are identified. (d) When these two pieces of bone are pulled toward the midline, there is evidence that the medial canthal ligaments are still attached to them. (e) A small double-T Luhr miniplate is now carefully bent at right angles on either side and attached to the small fragments of bone with two screws on either side. Note that the two fragments of bone with the attached miniplate are suspended across the nasoethmoid region. There is no bone around the bone fragments. (f) Placement of this miniplate has reapproximated the exact position of the canthal ligaments. (N = nose.) (g) The remainder of the reconstruction is completed by commencing with fixation of both zygomatic arches, establishing an outer facial frame. The nasoethmoid-orbital complex is now reconstructed with multiple miniplates. The frontal sinus is repaired and exenterated, and a galeal frontalis flap is inserted in addition to bone grafts. Note that when multiple plates are placed in a confined space, it is necessary to plan ahead and leave the anterior bone of the frontal sinus and frontal bone free of plates so that it can be used to apply the plate for subsequent nasal bone graft fixation. (f = frontal bone, Fs = frontal sinus.) (h) The nasal bone graft has now been placed and fixed with a long mini T-plate (arrow). (i) This postoperative x ray shows the three-dimensional reconstruction. (j) This lateral x ray shows the three-dimensional reconstruction with plates along the zygomatic arches and the miniplate that is carefully bent in a cantilever fashion to hold the nasal bone graft. (k) This axial CT scan through the orbits shows repair of the zygomatic arches and extensive deep orbital bone grafting in the orbital floor, extending back to the apex of the orbit (large arrow) and multiple grafts in the deep aspect of the medial walls (small arrows). (l) Appearance at three years with a one-stage correction. Note restoration of midfacial projection and contour and correction of facial width. There is slight asymmetry of the left orbit. (m) This close-up shows exact restoration of the nasoethmoid-orbital complex with extensive miniplate fixation and bone grafting. Note exact repositioning of the medial canthal ligaments and correction of traumatic telecanthus. (n) This inferior view shows reconstruction of the orbits with deep orbital bone grafting, which restored position without enophthalmos.

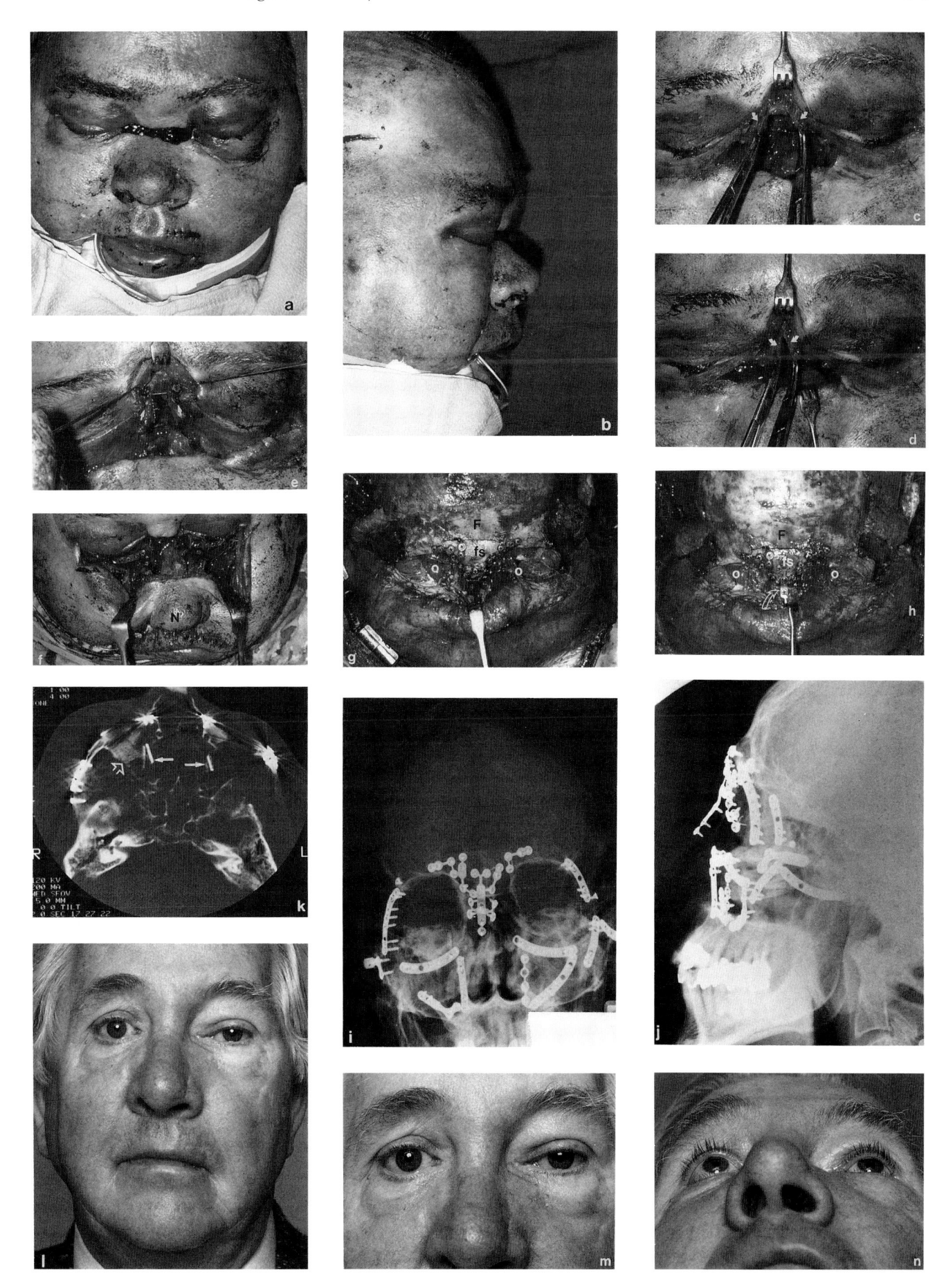

Rigid Fixation of Nasoethmoid-orbital Fractures

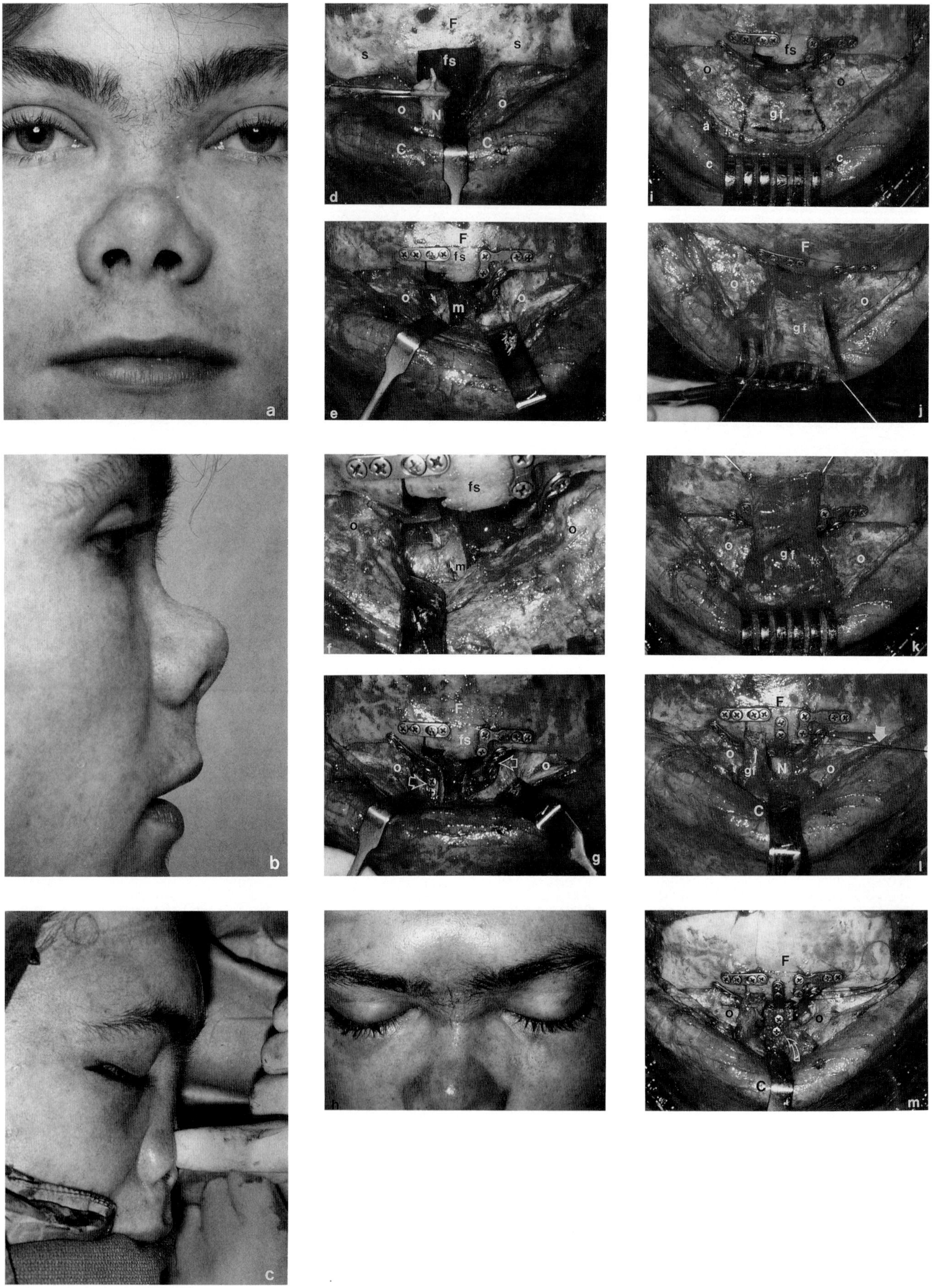
a
b
c
d
F
s
fs
s
o
N
o
C
C
e
F
fs
o
m
o
f
fs
o
m
o
g
F
fs
o
o
h
i
fs
o
o
gf
a
c
c
j
F
o
gf
o
k
o
gf
o
l
F
o
gf
N
o
C
m
F
o
o
C

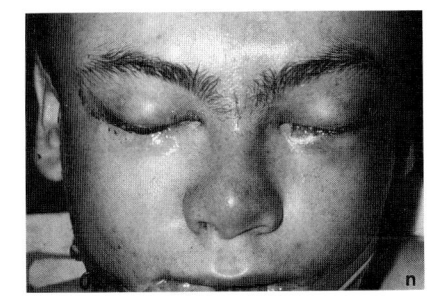

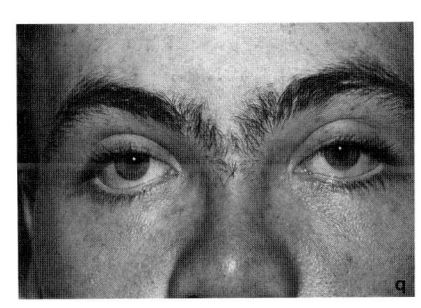

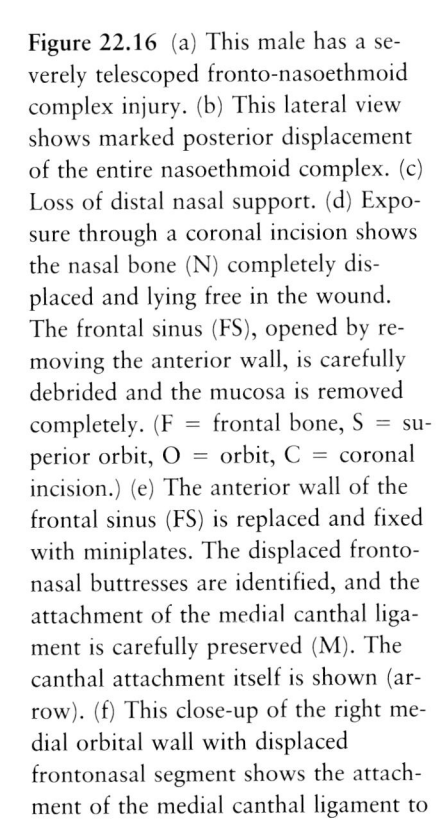

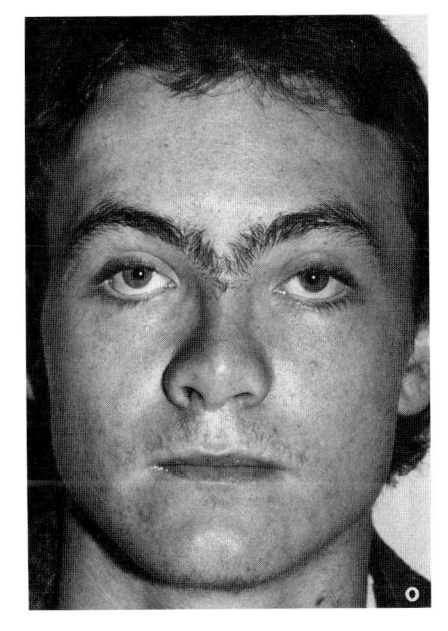

Figure 22.16 (a) This male has a severely telescoped fronto-nasoethmoid complex injury. (b) This lateral view shows marked posterior displacement of the entire nasoethmoid complex. (c) Loss of distal nasal support. (d) Exposure through a coronal incision shows the nasal bone (N) completely displaced and lying free in the wound. The frontal sinus (FS), opened by removing the anterior wall, is carefully debrided and the mucosa is removed completely. (F = frontal bone, S = superior orbit, O = orbit, C = coronal incision.) (e) The anterior wall of the frontal sinus (FS) is replaced and fixed with miniplates. The displaced frontonasal buttresses are identified, and the attachment of the medial canthal ligament is carefully preserved (M). The canthal attachment itself is shown (arrow). (f) This close-up of the right medial orbital wall with displaced frontonasal segment shows the attachment of the medial canthal ligament to the bone (white arrows). (g) Both frontonasal buttresses are reduced and carefully repaired with a miniplate on either side (arrows). (h) After application of the two plates, the medial canthal tendons have been exactly repositioned, restoring the intercanthal distance; the nasal bridge contour still has to be restored. (i) A galeofrontalis flap (GF) is planned with the base adjacent to the defect in the frontal sinus. (j) The galeofrontalis flap is raised. (k) The inferior aspect of the galeofrontalis flap with the base adjacent to the frontal sinus. (l) The nasal bone (N) is positioned and held in place with a mini T-plate. The galeofrontalis flap is tunnelled through a small window in the inferior portion of the frontal sinus. It is brought through into the frontal sinus and anchored to the opposite side over the bone grafts that are placed in the floor of the frontal sinus with a suture (large arrow). (m) The nasal bone graft provides contour and support to the nasal dorsum, but a split calvarial bone graft extending out into the nasal tip is now necessary to provide distal nasal support. Because the nasal bone has been previously stabilized with a miniplate superiorly, the nasal bone graft itself can be anchored to the underlying nasal bone with two lag screws (arrow). (n) On the operating table, repositioning of the nasoethmoid complex can be seen. (o) Appearance at three months shows exact restoration of the nasoethmoid-orbital region with restoration of medial canthal position. There is still tightness of the subciliary incisions, causing a slightly increased scleral show. (p) This lateral view shows restoration of nasal projection and contour. (q) This close-up view shows restoration of normal nasoethmoid-orbital anatomy. Note the exact restoration of intercanthal distance and the restoration of the normal anatomical configuration of the medial canthal region.

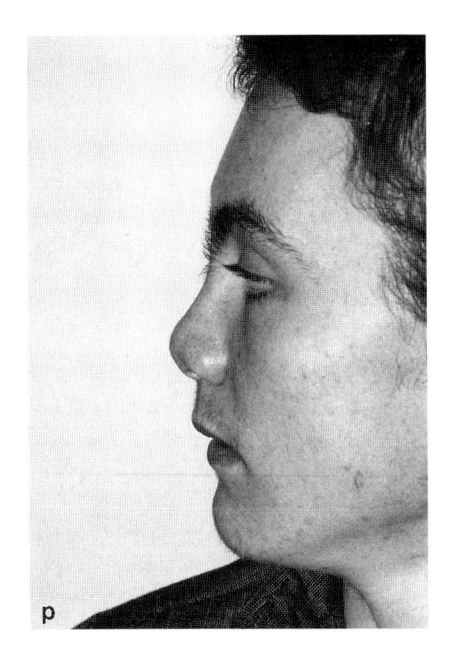

allows the screwhead to be countersunk without the fear of bone fracturing upon screw insertion.

Associated Cranial and Frontal Sinus Fractures

Multiple miniplates or microplates may be needed for concomitant cranial or anterior frontal sinus wall repair (see Figures 22.17 and 22.18). When applying these plates, care must be taken not to compromise plate fixation that may be required for subsequent frontonasal buttress repair or fixation of a nasal bone graft (see Figure 22.15f). Careful planning of plate positioning will allow subsequent use of additional plates for midfacial repair.

Internal Fixation in a Confined Space

When multiple comminuted and complex fractures occur in the fronto-nasoethmoid region, multiple plates and screws may be needed in a confined space. To facilitate their use, different techniques may be used:

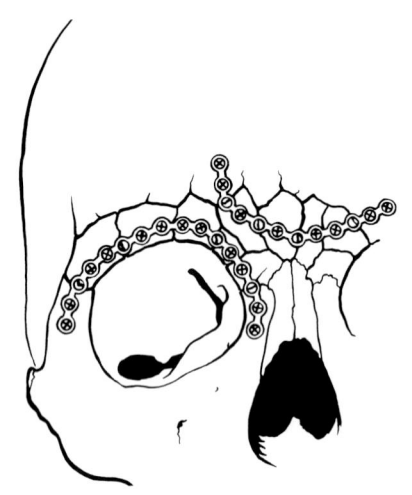

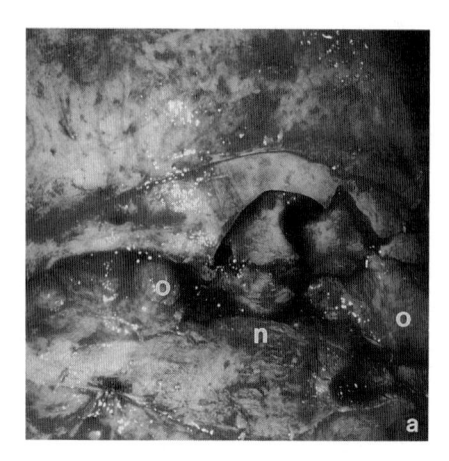

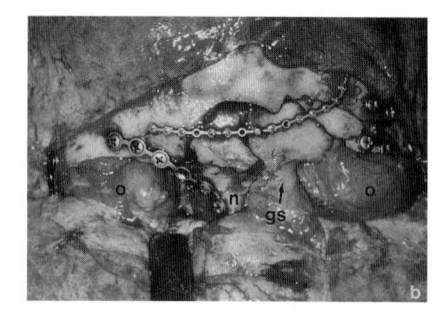

Figure 22.17 Artist's depiction of a typical fronto-naso-ethmoid complex fracture shows the ability of the mini-adaptive plate to be exactly contoured to comminuted fractures of the nasoethmoid-orbital, superior orbit, and frontonasal region. Plates are fixed to each stable ledge on either side, and then each fragment is fixed with one or two screws to the miniplate above.

1. *Screws through two plates.* In certain situations, two plates may be used at right angles to each other. Two or more screws may be used with one screw passing through two separate plates, thus allowing plating in multiple directions in a confined space.
2. *Plate jumping.* In a confined space, one plate may jump over another to allow fixation in more than one direction (see Figure 22.19).
3. *Microplates.* The combination of miniplates and microplates has facilitated the use of plating in a confined space. Severely displaced and unstable bone segments are repaired with miniplates, and the remainder are repaired with microplates and screws.

Reconstruction of the Medial Canthal Ligament

Reattachment of the medial canthal ligament may be necessary on one side or both. When bilateral transnasal wiring of the canthal ligaments is needed, a common technique is to pass a separate wire through each ligament, then to pass the wire transnasally and tie the two wires together over the nasal bone or, if used, the nasal bone graft. If there is any resorption of the underlying nasal bone or nasal bone graft, then the fixation of both canthal ligaments is lost (see Figure 22.20).

Fixation of both ligaments individually is preferable in a bilateral reconstruction. The wire is passed through the canthal ligament and then passed transnasally, as before. However, each canthal wire is now attached to a separate screw placed into the inferomedial aspect of the superior orbital margin (see Figures 22.19 and 22.20). This repair is now independent of the risk of resorption of nasal bone or bone graft.

The Nasolacrimal System

The management of possible injury to the nasolacrimal system in nasoethmoid-orbital fractures is controversial. Exploration, assessment, and repair of the nasolacrimal system at the time of initial fracture fixation have been recommended. However, the incidence of injury to and obstruction of the nasolacrimal system following these fractures appears to be less than previously presumed, and even in the most severe injuries the nasolacrimal system may escape injury. Eight of 46 patients (17.4%) in this series (Gruss and Hurwitz 1985) required dacryocystorhinostomy for persistent nasolacrimal obstruction. Cruse et al. (1980) reported 7 of 33 patients (21%) and Stranc (1970b) reported 5 of 25 patients (20%) with persistent obstruction of the nasolacrimal system. All 5 of Stranc's patients were in a group of 13 patients who were treated with closed reduction and external plating. Three of 5 patients treated

Figure 22.18 (a) Complex comminuted fractures of the fronto-naso-orbital complex. (N = nose, O = orbits.) (b) The nasoethmoid-orbital complex itself is repaired with a mini-adaptive plate (N = nose). A galeofrontalis flap (GF) has been inserted into the frontal sinus. The anterior wall of the frontal sinus, which is under the influence of minimal muscular forces, can be adequately repaired with a microplate.

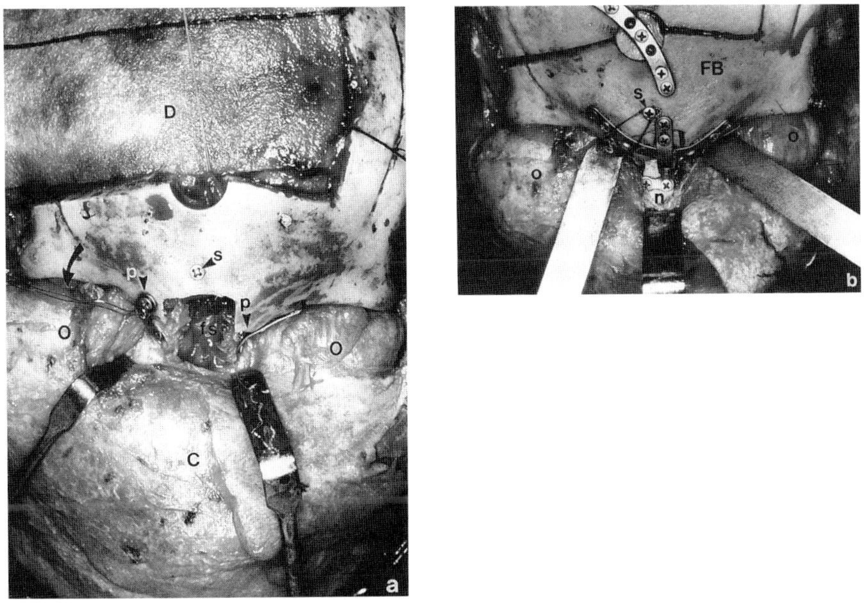

Rigid Fixation of Nasoethmoid-orbital Fractures

Figure 22.19 (a) In this patient with a complex displaced fronto-nasoethmoid complex fracture, the dural repair (D) has been completed. Plates (P) have now been applied to both upper portions of the frontonasal buttresses. The debrided frontal sinus (FS) can be seen. A separate screw (S) for the subsequent attachment of the transnasal canthopexy wire (arrow) can be seen. (O = orbit, C = coronal incision.) (b) The frontal sinus is repaired with a miniplate, and the nasal bone graft is fixed in place with another miniplate that jumps over the previous plate. The transnasal canthopexy wire is brought across the nose from the left side and anchored to the screw (S).

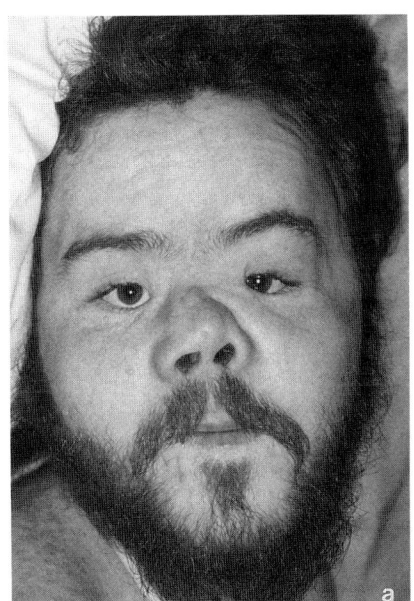

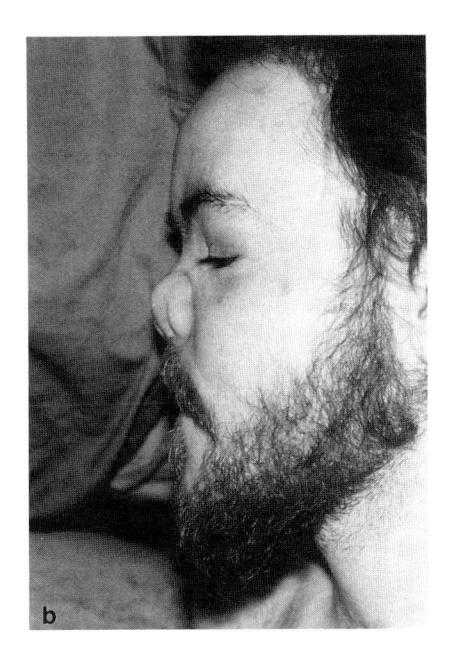

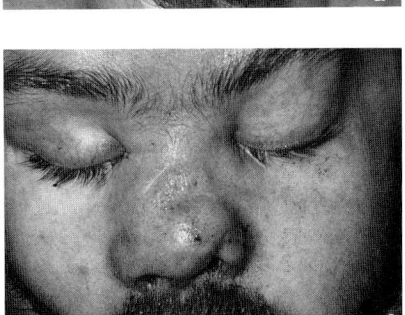

Figure 22.20 (a) This patient's complex nasoethmoid-orbital injuries were repaired with multiple miniplates and extensive bone grafting. Failure completely to clean out the frontal sinus resulted in infection of all bone grafts, resulting in loss of correction. When the medial canthal wires are passed transnasally and tied over the bone graft, this will result in loss of the medial canthal correction also if the underlying bone graft resorbs. (b) Loss of projection and contour of the nasoethmoid-orbital complex. (c) Each medial canthal tendon is identified through an external incision. A wire is inserted through the tendon and then passed transnasally. Each wire is attached to a separate screw in the frontal region (arrows). Thus any resorption of the subsequent nasal bone graft will not affect the positioning of the canthal tendon. (d) The transnasal canthopexy wires are anchored to each screw individually. (e) Initial correction obtained of each displaced medial canthal tendon.

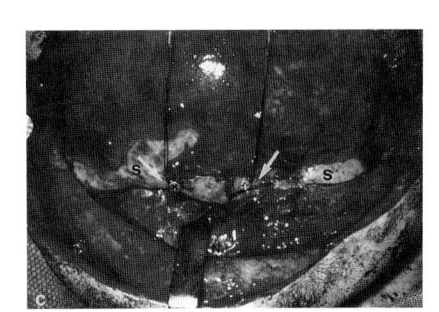

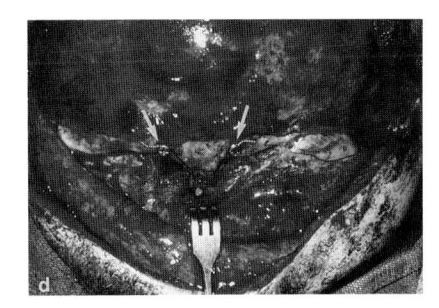

this way required a dacryocystorhinostomy for persistent nasolacrimal obstruction. Closed reduction of nasoethmoid-orbital injuries with compression plate fixation results in a greater incidence of nasolacrimal obstruction, probably because of external compression of the nasolacrimal system by unreduced bone segments or fragments. Open reduction and internal fixation of all fractures will minimize post-treatment deformity and complication. At the time of primary exploration, assessment of the status of the nasolacrimal system is difficult, and clinical recognition of actual injury or laceration is rare. Swelling of soft tissue and mucosa as well as bony displacement may produce apparent obstruction in the presence of a patent system. Attempts at assessment may damage an intact system or worsen damage already present. In the absence of clinically apparent laceration or damage, our policy has been not to attempt primary assessment or exploration of the nasolacrimal system. Full, delayed assessment is undertaken and secondary dacryocystorhinostomy is performed as needed (see Figure 22.21).

Specific Problems

An open, direct approach to nasoethmoid-orbital fractures, with meticulous reduction and internal fixation, is the treatment of choice. However, even with this approach, many of the severe injuries will obtain inadequate primary correction and often require numerous secondary procedures to correct post-treatment deformities. This is related to several factors. The invariable comminution of the medial orbital wall and orbital floor can be corrected only by primary bone graft replacement to prevent the likely occurrence of enophthalmos and diplopia (see Figure 22.2). The Type

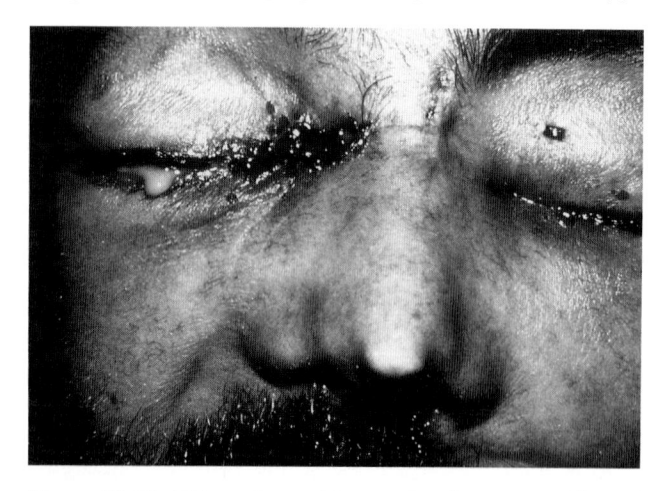

Figure 22.21 This patient with complex fronto-nasoethmoid injury presented at four weeks postsurgery with purulent drainage from the right nasoethmoid-orbital region. This was not indicative of an infection related to the bone grafting and internal fixation but was a result of a dacryocystitis and obstruction of the right nasolacrimal duct. Dacryocystorhinostomy after initial control of infection resulted in immediate resolution of the problem.

2 injury, with central maxillary crush and loss of distal nasal support, can be corrected only by primary nasal bone grafting. Severe comminution or bone loss in the frontal zygomatico-orbital or maxillary regions can be adequately stabilized only by immediate replacement of the missing or destroyed bone.

Although the Type 2C pattern of injury is similar in some respect to the classical Le Fort II or III injury, a differentiation should be made because the actual genesis of the injury, the detailed fracture pattern, and management are all different.

The most difficult injury to correct is the Type 2 injury with loss of distal nasal support. Extensive internal fixation combined with primary bone grafting may be necessary, even in the face of severe injury to the soft tissue of the skin or the nasal lining. Bone grafts, especially in the midface and nasal area, will maintain soft-tissue expansion and projection even if segments become exposed and partial resorption occurs. The failure to use bone grafts will cause soft tissue to shrink rapidly and will make subsequent reconstruction difficult and often inadequate.

Recognition of Type 4 injuries with oculo-orbital displacement or dystopia should result in repositioning and reattachment of the orbit in its correct position. Inadequate primary correction will result in severe oculo-orbital deformity, and this deformity may be difficult, or even impossible, to correct with secondary surgery.

Unexplained enophthalmos after adequate repair of the orbital floor due to injury to, and loss of the medial wall may be prevented by primary exploration and repair of damage to the medial wall with contoured bone grafts. When the entire medial orbital wall and orbital rim system has to be replaced by bone grafts, the medial canthal ligament on that side has to be wired directly into the bone graft. This will sometimes preclude optimal reconstruction of the medial canthal region, and residual deformity may occur. Traumatic telecanthus should always be corrected during the primary surgery.

SUMMARY

Nasoethmoid-orbital injuries can be classified into five types. The recognition and diagnosis of each fracture pattern will determine the correct choice of treatment. Open reduction and rigid internal fixation of these injuries with special attention to the medial canthal tendon-bearing bone fragment provides optimum repair. Craniofacial surgical techniques including immediate bone graft replacement of missing or severely comminuted bone allow one-stage reconstruction of even the most severe injuries.

BIBLIOGRAPHY

Converse JM, Hogan MV: Open sky approach for reduction of naso-orbital fractures. Plast Reconstr Surg 46: 396, 1970.

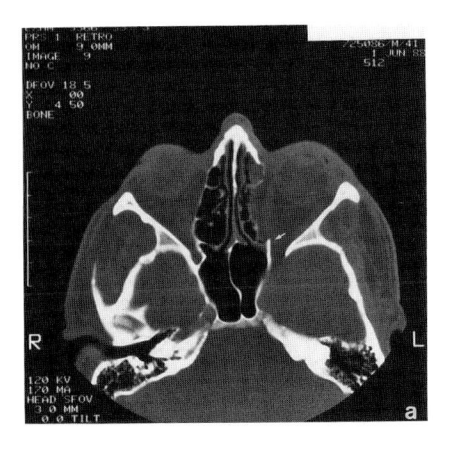

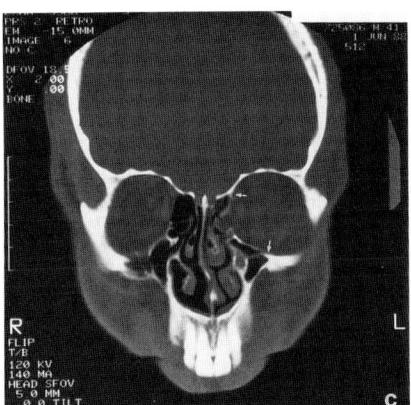

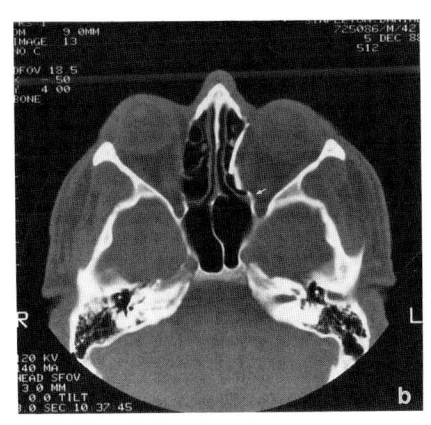

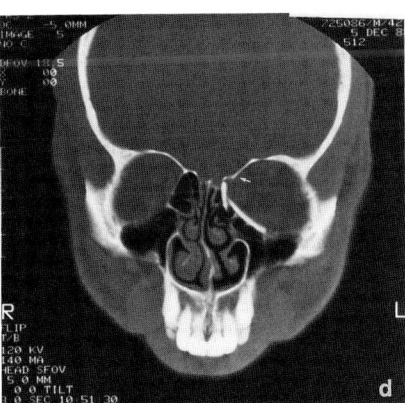

Figure 22.22 X rays of a patient with severe medial wall blowout fracture in association with a nasoethmoid fracture. (a) This axial CT scan shows a large defect in the medial wall. It is essential to identify this defect and replace it with a carefully contoured bone graft. Note that the medial rectus muscle is displaced into the defect. The small white arrow points to the posterior ledge onto which the bone grafts have to be placed. (b) This post-treatment x ray shows bone grafts placed to reconstruct the medial wall. These have been incorrectly placed; they do not extend far enough back onto the ledge. The bone grafts have prolapsed into the ethmoids, leading to a residual increase in orbital volume and enophthalmos. (c) This coronal CT scan shows the typical blowout fracture of the medial wall. Arrows point to the ledges onto which the bone graft must be placed. (d) This coronal CT scan shows the bone grafts placed to reconstruct the defect. Note that the bone grafts have not been properly placed onto the superior ledge, so that the upper bone graft has prolapsed into the ethmoids. Increase in left orbital volume can be seen.

Converse JM, Smith B: Naso-orbital fractures and traumatic deformities of the medial canthus. Plast Reconstr Surg 38: 147, 1966.

Cruse CW, Blevins PK, Luce EA: Nasoethmoid-orbital fractures. J Trauma 20: 551, 1980.

Dingman RO, Grabb WC, Oneal RM: Management of injuries of the naso-orbital complex. Arch Surg 98: 566, 1969.

Gruss JS: Fronto-naso-orbital trauma. Clin Plast Surg 9: 577, 1982.

Gruss JS: Nasoethmoid-orbital fractures: Classification and role of primary bone grafting. Plast Reconstr Surg 75: 303, 1985.

Gruss JS, Hurwitz J: The pattern and incidence of nasolacrimal injury in naso-orbital-ethmoid fractures. The role of delayed assessment and dacryocystorhinostomy. Br J Plast Surg 38: 116, 1985.

Gruss JS, Mackinnon SE, et al: The role of primary bone grafting in complex craniomaxillofacial trauma. Plast Reconstr Surg 75: 17–24, 1985.

Manson PN, Sargent L: Nasoethmoidal Orbital Fractures. Presented at the American Association of Plastic Surgeons, Annual Meeting, 1983.

Markowitz BL, Manson PN, Sargent L, Vanderkolk CA, Yaremchuk MJ, Glassman D, Crawley WA: Management of the medial canthal tendon in nasoethmoid-orbital fractures: The importance of the central fragment in classification and treatment. Plast Reconstr Surg 87: 843, 1991.

McCoy FJ: Fractures of the naso-orbital ethmoid complex. In Plastic and Maxillofacial Trauma Symposium. Georgiade ND (ed). St. Louis, Mosby, 1959.

Merville L: Multiple dislocations of the facial skeleton. J Maxillofac Surg 2: 187, 1974.

Merville LC, Real JP: Fronto-orbito-nasal dislocations. Scand J Plast Reconstr Surg 15: 287, 1981.

Morgan RF, Manson PN, Shack RB, Hoopes JE: Management of nasoethmoid-orbital fractures. Am Surg 48: 447, 1982.

Ramselaar JM, Van der Meulen JC, Bloem JJ: Naso-orbital fractures. Mod Prob Ophthalmol 14: 607, 1975.

Stranc MF: Primary treatment of naso-ethmoid injuries with increased intercanthal distance. Br J Plast Surg 23: 8, 1970a.

Stranc MF: The pattern of lacrimal injuries in nasoethmoid injuries. Br J Plast Surg 23: 339, 1970b.

Stranc MF, Robertson GA: A classification of injuries of the nasal skeleton. Ann Plast Surg 2: 468, 1979.

CHAPTER 23

Rigid Fixation of Orbital Fractures

Oleh M. Antonyshyn

Trauma to the orbit may result in significant facial deformity and visual dysfunction. Rehabilitation of the patient demands accurate preoperative assessment of the injury and early definitive reconstruction. Increasing sophistication in diagnostic imaging and recent innovations in surgical technique permit the realization of these goals.

CHARACTERISTICS OF ORBITAL FRACTURES

The orbit occupies a prominent position on the facial skeleton, and fractures of the bones composing the orbital rim and cavity are relatively common. The magnitude of these injuries varies greatly, ranging from simple, isolated blowout fractures to complete disruption of the bony orbit. The ability to distinguish between simple and complex orbital fractures provides the surgeon with a basis for optimal treatment.

Anatomic Considerations

The orbit may be regarded as a quadrilateral pyramid, with its base oriented forward, laterally, and downwards. This base consists of a circumferential rim of thick, resilient bone that serves to resist and dissipate impact forces. Further support is provided by buttresses in the contiguous facial bones, oriented into vertical and horizontal pillars. The orbital rim, therefore, presents an anterior abutment that reinforces and protects the skeletal framework of the orbital cavity.

The bony rim is divided into three anatomic segments. The frontal bone contributes to the supraorbital rim; the zygoma constitutes the inferolateral rim; and the body and nasal process of the maxilla compose the inferomedial rim. Although the impact tolerance of each of these individual bones is relatively high, the sutural articulations between them present areas of weakness that are predisposed to shearing.

The orbital cavity is composed of thin, delicate bone of the roof, medial and lateral walls, and floor. The inferomedial portion of the orbital cavity, further weakened by the close proximity of the ethmoid air cells and antrum, is particularly susceptible to injury.

The position of the ocular globe and its relationship to the skeletal framework of the orbit requires further consideration. The precise location of the ocular globe in three dimensions is determined by several factors: the relative volume of the orbital cavity and that of its soft-tissue contents, the configuration of the walls of the orbit, and the orientation and dimensions of the bony rim. Each of these must be appreciated and specifically addressed in reconstruction.

The coronal plane through the equator of the ocular globe divides the orbital cavity into anterior and posterior segments. It extends from the lateral orbital rim, through the center of the globe, to the medial orbital wall anterior to the lamina papyracea (see Figure 23.1). The pathological features and reconstructive requirements of fractures in these two segments are entirely different, and their anatomy is therefore discussed separately.

Anterior Segment of the Orbit

The anterior segment is defined as that part of the orbital cavity which is situated at or in front of the transverse axis of the globe. It comprises the bony rim

Rigid Fixation of Orbital Fractures 303

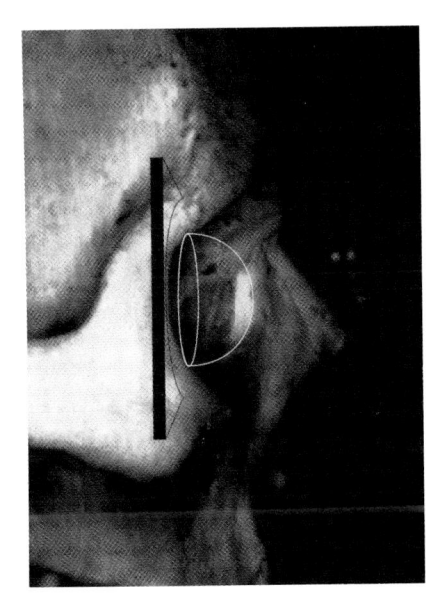

Figure 23.1 The coronal plane through the equator of the ocular globe divides the orbital cavity into anterior and posterior segments.

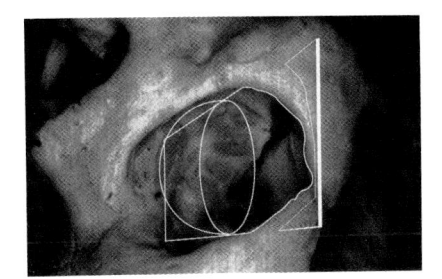

Figure 23.2 The anterior segment of the orbit is circumscribed by the anterior orbital floor, the medial wall anterior to the lamina papyracea, the supraorbital rim and floor of the frontal sinus, and the lateral orbital rim.

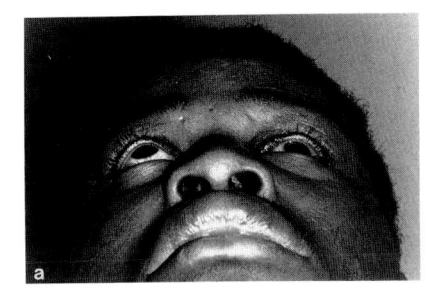

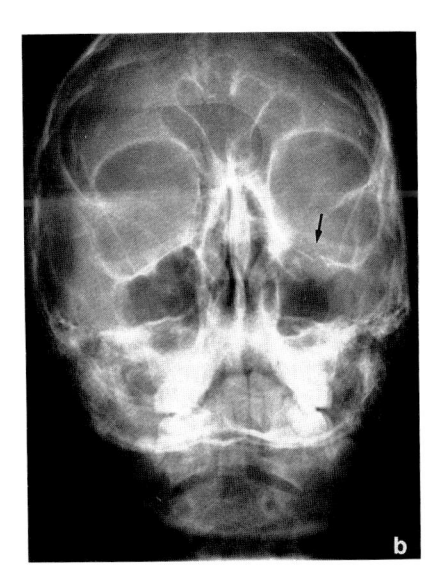

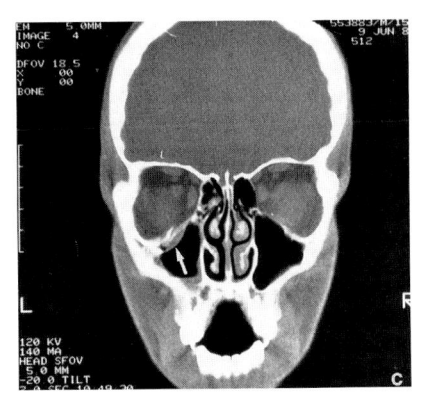

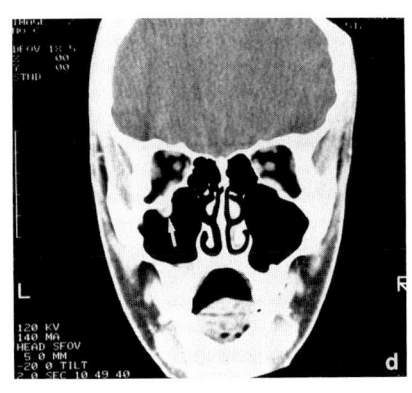

Figure 23.3 (a) This patient presented with muscle entrapment and enophthalmos of the left ocular globe. (b) This x ray shows the "Trap-door" fracture of the left inferior orbital rim. (c) This coronal CT scan through the anterior orbital segment shows the displaced hinge-like fracture of the orbital floor. (d) This coronal CT scan through the posterior orbit shows entrapment of muscle and soft tissue.

of the orbit and the anterior portions of the medial wall, roof, and floor (see Figure 23.2). In this region, both the medial wall and the floor of the orbit are concave in shape, and their junction is well defined.

Defects anterior to the axis of the globe generally do not cause significant changes in the volume of the orbital cavity and therefore do not alter the degree of ocular projection. These defects are usually seen in minor to moderate orbital trauma and can be repaired quite easily with autogenous or nonautogenous material. Post-traumatic enophthalmos is not likely to occur.

The one important exception to this rule is the anterior floor fracture that entraps the inferior rectus and inferior oblique muscles (see Figure 23.3). This is commonly a longitudinal fracture that runs posteriorly along the floor of the orbit toward the inferior orbital fissure. Although anterior to the axis of the globe, extraocular muscles entrapped within this narrow defect retract the globe, producing enophthalmos.

It is important to note that whereas the dimensions and configuration of the anterior orbital segment do not significantly affect the forward projection of the globe, they do determine ocular position in the coronal plane (see Figure 23.4). Poorly contoured grafts that do not duplicate the normal concavity of the anterior orbital floor are likely to cause superior globe displacement in the absence of enophthalmos or proptosis (see Figure 23.5). Displaced or malunited segments of the

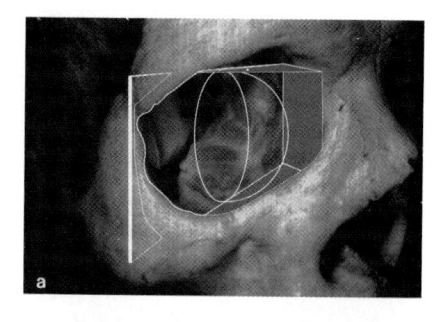

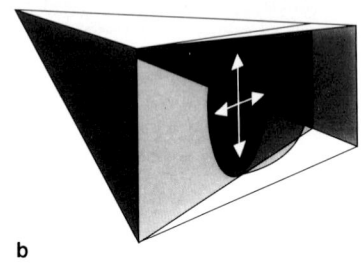

Figure 23.4 (a) The anterior segment of the orbit is a wedge-shaped space. (b) This schematic representation of the orbital pyramid shows that the dimensions and configuration of the anterior segment of the orbital cavity define the position of the ocular globe in the vertical and horizontal planes.

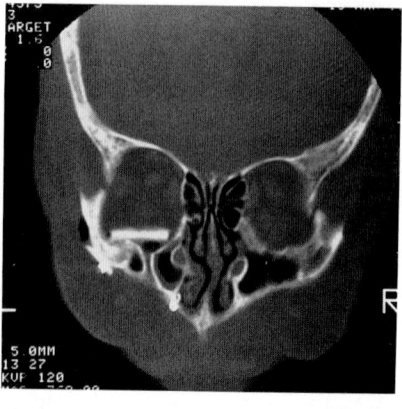

Figure 23.5 In the anterior segment of the orbit, the floor is concave (see uninjured right orbit). Poorly contoured grafts, as demonstrated in the left orbit, tend to elevate the globe.

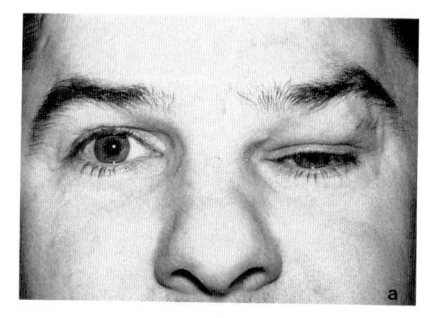

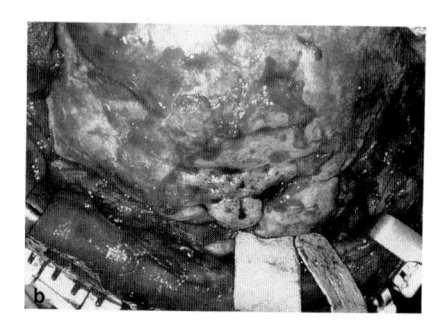

Figure 23.6 This patient has a malunited fracture of the supraorbital rim and contiguous roof. (a) The left ocular globe is displaced inferiorly. (b) The coronal flap is elevated. Segments of the supraorbital rim fracture are displaced inferiorly on the left.

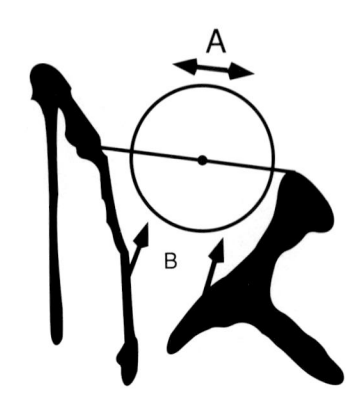

Figure 23.7 This axial cross-section of the orbit shows that the volume of the posterior segment of the orbital cavity (B) determines ocular projection. This volume is primarily influenced by the slope of the inferomedial orbital wall and the inclination of the lateral orbital wall.

orbital rim can result in ocular transposition in a transverse or vertical dimension (see Figure 23.6). Precise skeletal reconstruction at the level of the ocular axis is particularly important in ensuring accurate positioning of the globe.

Posterior Segment of the Orbit

The shape and volume of the orbital cavity posterior to the axis of the globe determine ocular projection in the anterior/posterior plane (see Figure 23.7). Within the posterior segment of the orbit, the medial wall is parallel to the sagittal plane; the lateral wall diverges at 45° and is entirely posterior to the axis of the globe.

Small changes in the orientation or position of the lateral wall profoundly affect orbital volume and globe projection. The lateral orbital wall is resilient and rarely comminutes. However, malrotation of the lateral wall due to poor reduction of a zygomatic fracture is frequently observed and is a leading cause of post-traumatic enophthalmos (see Figure 23.8).

Defects in the medial orbital wall are often overlooked. Isolated blowout fractures at this site cause an increased orbital volume posterior to the globe axis as well as enophthalmos. In rare instances, entrapment of the medial rectus muscle causes restricted ocular motility and retraction of the globe (see Figure 23.9).

Appreciation of the anatomic configuration of the junctional area between the medial wall and floor in the posterior third of the orbit is particularly important. The upper portion of the maxillary antrum produces a characteristic bulge in this region, obliterating the angle between the orbital floor and the medial wall. The inclination of this prominence in the inferomedial aspect of the orbital cavity is crucial in maintaining the for-

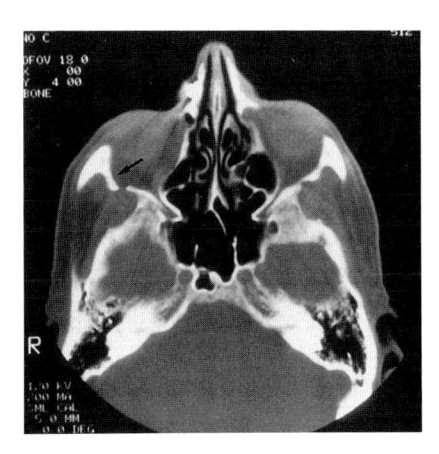

Figure 23.8 This patient presented with significant right enophthalmos following reduction and fixation of a zygoma fracture. The lateral orbital wall is rotated, and orbital volume is increased.

ward projection of the globe. Failure precisely to recreate this contour invariably leads to posterior globe displacement, even in the presence of small fractures (see Figure 23.10).

Etiologic Factors

Orbital injuries vary considerably in severity, according to the location and magnitude of impact forces. Low-velocity injuries, such as those resulting from personal altercation or a fall, generally result in simple, isolated fractures. The force of impact is effectively dissipated by the more resilient bony abutments of the orbital rim. The applied forces may be transmitted to the orbital cavity, resulting in a pure blowout fracture, or along bony processes to the sutural junctions, resulting in simple disarticulation with minimal comminution.

High-velocity injuries, such as motor vehicle accidents or industrial trauma, generate massive impact forces. These result in complex orbital fractures, frequently associated with panfacial fractures, multiple system trauma, and a relatively high incidence of injury to intraorbital soft tissues.

Pathologic Features

Simple orbital fractures are characterized by involvement of a single, isolated segment of the orbital rim or cavity. Adjacent facial bones generally remain intact. Fracture sites are classic, with disruption limited to well defined areas of weakness in the orbital rim, and particularly the sutural articulations. Comminution is absent, and displacement is minimal or moderate.

Complex orbital injuries are distinguished by the severity of skeletal disruption. Impact forces are so high that the component bones of the orbital rim fracture in multiple sites. Fracture fragments are grossly displaced and unstable. Concomitant injuries to the midface and craniofrontal region further predispose to instability. Extensive comminution and bone loss are prominent features.

Once the strong bony abutments of the orbital rim are disrupted, the thin, delicate bone composing the orbital walls offers little resistance to further trauma. Relatively unimpeded displacement of fragments of orbital rim fractures causes massive comminution of the contiguous roof, floor, or walls of the orbit.

Orbital trauma frequently results in a discrepancy between the volume of the orbital cavity and that of its soft-tissue contents. Enophthalmos is most commonly noted as a consequence. Fractures of the orbital rim and walls are blown out, causing a relative increase in the volume of the bony cavity. Defects in the orbital cavity permit escape of intraorbital fat and muscle, resulting in a relative diminution in the volume of orbital soft tissue and retrodisplacement of the globe.

Alternatively, fractures of the orbital rim or walls may be displaced inwardly, diminishing the orbital volume and causing proptosis of the ocular globe. These blowin fractures are uncommon, but they are important to recognize in view of the high incidence of associated injury to intraorbital contents and the necessity for immediate decompression.

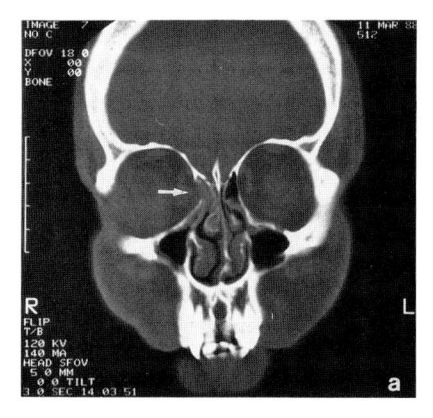

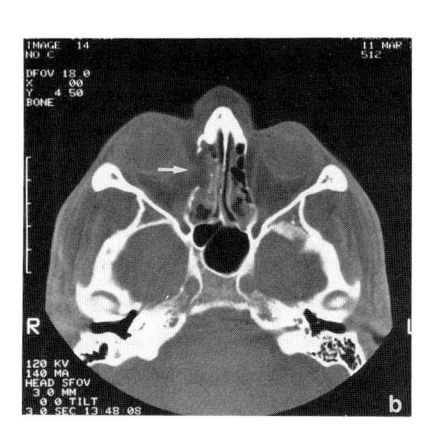

Figure 23.9 Medial wall blow-out fracture: (a) Coronal CT scan shows an isolated defect of the right medial orbital wall; (b) axial CT scan demonstrates entrapment of the medial rectus muscle.

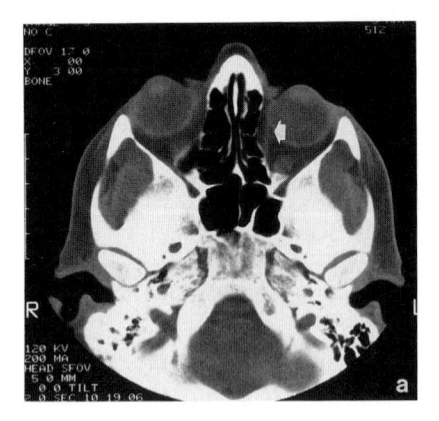

Figure 23.10 This patient with a soft-tissue facial injury presented three months later with progressive left enophthalmos. (a) This axial CT scan, high cut, shows a blowout fracture of the left medial orbital wall. (b) In this axial CT scan, low cut, note the complete loss of the maxillary sinus bulge in the left posterior orbit and the degree of globe retrodisplacement. (c) In this coronal CT scan through the anterior segment of orbit, anterior to the globe axis, the orbital cavity is intact. (d) This coronal CT scan through the posterior orbit shows loss of the normal prominence at the junction of the medial wall and floor of the left orbit, which produces a profound increase dimension of the in orbital cavity. (e) In this coronal CT scan through the orbital apex, note the prolapse of the contents through the bony defect in the left orbit.

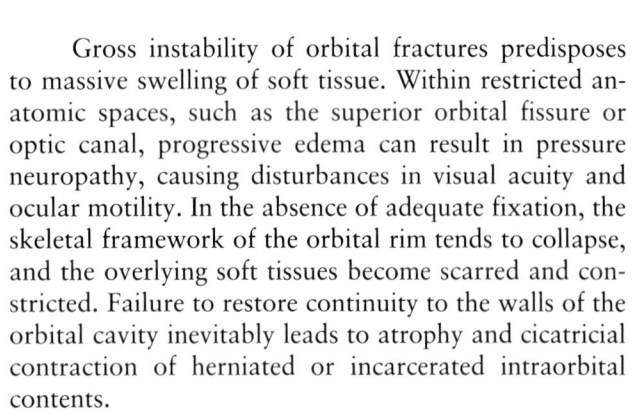

Gross instability of orbital fractures predisposes to massive swelling of soft tissue. Within restricted anatomic spaces, such as the superior orbital fissure or optic canal, progressive edema can result in pressure neuropathy, causing disturbances in visual acuity and ocular motility. In the absence of adequate fixation, the skeletal framework of the orbital rim tends to collapse, and the overlying soft tissues become scarred and constricted. Failure to restore continuity to the walls of the orbital cavity inevitably leads to atrophy and cicatricial contraction of herniated or incarcerated intraorbital contents.

Major orbital trauma, therefore, results in a deformity that becomes progressively more severe with time. Shrinkage and contracture of associated soft tissues amplifies the deformity and jeopardizes the results of secondary reconstruction.

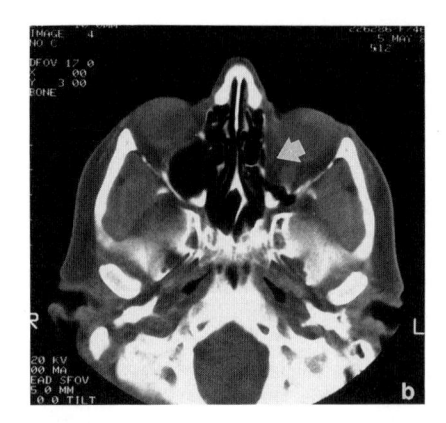

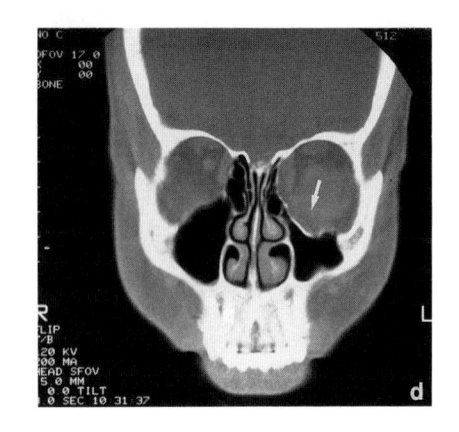

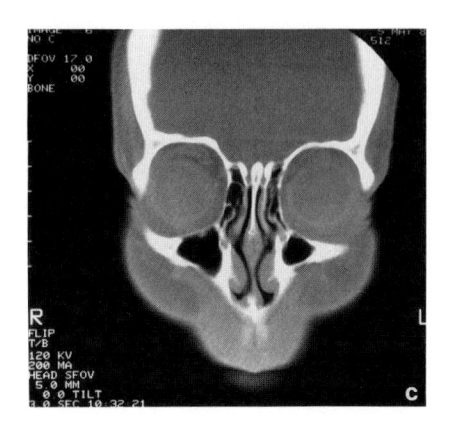

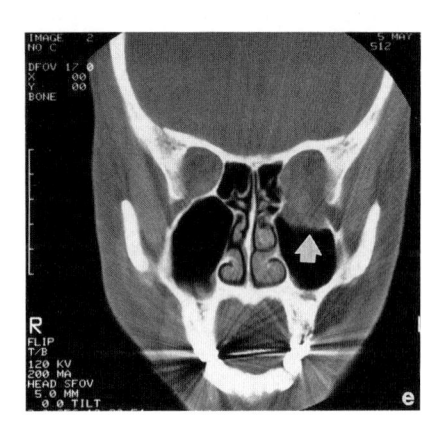

Clinical Features

Although the exact nature of underlying fractures cannot be adequately determined by physical assessment alone, simple and complex orbital injuries can often be differentiated on the basis of their clinical presentation. A history of high-velocity trauma and the presence of associated multisystem injuries and panfacial fractures should alert the surgeon to the possible presence of a complex orbital injury. Asymmetry in anterior and posterior global position (that is, proptosis and enophthalmos) identifies volumetric changes in the orbital cavity associated with blowin or blowout fractures. Displacement of the ocular globe in the vertical or transverse dimension indicates underlying positional changes in segments of the orbital rim. For example, disruption of the medial and lateral orbital rims and the zygomaticomaxillary region results in instability of the inferior two thirds of the orbit and inferolateral oculo-orbital displacement. When concomitant fractures involve the supraorbital rim, the entire bony orbit is displaced downward, producing a true orbital dystopia.

Associated injury to the contents of the orbital soft tissue should be anticipated and actively investigated. Jabaley (1975) documented ocular injuries in 29% of patients with orbital fractures. The injuries reported involved all anatomic segments of the eye, including the cornea, anterior chamber, lens and iris, posterior chamber, and retina. The frequency and degree of injury to orbital soft tissue is proportional to the severity of skeletal disruption. The direction of fracture displacement is also an important factor. The authors have noted a 12% incidence of globe rupture and a 10% incidence of superior orbital fissure syndrome in patients with blowin fractures.

PRINCIPLES OF MANAGEMENT

Conventional techniques of fracture management, although effective in the treatment of simple, isolated orbital injuries, have proven inadequate in the reconstruction of complex orbital trauma. Standard radiographs fail to demonstrate the degree of comminution or bone loss. Incomplete exposure of all involved skeletal regions further precludes accurate assessment of the bony injury and the subsequent anatomic reduction of fractures. Interosseous wiring techniques, particularly in comminuted areas, do not fix bone segments rigidly and frequently result in eventual bony collapse and soft-tissue shrinkage. Most important, failure to reconstruct defects of the orbital floor or walls predisposes to secondary problems, including enophthalmos, muscle entrapment, and diplopia.

Current management of complex orbital trauma aims to restore and maintain the normal anatomy of the craniofacial skeleton, thereby minimizing the secondary problems of massive edema, bony collapse, and soft-tissue shrinkage. Recent technical innovations and certain modifications in the surgical approach facilitate the attainment of these goals.

The limitations of preoperative assessment of orbital fractures have been largely overcome by the advent of computed tomography (CT) scanning. High-resolution axial CT scans clearly define thin elements and subtle defects of the orbital skeleton, and intraorbital soft tissues are visualized with unprecedented detail. Data obtained from serial transverse scans can be further reformatted to provide two-dimensional images in any plane or three-dimensional images from any perspective. The anatomic sites, displacement, and degree of comminution in orbital fractures can be precisely evaluated. Impingement or entrapment of soft tissues can be localized, and an optimal plan for management can be formulated.

Operative treatment of orbital injuries is performed as early as possible. In particular, clinical or radiological evidence of blowin fracture fragments impinging on the ocular globe or optic nerve necessitate immediate decompression (see Figure 23.11). Craniofacial surgical techniques are employed in the extended exposure of the facial skeleton to facilitate precise anatomic reduction of orbital fractures. Areas of extensive comminution or bone loss are reconstructed with primary bone grafts. Rigid internal fixation, using a com-

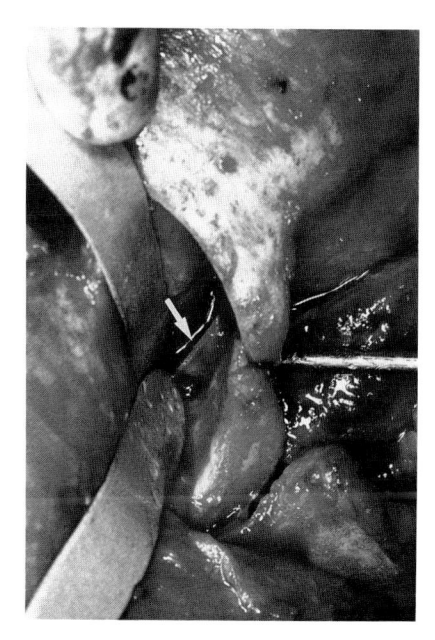

Figure 23.11 Impure lateral orbital blow-in fracture: Through a coronal approach, the periorbita is widely dissected to reveal a blowin segment of the lateral orbital wall impinging on the intraorbital contents.

bination of lag screws and miniplates, provides optimal stability in the reconstructed skeletal framework. This will result in the re-establishment of a normal craniofacial skeletal anatomy and will maintain soft-tissue expansion during the phase of healing. Use of these techniques will allow the repair of even the most severe injury in one stage and will prevent the development of secondary deformity.

METHODS OF FRACTURE FIXATION

The goal of primary reconstruction is to restore the normal anatomy of the orbit in three dimensions by accurately repositioning all fracture fragments and providing a functionally stable osteosynthesis. Stability is maintained if the sum of the static forces uniting the bone segments exceeds the sum of the functional forces acting on the bone. These functional forces comprise the various pressure, traction, and shearing forces generated by dynamic muscle action as well as progressive contracture of soft-tissue scar. With the exception of the action of the masseter muscle on the zygoma, the skeletal framework of the orbit is relatively isolated from significant functional stress. However, in the presence of gross disruption and comminution of the orbit, contraction of unsupported soft tissues and of scar tissue exerts a considerable force on orbital fracture segments. The requirements for stable skeletal fixation in the orbit therefore vary with the degree of skeletal disruption.

Fixation with Interosseous Wire

Fixation with interosseous wire relies on the static forces generated by the tension of the wire and by the friction between corresponding bone surfaces at the fracture site. An accurate anatomic reduction and a thorough adaptation of two broad apposing bone surfaces will result in sufficient friction to overcome the negligible functional forces acting on the orbit. Interosseous wire fixation is therefore restricted to the repair of simple, isolated orbital fractures resulting from low-velocity trauma. In the absence of comminution, bone deficiency, or associated fractures, a stable skeletal fixation can be obtained.

However, orbital injuries due to high-velocity trauma are frequently associated with significant comminution and actual loss of bone, which precludes precise apposition of bone fragments. Under these circumstances, wire ligatures provide insufficient immobilization of osseous segments. Progressive scar contracture exerts a continuous force on the reconstructed orbit, causing the interosseous wires to stretch and cut through drill holes. Eventual displacement and collapse of the skeletal framework is inevitable (see Figure 23.12). It is therefore important to recognize these more severe orbital injuries and to apply alternative means of fracture fixation in their repair.

Fixation with Miniplates

Miniature bone plates and screws permit a rigid, internal, three-dimensional fixation of skeletal elements. They are specifically indicated in the repair of complex orbital injuries. Multiple displaced and unstable osseous segments can be sequentially reduced and rigidly immobilized to re-establish normal craniofacial anatomy (see Figure 23.13). Areas of extensive comminution and small gaps in bony continuity can be bridged by contoured plates, producing a stable reconstruction that resists subsequent deformation by contracting scar tissue. Miniplate fixation is further indicated in the presence of associated fractures of the midface. The unopposed force of the masseter muscle, acting on a fractured zygoma, can displace the infero-

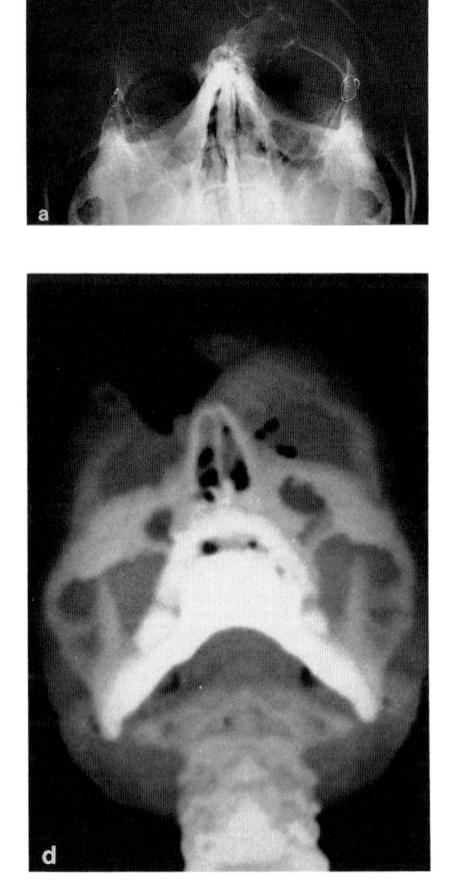

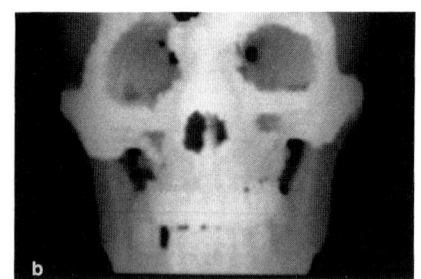

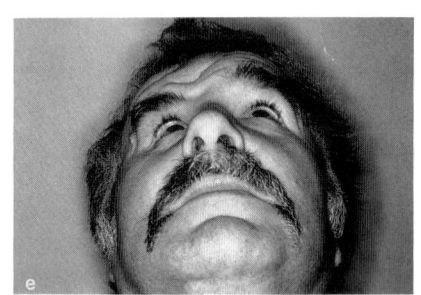

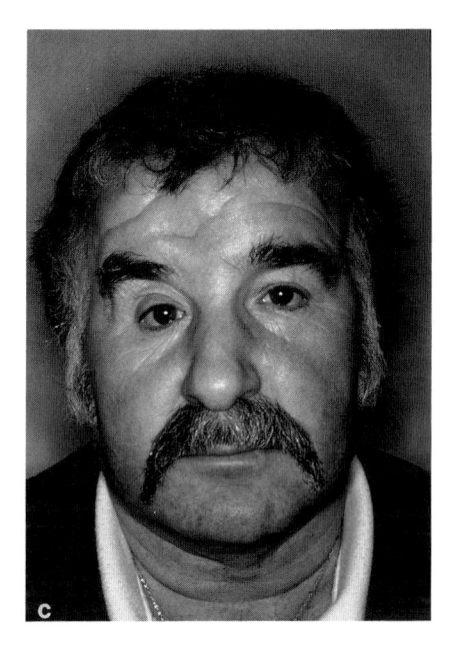

Figure 23.12 Late post-traumatic deformity of the right orbit: This high-velocity injury was initially treated by interosseous wiring of isolated fractures. (a) The facial x ray shows that a single interosseous wire at the right fronto-zygomatic suture fails to prevent diastasis at the fracture site and inferior displacement of orbital segments. (b) This three-dimensional CT illustrates inferomedial displacement of the right zygoma associated with collapse of the lateral buttress. (c) The resulting clinical deformity is characterized by right inferior oculo-orbital displacement. (d) This three-dimensional CT shows collapse of the zygomatic arch, resulting in a typical bowing deformity of the arch, which is associated with retrusion of the malar prominence. (e) The view from below demonstrates the degree of malar retrusion and enophthalmos.

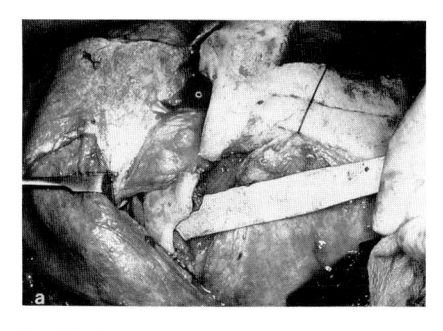

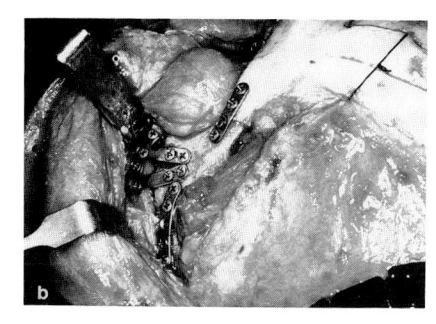

Figure 23.13 Complex left orbitozygomatic fracture: (a) The coronal flap is elevated to demonstrate fractures through the lateral orbital rim, malar body, and zygomatic arch; (b) miniplates and screws provide a rigid three-dimensional reconstruction.

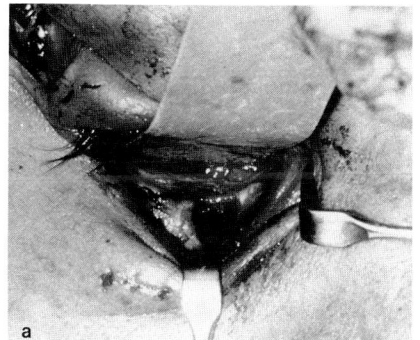

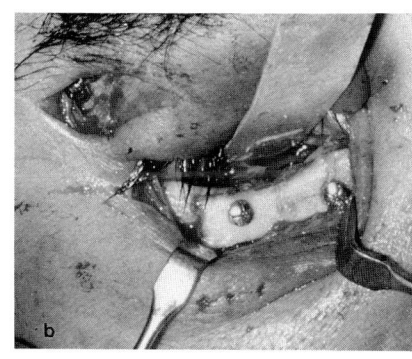

Figure 23.14 Onlay bone graft fixation technique:
(a) A defect in the right inferior orbital rim is shown.
(b) Reconstruction is performed using an oversized cranial bone graft, rigidly fixed to adjacent bone segments with lag screws.

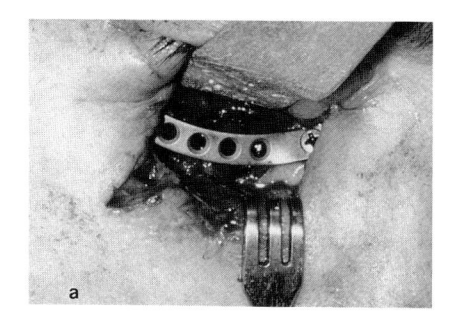

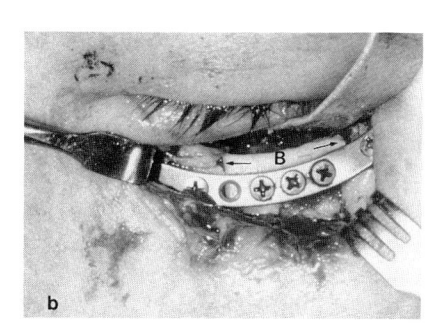

Figure 23.15 Inlay bone graft fixation technique: (a) A defect in the right inferior orbital rim is bridged by a long, curved miniplate. (b) A split cranial bone graft [B] is contoured to fit the defect precisely and then held rigidly in place with three screws.

lateral orbit down and out, resulting in enophthalmos. Similarly, extensive comminution of the maxillary buttresses exposes the inferomedial orbital rim to the functional stresses of mastication and predisposes to subsequent collapse.

Fixation with Bone Grafts

It is important to recognize that relapse has been documented in cases where miniplates have been used as the sole means of fixation in bridging large osseous defects. Osseous healing does not take place, and the tensile forces resulting from scarring and contracture of soft tissue can overcome the static forces generated by plate and screw fixation. Primary bone grafting is specifically indicated in this situation, both to speed osteosynthesis and osseous regeneration within the defect and to augment the stability of the reconstruction.

Bone grafts can be employed in a variety of ways in the fixation of orbital fractures. A simple technique uses interfragmentary compression of an onlay graft (see Figure 23.14). A slightly oversized corticocancellous bone graft is used as a rigid strut, spanning the skeletal defect and fixing the adjacent bone segments. At least two lag screws are used to secure the graft to each bony margin. The lag screw principle employs an unthreaded gliding drill hole in the proximal fragment (bone graft) and a threaded traction drill hole in the distal bone segment. As the screws are tightened, the graft is compressed to the skeletal margins of the defect, providing rigid internal fixation. Although extremely effective, this technique should be restricted to the reconstruction of buttresses and, in selected cases, the inferior orbital rim. Elsewhere, soft-tissue coverage is thin and contour irregularities will be obvious.

An alternative technique employs miniplates and inlay bone grafts for optimal restoration of contour, bony continuity, and stability (see Figure 23.15). A corticocancellous graft is carved to fit precisely into the osseous defect, flush with the adjacent bone surfaces. The graft is rigidly immobilized by multiple screw fixation to a miniplate bridging the defect.

SURGICAL APPROACH TO ORBITAL FRACTURES

The primary reconstruction of an orbital fracture involves multiple procedures, which are performed sequentially in an orderly, stepwise fashion. Although variations in technique are often dictated by the specific findings in each particular case, adherence to a standard operative protocol ensures that all pathologic features of orbital fractures are actively investigated, assessed, and treated.

Exposure

Adequate exposure implies that all fracture sites are directly visualized, such that each fracture fragment can be assessed in relation to neighboring segments and is freely accessible to mobilization and manipulation. The application of craniofacial techniques permits this extended exposure while protecting the contents of orbital soft tissue. This dissection must be performed prior to any attempts at fracture reduction or fixation. Visualization of all fractures through several incisions provides an appreciation of the overall fracture pattern in three dimensions and is a prerequisite to accurate reconstruction.

Reconstruction of the Orbital Rim

The orbital rim defines the circumference of the base of the orbital cavity and its location in relation to the contralateral orbit and the entire craniofacial skeleton. It further provides a supportive framework for the walls of the orbital cavity and the attachments of the canthal ligament. Accurate orbital reconstruction therefore begins with reconstitution of a stable orbital rim, providing it with its normal dimensions and placing it in its correct anatomical position.

Because each bony element affects the position of its neighbors, it is essential that fracture reduction proceed through an orderly sequence, starting from intact regions of the craniofacial skeleton. This orderly sequence permits a precise reassembly of the whole unit.

Supraorbital Rim

The craniofrontal region is composed of the most impact-resistant bone in the craniofacial skeleton. When fractures do occur, they tend to result in large bone segments with minimal comminution. This facilitates the precise anatomic realignment of parts. Proceeding from stable portions of the frontal cranium toward the orbital margin, the surgeon systematically reduces fracture fragments and fixes them with wire ligatures or miniplates. The correct spatial relationship of the supraorbital rim to the skull and contralateral orbit is thus ensured in three dimensions.

Fractures of the supraorbital rim itself are reassembled and rigidly fixed with a single curved miniplate. Bony defects must be repaired with carefully contoured bone grafts to reproduce both the concave surface of the orbital margin and the frontal prominence of the superciliary arch (see Figure 23.16). The reconstructed supraorbital rim now provides an index to the proper width of the orbit and a stable reference point for realignment of nasoethmoid and zygomatic fractures.

Lateral Orbital Rim

The zygoma is more resilient than the inferior and medial orbital rims, and the degree of fragmentation is generally less. More important, the respective articulations of the zygoma to the temporal, frontal, and sphenoid bone are oriented in three different planes. An anatomic reduction of the zygoma at each of these junctions ensures precise three-dimensional placement of the lateral orbital rim in relation to the skull (see Figure 23.17). Initial reconstruction of the superolateral orbital rim and zygomatic arch thereby establishes an outer facial frame, which serves as a stable reference for realignment and fixation of remaining fractures.

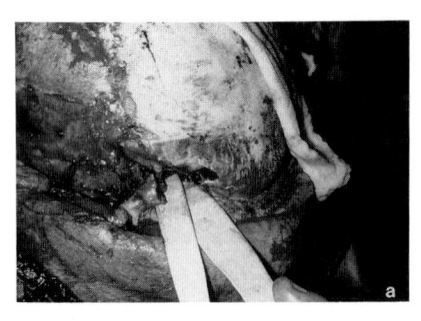

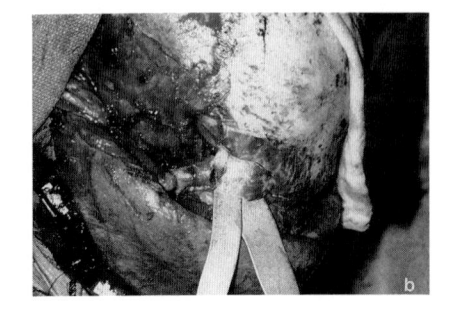

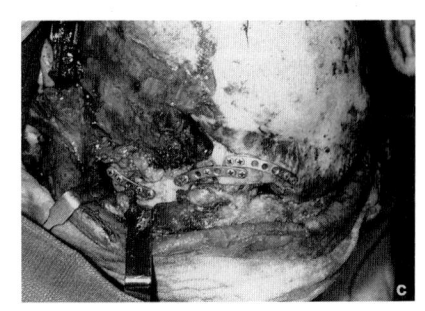

Figure 23.16 Reconstruction of the supraorbital rim: (a) The coronal flap is elevated to expose a bony defect in the right supraorbital rim. (b) A cranial bone graft is shaped to fit the defect precisely. (c) The completed reconstruction of superior and lateral orbital rims and the zygomatic arch is shown.

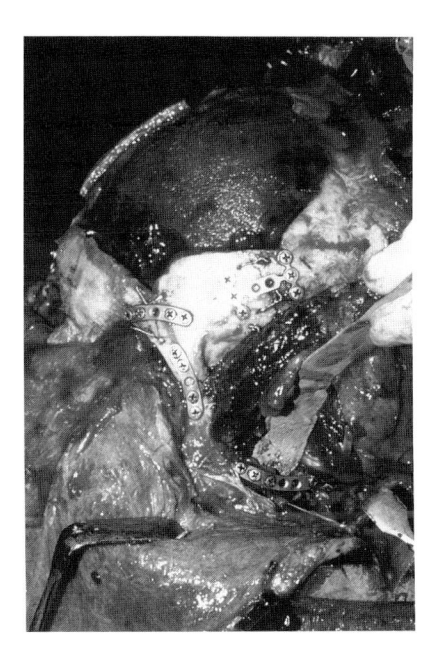

Figure 23.17 Anatomic reduction of the zygoma and supraorbital rim provides a stable outer facial frame and ensures a precise three-dimensional placement of the orbit in relation to the skull.

The excellent exposure that can be obtained in this area must be used to full advantage to ensure that the zygoma is repositioned in its proper relation to the cranium. Failure to do so predisposes to rotational deformity of the body of the zygoma and an exaggerated bowing or convexity of the reconstructed zygomatic arch. In addition to compromising the reduction of remaining fractures, inappropriate positioning of the zygoma results in an obvious orbital deformity associated with significant volumetric discrepancies in the orbital cavity, inadequate projection of the inferolateral orbit, and exaggerated facial width.

The arch of the zygoma projects directly forward in an almost straight line. An effort is made to recreate this normal contour as fracture segments along the arch are sequentially fixed to a long miniplate. Posteriorly, the arch is generally sheared off the zygomatic process of the temporal bone in an oblique fashion, and this fracture is consistently amenable to fixation with a single lag screw.

Fractures of the lateral orbital rim commonly occur through the fronto-zygomatic suture area. Although reduction of this fracture seems deceptively simple, it is important to consider that minimal deformation at this site may be associated with a pronounced rotational deformity of the zygoma. Accurate reduction of this fracture therefore requires simultaneous anatomic realignment of the fracture at the lateral rim and wall of the orbit. The lateral reduction of the orbital wall is viewed from within the orbital cavity, or, in difficult cases, it can be approached posteriorly following reflection of the temporalis muscle (see Figure 23.18). The direct apposition of the fractured zygoma to the frontal bone superiorly and to the sphenoid bone posteriorly ensures proper orientation. Fixation is generally provided by a single, curved miniplate along the lateral orbital rim.

Reconstruction of the superior and lateral orbital rims completes the outer facial frame. The vertical height and transverse width of the orbit are re-established. Rotational deformity is eliminated. A rigidly stabilized malar body provides a reliable skeletal reference for facial projection and a base for reconstruction of the inferior orbit.

Medial Orbital Rim

The medial orbital rims furnish an important anatomic landmark separating the orbital and interorbital spaces. This region is less resistant to trauma, and so skeletal disruption is more severe. Although comminution can be quite extensive in the bones of the nose, vomer, perpendicular plate, and labyrinths of the ethmoid, a central bone segment bearing the insertion of the medial canthal tendon is generally sheared off in

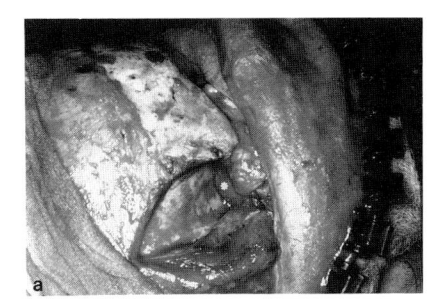

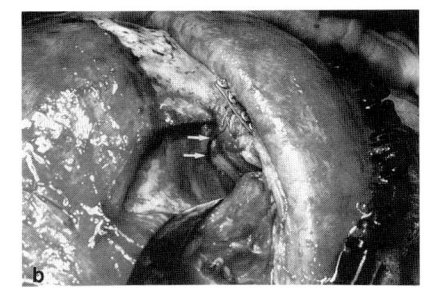

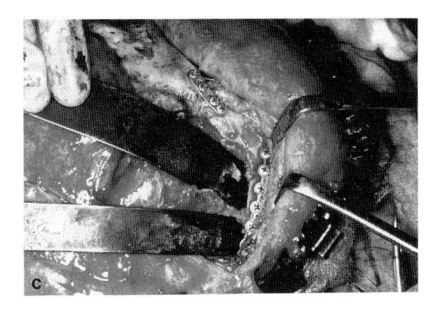

Figure 23.18 Reconstruction of the lateral orbit:
(a) The coronal flap is elevated, and the anterior temporalis muscle is reflected. Note the complete disruption of the zygoma with prolapse of orbital contents into the temporal fossa. (b) Anatomic reduction of the zygoma at the lateral orbital rim and at the sphenozygomatic fracture line (arrows) prevents rotational deformity of the lateral orbital wall. (c) Reconstruction of the zygomatic arch completes the outer facial frame.

one piece. This central fragment, the frontal process of the maxilla, and composes the superior extension of the nasomaxillary buttress, which in turn defines the medial orbital rim. When disrupted, this bony segment is generally displaced inferiorly and laterally.

Reconstruction of the medial orbital rim is based on the identification and accurate reduction of the central segment. Meticulous subperiosteal dissection delineates the margins of the bone fragment while preserving the insertion of the medial canthal tendon. Control of the central segment is obtained by grasping its inferior margin with bone-holding clamps via the intraoral or infraorbital incisions. The nasofrontal fracture is reduced anatomically while rotation of the fragment is manipulated to re-establish the intercanthal distance. A precisely contoured miniplate fixes the medial orbital rim to the glabella and supraorbital rim. Screws placed in the anterior wall of the frontal sinus provide a safe and reliable point of fixation to the cranial vault.

The reconstructed medial orbital rims define the transverse dimensions of the orbital and interorbital spaces and provide a rigid framework to guide and support bone graft reconstruction of the medial orbital walls. When the insertion of the medial canthal tendon is preserved, proper orientation of the central bone segment ensures restitution of the normal intercanthal distance and palpebral fissure width.

Inferior Orbital Rim

The inferior orbital rim is susceptible to extensive comminution and bone loss, frequently precluding accurate anatomic reduction of fractures. However, prior reconstruction of the outer facial frame and medial rim provides stable skeletal buttresses. Reconstruction of the inferior rim then becomes simply a matter of restoring bony continuity and contour across the intervening gap.

All fracture fragments are first identified and stripped of periosteum. Larger segments, which are amenable to fixation, are carefully approximated to bridge the skeletal defect. In the event of actual bone loss, cortical bone grafts are precisely carved and inlayed to provide a smooth contour. These multiple segments are then secured by a single seven-hole or nine-hole curved miniplate that spans the entire inferior rim. The miniplate is anchored peripherally by at least two screws, which are inserted into the zygomatic and nasomaxillary margins, respectively. All intervening segments are then rigidly stabilized by screw fixation to the miniplate.

Reconstruction of the Orbital Cavity

Reconstruction of the orbital cavity aims to restore the normal position of the ocular globe in all three dimensions and to ensure that there is no mechanical reconstruction to ocular motility. Following reconstruction of a rigid, circumferential bony margin at the base of the orbital pyramid, the roof, floor, and walls of the orbit must each be systematically re-explored. All defects are identified and obliterated in such a way as to restore both the volume and the shape of the orbital cavity.

Exploration of the orbital cavity entails subperiosteal dissection along remaining intact segments of the orbital walls toward areas of bony deficiency. Retraction of the periorbita then permits prolapsed orbital contents to be specifically identified and gently dissected free. It is essential that stable bony margins surrounding the defect be defined (see Figure 23.19). Direct visualization of lateral, medial, and posterior bony shelves ensures adequate retrieval of all herniated soft tissues and determines the size and shape of required bone grafts.

In the reconstruction of the orbital cavity, it is important to divide it conceptually into anterior and posterior segments in relation to the axis of the ocular globe. This axis extends transversely from the lateral orbital rim to the region just anterior to the lamina papyracea. At or anterior to this axis, defects in the orbital floor or medial wall may cause ptosis of the globe but are unlikely to result in enophthalmos. More important, bone grafts used in the reconstruction of this anterior segment of the orbit must be thin and precisely contoured to restore the normal concavity seen here. Bone grafts that are too bulky or inadequately contoured, or those that are allowed to project beyond the orbital margin, will result in displacement of the ocular globe in a vertical or transverse plane.

Posterior to the axis of the globe, volumetric changes within the orbital cavity affect the forward projection of the globe. It is important therefore not simply

Figure 23.19 Left orbital blowout fracture: (a) Following reconstruction of the orbital rim, subperiosteal dissection exposes the medial, lateral, anterior, and posterior shelves of the orbital floor defect. (b) In this close-up view, note that this defect involves the critical "bulge" area in the posterior orbit.

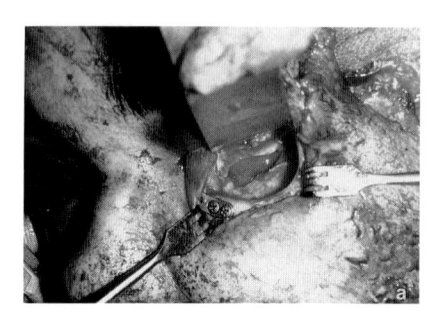

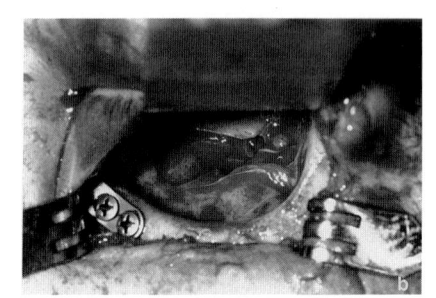

Rigid Fixation of Orbital Fractures 313

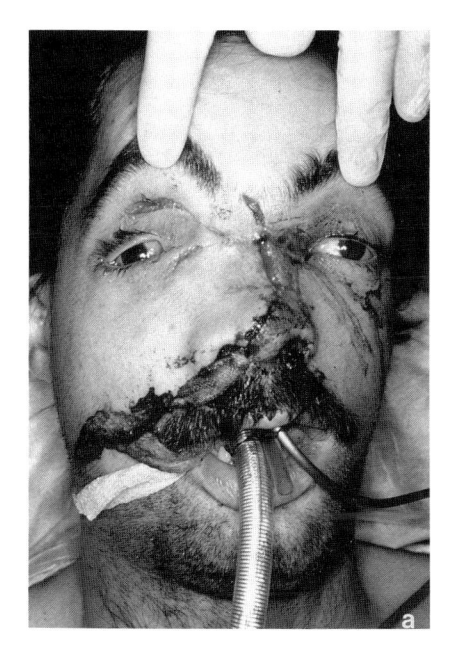

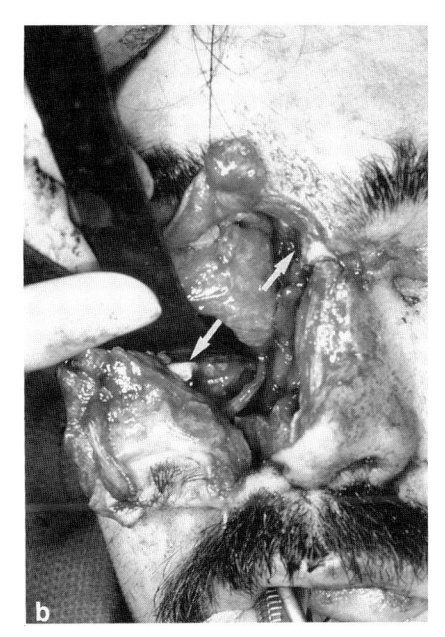

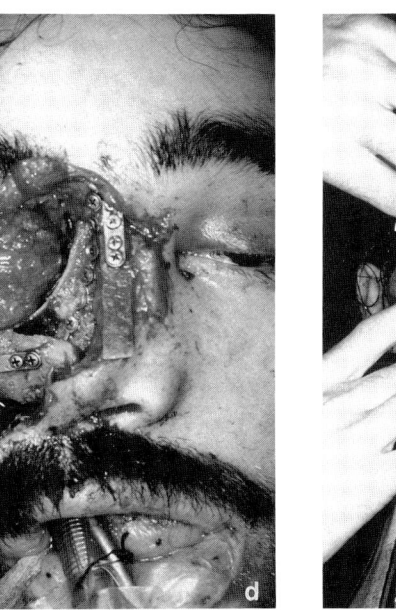

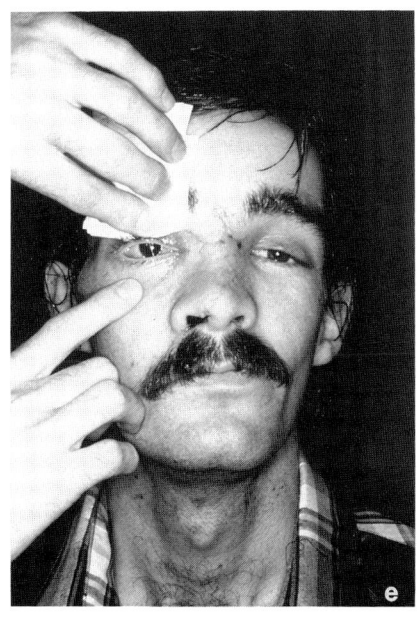

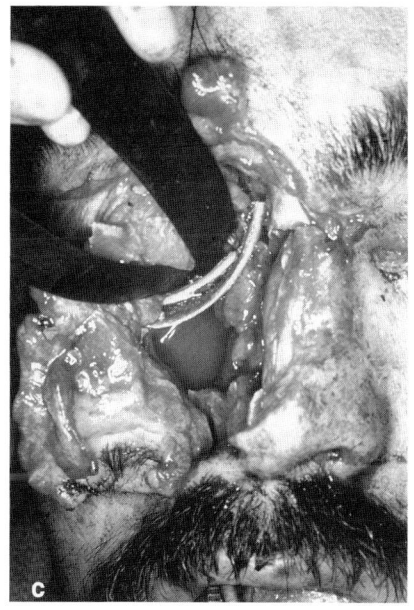

Figure 23.20 High-velocity compound injury to the right orbit: (a) This patient has a right inferolateral oculo-orbital displacement. Soft-tissue avulsion through the nose has been sutured at a peripheral hospital. (b) The right orbit is exposed through the laceration. Stable medial and lateral shelves (arrows) circumscribe a large defect involving the entire inferomedial orbit. (c) The orbital cavity was reconstructed with a rib graft. Grafts are stacked serially toward the orbital apex to recreate the upward slope of the floor. (d) The medial and inferior orbital rims are reconstructed with cranial bone grafts, which are fixed to adjacent bone with miniplates to provide a functionally stable orbital framework. (e) The early postoperative result demonstrates the symmetry of the ocular positions.

to obliterate skeletal defects in this area but to recreate the normal anatomic configuration as closely as possible. The orbital floor, for example, is sloped upward and medially in the posterior orbit to merge with the medial orbital wall. This creates a bony prominence immediately posterior to the ocular globe, pushing it forward. To reconstruct skeletal volume in this area, the posterior bony shelf must first be identified deep within the orbital cavity to establish the cant of the defect. Bone grafts are then stacked serially from anterior to posterior, thereby supporting each other and re-establishing the upward slope of the floor (see Figure 23.20).

The dimensions of the orbital wall defect are the primary criteria in selecting a suitable graft for reconstruction. The graft must be of sufficient size to obliterate the defect completely and to support the soft-tissue contents within the orbital cavity. Defects of moderate size are effectively bridged by split cranial grafts. Such grafts are ideally harvested from the temporoparietal region of the skull, where the curvature at the donor site approximates the contour of orbital wall segments. Larger defects, comprising two or more contiguous areas of the orbital cavity, such as the orbital floor and medial or lateral walls, are difficult to reconstruct with cranial grafts. Calvarial bone cannot be adequately contoured to duplicate the concave surfaces of larger segments of the orbital cavity. In these situations, split rib grafts are preferable. These are easily shaped to desired

Figure 23.21 Deformities can result from inadequate fixation of periorbital soft tissues. A patient is shown one year following primary reconstruction of a complex left orbito-zygomatico-maxillary fracture. (a) Symmetry in ocular projection and malar position indicates accurate skeletal reconstruction and successful restoration of orbital volume. (b) Similarly, in the AP view, symmetrical positioning of the ocular globes in a coronal plane is confirmed. However, failure to fix the soft tissues on the left results in ptosis of the cheek, mild ectropion, and scleral show. (c) Closer evaluation with a McCoy Trisquare (Padgett Instruments, Kansas City, MO) demonstrates the effects of canthal drift and gravitational displacement of soft tissues. These effects are left medial and lateral canthal dystopia, and increased height and inclination of the palpebral fissure.

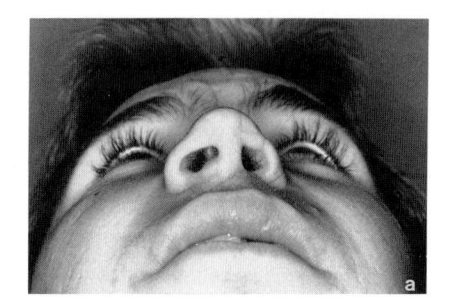

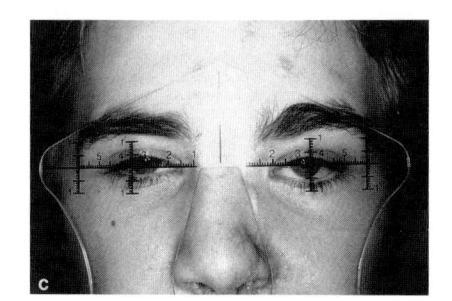

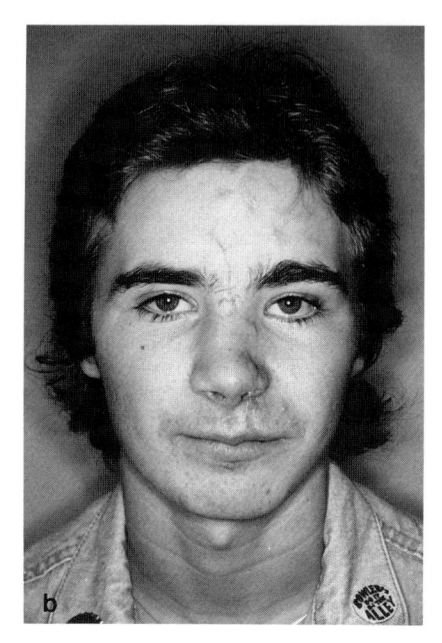

specifications with Tessier bone benders and can be fitted to any size or shape of defect.

As a rule, bone grafts within the orbital cavity are not fixed. Stable bony shelves surrounding the defect are used as buttresses to support the graft and to prevent outward displacement. The pressure exerted by the intraorbital contents then acts to tamponade the bone grafts and maintain them in position. Subsequent migration, extrusion, or displacement of bone grafts is only occasionally observed. In the rare circumstance where bony shelves are inadequate to support the bone graft, fixation to the orbital rim may be required. Both contoured miniplates and titanium mesh supporting trays have been employed for this purpose (see Chapter 24).

Fixation of Periorbital Soft Tissues

With the advent of rigid internal fixation and primary bone grafting, precise reconstruction of the orbital skeletal framework is readily accomplished. However, the periorbital soft tissues have all too often been neglected and simply allowed to "redrape," with the assumption that normal features will necessarily be obtained. Extensive subperiosteal stripping of the cheek and nasoethmoid region and detachment of canthal insertions, combined with postoperative fluid collection in subperiosteal spaces and gravitational pull on swollen, edematous soft tissues, predispose to deformity. Despite an excellent skeletal reconstruction and restoration of the normal position of the ocular globe, patients can present with medial or lateral canthal dystopia, ptosis of the soft tissues of the cheek, and ectropion associated with ptosis of the lacrimal sac and eversion of the puncta (see Figure 23.21). Prevention of these sequelae, and accurate placement and fixation of the periorbital soft tissues, pose the greatest challenges to the reconstructive surgeon and determine the extent to which orbital repair resembles normal facial features.

Medial Canthopexy

The insertions of the medial canthal tendons are reassessed following reconstruction of the bony orbit. In most cases, anatomic reduction of the central nasoethmoid bone segment ensures proper repositioning of the attached medial canthal tendon. However, persistent canthal dystopia indicates avulsion or attenuation of the tendinous insertion and necessitates a canthopexy.

The medial canthal tendon must first be reliably identified. This is best performed externally, through a small skin incision directly over the medial canthus. The white subcutaneous bands attaching to the tarsal plates can be easily located with minimal dissection. Once identified, the tendon should be grasped with forceps and retracted medially to ensure that its tension does bring the commissure to the required position. A 26-gauge wire is then passed through the tendon and retrieved on the deep surface of the coronal flap.

Selection of the correct point of fixation for the canthal tendon within the ipsilateral medial orbital wall can be difficult. Ideally, the avulsed tendon is anchored in an overcorrected position superior and posterior to the lacrimal crest. In the complex injury, however, the medial orbital wall is comminuted and the lacrimal crest may be deficient. If the contralateral medial canthus is intact, it is used as a guide for canthal positioning in the vertical and anterior/posterior planes. In the absence of any reference landmarks, as occurs in bilateral canthal avulsions associated with comminution, the point of medial canthal fixation can only be estimated. Under these circumstances, one aims to restore an intercanthal distance of 30 millimeters or less and to ensure symmetrical positioning of the canthi in all other planes.

In the presence of extensive comminution, the medial orbital wall is first reconstructed with a bone graft to provide a foundation for medial canthal repair. With use of a wire-passing drill, the canthopexy wires are brought through the bone graft and the nasal vault to the contralateral side. Distal fixation of the canthopexy wires must be secure. Simple ligature of wires over an intact skeletal frame or bone grafts in the contralateral orbit is insufficient. Progressive resorption of bone may allow the wires to pull through, resulting in recurrent telecanthus. We prefer to fix the wires to more rigid support structures. Where rigid skeletal fixation has been employed in the repair of nasoethmoid fractures, the canthopexy wires can be secured to adjacent miniplates or screws. Alternatively, a 4-millimeter screw can be placed in the midline glabellar region to offer a stable point of fixation for a medial canthopexy (see Chapter 22).

Canthal drift in the early postoperative period is the most frequent complication, particularly in those cases in whom the canthal tendon was avulsed. Causative factors include the anterolateral tensile forces across the palpebral fissure associated with orbicularis oculi muscle function and postoperative edema, subperiosteal hematoma, and seroma. These factors are extremely difficult to control. Paskert, Manson, and Iliff (1988) have advocated the use of nasal bolsters and transnasal wires to minimize swelling and hematoma and to aid redraping of the skin in the nasal orbital valley.

Lateral Canthoplasty

Lateral canthoplasty serves two primary functions. First, repositioning and fixation of the lateral canthal ligament determines the width and inclination of the palpebral fissure. This provides a more aesthetically pleasing result. Second, and more important, the lateral canthoplasty supports the lower eyelid and the orientation of the orbicularis sphincter superolaterally. Thus lateral canthoplasty can prevent postoperative lateral canthal dystopia, scleral show, and ectropion.

The lateral canthal ligament presents as a raphe within the orbicularis oculi muscle. It is identified and secured with a 3–0 stainless steel wire. The wire is then passed through a drill hole in the lateral orbital rim, placed immediately inferior to the fronto-zygomatic suture. In this fashion, the lateral canthus is fixed to the inner margin of the lateral orbital rim.

Advancement and Fixation of the Cheek

Following wide subperiosteal dissection of the midface, the soft tissues of the cheek are subject to gravitational inferior displacement. Failure to control this results in ptosis of the cheek and a relative soft-tissue deficiency over the malar prominence and infraorbital rim. More important, unrestricted traction on the lower eyelid predisposes to ectropion.

In the closure of the lower eyelid incision, we routinely identify the periosteal margin of the cheek flap. This facilitates superior advancement of the cheek soft tissues and their fixation to a drill hole or miniplate at the infraorbital margin. The cheekpad is thereby suspended over the malar prominence, and a tension-free closure of the subciliary incision is performed.

LONG-TERM RESULTS

The results of immediate post-traumatic orbital reconstruction were previously analyzed by the authors in a group of 49 complex orbital fractures (Antonyshyn 1989a). Patients underwent a detailed ophthalmological examination, and anthropometric evaluations of the position of the ocular globe and palpebral fissure.

Ocular Function

Ocular complications were generally related to the initial injury and were not influenced by the skeletal reconstruction. The one significant exception to this was previously noted in a review of orbital blowin fractures presenting with superior orbital fissure syndrome, where immediate orbital decompression was effective in providing resolution of ophthalmoplegia in four of five patients (Antonyshyn 1989b).

Strabismus, although common in the initial postoperative period, was documented in only 6% of patients on long-term follow-up. The majority of these cases were mild; patients reported diplopia only on extremes of gaze, and there was no objective evidence of restricted ocular motility.

Globe Projection

Enophthalmos presents as an obvious deformity if anterior globe projection is less than 12 millimeters or differs by more than 3 millimeters from the contralateral side, as measured by a Hertel exophthalmometer. Enophthalmos of this degree was documented in 14% of patients with complex fractures. In all cases, residual defects or deformity in the deep aspect of the orbital cavity, posterior to axis of the globe, were identified.

Specifically, failure to identify the posterior bony shelf of the orbital floor and to obliterate skeletal deficiencies completely in the deep inferomedial aspect of the orbital cavity was the most frequently observed problem. Prolapse of orbital contents into the ethmoid or maxillary sinuses at this site invariably resulted in significant retrodisplacement of the globe. The incidence of enophthalmos was also greater in those cases in whom conchal cartilage grafts were used to bridge orbital defects. Cartilage is felt to provide insufficient support to orbital contents in moderate and large defects and has therefore been abandoned in the reconstruction of complex injuries.

Ocular Position in the Coronal Plane

The position of the globe in a horizontal and vertical plane is determined by both the adequacy of support for orbital contents at or anterior to the axis of the globe and the relative volumes and locations of grafts in this area. Failure to taper or contour grafts sufficiently, particularly along the anterior segment of the medial orbital wall and floor will result in exaggerated superior or lateral displacement of the globe.

Canthal Relations

The average distance of the medial canthus to the midline in 49 reconstructed orbits was 16.3 millimeters, well within normal limits (Antonyshyn 1989a). However, it is important to note that asymmetry in the canthal positions is more visually disturbing than are mild degrees of telecanthus. Telecanthus is therefore considered a significant deformity if there is either an asymmetry of more than 2 millimeters or an absolute distance of 20 millimeters or greater from the midline. Telecanthus of this degree was noted in 12% of patients, and in each case this was attributed to canthal drift in the early postoperative period.

Although specific causative factors were often difficult to identify, canthopexy wires were observed to have pulled through at the proximal tendinous insertion or the distal bony fixation point.

Palpebral Relations

The relative positions of the medial and lateral canthi determine the width and inclination of the palpebral fissures. Mild degrees of malposition of the medial canthus in the vertical dimension produce very obvious deformities. A vertical asymmetry of the medial canthal position was noted in 4% of cases, and in 8% of patients an antimongoloid slant of the palpebral fissure was readily apparent. A discrepancy in palpebral fissure inclination associated with lateral canthal dystopia was further documented in 10% of patients.

Nasolacrimal Drainage

Epiphora was commonly observed in the initial postoperative period but was a persistent problem in only 6% of patients. Obstruction of the nasolacrimal duct was found to be the causative factor in two patients; the third patient developed epiphora secondary to cicatricial ectropion.

CONCLUSION

The routine application of craniofacial techniques, rigid skeletal fixation, and primary bone grafting permits accurate one-stage skeletal reconstruction of virtually any orbital injury. Long-term follow-up indicates that facial symmetry and the three-dimensional positioning of the ocular globe can be successfully re-established, provided that the normal skeletal anatomy of the orbital framework is reconstituted. Residual deformities generally are caused by technical errors in the reduction or fixation of orbital rim segments or in the contouring and placement of grafts within the orbital cavity. Most important, failure to reposition and fix the periorbital soft tissues can result in significant deformity, despite accurate skeletal reconstruction. An appreciation of the anatomy of the normal orbit and meticulous reattachment of the medial and lateral canthi and the cheek tissues optimize both the morphological and the functional results.

REFERENCES

Antonyshyn O, Gruss JS, Galbraith DJ, Hurwitz JJ: Complex orbital fractures: A critical analysis of immediate bone graft reconstruction. Ann Plast Surg 22(3): 220–233, 1989a.

Antonyshyn O, Gruss JS, Kassel EE: Blow-in fractures of the orbit. Plast Reconstr Surg 84(1):10–20, 1989b.

Gruss JS: Fronto-naso-orbital trauma. Clin Plast Surg 9:557, 1982.

Gruss JS: Naso-ethmoid-orbital fractures: Classification and role of primary bone grafting. Plast Reconstr Surg 75:303, 1985.

Gruss JS, Van Wyck L, Phillips JH, Antonyshyn O: The importance of the zygomatic arch in complex midfacial fracture repair and correction of post-traumatic orbitozygomatic deformities. Plast Reconstr Surg 85:878, 1990.

Jabaley ME, Lerman M, Sanders HJ: Ocular injuries in orbital fractures: A review of 119 cases. Plast Reconstr Surg (456):410–418, 1975.

Jackson IT: Classification and treatment of orbitozygomatic and orbitoethmoid fractures. Clin Plast Surg (116):77–91, 1989.

Paskert JP, Manson PN, Iliff NT: Nasoethmoid and orbital fractures. Clin Plast Surg 15(2):209–223, 1988.

Pearl RM: Surgical management of volumetric changes in the bony orbit. Ann Plast Surg 19(4):349–358, 1987.

CHAPTER
24

Reconstruction of the Internal Orbit Using Rigid Fixation Techniques

Michael J. Yaremchuk
Paul N. Manson

Alterations in the configuration of the bony internal orbit, rather than changes in the amount or character of its soft-tissue contents, are now known to be primarily responsible for posttraumatic enophthalmos. The anatomic reconstruction of the internal orbit can, therefore, predictably restore the position of the globe. Practically, this requires identification and replacement of the disrupted areas using adjacent intact bone as both a point of reference and one of stability for reconstruction. Injuries involving two, three, or four orbital walls are inevitably accompanied by distortion of the orbital rims, and this complicates this strategy. Limited exposure, fragile bony remnants, and the complex configuration of the internal orbit make accurate placement of grafts difficult and displacement common. Fortunately, the application of plate and screw concepts can obviate many of the problems intrinsic to internal orbit reconstruction. Custom metal implants can be contoured appropriately, fixated to stable portions of the orbit, and used to replace missing segments or, more commonly, can act as a stable construct for autogenous bone grafts. In addition to facilitating anatomic reconstruction, the use of implants decreases the amount of autogenous bone used, thereby lessening the effects of graft resorption and increasing the predictability of the end result.

ANATOMIC CONSIDERATIONS

The internal orbit may be conceptualized as a modified pyramid whose walls protect and support the globe. The walls vary in thickness, and their unique curvatures determine the patterns of fracture and subsequent deformity. The lateral wall consists of the substantial bone of the greater wing of the sphenoid and orbital process of the zygoma. The orbital roof, the medial wall, and floor can be divided into thirds based on bone thickness (see Figure 24.1). The anterior third consists of thick bone. Immediately behind the orbital rim, the anterior third of the orbit has a concave shape, and so the widest orbital diameter is approximately 1.5 centimeters within the orbital cavity. The posterior third also consists of thick bone with relatively flat walls (see Figure 24.2). The middle third consists of thin bone that acts as a crush zone, thus protecting the globe and optic nerve by absorbing impact forces. The floor medial to the infraorbital canal and the inferior portion of the medial wall is involved in the classic blow-out fracture. This area has a convex shape that produces a constriction behind the globe. Loss of this convexity transforms the internal orbital shape from pyramidal to spherical, increasing orbital volume and tending toward enophthalmos (see Figures 24.3 and 24.4).

When two to four walls of the anterior and middle orbit are disrupted, it is very difficult to find stable bone inferiorly, medially, and posteriorly on which to posi-

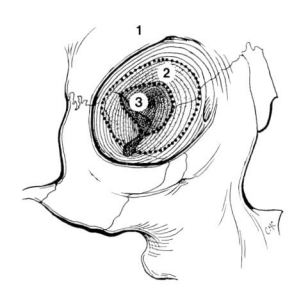

Figure 24.1 Orbit divided into concentric thirds based on bone thickness.

Figure 24.2 Left cadaver orbit with the middle third of the medial orbital floor removed. (a) Panoramic view. (b) Close-up shows a marked increase in bone thickness in the posterior third of the orbit.

Figure 24.3 Orbit with cross section showing the convex shape of the medial floor and medial wall in the middle third of the orbit. Fractures and loss of convexity increase orbital volume.

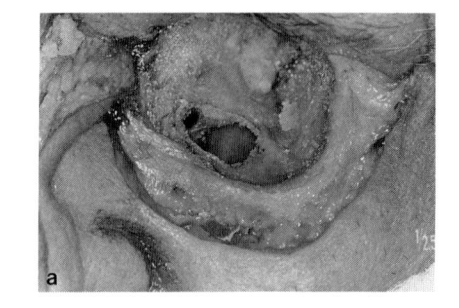

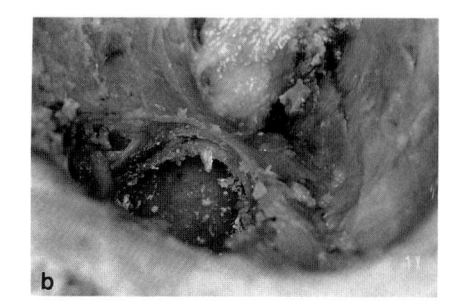

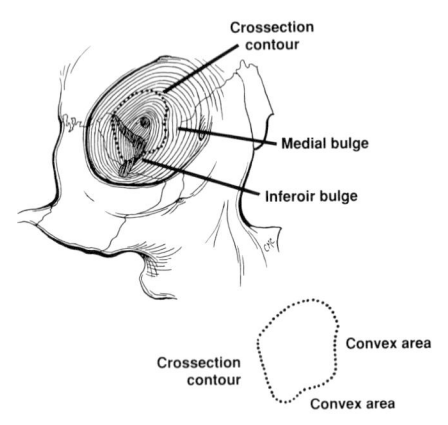

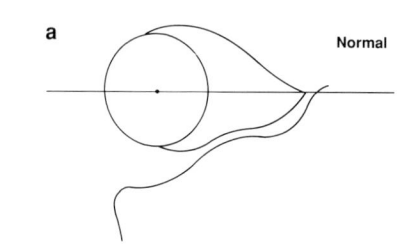

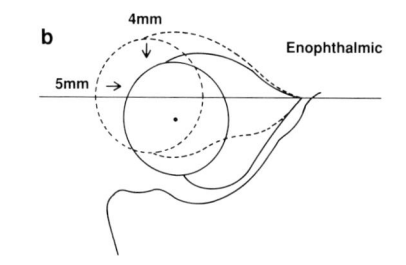

Figure 24.4 Sagittal section of orbit. (a) Intact. (b) Loss of convexity of the floor increases orbital volume and tends toward enophthalmos.

tion bone grafts when reconstructing the internal orbit. This lack of support explains the tendency for bone grafts to displace into the maxillary and ethmoid sinuses. In addition, the postbulbar constriction is difficult to reconstruct with bone grafts alone. Spanning the inferomedial portion of the internal orbit with metal implants provides a stable construct to allow accurate restoration of the anatomy of the internal orbital.

DIAGNOSIS

Patients with injuries to two, three, or four walls often present with obvious globe malposition. For these and more subtle injuries, plain x rays will confirm the presence of fractures but cannot define the extent of injury or the status of the orbital soft tissues. High-resolution computerized tomographic (CT) scanning is key in defining the injury to the orbit and surrounding structures. The ideal preoperative evaluation consists of both axial and coronal sections using both bone and soft-tissue windows. The information obtained is used to plan the surgical approach and the manner of reconstruction. Postoperative CT scans are helpful in defining the adequacy of reduction and accuracy of reconstruction. Both preoperatively and postoperatively, comparison of the orbits is useful.

Three-dimensional images are reconstructed or averaged from multiple two-dimensional images. The inevitable loss of detail limits the role of three-dimensional images in the evaluation of the inner orbit.

TREATMENT

The restoration of proper globe position requires exposure and anatomic reconstruction of all disrupted areas. Craniofacial approaches afford extended exposure of both the external and internal orbit. We prefer the blepharoplasty subciliary skin muscle flap to approach the orbital floor and lower medial and lateral walls. The coronal flap is used to approach the upper medial and lateral walls as well as the orbital roof. Extensive subperiosteal dissection of the lateral orbit will detach the lateral canthus which should be repositioned at closure. Extensive subperiosteal dissection of the lateral orbit will detach the lateral canthal tendon which should be repositioned at closure.

Reconstruction begins with the anatomic repositioning of the orbital rims. The position is stabilized with plates and screws. Because a small change in rim position leads to a large change in orbital volume, accurate rim positioning is an important first step in the reconstruction of the internal orbit. Keys in accurate

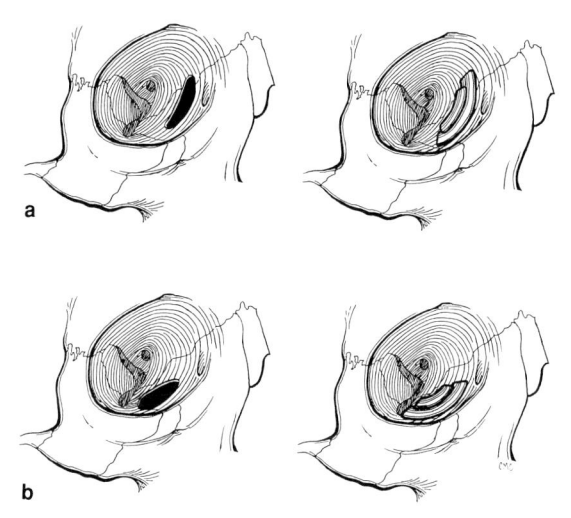

Figure 24.5 Diagram of defects of (a) the medial wall and (b) the floor reconstructed with grafts spanning the defects. Stable adjacent ledges make bone graft positioning relatively straightforward.

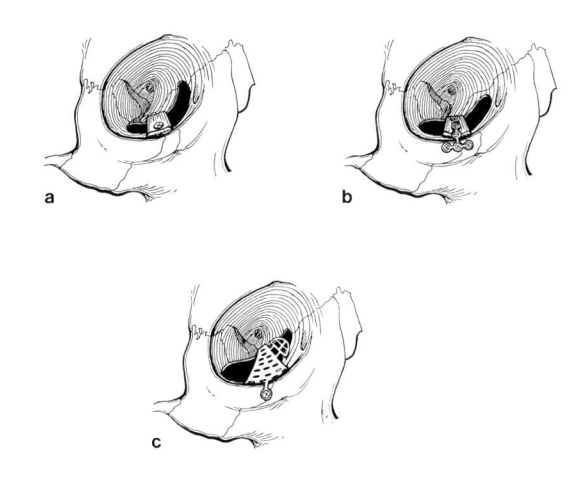

Figure 24.6 Large orbital defects spanned with: (a) bone graft fixated with lag screws, (b) bone graft supported with plates, (c) custom floor plate, which provides a stable construct on which to position a bone graft.

repositioning are the zygomatico-sphenoid articulation and the zygomatic arch. Unlike the narrow zygomatic frontal articulation, the zygoma's articulation with the sphenoid is a relatively long one, making edge-to-edge coaption more likely to reflect proper zygomatic positioning. Proper repositioning of the zygomatic arch assures restoration of facial width (which tends to be increased in these injuries) while, reciprocally, restoring malar projection.

The contents of the orbit are freed from the injured area by subperiosteal dissection. This is performed under loupe magnification, taking care to avoid damage to the lacrimal sac under the attachment of the medial canthus and the inferior orbital fissure. Ideally, intact landmarks should be identified as a basis for orientation and to provide stable constructs on which to position grafts (see Figure 24.5). In extensive injuries, the dissection can be exceptionally difficult. Identification of the posterior ledge is especially important for orientation. This ledge, usually 30 to 38 mm from the inferior orbital rim, may be unstable. Once the prolapsed contents of the orbit are removed from the maxillary ethmoid sinuses, temporarily interposing a piece of Silastic sheeting between the soft tissues and the area to be reconstructed is helpful. This maneuver prevents their falling back into the sinus thereby lessening their subsequent handling and allowing easier control during placement of the implant or graft. Once reconstruction is complete, the Silastic is removed.

Once the area to be reconstructed is defined, a variety of techniques may be employed effectively to divide the defect into smaller, more manageable areas. This includes the use of grafts secured with lag screws, plates, or custom-designed implants (see Figure 24.6). If custom implants will be used (see Figures 24.7 and

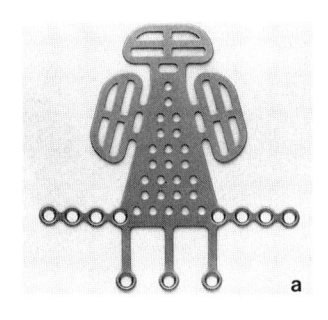

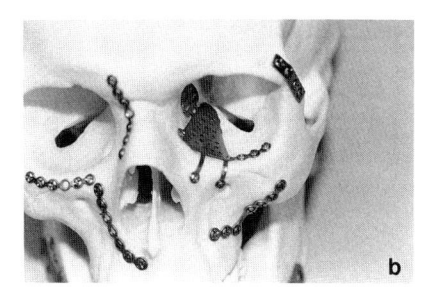

Figure 24.7 Titanium implants designed for internal orbit reconstruction. (a) This implant is designed with multiple flanges, allowing custom adaptation by bending or removal. (b) Implant in place in a dry specimen. It can be fixed to either the inner or outer aspect of the orbital rim using 1.5-millimeter screws.

24.8), an aluminum template may be adapted to simulate the necessary size and curvature. The properly adapted permanent implant is fixated to the inferior orbital rim or to the anterolateral internal orbit. The implant alone may be used to restore the internal orbital contour or, preferably, is used as a stable platform on which to place grafts (see Figure 24.9). Implants are particularly helpful in reconstruction of the convex inferomedial portion of the middle third of the orbit. Their

Figure 24.8 Vitallium implant designed for reconstruction of the internal orbit. (a) Large sheet of micromesh, which is adapted from (adjacent) microplate design. (b) Bending forceps used to contour the mesh. (c) Custom-cut and adapted mesh fixed to the intraorbital rim of a dry specimen using 0.8-millimeter screws.

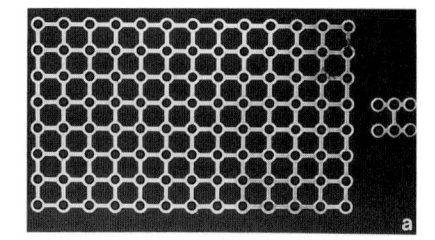

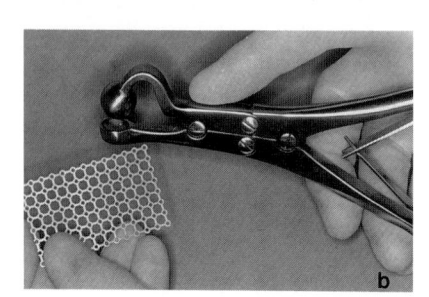

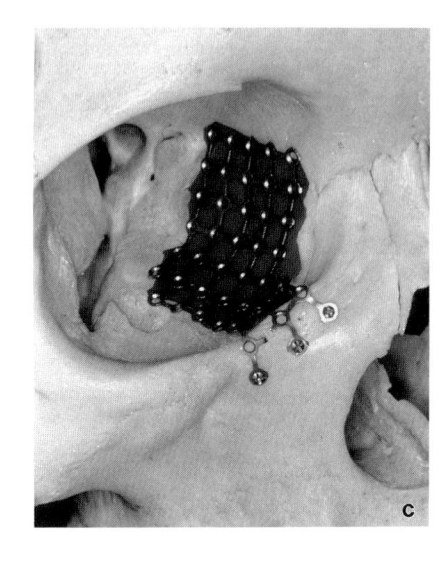

Figure 24.9 Pre- and postoperative x rays of patient who underwent internal orbit reconstruction to correct a traumatic enophthalmos. A Vitallium mesh plate was used to support cranial bone grafts. (a) Preoperative axial computerized tomogram shows blowout fractures of orbital floor and medial orbital wall. (b) Postoperative axial computerized tomogram shows reconstruction. Anatomy of internal orbit now mimics that on the right. (c) Lateral x ray shows position of floor plate.

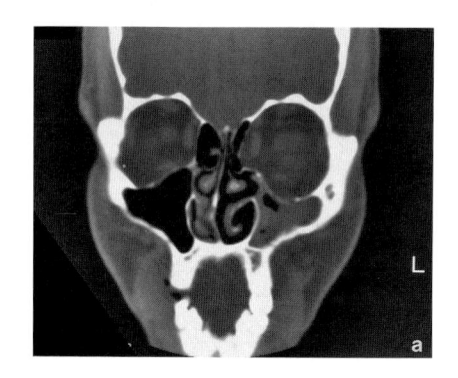

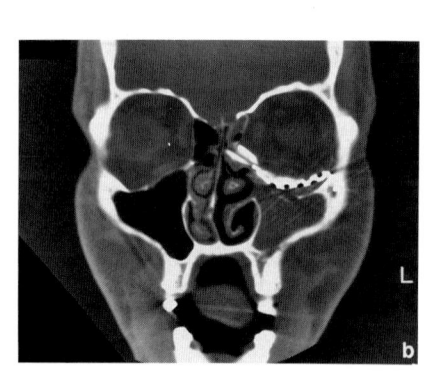

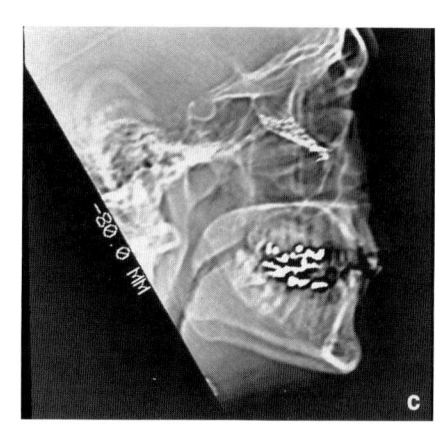

use in this area effectively transforms a single large defect into two smaller ones, which are easier to reconstruct. Metallic implants may be similarly used for late orbital reconstruction, which may require osteotomies for exposure and reconstruction.

RESULTS AND COMPLICATIONS

Metal implants have been used for both acute and late orbital reconstructions in over 75 cases. The infection rate, approximately 2%, has been associated with maxillary sinus obstruction. Despite the perforations in the implant, which may influence healing of orbital soft tissue, eye position and eye movement have not been adversely affected. Placement of bone grafts as an interface between the implants and the orbital soft tissue is recommended to avoid this problem. The persistence of grafts does not seem to be affected adversely when they are used in combination with implants.

Figures 24.10, 24.11, and 25.9 (Chapter 25) present cases in which implants have been used for reconstruction of the internal orbit.

CONCLUSION

Rigid fixation has proven to be an important adjunct in the reconstruction of the severely damaged internal orbit. It provides a stable support that otherwise

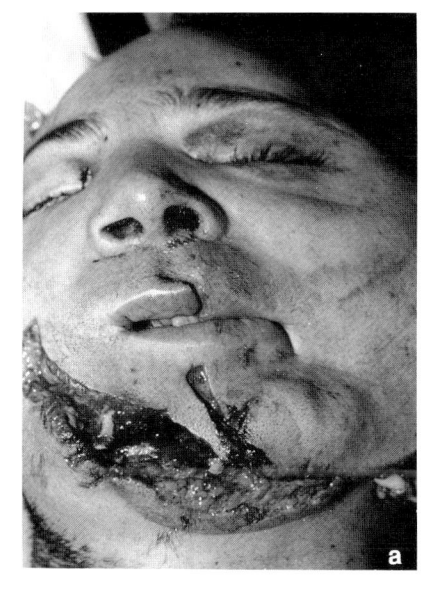

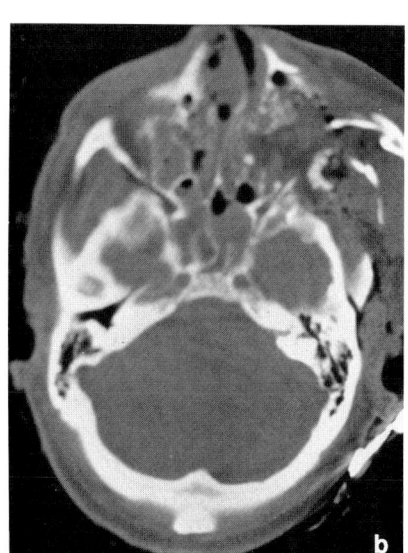

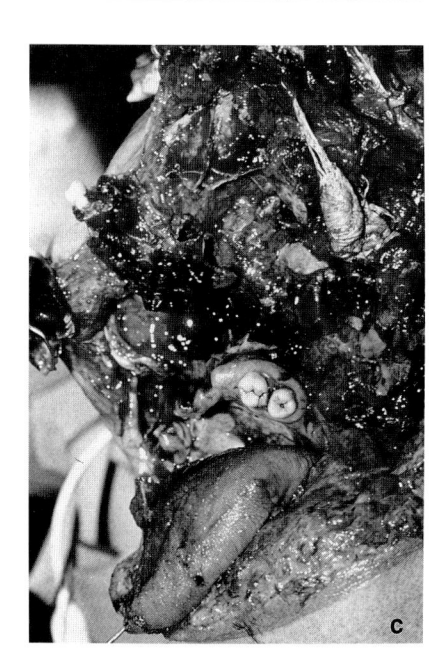

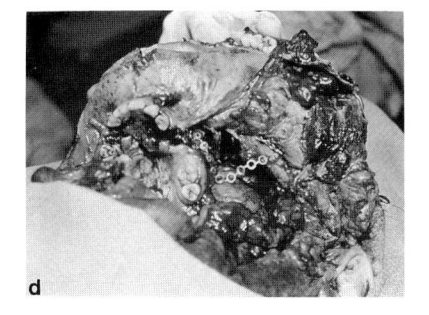

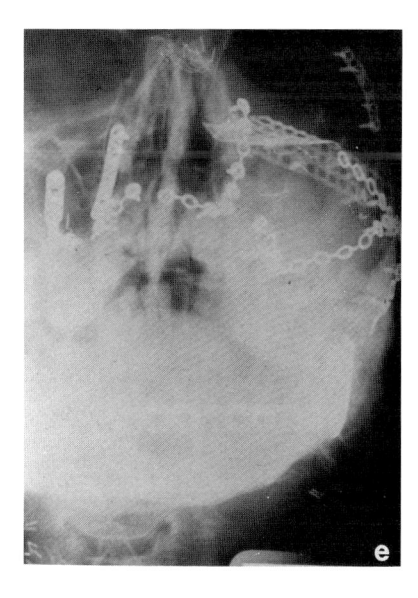

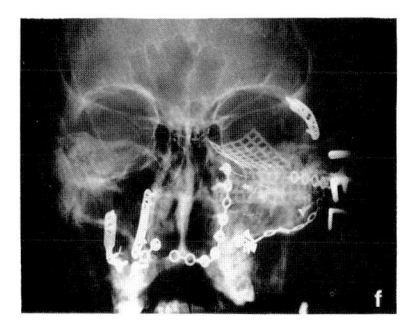

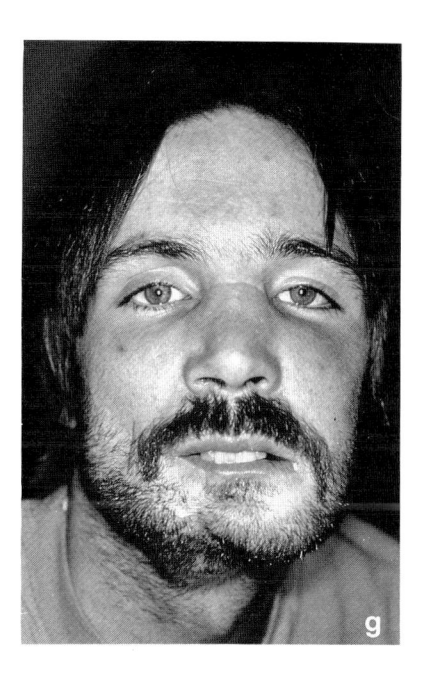

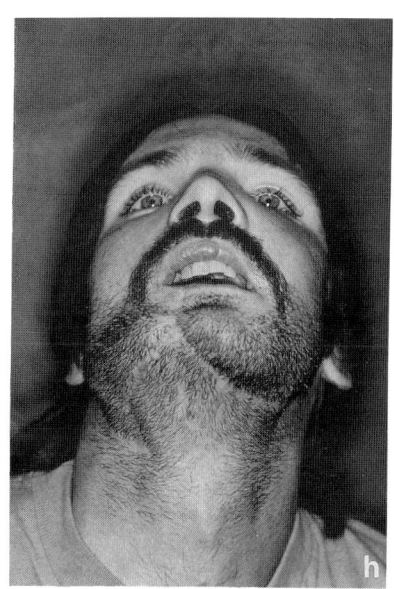

Reconstruction of the Internal Orbit Using Rigid Fixation Techniques

Figure 24.10 A devastating facial injury suffered in a motor vehicle accident. (a) Appearance on admission. (b) The axial CT showed marked disruption of the facial skeleton with three-wall orbital injuries. (c) Lateral view of face at the time of operation after the flap has been reflected to the patient's right to reflect common nasal, oral, maxillary, and orbital cavities. (d) Plate and screw reconstruction of the facial skeleton. TiMesh was used to reconstruct the floor. (e) Postoperative x ray, Waters view. (f) AP view. (g) Appearance two years postoperatively. (h) Worm's eye view.

Figure 24.11 (a) MVA victim with Le Fort and left three-wall injury. (b) CT view. (c) This intraoperative view shows marked disruption of the maxilla and lower orbit. (d) This intraoperative view shows a plate being attached to the infraorbital rim. (e) Appearance six months postoperatively, AP. Note increase in scleral show and displacement of cheek soft-tissue mass secondary to post-traumatic scarring and failure to resuspend cheek soft tissues. (f) Worm's eye view.

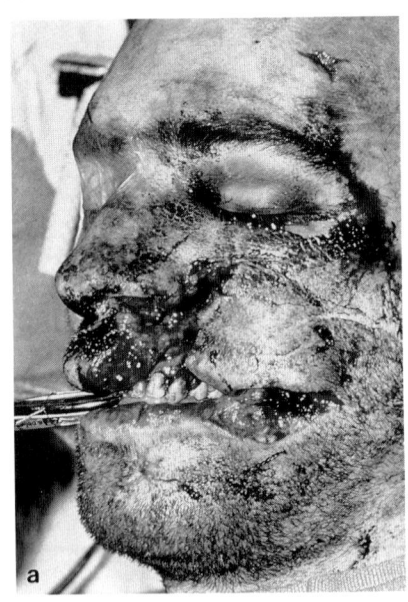

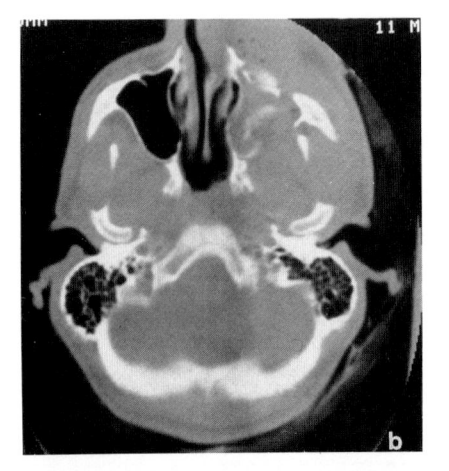

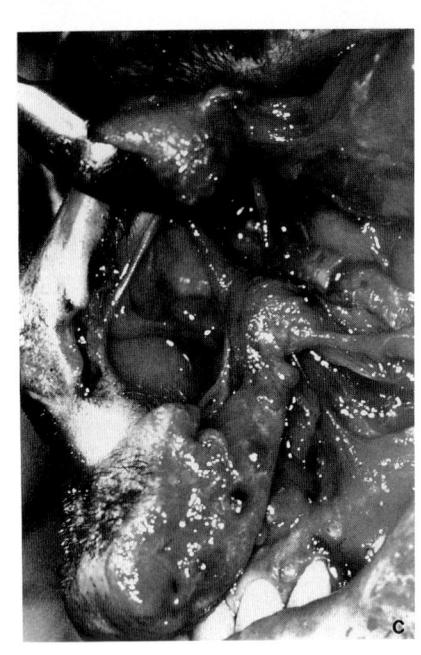

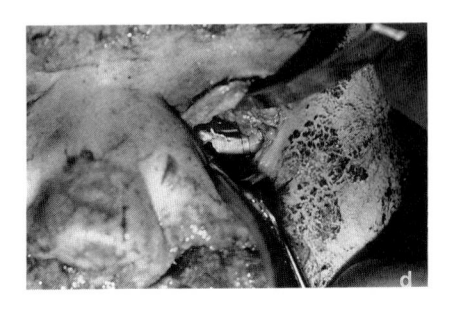

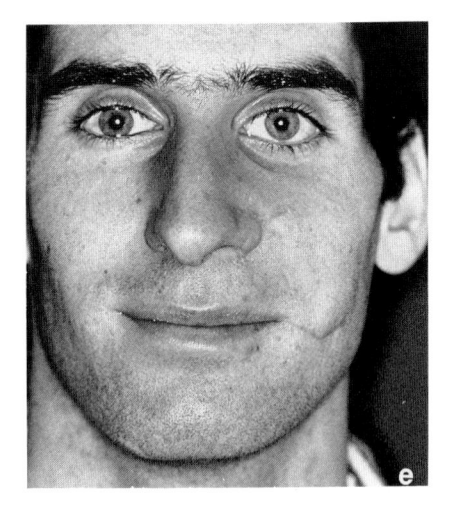

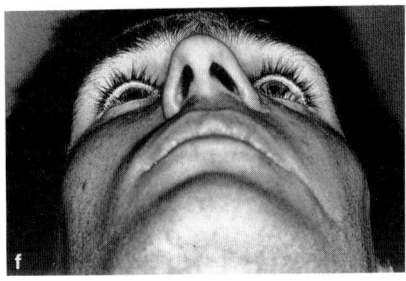

may be difficult or impossible to obtain. In effect, rigid fixation allows large defects to be converted into more easily manageable smaller ones.

BIBLIOGRAPHY

Bite U, Jackson IT, Forbes GS, et al: Orbital measurements in enophthalmos using three dimensional CT imaging. Plast Reconstr Surg 75:502, 1985.

Converse JM, Cole G, Smith B: Late treatment of blowout fractures of the floor of the orbit. Plast Reconstr Surg 28:183, 1961.

Glassman RD, Manson PN, Petty P, et al: Techniques for improved visibility and lid protection in orbital explorations. J Craniofac Surg 1:69, 1990.

Glassman RD, Manson PN, Vanderkolk CA, et al: Rigid fixation of internal orbital fractures. Plast Reconstr Surg 86:1103, 1990.

Kawamoto HK: Late post-traumatic enophthalmos: A correctable deformity? Plast Reconstr Surg 69: 423, 1982.

Manson PN, Clifford CM, Su CT, Iliff N: Mechanisms of global support and post-traumatic enophthalmos: I. The anatomy of the ligament sling and its relation to intramuscular cone orbital fat. Plast Reconstr Surg 77:193, 1985.

Manson PN, Grivas A, Rosenbaum A, Vannier M, Zinreich J, Iliff N: Studies on enophthalmos: II. The measurement of orbital injuries and their treatment by quantitative computed tomography. Plast Reconstr Surg 77:203, 1986.

Manson PN, Ruas E, Iliff N: Single eyelid incision for exposure of the zygomatic bone and orbital reconstruction. Plast Reconstr Surg 76:1, 1985.

Putterman AM, Stevens T, Urist MJ: Nonsurgical management of blow-out fractures of the orbital floor. Amer J Ophth 77:232, 1974.

CHAPTER 25

Rigid Fixation of Frontal Bone Fractures

Michael J. Yaremchuk
Paul N. Manson

A consensus has not been reached regarding the treatment of frontal bone fractures. A lack of unanimity exists for several reasons. Injuries to the frontobasilar area are relatively uncommon because high-energy forces are required for their production; hence few individuals have much experience in their treatment. Furthermore, this area is an anatomically complex one where multiple surgical specialties interface. The tendency has long been to segment treatment rather than to integrate the best possible management of the dura, sinuses, and fronto-orbital contour. The treatment regimen presented in this chapter is the one favored in our units. It addresses this area in a reliable, consistent manner; rigid fixation techniques are the key to restoring and maintaining the pre-injury anatomy.

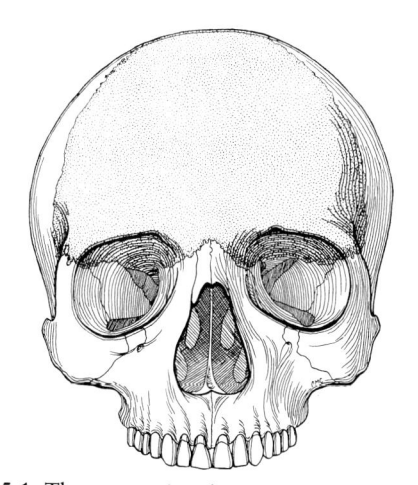

Figure 25.1 The anatomic relationships of the frontal bone.

ANATOMY

The frontal bone is the most anterior portion of the cranium. It forms the roof and portions of the medial and lateral walls of the orbit. In the superior lateral orbit it articulates with the greater wing of the sphenoid and the frontal process of the zygoma. In the medial orbit it articulates with the ethmoid, lacrimal, and frontal process of the maxillary bones. In the midline it articulates with the nasal bones. Laterally it articulates with the temporal bone and posteriorly, with the parietal (see Figure 25.1).

The anterior face of the frontal bone can be divided into central (frontal sinus) and lateral (fronto-temporo-orbital) regions (see Figure 25.2). The frontal sinuses are paired structures divided roughly into halves.

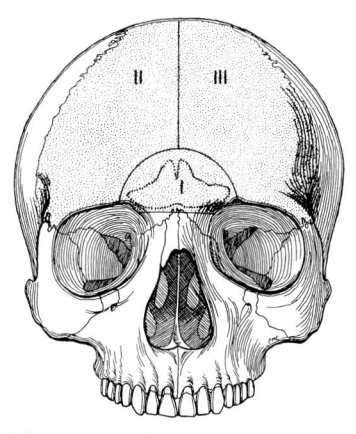

Figure 25.2 The anterior face of the frontal bone may be conceptually divided into central (sinus) (I) and lateral (fronto-temporo-orbital) (II,III) regions.

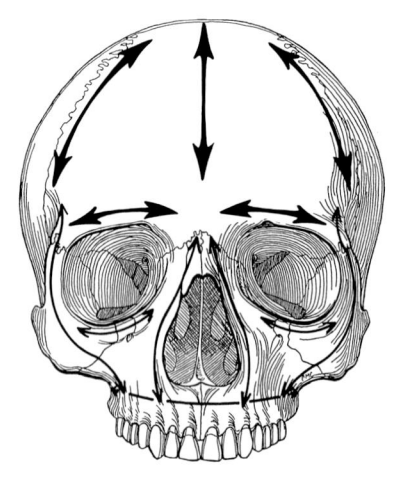

Figure 25.3 Similar to the face, the cranium has a structural framework, or buttresses, of thickened, folded, and therefore more dense, bone.

These sinuses lie between the inner and outer lamellae of the frontal bone. Their lesser thickness makes them more susceptible to fracture than the adjacent lateral temporo-orbital areas, which are composed of two thicknesses of bone. The supraorbital ridges, whose folded configuration makes for a considerable thickness of cortical bone, are buttresses of high resistance. The skull vault has a structural framework of thickened, folded, and dense bone between which are thin non–stress-bearing plates of bone that are protective in function. The arrangement of these arches and buttresses, together with the intensity and direction of impact, determines the fracture patterns of the skull (see Figure 25.3).

DIAGNOSIS

Suspicions of a frontobasilar fracture should be raised with any facial bruise or laceration, ocular injury, brain impairment, or fracture of adjacent facial bone. Frontal contusions, lacerations, and periorbital ecchymosis and hematoma may be signs of underlying fractures. Palpable deformities are prima facie evidence of fracture.

Radiographic examination is key in making the diagnosis. Waters, Caldwell, and lateral skull x rays are useful. However, bone overlap, suture lines, and vessel grooves may be misleading. Today, computerized tomography (CT) is the gold standard for diagnosis and assessment of injuries to the vault and the intracranial structures. Axial scans will reveal virtually all fractures save those of the orbital roof. This structure lies in an axial plane and is therefore best assessed with coronal views.

INDICATIONS FOR SURGERY

Surgical treatment of frontobasilar injuries may be undertaken to address dural tear or brain injury, to avoid early or late morbidity from frontal sinus dysfunction, or to avoid deformity. In our units, patients with pneumocephalus or cerebrospinal rhinorrhea accompanying a dislocated fracture of the frontal skull or a displaced posterior-wall sinus fracture undergo dural exploration and repair. Fractures involving the fronto-temporo-orbital area, not requiring neurosurgical intervention per se, are managed surgically if displacement will result in significant contour deformity or globe malposition. Fractures involving the frontal sinus are addressed if they are open or displaced, if they are associated with lateral fractures requiring repair, if they are associated with neurosurgical injury requiring intervention, or if they are shown to result in drainage dysfunction as evidenced by follow-up radiographic exam.

SURGICAL TECHNIQUE

Exposure

A bicoronal incision is preferred for its provision of unparalleled exposure for both neurosurgeons and craniofacial surgeons. It also provides access to cranial bone grafts, provides a panoramic view to compare for symmetry, and leaves an inconspicuous scar. Pre-existing lacerations, which rarely provide sufficient exposure without significant extension, are avoided unless the lacerations are so extensive as to compromise a potential bicoronal flap. We have been dissatisfied with the postoperative appearance of the eyebrow incision and therefore avoid its use. Neurosurgical exploration, if required, is usually done with the exposure and control provided by a frontal craniotomy and bone flap. Dural repairs are intended to provide a watertight seal.

Management of Frontal Sinus Fractures

The management of fractures involving the frontal sinus is controversial. With the exception of isolated anterior wall fractures where nasofrontal duct dysfunction is unlikely and whose therapy consists of replacing the fragments anatomically, our preference is based on the primary objective of isolating the cranial cavity from the nose and defunctionalizing the sinus (see Figure 25.4). In all cases this involves first removing or exenterating all sinus mucosa. This is done under loupe magnification using a high speed bur under constant irrigation to avoid leaving mucosal remnants or the potential for mucosal regrowth. The other common step is the mechanical isolation from the nose provided by a bone graft precisely sculpted to plug each nasofrontal duct. Only when the posterior wall is badly disrupted is it removed, thereby "cranializing" the frontal sinus. If it is intact, the sinus cavity is "obliterated" with autogenous bone. Depending on the size of the sinus and

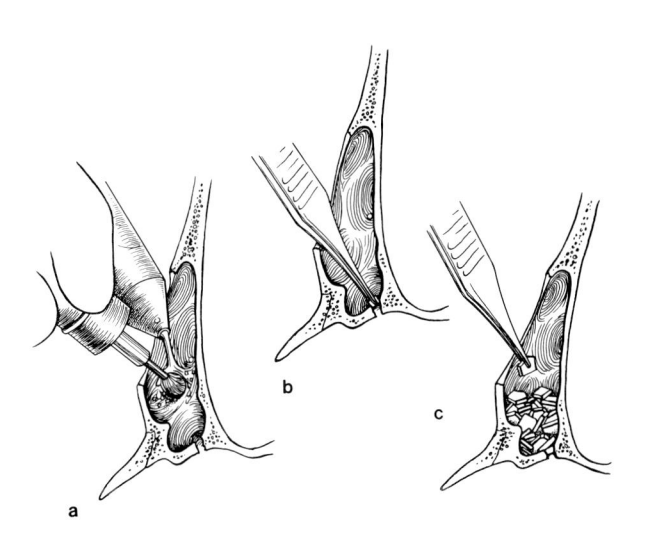

Figure 25.4 Surgical management of the frontal sinus. (a) Exenteration of sinus mucosa. (b) Plugging nasofrontal ducts with custom-fit graft plugs. (c) Obliteration of sinus with autogenous bone.

the amount of graft required to fill it, graft material consists of calvarial shavings or pieces of membranous bone from the iliac crest. We believe the bone that is not revascularized early has the potential for later replacement by the process of creeping substitution. It has never been our custom to use fat or alloplasts as obliterative materials. When the cranial base is severely disrupted, pericranial and galeal frontalis flaps can be useful in assuring a seal between the intracranial and nasal cavities. One should anticipate a slight depression at the frontalis muscle donor site. Implicit in this discussion of our approach is that no attempts are made to restore sinus function or nasofrontal duct patency.

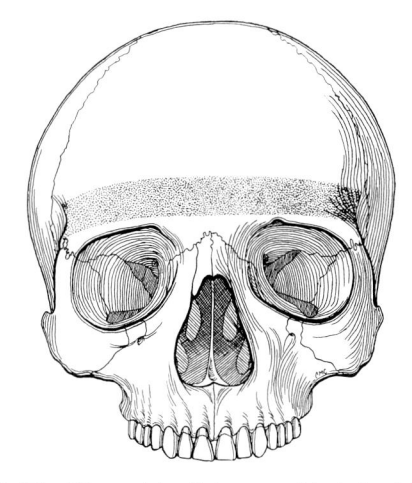

Figure 25.5 The "frontal bar" (supraorbital rims) is key in restoring pre-injury anatomy.

Reconstruction of Frontal Bone

The reconstructive goal is to restore the fronto-orbital contour to its pre-injury appearance. The safety of frontal bone replacement or acute bone grafting for replacement of severely comminuted segments is related to the condition of the overlying skin, the presence of "dead space," and sinus involvement. To avoid infection and problems with wound healing, the surgeon must establish a surgically clean wound with respect to skin, bone, and sinuses; then the frontal and paranasal sinuses must be effectively isolated from the intracranial dead space.

The "frontal bar" (supraorbital rims) is key in restoring the pre-injury anatomy in three dimensions (see Figure 25.5). In panfacial injuries, the temporal buttresses serve as guides for midfacial width and projection. Fracture segments are first linked with interfragmentary wires. When the final position is determined, it is maintained with rigid fixation. Without plate and screw fixation, multiply wired bone segments tend to sink posteriorly and inferiorly, thereby losing projection (see Figure 25.6). The loss of bone at fracture

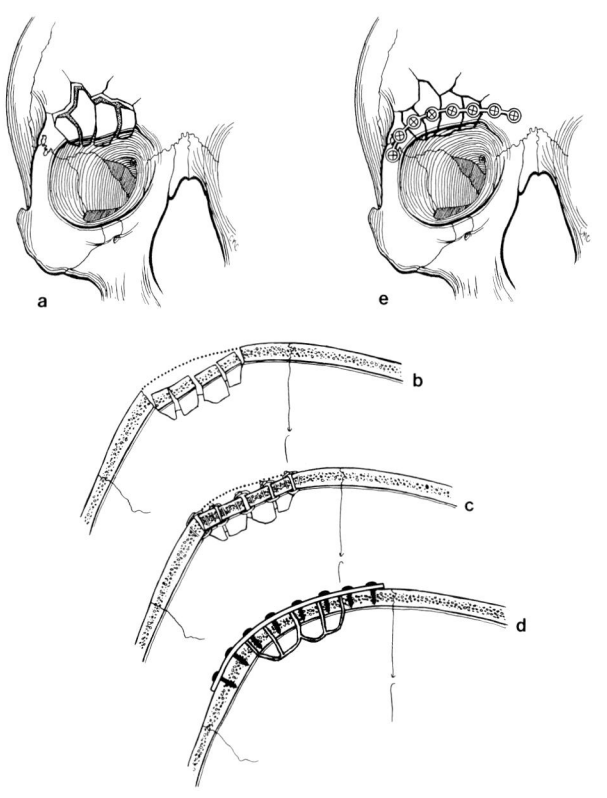

Figure 25.6 (a) Comminuted lateral frontal injury. (b) Axial view showing how comminuted fracture segments tend to collapse, thereby losing projection. (c) Interfragmentary wire fixation maintains alignment of fracture segments but fails to restore pre-injury projection. (d) Plate and screw fixation allows restoration and maintenance of frontal contour. Note that small gaps between fracture segments are maintained. (e) Frontal view.

Figure 25.7 Intraoperative view of comminuted depressed central and lateral frontal fractures. (a) Prior to reduction. (b) Because the fracture extended into the nasal frontal duct, the entire frontal sinus was exenterated and obliterated with calvarial bone after the nasofrontal ducts were plugged with custom-fit bone grafts. The comminuted fracture segments were replaced with calvarial bone harvested from the outer table and fixed with microplates.

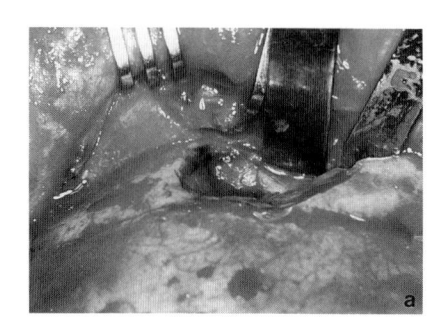

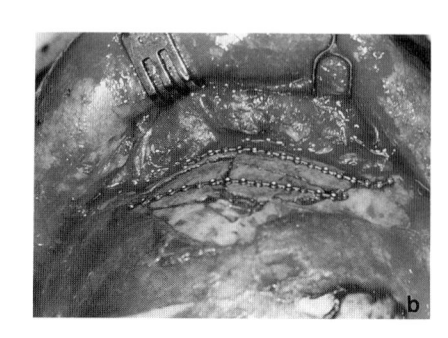

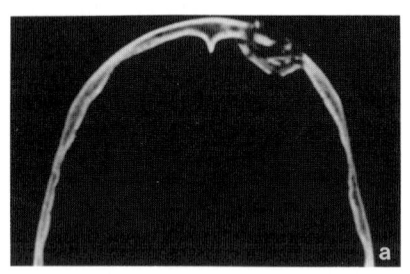

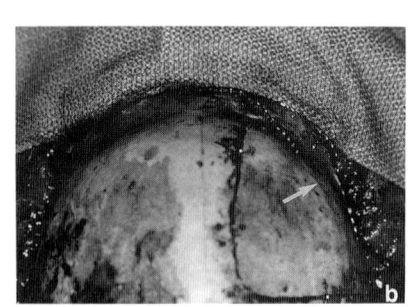

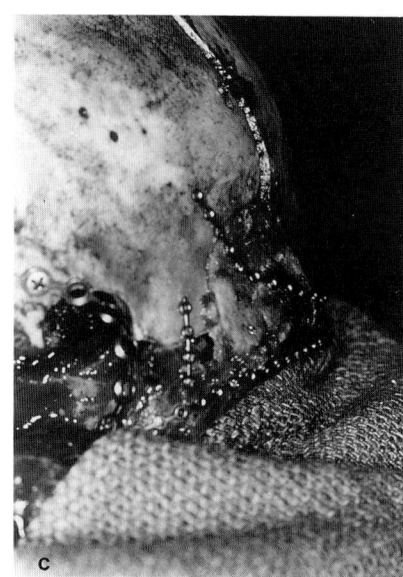

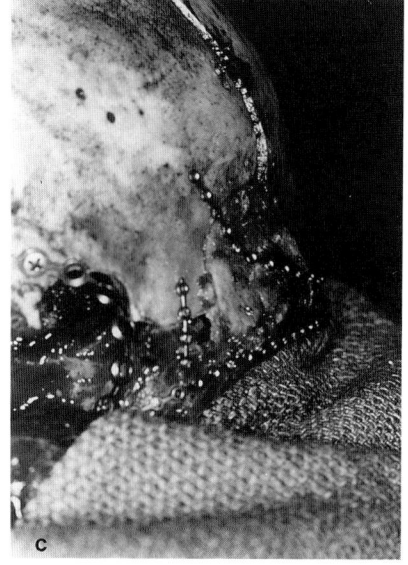

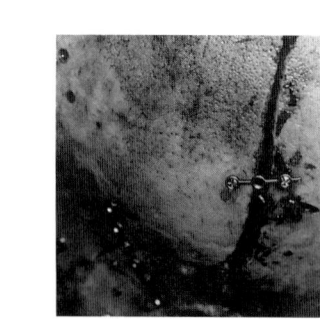

Figure 25.8 X-ray and intraoperative views of a finely comminuted lateral frontal injury. (a) Preoperative axial CT. (b) This panoramic view from above shows the overall symmetry of reconstruction obtained by replacing salvageable frontal bone fragments and replacing unusable portions with cranial bone obtained from the inner table of the frontal bone flap. (Arrow points to reconstructed area.) (c) This lateral view of reconstruction shows the use of microplates. (d) This close-up view of part (c) shows microlag fixation of onlay cranial bone grafts to restore frontal bossing. (e) This close-up shows frontal bone flap replacement fixated with microplate instead of wires. Three millimeter screws purchase the outer table to maintain the space created by a neurosurgical bone cut.

sites, and particularly by bone cuts made for neurosurgical exposure, decreases available bone length and aggravates this problem. Precise restoration of pre-injury contour usually requires realignment and fixation of fracture segments without bone to bone contact. When fracture segments are too small to be reassembled, they are replaced with autogenous bone harvested from the outer table of uninjured parts of the cranium, or from the inner table of bone flaps removed for neurosurgical access (see Figures 25.7, 25.8). Less commonly, ribs are harvested for reconstruction.

COMPLICATIONS AND LONG-TERM RESULTS

Clinical examples of frontal fractures managed by the above techniques are shown in Figures 25.9 and 25.10. Frontal sinusitis and mucocele are the most common complications after frontal bone fractures. Meningitis and brain abscess are the dread, but relatively uncommon, complications. Frontal sinusitis and mucocele may result when sinus mucosa continues to function in the face of an obstructed drainage system.

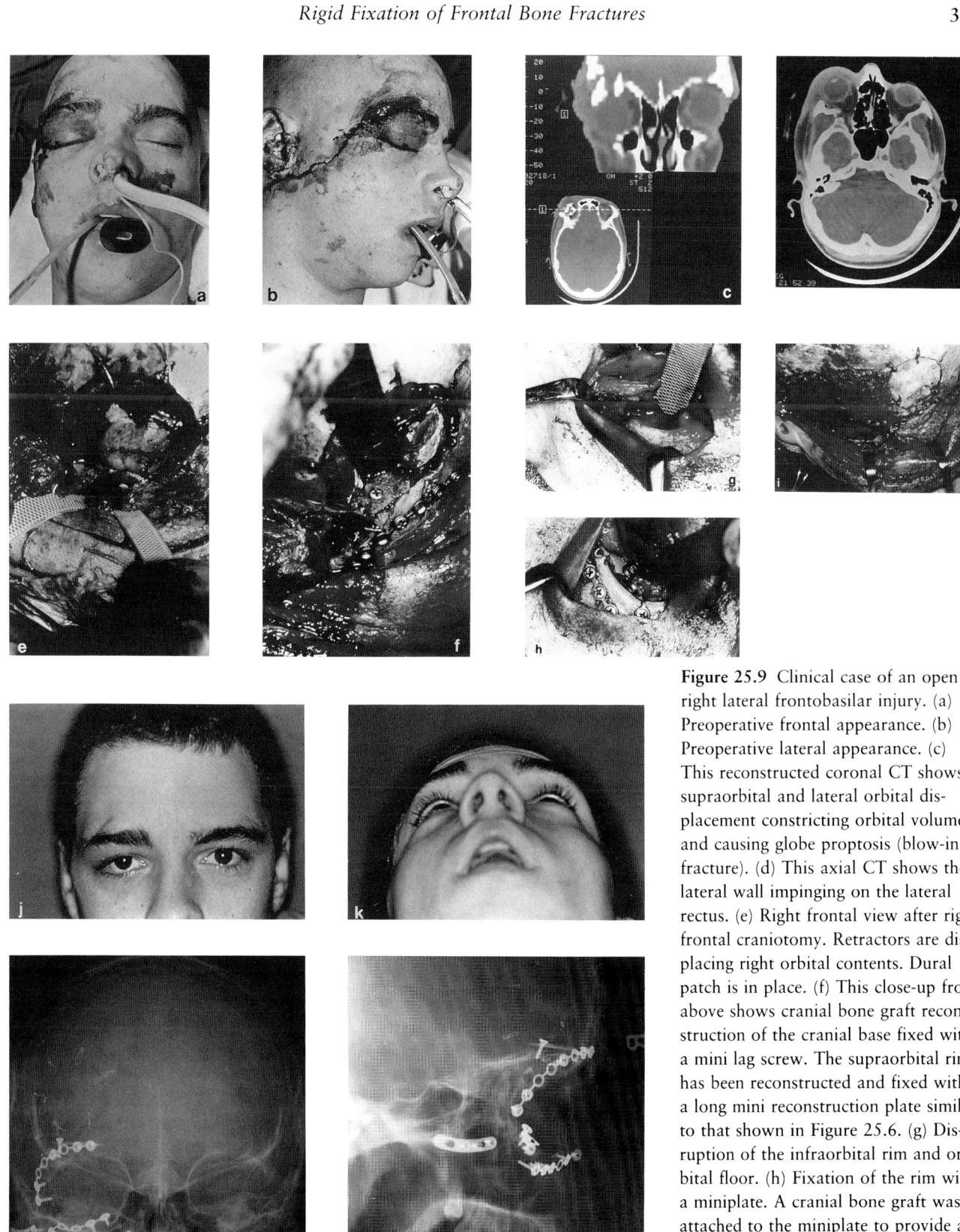

Figure 25.9 Clinical case of an open right lateral frontobasilar injury. (a) Preoperative frontal appearance. (b) Preoperative lateral appearance. (c) This reconstructed coronal CT shows supraorbital and lateral orbital displacement constricting orbital volume and causing globe proptosis (blow-in fracture). (d) This axial CT shows the lateral wall impinging on the lateral rectus. (e) Right frontal view after right frontal craniotomy. Retractors are displacing right orbital contents. Dural patch is in place. (f) This close-up from above shows cranial bone graft reconstruction of the cranial base fixed with a mini lag screw. The supraorbital rim has been reconstructed and fixed with a long mini reconstruction plate similar to that shown in Figure 25.6. (g) Disruption of the infraorbital rim and orbital floor. (h) Fixation of the rim with a miniplate. A cranial bone graft was attached to the miniplate to provide a stable platform to support floor grafts. (i) This panoramic view was taken after the frontal bone had been replaced. (j) Postoperative appearance, frontal view. (k) Postoperative appearance, worm's eye view. (l) Postoperative AP radiograph. (m) Postoperative lateral radiograph.

Figure 25.10 Case of central and lateral frontal fractures after MVA. (a) Preoperative appearance, frontal view. (b) Preoperative appearance, worm's eye view (note the discrepancy in brow position.) (c) This preoperative axial CT shows marked disruption of the anterior table of the frontal sinus. (d) Intraoperative view from above through the coronal exposure. (e) Close-up view of part (d). (f) Panoramic view after anatomic reconstruction and rigid fixation with microplates. The nasal frontal ducts and frontal sinus were obliterated with cranial bone after the sinus mucosa was exenterated. (g) Close-up lateral view of reconstruction. (h) Postoperative frontal view. (i) Postoperative lateral view. (j) Postoperative worm's eye view. (k) Postoperative AP x ray. (l) Postoperative lateral x ray.

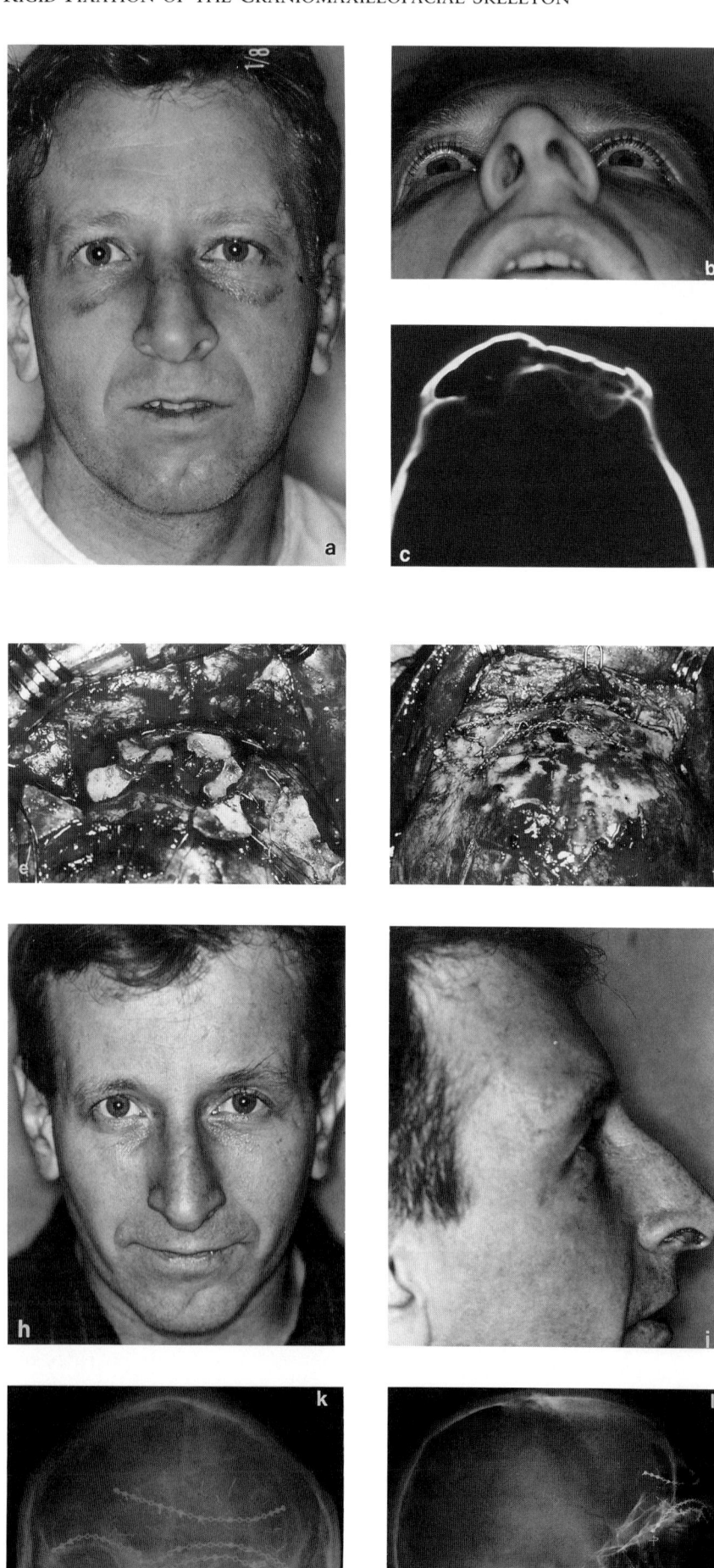

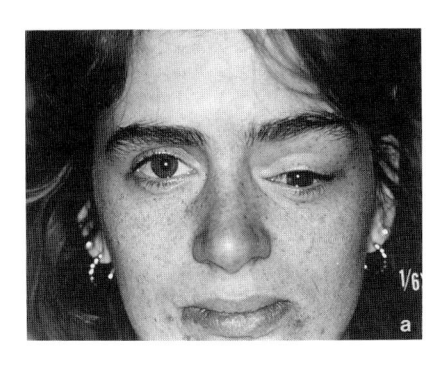

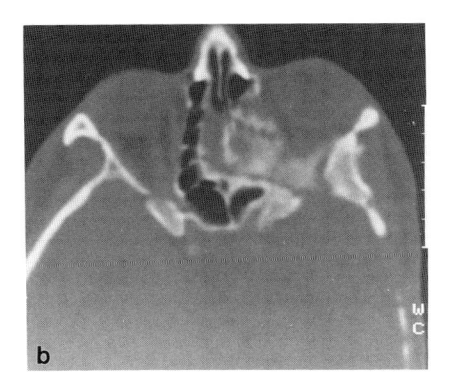

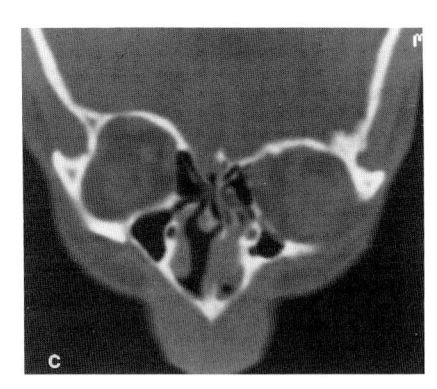

Figure 25.11 (a) This patient presented for secondary reconstruction of a lateral frontal injury. Note the inferior and anterior globe displacement. (b) This axial CT shows marked constriction of the internal orbit with globe proptosis from inferiorly displaced orbital roof fragments (blow-in fracture). (c) This coronal scan shows marked discrepancy of the orbital roof (frontal and sphenoid) position. Restoration of globe position will require intracranial and extracranial exposure.

Meningitis and brain abscess may occur if there is a communication with the frontal sinus. Using the protocol outlined above, in a series of approximately 80 patients with combined central and lateral injuries, we have found the incidence of acute infection to be 6% to 7% and for meningitis to be approximately 3%. Over a five-year period, no patients have returned with late infection or mucocele.

Aesthetic imperfections are related to the surgeon's technical skills and experience. Minor discrepancies in contour can usually be corrected with secondary reduction contouring or onlay augmentation. The most difficult problem to reconstruct secondarily is an inaccurate reconstruction of the orbital roof that causes downward displacement of the globe (see Figure 25.11). Correction of this deformity requires both extracranial and intracranial access. Temporal hollowing has been reduced but not eliminated by the careful reapproximation of the temporalis muscle to the lateral orbital rim.

SUMMARY

Optimal treatment of frontal bone fractures requires a close working relationship between the neurosurgeon and the plastic surgeon. Computerized tomographic scanning is ideal in the preoperative assessment of both brain and skeletal injuries. The bicoronal incision in most cases provides optimal exposure and minimal morbidity. Management of the frontal sinus will depend on the nature of its injury but should isolate the cranial cavity from the nasal cavity. Rigid fixation techniques and acute bone grafting provide the potential for near restoration of the pre-injury contour.

BIBLIOGRAPHY

Donald PJ: The tenacity of frontal sinus mucosa. Otolaryngol Head Neck Surg 87:557, 1979.

Donald PJ, and Ettin M: The safety of frontal sinus fat obliteration when sinus walls are missing. Laryngoscope 96:190, 1986.

Gruss JS, Pollock RA, Phillips JH, and Antonyshyn O: Combined injuries of the cranium and face. Brit J Plast Surg 42:385, 1989.

Larrabee WF, Travis LW, and Tabb HG: Frontal sinus fractures: Their suppurative complications and surgical management. Laryngoscope 90:1810, 1980.

Luce EA: Frontal sinus fractures: Guidelines to management. Plast Reconstr Surg 80:500, 1987.

Lynch RC: The technique of a radical frontal sinus operation which has given the best results. Laryngoscope 31:1, 1921.

Nadell J, Kline DG: Primary reconstruction of depressed frontal skull fractures including those involving the sinus, orbit, and cribiform plate. J Neurosurg 41:200, 1974.

Riedel: Totale Resektion der facialen und orbitales Stirnhohlenwand. In Handbuch der Hals-Nasen-Ohnen Heilkunder, Vol. 2. A. Denker, O. Kahler (eds). Berlin, Springer-Verlag, 1926, pp 806-808.

Stanley RB Jr: Fractures of the frontal sinus. Clin Plast Surg 16:115, 1989.

Wolfe SA, Johnson P: Frontal sinus injuries: Primary care and management of late complications. Plast Reconstr Surg 82:781, 1988.

CHAPTER 26

Rigid Fixation of Panfacial Injuries

Bernard Markowitz

The treatment of panfacial injuries has been revolutionized by the diagnostic and therapeutic advances adapted to facial-trauma care over the past two decades. In the past, management of complex facial fractures was marred by delayed treatment, inaccurate diagnosis, limited exposure, and inadequate stabilization. Facial disfigurement and functional derangement were frequent results. Currently, regional trauma care and the use of computerized tomography (CT), extended open reduction, immediate bone grafting, and rigid internal fixation make possible consistent restoration of the panfacial fracture patient's preoperative facial appearance and function.

DEFINITION

A panfacial injury is a fracture conglomerate that involves the upper, middle, and lower facial regions. Component fractures involve the nose, ethmoids, orbits, zygomas, maxilla, and mandible. Severe displacement and comminution of the bony architecture with extension to the frontal bone and palate are common.

Panfacial fractures occur subsequent to high-energy forces. Patterns of injury are dependent on the direction and force of impact. Central forces typically produce bilateral, comminuted, nasoethmoid-orbital, and Le Fort II fractures with symphyseal and bilateral subcondylar or angle fractures. Frontal sinus and sagittal fractures of the palate may be seen. Laterally directed impacts produce asymmetric nasoethmoid-orbital, midface (higher fracture level on impact side), and mandible fractures. Fractures of the frontotemporal region and maxillary tuberosity are seen with high-energy injuries.

ANATOMY

The adult craniofacial skeleton is composed of 22 bones surrounding the orbits, the pneumatized sinuses, and the nasal, cranial, and oral cavities. The facial skeleton is supported structurally by areas of confluent bony thickenings, or buttresses. These buttresses run vertically, transversely, and in an anteroposterior direction to maintain the facial dimensions of height, width, and projection (see Figure 26.1).

The vertical dimension is maintained by the anterior fronto-nasomaxillary buttresses medially and the fronto-zygomaticomaxillary buttresses laterally. Posterior facial height is dependent on the pterygomaxillary buttresses and the vertical portion of the mandible.

Facial width is divided into central and lateral zones (see Figure 26.2). Centrally, lower facial width is determined by the mandibular basal arch and alveolus,

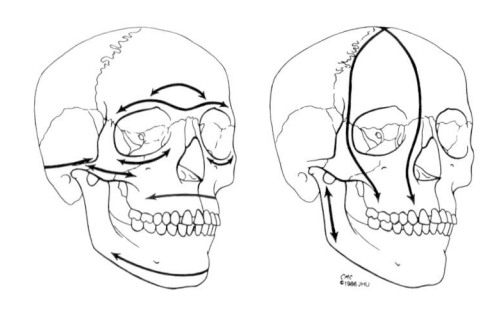

Figure 26.1 Facial proportions are maintained by the skeletal buttresses. (left) Width and projection are determined by identical buttress systems. (right) Facial height is established by the vertical maxillary buttresses anteriorly and by the condyle/ramus position posteriorly.

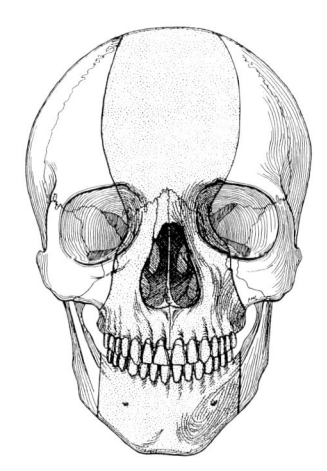

Figure 26.2 The critical dimension of panfacial fracture repair is facial width. To simplify the reconstruction, this region is divided into central and lateral zones. The frontal sinus, the nasoethmoid-orbital region, the maxillary and mandibular alveolus, and the horizontal mandible are central. The temporal portion of the frontal bone, the zygomatic complex, and the vertical portion of the mandible are lateral.

lower midface width by the maxillary alveolus, and upper midface width by the nasoethmoid-orbital complex. Laterally, the mandibular angles, the malar eminences, the zygomatic arches, and the external angular processes of the frontal bone are the determinants. This dimension is maintained by the frontal bar (supraorbital rims and glabella), the temporozygomaticomaxillary (infraorbital rim and zygomatic arch) buttress and the horizontal portion of the mandible.

In the midface, facial projection is dependent on the restitution of the frontonasomaxillary buttress and the zygomatic arches. In the lower face, projection is dependent on the length of the mandible from the angle to the symphysis and the relationship of the vertical mandible to the cranial base.

DIAGNOSIS

A careful history and physical and radiographic evaluation are crucial in establishing the component fracture patterns within the panfacial injury complex. Particular attention should be given to the patient's pre-injury appearance and occlusal relationships. Photographs, front and profile views, and dental records should be solicited to help guide the reconstruction.

The physical examination is performed in an orderly sequence. Static and dynamic inspection and palpation identify the soft-tissue, bone, and neurovascular injuries from the cranium to the mentum. Areas where injuries may be overlooked include the nasoethmoid region, the palate, and the eye.

A bimanual examination helps identify nasoethmoid-orbital fractures that require open reduction. Careful intraoral palpation identifies sagittal and tuberosity palatal fractures (not all palatal fractures have mucosal tears). The visual axis must be examined by the reconstructive surgeon prior to surgical intervention. Visual acuity, pupillary responses, and visual fields should be documented. When possible, all patients with complex craniofacial trauma should have a complete ophthalmologic evaluation.

CT has supplanted plain radiographs and tomography in the evaluation of facial trauma, except for that to the posterior or vertical portion of the mandible. The standard facial CT protocol implements 5-millimeter axial images with 2 millimeters of overlap. Coronal and sagittal reconstructions are most valuable in evaluating the orbits, anterior maxillary buttresses, and the vertical mandible. Three-dimensional CT scans are reconstructed from 1.5- to 3.0-mm axial images. Although their role in the care of acute facial fractures is still evolving, three-dimensional CT scans are an excellent teaching tool, and they may provide additional information not gained from the two-dimensional studies.

EVOLUTION OF TREATMENT PROTOCOL

Over the past decade, recommendations for treatment sequencing evolved from analysis of our results of acute panfacial repair and our post-traumatic patient population. General principles that positively affect management of complex facial fractures were delineated. These include (1) management of the complex facial fracture patient in a structured trauma center, (2) acute definitive fracture treatment (within 72 hours), (3) complete fracture exposure, (4) rigid internal stabilization, (5) primary bone grafting, and (6) the central zone concept.

Central Zone Concept

The reconstruction of normal facial proportions is simplified by dividing the fracture components into superior and inferior areas with central and lateral zones (see Figure 26.3). The area's boundary is the Le Fort I level. The central zone is composed of the bony elements that support the frontal sinus, nasoethmoid-orbital region, maxillary and mandibular alveolus, and horizontal portion of the mandible. The lateral zones are composed of the temporal portion of the frontal bone, the zygomatic complex, and the vertical portion of the mandible.

Stabilization of these complex facial disjunctions is initiated centrally. Beginning the reconstruction here allows the surgeon to address central facial width. In our experience the central face is the most difficult region to narrow acutely, and when this area is mismanaged irreparable secondary deformities arise. The lateral zones are then related and stabilized to the central core.

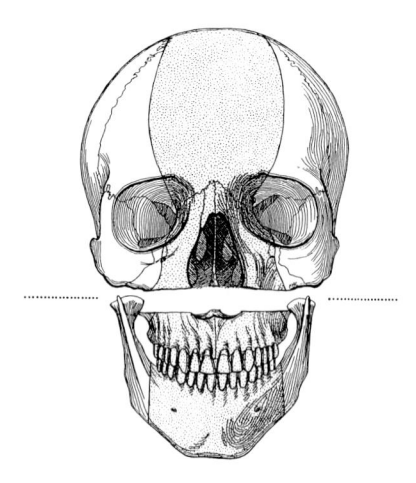

Figure 26.3 The central and lateral zones are separated at the Le Fort I level into superior and inferior divisions. Reconstruction may begin in either division.

This sequencing of panfacial fracture management has allowed us to re-establish accurately the difficult dimension of facial width both centrally and laterally. When facial width is successfully controlled, projection is reciprocally restored and subsequent reproduction of facial height is easily achieved.

It is recognized that adherence to this sequence is not inviolate. Equally good results are obtained by Gruss and Phillips (Chapter 20) who prefer to initiate reconstruction with reduction and stabilization of an outer facial frame using zygomatic arch reduction as the basic reference. Both approaches recognize and address the difficulties in three-dimensional reduction when there is a paucity of stable anatomic reference points.

SEQUENCE OF TREATMENT

Although the majority of patients who sustain panfacial injuries are victims of multisystem trauma, many are candidates for acute facial fracture repair. Contraindications to acute management are cardiopulmonary instability, coagulopathy, and severe neurological insults with intracranial pressure recordings of greater than 15. Once the multisystem injuries are evaluated and treated, the head and face are prepared for surgery. A strip of hair may be shaved 5 to 8 cm behind the hairline for a coronal incision. The oral cavity should be cleansed with antiseptic solution (Betadine/peroxide/normal saline). The lacerations should be scrubbed, and foreign bodies should be removed. The lacerations are closed after the facial fracture is stabilized.

Inferior Division

Central Zone

The Occlusion The operative procedure is initiated with the restoration of pre-injury occlusal relationships. Masticatory function can be predictably re-established if the articulatory pattern is precisely re-aligned and stabilized in three dimensions. To achieve this result, the occlusal surface of the mandible is keyed to the maxilla. These relationships are more difficult to identify in the presence of comminuted maxillary fractures. Old dental records, pre-injury photographs, and wear facets are used as guides. When palatal fractures (sagittal or tuberosity) are present, rigid stabilization—when possible—serves as a means to obtain the best anatomic reduction of the maxilla. This stabilization limits central facial width and serves as a template for mandibular articulation.

A throat pack is placed, and the oral cavity is again cleansed with saline solution. Alginate impressions are taken from which models are constructed. The models are cut, stabilized, and articulated to recreate the patient's pre-injury occlusion. Models serve as templates for splint fabrication and as guides for establishing the occlusal relationship in MMF.

Erich arch bars are placed along the upper and lower dental arches. The arch bar is stabilized with 24-gauge circumdental stainless steel wires that extend from the canines to the posterior molars. The arch bars serve as tension bands for fractures through the maxillary and mandibular alveolus and provide abutments for MMF. Pyriform aperture, transpalatal and circummandibular wires may be required to augment the stabilization of arch bars or to secure splints when dentition is lacking or absent.

Rigid stabilization of palatal fractures is performed through mucosal lacerations or incisions placed over the fracture sites. The oral mucosa is elevated only enough to allow placement of a two-hole mini-fragmentation plate; one hole is placed on each side of the fracture. Two plates are placed along one side of the fracture and stabilized with screws 2 millimeters in diameter. The fracture is reduced and stabilized when a screw is placed on the opposite side of the fracture (see Figure 26.4). Stabilization at the pyriform aperture and maxillary buttress level is subsequently achieved.

When palatal stabilization is necessary and rigid fixation is not applicable, a palatal splint is applied. The palatal splint, fabricated from the model, is stabilized to the palatal dentition and previously placed arch bar with 26-gauge stainless steel wires. At this time, lingual splints, which are used when the horizontal mandible is comminuted, are secured to the mandibular dentition. The fractures are always reduced before the wire is tightened (see Figure 26.5).

The operative procedure may next address the central zone of the lower or upper face. Fracture comminution, neurosurgical intervention, and other factors help determine the next stage in reconstruction. Our usual preference is to complete the mandibular reconstruction before moving on to the upper face.

The basal portion of the horizontal region of the mandible is exposed via an intraoral incision; care must be taken to leave an adequate cuff of mucosa for closure. External lacerations may also be used for expo-

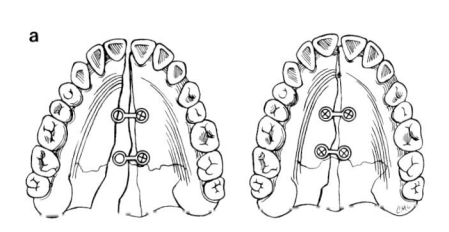

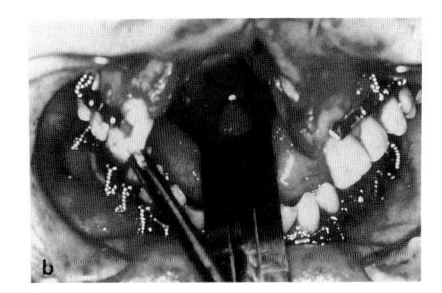

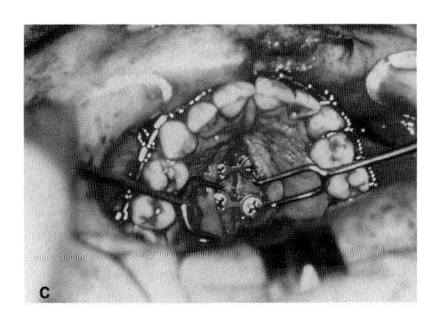

Figure 26.4 Rigid fixation of a sagittal palate fracture. (a) Mini-fragmentation plates are used for stabilization. Both two-hole plates must be placed on one side of the fracture before it is reduced and further stabilized. The fixation is supplemented by the arch bar, pyriform aperture, and maxillary buttress plates. (b) Sagittal palate fracture. (c) After stabilization, the maxillary alveolar width is restored. This provides an accurate template to which the mandibular reconstruction is related.

sure. Fracture segments are aligned by placement of figure-eight interosseous wires along the basal bone. Reduction forceps are an alternative when external lacerations or incisions are used for reduction, but they are too large and cumbersome to be used through the intraoral approach. Rigid fixation is achieved by mandibular plates stabilized with 2.7-millimeter screws. An attempt is made to place at least three screws on each side of the fracture. When the horizontal mandible is comminuted or multiple fracture segments are missing, a mandibular reconstruction plate is indicated. Care must be taken not to compress these fractures; compression may cause occlusal abnormalities and angle splaying.

Lateral Zone

Vertical Portion of the Mandible The treatment of angle fractures varies with the degree of comminution in that region and the status of the remaining mandible. As a rule, comminuted fractures are exposed via external approaches and require more intricate stabilization techniques than do simple fractures that are intraorally exposed. Prior to rigid stabilization the fractures are aligned with interosseous wires. Isolated simple angle fractures that "lock into" reduction may be stabilized by a mini-reconstruction plate along the external oblique line stabilized with 2-millimeter screws or a 2.7-millimeter lag screw. Comminuted fractures, or those associated with complex injuries in other mandibular regions, are stabilized with mandible plates along the angle's basal border. A combination of mini-reconstruction plates, along the basal border and external oblique ridge (tension band), also provides acceptable fixation. At least two screws per distal and proximal fracture segment are required for adequate stability (see Figure 26.6).

An aggressive approach is taken when subcondylar and ramus fractures are managed in the context of the panfacial crush. Open reduction is performed when

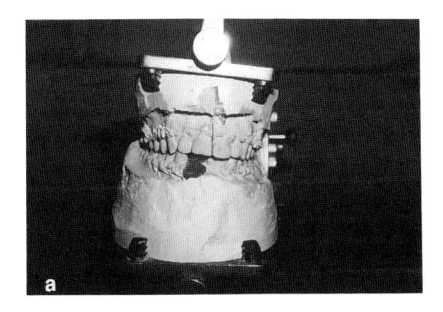

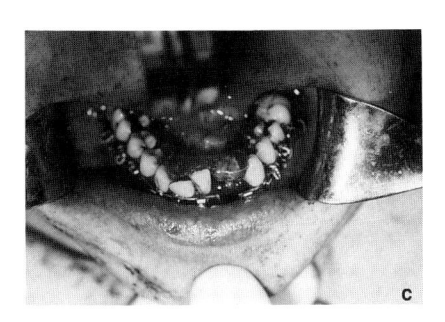

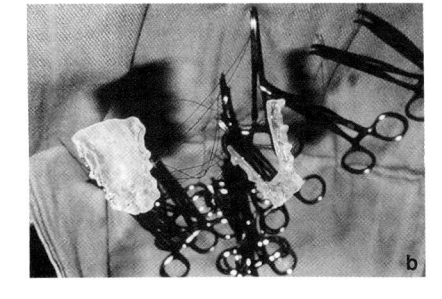

Figure 26.5 When the palatoalveolar and mandibular alveolar structures are comminuted, the addition of splint support is recommended. Palatal and lingual splints are fabricated from models that have been cut and anatomically aligned to recreate the pre-injury occlusion. (a) An articulated model. (b) Splints prepared for placement with 26-gauge wires. (c) Lingual splint in place.

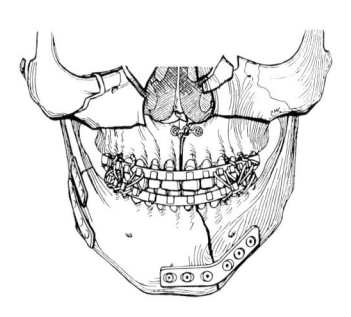

Figure 26.6 Completed lower facial reconstruction. Due to the dynamic masticatory forces, most mandible fractures are stabilized using mandibular plates with biocortal screws.

fracture dislocation is severe or when posterior facial height is reduced and anterior relationships are questionable. In this case a partoid type incision is used for exposure. Preauricular extension is required for those fractures that are more proximal to the cranial base. Stabilization is performed using a mini-reconstruction plate. An attempt is made to place two 2-millimeter screws per fracture segment.

Superior Division

Central Zone

Cranial vault fractures are managed in collaboration with the neurosurgeon. As the fracture and craniotomy bone fragments are elevated they are stripped of all necrotic debris and oriented for reconstruction. The fragments are repositioned with wires and stabilized with mini- or micro-fragmentation plates. The calvarium's inner table provides an excellent source of material for bone grafts. It is split with sagittal saws and osteotomies.

The upper craniofacial skeleton is exposed through lacerations and coronal, subciliary, and maxillary gingivobuccal sulcus incisions. The status of bony disjunction and comminution is assessed, and the fracture segments are linked with interosseous wires. Stabilization proceeds superiorly and centrally through the frontal bone and naso-ethmoid region.

The frontal sinus is exenterated, excluded, and obliterated when displacement of the anterior wall and fractures of the posterior wall are associated with significant mucosal damage and obstruction of the nasofrontal duct. Cranialization is performed when the posterior wall is comminuted.

Exenteration is achieved by removing all sinus mucosa with a Freer elevator and lightly burring the entire sinus cavity under loupe magnification and saline irrigation. The frontal sinus is then excluded from the nasal cavity using form-fit calvarial bone plugs. Pericranial and galeofrontalis flaps are used when the sinus floor is destroyed and are more frequently employed when the frontal sinus is cranialized. Cancellous bone grafts from the iliac crest are used to obliterate the frontal sinus dead space.

The treatment of nasoethmoid-orbital fractures is predicated by the status of the central fragment of the injury complex (the medial orbital rim where the medial canthus attaches). Single-fragment injuries are reduced and stabilized superiorly at the nasofrontal junction and inferiorly at the infraorbital rim and nasomaxillary buttress. Mini- and micro-fragmentation plates utilizing 0.8- to 2-mm screws are employed for fixation. Care is taken to avoid placing the plate in the anterior naso-orbital valley. Comminuted fractures require transnasal wiring to narrow and stabilize the interorbital distance prior to rigid fixation. The medial canthus is detached only when severe comminution of the medial orbital wall precludes its adequate restoration. In such a case the medial canthus is stripped and repositioned in a posterior, superior direction with transnasal wires (see Figure 26.7).

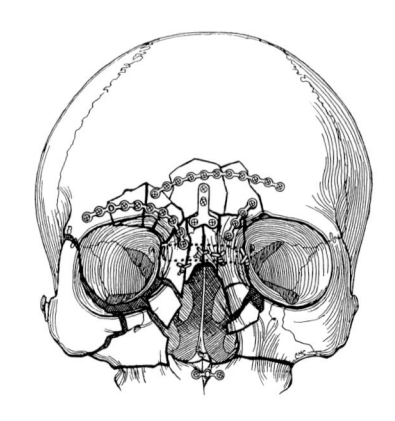

Figure 26.7 The central upper craniofacial skeleton is stabilized after the frontal sinus is appropriately managed. When nasoethmoid-orbital fractures are comminuted, narrowing of the interorbital space is best achieved with transnasal wires. Superior and inferior stabilization is achieved with plate and screw fixation.

Lateral Zone

Zygomatic Orbital Complex The zygomatic complex is related centrally to the medial orbit at the inferior and superior orbital rims. Intraorbitally, the lateral portion of the orbital plate of the zygoma is aligned with the greater wing of the sphenoid. We have found this relationship to be the best guide to an anatomic reduction of the zygoma. When the zygomatic complex is significantly displaced posteriorly in the presence of a severely comminuted zygomatic arch, the coronal incision is extended inferiorly and the arch is exposed. Interosseous wires are used to reduce the fracture segments prior to rigid fixation.

Stabilization proceeds from the zygomatic arch to the inferior orbital rim. The superior orbital rim and the fronto-zygomatic suture are then stabilized. The arch is stabilized with a mini-fragmentation plate using 1.5- to 2.0-mm screws. Remember that the zygomatic arch is not a true arch but is flattened in its middle portion. The orbital rims are stabilized with micro-fragmentation plates using 0.8-millimeter screws. These plates are particularly useful when multiple small bone fragments require precise alignment. The fronto-zygomatic suture is then stabilized with a mini-reconstruction plate using 2.0-millimeter screws. Although not always possible, two screws should be placed on the most distal and proximal bone fragments spanned by the plate (see Figure 26.8).

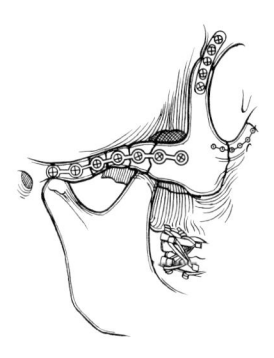

Figure 26.8 The key to the restoration of lateral facial width and projection is the zygomatic arch. Its exposure, reduction, and fixation is the initial step in the reconstruction of the lateral zone.

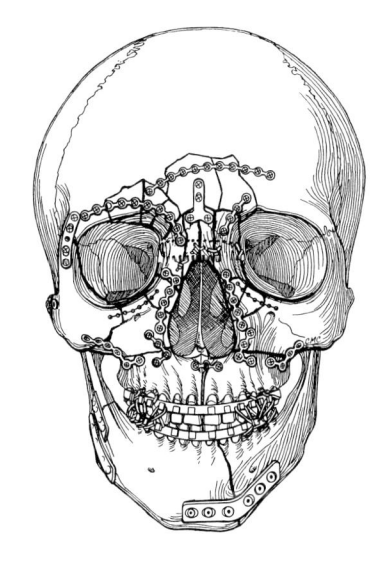

Figure 26.9 The lateral zones are related centrally, and facial height is restored at the Le Fort I level. Bone grafting, when indicated, completes the rigid stabilization.

Le Fort I Level The Le Fort I level, previously exposed through a maxillary gingivobuccal sulcus incision for alignment of the zygomatic and naso-orbital complex, is stabilized to re-establish the vertical dimension. Comminution and bone loss at this level is frequent, but at least one of the four anterior buttresses is sufficiently intact to guide reconstruction of midfacial height. A straight 20- to 30-mm mini-adaptation plate is used with 2-millimeter screws to stabilize the nasomaxillary buttress. Angular 90° or 110° mini-adaptation plates are usually applied to the zygomaticomaxillary buttress (see Figure 26.9).

Bone Grafting Throughout the reconstruction procedure, the extent of bone loss and comminution is assessed and plans are established for bone grafting. The calvarium is the preferred donor site, but rib and iliac bone are good alternatives. Calvarial grafts may be harvested as split cortical grafts, leaving the pericranium intact, or as complete internal or external table grafts. Rib grafts are split and may be harvested with cartilage (costochondral grafts). The iliac bone provides an excellent source of cortical and cancellous bone graft.

Form-fit calvarial bone plugs are placed in the nasofrontal ducts and, if necessary, along the entire floor of the frontal sinus to exclude the sinus from the nasal cavity. The sinus is obliterated using cancellous bone from the cranium diploic space or more commonly from the iliac crest. Split calvarial or cortical grafts from the ilium are used to reconstruct the anterior table of the frontal sinus.

Split calvarial or rib grafts are used for the nasal dorsum. Fixation is achieved with lag or tandem screws or with miniplates and microplates and screws. Costocartilage grafts are used when caudal support is needed.

Orbital defects are best managed using split cortical calvarial grafts (leaving pericranium attached) or split rib grafts. These grafts allow for precise contouring and may be placed behind the infraorbital rim without fixation when moderate size defects are grafted. Larger defects, defects of the lateral wall, and orbital roof defects should be rigidly stabilized with mini- or microfragmentation systems. Another alternative for repair of smashed orbit is the orbital reconstruction plate. This plate is stabilized to the infraorbital rim and spans the orbital defect along the floor to the posterior limit of the injury. Contoured medially and laterally, it provides a stable platform for graft placement.

Gaps in the bony continuity of the facial buttresses are spanned mini- or microplates. Screw holes over the areas of bone deficiency allow for precise alignment and stabilization of the form-fit grafts.

Repair of Soft Tissue To prevent the inferior migration and sag of the facial soft tissues, successful resuspension is achieved by careful management of the subcutaneous layers at specific sites.

The coronal incision is closed in two layers (galea and scalp). Care is taken to reapproximate the periosteum over the frontal process of the zygoma and the zygomatic process of the frontal bone to the deep temporal fascia. This prevents temporal depressions and brow ptosis. The medial canthus is repositioned as the naso-orbital complex is stabilized, and the lateral canthus is reattached near the fronto-zygomatic suture. A layered closure of the periosteum and orbicularis oculi muscle is performed in the lateral extension of the subciliary incision. The malar cheek pad is sutured to the inferior orbital rim, and a layered closure (muscle and mucosa) of the gingivobuccal sulcus incisions is performed.

Figure 26.10 Panfacial injury subsequent to a MVA. The fracture pattern included the anterior and posterior wall of the frontal sinus, the nasoethmoid orbital region, right Le Fort II, left Le Fort III, maxillary alveolus symphyseal region, and the bilateral subcondylar region. (a and b) Preoperative appearance. Not the wide, retruded long face typical of the untreated patient. (c and d) Representative axial CT images from the region of the nasofrontal junction and the midface. (e–h) Postoperative appearance and function two years after injury.

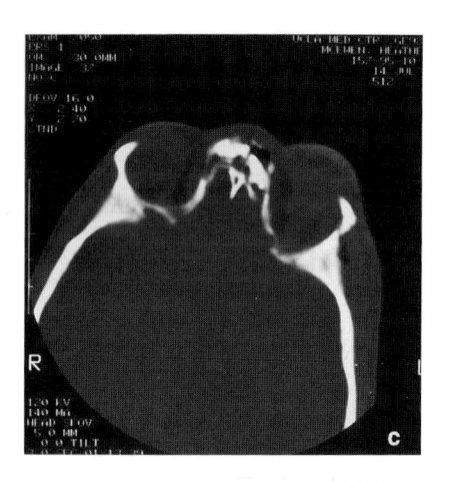

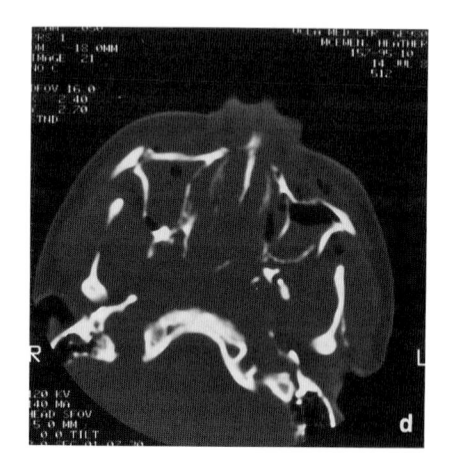

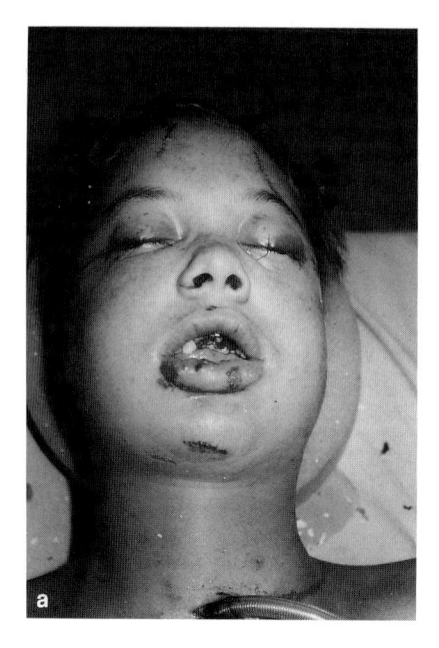

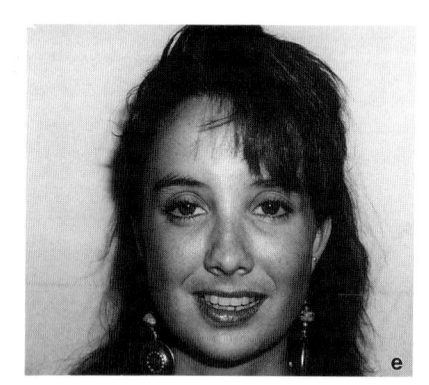

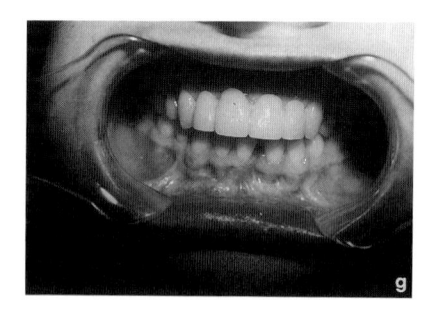

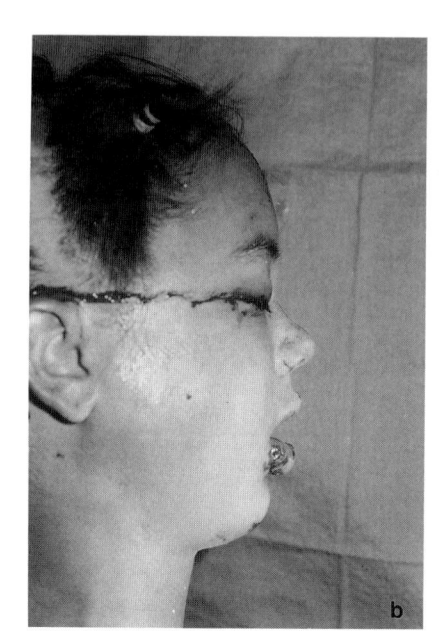

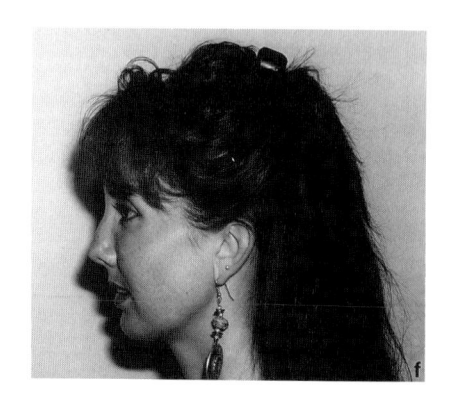

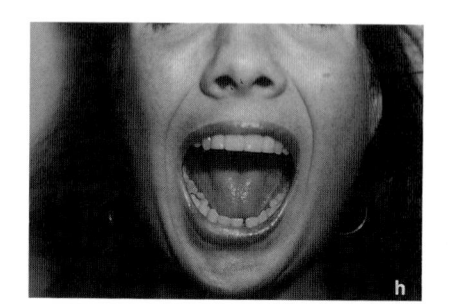

COMPLICATIONS AND LONG-TERM RESULTS

Acute treatment of panfacial fractures with extended exposure, rigid internal fixation, and primary bone grafting has actually decreased the overall morbidity and improved the long-term results when compared to management using closed techniques (see Figure 26.10). Acute infectious complications occur in approximately 10% of patients. Facial cellulitis and purulent drainage from the suture lines may represent deep-tissue processes. Subcutaneous abscesses or frontal, ethmoid, or maxillary sinusitis must be expeditiously diagnosed and treated with intravenous antibiotics and drainage. In these situations, early aggressive treatment helps avoid necrotizing infections, which may result in bone loss and plate and screw loosening prior to bone healing.

Secondary reconstructive procedures for malocclusion, enophthalmos, and soft-tissue deformities are necessary in 1%, 5%, and 12%, respectively, of the panfacial fracture patient population.

SUMMARY

Advances in facial trauma management now enable the surgeon to define and to reconstruct complex panfacial injuries with restoration of preoperative form and function. An organized approach to these injuries begins at the maxillary and mandibular arches with progression to the vertical mandible. Next, the naso-orbital ethmoidal complex is stabilized to the cranium and bone grafted where necessary. The zygomatic complex is related medially and then internal orbit reconstruction performed. Facial skeletal reconstruction is completed at the Le Fort I level.

In our experience, adherence to this protocol optimizes the result, even in the most severe injuries.

BIBLIOGRAPHY

Glassman RD, Manson PN, Vanderkolk CA, et al: Rigid fixation of internal orbital fractures. Plast Reconstr Surg 86:1103, 1990.

Gruss JS: Fronto-naso-orbital trauma. Clin Plast 9:577, 1982.

Gruss JS, Mackinnon SE, Kassel ED, et al: The role of primary bone grafting in complex craniomaxillofacial trauma. Plast Reconstr Surg 75:17, 1985.

Gruss JS, Mackinnon SE: Complex maxillary fractures: Role of buttress reconstruction and immediate bone grafts. Plast Reconstr Surg 78:9, 1986.

Gruss JS, Van Wyck L, Phillips JH, Antonyshyn O: The importance of the zygomatic arch in complex midfacial fracture repair and correction of post traumatic orbitozygomatic deformities. Plast Reconstr Surg 85:878, 1990.

Kelly JK, Manson PN, Vanderkolk CA, Markowitz BL, Dunham CM, Rumley TO, Crawley WA: Sequencing Le Fort fracture treatment (organization of treatment for panfacial fractures). J Craniofac Surg 1:168, 1990.

Manson P: Some thoughts on the classification and treatment of Le Fort fractures. Ann Plast Surg 17:356, 1986.

Manson P, Crawley WA, Yaremchuk MJ, et al: Midface fractures: Advantages of immediate extended open reduction and bone grafting. Plast Reconstr Surg 76:1, 1985.

Manson PN, Hoopes JE, Su CT: Structural pillars of the facial skeleton: An approach to the management of Le Fort fractures. Plast Reconstr Surg 66:54, 1980.

Manson PN, Markowitz BL, Mirvis S, Dunham M, Yaremchuk M: CT based diagnosis of facial fractures. Plast Reconstr Surg 85:202, 1990.

Manson P, Shack B, Leonard LG, et al: Sagittal fractures of the maxilla and palate. Plast Reconstr Surg 72:484, 1983.

Markowitz BL, Manson PN: Panfacial fractures: Organization of treatment. Clin Plast Surg 16:105, 1989.

Merville L: Multiple dislocations of the facial skeleton. J Maxillofac Surg 2:187, 1974.

Merville LC, Derome P: Concomitant dislocations of the face and skull. J Maxillofac Surg 6:2, 1978.

Zide MF, Kent JN: Indications for open reduction of mandibular condyle fractures. J Oral Maxillofac Surg 41:89, 1983.

CHAPTER 27

Rigid Fixation of Complex Gunshot Wounds

Joseph S. Gruss

Severe facial gunshot wounds, produced by high-velocity rifles or shotgun blasts, present a formidable challenge to the reconstructive surgeon. Damage to or loss of bone and soft tissue is often complicated by concomitant injuries to the nasal passages, orbits, and oral and cranial cavities.

Traditional management of these wounds dictates initial debridement and closure of the soft tissues combined with external fixation of the remaining maxillary and mandibular bone segments. Definitive bone replacement is delayed until soft-tissue replacement is completed. However, in most cases, this multistage therapy is seriously compromised because loss of the underlying bone prevents maintenance of midfacial soft-tissue expansion.

The treatment of complex facial fractures has been facilitated by the use of craniofacial surgical techniques, extended open reduction, rigid internal fixation with plates and screws, and the replacement of severely damaged or missing bone with immediate bone grafting. The successful application of these techniques to the management of severe gunshot wounds to the face, which has facilitated continued evolution and refinements in methods of reconstruction of bone and soft tissue, forms the basis of this chapter.

Few authors to date have supported the concept of primary, definitive reconstruction of soft tissue or reconstruction of bone and soft tissue in the treatment of complex gunshot wounds to the face. The generally accepted methods of secondary delayed reconstruction necessitate multiple operations over an extended period. Even though the position of mandibular bone segment and expansion of lower facial soft tissue can be maintained by external fixation devices, expansion of midfacial soft tissue cannot be maintained by these devices alone. Frequently, failure to reconstruct the underlying bony skeleton will result in rapid shrinkage of soft tissue, especially in the midface, making adequate secondary bone reconstruction difficult and sometimes impossible. Our experience in the treatment of 37 patients has demonstrated that early three-dimensional bone replacement, particularly in the midface, will maintain soft-tissue expansion during the healing phase. Even though bone grafts in the midface may become exposed into the nasal or oral cavity or externally, they will still maintain soft-tissue expansion for a prolonged period as long as they remain rigidly fixed in place. These bone grafts, acting as an internal splint, can then be replaced with a definitive bone graft at a later stage.

PRINCIPLES OF RECONSTRUCTION

General Principles

The principles of immediate wound care, with conservative debridement of bone and soft tissue, have been previously delineated (see Chapter 16). Only small pieces of bone, devoid of periosteum, are removed. In the less severe injury, involving mainly bone disruption with minimal injury to soft tissue, immediate, definitive repair of bone and soft tissue can be accomplished. In more severe injuries, with extensive injury to or loss of bone and soft tissue, the immediate debridement is followed by further debridement as necessary. Within seven to ten days, delayed primary definitive reconstruction and replacement of missing midfacial bone and soft tissue is performed. Late repair then involves scar revision, oral commissure creation, total nasal reconstruction utilizing forehead skin, and bony mandibular reconstruction.

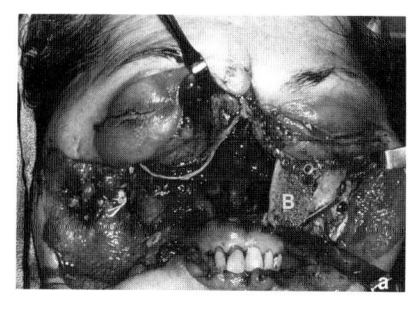

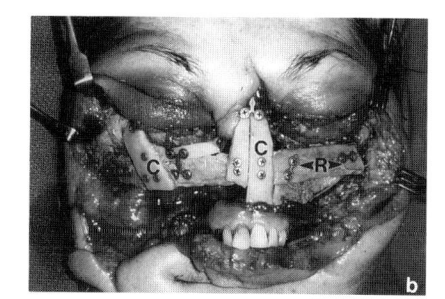

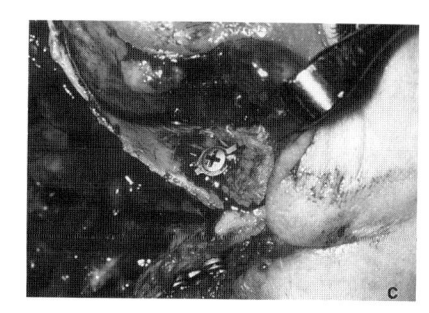

Figure 27.1 (a) Method of bony replacement with extensive midfacial bone loss. Contoured split rib grafts replace missing orbital walls and rims following the establishment of correct facial width with the zygomatic arch and body stabilization with miniplates. Split calvarial bone graft (B) extends from the left orbital rim and is lagged into the hard palate (arrows) to re-establish correct midfacial height. (b) A full-thickness rib graft (R) spans across the maxillary defect. Note that small segments of miniplate are used as washers underneath the screwheads to prevent cracking of the rib cortex when screws are inserted (arrows). Split calvarial bone struts (C) are bridged from the nasoglabellar region down to the maxillary bone graft and from the right orbital reconstruction down to the bone graft. These calvarial bone grafts are rigidly fixed with lag screws, which can be countersunk into the thick cortical outer plate. No washer is necessary for fixation in a split calvarial bone graft. The bony scaffold is totally restored prior to coverage with free-vascularized soft-tissue flap. (c) A lag screw with a washer (one hole of a mini-adaptive plate) is used to stabilize a split rib graft in an orbital reconstruction.

Specific Principles

Midfacial Bone

Extended craniofacial exposure combining a coronal incision, lower eyelid incisions, and the open wound allows access to the upper craniofacial skeleton. Exposure of the zygomatic arch is critical to facilitate adequate repair. All fractures are delineated, and stable areas of the craniofacial skeleton are identified. These fractures are then reduced and stabilized with miniplates and screws. Once the fractures are repaired, areas of bone destruction are replaced with bone grafts to provide a midfacial scaffolding for support of soft tissue or subsequent replacement of the flap. When bone loss is confined mainly to the central midface, repair is commenced with the zygomatic arch and the lateral orbital rim. This reconstructs an outer facial frame with the correct facial width. The exact amount of missing midfacial bone is now assessed. Minor areas of bone loss are replaced by split calvarial bone grafts. Moderate to extensive areas are replaced by a combination of split calvarial bone and rib grafts.

Segmental deficits in the orbital rims are reconstructed with split calvarial bone. Extensive deficits involving contiguous lateral, inferior, or medial rims are replaced with contoured split rib grafts. Once the orbital rim is reconstructed, deep orbital exposure and bone grafting, using either calvarial or rib grafts, replaces the missing orbital wall. This facilitates reconstruction of the correct orbital volume. Transnasal wiring of the medial canthal ligaments through the reconstructed medial rim is usually necessary to correct the traumatic telecanthus.

Maxillary bone loss is replaced with a full-thickness rib graft that extends between both previously stabilized zygomatic bodies. The missing nasal, nasoethmoid, and upper maxilla is replaced with rib or calvarial bone that extends between the frontoglabellar region above to the full-thickness rib graft below (see Figures 27.1 and 27.2). This bone replacement provides a three-dimensional scaffold for midfacial support. The upper portion of the bone graft acts as a base for late nasal bone grafting at the time of definitive nasal re-

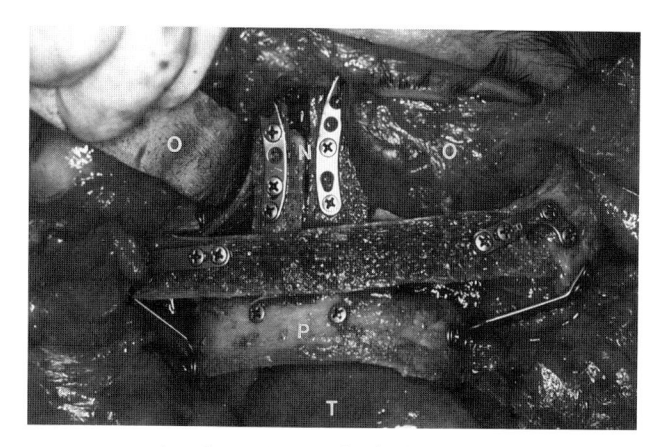

Figure 27.2 An alternative method of midfacial bony reconstruction is shown using rib and calvarial bone grafts (O = orbits, N = nasoglabellar, T = tongue). Separate rib grafts reconstruct the maxilla (M) and anterior palate (P). Bone grafts from the nasoglabellar region are linked to midfacial bone grafts in a three-dimensional fashion.

construction. Additional midfacial support can be obtained by bridge grafts from the orbital rims above to the full-thickness rib graft below.

Although calvarial bone grafts are now the invariable source of bone in the management of acute facial fractures, they are difficult to bend and to obtain in segments of sufficient length. In gunshot wounds with extensive bone loss, combinations of calvarial and rib or iliac grafts are usually needed. Split rib grafts can be bent to replace contiguous areas of the orbital rims and walls; and long, full-thickness rib grafts are ideal to bridge across the midface for maxillary replacement. All bone grafts, except in the reconstruction of the deep orbit, are rigidly fixed with lag screws or miniplates. Split calvarial bone is ideally fixed with lag screws due to its thick cortical layer. Lag screw fixation of rib or iliac bone may fracture the more fragile outer cortex and may have to be reinforced with a washer, which can be obtained by cutting one or two holes from a mini-adaptive plate (see Figure 27.1c). Fracture segments should be accurately reduced and stabilized with miniplates to provide three-dimensional stability. Only then can the exact amount of missing bone be accurately assessed and replaced.

Mandible

Injury to the mandible may result in unilateral, bilateral, segmental, or comminuted fractures, or fractures with bone defects. Combinations of injury types are frequently seen. Use of remaining tooth-bearing segments of the maxilla and mandible enables establishment of the correct occlusion with interdental wiring. Fractures without comminution, segmentation, or defect are repaired whenever possible with mandibular compression or reconstruction plates. Initial restoration of the contour of segmental or comminuted fractures is provided by miniplates and lag screw fixation. Final, definitive stabilization is provided by long, contoured reconstruction plates extending from stable bone on each side; separate screws are placed into each intervening segment (see Figure 27.3).

Fractures with bone gaps are bridged by reconstruction plates, which are anchored at each end with a minimum of four screws (see Figures 27.4, 27.5, 27.6, and 27.7). Primary bone grafting for mandibular defects is rarely indicated because the reconstruction plates will maintain the bone gap until soft tissue (particularly the intraoral lining) has healed, allowing safe, delayed bone reconstruction.

Although primary bone graft reconstruction of the midface is the cornerstone of repair and has few major complications, primary bone replacement of mandibular defects has an unacceptably high rate of complication. Because the mandibular repair lies in the path of the salivary stream, even minor degrees of exposure or contamination from the oral cavity will lead to severe infection, necessitating the removal of bone grafts. This rarely occurs in the midface. In addition, in our experience, primary bone grafts for traumatic mandibular defects are unpredictable and have a high incidence of significant resorption even if infection does not arise. The position of the mandibular bone segments can be readily maintained by the use of strong, three-dimensionally bendable reconstruction plates, rigidly fixed to the bone stump at either end. These plates act as a spacer until soft tissue has healed completely. Definitive bone reconstruction can then be accomplished through an external approach with maintenance of the intraoral seal. In defects of up to 3 or 4 centimeters, conventional iliac cancellous bone grafting is used (see Figures 27.4 and 27.5). When the defect is larger, this type of bone grafting has proven unpredictable, and free vascularized bone grafting provides optimal reconstruction (see Figure 27.6). It is always essential eventually to bridge a mandibular bone defect with bone, because a plate alone will not maintain adequate stability against the continued forces of mastication. In two cases, failure to do this resulted in plate loosening and infection 18 to 24 months after initial plate reconstruction. Once bony continuity has been established, the plate is then removed at 3 to 6 months to allow functional stresses across the mandible to maintain bone graft volume.

Reconstruction of Soft Tissue

Once reconstruction of midfacial and mandibular bone is complete, reconstruction of soft tissue can be completed by direct-closure, local, regional, or free-vascularized flaps. These include forehead, scalp, deltopectoral, and pectoralis major flaps; free-vascularized rectus abdominis-muscle; and musculocutaneous, gracilis, and omental flaps.

In certain patients, significant bone and soft tissue may be lost following severe gunshot wounds to the face produced by high-velocity rifles or shotguns. Following reconstruction of a midfacial scaffold with bone grafts and the mandibular arch with plates, there are large deficits of lining in the palate and upper buccal sulcus, the floor of the mouth, the lower buccal sulcus, and laterally the cheeks. These deficits are frequently combined with significant loss of external coverage in the midface and lower face. These defects, involving multiple sites and surfaces, are difficult and usually impossible to reconstruct adequately by conventional flap techniques or with multiple free-vascularized flaps of skin and muscle. A free-vascularized omental flap can be wrapped around all bone grafts and plates and reconstruction of multiple sites and surfaces with one flap is possible (see Figure 27.7).

The greater omentum is an intra-abdominal organ that protects the abdominal viscera and aids in localization and resolution of peritonitis. The omentum is frequently used to protect or reconstruct other intra-abdominal structures, such as the stomach, duodenum, liver, and urological system. It has been mobilized on a vascular pedicle for coverage of chest wall defects, protection of exposed vessels, and the treatment of lymphedema. Free omental transplantation with microvascular anastomosis has been used for the treatment of mandibular osteoradionecrosis, reconstruction of scalp defects, correction of hemifacial atrophy, reconstruction of the face, reconstruction of the oral cavity and pharynx, and the treatment of lower extremity osteomyelitis after trauma. Arnold (1980) reported its use in combination with adjacent gastric mucosa in the reconstruction of a massive craniofacial defect after a close-range shotgun blast.

Rich in blood vessels and lymphatics, the omentum is a powerful defense against infection. The surface peritoneum readily accepts a split-thickness skin graft. The whole omentum will survive on its blood supply from either the right or left gastroepiploic vessels, al-

Figure 27.3 Woman with accidental gunshot wound to the left side of the face. (a) The massive bursting wound of facial soft tissues is shown. (b) Multiple segmental fractures of the mandible are seen extending from the left condyle (C) to the midline. (c) Mandibular contour is restored by multiple interosseous wire and lag screw fixation. This fixation is inadequate to maintain adequate stability. (d) Final stabilization is provided by a long, prebent, angled reconstruction plate. The upper screw is placed into the condyle (arrow), and plate extends to the midline in order to bridge all fracture segments. Individual screws are inserted from the plate into intervening segments. A miniplate aids fixation at the upper border of the mandible. (e) Simple soft-tissue closure has been performed without revision. Note the healing and the maintained soft-tissue expansion following correct and rigid reconstruction of underlying bone. (f) Mandibular function has been restored. The persistent left facial palsy required subsequent reconstruction with cross-facial nerve grafts and a free muscle flap.

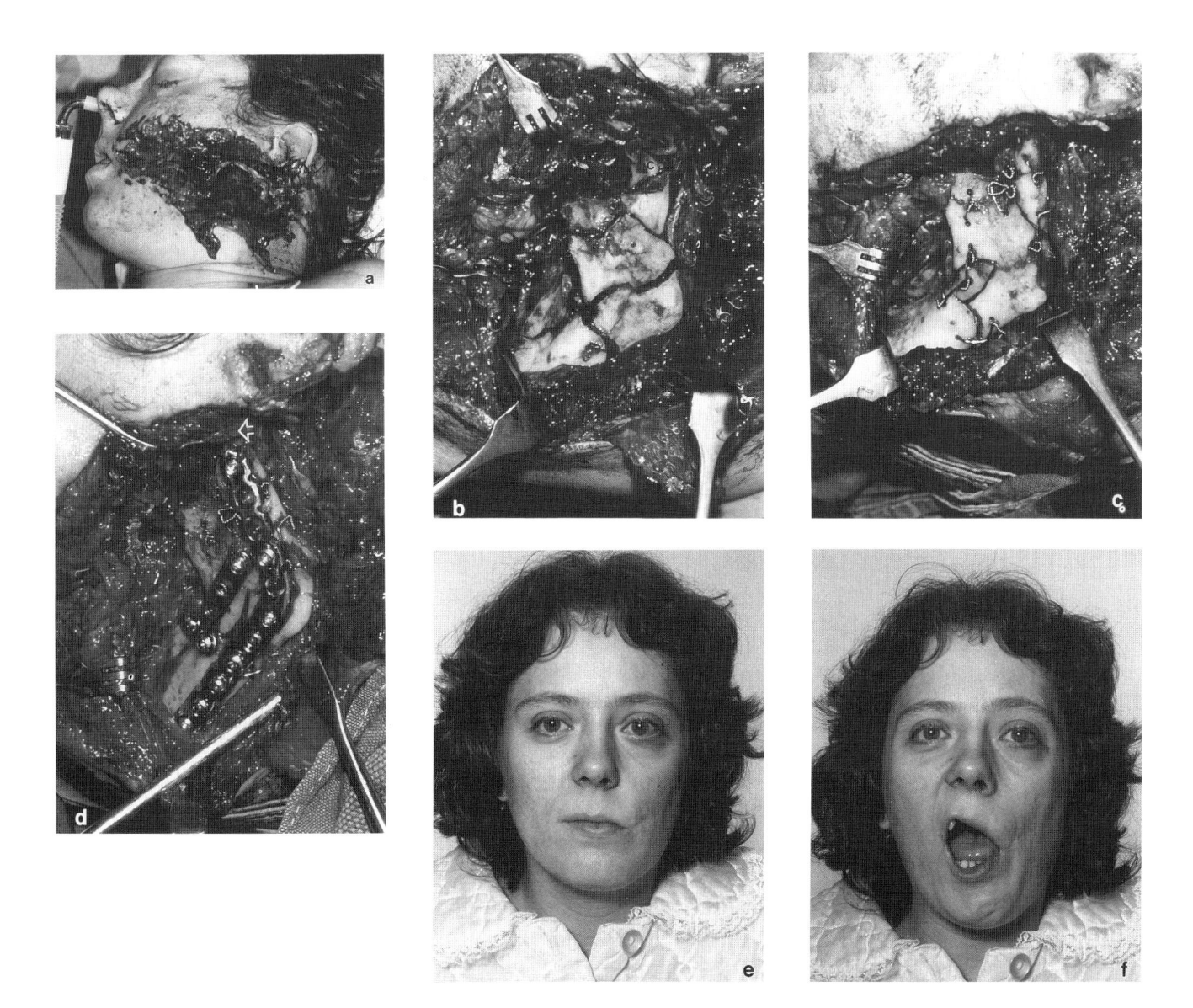

Figure 27.4 Severe gunshot wound of the mandible and midface. (a) The entrance wound is below the mandible, and the exit wound is in the midface. Disruption of midfacial bony and soft-tissue structures extends up into the frontal sinus with severe traumatic telecanthus. (b) The cheek flaps are retracted to show complete destruction and bone loss of all nasoethmoid-orbital, nasal, and anterior maxillary bony structures. (c) Missing orbital and nasoethmoid bone is replaced with contoured rib grafts. A full-thickness rib graft replaces the missing maxilla. (d) The mandible exposed through the upper neck incision communicating with the entrance wound reveals multiple complex segmental fractures of the mandible, extending from angle to angle. (e) Multiple mandibular fractures are reduced, and contour is restored with a combination of lag screws and interosseous wires. Final stabilization is provided by a strong reconstruction plate, which extends from the right angle to the left posterior body. Separate screws are placed into each intervening segment. (f) This panorex x ray shows the reconstruction plate combined with interosseous wires and lag screws. (g) Appearance at three months after one operation. The midfacial bone has been replaced by a full-thickness bone graft that extends from zygoma to zygoma. The medial and inferior orbital walls and rims are replaced by contoured split rib grafts. The central bone underlying the nasal base is restored with rib graft reconstruction. Each medial canthal ligament is wired separately through the medial wall reconstruction and passed transnasally. Note the restoration of soft-tissue projection and contour without shrinkage. The small sinuses present on the right cheek and under the chin are not indicative of infection; rather, they are due to extrusion of bony sequestra and small pieces of shot. Recurrent small sinuses such as these commonly arise in these cases and are not an indication for exploration and removal of bone grafts or internal fixation devices unless the grafts or devices are obviously loose. (h) Tissue expansion of forehead skin allows the use of an 8-centimeter-wide forehead flap for total nasal reconstruction. (i) Midfacial appearance at seven years is shown following total nasal reconstruction with tissue-expanded forehead skin wrapped around a split calvarial bone graft. Note restoration of the correct intercanthal distance, medial canthal anatomy, and midfacial projection and contour. The philtral region of the upper lip has been reconstructed by an Abbe flap from the lower lip. (j) This close-up view of the midface shows restoration of the contour and anatomy of the midfacial and nasoethmoid-orbital regions. Midfacial soft tissues have retained normal contour and consistency following expansion by underlying bony scaffold reconstruction. (k) Restoration of normal facial contour and appearance and normal function of the mandible. (l) This inferior view shows restoration of normal midfacial projection and width with bone graft supporting ultimate total nasal reconstruction. Oculo-orbital position is restored without enophthalmos following extensive deep orbital reconstruction with bone grafts. (m) This lateral view shows restoration of midfacial projection. (n) The patient has been fitted with functional dentures in both upper and lower jaws.

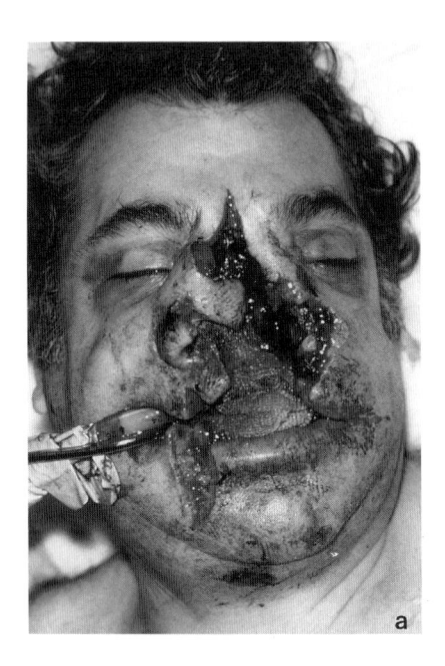

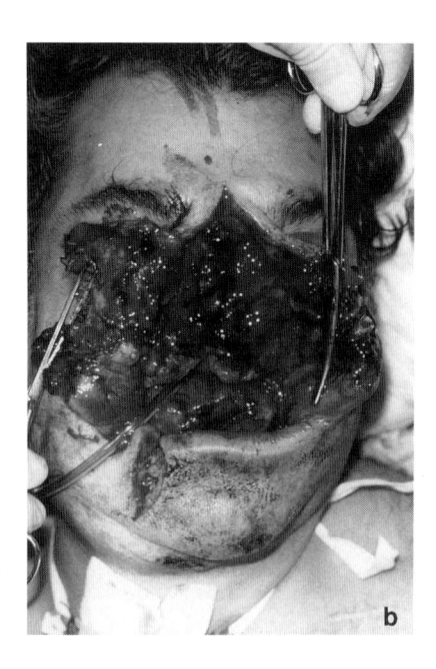

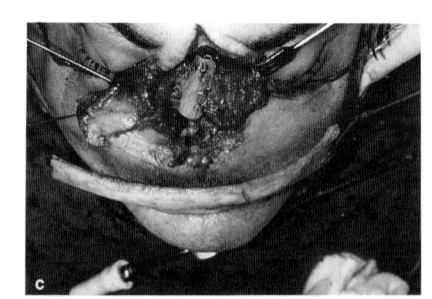

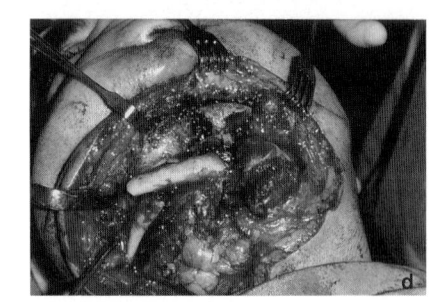

Rigid Fixation of Complex Gunshot Wounds

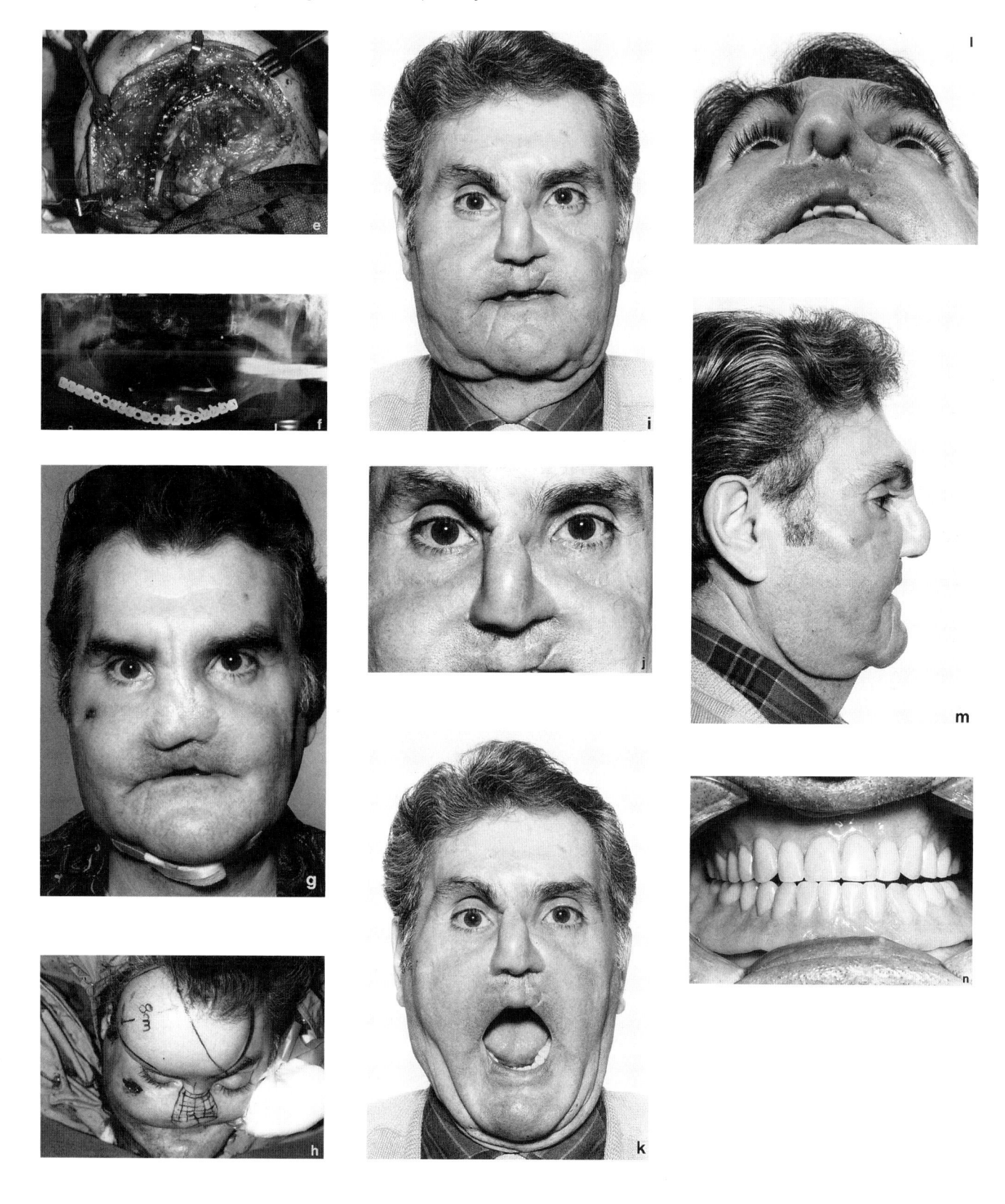

Figure 27.5 Patient with extensive shotgun blast to the mandible and midface following a suicide attempt. (a) The entrance wound in the neck and the exit wound in the left midface are shown. The left orbit and its contents have been destroyed. (b) Retraction of skin flaps demonstrates severe injury to bone, with massive destruction of all midfacial bone. Extensive injury is seen to the soft tissue of the floor of the mouth, the tongue, and the hard and soft palates. There is total bony loss of the maxilla, the nasoethmoid-orbital region, and the entire left orbit. (c) The missing orbit is reconstructed with a contoured split rib graft. A full-thickness rib graft reconstructs the maxilla and extends between both zygomas (R). Further struts are placed between the orbital and maxillary reconstruction. Missing nasal bone is replaced with a costochondral graft (C). A midline forehead flap will reconstruct the soft-tissue deficit in the left orbital region and cover the bone grafts. (d) A midline forehead flap covers the bone grafts. (e) The fracture of the right mandible is repaired with an A-O compression plate (small arrows). The fracture deficit in the left mandibular body is bridged by a strong reconstruction plate; five screws are placed in the anterior segment and four screws in the ramus. A bony gap is left, and no primary bone graft is used (large arrows). (f) At three months, once the intraoral lining is healed, a 4-centimeter-long bone gap in the left mandibular body is bridged by a conventional cancellous bone graft, which is packed into the gap underneath the plate and molded to the shape of the missing mandible (arrows). (g) The compression plate is placed on the right to allow fracture healing, and the reconstruction plate is placed on the left to provide continuity restoration across mandibular gap. (h) The mandibular reconstruction plate is removed at seven months to allow functional stresses across the bone graft and subsequent hypertrophy. Note the perfect bony restoration across the previous mandibular gap. (i) The full-thickness bone graft used for maxillary reconstruction became exposed in the intraoral cavity. It was left in situ for 10 months, while it acted as an internal splint to maintain midfacial soft-tissue expansion. The graft was subsequently removed and replaced with another full-thickness rib graft and covered with local mucosal flaps. Unchanged appearance of rib graft at 10 months, with no resorption, can be seen. (j) Appearance at eight years after reconstruction. Note the restoration of midfacial width and projection without soft-tissue shrinkage. A left orbital prosthesis is in place. (k) Mandibular function is restored; glasses provide camouflage. (l) This lateral view shows restoration of the midface and mandibular projection. The upper lip is retruded because of difficulty in fitting a conventional denture. Patient has refused osseointegrated implants.

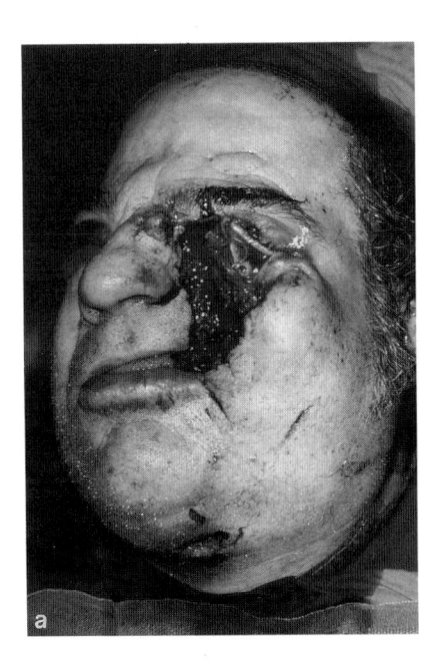

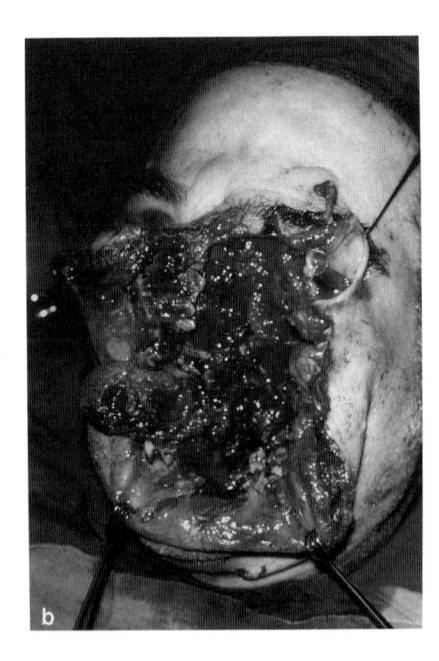

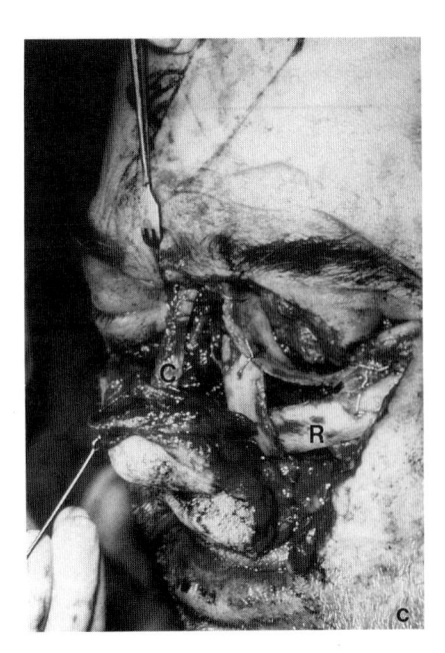

Rigid Fixation of Complex Gunshot Wounds   345

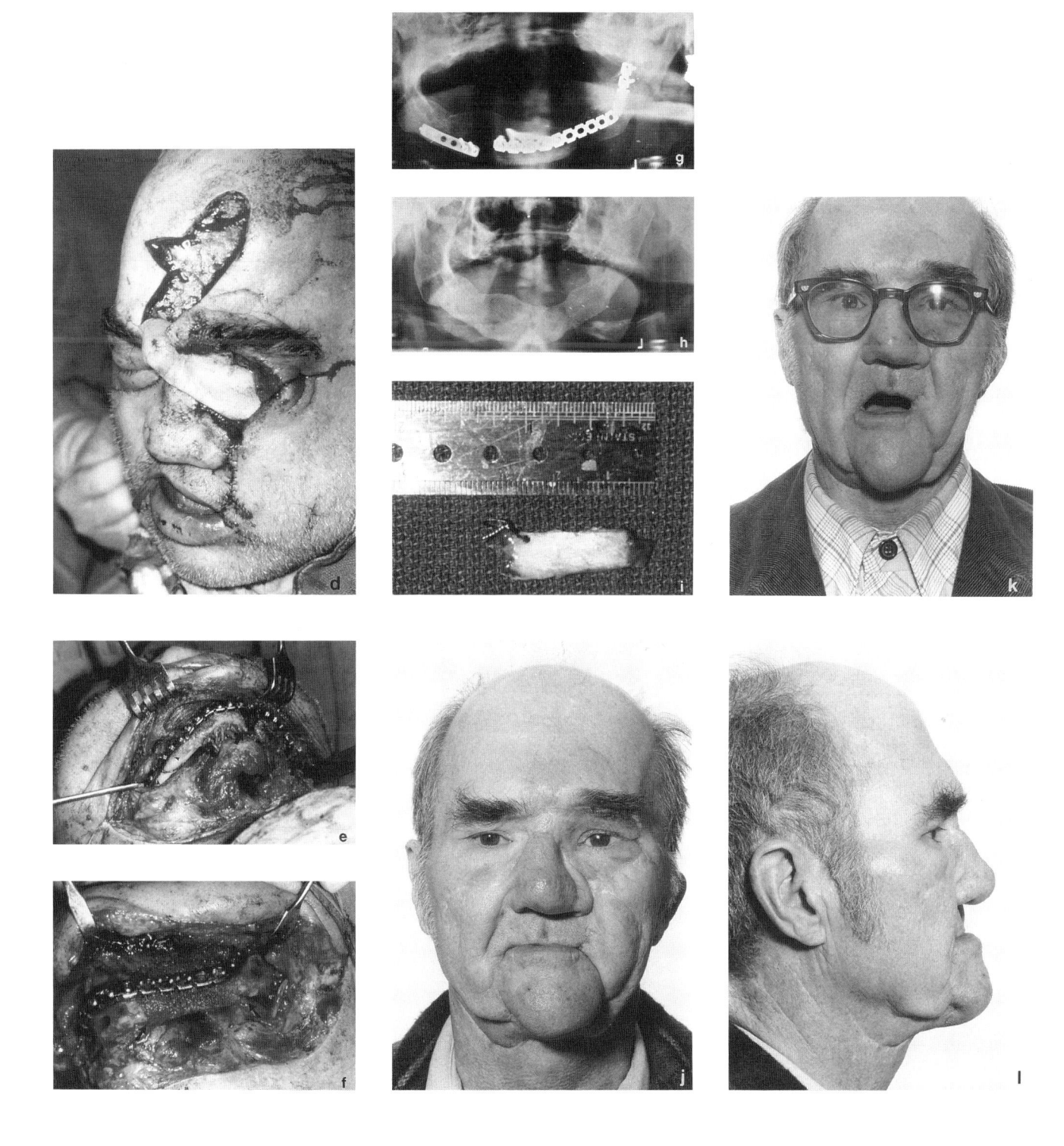

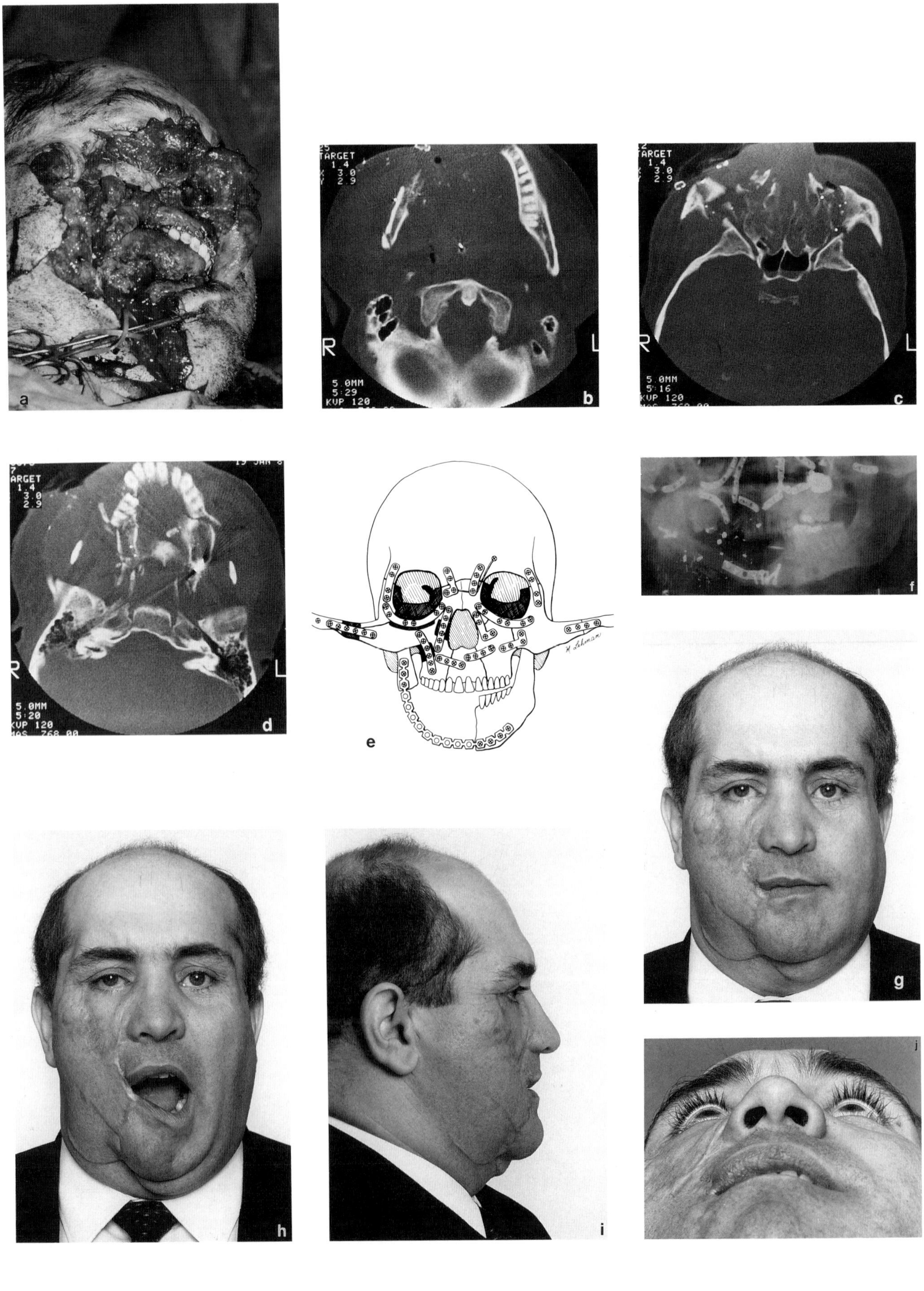
a
TARGET
1.4
R
L
5.0MM
5:29
KVP 120
b
TARGET
1.4
R
L
5.0MM
5:16
KVP 120
c
TARGET
1.4
3.0
2.9
R
L
5.0MM
5:20
KVP 120
d
e
f
g
h
i
j

Figure 27.6 (a) Very complex lower and midfacial gunshot injury following a suicide attempt is shown. Extensive bursting injury to soft tissue can be seen, particularly involving the right side of the face. (b) This CT scan of the mandible shows bone loss from the left body to the right angle. (c) This CT scan through the maxilla shows extensive destruction and loss of bone. (d) An axial CT scan through the lower maxilla and palate reveals multiple comminuted segmental and sagittal fractures of the maxilla and palate. (e) Artist's drawing of reconstruction. Reconstruction is commenced by rigid fixation of the orbitozygomatic complex and zygomatic arches, restoring an outer facial frame with correct facial width and projection. The remainder of the midfacial reconstruction is completed with extensive use of miniplates and bone grafts (shaded). Note extensive and deep bone grafting in both orbits. The mandibular gap is bridged by a long reconstruction plate after establishment of the correct occlusion of the remaining dentulous bone segments. (f) At seven months, the mandibular bone gap is replaced by a free-vascularized radial forearm flap. Its radius is fixed with lag screws and a compression plate anteriorly (performed by Dr. J.B. Boyd). (g) Appearance at one year shows maintenance of soft-tissue expansion. (h) Appearance at one year shows excellent restoration of mandibular function and maintenance of correct occlusion. Correct facial width and projection have been restored. (i) This lateral view shows restoration of projection and height of the midfacial and mandibular areas. (j) The inferior view shows restoration of correct facial width, zygomatic projection, and ocular orbital position. No enophthalmos or diplopia is apparent. Depression of the right zygomatic body is due to soft-tissue atrophy following extensive injury in this area.

lowing its reach to be extended. Further extension is obtained by dividing the omentum and making use of the anastomoses of the vascular arcades. The size of the human omentum and methods of lengthening it for transplantation have been extensively studied.

The omentum is isolated on the right gastroepiploic artery and vein and anastomosed to the left or right facial artery and vein. A hole is then made in the center of the omentum to accommodate the oral cavity, leaving the vascular arcades in a peripheral circular pattern. The omentum then provides circumferential coverage of the mandibular reconstruction, reconstructing the floor of the mouth. It is then tunneled in a circle through both cheeks into the midface and upper face. The omentum then provides for reconstruction of deficits in the hard palate and upper buccal sulcus. It is then wrapped around all zygomatic, orbital, and midfacial bone grafts and used to fill dead space in the maxillary and ethmoid sinuses. Tunneled into the nasoglabellar region the omentum can be used to cover nasal bone grafts and obliterate the frontal sinus; it shows a remarkable ability to adhere to bone grafts and obliterate dead space. It can be mobilized to cover bone grafts placed for secondary nasal reconstruction with tissue expanded forehead skin.

Any externally or intraorally exposed areas of omentum are covered primarily with mesh-split skin grafts. Graft take is usually rapid. Mesh skin grafting is essential to allow for possible leakage of lymph fluid.

Limitations of the use of omentum are the necessity of laparotomy and the technical difficulty of microvascular surgery. In addition, the omentum may shrink, may increase in bulk after weight gain, and will sag readily under the influence of gravity. It should not be used to provide contour or bulk. Carefully shaped and contoured bone grafts should provide the correct craniofacial scaffold; omentum should be used purely to cover and fill dead space. Sagging may be prevented by careful wrapping of all bone grafts with the omentum.

Early restoration of a midfacial bony scaffold and the prevention of soft-tissue contraction facilitate secondary reconstruction. Success of total nasal reconstruction with expanded forehead skin, wrapped around further bone grafts, is ensured due to the previously reconstructed bony base of the nasoglabellar region (see Figure 27.4). Scar revision is aided by the lack of significant deformation and contracture of soft tissue.

BIBLIOGRAPHY

Arnold PG, Irons GB: One stage reconstruction of massive craniofacial defect with gastromental free flap. Ann Plast Surg 6:26, 1980.

Broadbent TR, Woolf RM: Gunshot wounds of the face: Initial care. J Trauma 12:229, 1972.

Brown RG, Nahai F, Silverton JS: The omentum in facial reconstruction. Br J Plast Surg 31:58, 1978.

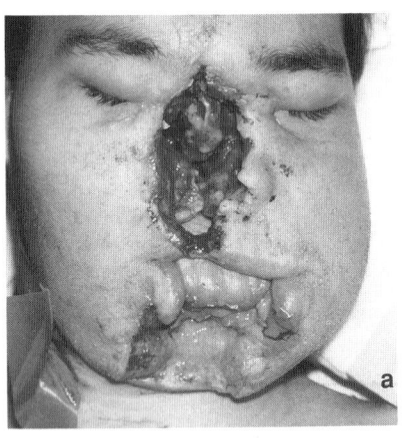

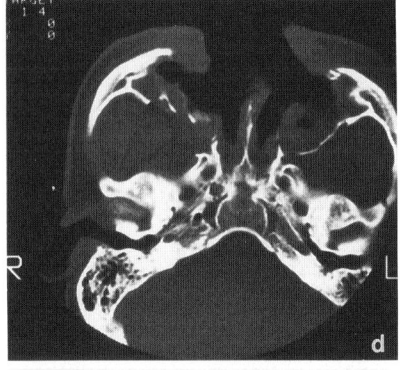

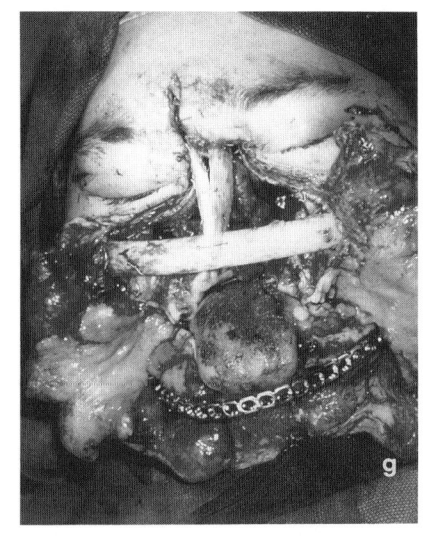

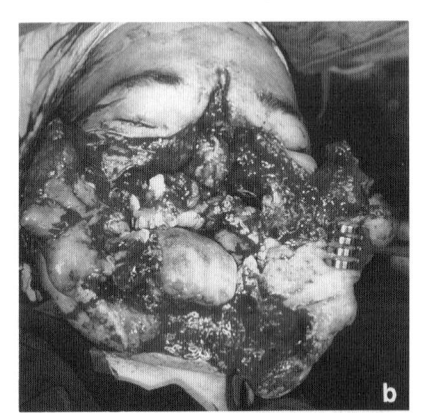

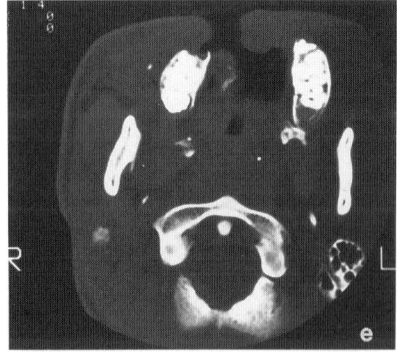

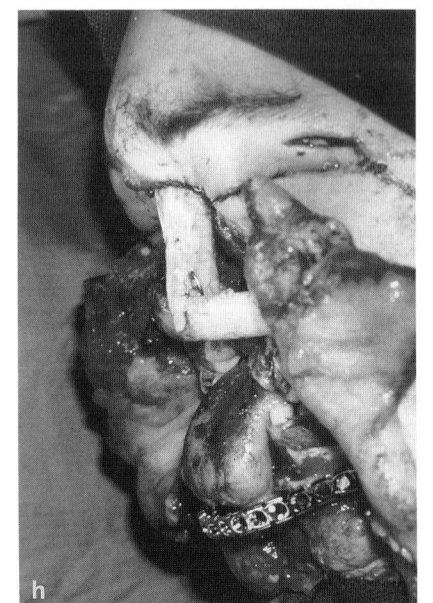

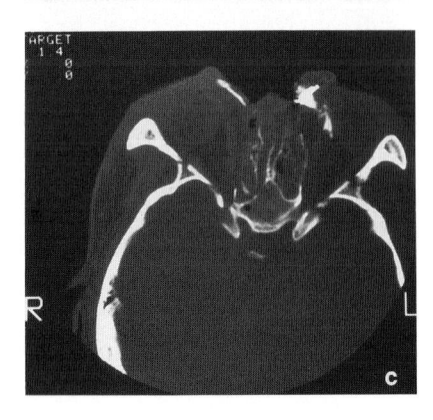

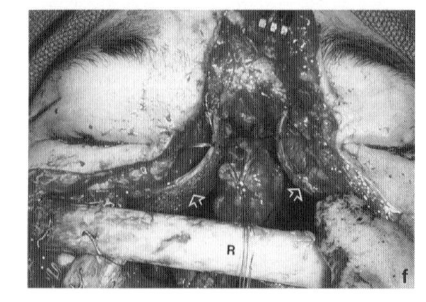

Figure 27.7 (a) This male has massive destruction of lower and midfacial soft tissue and bone following an accidental gunshot wound with a high-velocity hunting rifle. Large amounts of soft tissue loss in the naso-ethmoid and midface areas, as well as in the lower lip and chin, can be seen. (b) Reflection of the remaining skin flaps reveals extensive destruction and bone loss involving the entire nasoethmoid-orbital region, bilateral medial and inferomedial orbital rims, maxilla and hard palate, floor of mouth, and mandibular bone from posterior body to posterior body. (c) This axial CT scan through the orbits shows the extensive bone loss of the medial orbital walls and rims and the nasal bones. (d) An axial CT scan shows extensive bone loss of the central midface and maxilla. (e) This axial CT scan shows extensive bone loss of the hard palate. (f) Total reconstruction is shown of the missing medial and inferior orbital rim and wall with carefully contoured and bent split rib grafts (arrows). A full-thickness rib graft reconstructs the maxilla (R). Bilateral wires passed through the medial canthal tendons can be seen passed through the rib grafts to correct the telecanthus and re-establish the correct medial canthal position. (g) The three-dimensional reconstruction with a full-thickness rib graft spanning the maxillary gap is shown. The rib graft is anchored on either end to the residual zygoma. Split rib grafts run from the nasoglabellar region down to the full-thickness grafts. All this produces a three-dimensional reconstruction of the missing midfacial bone. A strong reconstruction plate bridges the mandibular gap running from posterior body to posterior body. (h) This lateral view shows the three-dimensional projection produced in the midface and mandible prior to soft-tissue coverage. (i) The mandibular plate has been covered circumferentially with long strips of cancellous bone from the hip (M). The omentum has now been anastomosed to

the left facial artery and vein. A hole is made in the center of the omentum, and it is now ready to be tunneled circumferentially through both cheeks (C) into the upper face. (T = tongue, N = nasoglabellar region.) (j) Omentum can be seen tunneled through a separate incision in both cheeks (C). It has been wrapped circumferentially around the mandibular reconstruction (M), anchored into the missing floor of the mouth, anchored into the missing palate and upper buccal sulcus, and then tunneled circumferentially to wrap all the bone grafts in the midfacial reconstruction (MX). The omentum is also tunneled up into the nasoglabellar region (N) to seal off the frontal sinus and is used to pack the ethmoid and maxillary sinuses on both sides (S). (T = tongue.) (k) Remaining soft tissues are repaired, and all exposed areas of omentum are covered with mesh split skin grafts. Note the mesh split skin grafts extending into the floor of the mouth and upper buccal sulcus. (l) Primary healing of initial reconstruction is demonstrated with no drainage or infection. A rectangular tissue expander has been placed in the forehead and expanded to provide skin for subsequent total nasal reconstruction. (m) Five years after reconstruction, the tissue-expanded forehead skin has been wrapped around a split calvarial bone graft. There is excellent function of both the upper and lower jaw. Lack of shrinkage and scarring of midface and lower facial soft tissue can be seen. There is slight enophthalmos of the right eye and asymmetry of the medial canthal regions, but the patient has normal binocular vision without diplopia. He has declined to have further soft tissue correction in the midfacial region. (n) This lateral view demonstrates restoration of good midfacial projection. (o) The patient has been fitted with functional dentures on both reconstructed upper and lower jaws.

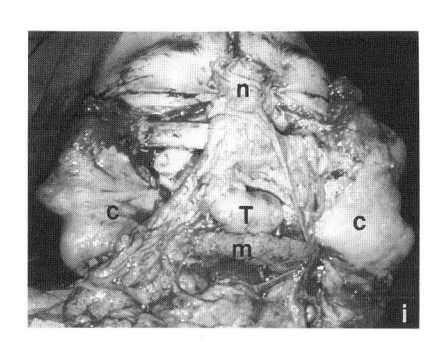

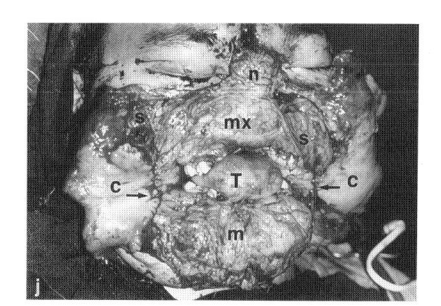

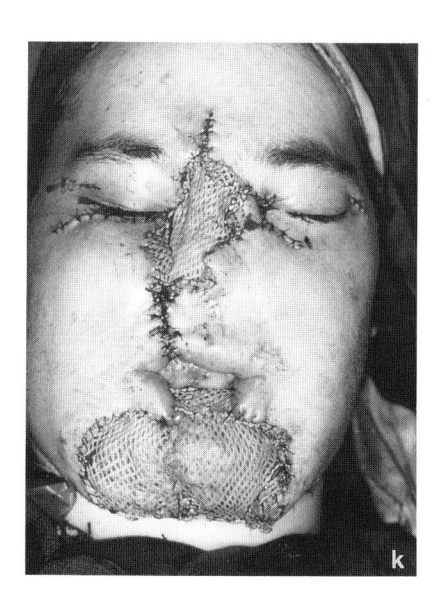

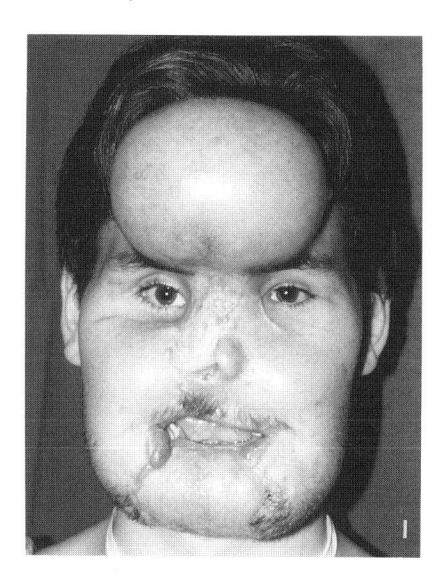

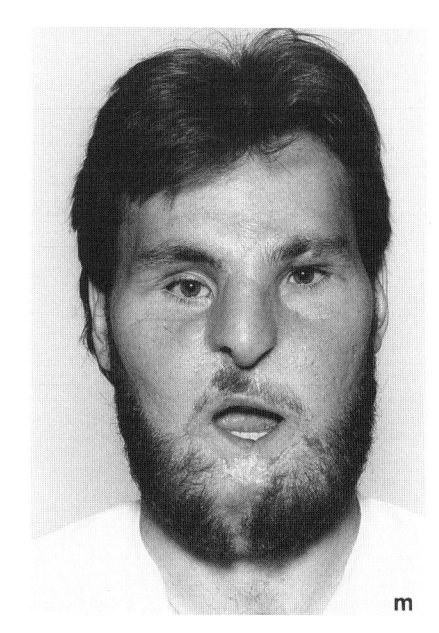

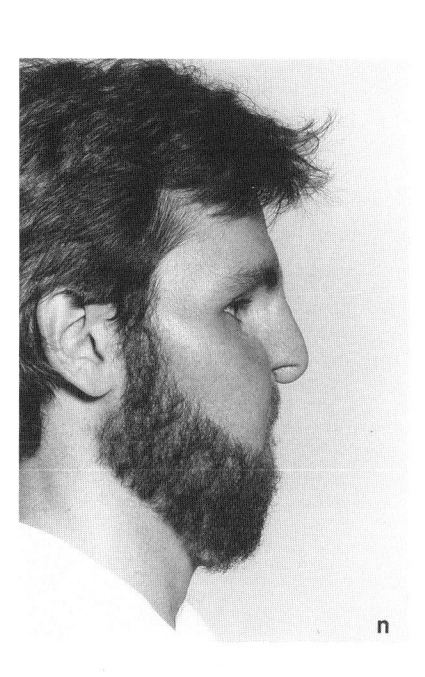

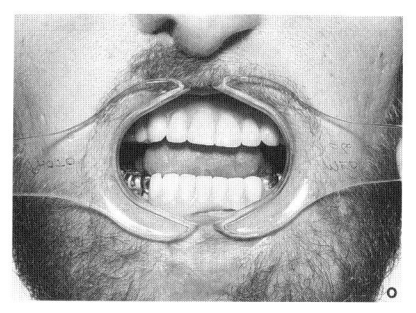

Das SK: The size of the human omentum and methods of lengthening it for transplantation. Br J Plast Surg 29:170, 1976.

Finch DR, Dibbell DG: Immediate reconstruction of gunshot injuries to the face. J Trauma 19:965, 1979.

Gruss JS: Internal fixation in facial fractures. In Current Therapy in Plastic and Reconstructive Surgery. Marsh J (ed). Toronto, Decker, pp 113–119, 1989.

Gruss JS, Phillips JH: Complex facial trauma: The evolving role of rigid fixation and immediate bone graft reconstruction. Clin Plast Surg 16:93, 1989.

Gruss JS, Pollock RA, Phillips JH, Antonyshyn O: Combined injuries of the cranium and face. Br J Plast Surg 43:385, 1989.

Gruss JG, Antonyshyn O, Phillips JH: Early definitive bone and soft tissue reconstruction of major gunshot wounds of the face. Plast Reconstr Surg 87:436, 1991.

Moore AN, Winslow P: Initial care of shotgun wounds of the face. Am Surg 31:321, 1965.

Phillips JH, Rahn B: Fixation effects on membranous and endochondral onlay bone graft resorption. Plast Reconstr Surg 82:872, 1988.

Schmoker R: Mandibular reconstruction using a special plate. J Maxillofac Surg 11:99, 1983.

Spiessl B: Internal Fixation of the Mandible. Berlin, Springer-Verlag, 1989.

Spira M, Hardy SB, Biggs TE, Gerow FJ: Shotgun injuries of the face. Plast Reconstr Surg 39:449, 1966.

CHAPTER 28

Complications in the Rigid Fixation of Midface Fractures

Leon A. Assael

Although fracture stability may be provided by rigid internal fixation, it is up to the surgeon to ensure that it be applied in a completely satisfactory manner. The main disadvantage of this technique has been in its application. As compared to conventional methods, rigid internal fixation is a technically demanding, complicated, and unforgiving method of treating midface fractures. To develop and maintain expertise in its use requires a detailed knowledge of theory and method as well as ongoing clinical experience. Nowhere is this more manifest than in complications that might occur when this technique is used in the treatment of midface fractures. Poor results in the treatment of midface fractures have two fundamental causes. First is the inability to restore the three-dimensional anatomy, and second is the inability to maintain the restoration because of flawed technique in plate and screw application.

ETIOLOGY OF CLINICAL COMPLICATIONS

Inadequate Reduction

A fundamental cause of poor results in the treatment of midface fractures is not unique to the use of plate and screw stabilization of the fracture but stems from the malalignment of the fracture segment. This failure to restore pre-injury form may result in changes in the functions of the masticatory apparatus, airway, oculo-orbital structures, and nervous system. These changes may cause functional deficits in chewing, speech, respiration, vision, somatic sensation, and muscular function. Failure to restore form may also produce significant esthetic deficits with only small malpositions of bone.

Because midface structures have a complex three-dimensional shape and therefore a more complex relation with the other structures, restoration of pre-injury form in the midface is far more complicated than in long bones. A structure that relates with several others may be reduced at one articulation but not necessarily at the others. For example, because the fronto-zygomatic suture has a relatively small interface, an apparent clinical reduction there may coexist with a gross malalignment at the inferior orbital rim because tiny discrepancies in reductions at one point are increasingly manifest as one proceeds from this pivotal point. Midface fracture should therefore be exposed sufficiently to allow anatomic alignment at all articulations.

The dental occlusion is not tolerant of even the smallest changes in anatomic form. The proprioceptive ability of the periodontal ligament is so discriminating that occlusal changes of less than 100 microns can be detected by the patient as a "change in bite." Movements of less than 1 millimeter can disarticulate the entire occlusion (see Figure 28.1). Although remodeling and slow movement of the teeth are capable of producing delayed compensation for some of these discrepancies, many cannot be corrected without subsequent surgical treatment—particularly where rigid fixation has been employed.

The main etiology of malocclusion of the teeth subsequent to rigid internal fixation is the failure of the surgeon to establish the occlusion adequately prior to the placement of fixation. Establishment of the pre-injury occlusion with MMF is the key initial step before the placement of stable fixation in the midface. If the condyles are not in the fossae or there is an associated condylar fracture, the establishment of correct occlusion may not represent a correct functional position. When

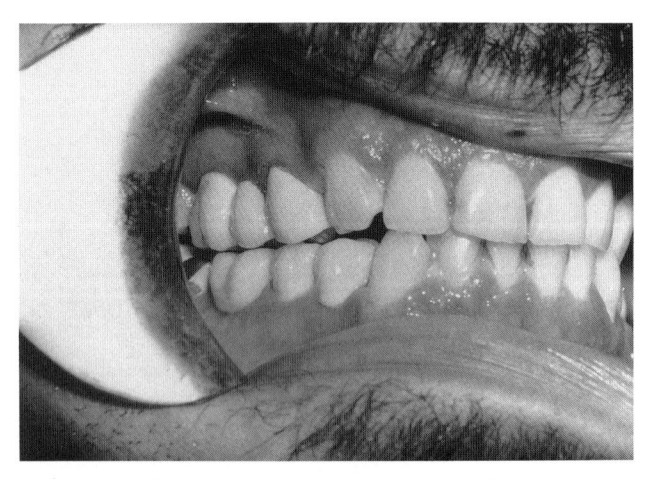

Figure 28.1 A post-treatment malocclusion following a midface fracture. Note that although the maxilla is retropositioned only 1 millimeter, the posterior occlusion is entirely disarticulated.

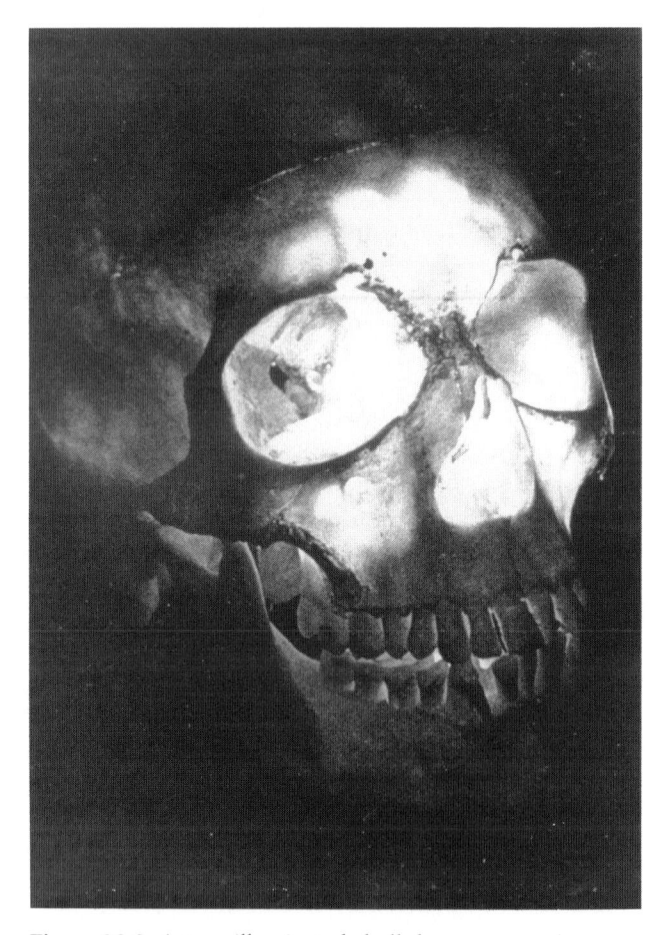

Figure 28.2 A transilluminated skull demonstrates the supporting buttresses of the midface. These include the palate, alveolus, piriform rim, nasomaxillary complex, zygomatic buttress, infraorbital rim, frontal process of the zygoma, and zygomatic arch. Plates placed in these locations will most reliably key into pre-injury form and will best resist functional forces.

the fixation is released, a malocclusion may be noted. Alternatively, the malocclusion may be noted only in function.

The restoration of midfacial width is first dependent on the accurate reduction of fractures of the mandibular corpus. Open reduction and rigid fixation of these fractures will prevent lateral splaying of the mandible, which will be magnified in the midface. Checking the lingual cortical plate for reduced fractures of the mandibular symphysis is especially important to prevent this problem. If the palate is split, the use of a dental splint may help prevent the unseating of the palatal cusps in MMF. If the palatal cusps are out of contact, the facial width will be increased, often with clinically noticeable widening of the upper midface. Postoperative distortion and dental occlusion should be looked for at the completion of the operation by removing the MMF and placing the mandible in its presumed pre-injury relationship with the maxilla. Unlike the situation with less rigid, conventional means of midface stabilization, the bony position cannot change significantly to accommodate occlusal discrepancies. Furthermore, postoperative movement should not be counted on to correct the occlusal discrepancies. The best time to correct a malocclusion is during the initial operation.

A frequent complication in the treatment of midface fractures is the failure to restore and maintain the pre-injury vertical, anterior/posterior, and transverse dimensions of the face. The vertical dimension may be lost if there is comminution at the supporting buttresses. This comminution eliminates the "key" that will guide the placement of plates (see Figure 28.2). The use of preoperative and postoperative cephalometric evaluation will offer objective data as to the deficits and restoration of vertical position (see Figure 28.3). Preoperative coronal CT scans will give information as to which buttresses are sufficiently intact to permit anatomic reduction. Careful evaluation at the time of surgery, along with a thorough understanding of the fracture morphology, will nearly always obviate the possibility of losing the vertical dimension. It is useful to note that midface fractures do not avulse bone. The pieces of the comminuted puzzle are present, waiting to be restored. The anatomic restoration of a single zygomatic buttress or piriform rim is enough to provide a "key" against which the entire vertical dimension of the midface can be restored.

The restoration of the anterior/posterior and transverse dimensions of the midface depends on the placement of a normal dental occlusion against an intact or restored mandible. This portion of the procedure, which includes the treatment of mandible fractures, should be carried out prior to restoration of vertical dimension. The restoration of the vertical dimension at the Le Fort I level must also follow the establishment of reduction of any displaced zygoma or nasomaxillary complex.

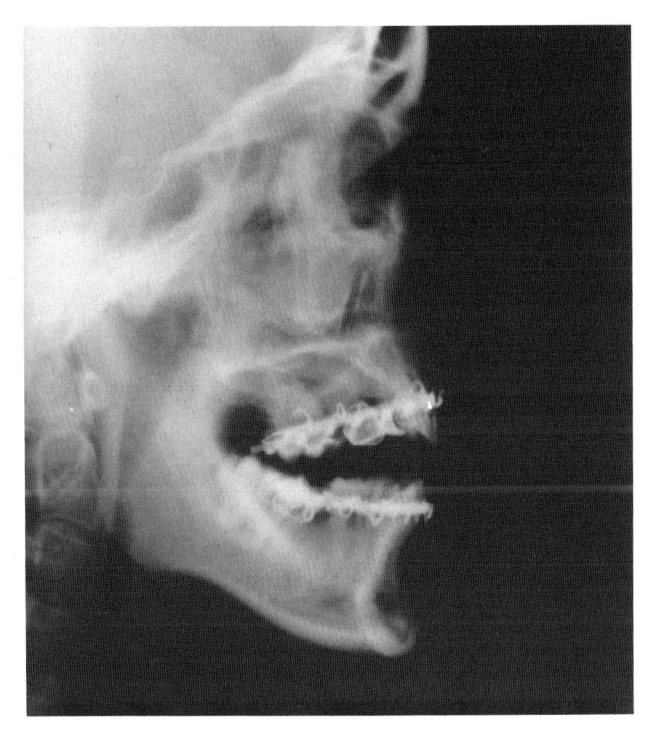

Figure 28.3 Preoperative lateral cephalogram in a patient with a Le Fort III fracture. Note the open bite, intrusion of the anterior midface, and alteration of the palatal plane.

Improper Fixation Technique

Given that the surgeon has appropriately realigned the skeletal anatomy, the most common error in rigidly fixating midface fractures is failure to adapt the plate passively to the bones to be fixated. Once the MMF is removed, the preapplication contour of the plate will determine the position of the attached bone. The subsequent inevitable movement of the bone will distort the occlusion if the segment is attached to the dentition. If the segment is not attached to the bone, movement of the bone will have some affect on midface contour. Fixation that is inadequate to resist functional force may produce additional complications. These include infection, nonunion, and bone malposition. Fixation forces must be sufficient to resist all functional forces. If a functional force exceeds fixation forces even briefly, bones will displace and fixation will fail. Loose hardware, contamination, and interfragmentary mobility will combine to produce infection. Because the forces on the maxillary dental arch are mainly directed cephalad, the buttressing effect of the malar eminence and piriform rim is vital in preventing the loss of fixation. Bone contact in these areas will assist the plates in preventing movement of the maxilla. If comminution is present, the fixation alone may not ensure undisturbed healing. The use of autogenous bone grafts may be necessary to re-establish the portion of functional load that the bone must sustain. In general, defects greater than 1 centimeter at supporting buttresses are filled with bone grafts.

RECOGNITION OF COMPLICATIONS

After therapy using rigid internal fixation of a midface fracture, the best time to correct a suboptimal result is in the early postoperative period. However, if not immediately manifest as a malocclusion, treatment inadequacies may be difficult to detect in the early postoperative period. Tissue edema and emphysema prevent an accurate assessment of the final position of the soft-tissue structures over the facial skeleton. Hence the final position of the globe in the orbit, nasal and malar contour, ratio of lip to tooth, mandibular plane angle, and other important soft-tissue features may be obscured in the early clinical examination.

The use of postoperative cephalometric evaluation will offer objective measurement regarding the support of the soft-tissue drape of the face. The facial height and projection may be measured according to norms to assure that the supporting buttresses of the midface have been accurately restored. Facial symmetry can be evaluated both clinically and with the assistance of a posterior/anterior cephalogram.

The postoperative assessment of orbital volume and the resulting position of the globe may be obscured by several factors. Postoperative edema and orbital emphysema may temporarily place the globe in an anterior position in the orbit. If there is displaced orbital tissue, late cicatrization may displace the globe posteriorly and inferiorly. If the postoperative assessment of orbital volume is in question, postoperative CT scanning with objective measurements of orbital size will offer additional information.

MANAGEMENT OF COMPLICATIONS

Treatment Planning

Dental malocclusion following rigid internal fixation of a midface fracture must first be examined with careful scrutiny as to its etiology. Diagnostic dental casts, radiographic imaging, and clinical evaluation are the mainstays of diagnosis.

In clinical evaluation, the surgeon determines the type of malocclusion in evidence. The malocclusion may be characterized by the deviation noted from normal maxillary position. Disorders in the vertical dimension will result in open bite or overclosure. Anterior/posterior malposition will cause excessive overjet (Class 2) or a horizontal maxillary deficiency (Class 3) malocclusion. Deviation of the dental midline off center may be produced by lateral displacement of the maxilla. Malocclusions may be pre-existing, or they may be the result of trauma. Clues as to the etiology of a malocclusion can be seen in the wear facets of teeth. An open bite that disarticulates the occlusion as the result of a single premature contact creates a wedge-shaped opening that is generally the result of trauma (see Figure 28.4). Teeth that have always been in open bite will often have persistent mammelons.

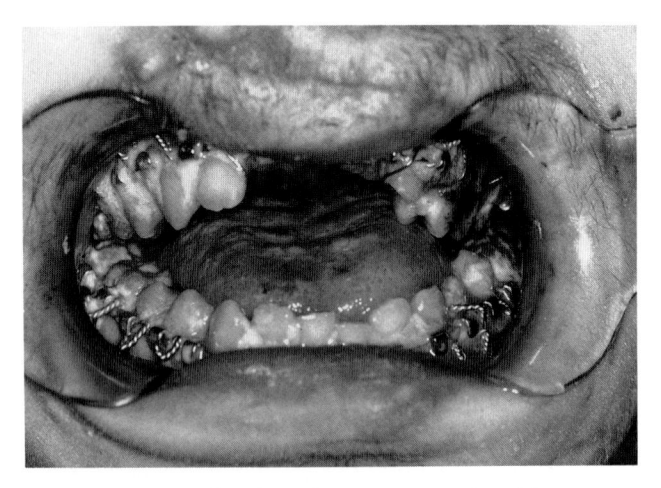

Figure 28.4 A wedge-shaped open bite produced by a Le Fort II fracture. Note the wear facets on the cuspids and incisors; these indicate this malocclusion was not pre-existing.

Clinical evaluation of the dental occlusion must always be correlated with facial analysis. Dental midlines generally should correspond closely to facial midlines. Discrepancies in midline with an otherwise normal occlusion may be due to misplacement of fixation in a panfacial fracture. Evaluation of the facial features may show a canting of the lips and deviation of the mandible. Open-bite and Class 2 malocclusion in the post-trauma patient are often associated with retrognathia, lip incompetence, and a high angle of the mandibular plane. Loss of the vertical dimension of the midface with a Class 3 overclosed bite is often associated with eversion of the lip, depression of the columella, loss of nasal tip projection, and paranasal deficiency.

In the patient with a postoperative occlusal, esthetic, or functional deficit, evaluation of dental casts and a cephalogram is helpful in determining etiology and planning treatment. Diagnostic dental casts should be evaluated to verify the pre-injury dental occlusion, to examine the postoperative condition, and to plan for optimal correction. Postoperative malocclusion is often complicated by compensatory orthodontic movement of the teeth. Malunion of fractures within the dental arch may also prevent the interdigitation of the dental casts. Casts should be mounted on a semianatomic articulator with a face bow transfer so that findings can be correlated with the cephalogram. Appropriate analysis will identify and quantify postoperative deficits.

Examination of pre-injury photographs of the patient may offer detailed information regarding the traumatically induced deficits present. This may be particularly useful when the patient's facial projection, height, or width is in question without an associated functional alteration. Evaluation of nasal morphology including alar width and tip projection may also be assisted by pre-injury photographs. In the case where a dentofacial deformity may have been pre-existing, the evaluation of the photographs may offer a clue as to what the natural occlusion and symmetry might have been.

The patient with associated deficits in the upper midface, orbit, airway, and nose may receive optimal correlation with clinical findings by the use of CT scans with three-dimensional reconstruction. The location of deficits in the supporting buttresses of the face and orbit may be quantified and integrated with clinical diagnosis. Objective data on the position of the globe and orbit may also be obtained with the ophthalmometer and the use of facial moulage. By quantifying deficits, a treatment plan can be formulated that will precisely correct each problem.

Early diagnosis of malpositioned segments of the midface may help avoid the need for secondary osteotomy. Surgical intervention within four weeks of injury usually permits immediate repositioning and refixation of all segments. Because small segments of bone may undergo early resorption, bone grafting may be necessary to reconstitute the buttresses of the midface. Selective sites of osteotomy may be necessary in the four to eight week postinjury phase in order to remobilize fractured segments. Cases in which malunion has occurred greater than eight weeks post injury are probably best managed with conventional osteotomy techniques.

Repositioning of the fractured segments of bone is not the only means whereby an esthetic or functional deficit may be corrected. Compensatory change in associated structures may be utilized to overcome the underlying deficit. This is an especially helpful treatment philosophy where discrepancies are small. For example, orthodontics and restorative dentistry may correct a small malocclusion due to a malpositioned maxilla, and alloplastic augmentation may correct small contour deficits. The problem in these compensatory techniques arises when they are used to mask problems that are beyond their ability to correct. A deficit must be carefully quantified before a treatment plan is formulated.

A problem list and treatment plan are formulated below for a patient who is evaluated 6 months after being treated for Le Fort III and comminuted mandible fractures with rigid internal fixation. The problem list describes, to the most objective extent possible, all of the deficits seen in a particular patient. The treatment plan specifically addresses in turn each of this patient's deficits.

Problem List

1. Skeletal deficits (see Figure 28.5).
   a. The maxilla is displaced posteriorly 12 millimeters, superiorly 16 millimeters at the piriform rim, and laterally 5 millimeters to the right.
   b. The mandible corpus is displaced posteriorly 7 millimeters and to the right 3 millimeters.

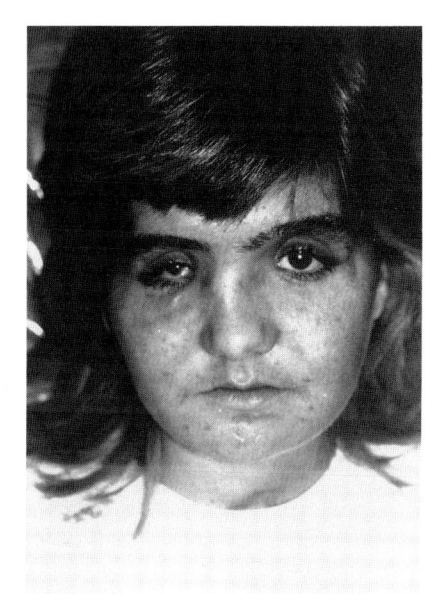

Figure 28.5 A patient's status after rigid internal fixation of a Le Fort II fracture and mandible fracture. Note severe loss of the vertical dimension, nasal septal deviation, malar deficiency, telecanthus, and enophthalmos.

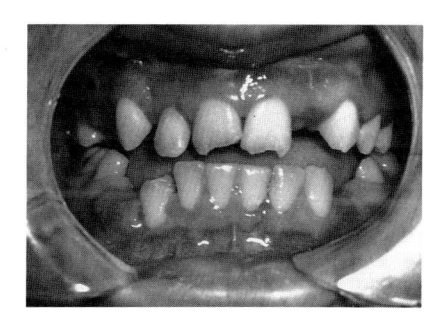

Figure 28.6 Malocclusion of the patient in Figure 28.5. Note the wedge-shaped open bite, stepped mandibular dental arch, and pre-existing wear facets.

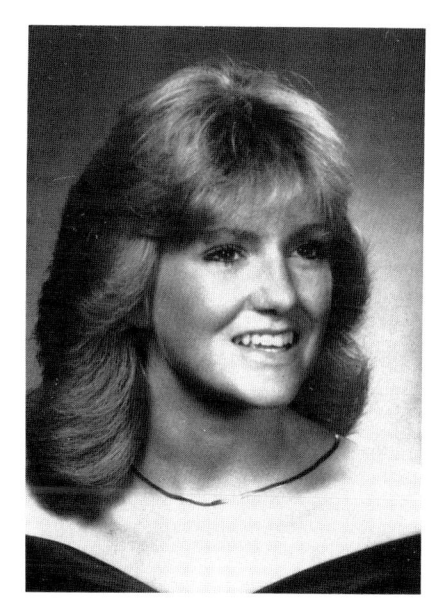

Figure 28.7 A pre-injury photograph of the patient in Figure 28.5 shows the normal vertical dimension, lip to tooth ratio, and mandibular plane angle. Anterior projection of the face including mentum, malar, columella, and nasal dorsum are all excellent.

   c. The mentum is crushed, with loss of 12 millimeters in height and 5 millimeters in anterior projection.
   d. The right zygoma displaced posteriorly 10 millimeters and inferiorly 10 to 15 millimeters.
   e. The right enophthalmos is displaced posteriorly 5 millimeters, inferiorly 7 millimeters, and medially 3 millimeters.
   f. Right lateral and right medial canthi malpositioned.
   g. The nasal tip is 4 millimeters to the right with deviated septum; the alar base is displaced to 36 millimeters in width.
   h. Dental malocclusion is present, with apertognathia of 6 millimeters, Class 3 4 millimeters. Deviation of dental midlines maxillary incisor 4 millimeters right, mandibular incisor 2 millimeters right (see Figure 28.6).
2. Functional deficits
   a. Diplopia is seen in upward and left lateral gaze.
   b. The right nasal airway is obstructed.
   c. Anesthesia is found in the right infraorbital and bilateral mental nerves.
   d. Mandibular hypomobility is present to 20 millimeters.
   e. Speech articulation is difficult.

The skeletal deficits noted were quantified with the assistance of pre-injury photographs (see Figure 28.7).

Treatment Plan

(See Figures 28.8, 28.9, and 28.10.)

1. Maxillary Le Fort I osteotomy for advancement, downgrafting, and rotation
2. Mandibular osteotomy for advancement
3. Genioplasty for advancement and downgrafting
4. Right malar osteotomy for advancement and elevation
5. Right orbital reconstruction for enophthalmos and diplopia
6. Septorhinoplasty

The order of treatment for corrective surgery should be formulated with attention to not undoing previous correction with a subsequent procedure. For example, a planned maxillary osteotomy should precede septorhinoplasty. Ocular muscle surgery should be accomplished after restoration of the orbit. If simultaneous correction of a series of problems is planned, the sequence of the procedure may well have a significant impact on the result. A general scheme is presented below for the simultaneous restoration of esthetic and functional deficits following midface trauma.

Repositioning of the maxillary dental arch against an intact or restored mandible is a good way to begin. This provides an anatomic key that restores the anterior/posterior and transverse dimensions of the midface. Correction of the position of the zygomas follows. The position of the zygomatic arch and infraorbital rim may be evaluated to prevent overrotation of the malar em-

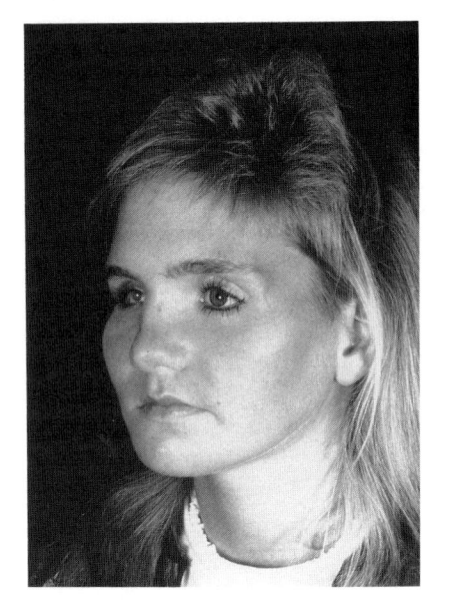

Figure 28.8 Clinical photographs of the patient in Figure 28.5 after maxillary and mandibular osteotomies to correct facial height, projection and dental occlusion. Enophthalmos has not been repaired (oblique view).

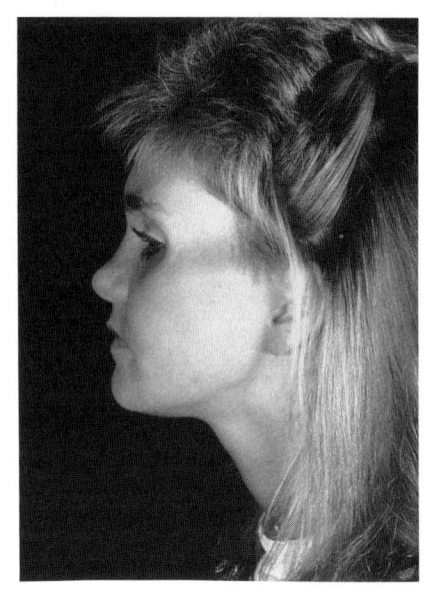

Figure 28.9 Postoperative lateral view.

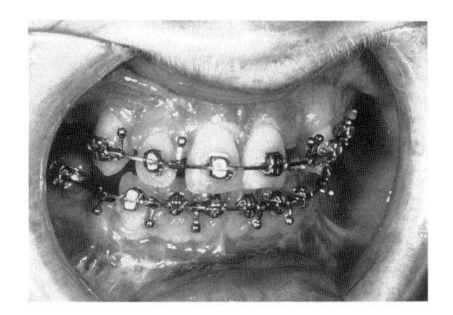

Figure 28.10 Postoperative occlusion.

inence. The vertical dimension of the midface can then be restored at the zygomatic buttresses. Correction of the medial orbital rim and orbital walls may then follow. Corrective nasal surgery can then be accomplished against the restored midface. The use of rigid internal fixation will permit the replacement of the naso-tracheal tube with an oral-tracheal one. Finally, soft-tissue procedures may be carried out against a restored osseous infrastructure.

SUMMARY

Complications in the management of midface fractures with rigid internal fixation are most often due to malaligned fracture segments or improper application of plates and screws. Preoperative assessment of the injury, including careful objective review of the clinical examination, imaging, dental casts, cephalometrics, and pre-injury photographs, is helpful in planning for optimal correction. Rigid internal fixation of midface fractures must fix facial bones in their pre-injury position and provide fixation forces that will exceed functional forces at all times. An ability to accurately execute rigid internal fixation procedures is necessary to produce satisfactory results. If postoperative assessment of the patient reveals persistent deficits, a comprehensive analysis is necessary to quantify the problems, determine their etiology and formulate a treatment plan. As in initial surgical management, good results in secondary reconstruction depend on careful analysis and attention to detail.

BIBLIOGRAPHY

Bell WH, Profitt WR, White RP, Jr: Surgical Correction of Dentofacial Deformities, Vol 1 and 2. Philadelphia, Saunders, 1980.

Hotte H: Orbital Fractures. Springfield, Thomas, 1970.

Kruger E, Schilli W (Eds): Oral and Maxillofacial Traumatology, Vol 1 and 2. Chicago, Quintessence, 1986.

Manson PN, Clifford CM, Su CT, et al: Mechanisms of global support and post traumatic enophthalmos: The anatomy of the ligament sling and its relationship to intramuscular cone orbital fat. Plast Reconstr Surg 77:193-207, 1986.

Manson PN, Grivias A, Rosenbaum A, et al: Studies on enophthalmos II: The measurement of orbital injuries and their treatment by quantitative computed tomography. Plast Reconstr Surg 77:203-214, 1986.

Rowe NL, Williams J: Maxillofacial Injuries. Edinburgh, Churchill Livingstone, 1985.

Spiessl B: New Concepts in Maxillofacial Bone Surgery. Berlin, Springer-Verlag, 1976.

CHAPTER 29

Craniofacial Osteotomies and Rigid Fixation in the Correction of Post-traumatic Craniofacial Deformities

Joseph S. Gruss

Over the past decade, the treatment principles of craniomaxillofacial injuries in patients sustaining multiple trauma have been outlined by several authors. The standard principles of craniofacial exposure, rigid internal miniplate fixation, and primary bone grafting in acute facial trauma have been well documented.

Current management of complex craniomaxillofacial trauma consists of early (within two weeks of injury) exposure of all fracture fragments and the restoration and maintenance of the normal anatomy of the craniofacial skeleton by use of rigid internal fixation techniques. Preoperative computerized tomographic (CT) scans are routinely employed in all facial fractures; their use allows precise delineation and identification of fracture patterns. Primary bone grafting is indicated for comminuted or missing bone. The utilization of these techniques allows for a single-stage repair of most injuries and has not been demonstrated to be associated with a significant increase in the rate of infection.

Failure to diagnose craniomaxillofacial injuries and inappropriate application of the techniques of internal fixation and bone grafting are associated with the establishment of post-traumatic secondary facial deformities. Common mistakes made in acute facial trauma repair include inadequate exposure and reduction of midfacial and mandibular fractures. The use of suspension wires in comminuted Le Fort fractures of the maxilla may lead to midface collapse and malocclusion. Inadequate repair of orbitozygomatic fractures can result in late enophthalmos and vertical oculo-orbital dystopia. Failure to repair defects of the orbital wall and insufficient orbital bone grafting may also produce these deformities. The significance of nasoethmoid-orbital injuries is often underappreciated. Enophthalmos and telecanthus can arise from failure to reposition the medial orbital walls and the medial canthal ligaments. Characteristic nasal deformities associated with nasoethmoid-orbital fractures with a central maxillary crush may be present if nasal projection is not restored. Midface and orbitozygomatic projection and contour will be restored inadequately unless the role of the zygomatic arch in the treatment of these fractures is understood.

Lack of recognition of the severity of these injuries and failure to understand the principles of reconstruction will compromise outcome and may result in these secondary facial deformities; once established, they are difficult to correct. The most common deformities are enophthalmos, vertical ocular dystopia, malar flattening with or without orbital dystopia, increased facial width across the arches, increased width and collapse of the nasoethmoid-orbital region, telecanthus, and occlusal problems related to maxillary and mandibular injuries. Establishment of an anatomic three-dimensional skeletal framework prior to the onset of soft-tissue scarring and cicatricial contracture is the key to prevention of post-traumatic secondary craniofacial deformities. Maintenance of soft-tissue expansion by the underlying bone can be achieved only with early intervention. In the post-traumatic, established, secondary facial deformity, soft-tissue distortion from contracted underlying scar tissue and adherence to bony depressions and defects is the limiting factor in late facial reconstruction.

Historically, the treatment of common orbitozygomatic and nasoethmoid-orbital deformities consisted chiefly of onlay bone grafting. Seemingly adequate correction was often followed by progressive relapse. The

Table 29.1 Principles of Repair

Bony Deficit
Segmental depression
    Onlay bone graft
Segmental deficit
    Inlay bone graft

Bony Malposition
Anatomically normal
    Osteotomy
    Reposition bone
    Stabilize with miniplates
    Bone grafts fill gaps
Anatomically abnormal
    Rebuild totally with bone grafts

---

use of bone grafts to maintain the position of osteotomized bone segments is frequently unsuccessful due to continued tension produced by the scarred soft tissue; this continued tension causes resorption of bone grafts and relapse.

In this chapter, we present a logical, simplified approach to the correction of regional secondary deformities and details of the essential principles of repair. Emphasis is placed on the important role of the zygomatic arch in establishment of correct midface width and projection. The expanded roles of craniofacial exposure, segmental osteotomies, and bony repositioning rigidly fixed with miniplates combined with bone grafts have revolutionized care in these complex cases. Craniofacial osteotomies using intracranial/extracranial approaches recreate the original fracture pattern and can now be rigidly fixed in their new position with miniplates, thus preventing late relapse. We have formulated a graduated approach to the correction of regional bony post-traumatic secondary deformities. Bony depressions are corrected by onlay grafts, rigidly fixed with lag screws. Malposition of anatomically normal bone is corrected by osteotomy and repositioning. Anatomically abnormal bone is corrected by total reconstruction with bone grafts (see Table 29.1).

SECONDARY FACIAL DEFORMITY
Principles of Repair
General

Treatment of established post-traumatic facial deformities employs the same principles used in the acute situation: direct exposure of the fractures through an extracranial approach and, when appropriate, combining this with an intracranial approach. The use of miniplates and lag screw techniques provides rigid internal fixation and therefore primary bone healing of osteotomy sites and bone grafts. The orbit is an exception to these principles, as outlined below.

Exposure

The coronal incision is used for access to the supraorbital and lateral orbital rims, the nasoethmoid-orbital region, and the zygomatic arch. Direct access to the entire craniofacial skeleton can be obtained by combining this approach with subciliary incisions and an upper buccal sulcus degloving incision. Previous lacerations may also be employed for access. Direct exposure of the injury site allows for accurate evaluation of the exact fracture pattern and the positions of involved bony fragments. Only then can a logical plan for reconstruction be applied. All incisions are linked to each other with subperiosteal dissection.

It must be noted that following extensive subperiosteal stripping of the orbital, zygomatic, and maxillary regions, the loss of soft tissue attachments to the underlying bone will result in sagging of these tissues due to gravitational pull. This will accentuate underlying bony prominences and malunions and will contribute to loss of anterior malar projection. In order to prevent this, it is important to resuspend these soft tissues from underlying stable bony structures. The inferior orbital rim, fronto-zygomatic region, and deep temporal fascia may be used for this purpose. A strong, absorbable suture may be placed through drill holes or miniplates in these regions.

In addition, reattachment of the lateral canthal ligaments through separate drill holes in the lateral orbital wall facilitates resuspension of the lower eyelid, further reducing the incidence of lower-lid ectropion and lateral canthal deformity.

Free autogenous bone grafts are the material of choice for reconstruction. Cortical or corticocancellous bone provides stability and stimulates formation of new bone through induction of osteogenic precursors at the recipient site and by cellular elements in the graft. Split calvarial bone, rib, and iliac crest may be used for this purpose, but membranous bone from the skull is usually preferred due to its low donor site morbidity and availability. Inability to bend cranial bone for contouring to large curved surfaces remains its main disadvantage.

Bone graft must be rigidly immobilized to prevent shearing forces and to allow vascular ingrowth. Immobilization may be achieved by multiple screw fixation to a miniplate or using the lag screw technique. The orbit remains the exception to this rule: reconstruction of defects of the orbital wall is achieved by the insertion of carefully contoured calvarial bone grafts supported by bony shelves surrounding the defect. Pressure generated by intraorbital contents tamponades the bone grafts and maintains their position.

Method of Fixation

Post-traumatic facial deformities are associated with secondary cicatricial contracture that must be overcome if anatomic restoration of the skeletal framework is to be maintained. Fixation of osteotomized bony segments must therefore be rigid enough to withstand deformation from these forces and from pressure, traction, and shearing forces generated by dynamic muscle action.

Fixation by Interosseous Wire

Fixation by interosseous wire relies on the static forces generated by the tension of the wire and by the friction between corresponding bone surfaces at the fracture/osteotomy site. In the acute situation, the use of interosseous wires is primarily indicated in the repair of low-velocity, isolated orbital fractures without comminution or bone deficiency. However, in reconstruction of the post-traumatic secondary deformity, this method, which provides insufficient immobilization of the bony segments, cannot be used to bridge bony gaps; an alternative means of bony fixation is therefore needed.

Miniplate Fixation

Miniplates and screws are used to provide rigid internal fixation of the facial skeleton. Self-tapping screws should be employed in the upper and midface regions, where the bone is thin. Following precise contouring, miniplates are fixed to the underlying bone, allowing for placement of at least two screws in intact bone on either side of the fracture/osteotomy site. Drill holes must be placed precisely in the centric screw hole position to avoid compression and associated displacement of the osseous segments. Around the orbit, thinner (1.5-millimeter) miniplates or microplates may be applied in order to avoid palpation through the overlying skin.

Relapse has been documented in situations in which miniplates have been used as the only means of bridging large bone gaps. Due to the lack of new bone formation, tensile forces from dynamic muscle pull and soft-tissue scarring can overcome static forces resulting from plate and screw fixation. In situations with bone gaps greater than 5 millimeters, primary bone grafting should be performed for the reasons cited above. Bone grafts should be fixed to the miniplate with screws or to the underlying stable bone with lag screws. Because the graft can rotate around a single lag screw, more than one lag screw is usually required for adequate fixation. Research has shown that rigid fixation of bone grafts significantly inhibits resorption. Bone grafts should be carefully contoured to fit precisely into the osseous defect. Once grafts are rigidly fixed, they may be further contoured in situ with a drill and bur and copious irrigation.

Specific Principles

The successful management of post-traumatic facial deformities relies on accurate assessment of the state of the underlying skeleton. Clinical and radiologic assessment will allow the reconstructive surgeon to determine the nature of the bony facial deformity, which may be broadly classified into a bony deficit and/or a bony malposition (see Table 29.1). Treatment protocols may be designed based on these deformities as they pertain to specific anatomic regions.

Bony deficits exist as either a segmental deficit or depression, or they may involve the entire bone (see Figure 29.1). Treatment of such problems involves the use of autogenous bone graft, which is employed as either onlay or inlay grafts and is rigidly fixed using lag screws or miniplate techniques. The management of bony malpositions depends on whether the involved bone is anatomically normal or is abnormal due to segmental fractures. Specifically, anatomically normal bone (without segmental fractures) that is malpositioned may be treated with osteotomies at the fracture sites, repo-

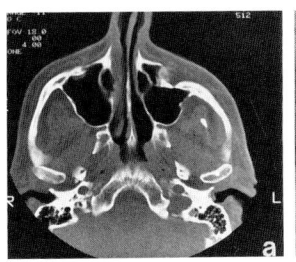

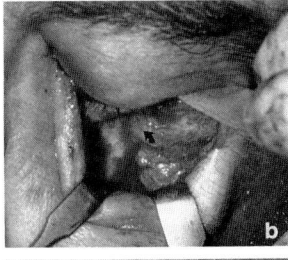

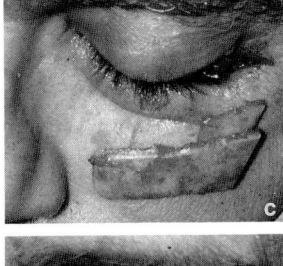

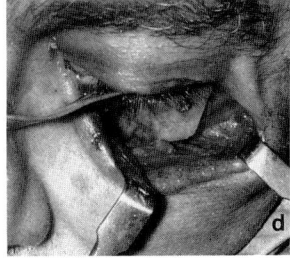

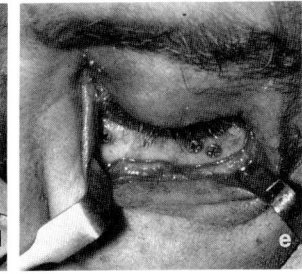

Figure 29.1 Patient with segmental depression of the zygomatic body and anterior maxillary wall. (a) This axial CT scan demonstrates segmental fracture with bone loss. (b) Exposure through a subciliary muscle splitting incision. The arrow identifies the segmental depression. (c) Plan of reconstruction using sandwich split calvarial bone grafts. (d) The calvarial bone graft is wedged into a narrow portion of the defect and fixed with a lag screw. (e) A larger piece of bone graft bridges the orbital rim and zygomatic body overlying the previously placed bone graft; it is fixed with three lag screws.

sitioning, and rigid internal fixation. Recreation of the fracture pattern allows malunited bone to be aligned anatomically.

Malpositioned anatomically abnormal bone cannot be treated in this way; it must be totally rebuilt using autogenous bone grafts. Bone grafts are used only to bridge bone gaps already bridged by miniplates, in order to promote osteosynthesis. Prior to miniplate fixation, osteotomies were stabilized with wires and bony gaps were bridged with bone grafts, which were used to hold osteotomized segments in their new position. As scarred and deformed soft tissues healed, bone grafts would resorb and, combined with inadequate fixation using interosseous wires, this would lead to relapse of correction in the majority of cases. Bone grafts, therefore, should not be used to maintain the position of osteotomized segments.

Specific Deformities

Enophthalmos

Post-traumatic enophthalmos has been demonstrated to be almost entirely due to displacement of the orbital walls with enlargement of the bony orbital cavity. Fat atrophy is not a prominent feature in most patients with post-traumatic enophthalmos. Enophthalmos may result from a pure blow-out fracture with an intact orbital rim, but it is more commonly associated with malpositioned orbitozygomatic complex fractures with resultant increased orbital volume. This deformity may be associated with ocular dystopia and sometimes with true orbital vertical dystopia. Characteristic areas of bone loss are seen at the junction of the floor and medial wall, the lamina papyracea, the lateral orbital wall, and on the posterior aspect of the medial wall, where ethmoid air cells bulge into the orbit.

Procedures designed to treat post-traumatic enophthalmos aim to restore the shape and position of the orbital soft tissue by mobilization of soft tissues and bone reconstruction to restore orbital volume. Of paramount importance in this endeavor is adequate exposure. Coronal and subciliary incisions are used to obtain 360° circumferential subperiosteal dissection of the orbit down to the orbital cone. The lateral canthal ligament may be stripped from its insertion into Whitnall's tubercle in order to facilitate exposure and is later reconstructed. Additional exposure may be obtained by marginal osteotomies along the inferior, superior, and lateral orbital rims or at the fronto-zygomatic suture.

Reduction of all herniated periorbital contents is necessary to restore orbital volume and prevent entrapment of globe motion. All orbital defects are identified and surrounding bony shelves are delineated. Reconstruction of these defects is undertaken using autogenous cranial bone graft, carefully contoured to fit exactly into the existing defects. These grafts are stabilized by being placed on delineated bony shelves; their position is maintained through pressure exerted by the intraorbital contents.

Once the deficits in the orbital wall are reconstructed, correct orbital volume and contour are produced by the use of smaller grafts and chips placed behind the globe axis in the medial, inferior, and lateral orbit. Special attention is given to reconstruction of the inferomedial sinus bulge, which is critical for the maintenance of correct globe position. Bone paste, collected when cranial bone is harvested, is then used for final contouring (see Figures 29.2 and 29.3).

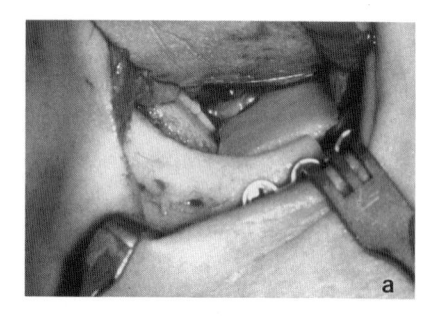

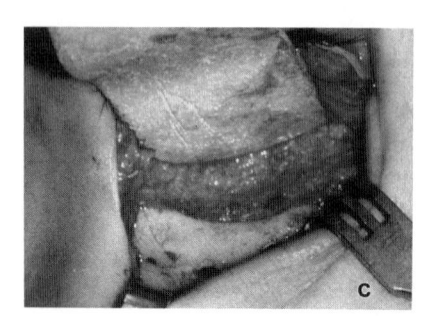

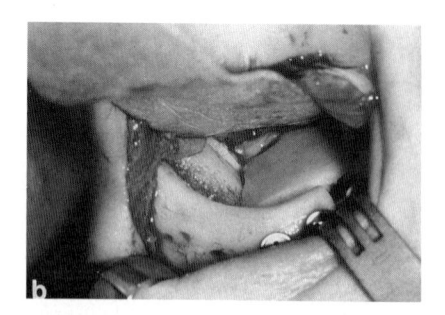

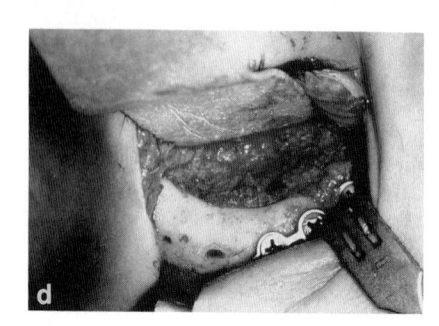

Figure 29.2 Methods of bone graft reconstruction in enophthalmos correction. (a) Split calvarial bone grafts wedged into place. Bone grafts are stacked one against the other to try to recreate the natural curvatures of the missing orbital walls. Bone grafts are supported posteriorly on remaining bony ledge (arrow). Prior osteotomy has been performed of the orbitozygomatic complex. The miniplate can be seen at the infraorbital rim. (b) Close-up view of orbital bone grafts extending back into the orbital apex, where they are being wedged on the posterior ledge. (c) Final contouring and volume adjustment is obtained by packing chips into the orbit and moulding with bone dust. (d) Close-up view of orbital contouring with bone chips and compressed bone paste.

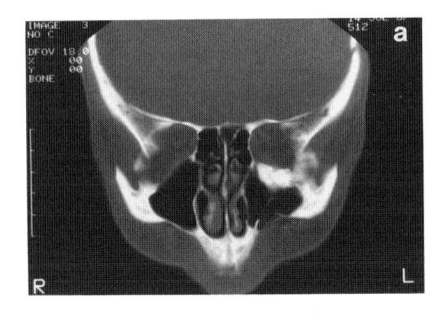

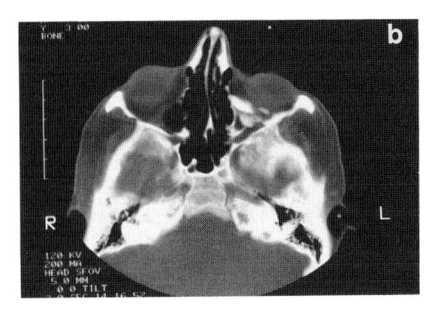

Figure 29.3 (a) This coronal CT scan of the orbit shows the method of bone graft reconstruction used to try to re-create the pre-injury contour of the orbit, to reconstruct the inferomedial maxillary sinus bridge, and to restore the correct orbital volume. (b) This axial CT scan shows the position of the deep orbital bone grafts, situated behind the axis of the ocular globe.

In extensive three- and four-wall bony deficits extending back to the optic canal, bone grafts placed on an inadequate posterior ledge may displace, causing the orbital volume to increase once again. The bone grafts may have to be stabilized with miniplates or microplates to the orbital rim or held in place with specially designed orbital floor plates or meshes.

Orbitozygomatic Deformity

Inadequate initial treatment of a displaced orbitozygomatic injury will result in a characteristic deformity. There is a decreased anteroposterior projection of the zygomatic body, associated with increased facial width due to collapse and bowing of the zygomatic arch and concomitant rotation of the zygomatic body. Increased orbital volume results in enophthalmos. Bone loss of the thick lateral orbital wall is uncommon in acute injuries; yet a bone gap is invariably present following inadequate treatment due to rotation and displacement of the lateral orbital wall and rim. Orbital and/or ocular dystopia, diplopia, and decreased sensation in the infraorbital nerve may be present. Treatment of enophthalmos may be carried out in conjunction with correction of the orbital and zygomatic deformity. As outlined previously, the basic principle of successful correction relies on the determination of whether the deformity is the result of bony deficit or bony malposition.

Bony deficits result from severe comminution and subsequent resorption of small bony fragments (bone loss), or from displacement by soft-tissue cicatricial contracture, and extensive fibrosis prevents satisfactory anatomic replacement of these segments (bone depression). Segmental bone loss along the orbital rims, zygomaticomaxillary buttress, and zygomatic temporal suture is replaced with autogenous split calvarial inlay bone graft and rigidly held with miniplate or lag-screw fixation techniques. Bony deficits due to segmental bone depression are corrected with onlay bone grafts fixed with lag screws. Care must be taken to choose the correct size of graft because bony gaps between graft and recipient site will delay osteosynthesis. Bone grafts may be contoured in situ using a bur when fixation is complete. Partially overdrilling the entry hole (proximal cortex) enables countersinking of screwheads; countersinking increases the rigidity of fixation and avoids palpation through the skin. Calvarial bone graft lends itself well to this purpose due to the thick cortical layer. Because rib and iliac bone grafts have thin cortices, countersinking may weaken these grafts if not done very carefully. An alternative technique to ensure fixation involves the use of a washer made from one hole of a mini-adaptive plate (see Figure 27.1c). Grafts may also be sandwiched and stacked in layers to augment facial prominence, that is, at the orbital rims and body of the zygoma.

The treatment of orbitozygomatic deformities secondary to bony malposition depends on the structure of the bone. Malunion with anatomically normal bone (minimally displaced or with no segmental fractures) is corrected by recreating the fracture pattern and repositioning the bone. Specifically, extended exposure and orbitozygomatic osteotomies may be performed at the fronto-zygomatic suture, at the inferior orbital rim, at the lateral maxillary buttress, and along the zygomatic arch. Extended exposure and orbitozygomatic osteotomies allow mobilization of the entire complex and facilitate deep orbital exploration.

Accurate re-establishment of the correct position of the zygomatic arch, the body, and the orbital rims helps restore the correct orbital volume and, combined with deep orbital bone grafting, corrects enophthalmos. The outwardly bowed and deformed zygomatic arch commonly requires an osteotomy to re-establish its correct anatomic configuration. This may be performed as a greenstick osteotomy and rotated inward using the greenstick as a hinge (see Figure 29.4). A common mistake is to create a gentle curve along the arch. It is important for satisfactory correction to appreciate that the anatomic shape of the zygomatic arch is a slope. Long adaptive miniplates are used to stabilize this osteotomy and to bridge the invariable bone gap at the zygomatic-temporal suture. Miniplates are also applied at the fronto-zygomatic suture, lateral maxillary buttress, and inferior orbital rim to provide four-point fixation and, thus, three-dimensional stability. Autogenous bone grafts are then used along bone gaps in the arch and along the lateral maxillary buttress if the gap is large enough (greater than 5 millimeters). Onlay grafts may be used to augment the anterior maxillary wall if the wall is depressed and if concomitant correction of orbital wall defects is performed (see Figures 29.5, and 29.6).

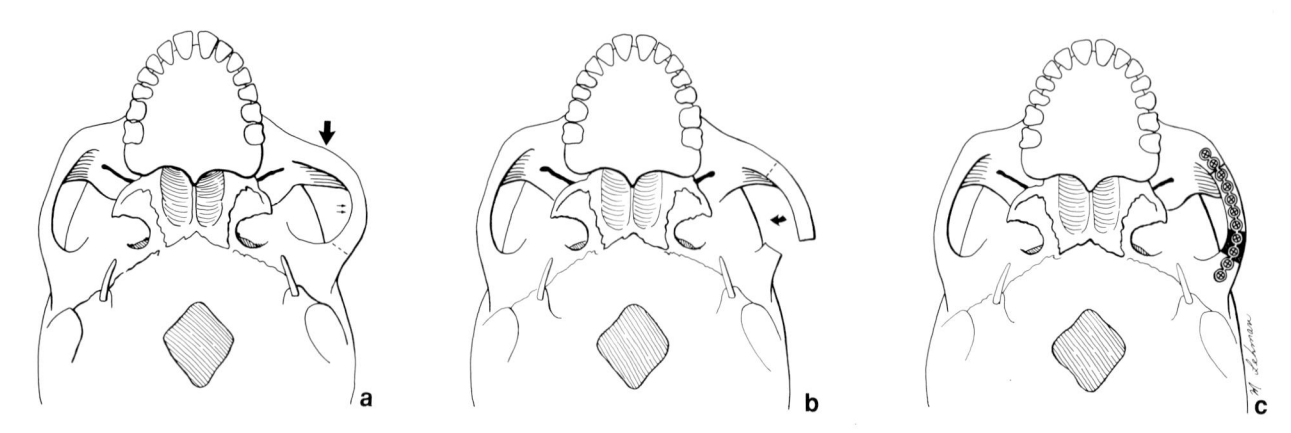

Figure 29.4 A method of osteotomizing the zygomatic arch. (a) Characteristic depression of the zygomatic body and outward bowing of the zygomatic arch. (b) Once the entire orbitozygomatic complex has been osteotomized at the frontozygomatic suture line, the infraorbital margin, the lateral maxillary buttress, and the zygomatic arch, it is repositioned. The outward bowing deformity of the zygomatic arch is now accentuated. This requires a compensatory greenstick osteotomy to recreate the correct curvature of the arch. (c) The compensatory osteotomy having been performed, the variable posterior defect in the arch plus osteotomy is bridged with a long mini-adaptation plate. The bone gap in the zygomatic arch is replaced with a small calvarial bone graft, which is fixed to the miniplate with two screws.

Figure 29.5 This woman has very severe post-traumatic deformities of the face following complex naso-orbito-ethmoid and right orbitozygomatic injuries. Treatment consists of osteotomy and repositioning of malpositioned bone segments as well as bone grafting of bone defects. (a) Widening of the naso-ethmoid region; flattening of the nasal bridge; very severe fibrotic, immobile enophthalmos; and flattening of the right zygomatic body with widening of the right facial diameter through the zygomatic arch are shown. (b) This inferior view shows flattening of the zygomatic body and widening of the right side of the face through the arch. Extremely severe fibrotic enophthalmos can be seen. (c) This axial scan shows extensive destruction of the right orbit with loss of the sinus bulge in the posterior medial orbit and large defect in the lateral orbital wall. Bowing, telescoping, and shortening of the zygomatic arch can be seen with depression of the zygomatic body. (d) Marked depression of the zygomatic complex, almost adjacent to the mandible, can be seen. Failure to reduce the zygomatic complex and an attempt at camouflaging the deformity with a rib graft placed over the zygomatic complex can be seen. Following initial stabilization, this patient could open her mandible only 3 millimeters. At subsequent surgery, complete bony ankylosis of the zygomatic body to the coronoid process of the mandible was found. (e) Extensive exposure of the entire craniofacial skeleton through a coronal incision can be seen. The incision is extended down in the preauricular region and gives a view of the entire orbit (o), zygomatic body (zb), zygomatic arch (za), and maxilla (m) to the midline, as well as the temporomandibular joint (t) and the entire right mandible to the midline. The depressed zygomatic body with bony ankylosis to the mandible (ZB) can be seen, as well as the rib graft (r) used to try to camouflage the depression. (TM = temporalis muscle, c = coronoid process.) (f) Release of the bony ankylosis allows osteotomy of the entire orbitozygomatic complex. (ZA = zygomatic arch, ZB = zygomatic body). Release of the left temporomandibular joint (T) and coronoid process was necessary as well. (g) Accurate repositioning of the orbitozygomatic complex and reconstruction of the zygomatic arch, using miniplates. Split calvarial bone graft (arrows) replace the bony gap in the arch; it is fixed with two screws to the overlying plate. (h) Repositioning of the orbitozygomatic complex at the infraorbital margin with a miniplate. Extensive bone graft reconstruction of the orbit can be seen following extensive subperiosteal dissection of the ocular globe. The globe was found wedged into the maxillary antrum. (i) The split calvarial bone graft to the nose is fixed in place with three lag screws and a right transnasal canthopexy wire prior to fixation (arrow). (O = orbits, F = frontal bone.) (j) This coronal CT scan shows extensive bone graft reconstruction of the medial orbit, the floor, and the lateral orbit. Most bone grafts have been placed behind the axis of the globe. (k) This axial CT scan demonstrates the position of the orbital floor bone grafts. Grafts extend right back to optic canal. (l) Three-dimensional reconstruction of the orbitozygomatic complex with repositioning of the zygomatic body and reconstruction of the arch. Note that despite osteotomies and reconstruction, the arch is still slightly wide because of the uncorrected sagittal fracture at the temporal bone articulation and the thickness of the miniplate. (m) Appearance at one year. Note the restoration of facial projection and width and right eye position. However, fibrotic enophthalmos prevents sufficient motion to the right eye. Significant diplopia persists. (n) This inferior view shows restoration of zygomatic projection and contour and correction of enophthalmos. Unnatural appearance of ocular globe can be seen. As predicted by axial CT the arch remains slightly bowed. (o) This lateral view shows the restoration of projection of the nasal contour.

Post-traumatic Craniofacial Deformities

Malpositioned orbitozygomatic injuries with anatomically abnormal bone (segmental and comminuted fractures or bone loss) will need to be totally rebuilt if the bone has been sufficiently comminuted. Split calvarial bone is difficult to bend, and therefore split rib may be used occasionally for orbital reconstruction. The principles of reconstruction are similar to those described above (see Figure 29.7).

Combined Nasoethmoid and Le Fort Deformities

Combined nasoethmoid-orbital and Le Fort, or orbitozygomatic, fractures are managed with wide exposure and osteotomies to recreate the fracture pattern. The nasoethmoid-orbital bones are repositioned and rigidly fixed with miniplates, thus allowing the segments in the orbitozygomatic complex and maxilla to

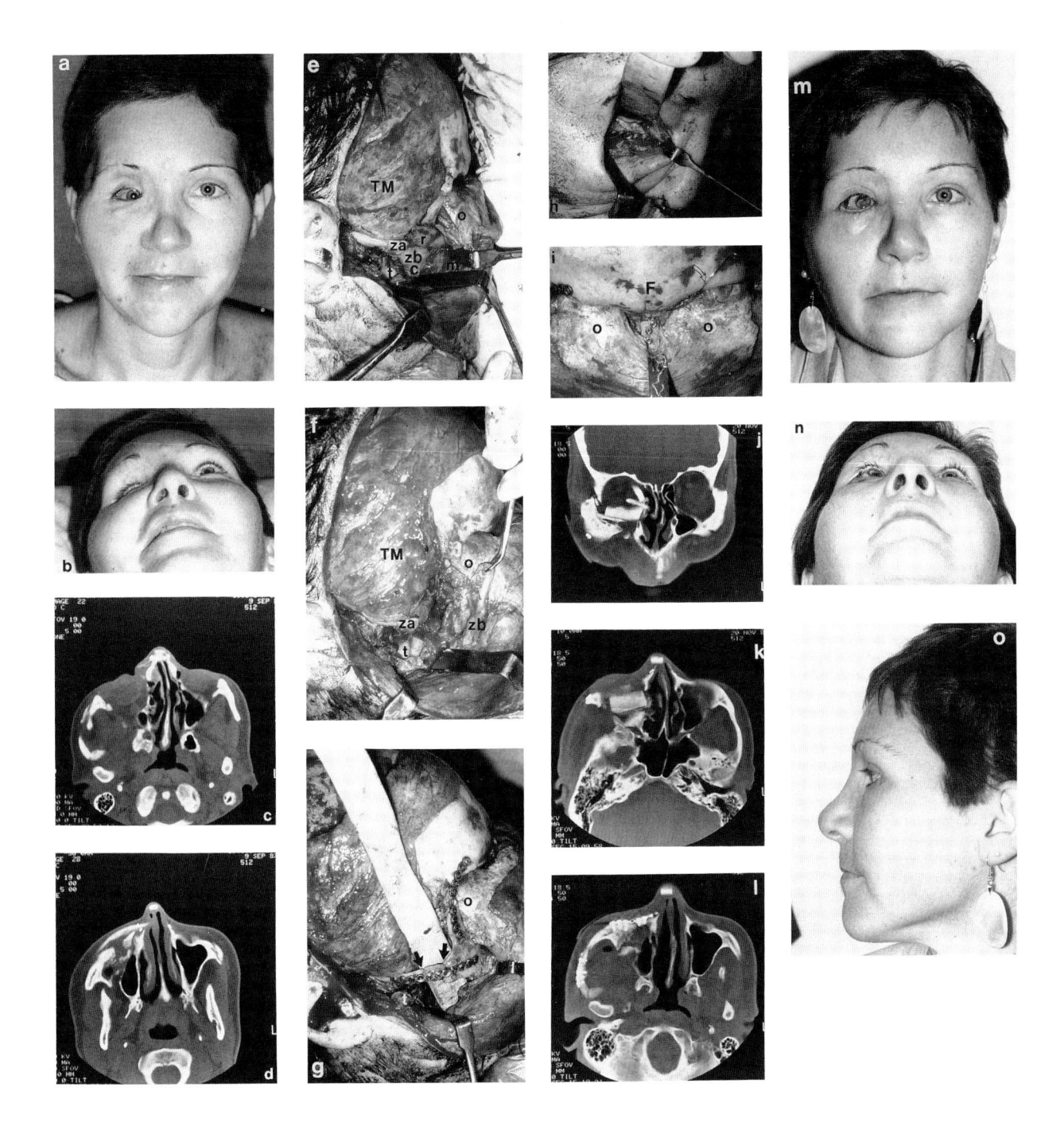

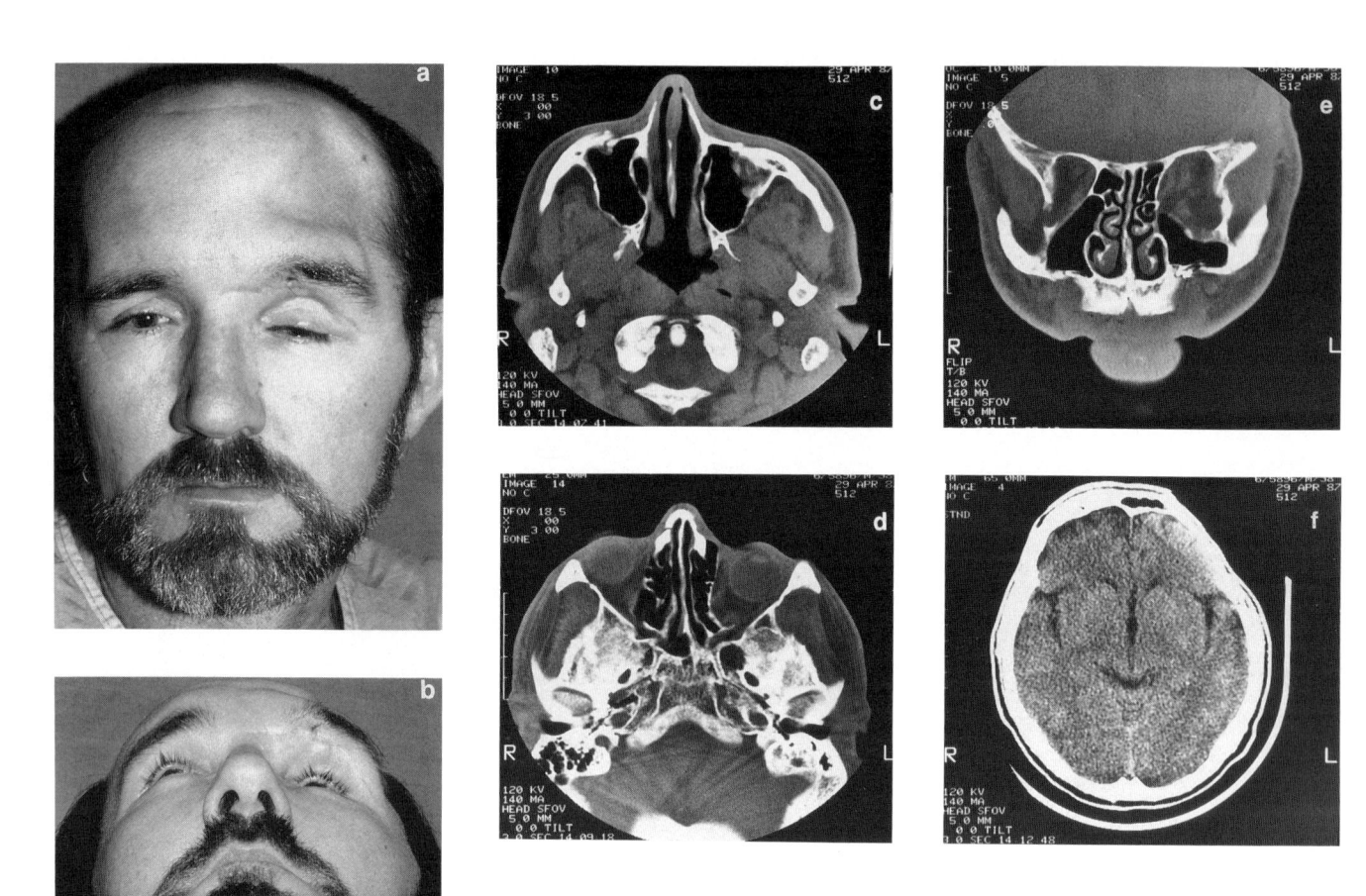

Figure 29.6 (a) This patient has untreated complex craniofacial injuries. He is blind in his right eye and is enophthalmic in his seeing eye. Extensive cranial defect can be seen. (b) This inferior view shows the deformity characteristic of significant enophthalmos, widening of the left zygoma, and flattening of the zygomatic body. Characteristic outward bowing of the zygomatic arch can be seen. (c) This axial CT scan confirms the findings of part (b), showing characteristic depression of the zygomatic body and outward bowing of the arch. (d) This axial CT scan shows the marked increase in orbital volume on the left. (e) This coronal CT scan shows the marked increase in orbital volume with loss of characteristic sinus bulge in the inferomedial wall. (f) Large cranial bone defect. (g) Artist's drawing depicts multiple craniofacial osteotomies. In order to preserve eyesight in the only seeing eye, a combined intracranial/extracranial approach is performed. The supraorbital margin is osteotomized. In combination with an orbitozygomatic osteotomy, the entire orbital rim is thus removed, allowing adequate dissection of the enophthalmos. A template is taken of the cranial defect and applied to the right side of the skull, where a full-thickness bone graft is harvested and split in two. The outer table is placed back, and the inner table is used for cranial reconstruction on the opposite side. (h) Access to the deep orbit after the supraorbital margin (SO) and roof have been removed. (O = orbit, T = temporalis muscle.) (i) Excellent access into the inferior medial orbit after completing orbitozygomatic osteotomy. (j) The superior orbital rim (SO) and orbital roof are repositioned and rigidly fixed back into place with miniplates and lag screws (arrow). (k) The initial repositioning of the zygomatic body shows the characteristic residual bowing of the zygomatic arch (Z) and posterior defect (arrows). (l) Compensatory greenstick osteotomy of the anterior arch (large arrow) restores correct contour of the arch. Split calvarial bone graft (BG) fills in the posterior arch gap (small arrows). (m) Inferior orbital rim (OR) osteotomy rigidly fixed with a miniplate. Extensive bone grafting to the deep orbit can be seen (B). (n) Osteotomy of the zygomaticomaxillary buttress is stabilized with miniplates. (o) Right frontal bone flap is split into inner (IT) and outer tables (OT). (p) The split inner and outer tables are now anchored into the donor and recipient defects with miniplates. (F = frontal.) (q) Artist's diagram of final reconstruction and repositioning of the supraorbital margin, orbitozygomatic complex, and cranial bone reconstruction of the cranial defect. All bone grafts and bone flaps are fixed rigidly in place with miniplates and screws. (r) Final reconstruction with correction of enophthalmos and orbitozygomatic injury. Residual soft-tissue problems in the left upper eyelid and temporal region can be seen. (s) This inferior view shows perfect restoration of orbitozygomatic projection with ocular position.

Post-traumatic Craniofacial Deformities 365

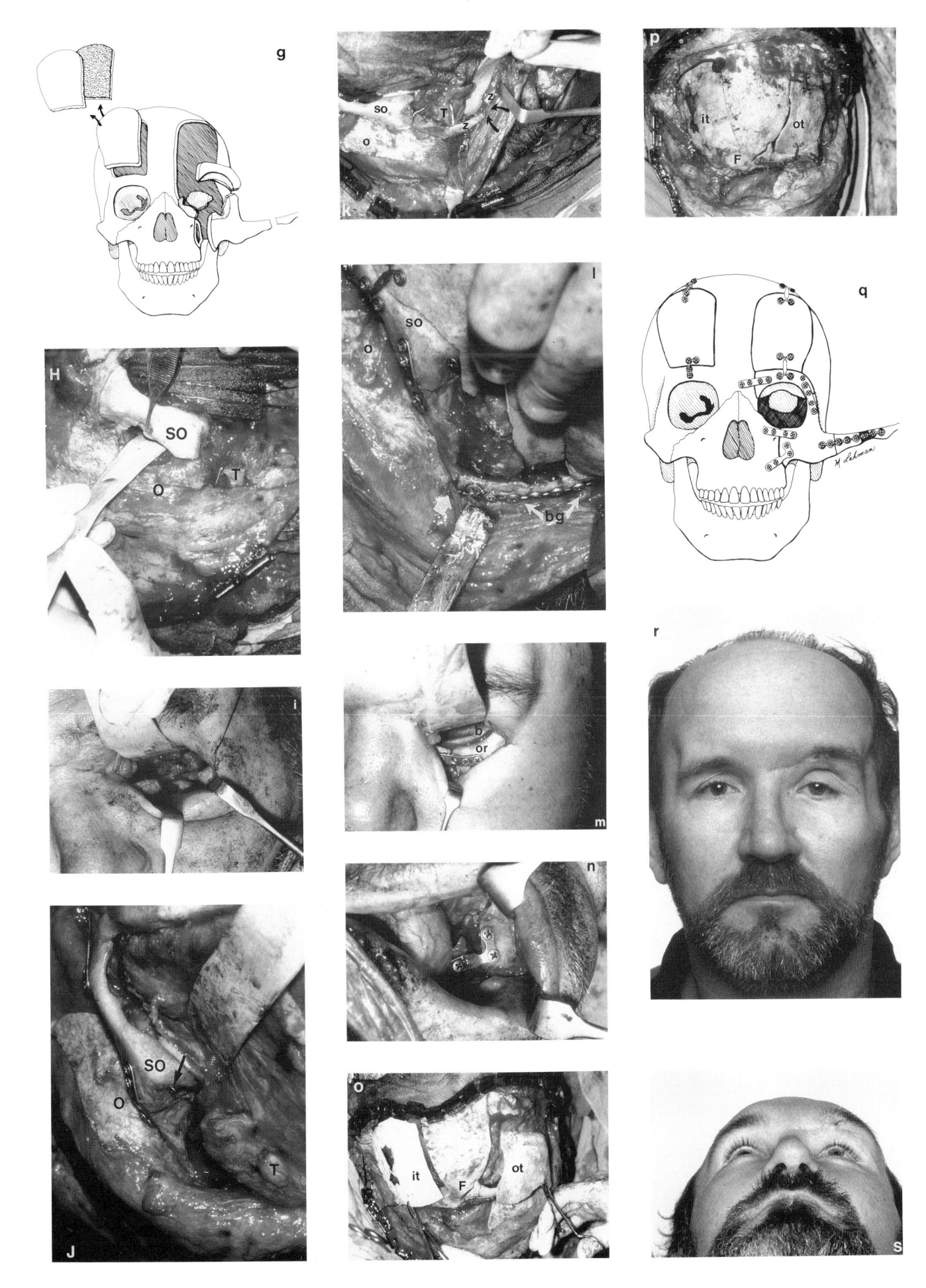

Figure 29.7 This patient has complex comminuted left orbitozygomatic injury and severe enophthalmos.
(a) Appearance with severe enophthalmos and flattening of the zygoma. (b) At exploration, it is found that the entire obitozygomatic complex has been destroyed. Anatomically abnormal bone precludes the ability to osteotomize and reposition. (c) Exposure of the orbitozygomatic complex through a coronal incision shows absence of the lateral orbital rim and wall (arrow) and severe anatomical abnormality of the zygomatic body and arch. (Z = arch, SO = superior orbit, T = temporalis muscle, O = orbit.) (d) Harvesting of multiple split calvarial bone graft strips from the intact skull. (e) Multiple strips harvested. (f) Reconstruction is commenced by reconstruction of the lateral orbital wall with a split calvarial bone graft held in place with a miniplate (lo). (g) A further bone graft is now placed over the first to reconstruct the lateral orbital rim (OR), and a long bone graft is used to reconstruct the zygoma (ZA). Further onlay grafts are placed over the zygomatic body (ZB). All grafts are fixed with miniplates or lag screws. (h) Extensive onlay bone grafts are used on the inferior orbital rim and anterior maxilla. All grafts are rigidly fixed with lag screws. (i) Intraoperative view at 1½ years, at the time of secondary bony contouring and soft-tissue correction. Note that all grafts have retained almost perfect volume. (j) Appearance at two years with correction of enophthalmos and bony reconstruction. Unfortunately, soft-tissue atrophy has resulted in less than adequate contour restoration. Proplast implants were subsequently placed in the left temporal hollow and the hollow in the cheek. (k) This inferior view shows perfect correction of enophthalmos and zygomatic position. (l) This lateral view shows restoration of good bony contour and ocular globe position. Soft-tissue scarring and atrophy can be seen.

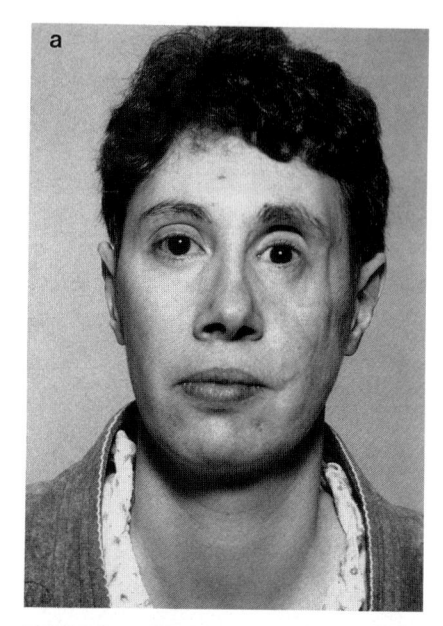

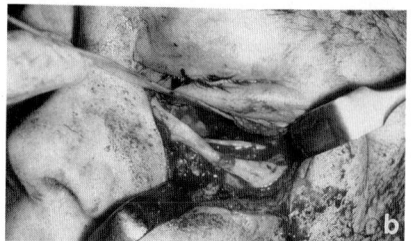

be reduced and fixed in their correct anatomic position. Ancillary procedures, such as dacryocystorhinostomy, for nasolacrimal duct obstruction are performed if necessary.

Specific treatment of post-traumatic maxillary deformities requires the assessment of associated bony injuries. Isolated maxillary deformities (Le Fort I and II) consisting of retrusion and loss of vertical height may be treated with Le Fort I osteotomy and maxillary extrusion. Maxillary injuries combined with other fractures (that is, Le Fort III and IV, nasoethmoid-orbital injuries) are not satisfactorily managed with standard Le Fort III osteotomies due to bony malposition of the nasoethmoid-orbital and orbitozygomatic regions. In these cases, multiple segmental osteotomies in a Le Fort III pattern are made to recreate all major fractures and reposition segments. This involves bilateral orbitozygomatic osteotomies, nasoethmoid-orbital osteotomies, and Le Fort I osteotomies (see Figure 29.8).

Careful assessment of both zygomatic arches is the key to restoring adequate midfacial width and projection. In unilateral Le Fort III fractures (as in unilateral orbitozygomatic injuries), the injured and uninjured arches can be compared and the degree of depression or outward bowing can be accurately assessed on the axial CT scan. In bilateral injuries, accurate assessment of arch projection may be difficult because both arches may be depressed or bowed. Recognition of this important and common finding by comparison with normal arch radiographs or a normal skull will facilitate accurate restoration of bilateral arch projection.

Repair commences with repositioning and reconstruction of the zygomatic arch and lateral orbital rim, producing an outer facial frame with correct anteroposterior projection and transverse facial width. The nasoethmoid-orbital region is now repositioned and stabilized within the outer facial frame to complete the reconstruction of the upper facial frame; this reconstruction is independent of occlusion. Miniplate fixation of the nasofrontal buttress and inferior orbital rim allows exact repositioning of the medial orbital rim and the attached medial canthal ligament, thus correcting traumatic telecanthus. The lower facial frame is now reconstituted by establishing accurate MMF to restore occlusion in combination with reduction and fixation of the four anterior maxillary buttresses. When an edentulous maxilla is present, accurate reconstruction of the lateral and upper face allows anatomic reconstruction of the medial and lateral maxillary buttresses without the need for MMF. All osteotomy sites are repaired with miniplates, and autogenous bone graft is used to fill bone gaps.

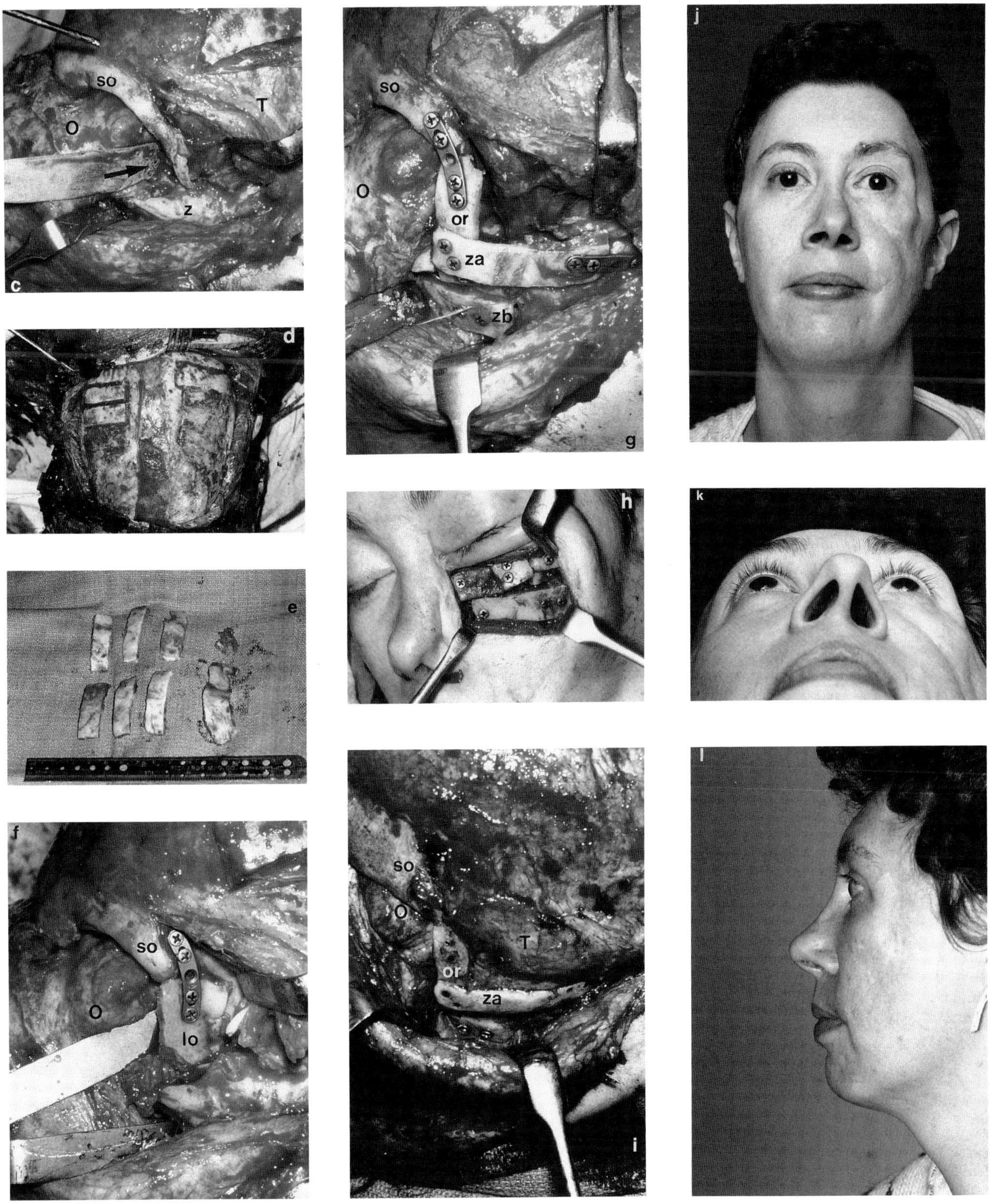
c
so
T
O
z
d
e
f
so
O
lo
g
so
O
or
za
zb
h
i
so
O
T
or
za
j
k
l

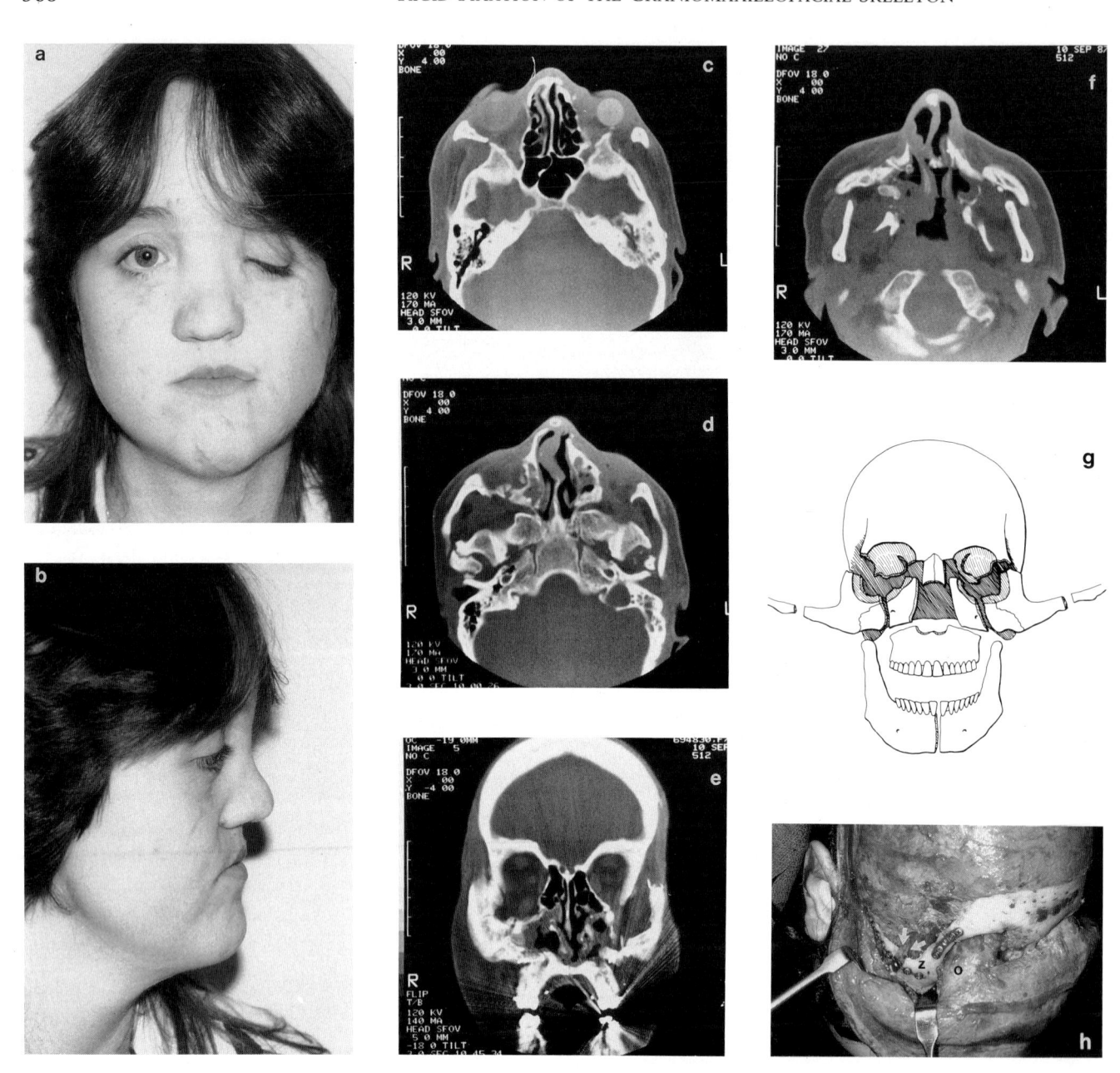

Figure 29.8 (a) This 18-year-old woman has very severe post-treatment facial deformity following severe Le Fort III mandibular and naso-ethmoid injuries. She was kept in MMF for nine months because of fear of nonunion of the maxilla. She has lost her left eye, and the ocular prosthesis has prolapsed into the temporal fossa due to loss of orbital bone. She is enophthalmic in her only seeing eye. (b) This lateral view shows severe midfacial retrusion following Adams suspension. There is a severe malocclusion with anterior open bite deformity and mandibular collapse. (c) This axial CT scan shows severe dislocation and depression of the left lateral orbital wall, with the ocular prosthesis protruding laterally into the temporal fossa. (d) The characteristic posterior telescoping of both zygomatic arches, which have been sheared off at their attachment to the temporal bone posteriorly is shown. The entire midface and zygomas are depressed. (e) This coronal CT scan shows marked deformity of the entire midface, with outward splaying of both zygomas and zygomatic arches and massive bone loss in both orbits. (f) This axial cut through the maxilla and the mandibular rami shows massive loss of midfacial bone with retrusion of the maxilla as well as the zygomatic bodies, which are placed close to the mandible coronoid process on either side. (g) Bony correction involves reosteotomizing the entire craniofacial skeleton, recreating the fracture pattern in a segmental Le Fort I, II, and III pattern. This involves bilateral orbitozygomatic, bilateral nasoethmoid, and Le Fort I osteotomy in a subcranial fashion. In addition, osteotomy through the symphyseal region through the old fracture site enables expansion of the mandible. (h) Initial stabilization of both zygomatic arches using a long mini-adaptive plate across the arch and a mini-compression plate at the fronto-zygomatic suture line. The gap in the zygomatic arch following expansion of the zygoma (Z) can be seen (arrows).

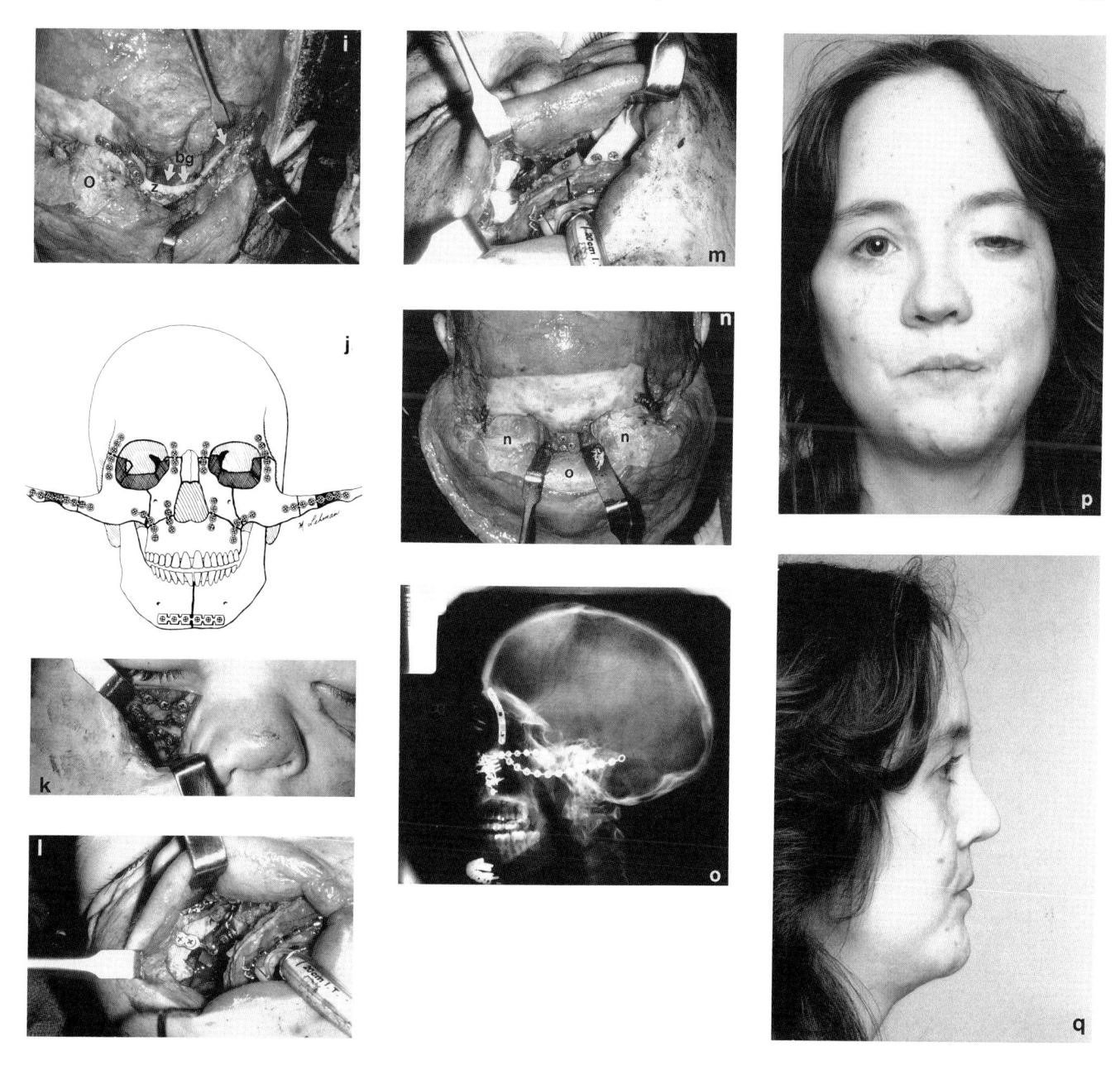

(i) Zygomatic arch stabilization on the left side with compression plate fixation at the fronto-zygomatic suture line. This establishes an outer facial frame with the correct facial width and projection. Bone graft (BG) has replaced the gap in the osteotomized arch (arrows). The small arrow points to the compensating greenstick osteotomy. (j) Stabilization of the nasoethmoid osteotomy and stabilization at the Le Fort I level using miniplates. The correct occlusion is established, and the mandibular expansion osteotomy is stabilized using a strong reconstruction plate to maintain the expansion through the osteotomy. Extensive bilateral deep orbital bone grafting is seen. (k) Fixation of multiple osteotomies of the nasoethmoid and maxilla. Pre-existing lower eyelid incisions were used. (l) Stabilization with multiple miniplates at the Le Fort I level. (m) Application of extensive onlay bone grafting overlying miniplates in the maxilla to further augment the contour of the midface. Note that all bone grafts are stabilized with lag screws. Note the separate bone graft placed in the region of the anterior nasal spine to augment this region (arrow). (n) Application of onlay bone graft to the nasal region (N), fixed in place with three lag screws. Extensive bone grafting to both orbits (O) is performed to correct the enophthalmos. (o) This lateral x ray shows the extension of long mini-adaptive plates from the base of the skull onto the zygomatic body on both sides to establish the correct outer facial frame. (p) Improved appearance at one year. Note the restoration of correct facial width and projection. The left ocular prosthesis, which had been enlarged due to the inadequate orbit, is now too large for the socket and has to be made smaller. (q) This lateral view shows the restoration of facial projection.

SUMMARY

Post-traumatic craniofacial deformities may result from failure to diagnose craniomaxillofacial injuries or from less than adequate repair. The skeletal deformities may be corrected by procedures employing extended craniofacial exposure, segmental osteotomies and bony repositioning. A graduated approach to the correction of regional bony post-traumatic deformities has been formulated. Bony depressions are corrected by onlay grafts, rigidly fixed with lag screws. Malposition of anatomically normal bone is corrected by osteotomy and repositioning. Anatomically abnormal bone is replaced with bone grafts. The use of rigid fixation techniques prevents the late skeletal relapse seen with previous techniques. In the established post-traumatic deformity, soft tissue distortion from contracted underlying scar tissue and adherence to bony depressions and defects is the limiting factor in restoring the pre-injury appearance.

BIBLIOGRAPHY

Antonyshyn O, Gruss JS: Complex orbital trauma: The role of rigid fixation and primary bone grafting. Adv Ophthal Plast Reconstr Surg 7:61, 1988.

Antonyshyn O, Gruss JS, Galbraith DJ, Hurwitz JJ: Complex orbital fractures: A critical analysis of immediate bone graft reconstruction. Ann Plast Surg 22:220, 1989.

deVisscher JGAM, Van der Wal KGH: Medial orbital wall fracture with enophthalmos. J Cranio-Max Fac Surg 16:55, 1988.

Gruss JS: Fronto-naso-orbital trauma. Clin Plast Surg 9:577, 1982.

Gruss JS: Nasoethmoid-orbital fractures: Classification and role of primary bone grafting. Plast Reconstr Surg 75:303, 1985.

Gruss JS: Complex nasoethmoid-orbital and midfacial fractures: Role of craniofacial surgical techniques and immediate bone grafting. Ann Plast Surg 17:377, 1986.

Gruss JS, Mackinnon SE: Complex maxillary fractures: Role of buttress reconstruction and immediate bone grafts. Plast Reconstr Surg 78:9, 1986.

Gruss JS, Mackinnon SE, Kassel EE, Cooper PW: The role of primary bone grafting in complex craniomaxillofacial trauma. Plast Reconstr Surg 75:17, 1985.

Gruss JS, Phillips JH: Complex facial trauma: The evolving role of rigid fixation and immediate bone graft reconstruction. Clin Plast Surg 16:93, 1989.

Gruss JS, Pollock RA, Phillips JH, Antonyshyn O: Combined injuries of the cranium and face. Br J Plast Surg 42:385, 1989.

Jackson IT, Somers PC, Kjar JG: The use of Champy miniplates for osteosynthesis in craniofacial deformities and trauma. Plast Reconstr Surg 77:729, 1986.

Kawamoto HK: Late posttraumatic enophthalmos: A correctable deformity? Plast Reconstr Surg 69:243, 1982.

Manson PN, Clifford CM, Su CT, Iliff NT, Morgan R: Mechanisms of global support and posttraumatic enophthalmos. Plast Reconstr Surg 77:193, 1986.

Manson PN, Crawley WA, Yaremchuk MJ, Rochman GM, Hoopes JE, Franch JH: Midface fractures: Advantages of immediate extended open reduction and bone grafting. Plast Reconstr Surg 76:1, 1980.

Manson PN, Hoopes JE, Su CT: Structural pillars of the facial skeleton: An approach to the management of Le Fort fractures. Plast Reconstr Surg 66:54, 1980.

Manson PN, Shack RB, Leonard LG, Su CT, Hoopes JE: Sagittal fractures of the maxilla and palate. Plast Reconstr Surg 72:484, 1983.

Phillips JH, Rahn B: Fixation effects on membranous and endochondral onlay bone graft resorption. Plast Reconstr Surg 82:872, 1988.

Thaller SR, Zarem HA, Kawamoto HK: Surgical correction of late sequelae from facial bone fractures. Amer J Surg 144:149, 1987.

CHAPTER 30

The Use of Rigid Fixation in Secondary Post-traumatic Cranio-orbital Reconstruction

Ian T. Jackson

The pattern of a fracture in the cranio-orbital area can be classified as

cranial,
supraorbital,
glabellar,
nasoethmoid-orbital,
orbitozygomatic, or
orbital.

Fractures may occur alone or in combination. Unless the fracture is diagnosed and analyzed properly, exposed satisfactorily, and treated adequately, deformity and functional problems will arise. Although achieving an optimal anatomical result may be difficult, the chance of reversing the associated functional defects is frequently very slim.

ANATOMY
Cranial

The cranial deformity usually is caused by a depressed fracture, frequently a comminuted one. In spite of all evidence to the contrary, loose skull fragments may have been removed when the original trauma was treated; alternatively, due to insufficient fixation, bony fragments may have been displaced, producing surface irregularity.

Supraorbital

Most frequently the supraorbital deformity is a result of an injury that is part rotational and part impaction. Such an injury causes flattening and irregularity of the rim, which leads to downward displacement of the eye. The orbital roof may be displaced upward or downward, or it may be absent. The lateral portion of the anterior wall of the frontal sinus may be displaced inward. Portions of the supraorbital rim may have been removed at the initial procedure.

Glabellar

An inward fracture in the anterior wall of the frontal sinus results in an irregularity of the glabellar area. Bone may be missing, and a connection may be established between the extradural space, the frontal sinus, and the nasopharynx, depending on the extent and position of the original trauma.

Nasoethmoid-orbital

Inadequate treatment of a nasoethmoid-orbital fracture leads to one of the most complex anatomic problems seen in the facial area. The fragment has usually been rotated caudally, laterally, and/or posteriorly. This leads to flattening, irregularity, and asymmetry of the nasal bridgeline, bony telecanthus with downward displacement of the medial canthal ligament, enophthalmos due to absence of the medial wall, and oculoorbital dystopia. The fracture may be comminuted and displaced in any area.

Orbitozygomatic

The orbitozygomatic fracture, a common one, may be displaced as a block or may be comminuted. It is usually always treated at the time of the initial injury, but often the full extent and complexity of the fracture is not appreciated. In such a case, inadequate correction causes the deformity to recur.

The most frequent displacement in the orbitozygomatic fracture is lateral, caudal, and posterior. There is cheek flattening with irregularity of the lateral and orbital rims at the fracture sites. This is accompanied by lateral displacement of the fracture at the zygomaticomaxillary buttress. The lateral orbital wall is crushed by the displacement, and the orbital floor may be traumatized. Interesting and significant displacements are seen on the zygomatic arch. Two fractures are usually present, accompanied by telescoping of the fragments. The telescoping takes place because of the posterior displacement of the bony block. It causes characteristic widening of the face in this area.

Orbital

Isolated orbital fractures are rare, and consequently to be called upon to reposition orbital rim segments is unusual. Displaced orbital rim segments are usually a part of a more extensive orbital fracture. When a segment is displaced, it is in the lateral or infraorbital rim.

The lateral rim segment is usually displaced posteriorly and laterally. The inferior rim segment is usually displaced caudally and posteriorly; corresponding displacements of the lateral orbital wall and orbital floor are present.

DIAGNOSIS

The presence of deformity is obvious and palpable. Any displacement of the eye vertically, horizontally, or anteroposteriorly is noted. The position of the canthi is determined and compared with the contralateral side if this is uninvolved. Disturbance of tear drainage is investigated, as is double vision. Eye movement is observed. The position of the nose and nasal septum and the airway patency is examined. In the case of the orbitozygomatic fracture, the contour and position of the zygomatic arch are scrutinized, and particular attention is paid to prominence of the arch and the resultant facial widening. This feature indicates the displaced position of the orbitozygomatic fragment. Intraoral palpation of the zygomaticomaxillary buttress is advocated, because the magnitude of displacement and deformity in this area is a direct and accurate indication of what has happened to the bony fragment. It is wise to check for limited mouth opening and reduced or absent sensation over the distribution of the infraorbital and supraorbital nerves.

RADIOLOGIC INVESTIGATIONS

Standard facial bone radiographs are usually taken; they are certainly useful in obtaining a quick survey of the situation. These studies do not give a true picture of the extent of the damage; because of this, tomography was used in the past. This necessitated considerable doses of radiation and was not used unless there were specific indications; at present, this investigation is no longer recommended.

The main radiologic method of assessing these deformities is by computerized axial tomography (CAT) scan. If this scan is taken in the coronal and axial planes, a great deal of information can be obtained. The position of the orbital wall floors, orbital rims, and cranium can be accurately shown. If there are capabilities for reformatting the long axis of the orbit, a very clear representation of orbital floor damage and globe position can be obtained.

A more recent development has been three-dimensional imaging. The initial CAT scan cuts are taken, preferably at 1.5 millimeters; the appropriate software converts these slices into three-dimensional images. These images give a graphic representation of the anatomic deformity.

A specific program can cut these reformatted images and come up with a standard CAT scan image that is in the exact plane chosen. When this is done, traumatized areas of the skull and facial skeleton—for example, the orbits—can be compared for change in volume, position, and so on.

Another development is interactive planning; with this technique, the images are produced on the screen of a work station, instead of or in addition to hard copies. These images enable measurements of volume, distance, and area to be determined. By a technique of mirror imaging, variations from normal position, volume, and area can be accurately assessed. Furthermore, with a cursor the image of the displaced fragment or fragments can be cut out and placed in the correct anatomic position. When this is done, bone defects open up, allowing a degree of preplanning of bone graft size and position. This technique also helps in deciding whether to perform an osteotomy or an onlay bone graft. This interactivity may also give some indication of where to apply plates and of what size plate to use.

TREATMENT

Cranial

Standard noncompression plates are not usually applied on areas not covered by hair. More frequently microplates (a product of Howmedica, 359 Veterans Blvd., Rutherford, N.J.) (Luhr 1988) are used, especially in children, because they give adequate stability without being unduly palpable or visible. Because plates are not usually removed, the screwheads can be considerably flattened with a contouring bur. It is easy to decide what length of screw to use because the thickness of the skull is visible. In replacement of bone under the hair-bearing scalp, standard noncompression miniplates can be used; and again the screwheads are flattened as described above. If two or more portions of skull are being used to reconstruct a skull defect, a miniplate of correct size is taken and molded to the contours of the corresponding area on the nontraumatized skull. The plate is adjusted slightly and the portions of bone are arranged in such a way that when applied on top of the plate, the bone obtains the correct shape. In this way, the plate lies inside the cranium. Screws are inserted and usually penetrate the outer cranial layer. The points are contoured flush with the surface with a contouring bur (Jackson 1988) (see Figure 30.1). The recontoured fragment is now solid and of good shape; the size is adjusted as necessary, and the fragment is inserted into the skull defect and fixed with miniplates, microplates, or wires.

It must be said that apart from the situation mentioned above, the skull is usually fixed with wire, or in young children, with nonabsorbable suture material. The latter is used in preference to wire, which is palpable through the child's thin scalp.

Supraorbital

Although an osteotomy to correct a supraorbital rim deformity is frequently stabilized with wire, multiple fragments are initially stabilized on their intracranial aspect on a side table with contoured miniplates or microplates as described above. If the roof is also to be reconstructed, a contoured plate is applied on the intracranial or extracranial surface from the supraorbital rim to the roof; all penetrating screw points are contoured off (see Figure 30.2). This reconstructed rim and roof fragment is placed in position and adjusted as necessary. It may be stabilized with wires or microplates on the anterior surface of the rim, or with miniplates on the undersurface of the rim. The thick sub-eyebrow tissue is excellent for hiding any contour deformity caused by the underlying plates.

A further method of plating, occasionally employed, is to place the plate on the cut edge of the supraorbital area. When the bone segment is inserted, the plate and screws, the heads of which have been contoured flat, are now invisible and not palpable.

If the screws penetrate the thin outer wall of the frontal sinus, there is concern about the possibility of infection. In this situation, it is preferable to remove the mucosal lining of the sinus prior to fragment stabilization and fill the sinus with a well vascularized galeal frontalis myofascial flap (Jackson 1986b).

Glabellar Region

In the glabellar region, wire fixation is used most frequently; but again, if several osteotomy fragments are present, a plate is placed on the cranial aspect or on the osteotomy edge (see Figure 30.3). Lateral stabilization is obtained by plating on the orbital aspect of the supraorbital rim and to the bony nasal pyramid if this

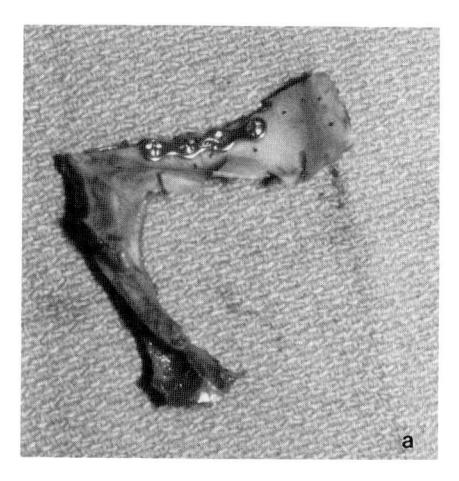

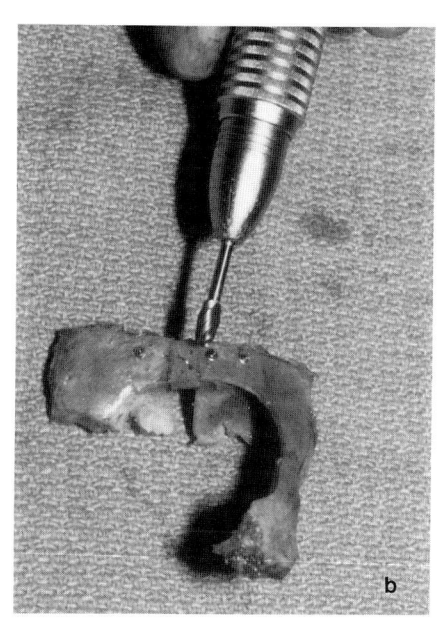

Figure 30.1 (a) A miniplate has been applied to the inner surface of the supraorbital rim. (b) The protruding points of the screws are being ground down flush to the bone with a contouring bur.

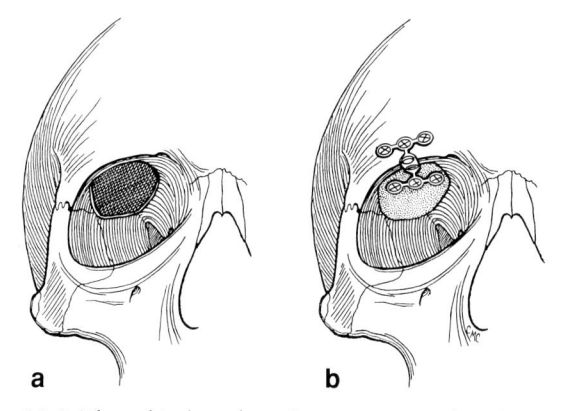

Figure 30.2 The orbital roof can be reconstructed with a plate applied to the supraorbital rim and contoured over into the roof. Prior to inserting this bone graft, the screws on the superior surface—that is, the intracranial surface of the bone graft—will be contoured off. A microplate is ideal for this procedure.

Figure 30.3 (a) It is possible to apply a plate to the cut surface of the cranium and get good stability. This can be seen when a supraorbital osteotomy or fracture is dealt with. (b) This plate is hidden in the fracture site or the osteotomy site; cranial bone dust packed around it will ensure good healing and covering of the plate.

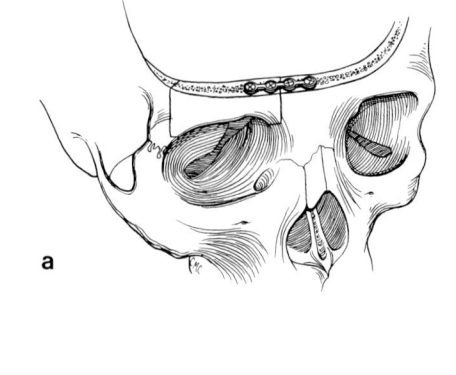

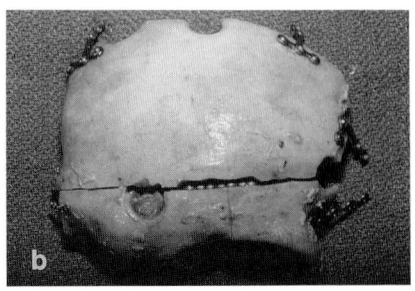

Figure 30.4 (a and b) The method of insertion of a galeal frontalis flap. The flap is turned down from the back of the coronal flap. It is taken through a defect in the medial wall of the orbit. This is the so-called "letter-box" technique. (c) A severe supraorbital roof fracture is repaired with the insertion of a split-thickness skull graft. (d) The split-thickness skull graft of part (c) is in place, and another split-thickness skull graft is being inserted into the lateral wall of the orbit. (e) In order to close the nasal pharynx from the extradural space, a galeal frontalis flap has been raised. (f) The flap has been "mailed" through the bony defect into the frontal sinus to seal off the potentially disastrous connection with the oronasal pharynx.

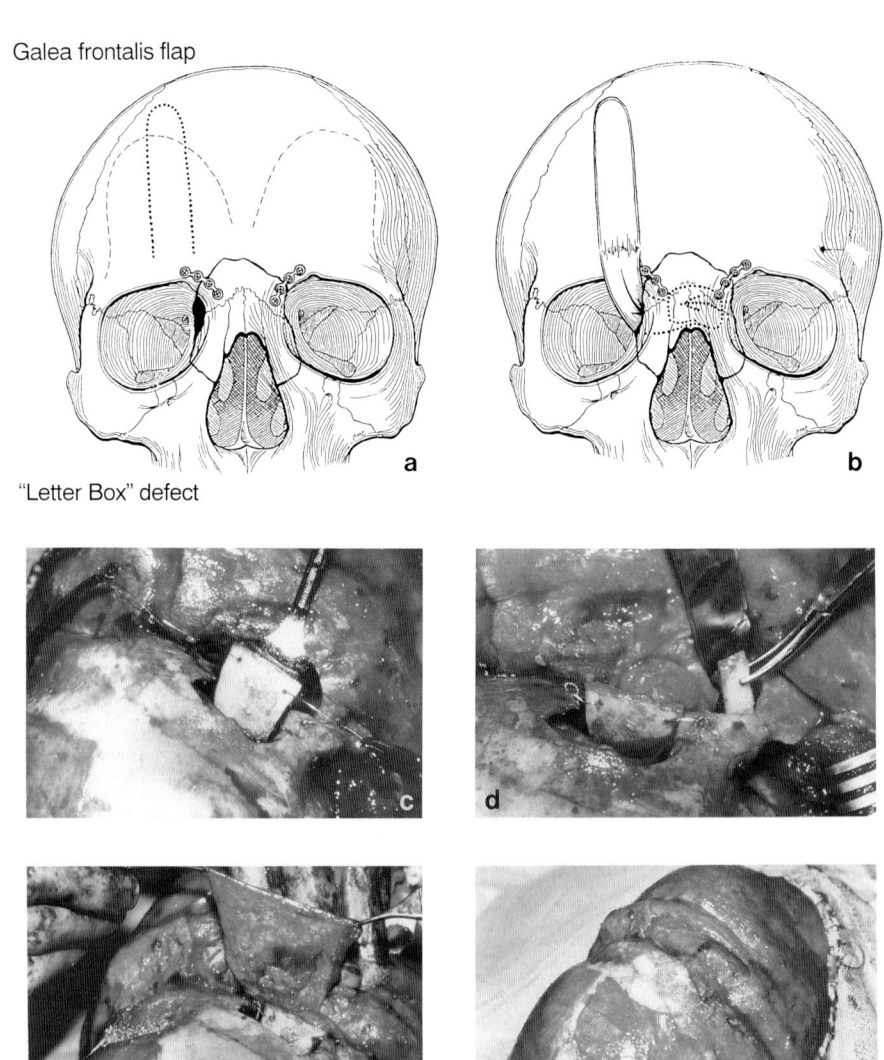

is stable. Precautions similar to those described above are taken if there is any concern in relation to the frontal sinus. The galeal frontalis myofascial flap can be taken into the sinus through a hole in the supramedial portion of the orbit; this is the "letter box" technique (see Figure 30.4).

Nasoethmoid-orbital

As with all other fracture deformities of the upper face, the nasoethmoid-orbital deformity is approached by a coronal flap. In addition, a lower lid subciliary incision is usually necessary to explore the infraorbital rim deformity.

The osteotomy required to reduce the segment begins at the base of the nose and is taken down the center of the bony nasal pyramid, and to the medial wall and floor. It continues across the infraorbital rim at the area of the infraorbital nerve foramen and finally is taken transversely to the pyriform aperture.

The segment is mobilized and fixed with a miniplate or microplate on the orbital aspect of the supraorbital rim and medial wall. A small plate is placed on the external aspect of the infraorbital rim. The lengths of these plates are determined by the presence or absence of multiple osteotomies. In some cases a very long miniplate will be contoured in such a way that it spans and stabilizes the entire segment (see Figure 30.5).

Should a bone graft be necessary to provide adequate nasal projection, rigid fixation is desirable. A dorsal pocket is created from the glabellar area to the nasal tip; and an outer table or full-thickness skull graft, as indicated, is taken from the temporoparietal region. It is contoured and inserted into the pocket to obtain the ideal nasal bridgeline. To obtain optimal stability, an L plate or two lag screws are necessary; in children, microscrews have been used. Countersinks are made in the bone graft with the contouring bur, and the screws are inserted. Overtightening can be disastrous and may cause loosening of the screws or fracture of the graft, or the screws may cut through the graft completely.

When a graft in the medial orbital wall is necessary to reconstruct any resulting defect following the osteotomy, it is usually taken from the skull; a split-thickness graft, it is not stabilized. If it is necessary to fix the graft, this may be done by contouring a plate from a stable portion of the orbit or nose. The plate is then screwed onto the graft in the proper position (see Figure 30.6). The graft and plate are then put in position, and the projecting portion of the plate is contoured further, if necessary, and fixed to the relevant stable bone with screws.

Orbitozygomatic

After exposure of the orbitozygomatic segment by the coronal approach, it is usually decided that a subciliary incision will be necessary. The zygomatic arch is carefully inspected to assess whether one or two osteotomies will be required to obtain a normal contour. This will probably have been ascertained prior to surgery from the three-dimensional imaging, particularly if the ability to do interactive planning is available.

The bone segment is osteotomized. The correct shape of the arch is obtained by taking a long miniplate and contouring it to the nondeformed arch on the contralateral side.

The main bone fragment and the arch fragments are plated; overlap is left for fixation to the stable posterior portion of the arch. This is performed on the superior edge of the arch, if possible, to ensure that the plate and screws are not palpable (see Figure 30.7). This will be further ensured by reapplication of the temporalis muscle.

The fronto-orbital portion of the osteotomy is now plated vertically on the temporal aspect of the lateral orbital wall (see Figure 30.8). The infraorbital rim is plated on its anterior aspect with a mini or microplate.

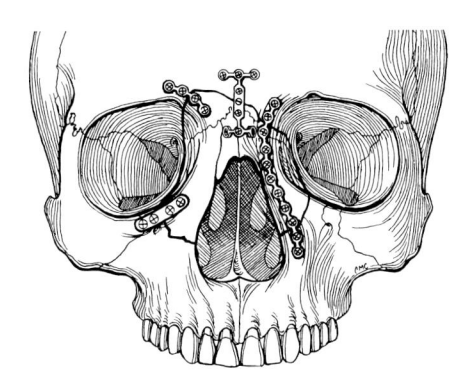

Figure 30.5 The use of a long plate to stabilize a fronto-orbital ethmoid fracture is shown.

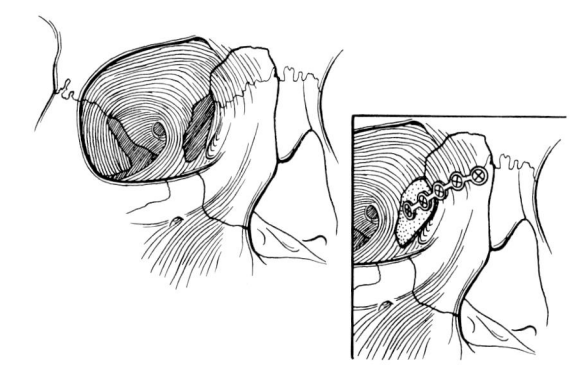

Figure 30.6 The use of a miniplate to reconstruct the medial wall of the orbit is shown. The new microplates are better suited to this than are the conventional miniplates.

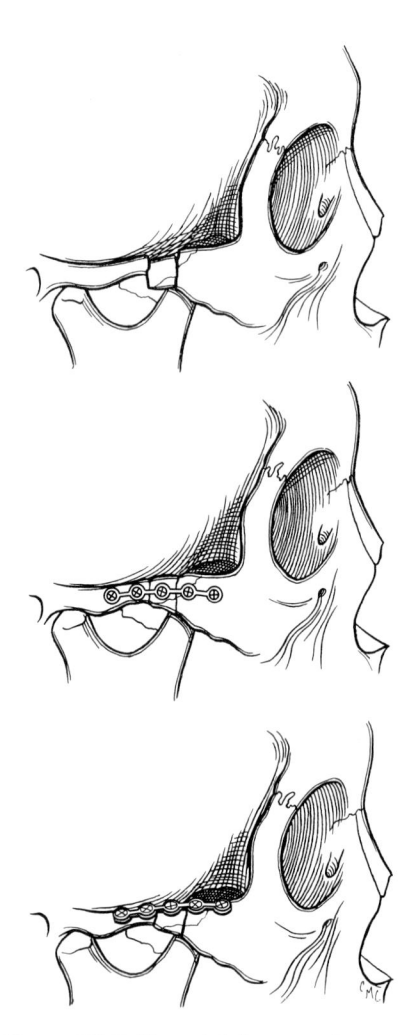

Figure 30.7 The miniplate or microplate can be placed on the upper surface of the zygomatic arch rather than on the lateral aspect. This is particularly important if a microplate is used, because the screws may be palpated through the cheek.

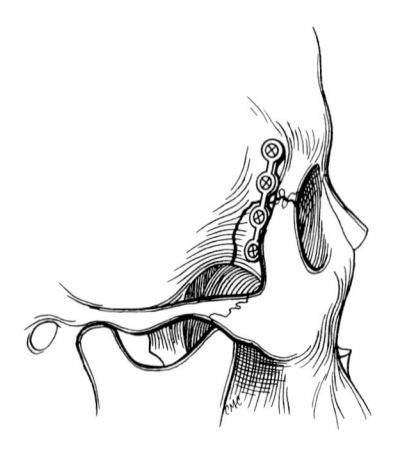

Figure 30.8 The use of a vertical plate hidden by the temporalis muscle to stabilize an orbitozygomatic fracture is shown.

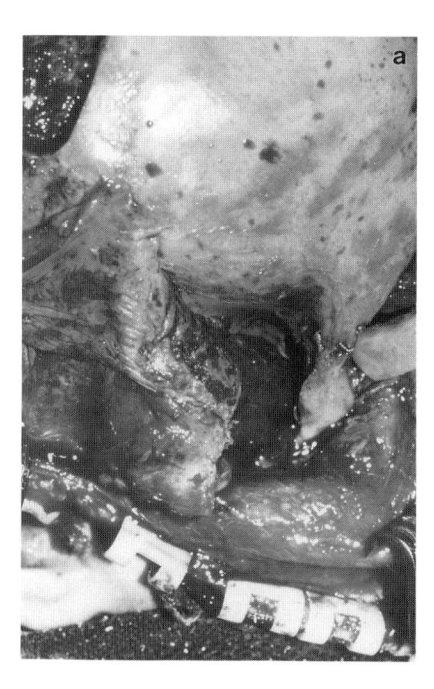

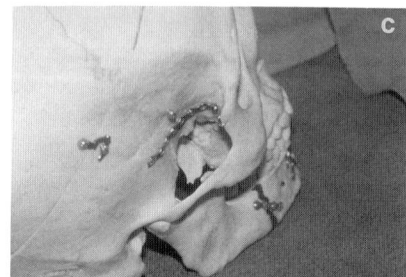

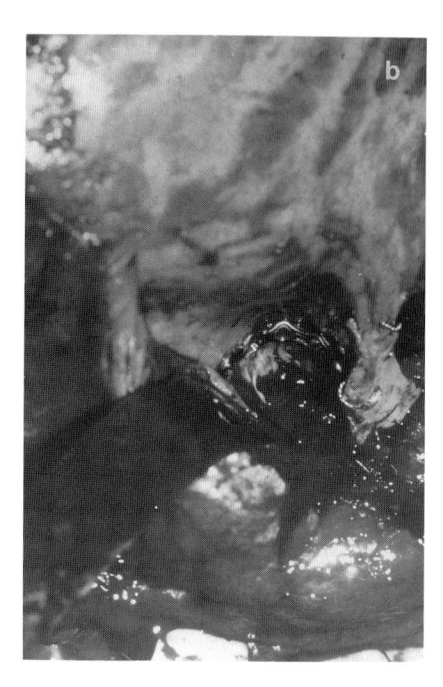

Figure 30.9 (a) This defect in the lateral orbital wall is associated with a severely comminuted orbitozygomatic fracture. A bone graft is being inserted into the lateral orbital wall. (b) A miniplate, inserted from the temporal bone to the lateral orbital rim, holds the fracture in position and stabilizes the bone graft. (c) This plate is demonstrated on the dry skull.

When this has been accomplished, there is usually a defect in the lateral orbital wall. A long plate is now contoured and is taken from the temporal area across the defect and onto the lateral orbital wall. An accurate cranial bone graft is cut and placed in the defect and is held by screws through the plate. As these screws are tightened, the graft comes into the perfect anatomic position (Jackson 1986a), achieving absolute stable fixation of the osteotomized segments (see Figure 30.9). Care should be taken when inserting the screws in the temporal bone area; 5-millimeter screws are best. Even then there is occasionally a leak of cerebrospinal fluid, but no problems have resulted from this. All screws penetrating the orbit are smoothed off flush with a contouring bur.

Should it be necessary to place an onlay graft on the lateral orbital rim or malar region, this is preferably held by two lag screws that are countersunk in the manner described above. The grafts are placed as taken and are then adjusted by in situ contouring (Shaw 1987) after they have been stabilized by countersunk lag screws; again, miniscrews are used in adults and microscrews in children.

Orbital

Segmental

In rare segmental displacements of the lateral or infraorbital rim, wire fixation is usually satisfactory, because instability and later recurrence of displacement of the corrective osteotomy is not a problem. If plate fixation is considered desirable, this may be achieved on the temporal aspect of the lateral orbital rim or on the anterior surface of the inferior orbital rim.

Depending on the size of the fragment, a long plate is usually satisfactory. Again any points penetrating into the orbit are smoothed off flush with a contouring bur.

Orbital Displacement

In rare cases, the original trauma can cause an inferior orbito-ocular dystopia. There may be a degree of lateral or medial dislocation, but this is unusual. To elevate the orbit, an intracranial exposure is necessary, and a "box" osteotomy is performed to raise the whole orbit. Bone is removed from the free margin superiorly to achieve the correct superior shift.

Solid fixation may be obtained by wiring in the frontal area or by microplates. Additional fixation is obtained with contoured plates from the temporal skull to the lateral orbital wall. A small plate is usually placed on the osteotomy at the anterior portion of the zygomatic arch. This combination of plates makes further stabilization unnecessary. An unstabilized cranial bone graft is placed on the orbital floor to raise the eye into its correct position.

COMPLICATIONS

My experience, which began using the very primitive plates of the early 1970s, shows that plates placed in the upper face, even for acute trauma, have been relatively free of complications. In the temporal or forehead area, poorly placed plates occasionally are palpable. They may be visible, especially in children, but this is rare. On two occasions, the plates have been removed at the patient's request. This does not happen today for several reasons: The plates are placed in less obvious positions; the screwheads are contoured almost flat; and microplates are being used in children with increasing frequency.

In many hundreds of plates placed for post-traumatic deformity corrections, we found two sinuses that led down to loose screws. The screws were removed and the plates left in situ, after which the sinuses healed without further intervention.

In several cases referred to us, after osteotomies and plating or after acute trauma correction with plating, insufficient correction of the deformity has been achieved. This is a considerable problem since it requires re-exploration, recreation of the osteotomies, and replating. This problem emphasizes an absolute rule in plating: Any imprecision in plate application can result in a considerable skeletal deformity.

Occasionally the question is raised as to possible complications resulting from the combined use of wire and plates, because these may be made of different metals. In our experience, their use has never been a source of any complications and we do not hesitate to use them in combination.

LONG-TERM RESULTS

In a practice that began in Europe, where plate and screw fixation has been commonplace for many years (Shaw 1987), our follow-up has now extended for 19 years. Initially, combinations of plates and wire were used because specialized plates did not exist. It was only in the late 1970s that plate design became more sophisticated. There is no doubt that rigid fixation results in virtually no relapse and there is better bone graft take. In post-traumatic cases, we have not had to reposition any corrected segment. Occasionally, an onlay bone graft may be required in the malar area, probably because the malar shape has altered as a result of the trauma and was insufficiently corrected at the time of the osteotomy.

A similar situation has been seen in post-traumatic osteotomies in children, although the numbers are small. On the other hand, the follow-up is significant, usually going beyond the time of active facial growth and development.

An interesting expansion in the technique of correction of post-traumatic facial deformity has been the repositioning of the displaced facial mask at the subperiosteal and subcutaneous levels. In addition, the masseter is repositioned on the zygomatic arch. The mask is stabilized by sutures through drill holes on the osteotomized segment. This can be done because of rigid stability of the segment and the consequent lack of concern about relapse due to the forces generated by the repositioned soft tissue.

NUANCES IN TECHNIQUE

Several points about rigid fixation on the upper face must be emphasized. Compression plates are not necessary; screws should be self-tapping and should be countersunk when used as lag screws. As with any other area, a loose screw should be removed and an emergency screw inserted if necessary for stabilization; otherwise, the hole can be left empty.

Bone defects should be grafted accurately and the grafts stabilized by plates if possible. This is best accomplished by creating the defect and placing a plate across it to maintain it. The graft can then be placed; and as the screws are inserted, the graft approximates to the plate and comes to lie exactly in the correct position within the gap.

Plates should be placed to counteract relapsing forces, for example, from the temporal bone to the lateral orbital wall and along the zygomatic arch.

If possible, the segment to be replaced is prefabricated. This is done on a side table with an accurate pattern, and information obtained from interactive planning with three-dimensional imaging, if available is used. It is then very simple to place the segment in position and stabilize it as described. One should not be afraid to plate on the intracranial aspect of the reconstructed segment; this practice has been virtually routine in many post-traumatic and congenital deformities for several years.

Plates should be hidden, if possible; fortunately, many can be covered by the temporalis muscle and many can be placed inside the orbit or the cranium or within the osteotomy cut.

If these rules are applied, stabilization of the face in any situation—be it acute trauma, post-traumatic deformity, or congenital deformity—can be virtually complication-free and extremely stable.

REFERENCES

Jackson IT: Orbital Hypertelorism. In Plastic Surgery in Infancy and Childhood. Mustarde JC, Jackson IT (eds). London, Churchill Livingstone, 28:467-498, 1988.

Jackson IT, Adham MN: Metallic plate stabilisation of bone grafts in craniofacial surgery. Br J Plast Surg 39:341-344, 1986a.

Jackson IT, Adham MN, Marsh WR: Use of the galeal frontalis myofascial flap in craniofacial surgery. Plast Reconstr Surg 77:905-910, 1986b.

Luhr H-G: A micro-system for craniomaxillofacial skeletal fixation. J Cranio-Max-Fac Surg 16:312-314, 1988.

Shaw KE, Jackson IT, del Pinal Matorras F: In situ contouring of cranial bone grafts. Eur J Plast Surg 10:144-146, 1987.

CHAPTER 31

The Use of Rigid Fixation in Post-traumatic Maxillary and Mandibular Reconstruction

Steven R. Cohen
Henry K. Kawamoto, Jr.

When confronted with well established post-traumatic deformities, as opposed to acute injuries, the surgeon must address the problems of nonunited or malunited bone, absent parts, and irreversible scar contracture. Although the distortion may be complex and difficult, an orderly analysis of component parts will aid in planning a solution. Also, unlike in the acute situation, the luxury of time is available to study the details of the problem and formulate an appropriate treatment plan.

Whenever possible, the primary goals of reconstruction should be to (1) restore normal and anatomic bone alignment, (2) re-establish the underlying skeletal support prior to addressing soft-tissue abnormalities, and (3) replace missing tissues with like tissue. Restoring the normal bony architecture should be the primary consideration unless the quantity or quality of the soft-tissue envelope is inadequate to protect the osseous reconstruction. Ultimately, whatever the etiology of facial disfigurement, successful correction of the deformity requires the surgeon to realign discontinuous osseous fragments into the normal contours of the human face. Rigid internal fixation with plates and screws has facilitated this task.

ANATOMY

The management of acute maxillary and mandibular fractures requires an understanding of the patterns of fracture fragments. By the same token the treatment of post-traumatic deformities mandates a knowledge of functional bony units and stable elements of the craniofacial skeleton to construct an integrated plan of treatment.

The Maxilla

Although little can be added to Le Fort's original descriptions of the patterns of midface fractures, it should be emphasized that the majority of maxillary fractures are severely comminuted, consisting of combinations of Le Fort types. The standard classification of Le Fort fractures, based on the level of the most superior fracture site, makes no reference to comminution, the fracture bearing the teeth, or the pattern of fracture fragments (see Figure 31.1).

In Manson's (1980) article on the structural pillars of the facial skeleton, Le Fort II fractures were the most commonly observed (42%). Le Fort I fractures were found in 30% of patients, and Le Fort III fractures were seen in 28%.

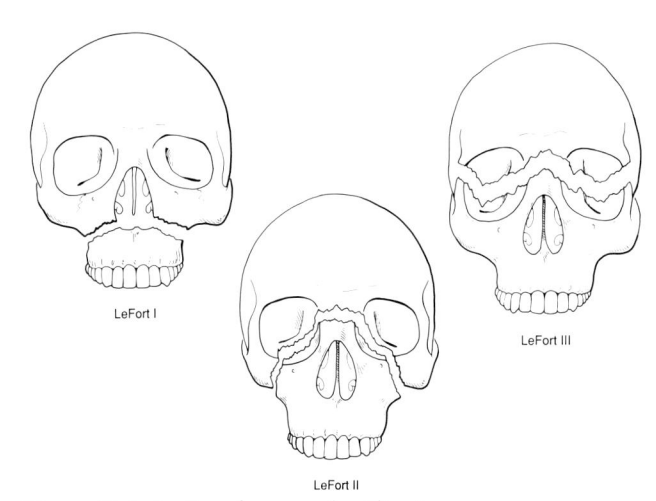

Figure 31.1 Le Fort fracture classifications.

Figure 31.2 (a) Frontal and (b) lateral photographs of a 25-year-old male with late post-traumatic facial deformities following severe midface fractures sustained in a motor vehicle accident. Note the coronal incision from the initial management of facial fractures. Treatment left the patient with moderate midface retrusion secondary to cephalad displacement of the maxilla. Note the overclosed mandible, which leads to a pseudo-prognathic appearance and shortening of the middle third of the face. Occlusion (not shown) was class III.

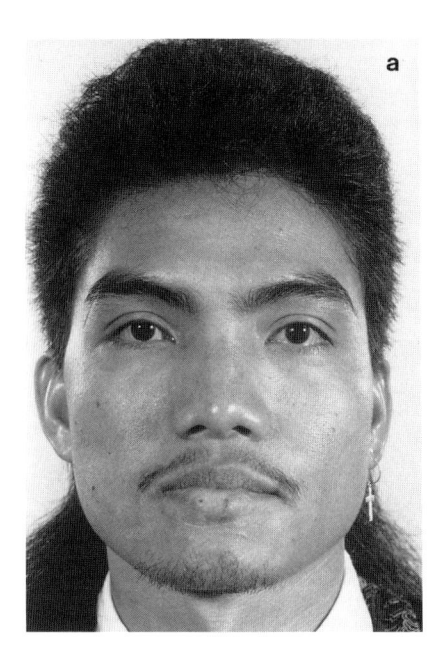

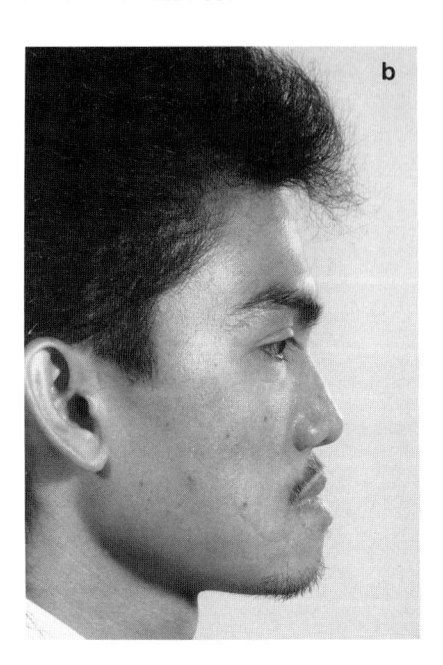

The maxilla, unlike the mandible, has few sites of origins to muscles sufficiently powerful to displace fracture fragments. Displacement therefore is less marked and generally occurs in an inferior, lateral, and inferior, or in a lateral and posterior direction. Displacement with impaction is less common in the maxilla than in the mandible. The external pterygoid accounts in part for the retrodisplacement of the maxilla. The open bite in fractures of the maxilla is related to the downward pull of the internal pterygoids, which leads to a backward tilting of the maxilla.

Following fracture treatment, midface elongation is seen more rarely than midface compression. Midface elongation is probably limited by the presence of intact periosteum and muscular attachments across fractured segments. Comminution in midface fractures tends to lead to retrusion accompanied by reduction in midfacial height. Failure to reduce the maxilla appropriately may cause permanent changes in the contour and outline of the face. The classic post-traumatic deformity of the malunited maxilla leaves the patient with a shortened, retruded maxilla with or without retropositioned maxillary dentition. An anterior open bite may be present, or overclosure of the mandible may lead to a pseudo-prognathic appearance (see Figure 31.2).

The Mandible

Distraction, migration and motion of mandibular fracture fragments is influenced by (1) the direction of muscle pull, (2) the direction and bevel of the fracture, (3) the presence or absence of teeth, (4) the extent of soft-tissue injury, and (5) the direction and intensity of the traumatic force. In fractures of the mandible the geniohyoid, myohyoid, and digastric (anterior muscle group) muscles tend to displace the anterior mandibular fragment downward and inward (see Figure 31.3).

The actions of the muscles of mastication on mandibular fractures also determine displacement of bony segments (see Figure 31.3). The masseter's pull on the angle of the mandible is upward, and the temporalis pulls the coronoid process upward and backward. The external and internal pterygoid muscles tend to pull the ramus inward and slightly upward. Because of the sandwiching effect that the masseter muscle and pterygoid muscle have on the body of the mandible, displacement in this region is rare. With condylar neck fractures the action of the pterygoids is to tip the condylar head forward and anterior. This causes loss of posterior ramal height and anterior open bite deformity. Knowledge of the forces and vectors of pull of these muscles leads to a better appreciation of the possible combinations of late deformities of the mandible.

Malunion and Nonunion of Maxillary and Mandibular Fractures

Bone heals as a result of a series of complex and predictable histopathologic events that resemble embryonic osteogenesis. Immediately upon fracture the blood supply to regional osteocytes is disrupted. Loss of vascular continuity, as well as direct trauma, leads to osteocyte death. Extravasated blood clots produce a fracture hematoma at the bone ends. Within hours, an inflammatory response is observed. Periosteal cellular activity follows, and medullary capillary buds invade the fracture hematoma. The extraosseous blood supply from surrounding soft tissue and periosteum also participates in neovascularization, playing an important role in fracture healing. As the capillary buds mature, fibro-

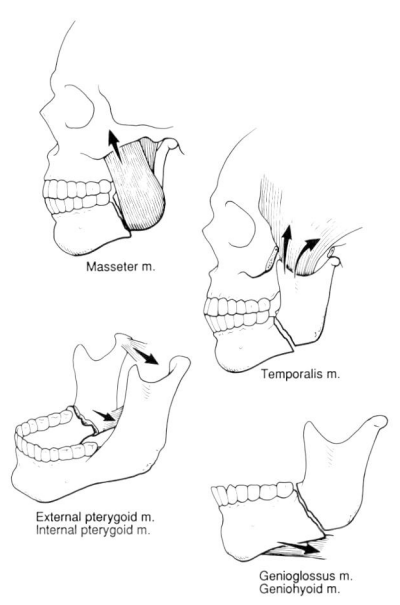

Figure 31.3 Muscle function influences the degree and direction of displacement of fractured mandibular segments. The posterior group of muscles is commonly referred to as the "muscles of mastication." The muscles of mastication are the temporalis, masseter, and the medial (internal) and lateral (external) pterygoid muscles. The overall function of this group is to move the mandible in the upward, forward, and medial direction. The anterior or depressor group of mandibular muscles are the geniohyoid, genioglossus, mylohyoid, and digastric muscles. When the mandible is fractured, these muscles displace the fractured segments downward, posteriorly, and medially.

blasts appear and collagen synthesis begins. Osteoclasts which resorb necrotic bone comingle with osteoproginator cells and osteoblasts.

Bony union then proceeds by one of two different mechanisms: primary union or secondary union. *Primary union* takes place when bone heals without a cartilaginous intermediary phase. When the fracture is immobilized by rigid compressive fixation with tight abutment of bone ends, direct appositional bone formation takes place without a cartilaginous intermediary. *Secondary union*, the more common process, involves an endochondral phase.

Nonunion of a fracture denotes absence of histologically identifiable osteogenic tissue between fracture segments. Nonunion may occur in one of three forms: (1) fibrous and/or fibrocartilaginous bridging of the fragments, (2) pseudoarthrosis with fibrocartilage capping of the fracture ends, or (3) persistence of distracted fracture segments. Nonunion implies that the injured bone ends are mobile and will not progress to osseous consolidation. *Delayed union* is defined by retarded bony consolidation; *malunion* implies healing of bone fragments in nonanatomic positions.

Etiologic factors causing nonunion or malunion may be either local or systemic. Local factors include insufficient blood supply, inadequate reduction of fracture fragments, ineffective fixation, recurrent trauma, and infection. Systemic factors, which are protean, include general metabolic disorders, nutritional deficiencies, the patient's age, effects of various medications, and primary diseases of bone.

Malunion of maxillary fractures in patients who have undergone initial fracture treatment usually arises because of insufficient duration of immobilization, severity of injury, and lack of availability of adequate surgical expertise. Potential problems and adverse variables in healing of mandibular fractures do not differ significantly from those associated with maxillary fractures. The exact incidence of nonunion and malunion of mandibular fractures is difficult to estimate but probably is under 5% of total cases. The incidence of nonunion is higher in edentulous mandibles. The prevalence of midface deformities following fracture is more difficult to pin down.

Influence of Growth and Development: Pediatric Trauma

Although the child's face generally is resilient and recovers from trauma without adverse sequelae, certain injuries, if they occur within specific time periods, may have a detrimental effect to craniofacial growth and development. Post-traumatic growth disturbances generally involve deficiencies, but on rare occasions excessive growth may be seen.

Although both maxillary trauma and mandibular trauma place the many dental follicles in a precarious position—such traumas may lead to delayed eruption or maleruption, as well as to other consequences of injury—by far the most feared complications of mandibular fractures in children are those occurring to the condylar region. Conservative treatment generally is indicated, and most children do well. Unfortunately, damage to the mandibular condyle and temporomandibular joint (TMJ) structures may lead to fibrous or bony ankylosis accompanied by resultant mandibular growth disturbances.

Although some follow-up studies indicate that as many as 25% of children may demonstrate deficiencies in mandibular growth following condylar fractures, this estimate is probably high. However, it should be remembered that up to 10% of all severe mandibular deficiencies or asymmetries may be traced to growth disturbances related to trauma during childhood.

Maxillary trauma leading to late growth disturbances is extremely rare, although cases of severe midface deficiencies have been reported. Some surgeons have speculated that the common denominator of late maxillary deformities in these patients has been a fracture involving midline structures such as the ethmoids and the nasal septum.

DIAGNOSIS AND CLINICAL ASSESSMENT

The diagnosis of post-traumatic deformity of the maxilla and mandible is usually quite obvious. Patients enter the office carrying with them pre-injury photographs and a remembrance of their lost appearance. For those patients with severe midface deformities, the image in the mirror is cracked and broken and reminds them daily of their devastating alteration.

In addition to an appreciation of the psychological needs of the patient, a proper preoperative evaluation includes a detailed history and topographical appraisal of the patient's facial deformities. The circumstances and mechanism of the injury should be ascertained. The date of the injury is also important in that additional abnormalities may accrue over time. There may be occlusal drift as well as changes arising as a result of growth. Prior reconstructive surgery and the use of any alloplastic materials should be determined.

The key to treatment planning is in establishing a correct diagnosis. It is primarily on the basis of physical examination and the assessment of facial form that the full deformity becomes apparent and an initial treatment plan may be devised. Various diagnostic aids such as cephalograms, panoramic radiographs, facial photographs, study models, and other measurements are helpful in confirming the preliminary diagnosis.

Frontal Analysis

Symmetry, balance, and morphology are studied in the frontal plane (see Figure 31.4). The upper third of the face begins at the hairline and terminates at the eyebrow. General shape and symmetry of the calvarium—specifically the temporal areas, frontal region, and eyebrows—are observed for abnormalities.

The middle third of the face, which begins at the eyebrows and ends at the subnasale, includes the eyes and orbits, nose, cheeks, and ears. Beginning with measurements of intercanthal and interpupillary distance, the eyes and orbits are examined. Vertical symmetry of the medial and lateral canthi is noted. The nose is studied for form and symmetry. When deformities are present, their specific anatomic location is recorded.

Evaluation of the cheeks consists of assessment of the malar eminences, infraorbital rims, and paranasal areas for normal projection and symmetry. Evaluation is supplemented by viewing the patient from both the submental and vertex views.

The lower facial third begins at the subnasale and ends at the menton. When "ideal" aesthetics exist, the vertical length of the lower third of the face is approximately equal to that of the middle third. In addition, the relation between the vertical distance from the subnasale to the upper lip stomion and the distance from the stomion to the soft-tissue menton is a ratio of about 1:2. The relation between the vertical distance from the subnasale to the vermilion-cutaneous margin of the lower lip and that from the vermilion-cutaneous margin of the lower lip to the soft-tissue menton is a ratio of about 1:1. Disparities in these relations define the precise nature of lower-third facial imbalances. Measurements should be made with the facial musculature at rest.

The lips, which are extremely important in overall aesthetics of the face, should be evaluated in repose and during animation (see Figure 31.4). At rest, an interlabial separation of up to 3 millimeters is present. The width of the lips from commissure to commissure is roughly equal to the interpupillary distance. In repose, the maxillary incisors show 3 to 5 mm beneath the upper lip. There is usually less exposure in males than in females. At rest the lower teeth are seldom seen. Display of the lower teeth may be an indication of inadequate lower-lip support secondary to chin deficiency in the sagittal plane, severe mandibular dentoalveolar protrusion, or hypotonicity of the lip. During animation, symmetry is the most important factor in producing an aesthetic smile. In post-traumatic patients differentiation between asymmetry caused by facial-muscle dysfunction and one caused by intrinsic lip deformity or a skeletal and/or dental abnormality is important.

The dental midlines should align with one another and with the facial midline. When the midline has shifted establishing whether this shift is maxillary, mandibular, or both is important. Finally, the chin is evaluated for symmetry, vertical relations, and shape.

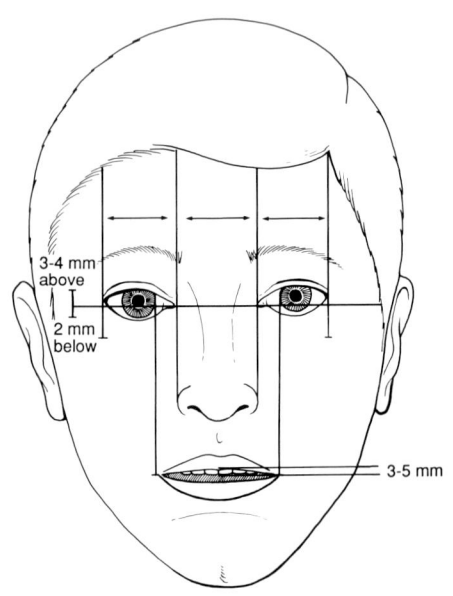

Figure 31.4 Analysis of the frontal plane of the face determines its symmetry, balance, and morphology.

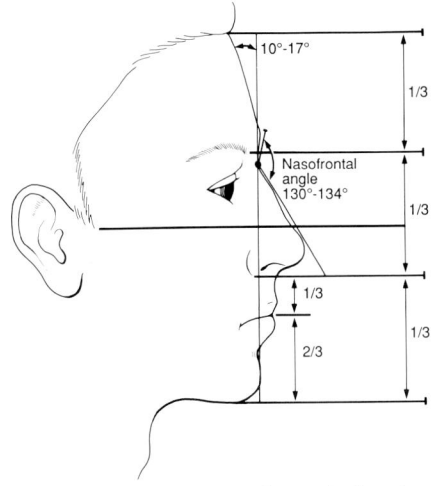

Figure 31.5 Profile analysis is performed after frontal analysis.

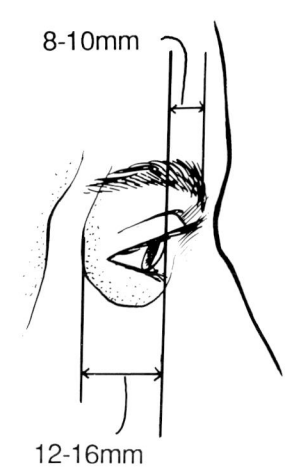

Figure 31.6 The relationship of the anterior cornea to the anterior projection of the supraorbital rim and to the posterior edge of the lateral orbital rim is shown.

Profile Analysis

After frontal plane analysis, profile analysis should be performed (see Figure 31.5). Again, the face is broken into thirds. The normal forehead has an anterior slope from superior to inferior, with accentuation at the superior orbital rims. The superior orbital rims are evaluated as they relate to the globes. The globes in profile are used as fixed reference points (see Figure 31.6). Normally, the superior orbital rims project 8 to 10 mm beyond the most anterior projection of the globe. When variations in the shape of the forehead and position of the superior orbital rims exist, frontal bossing must be differentiated from supraorbital hypoplasia.

Analysis of the middle third of the face consists of sequential examination of the nose, cheek, and paranasal regions. The nose generally exhibits a distinct angle at the junction of the forehead and nasal bridge. Following severe midfacial trauma, this angle may be excessive, absent, or displaced (see Figure 31.7).

The nasal bridge at the glabella projects 5 to 8 mm anterior to the globes. The nasal dorsum is evaluated for convexity or concavity in profile. The nasolabial angle is assessed—the normal angle is between 90° and 110°—and the nasal tip is inspected.

The cheeks and orbital rims are then evaluated in profile relative to the globes. The infraorbital rims generally project 0 to 2 mm in front of the most anterior projection of the globes, and the lateral rims lie 8 to 12 mm behind that point (see Figure 31.6).

In established cases of enophthalmos, the eye examination should include assessment of visual acuity, visual fields, extraocular muscle function, and the integrity of the infraorbital nerve. The results of forced duction testing and Hertel exophthalmometry should be recorded. If the lateral orbital rims are intact, corneal projection can be measured from these benchmarks. If the lateral orbital rim is displaced, the patient should

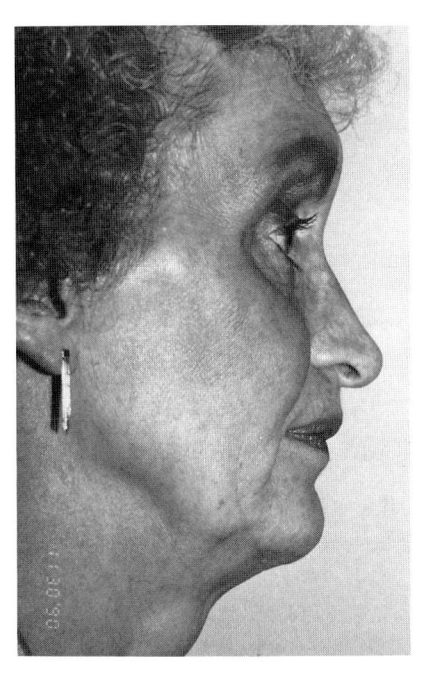

Figure 31.7 This 62-year-old woman suffered Le Fort III and nasoethmoid-orbital fractures 25 years prior to this lateral photograph. Note disruption of the nasofrontal angle, accompanied by loss of nasal dorsal projection and accentuation of the glabella.

be examined from the basal or vertex position with the nasion or intact superior orbital rim used as a reference in comparison to the normal eye (see Figure 31.8).

Enophthalmos of 3 to 4 mm will cause deepening of the supratarsal fold, narrowing of the palpebral fissure, and pseudoptosis of the upper lid. The position of the medial and lateral canthi should be noted, as well as the contour of the malar eminence.

The cheeks usually exhibit a convex appearance from the infraorbital rims to the level of the commis-

Figure 31.8 (a) Frontal and (b) submental view of a patient with left enophthalmos. Note the lack of malar projection, which is best seen in the submental view.

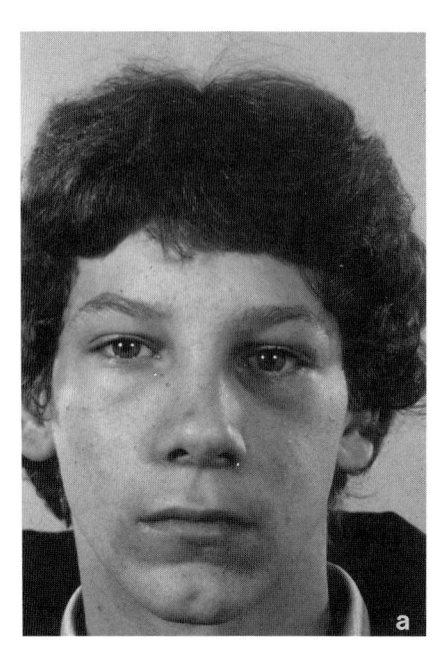

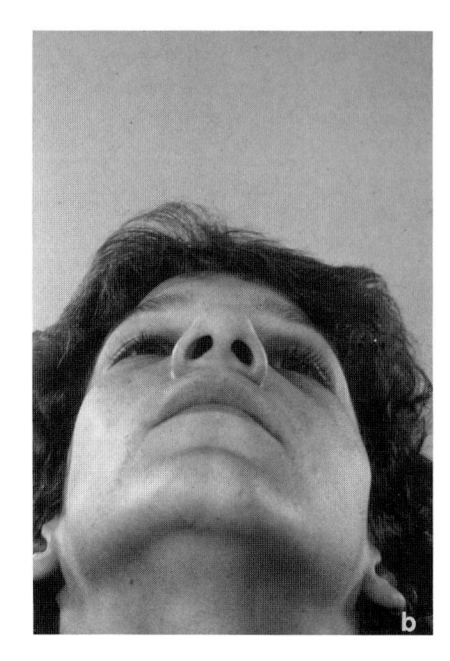

sures of the mouth. Significant asymmetry of the malar regions may exist when a malunited zygoma fracture is present. Inferior, lateral, and/or posterior displacement of the malar complex is the most common finding (see Figure 31.8). Paranasal areas are normally convex, but with midface deficiencies or retrusion, concavities may be apparent. In the patient with severe midface retrusion, the paranasal regions should be evaluated with the mandible at rest to eliminate soft-tissue posturing effects.

The lower third of the face includes the lips, labiomental fold, chin, and neck. Normally, the upper lip projects slightly anterior of the lower lip in repose. Lip position is related to the underlying dental support. Protrusion or retrusion of each lip may be indicative of underlying occlusal-skeletal abnormalities. The labiomental fold is assessed for depth. Lack of a labiomental groove detracts from chin definition. Chin projection is related to the middle third of the face as well as to the entire facial profile to determine whether balance in the sagittal plane is adequate.

Photography

Pre-injury photographs are perhaps the most valuable guides in mapping an operative plan. As with acute facial trauma, realization of the three-dimensional architecture of the face is crucial for restoration of pre-injury appearance and function. Thus facial height, width, and projection are evaluated on pre-injury pictures if they are available.

Properly oriented preoperative photographs can also be of great help. Perhaps, due to the two-dimensional nature of the image, photographs act like a mirror and accentuate the distortions and asymmetries that may elude the observer when a subject is examined directly at the initial office visit. Although restoring a face to its pre-injury state might not be possible, prior photographs provide a tangible goal for the surgeon.

Radiologic Workup

Clear radiographs of the skull are universally available, but their value is diminished by variable orientation of the patient. Thus lateral and PA cephalograms are more informative than radiographs because of the strict standards under which they are taken. Cephalometry is an excellent tool for monitoring progress and studying specific sagittal changes produced by treatment.

Cephalometric radiographs should be taken with the teeth in centric occlusion and the lips in repose. Centric occlusion is used in all instances except (1) when there is a clinically significant difference between centric occlusion and centric relation and (2) in the patient with true vertical maxillary deficiency. The second exception may apply to the patient with midface trauma in whom shortening of the maxilla arises secondary to posterior and cephalad telescoping of the midface. In such patients, the cephalometric radiograph must be taken with the mandible in rest position to study freeway space, permit assessment of the relationship of the upper teeth to the lip, and to study the true relations of the maxilla and mandible. Confirmation of the TMJ within the glenoid fossa ensures that the cephalogram has been taken in centric relation.

Computerized tomography (CT) and three-dimensional imaging have greatly contributed to visual assessment of the traumatized face. CT scans provide more accurate information than do plain films and tomograms. They are especially informative in studying periorbital and midfacial regions. The high resolution, narrowly collimated (1 to 3 mm) CT scans through areas

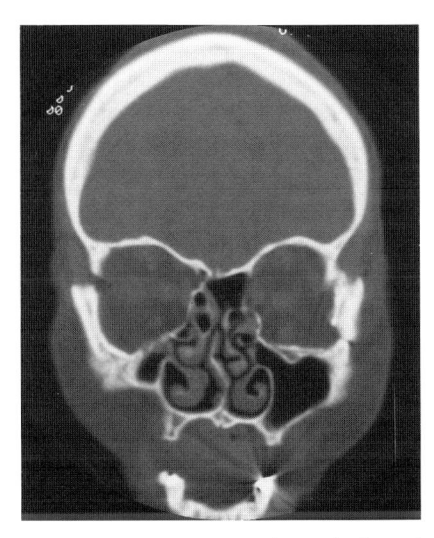

Figure 31.9 This coronal CT scan through the orbits demonstrates bilateral zygomatic fractures with displacement.

of injury allow visualization of fragments; assessment of the degree of bony displacement; and, in some cases, definition of soft-tissue disruption beyond that possible with conventional radiography (see Figure 31.9). A major advantage of CT scanning is its flexibility of data manipulation. A single axial CT study in a patient with post-traumatic craniofacial trauma may be reformatted to coronal, sagittal, parasagittal, and three-dimensional projections. Three-dimensional projection may aid in evaluating midface asymmetry, especially when the initial injury consisted of a hemi-Le Fort type fracture or a combination of Le Fort fracture patterns. Also, three-dimensional scanning of the mandible may provide a better "sense" of the post-traumatic deformity.

Finally, panoramic, or full-mouth, peri-apical radiographic evaluation provides excellent information about the dentoalveolar structure and their basilar support. The surgeon should be particularly aware of the high incidence of post-traumatic dental problems, such as insensate teeth, peri-apical abscesses, retained roots, and periodental pathology. It is generally preferable not to make a definitive diagnosis of general dental problems or periodontal disease but to refer patients to their dentist prior to undertaking surgical correction.

Occlusal Evaluation and Dental Casts

Functional and static occlusal evaluation should be performed. The former is completed by evaluating the patient and the latter by analysis and manipulation of hand-held dental models.

The objective of functional evaluation is to determine the compatibility between centric occlusion and centric relation and to assess tooth wear. Failure to appreciate inconsistencies in centric occlusion and centric relation may lead to significant errors in treatment planning. In addition, tooth attrition is assessed.

Static evaluation is performed on anatomically oriented models. Arch form, symmetry, missing teeth, and over-erupted teeth are noted. Any cant to the occlusal plane is recorded. Angle classification is observed for both molar and canine teeth. Incisor overjet and overbite are noted.

Transverse relationships, including coordination of the upper and lower midlines and buccal or lingual cross-bites, are then evaluated. When a class II or class III malocclusion is found, it is important to note the existing transverse relations when the models are placed into class I occlusion. The true nature of any transverse abnormality is revealed, and the need for segmentation of the maxilla can be determined.

Assessment of tooth-mass problems is especially important in treating late deformities arising after childhood injury. The simplest method to assess possible anterior tooth-mass discrepancy involves evaluation of the lateral incisors. If the upper lateral incisors are not larger than the lower lateral incisors, there is a good chance an anterior tooth-mass problem is present. When the teeth are relatively well aligned, another method is to hold the models so that a normal incisor relation is simulated and determine whether the distal of the upper lateral incisor reaches the middle of the lower canine. If it does, tooth mass is probably normal. If it does not, the upper incisors are probably too small in relation to the lower incisors.

Properly oriented dental casts are useful when the jaws are malaligned. They are used not only to study occlusion but also for model surgery and splint construction.

TREATMENT

Surgical Exposure

As with acute facial injuries, with well established post-traumatic deformities, there is no substitute for exposure in accomplishing successful anatomic restoration of the bony skeleton. Only a few incisions need be mastered to gain access to the entire craniofacial skeleton. Approaches are similar to those used in the management of acute trauma. Opening a pre-existing scar can be considered. However, greater exposure is frequently called for if the fracture is to be recreated and skeletal parts are to be repositioned. Thus the final choice of incisions will be determined by the location and type of deformity.

Skeletal Reconstruction: Bone Grafts

Whenever feasible, large malunited and malpositioned segments of the craniofacial skeleton should be returned to their anatomic location. Camouflage-onlay techniques should be used only when the endpoint is cosmetic and the deformity is not great. Autogenous bone is the preferred building material. The traditional donor sites are the rib cage, ileum, and calvarium.

Calvarial bone grafts are thought to have the advantages of a lower rate of resorption, minimum morbidity, a hidden scar, and proximity to the recipient site. The material can be harvested as shavings, chips, split grafts, or full-thickness grafts to suit the reconstruction. Their principal disadvantage is the brittleness of the cortical plate, especially in the older patient; their brittleness makes contouring the grafts difficult.

In the treatment of late deformities of the maxilla and mandible, calvarial bone has been used as onlay grafts to the nasal dorsum in patients with dish-face deformities, as inlay grafts to reconstruct osteotomy gaps, and as onlay grafts to refine or camouflage midfacial asymmetries and contour deformities.

When using calvarial bone grafts to the nasal dorsum, we prefer to attach a strong Y-plate to the nasal graft in vivo. Two screw holes are placed through the footplate of the Y and into the nasal bone graft. The plate is then bent to the appropriate angle at the junction of the Y and footplate. The angle is determined by a combination of aesthetic requirements as well as an estimate of the adequacy of soft-tissue coverage. With the plate attached, graft is inserted through the dissected pocket out to the nasal tip. To facilitate expansion of the pocket, several radial incisions in the periosteum and scar are made with a 15 blade. When possible, we prefer to bring the alar cartilages over the end of the graft at the tip. This may require a separate degloving of the nose via a columella incision and open rhinoplasty technique. The Y-plate is then fixed to the frontal bone of the calvarium. Alternatively, one or two lag screws may then be used to fix the graft to the nasal dorsum, wedging the graft into the nasofrontal angle.

When calvarial bone is used to close gap osteotomies, the gap distance may be measured with a small caliper; and the bone may be marked and cut to the appropriate size, wedged into the gap underneath a pre-existing plate, and tandem screwed to the plate. Onlay bone grafts may be stabilized by lag or positioned screws. When small contour deficiencies are dealt with, bone chips may be used, the skin envelope may be replaced, and the small chips can be massaged into position under the cutaneous flap.

For post-traumatic deformities of the orbital floor and medial wall, satisfactory access can usually be gained by way of a lower-eyelid incision, with the addition of a medial upper-eyelid incision if necessary. A transconjunctival approach can also be considered. A subperiosteal dissection is begun on the intact bone, working toward the defect. The *posterior edge of the defect must be identified*; otherwise, the exploration will be inadequate. The prolapsed soft tissue is returned to the confines of the orbit.

A thin shaving of calvarial bone is harvested with the periosteum attached. The calvarial bone gathered in this manner will be curved by the microfractures that are produced by the sharp osteotome during removal.

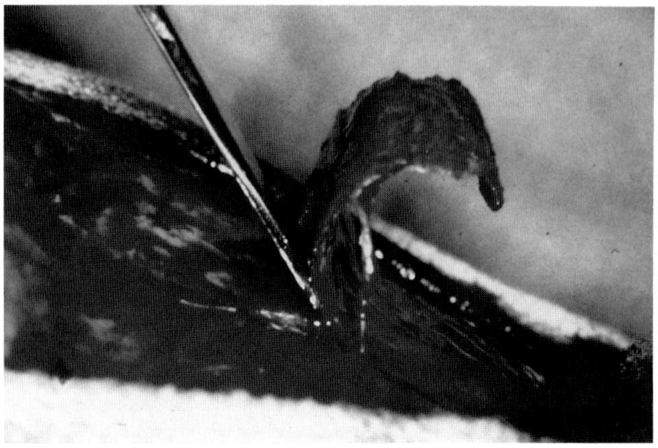

Figure 31.10 A split-thickness calvarial bone graft is shown with periosteum attached to control microfractures. This technique is most useful for obtaining bone to graft defects of the orbital floor and walls.

The periosteum will hold the microfractured pieces together and also provides a gliding surface (see Figure 31.10).

Iliac bone grafts may be necessary when large amounts of bone are required or when sizable blocks of corticocancellous bone is needed to fill osteotomy gaps.

Bone grafts may also be needed in the treatment of late mandibular deformities following trauma. For mandibular nonunion, initial treatment may require debridement of necrotic and/or infected bone and placement of an external fixation apparatus to maintain mandibular height, length, and projection. Following adequate treatment and re-establishment of good soft-tissue covering, the fracture fragments may be reunited, and cortical bone from the ilium can be packed along the fractured site while the fragments are rigidly stabilized with larger compression plates. True bony gaps in the mandible will require interposition of corticocancellous bone grafts.

Of the available alloplastic materials, hydroxyapatite holds the most promise. One should proceed with caution, however, in using this material in the reoperative situation, because scar tissue and open cavities may be less tolerant of foreign bodies and more prone to infection.

Maxillary Reconstruction

A maxillary fracture can be malunited in any position but most frequently is driven posteriorly and telescoped cephalad. The result is midface retrusion and vertical maxillary shortening. The mandible may look overclosed and give the appearance of prognathism (see Figure 31.2). However, when the mandible is in centric relation, the SNB angle may be normal. If complex fractures of the midface are present along with combinations of Le Fort fracture types, bone loss, and significant asymmetry, then normal relationships are difficult to restore by adhering to the principles of elective orthognathic surgery. In these complex cases, recreation of the injury by way of refracture and repositioning is necessary. In symmetric situations without midline shift or rotational abnormalities, more straightforward principles of elective orthognathic surgical treatment can be applied.

Panorex x-rays are perused and the patient's expectations are solicited. A radiologic work-up that includes cephalograms, panorex, and CT scans is specifically tailored to the patient's deformity. Dental models are helpful in planning and are essential to enable restoration of the original occlusion when the maxilla must be divided into multiple segments. Consultation with an orthodontist in these cases is advisable, because the bite often needs fine tuning prior to surgical therapy. Using hand-held dental models and bringing the teeth into class I relationships both anteriorly and posteriorly can help the surgeon to begin to get a sense of transverse maxillary deficiencies. Such discrepancies in the transverse width of the maxilla in relation to the width of the mandible may arise after sagittal fractures of the hard palate are treated inadequately. In cases where the palate has collapsed, lingual crossbite will be apparent. With the dental models in hand, one can rotate the teeth from side to side to determine whether a segmentation procedure will be necessary to correct the transverse discrepancy.

Not all cases of late maxillary deformities will require refracture and reposition techniques or Le Fort type osteotomies for correction. In milder cases where cosmetic correction is the desire, onlay bone grafting may be sufficient to camouflage contour deformities. Options should be carefully discussed with the patient, and realistic goals should be outlined.

It should also be remembered that many post-traumatic bony deformities are complex and extended. The term "post-traumatic midface-maxillary deformities" is therefore a somewhat artificial classification. Nasoethmoid-orbital, zygomatic, frontobasilar, and mandibular fractures may co-exist; and surgical planning requires an organized and methodical approach. Other chapters are devoted to rigid fixation of these aforementioned fracture sequences; we confine the following discussion to the malar-midface region.

Le Fort I Deformities

Le Fort I fractures account for 30% of maxillary fractures. Post-traumatic deformities associated with "pure" Le Fort I fractures are probably not as common as those associated with Le Fort I fractures that are components of more extensive injuries. Thus, in practice the isolated Le Fort post-traumatic deformity is rare. When it does arise, abnormalities are more likely to be restricted to the occlusion and the aesthetics of the lips and nasal area.

Establishment of a sound preoperative diagnosis is important. Show of the upper teeth, discrepancies in the dental midline, cant of the occlusion, inclination of one or more upper incisors, appearance of the nasal tip, and width and support of the alar base should all be assessed.

If a Le Fort I osteotomy is decided upon for correction of established post-traumatic deformities, an incision is made approximately 5 to 10 mm above the mucogingival junction, extending around the dental arch from first molar to first molar. The mucosa is elevated from the maxilla, and the dissection is continued posteriorly to the pterygopalatine junction. The nasal mucosa is lifted off the nasal floor and dissected a short distance up the lateral nasal wall and septum.

The horizontal portion of the osteotomy, including the lateral nasal wall and septum at the level of the nasal floor, is performed with a reciprocating saw. The level of the osteotomy should be at least 3 to 5 mm above the apices of the dental roots and even higher if plate and screws are to be used. A curved thin osteotome is used to separate the pterygopalatine junction. The maxilla can then be downfractured, mobilized, and moved to its pre-injury position. A previously fabricated occlusal splint is inserted, and the patient is placed in maxillo-mandibular fixation (MMF), generally with dental elastics. Alternatively, 24 or 26 gauge wire can be used.

If the mobile Le Fort I dentoalveolar segment is to be inferiorly repositioned, the medial canthus is tattooed with methylene blue. A vertical reference distance using this landmark is recorded. This may be the vertical distance from the medial canthal tattoo mark to the upper incisal edge of a central or lateral incisor; or to the interdental gap between the upper central and lateral incisor; or to the arch bar itself. The maxilla is then moved downward into the desired position, and the vertical distance from the aforementioned locations is remeasured. The difference between these distances represents the amount of inferior repositioning necessary to lengthen the shortened and telescoped midface.

Rigid osteosynthesis is then accomplished by placing plates and screws at the zygomaticomaxillary buttress and at the nasomaxillary buttress. Two screw holes on either side of the osteotomy for each metal plate are absolutely necessary. Bone grafts from the ileum or calvarium are used to fill osteotomy gaps (see Figure 31.11).

The patient is then released from MMF, and the mandible is brought passively into occlusion. Mandibular motion should be smooth and should achieve intercuspation without interferences into the planned occlusion. Any deviation from this may indicate that rigid fixation of the maxillary osteotomies was inadequately carried out while one or both of the mandibular condyles were displaced from the glenoid fossae. In this

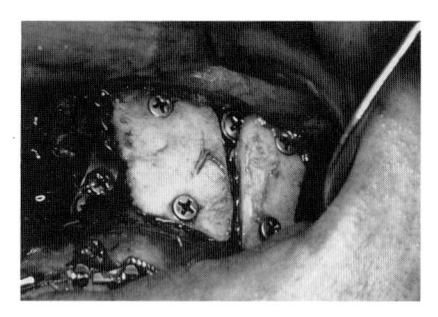

Figure 31.11 This intraoral view shows the maxilla inferiorly repositioned and advanced. The plate is placed across the nasomaxillary buttress, and bone grafts are lag-screwed into position across the osteotomy gap.

situation one can remove the two screws on the superior maxilla, leaving the plate and screws attached to the inferior segment. MMF is then replaced, and care is taken to position the condyle back into the glenoid fossa. If titanium plates, which have a lower profile and are more flexible, have been used, it is generally possible to recontour the plate without removing it, and the upper holes can be redrilled and screws replaced. When Vitallium minifragment plates, which have a higher profile and are somewhat less malleable, have been employed, it is necessary to remove and rebend the plate to allow precise adaptation to the bone.

When the maxilla must be divided into multiple segments, this can be performed from above with the

Figure 31.12 (a,c,e) Preoperative and (b,d,f) post-treatment photographs show a 47-year-old woman who suffered severe panfacial injuries and had undergone six prior reconstructive attempts by other surgeons, including refracture and repositioning of the mandible. She presented to us with a displaced zygoma, enophthalmos of the prosthetic right eye, nonunion of the maxilla with malocclusion and a cant (e). A five-stage reconstruction was performed: Stage 1 (4/87) consisted of refracture, repositioning of the right zygoma, a right sagittal split to rotate the mandible, Le Fort I osteotomy, and a cranial bone graft to the nose. Stage 2 (10/87) consisted of a rhinoplasty with tip refinement, additional cranial bone grafts to the nose, genioplasty, subperiosteal facelift, and a right lateral canthopexy. Stage 3 (3/88) consisted of a conchal cartilage graft to the nasal tip and alar rims, FTSG (full-thickness skin graft) from the left upper lid to the right lower lid, and a wedge resection of the right lower lid. Stage 4 (11/88) consisted of Fasanella/Servat ptosis repair of the right upper lid and creation of a right superior palpebral fold. Stage 5 (3/90) consisted of a free palate graft to the conjunctiva of the right lower lid for increased lining.

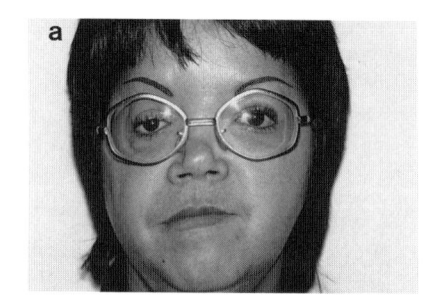

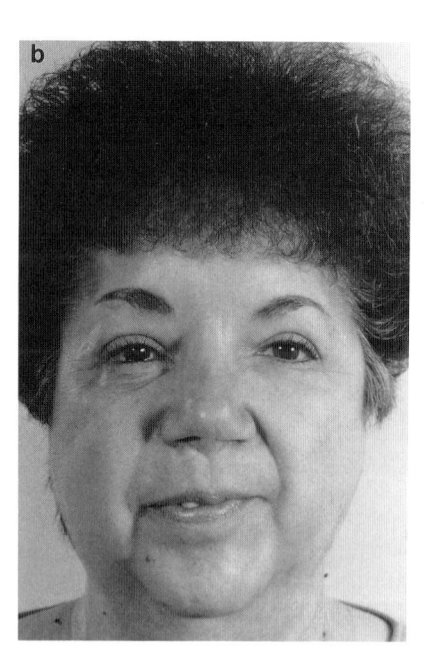

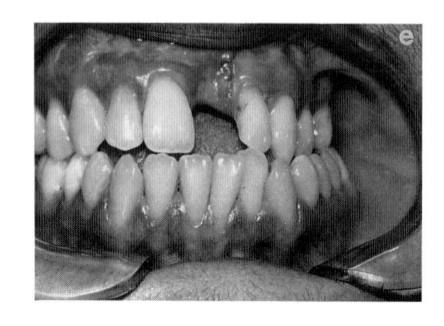

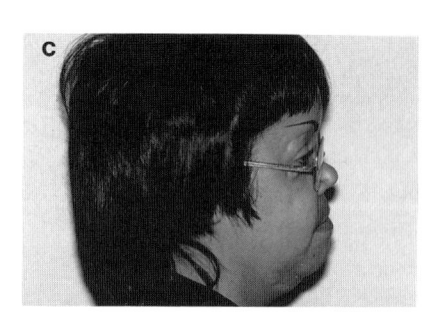

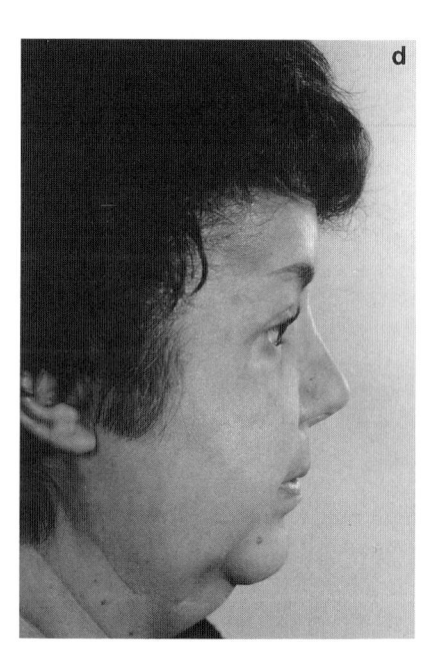

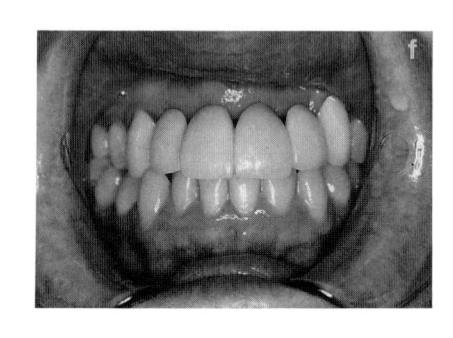

maxilla in the downfractured position. Care is exercised to preserve the integrity of the palatal mucosa in order to maintain the blood supply to what is now a composite flap of bone, teeth, and mucosa. An occlusal splint, prefabricated on dental models, is required to orient the multiple segments. Again, the patient is placed into MMF and rigid fixation with plates and screws, except now at the pyriform rim a U-shaped minifragmentation plate may be employed that has two screw holes on the superior maxillary segment, two screw holes on the inferior maxillary segment, and one or two screw holes placed across the anterior segment from either side. When the palate has been split widely to re-expand the maxillary arch, this osteotomy gap must also be bone grafted. It should be remembered that relapse in the transverse dimension is not prevented by the aforementioned techniques of rigid fixation. The maxillary splint must therefore be left ligated to the upper arch bar. Early reconstitution of the previously segmented maxillary arch wire is performed to help retain the maxillary arch in its expanded position. For more detailed information regarding the technique of treating Le Fort I fractures, the reader is referred to Chapter 33 (see Figures 31.12 and 31.13).

Le Fort II Deformities

Le Fort II osteotomy is rarely performed in elective orthognathic surgery. Even in post-traumatic maxillary deformities, Le Fort I osteotomy combined with paranasal onlay bone grafting and nasal bone grafting may be sufficient to correct mild or even moderate midface deformities without the need for a Le Fort II osteotomy. However, it should be noted that Le Fort II fractures are the most commonly observed of the Le Fort fractures in large series. Thus at times re-creation of the original fracture may require a Le Fort II type osteotomy.

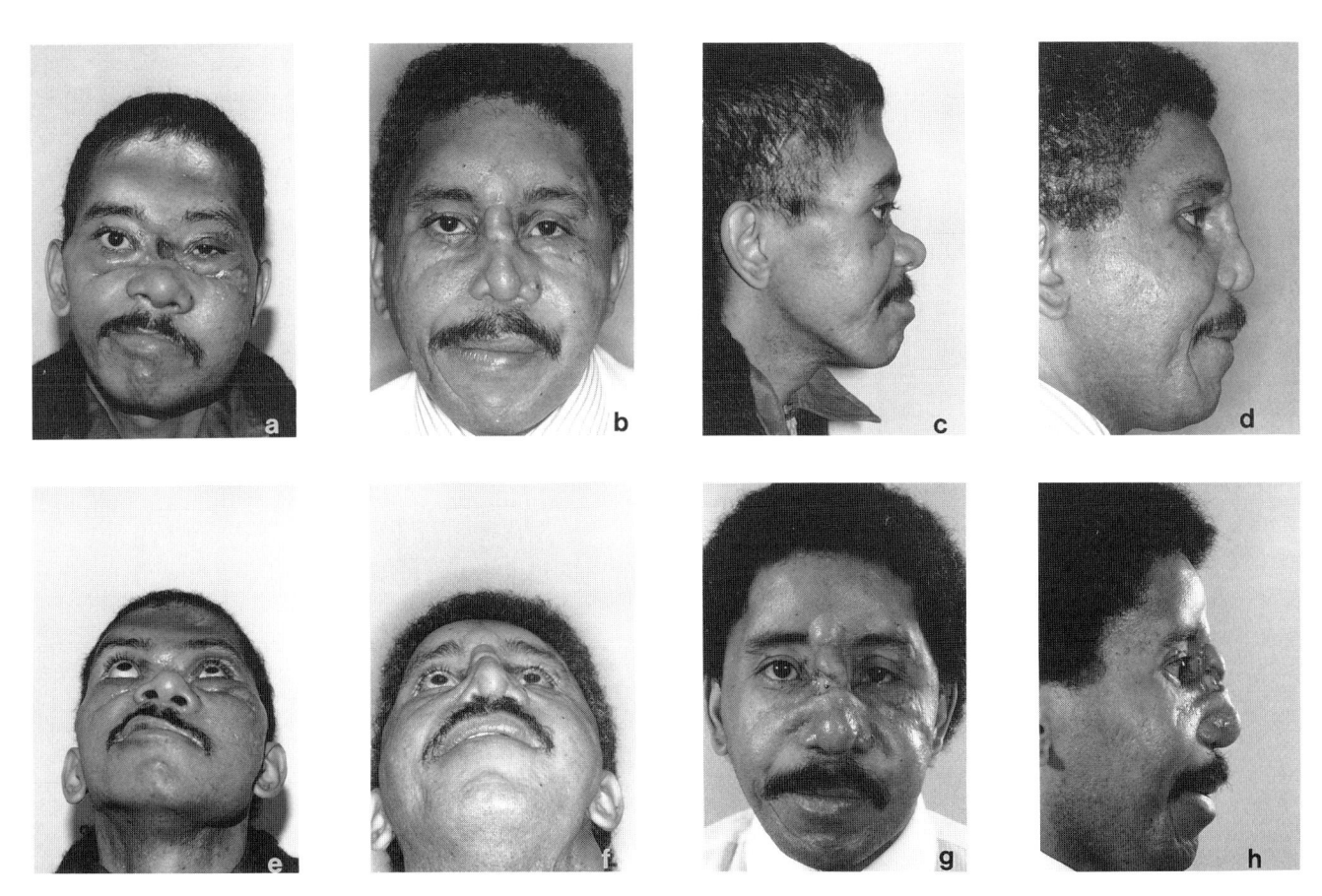

Figure 31.13 (a,c,e) Preoperative and (b,d,f) post-reconstructive photographs show a 29-year-old male with severe post-traumatic facial deformities. A prior reconstructive attempt resulted in infection and loss of bone grafts placed to the frontal region. Note collapse of the forehead in the lateral view. Following control of infection, the patient underwent 14 reconstructive procedures to obtain the present result. Initially, split rib grafts were placed to the forehead and a forehead flap was used for nasal coverage. Because of severe transverse collapse of the maxilla, a segmental Le Fort I osteotomy with iliac bone grafting was necessary. The Le Fort I was repeated for a transverse relapse two years later. Bone grafts to the nose needed to be replaced five times because of infection and/or exposure (g,h). The patient still requires additional refinements.

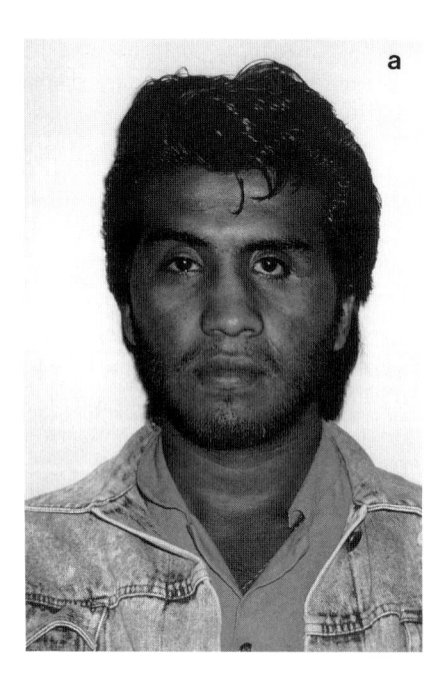

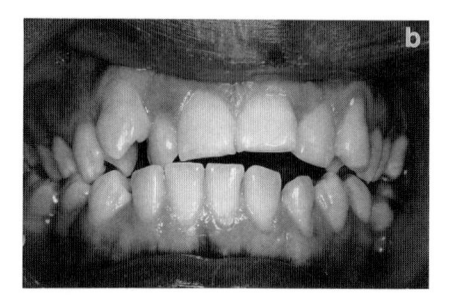

Figure 31.14 (a) Post-traumatic facial deformity in a 20-year-old male is shown. Note deviation of the nasal root. (b) Intraoral exam reveals a shift of the maxillary dental midline toward the right. Le Fort II type osteotomy is indicated to derotate the nasal pyramid and reposition the maxillary dental midline.

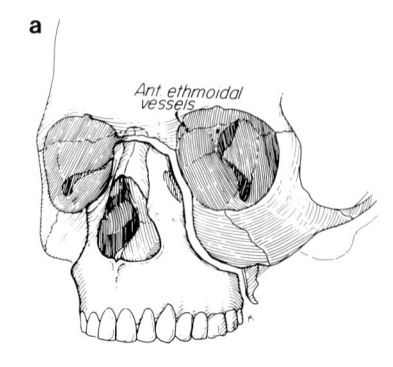

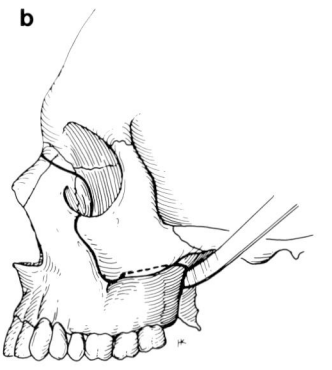

Figure 31.15 Le Fort II osteotomy lines: (a) oblique view, (b) sagittal view.

Our indications for this osteotomy are (1) nasomaxillary hypoplasia limited to the medial inferior orbital rims and paranasal areas and (2) lateral deviation or rotational abnormalities of the nasal pyramid with or without unilateral telecanthus (see Figure 31.14).

In these situations the entire maxilla, the nasofrontal junction, and the superior aspect of the medial orbital walls are exposed sufficiently to enable identification of the anterior ethmoidal vessels. Le Fort II osteotomy is performed by separating the nasal bone from the frontal process with a reciprocating saw placed parallel to the medial orbital walls below the level of the anterior ethmoidal vessels. Osteotomies are then performed along the nasomaxillary buttresses medial to the nerve; these osteotomies are then flared outward to the zygomatic maxillary buttresses to complete the pyramidal osteotomy (see Figure 31.15). The pterygopalatine junctions are then separated with an osteotome, and Rowe-Killey forceps are used to rock the Le Fort II segment forward. A double-balled septal osteotome is inserted through the nasofrontal osteotomy and used to separate the septum from the vomer. The pyramidal segment is then downfractured and mobilized. Proper vertical dimensions are established, and the patient is placed in MMF by way of a previously fabricated occlusal splint.

Because the medial canthus is mobile, a reference point on the frontal bone is marked by placement of a single screw. Vertical and sagittal dimensions are established, and the Le Fort II segment is rigidly stabilized by bilateral, large H-plates, placed across the zygomaticomaxillary buttresses and properly adapted fragmentation plates placed across the inferior orbital rim. A strong Y-plate across the nasofrontal osteotomy completes the fixation process. Bone grafts are inlaid at the osteotomy sites when gaps are present.

Hemipalatal fractures may occur in as many as 11% of Le Fort II fractures. It is therefore imperative that preoperative assessment include dental models to detect abnormalities in transverse dimensions of the maxilla. Also, because the medial and inferior orbital walls will frequently be involved in a Le Fort II fracture if enophthalmos is present or if refracture techniques leave significant gaps in the medial wall of the orbit or the orbital floor, bone grafting will be necessary. Determination of the need for a bone graft to the nasal dorsum can generally be done preoperatively and confirmed in the operating room if inadequate projection is not obtained by repositioning the Le Fort II fragments.

Preoperative assessment of any post-traumatic deformity should always include global aesthetic evaluation. In this way, procedures that may ultimately enhance facial appearance can be added to the overall treatment plan.

Le Fort III Deformities

It has been emphasized many times in the trauma literature that Le Fort III fractures are not pure. Le Fort I fragments are present in up to 80% of Le Fort III fractures. Associated mandibular fractures are found in as many as 50% of patients, and bilateral zygomatic fractures and nasoethmoid fractures frequently are present. In addition, palatoalveolar fractures are seen in as many as 17% of cases. Therefore, the surgeon must detect the subtleties of the facial deformity prior to operation. As stated throughout this section, elective or-

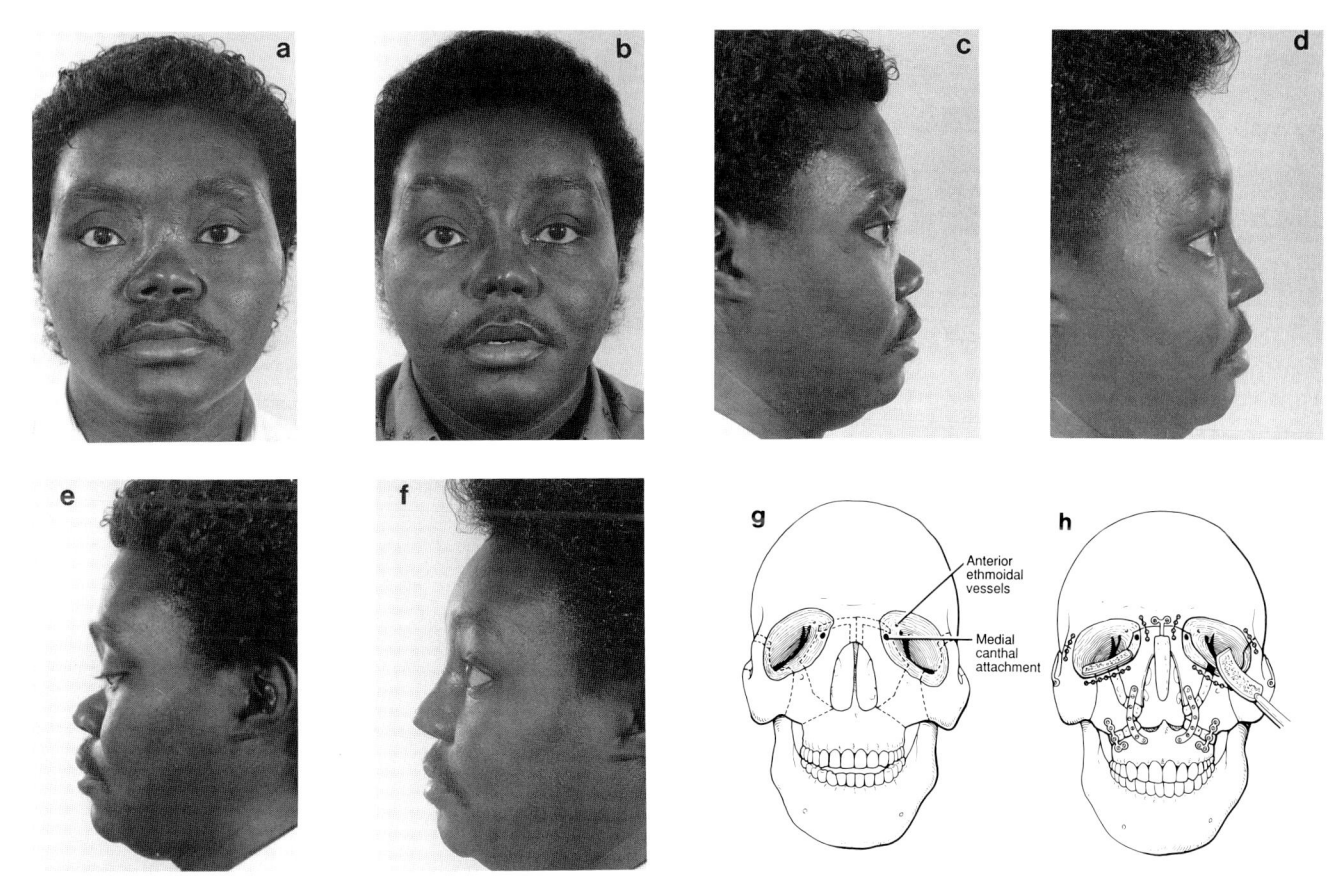

Figure 31.16 (a,c,e) Preoperative and (b,d,f) postoperative photographs show a 26-year-old male who underwent a two-stage reconstruction of severe post-traumatic deformities consisting of bilateral telecanthus, bimalar displacement, nasal retrusion, and shortening of the midface. (g,h) Artist's composite of total reconstruction. Stage 1 consisted of refracture, repositioning of both zygomas, and Le Fort I inferior repositioning. Stage 2 consisted of bilateral medial orbital osteotomies and a cantilever cranial bone graft to the nose.

thognathic principles must yield to refracture techniques. Only in this manner may one accurately recreate the original injury and attempt to reposition the fracture segments into their pre-injury positions.

A true Le Fort III osteotomy is rarely indicated in the post-traumatic patient (see Figure 31.16). Instead, refracture and repositioning of both zygomas along with lateral canthopexies, medial canthopexies (or medial orbital osteotomies), bone grafting of the orbital floor and walls, and a cantilever nasal bone graft may be performed in conjunction with a Le Fort I osteotomy to advance and inferiorly reposition the midface. In such cases, the upper craniofacial skeleton, the zygomatic arches, the zygomatic bodies, and the lateral walls of the orbit are approached via a coronal incision. An upper gingivobuccal sulcus incision exposes the remaining midface. Subciliary or transconjunctival incisions are usually necessary. Normally straight (rather than bowed) until it reaches the body of the zygoma, the zygomatic arch may need to be refractured in multiple small segments.

Identification of the intact bony edges of the original fracture is of the utmost importance to ensure that the entire defect is displayed. The periorbita is degloved to the posterior limits of the bony destruction.

If the zygomas are to be repositioned, the attachments of the temporalis and masseter to the zygoma are sharply divided to allow free movement of the zygoma. Additional exposure to the zygomaticomaxillary buttress is attained via an intraoral maxillary vestibular incision. The fracture is then re-created with a reciprocating saw. The orbital framework is anatomically reduced and fixed. Formerly, only interosseous wires were used and the zygoma was fixed in an overcorrected superior and medial direction prior to bone grafting. With the advent of miniplate and screw fixation to increase stability, as well as cranial bone grafts—which undergo less resorption than endochondral bone—anatomic alignment is attained during the operation and maintained postoperatively. Usually, miniplates at the fronto-zygomatic, inferior orbital rim, and zygomatic arch osteotomies provide adequate fixation.

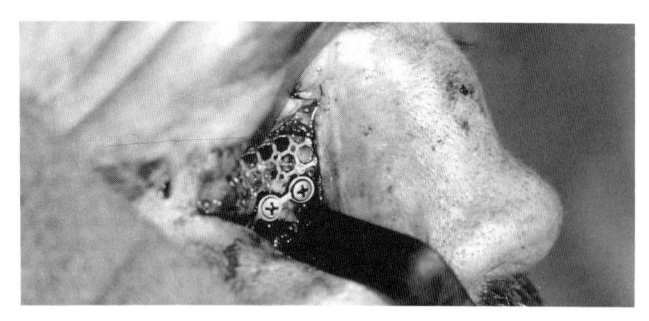

Figure 31.17 For an extensive bony defect, Vitallium mesh used to reconstruct the orbital floor.

Defects of the orbital floor, medial and lateral orbital walls, and zygomatic arch are obliterated with autogenous bone graft. To thrust the globe forward effectively, it is absolutely essential that the bone grafts be placed behind the mid-coronal plane of the globe. Bone grafts are stacked in layers to allow for slight anterior overcorrection of the globe's position. The contour of the normal orbital walls must be kept in mind when the orbit is reconstructed—especially the acute superior angulation of the medial orbital floor as it joins the medial orbital wall. The position of the bone graft is usually maintained by closure of the periorbita alone, but microfragmentation plates—or in some cases when the orbital floor is extensively destroyed, Vitallium mesh—may be employed (see Figure 31.17). It is also important to bone graft any defects of the anterior maxilla to prevent soft-tissue retraction into the gaps and subsequent depressions of the cheek.

To treat associated unilateral or bilateral posttraumatic telecanthus and/or hypertelorbitism, we currently favor a medial orbital osteotomy that leaves the canthal ligament attached to the central fragment and repositioning the entire medial orbital wall, along with its attached canthus, into the desired position (that is, generally posterior and superior) (see Figure 31.16). This maneuver essentially re-creates the nasoethmoid-orbital fracture and repositions the canthus-bearing fragment. When this procedure is performed unilaterally, the lateral aspect of the nasal bone frequently needs additional onlay bone grafting. Lateral canthopexies are performed in the usual fashion. The cantilever nasal bone graft, if required, is placed as previously described.

A Le Fort I osteotomy is performed, re-establishing vertical height. Bone grafts are used in any of the osteotomy gaps. For surgical steps involved with elective surgery to manage Le Fort III fractures, the reader is referred to Chapter 34.

MANDIBULAR RECONSTRUCTION

Assessment of a malunited mandible begins with clinical evaluation of occlusion. Dental models and a panoramic radiograph supplement the examination. Consultation with an orthodontist may add valuable information and help. When the dental arch is disrupted, model surgery is required to realign the segments and fabricate a dental splint.

A fractured mandible is continually subjected to powerful displacing forces in addition to that of the initial traumatic impact. The muscles of mastication insert on the lower jaw. Their distorting vectors are influenced by the pull of the suprahyoid muscles. Failure to neutralize these forces effectively is a major contributor to malunion. Similar forces are at play in the secondary treatment of mandibular fractures.

Although the mandible is often fractured in more than one location, for the purpose of discussion we cover the various regions separately. The basic concepts can be integrated to treat the mandible as a whole.

An intraoral approach can be used in most instances. Proper instrumentation, similar to that used in orthognathic surgery, is important for exposure. Preauricular and submandibular external incisions are occasionally needed and should be placed in natural skin creases.

Re-creation of the fracture is usually the treatment of choice for malunited fractures of the symphyseal and body regions (see Figure 31.18). The mobilized segments are placed into a prefabricated splint, and occlusion is restored with MMF. The reduction is further stabilized with interosseous wires or plates and screws. When rigid compression plates and screws are used, continued MMF can be eliminated after the desired occlusion is established. The same guidelines for rigid fixation of acute mandibular fractures should be followed in the post-traumatic patient. The more oblique the line of refracture, the longer the plate and the more screw holes on either side of the fractured site should be utilized. In addition, whenever feasible the plate is placed perpendicular to the fracture line.

In keeping with the principle of conservative management of most fractures around the condylar region, less than ideal anatomic reduction is acceptable. Fortunately, patients are able to compensate and tend to do well despite the lack of perfect alignment. This is especially true in the case of unilateral fractures, unless healing is complicated by an open bite or subsequent ankylosis. When secondary correction for unilateral fracture of the condylar region is required, the approach is similar to that used for a ramus or angle fracture. In addition to the sagittal split procedure, an oblique or vertical osteotomy of the ramus can be used. The main problem is the propensity for relapse. The shortened strong muscles of mastication tolerate poorly the stretching forces that are generated when the height of the ramus is restored. Thus a tendency for the mandible to deviate toward the affected side remains, causing premature occlusion in the molar region.

The risk of regression is worst in established bilateral condylar fractures. Height of the ramus is

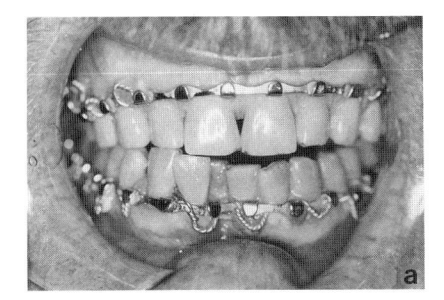

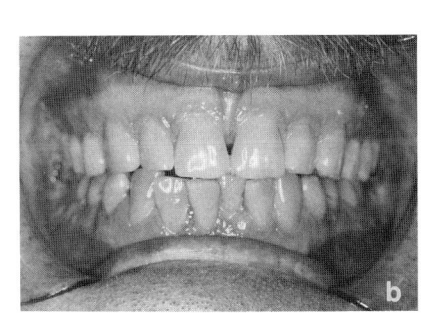

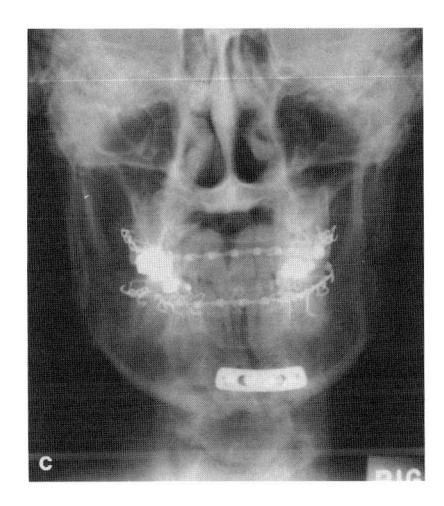

Figure 31.18 (a) Preoperative view shows a malunited parasymphyseal mandibular fracture. (b) Postoperative view shows the effect of refracture and repositioning. (c) This radiograph shows the position of the Vitallium plate used to stabilize the osteotomy site.

compromised, and the entire mandible is displaced posteriorly. The consequence is anterior open bite. Ramal sectioning procedures can be considered, but the relapsing forces are particularly strong and may be difficult to conquer. A more reliable treatment alternative is to close the open bite by using a Le Fort I osteotomy with posterior intrusion of the maxilla and to camouflage the mandibular recession with an osseous advancement genioplasty. This may not be adequate if the ramus is severely shortened. For unusually complex condylar fractures, joint replacement with a costocartilage graft is an alternative. However, unless there is progression to ankylosis, the need for condylar replacement is rare.

Liberating an ankylosed TMJ is a taxing mission. Intubation for anesthesia is treacherous, even with the aid of fiberoptic instrumentation. Tracheostomy should therefore always be available. At surgery, the path of the facial nerve should be respected when the obliterated joint is approached through a preauricular incision. The osseous proliferation can be massive, making dissection and bony separation difficult. Depending on the extent of destruction, various means to maintain movement have been proposed.

Because of the strong tendency toward recurrence of ankylosis, a wide-gap ostectomy has been advised. However, an undesirable shortening of the ramus is a result of this technique. Partially to offset this deficiency, large blocks of alloplastic material have been inserted. However, introduction of a foreign body that accommodates movement is often not well tolerated by the already damaged tissues. Artificial joints have also been inserted, but the threat of extrusion is forever present, because the interface between the implant and the remaining mandible is mechanical and the forces of mastication are tremendous. Therefore, in the ideal operation autogenous materials are used to restore movement and preserve the vertical dimension of the ramus.

When pathologic ossification is limited, linear resection may suffice. A key step in the dissection is first to locate the meniscus. Although this is sometimes impossible, it is worth trying. The soft tissues are stripped from the ramus, and the joint is separated to its maximum extent. An inferiorly based flap of temporoparietal fascia is turned into the gap and wrapped around the condylar stump. A free fascial graft may also be used to cap the new condylar post. In this case, MMF is contraindicated, and early, active movement of the mandible and physical therapy are rigorously encouraged.

More frequently, the joint is totally obliterated by a mass of bone. Resection of the pathologic overgrowth leaves a considerable gap, which is best spanned by an autogenous costocartilage graft. Rigid fixation of the graft with lag screws may avoid the need for MMF. Considerable distortion of the maxillofacial skeleton often accompanies TMJ ankylosis, especially when the injury is sustained early in life. With adaptation of craniofacial surgical principles, extensive freeing of the mandible from its soft-tissue restraints, and intensive post-immobilization physical therapy, a one-stage correction is possible.

Associated Procedures

Reoperative surgery after facial fractures can be a difficult task, and various adjuvant maneuvers may be necessary to obtain a satisfactory result. Soft tissue is frequently the limiting factor. Careful consideration therefore should be given to scar revision, either at the time, or after, bony fragments are replaced in their normal anatomic positions.

Fatty atrophy of the subcutaneous tissues may have occurred, and even under the best circumstances correction may be difficult. At present, the histopathology and pathogenesis underlying the sometimes tenacious scar formation associated with these post-traumatic deformities are unknown.

Every attempt is made to cover plates and screws with periosteum. In selected cases, midfacial periosteal covering may be resuspended to an available bony ledge—as in a subperiosteal facelift—to correct cheek ptosis, which may be associated with fractures of the zygoma. Dynamic and adynamic correction of facial nerve palsies may also be indicated. Accordingly, browlift can be combined with coronal flap closure if frontal nerve palsy is present. In some cases ingenious use of facial prosthetics may enhance ultimate outcome.

It is not uncommon for patients suffering midfacial fractures to present with both paresthesias and hyperesthesias. Positive Tinnel's signs may be elicited over the inferior orbital nerve, the mental foramen, and along the distribution of the supratrochlear and supraorbital nerves. Although the results are extremely variable, one should consider decompression of involved nerves at the time of skeletal corrections.

COMPLICATIONS

Certain complications are common to all surgical procedures; others are specific to particular operations. Little information is available on the complication rate following repair of late sequelae from midface and mandibular fractures. In one large series of 133 patients who underwent various procedures for correction of late sequelae of facial bone fractures, a complication rate of 15% was reported. This study, however, did not specifically address complications related to correction of post-traumatic maxillary or mandibular deformities. Moreover, within the reported 15% complication rate, residual deformity was included.

Complications seem to arise more frequently in correction of post-traumatic deformities than in elective orthognathic surgery. This primarily reflects the difficulty involved in reconstruction within contaminated and scarred beds.

Small areas of uncovered bone generally heal in spite of exposure to the oral cavity. Debridement may be carried out in the office to hasten healing by secondary intention. Persistent osteitis and spreading osteomyelitis are rare complications, especially if the patient is maintained on antibiotic therapy during the period of healing.

Provision of soft-tissue coverage is one of the major concerns in reoperative surgery. The literature contains little documentation concerning treatment of exposed plates and screws. It has been our clinical experience that when infection is well controlled and minor exposures of hardware are seen, generally the plate can be left and healing will follow. However, when bony fragments are grossly unstable and plates and screws are mobile, formal debridement should be performed and hardware should be removed.

Malunion of bone is caused by faulty reduction or by inadequate fixation, which causes slippage of bony fragments. Generally, malunion can be avoided by careful intraoperative planning. Delayed union and nonunion are the result of absence of bony alignment and poor impaction of fragments of bone. Poor fixation of fragments, failure to close large osteotomy gaps with appropriate bone grafting, and lack of control of masticatory musculature are leading causes of these complications. Adequate rigid fixation is imperative. In cases of nonunion, re-exposure of nonunited bone, excision of fibrous tissue between fragments, and insertion of corticocancellous bone grafts are warranted.

Exposure of or injury to tooth roots or tooth root exposure may cause loss of teeth. Preoperative dental work-up is indicated in all patients undergoing surgery for late sequelae of maxillary and mandibular fractures. Periapical abscesses should be resolved prior to corrective surgery. In contrast, endodontic procedures may be performed either before or after jaw surgery.

Fortunately, major maxillary bone loss is extremely rare. Adequate circulation is derived from both the gingiva and the mucosa of the palate. In addition, intramedullary vasculature courses through the maxilla. When single-segment maxillary surgery is performed there is generally little concern about tissue ischemia. However, in the reoperative situation, when extensive scarring may be present in both the palate and gingiva, care must be taken in designing incisions for exposure and in contemplating segmentation of the maxilla.

Internal rigid fixation with miniplates and screws, as already mentioned, is a significant advance in treatment of late deformities. One of the major disadvantages of miniplates and screws is the increased operating time required for precise contouring and exact positioning of the plates. In jaw surgery the single most important intraoperative consideration for successful use of rigid fixation is the release of MMF once the jaws have been rigidly immobilized. This allows the surgeon to ascertain whether the mandibular condyles were correctly positioned at the time of bony fixation. If upon release of MMF the mandible does not occlude properly with the maxillary dentition or the surgical splint, rigid fixation must be dismantled and new drill holes must be placed.

It is our practice to use only light guiding elastics at the termination of surgery (see Figure 31.19). Within the first 24 hours of surgery it is important that the anatomic relationship between the condyle and glenoid fossa, established at the termination of surgery, is unchanged. If the patient is able to reproducibly and comfortably obtain proper occlusion without mandibular translation, one can assume that the condylar position established at surgery is correct. However, if the patient is unable to occlude properly, condylar distraction probably existed at the conclusion of surgery and the patient should be returned to the operating room as soon as possible.

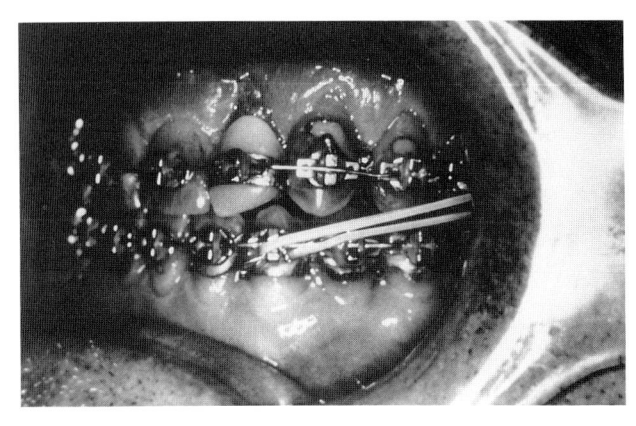

Figure 31.19 Intraoral photograph shows a patient's occlusion following a Le Fort I osteotomy. Note the class III"ish" malocclusion at the canine position. Dental elastic has been placed to pull the mandibular segment posteriorly while simultaneously drawing the maxillary segment mesially.

LONG-TERM RESULTS

One must take a pragmatic view of the correction of late sequelae of fractures of the maxilla and mandible. In general, it is fair to say that occlusion can definitely be improved and is usually stable, especially in the era of plate and screw fixation. In addition, transverse, sagittal, and vertical skeletal proportions can generally be re-established by refracture osteotomies and repositioning techniques. However, for the patient with facial disfigurement, release from the prison of his or her deformity is the ultimate desire. In a previous report from our institution, it was found that multiple operations were often necessary to achieve a final result (Resnick and Kawamoto, 1989). When this so-called "final" result was carefully evaluated, residual abnormalities were frequently revealed. Ultimately, the limiting factor in obtaining a "near perfect" result is the status of the soft tissues. Soft tissue injured by repeated scarring and neurologic losses will compromise the best bony repair.

BIBLIOGRAPHY

Bell WH: Le Fort I osteotomy. In Surgical Correction of Dento-Facial Deformities. Bell WH, Proffit WR, White RP (eds). Philadelphia, W.B. Saunders, 15-44, 1985.

Dingman RO, Harding RL: Treatment of malunited fractures of facial bones. Plast Reconstr Surg 7:505, 1951.

Hardesty RA, Marsh JL: Malunion and nonunion. In Facial Fractures. Habal MD, Ariyan S (eds). Toronto, B.C. Deckers, 195-229, 1989.

Kawamoto HK Jr: Correction of established traumatic deformities of the facial skeleton using craniofacial principles. In Facial Injuries. Schultz RC (ed). Chicago, YearBook Medical Publishers, 601-630, 1988.

Kawamoto HK Jr: Simplification of the Le Fort I osteotomy. Clin Plast Surg 16:777, 1989.

Manson PN, Hoopes JE, Su CT: Structural pillars of the facial skeleton: An approach to the management of Le Fort fractures. Plast Reconstr Surg 66(1):54-61, 1980.

Markowitz BL: Complex midfacial injuries. In PSEF Instructional Courses, Vol 3, Russell R (ed). CV Mosby Co, in press.

Merville LL, Derome P, Saint-Jorre G: Fronto-orbito-nasal dislocations: Secondary treatment of sequelae. J Maxillofac Surg 11:71, 1983.

McCoy FJ, Chandler RA, Crow ML: Facial fractures in children. Plast Reconstr Surg 37:209-215, 1966.

McGuirt WF, Salisbury TL: Mandibular fractures: Their effect on growth of dentition. Arch Otolaryngol, Head Neck Surg 113:257-261, 1987.

Mullikan JB, Kaban LB, Murray JE: Management of facial fractures in children. Clin Plast Surg 4(4):491-501, 1977.

Ousterhout DK, Vargervik K: Maxillary hypoplasia secondary to midfacial trauma in childhood. Plast Reconstr Surg 80:491-497, 1987.

Polayes IM: Facial fractures in the pediatric patient. In Facial Fractures. Habal MB, Ariyan S (eds). Toronto, B.C. Decker, 257-288, 1989.

Proffit WR, Epker BN: Treatment planning for dentofacial deformities. In Surgical Correction of Dento-Facial Deformities. Bell WH, Proffit WR, White RP (eds). Philadelphia, W.B. Saunders, 155-199, 1980.

Proffit WR, Vig KWL, Turvey TA: Early fractures of the mandibular condyles: Frequently an unsuspected cause of growth disturbances. Am J Orthod 78:1-24, 1980.

Resnick JI, Kawamoto HK Jr: Traumatic enophthalmos. In Facial Fractures. Habal MB, Ariyan S (eds). Toronto, BC Decker, 155-169, 1989.

Steidler NE, Cook RM, Reade PC: Residual complications in patients with major middle third facial fractures. Int J Oral Surg 9:259-266, 1980.

Tessier P: Total osteotomy of the middle third of the face for fascio-stenosis or for sequelae of Le Fort III fracture. Plast Reconstr Surg. 48:553, 1971.

Thaller SR, Zarem HA, Kawamoto HK Jr: Surgical correction of late sequelae from facial bone fractures. Am J Surg 154:149-153, 1987.

CHAPTER 32

The Role of Plate and Screw Fixation in the Treatment of Pediatric Facial Fractures

Jeffrey C. Posnick

The management of facial fractures, whether in children or adults, usually follows the dictum "form equals function." Therefore, the goal is early re-establishment of pre-injury bony anatomy with fixation that is adequate to allow for bony healing and rapid return of normal function with limited morbidity. Patients who are considered too ill to undergo optimum early management of their facial injuries may require endotracheal intubation or tracheostomy to bypass the airway. However, in children, tracheostomy should be avoided whenever possible (Bridges 1966, Crysdale 1987). In addition, such patients may require a nasogastric tube or gastrostomy to replace oral feedings.

Pediatric trauma presents special problems that differ from those seen in adults (Kissoon 1990). This is also true of injuries sustained to the facial bones. Children with facial fractures have different overall fracture fixation needs and must not be viewed as small adults with small jaws (Schultz 1988). Before definitive fracture management can be undertaken, consideration must be given to pre-existing conditions, such as asthma, blood dyscrasias, and congenital anomalies, as well as to multiple-system trauma (for example, brain or abdominal injury).

When options for fracture fixation are available, the method used for each fracture is determined by the patient's total treatment plan. This must be individualized to accommodate overall healing of multiple facial fractures and timely restoration of normal upper-airway breathing, swallowing, and chewing. The options for fracture stabilization can vary from a soft diet alone to closed reduction with arch bars and maxillo-mandibular fixation (MMF) to open reduction with direct wire fixation or stable plate and screw fixation with mini- or microplating systems.

When the temporomandibular joint has been injured (that is, a condyle fracture), early restoration of function is important to prevent ankylosis. In the case of dentoalveolar fractures, prompt reduction and immobilization are mandatory. Iatrogenic injury to the sensory nerves of the face (that is, the supraorbital, infraorbital, and inferior alveolar-mental nerves) must be avoided, and fracture nerve compression must be relieved (Posnick, 1990). In children, particular care must be taken to avoid injury to the developing tooth buds and to promote continued normal growth and development of the jaw.

If placement of plates and screws is used, additional decisions must be made. A choice must be made as to what metal (that is, titanium, Vitallium, or stainless steel) will be used, whether self-tapping screws or tapped screws will be used, whether the tension-band concept should be applied, whether screw placement will be bicortical or unicortical, and what thickness of plate (that is, full reconstructive plate, fracture plates, miniplates, thin plates, or microplates) will be used.

In this chapter we attempt to explain a philosophy for the management of pediatric facial fractures based on the region of the craniofacial skeleton injured, the presence or absence of multiple facial fractures and in what combination, the patient's age, and the multiple-system injuries sustained.

PEDIATRIC FACIAL FRACTURES: A TEN-YEAR REVIEW FROM THE HOSPITAL FOR SICK CHILDREN

A retrospective chart review was carried out at The Hospital for Sick Children (HSC) in Toronto to study the demographics of pediatric facial fractures

Table 32.1 Pediatric facial fractures

Etiology	
• Vehicle/Passenger	60
• Vehicle/Pedestrian	33
• Bicycle	22
• Fall	53
• Sport	65
• Altercation	28
• All-terrain Vehicles	6
• Other	69
	N = 336

Table 32.2 Pediatric facial fractures

Associated Injuries	
• Head	55
• Ocular	17
• C-Spine	1
• Thorax	5
• Abdomen	4
• Extremity	22
• Other	9
	N = 113

Table 32.3 Pediatric facial fractures

Regions Fractured	
• Orbit	57
• Zygoma	32
• Nose	175
• Midface	27
• Mandibular	148
• Dentoalveolar	25
	N = 464

Table 32.4 Pediatric facial fractures

Mandible	
• Condyle	58
• Ramus	15
• Coronoid	1
• Angle	16
• Body	17
• Parasymph./Symph.	41
	N = 148

treated from 1979 through 1988 (Smith, Posnick et al., 1989). Medical records, emergency charts, radiographic reports, operative notes, and clinic notes were examined to identify patients who had sustained acute trauma requiring admission to the hospital.

The chart review identified 336 patients, of whom 227 were male. They ranged in age from 10 months to 16 years, with a mean age of 10 years. The greatest frequency of facial fractures occurred from May through August. Table 32.1 shows the varied etiologies of the fractures sustained.

These patients also had 113 concurrent injuries to other body regions, the distribution of which is shown in Table 32.2. Fifty-five patients had associated head trauma; of these, 22 (40%) sustained skull fractures. Seventeen had associated ocular injuries; six blind eyes, six eyes with reduced visual acuity, and two eyes with residual diplopia were found. Only one patient had associated cervical spine injury. The high incidence of head and ocular trauma with a low incidence of cervical spine and abdominal trauma is interesting in contrast to observations in adults with facial trauma.

The facial fractures were broken down by region as follows: orbit, zygoma, nose, midface, mandibular area, and dentoalveolar area (see Table 32.3). Of the 336 patients sustaining facial fractures, 234 had single fractures, 42 had multiple fractures at a single site (that is, condyle and parasympheseal of the mandible), and 60 had multiple fractures at multiple sites (that is, mandible, maxilla, zygoma, and so on). A breakdown by region of the mandibular fractures sustained is shown in Table 32.4. Associated soft-tissue injuries, most of which consisted of facial abrasions and lacerations, were found in 25% of the patients. Various reported studies have discussed pediatric facial fractures (Frief 1954, Graham 1960; McCoy 1966, Rowe 1968, Bales 1972, Hall 1972, Waite 1973, Bernstein 1974, Hall 1974, Kaban 1977, Adekeye 1980, Fortunato 1982, Manson 1988).

Classification System

In Ontario, HSC is a major level-one pediatric trauma center for a population of 8 million. Recently, we have introduced a computerized prospective patient registry for craniomaxillofacial trauma. Data are gathered to indicate demographic information and trauma status (that is, bony fracture, associated injuries, visceral injury, and soft-tissue injuries). Our team has developed a classification for bony fractures that includes the cause of the trauma event, initial airway management, radiographic investigations obtained, fracture type, fracture treatment, and early and late complications. It is our hope that gathering this information prospectively will enable us to do more complete periodic analyses.

Surgical Anatomy

Maxillofacial trauma is much less common in younger children than in adolescents and adults. The comparative immunity of children to facial fractures is a result of environmental, physical, and craniofacial anatomic factors (Nahum 1975).

Before age five, most children have a relatively protected existence because of close parental supervision and in spite of their spontaneous, curious spirit and general lack of caution (Rowe 1968). Although falls are frequent, they usually occur from minimal height and the momentum gained by the child's small body is of low velocity. As a result, the low impact force can usually be absorbed by the generally well-padded skin, elastic skeleton, and cartilaginous growth centers between the bones.

After age five, children begin to participate in events at school, contact sports, and bicycling. Height, weight, and muscular development increase and are often combined with a more competitive and aggressive attitude, which leads to more frequent falls from greater heights and more severe, direct facial trauma.

For the first several years of life, the cranium is relatively large, having a prominent forehead that is unprotected by a frontal sinus. Development of the frontal sinus is somewhat variable but does not begin until after one year of age and until five years of age is only minimally visible on radiographs. By age six, a definitive frontal sinus cavity is present. There is a lack of maxillary and ethmoid sinus development as well as limited dental development. As a result, downward projection of the face is minimal in infancy and early childhood. These factors result in a high ratio of skull to face, leaving the frontal bones and brain relatively exposed to trauma while the facial bones are protected.

From the time of birth until skeletal maturity, the size of the cranium increases fourfold and the size of the facial bones increase tenfold (see Figure 32.1). Approximately 80% of postnatal growth of the cranial vault is complete by age two, and 85% of orbital growth is complete by age five. In contrast, the jaws are small at birth, through infancy, and during much of childhood. The maxilla is not separated from the cranial base by well pneumatized air sinuses, as in later life. The condylar process is well vascularized; its neck is thick and short, making it an uncommonly strong site of the mandible when contrasted to its shape and limited strength later in childhood and in adolescence. The basal bone of the jaws grows rapidly in childhood and has a high metabolic rate and a high ratio of cancellous bone to cortical bone. Both of these factors result in greater elasticity to the jaws, leading to more greenstick and nondisplaced fractures in childhood than are seen in adulthood. In children, the periosteum is extremely osteogenic, and this leads to early bony union and active remodeling of the healed bone over time.

During the first few years of life the crowns of the developing permanent teeth are incompletely formed, and the ratio of tooth to bone is relatively low. Later, the presence of a mixed deciduous and permanent dentition results in a high tooth-to-bone ratio; this encourages fracture through the developing tooth crypts. In adults, a sharp angular pattern is usually seen in mandibular fractures, whereas in children there is usually an irregular fracture line because the bone shears between the crypts of the developing teeth.

In late childhood and in adolescence the development of the maxillary antrum and other paranasal sinuses is a major factor in the shift of facial bone fractures toward the zygomatic bones and Le Fort (midface) fractures.

Airway Management

The first step in managing a traumatized patient is to ensure a patent airway. An adequate spontaneous or assisted airway must be established and maintained throughout fracture healing.

When an artificial airway is required, endotracheal intubation is almost always possible and in pediatric patients is preferred to a tracheostomy. A tracheostomy, with its associated complications in children, is selected only as a last resort (Bridges 1966, Crysdale 1987). Possible indications for tracheostomy are for long-term management of central nervous system impairment, management of a direct tracheal injury, need to maintain adequate pulmonary toilet, and situations in which the larynx cannot be intubated with endotracheal procedures.

PRINCIPLES OF TREATMENT BY REGION

Fractures of the Cranial Vault, Supraorbital Rim, and Lateral Orbital Rim

Thorough evaluation with computerized tomography (CT) scanning, neurosurgical assessment, and ophthalmologic consultation must be performed. Unless direct lacerations give adequate exposure, a coronal in-

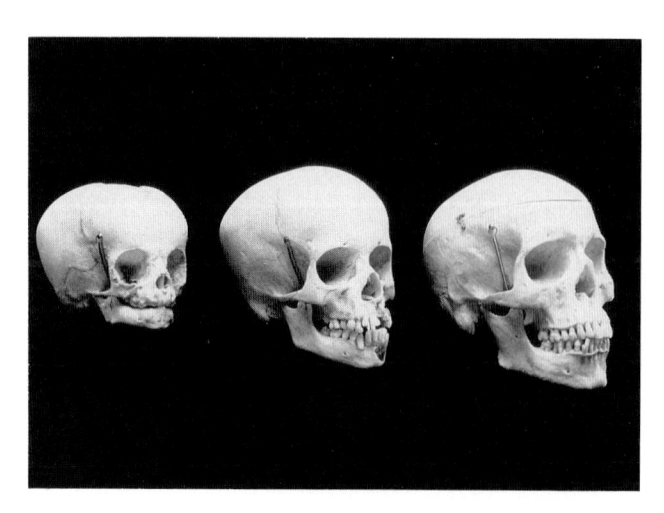

Figure 32.1 Dry skulls of various ages are demonstrated in oblique view. The skulls are age approximately 6 months, 11 years, and 20 years.

cision is usually made to provide the necessary exposure for fracture treatment. A thorough subperiosteal dissection of the fracture region with complete exposure out to the region of normal anatomy is generally required. Fixation is achieved with either direct transosseous wires or bone plates (mini or micro) as indicated. In most situations when bony defects are present, primary bone grafting with autogenous cranial bone is preferred to secondary bone grafting. A combined procedure is carried out with the neurosurgeon if intracranial exposure is required as part of the trauma management or if exposure is needed for fracture reduction.

Naso-fronto-ethmoid Fractures

Preoperative assessment, incisions, dissection, and fixation for naso-fronto-ethmoid fractures are similar to those required for combined cranial vault and orbital rim fracture. Plate and screw internal fixation and primary cranial bone grafting are used to achieve and maintain anatomic reduction and adequate fixation to permit bone to heal in its pre-injury location. If the medial canthal ligament is displaced, it is usually attached to a bone fragment. In most cases, repositioning and immobilization of the medial canthal ligament and bone fragment is accomplished without the use of a more aggressive medial canthopexy procedure. Formal medial canthopexies often add to an unnatural appearance. Careful dissection is essential to avoid iatrogenic injury to the nasolacrimal apparatus.

Before age five, which is when most pediatric skull and upper orbital trauma occurs, the frontal sinus is minimally developed. When the frontal sinus is injured and displaced, anterior table fractures should be anatomically repositioned and stabilized if a cosmetic deformity would otherwise result. Depending on the extent of sinus fracture, the mucous membranes may require debridement with maintenance of a patent nasofrontal duct. If the posterior table of the frontal sinus is also fractured, neurosurgical consultation is needed to determine whether the posterior table (cranialization of the sinus) should be removed and the nasofrontal duct closed off. The possible growth disturbance to the supraorbital ridge must be considered if the frontal sinus is injured or debrided at an early age (prior to bony maturity).

Le Fort I, II, and III Fractures

Le Fort type fractures usually occur in older children and adolescents and should be treated with open reduction and internal fixation as required to achieve anatomic restoration. Closed reduction is often preferred in younger children to avoid injury to the unerupted permanent dentition.

When open reduction is considered necessary, a maxillary circumvestibular mucosal incision provides excellent exposure to the fractures through the zygomatic buttress, anterior maxillary wall, and piriform nasal aperture regions. Care must be taken to avoid injury to the infraorbital neurovascular bundle. When access to the combined areas of the zygomatic arch, fronto-zygomatic suture, and supraorbital ridge is required, a coronal incision allows the necessary added exposure.

The goals of midface and zygomatic fracture fixation in children is to restore normal anatomy and to immobilize the segments for fracture healing. In cases of greenstick or nondisplaced fractures, a soft diet and rest alone are often adequate. As in adults, bone grafts and mini- and microplate and screw fixation is often preferred to manage displaced fractures.

Zygomatic Complex Fractures

The most common physical findings in a zygomatic complex fracture are periorbital ecchymosis and subconjunctival hemorrhage. Treatment is similar to that in adults. If a comminuted zygomatic arch fracture is associated with a zygomatic complex fracture, a coronal incision is combined with intraoral and subciliary incisions to give full exposure for reduction and fixation.

When minimally displaced or incomplete zygomatic complex fractures are present but are believed to require open reduction and internal fixation (ORIF), local incisions (that is, lateral brow, subciliary, lower lid, conjunctival, and intraoral) can be used for exposure to avoid a coronal incision. Bony grafts, direct wires, or plate and screw fixation can then be applied.

Blowout Fractures

Blowout fractures may occur as isolated events involving one or more orbital walls. They may also be associated with more complex fractures (that is, naso-fronto-ethmoid, cranial-vault, supraorbital ridge, zygomatic complex, Le Fort II, or Le Fort III).

A thorough ophthalmologic assessment is mandatory, and urgent treatment of associated ocular trauma must be instituted. An adequate CT scan must include coronal cuts for a complete orbital evaluation to determine whether orbital exploration and repair should be undertaken. Visualization of all four orbital walls on the preoperative CT scan is important to ensure that all blowout or blowin fractures are recognized and treated with appropriate soft-tissue repositioning and bony reconstruction (Messinger 1989). Manson (1986) outlined the mechanism of injury, surgical anatomy, and general indications for surgical intervention in blowout fractures. Because the complications of entrapment, enophthalmus, and diplopia are difficult to treat later, early evaluation, recognition of patients at high risk, and surgical intervention are mandatory.

If left untreated, blow-out fractures heal rapidly in children and result in cicatrization of the herniated contents of the orbital. When indicated, early exploration, repositioning of infraorbital soft-tissue, and reconstruction of orbital walls to appropriate dimensions and volume with autogenous bone is preferred.

Nasal Fractures

The growth of the nasal septum is often considered to be a major factor in development of the midface (Moss 1968, Bergland 1974). In theory, severe trauma to this region in childhood could retard normal growth potential, resulting in a saddle nose deformity and total midface deficiency. However, although the nasal area is the most frequently fractured part of the face in children, extensive retardation of midface growth is rarely documented.

Nasal fractures are often treated inadequately; as a result, late deformity with functional symptoms is seen in a high percentage of patients. Late problems include a deviated pyramid, nasal dorsal hump, and septal deformity with resulting partial nasal obstruction. Perhaps the most common pitfall in treating nasal fractures is the failure to recognize fractures that extend outside the nose (Manson 1988). Adjacent fractures often include the maxilla, orbit, frontal sinus, or frontal bone regions.

Despite surgical manipulation residual malalignment of nasal bones may be masked by edema. Laterally deviated greenstick fractures are the most common fractures found in the pediatric population. If closed reduction is carried out, completion of the fracture by manipulation is mandatory to avoid the problem of incomplete reduction.

A septal hematoma is more likely to arise after nasal trauma in children than in adults. This complication must be looked for, and if it is identified drainage must be instituted to prevent septal necrosis and perforation.

Principles of Mandibular Fracture Repair

The pediatric facial skeleton presents a unique and changing anatomy that resembles that in the adult in some ways but not in others (MacLennan 1957, Khosla 1971, Morgan 1975, Lehman 1976, Moss 1988, Jones 1988). The child's mandible is almost completely filled with teeth in various stages of development; this fact affects mandibular fracture patterns. Trauma of the fracture may injure the developing tooth buds, but overzealous and misdirected open reduction and fixation techniques also may injure the tooth buds.

When internal fixation techniques are required, either direct interosseous wire fixation or plate and screw fixation (miniplates or microplates) must be applied carefully so that drill holes are located at or close to the mandibular inferior border to avoid the developing teeth. If this basic principle is followed, the application of fixation will not cause iatrogenic injury to the teeth.

In general, loose teeth and alveolar fractures should be supported with surgical immobilization until bone union has occurred (4 to 6 weeks) (Gelbier 1967, Andreason & Ravn 1971, Lu 1973). Treating these dentoalveolar fractures with a soft diet alone is rarely adequate. If the involved deciduous teeth are approaching the time of natural exfoliation and are not attached to alveolar bone, extraction, rather than reduction, is the procedure of choice.

The general principles of treating mandibular fractures are the same in children and adults: fixation of the bony fragments in their pre-injury pattern, placement of the teeth in their pre-injury occlusion, and establishment of stabilization until union has occurred. For problems of occlusion, a degree of flexibility exists in the child which is not present in the adult. When the primary dentition exfoliates and the permanent dentition erupts, minor occlusion discrepancies may be self-correcting or at least amenable to orthodontic alignment. This should not be viewed as an excuse for sloppy technique.

As a result of the greatly increased osteogenic potential of the mandible, union is often completed within two to four weeks, with the fragments becoming sticky in as little as three to four days. For these reasons early, definitive treatment is the rule. Specific fracture treatment recommendations vary with the type of fracture (that is, greenstick or complete), the location of the fracture (that is condyle or body), age of the patient, presence of other facial fractures, and presence of other associated systemic injuries.

In addition to efforts to obtain normal occlusion, thought must be given to future impairment of the developing dentition or the temporomandibular joints (TMJ), and the effect on mandibular range of motion.

Condylar Process

The treatment of fractures of the mandibular condylar process remains controversial (Chalmers 1947, Walker 1957, Rowe 1960, Walker 1960, Rakower 1961, Kaplan 1962, Thomson 1964, Anderson 1965, MacLennan 1965, Boyne 1967, Coccaro 1969, Gilhuus-Moe 1969, Leake 1971, Campbell 1975, Schettler 1975, Winstanley 1978, Proffitt 1980, Zide 1989). Although most authors advocate a conservative approach, a few prefer more aggressive open reduction techniques (Zide 1989, 1983).

The condylar head is an important growth center of the mandible, which is the last facial bone to complete its growth and development. Usually mandibular growth is complete in girls by age 14 to 16 and in boys by age 16 to 18. Injury to the condylar head before these ages may lead to growth retardation, which leads to facial asymmetry and malocclusion.

It is likely that the condylar growth center does not maintain a constant low level of activity but rather yields high growth rates at very specific intervals (Schultz 1988). From birth to age 12, the face undergoes continual growth, but the velocity of that growth varies with age. Up to six months of age, facial growth is very rapid, whereas from six months to 4 years it is relatively slow. Rapid growth returns between ages 4 and 7, and then slower growth is seen between ages 9 and 15. The last facial growth phase, between ages 15 and 19, primarily affects the mandible. It is likely that condylar injury (fracture or compression) before age 3 will result in significant mandibular growth distortion, whereas such injury after age 12 will have little overall effect on growth. Between these age ranges, a wide spectrum is seen (Schultz 1988).

It is important to recognize that secondary growth distortion may arise once the mandible is affected. This is most commonly seen in the maxilla, with canting of the occlusal plane and shifting of the maxillary dental midline off the facial midline. Growth distortions may be seen in the nasal septum, nasal bones, zygoma, and even the orbit.

When considering condylar fractures and their treatment, it is important to recognize that not all condylar fractures are the same. They may be either intracapsular or extracapsular, displaced or nondisplaced, of the medial or lateral pole, open or closed, or of the low condylar neck or high condylar neck. When a complete fracture of the condylar process occurs, the fracture segment is generally dislocated anteriorly and medially. Dislocation of the fractured segment is the direct result of muscle spasm of the lateral pterygoid muscle, which originates on the lateral pterygoid plate and inserts on the condylar head.

With dislocation of the condylar fragment, there is a loss of posterior facial height on the affected side, causing premature contact of the posterior teeth on the fracture side. With wide vertical opening or protrusive excursion, the mandible shifts to the side of the fracture.

On radiographic examination the fracture fragment may be visualized in its displaced location. The surgeon, who naturally wants to restore anatomy and function, is therefore tempted to suggest ORIF on a regular basis. However, the treatment options for fractures of the condylar process will vary depending on the location of the condylar fracture. For example, it is not possible to perform an ORIF on an intracapsular medial pole fracture of the condylar head. Similarly, because visualization and dissection are difficult, high condylar neck fractures are poor candidates for ORIF. Low condylar neck fractures (extending into the ramus) may be suitable for ORIF, but unfortunately they make up only a small proportion of condylar fractures. Overzealous attempts at surgical exploration with combined preauricular-coronal, submandibular, and intraoral incisions for condylar exposure, fracture reduction, and fixation often result in incomplete fracture reduction, devascularization of the condylar head, and injury to branches of the facial nerve. Furthermore, it has not been clearly demonstrated that a lower incidence of growth disturbance, TMJ ankylosis, or malocclusion can be achieved through open reduction techniques when they are compared to more conservative treatment measures.

I use the following indications for exploration of condyle fractures: (1) lateral displacement of the proximal fracture segment, (2) presence of a foreign body in the joint capsule, (3) fracture with dislocation into the middle cranial fossa and clinical disability, (4) inability to open or close the mouth because of the mechanical blockage of the fractured segments, and (5) a low condylar neck (ramus) fracture with displacement and dislocation.

In addition to these indications for exploration of condyle fractures, if ORIF is to follow, the assumptions are that the fracture is extracapsular, its location is low in the condylar neck, the condylar head is not split (bipolar fracture), functional disability would be likely without ORIF, and an ORIF technique would be likely to limit functional disability. Bilateral condylar fractures with or without midface fractures are not in themselves indications for ORIF unless the above indications are met. If the conservative approach is selected for condylar fracture treatment maxillo-mandibular (MMF) may be useful for the patient's comfort, encouraging soft-tissue healing, relieving muscle spasm, and limiting the conversion of greenstick or a minimally displaced fracture into a complete or fully displaced one. Approximately two weeks of MMF is enough time to accomplish these goals and yet allow early controlled range of motion to limit the likelihood of developing TMJ ankylosis.

When a condyle fracture is present and there is a need to limit MMF, the fixation technique for additional fractures must be carefully selected. For example, if parasymphyseal and condylar fractures have occurred, a more stable form of internal fixation may be selected for the parasymphyseal fracture so that MMF can be released early, as would be preferred for the condylar fracture.

The importance of looking for a condylar fracture in the growing patient who has sustained facial trauma cannot be overstated (Thomson 1964). Not only can TMJ ankylosis occur as an early complication but also long-term follow-up will be required by the surgeon and orthodontist to monitor growth and development. Later, some patients will require a combined orthodontic and surgical approach (that is, Le Fort I osteotomy, bilateral sagittal split osteotomies of the mandible, and genioplasty) to restore facial contour and occlusion. Whether orthodontic activators or functional appliances have a role to play in the management of condylar fractures after injury remains controversial (Harvold 1975).

Body Fractures

Body fractures of the mandible usually have favorable muscle force, so closed reduction with MMF will suffice (two to four weeks in children). In the very young or in situations of simple greenstick or nondisplaced fractures, a soft diet alone may provide adequate treatment. Mini- or microplate and screw fixation may be selected if MMF is to be avoided.

Parasymphyseal and Symphyseal Fractures

Even with closed reduction and MMF techniques, the muscle forces on parasymphyseal fractures tend to displace the fracture during the healing process. Often a small dental gap (step-off) arises between the two teeth adjacent to the fracture site. In the primary or early mixed dentition, this gap should not cause significant long-term problems. If a parasymphyseal fracture is associated with other facial fractures, such as a condylar fracture, a more stable form of fixation (plate and screw fixation) may be advisable to allow for early mobility of the condylar fracture and to limit problems of TMJ ankylosis.

Dental Alveolar Fractures

Anterior teeth usually bear the brunt of accidental injury; however, alveolar supporting structures are frequently involved (Gelbier 1967, Andreason 1971, Lu 1973). Individual teeth may be luxated, partially or totally avulsed, or impacted.

Minor luxations that are easily returned to a stable position may not require splinting. Teeth that have been significantly loosened should be returned to their normal position in the alveolar arch and stabilized as soon as possible. Severely luxated teeth associated with alveolar fractures can be difficult to return to a stable anatomic position after hematoma formation. Controlled digital force is required to accomplish reduction.

Reimplantation of avulsed teeth is generally regarded as a temporary measure, but it may prove useful. The tooth usually reattaches, although it may be lost after 5 or 10 years because of late root resorption or ankylosis.

Methods of stabilizing dentoalveolar fractures involve acrylic splints, wires, and arch bars. The newer acid-etch technique is now becoming popular. Plate and screw fixation has little or no role in the management of dentoalveolar fractures. Regardless of the stabilization technique selected, the splint must meet specific criteria, which include being easily fabricated, maintaining only passive force on the teeth, not irritating the soft tissues, allowing normal occlusion to be maintained, permitting good oral hygiene, allowing access for subsequent endodontic treatment, and being easily removable.

Maxillo-Mandibular Fixation in the Pediatric Patient

There are many misconceptions about the possibility of performing MMF in pediatric patients (see Figure 32.2). The newborn is edentulous, and the first

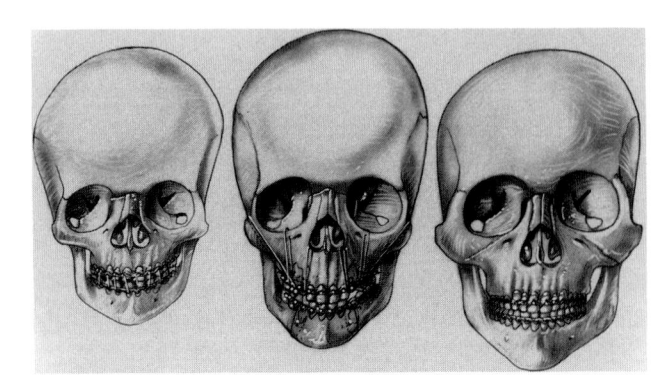

Figure 32.2 Three skulls of various ages (2 years, 6 years [mixed dentition], and 12 years, [adult dentition]) are shown. Different methods of direct wire fixation are demonstrated. These include arch bars and MMF, and circomandibular, circumzygomatic, infraorbital, and piriform sinus skeletal fixation.

primary teeth erupt by six months of age. By about age two, the primary dentition is complete, with 5 teeth in each quadrant (20 total). The primary dentition provides a stable foundation for MMF if it is healthy and complete and there are no severe or multiple carious lesions or root resorption resulting from the underlying developing permanent tooth buds. When the patient has a full complement of deciduous teeth (at age two), MMF is accomplished with standard arch bars and circumdental wires; all 20 teeth can be used as needed.

The stability provided by the primary dentition begins to wane by age 5½ to 6, when the development of permanent tooth buds gradually leads to resorption of their overlying primary teeth. This process continues until age 12, when the permanent dentition is complete (except for the third molars). Consequently, the application of MMF can present special problems between ages 5½ and 12 (mixed dentition phase), but only rarely is MMF impossible. Elaborate cast cap splints are not needed. Skeletal fixation wires—for example, circummandibular or circozygomatic—and wires at the infraorbital rim, anterior nasal spine, or piriform aperture can be used easily to give the extra support required for arch bar stabilization and the application of MMF.

CASE REPORTS

Case 1

An 11-year-old boy sustained multiple facial trauma when the all-terrain vehicle in which he was riding overturned. His injuries included a left intracapsular condyle fracture, a right low condylar neck fracture, a right parasymphyseal fracture of the mandible, dentoalveolar injuries, and multiple facial lacerations (see Figure 32.3).

Erich arch bars were applied under general anesthesia to stabilize his dentoalveolar fractures. His jaws

Pediatric Facial Fractures

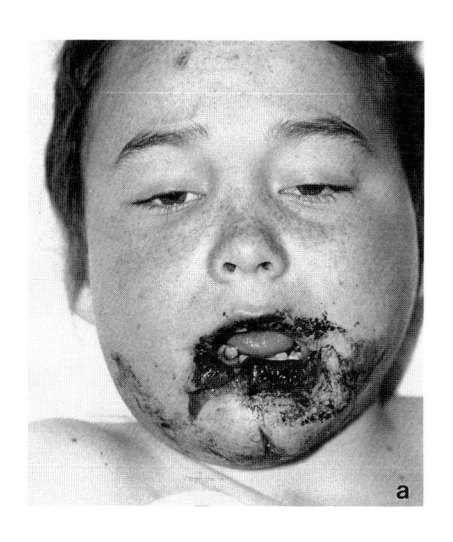

Figure 32.3 This 11-year-old boy sustained multiple facial trauma, including a left intracapsular condyle fracture, a right condylar neck fracture, a right parasymphyseal fracture of the mandible, dentoalveolar injuries, and multiple facial lacerations. (a) Frontal view of face before fracture reduction. (b) This CT scan demonstrates the left intracapsular condyle fracture and right condylar neck fracture. (c) This CT scan demonstrates the displaced right parasymphyseal fracture. (d) Intraoral view shows the displaced right parasymphyseal fracture of the mandible. (e) Intraoral view shows the reduced right parasymphyseal fracture of the mandible, fixation with titanium bone miniplate and screws, and MMF. (f) Intraoperative view shows the ORIF right condyle fracture of the mandible through the submandibular incision. Fixation was done with a titanium miniplate and screws. (g) Six months later, 40 millimeters of vertical opening is shown. (h) Oblique view of face six months after injury. (i) Occlusal view six months after injury. (j) Postoperative panorex demonstrates good reduction of fractures.

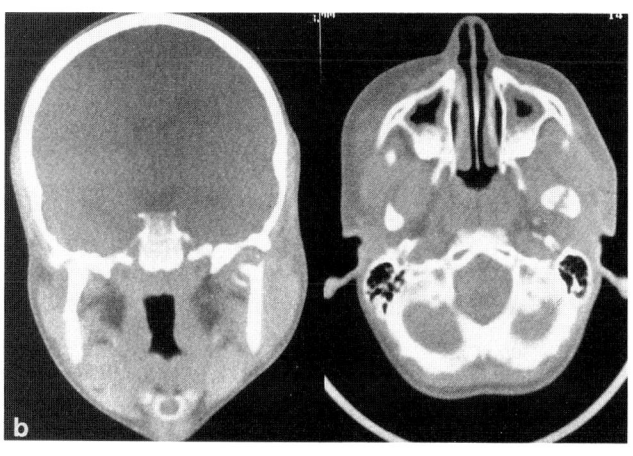

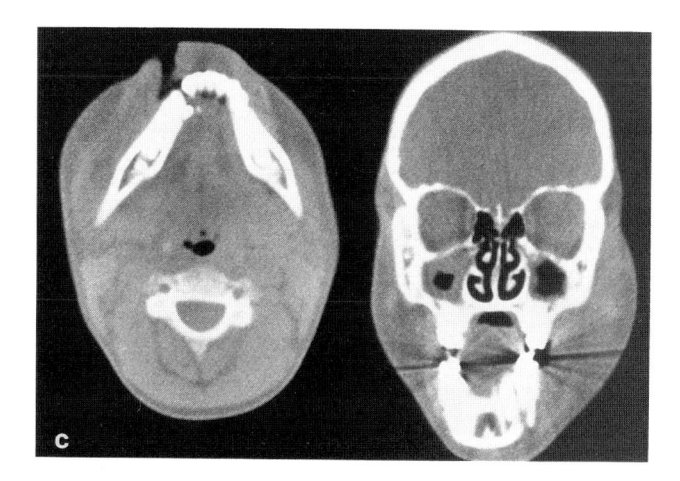

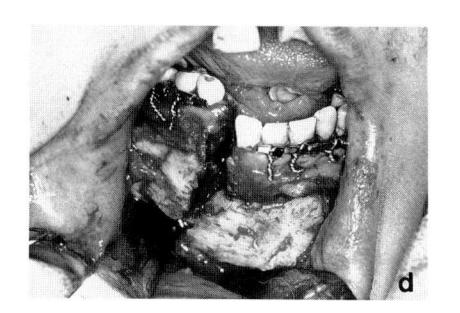

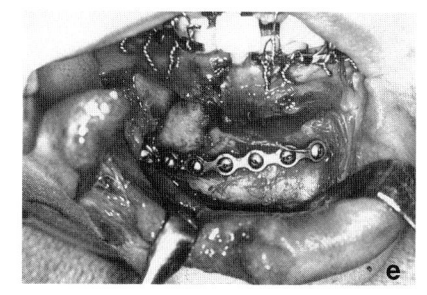

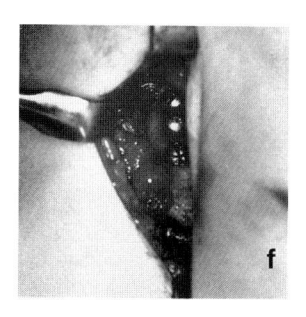

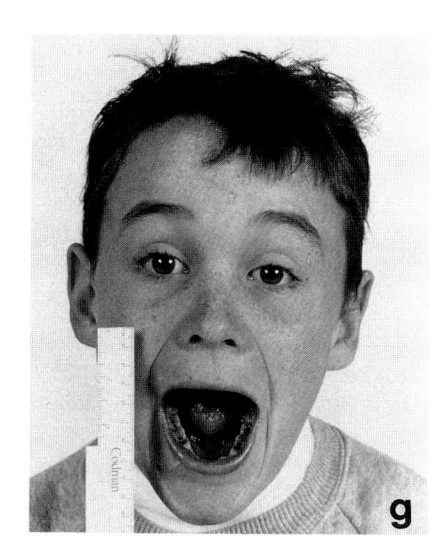

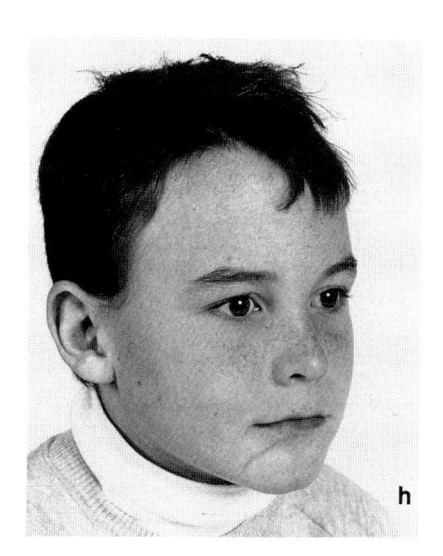

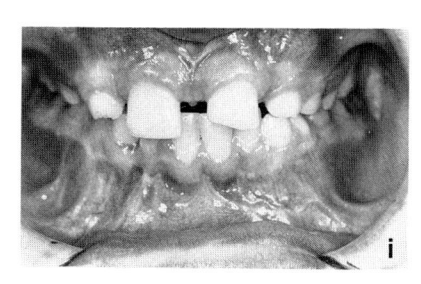

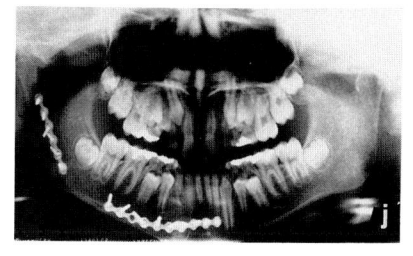

were then wired together in their pre-injury occlusion. He underwent ORIF of the right parasymphyseal fracture of the mandible with application of a miniplate at the inferior border of the mandible through an intraoral vestibular incision. The low condylar neck fracture was also treated with ORIF by means of a miniplate placed through a small submandibular incision. The jaws were wired together; the wires remained in placed for one week.

One week after surgery, progressive physiotherapy was instituted. This patient has maintained a good range of motion without evidence of ankylosis or major occlusal discrepancies.

Critique

When plate and screw fixation is used, care must be taken to regain the pre-injury dental relationship on each arch first, before MMF is applied, so that the upper and lower teeth occlude in their pre-injury position. Only then can the exposed mandibular and maxillary fractures be further reduced and stabilized.

In general, the degree of fixation required to achieve stability in the growing mandible is less than that in the adult. When plate and screw fixation is used, miniplates with bicortical screw placement are usually adequate. These are combined with an arch bar secured as a tension band across the tooth-bearing fracture site. The heavier fracture plates or mandibular reconstructive plates are not required and would only add unnecessary bulk while increasing the risk of injury to developing tooth buds. Depending on the patient's age and extent of fractures, microplates and screws may give adequate stability. When internal fixation is used in the developing mandible, drill holes and screw placement must be close to the inferior border to prevent injury to the tooth buds and to allow plate fixation in the thickest portion of the mandible.

I generally prefer a noninvasive approach to the management of condyle fractures of the mandible. A short period of MMF usually relieves muscle spasm and allows time for soft tissue to heal. Early progressive range of motion is instituted to limit possible ankylosis problems. Elastics may be used to encourage an even bite and to re-educate the centric occlusion, thereby limiting any centric relation and centric occlusion discrepancy.

In this case, the patient's right condylar neck fracture was low and was essentially located in the ramus region of the mandible. It was therefore amenable to open reduction with miniplate internal fixation. His left condyle fracture was intracapsular and therefore not in a location that is surgically approachable. Through the use of stable fixation techniques for both the right condyle and right parasymphyseal fractures, it was possible to mobilize him early without concern for right condylar dislocation or parasymphyseal fracture malunion.

He regained early function and has maintained a good vertical range of motion.

Because growth disturbance may result, careful follow-up by the surgeon and orthodontist is required.

Case 2

A three-year-old boy sustained multiple traumas in a motor-vehicle accident. These included cerebral concussion, facial fractures, and an open femur fracture (see Figure 32.4). His Glasgow coma index was only 5. In the emergency room, a nasotracheal tube was positioned for airway protection. A Richmond screw was placed to monitor his fluctuating intracranial pressure. His open femur fracture was managed on the second day after the injury, but his facial fractures were not treated initially.

He sustained a greenstick fracture in the left angle of the mandible and a badly displaced fracture of the right angle of the mandible which was open into the mouth and markedly mobile. By the tenth day after the injury, his brain injury had stabilized to the point where he could be taken back into the operating room for management of his mandibular fractures. To avoid a tracheostomy, it was necessary to limit MMF because pulmonary toilet was a problem in this partially comatose child.

Erich arch bars were placed on the upper and lower jaws to stabilize multiple dentoalveolar injuries. The boy's jaws were then wired together in their pre-injury occlusion, which was in fact an open-bite deformity produced by thumb sucking. A submandibular incision was made to expose the mobile angle of the mandible fracture. The fracture was reduced, and a titanium miniplate and screws were placed at the inferior border for stable internal fixation. His jaws were unwired, and the occlusion was checked and found to be even. Because it was not necessary to wire his jaws together, a tracheostomy was avoided.

Two days later he was extubated and then transferred from the intensive care unit to the ward, where he recovered over the next several weeks. Although some residual brain damage remained, he was discharged in the care of his parents.

Critique

Taken in isolation, this mandibular injury could have been managed with a direct intraosseous wire at the fracture site and MMF. However, with the multiple-systems trauma, including cerebral injury and the need for pulmonary toilet, the use of stable fixation was necessary to allow for postoperative airway management and to avoid the need for tracheostomy.

When a bone miniplate is used in this situation, it must be placed as close to the inferior border as possible to avoid injury to the tooth buds. With care and caution

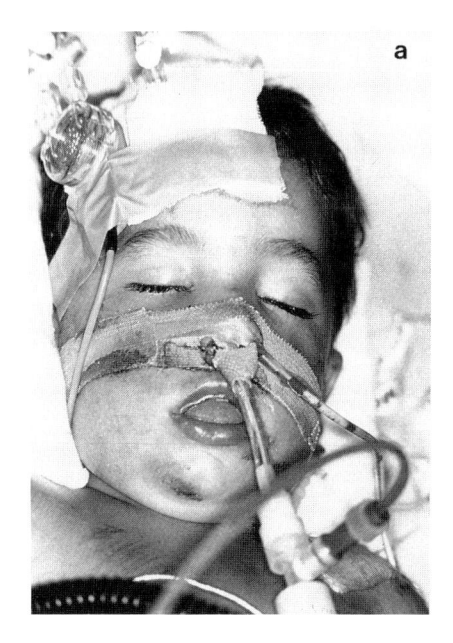

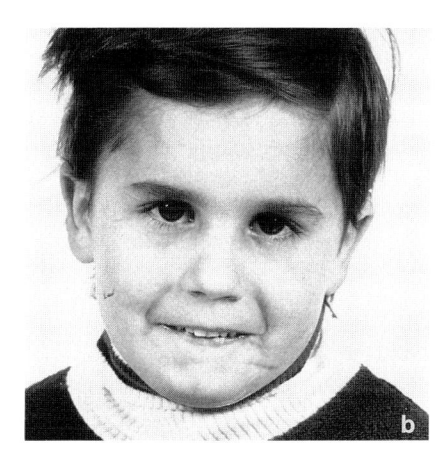

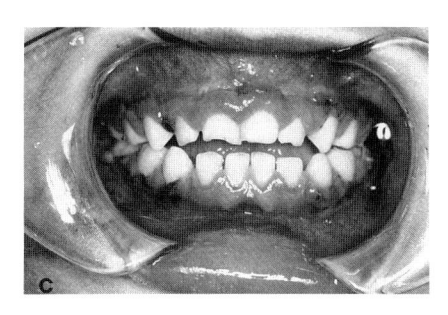

Figure 32.4 This three-year-old boy sustained multiple traumas in a motor-vehicle accident, including cerebral concussion; an open femur fracture; and facial fractures, including a greenstick fracture of the left angle of the mandible and a displaced fracture of the right angle of the mandible. (a) The patient has a nasotracheal tube with a Richmond screw for monitoring intracranial pressure before facial fracture reduction. (b) Frontal view six months after fracture repair. (c) Occlusal view six months after repair. His pre-injury occlusion, an anterior open-bite deformity due to thumbsucking, remains. (d) CT scan demonstrates the greenstick fracture of the left angle of the mandible and the displaced fracture of the right angle of the mandible. (e) Postoperative plain radiographs demonstrate miniplate and screw fixation of the right angle of the mandible.

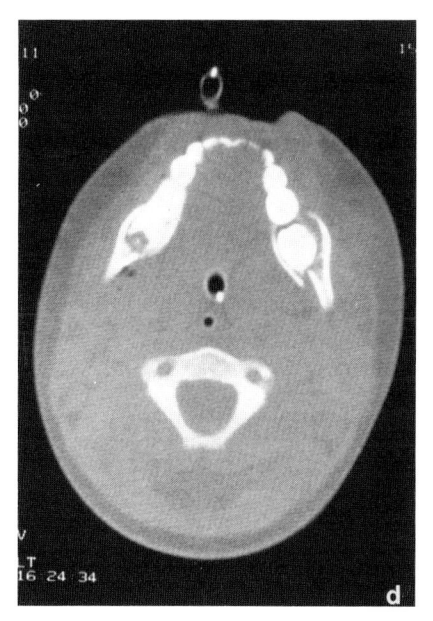

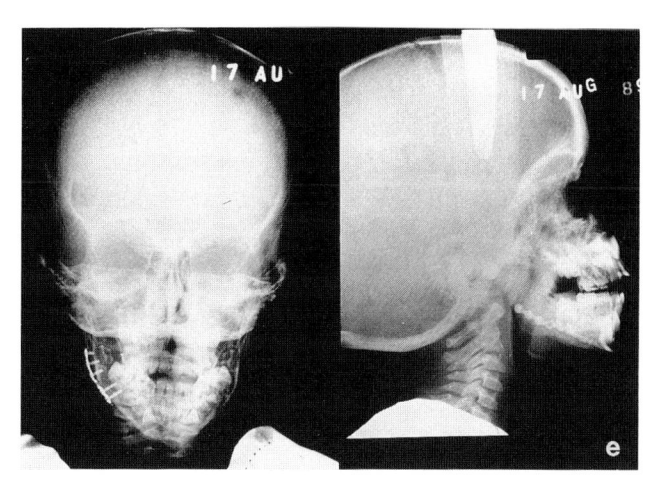

this complication can be avoided. I have not found it necessary to use compression plates or heavier reconstructive or fracture plates for this type of fracture in this age group. Whether bone plates placed on the mandible at such an early age should be removed after bone healing to prevent growth distortions is open to question. The potential for a degree of growth retardation arising from the injury itself may preclude our answering this question.

Case 3

An eight-year-old boy sustained multiple trauma in a motor vehicle accident. These included multiple facial fractures, lower extremity fracture, and soft-tissue loss over the dorsum of the foot (see Figure 32.5).

He was intubated in the emergency room and after radiographic evaluation was taken to the operating room for simultaneous management of his lower extremity injuries and facial fractures. Radiographs revealed a bilateral parasymphyseal fracture with a free-floating symphyseal unit. He had severe maxillary and mandibular dentoalveolar trauma, including loss of his four maxillary incisors and mandibular right canine tooth. A left intracapsular condylar fracture of the mandible was also present.

Erich arch bars were placed to stabilize his salvageable teeth and alveolar fractures, and MMF was established in his pre-injury occlusion. Access was gained to the inferior border of his mandible through his open-chin laceration. After the comminuted bilateral parasymphyseal fracture was reduced, a long miniplate was

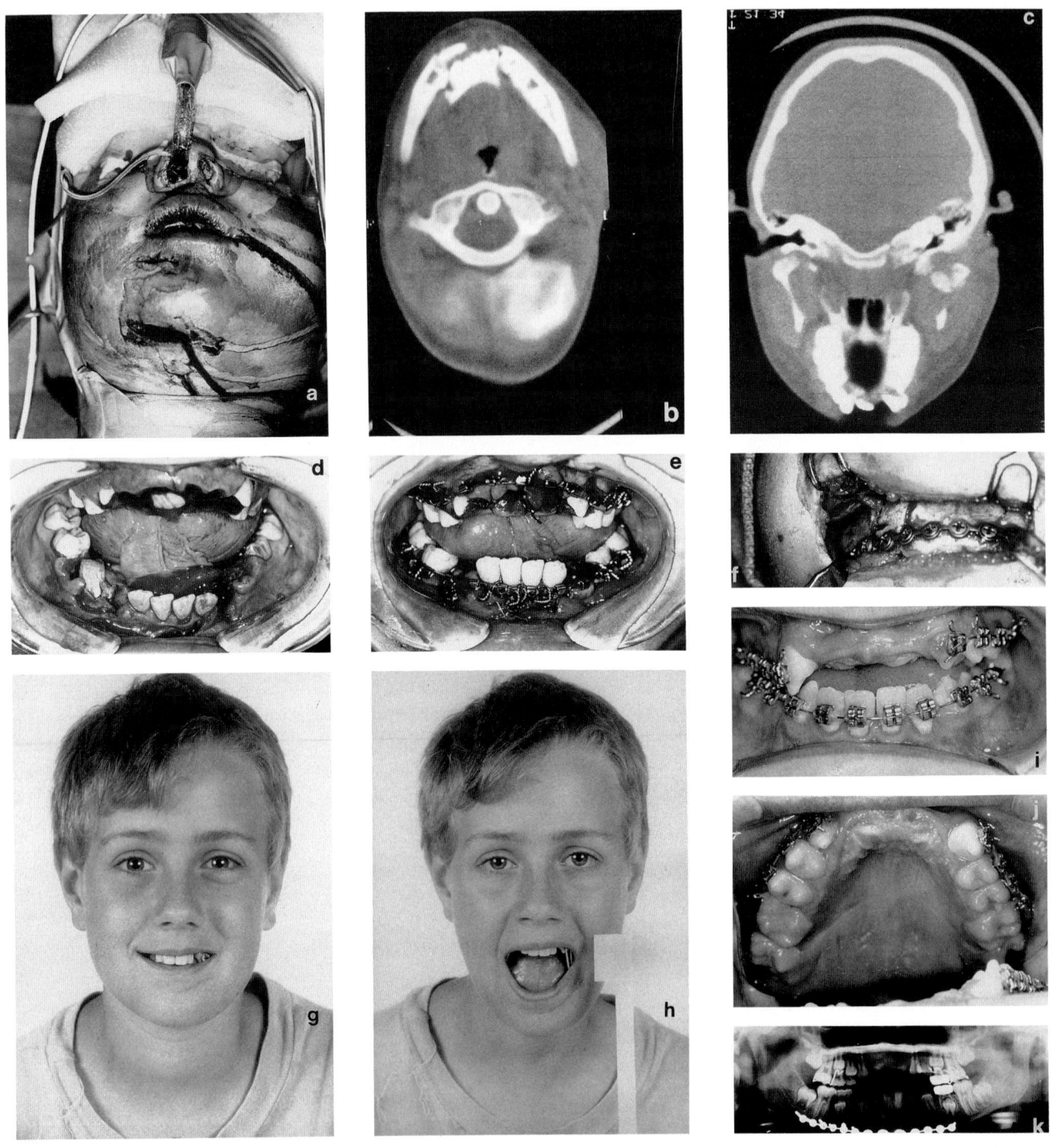

Figure 32.5 This eight-year-old boy has two fractures of the lower extremity and soft-tissue loss over the dorsum of the foot, resulting from a motor-vehicle accident. Facial fractures include maxillary and mandibular dentoalveolar injuries, and bilateral comminuted parasymphyseal and left intracapsular condyle fractures of the mandible. (a) The patient has a nasotracheal tube with central venous line in the neck. At this time, he was taken directly to the operating room. (b) CT scan demonstrates free-floating symphysis of the mandible. (c) CT scan demonstrates displaced intracapsular condyle fracture of the left mandible. (d) Intraoperative occlusal view, before fracture reduction. (e) Intraoperative occlusal view, after reduction of dentoalveolar fractures. (f) Intraoperative view through chin laceration shows reduced comminuted parasymphyseal fractures of the mandible. A long miniplate with screw fixation is in place. (g) Frontal view three years after repair shows maxillary partial denture in place. (h) Frontal view three years after repair demonstrates normal vertical opening. Orthodontic braces are in place. (i) Occlusal view three years after repair. (j) Palateal view three years after repair shows maxillary partial denture in place. (k) Panorex one year after repair demonstrates the long miniplate along the inferior border of the mandible.

placed at the inferior border to stabilize his mandible. All lacerations were closed. MMF was released, and his occlusion was checked and found to be satisfactory. The fractures were stable. He was taken to the intensive care unit with the jaws unwired. He was extubated the following day. He had to return to the operating room for dressing changes of his lower extremity until a skin graft was placed. His facial fractures healed uneventfully, and he has maintained a good vertical opening. Because he lost his four incisor teeth, he now has a partial denture in the maxilla. Orthodontic treatment and fixed prosthetic dental rehabitation within endosseal implants is planned for the future.

He is being followed at intervals by his surgeon, orthodontist, and prosthodontist: Further surgical intervention may be required because of limited jaw growth.

Critique

The use of plate and screw fixation in a situation like this not only ensures adequate reduction of the mandibular fractures but also limits the incidence of postoperative infection and TMJ ankylosis. In the multiple-trauma patient who will be bedridden for a time, it also ensures easier management of the airway and improves oral caloric intake. With his need to return to the operating room for multiple-dressing changes over several weeks, the only alternative to plate and screw stable fixation of his facial fractures would have been MMF and then a tracheostomy.

Case 4

A five-year-old girl had sustained bilateral intracapsular condyle fractures of the mandible when she fell down a flight of stairs 1 year before she was seen at HSC (see Figure 32.6). These fractures were not recognized or treated until her arrival six months after initial surgery. She was unable to open her mouth more than 2 millimeters. A CT scan confirmed the presence of bilateral ankylosis of the condyles to the zygomatic arches and glenoid fossa.

Two costochondral rib grafts were harvested from the right chest. Coronal and bilateral Risdon neck incisions were made. The ankylosis was identified through the coronal incision. With both an oscillating saw and a reciprocating saw, the bony ankylosed condylar heads were excised, and the glenoid fossa was carefully cleaned out with a rotary drill. Range of motion of the mandible improved immediately to 35 millimeters. The occlusion was then re-established with Erich arch bars and MMF.

The harvested costochondral rib grafts were inset and secured to the residual ascending rami of the mandible with bone miniplates and screws. Intraoperatively the MMF was released and the occlusion was checked. After soft-tissue healing, the jaws were unwired at two weeks; an immediate vertical opening of 35 millimeters was obtained. The girl remained on a wired jaw diet for six weeks, but range of motion was encouraged. Now, one year later, she has maintained a good vertical opening.

Critique

Ankylosis of the TMJ is a severe complication of a condyle fracture. Fortunately, it is not seen frequently, although its true incidence is not known. Once bony ankylosis has occurred, one cannot expect spontaneous improvement and a conservative approach will not solve the problem. It is necessary to remove the ankylosed bone and then reconstruct the joint. Costochondral bone grafts are probably the best choice at present. The use of plate and screw fixation for stabilization of these grafts has greatly improved the outlook of TMJ ankylosis management. If an attempt is made to achieve stable fixation of the rib graft with bicortical or lag screws alone, the graft is likely to splinter, preventing adequate stabilization. If a titanium miniplate is used over the bone, the compression forces are spread out and the splintering problem is minimized. The use of a heavier reconstructive plate is not needed in this age group.

These innovations in graft fixation overcome the need to wire the jaws together for an extended period. Early range-of-motion exercises can be initiated, and the incidence of postoperative infection and recurrence of ankylosis should be diminished.

Further growth disturbance with an asymmetric mandibular retrognathism must be anticipated when joint reconstruction is required in this age group. Long-term follow-up with both the surgeon and the orthodontist is therefore mandatory.

Case 5

This 14-year-old boy was accidentally kicked directly in the face during a high school soccer game. He sustained combined Le Fort I and II fractures with bilateral orbital floor blowout fractures resulting in an anterior open-bite deformity and diplopia (see Figure 32.7).

When he was taken to surgery, Erich arch bars were placed on the upper and lower jaws. Maxillary circumvestibular, intraoral, and bilateral lower-eyelid incisions were made to expose the fractures. Tessier disimpaction forceps were placed, and the Le Fort I and II fractures were reduced. MMF was then applied to achieve his pre-injury occlusion. Bone miniplates were placed vertically through the intraoral incisions at each zygomatic buttress and each piriform aperture, and horizontally at each infraorbital rim through the lower eyelid incisions. When MMF was released intraoperatively and the occlusion was found to be stable, the herniated intraorbital contents were repositioned from the max-

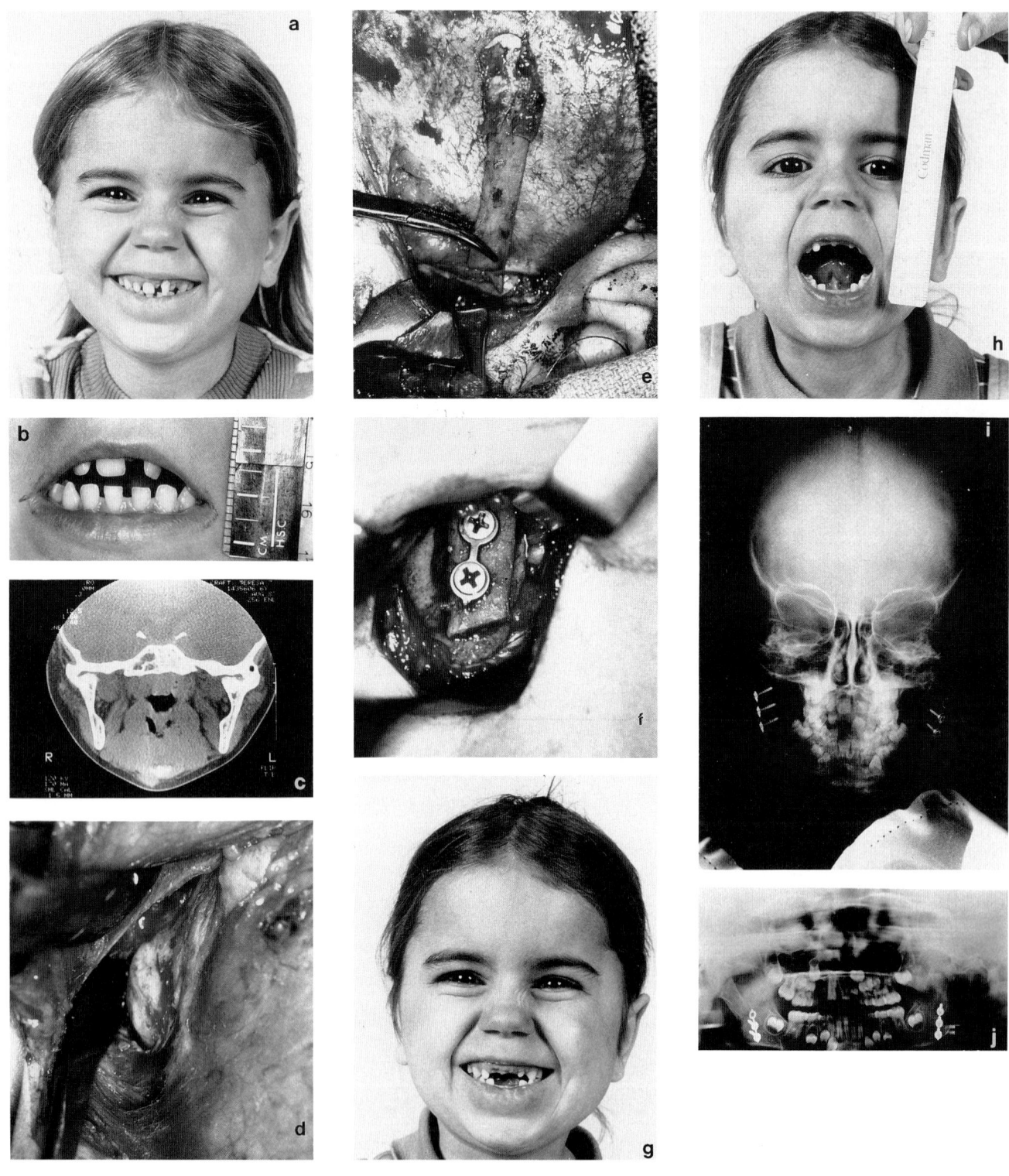

Figure 32.6 This five-year-old girl has bilateral intracapsular condyle fractures of the mandible, resulting in bilateral TMJ ankylosis. (a) Frontal view before ankylosis release. (b) Maximum vertical opening of 2 millimeters. (c) Coronal CT scan demonstrates bilateral bony fusion of the condyles to the zygomatic arches and glenoid fossa. (d) Intraoperative close-up of the condylar head fused to the zygomatic arch is seen through the coronal incision. (e) Costochondral rib graft is inset through the coronal incision to reconstruct the ascending ramus and condylar head. (f) Intraoperative view through the Risdon incision demonstrates the costochondral graft fixed to the mandible with miniplate and screws. (g) Frontal view one year after reconstruction shows stable occlusion. (h) Frontal view demonstrates adequate vertical opening. (i) Plain radiograph one year after reconstruction demonstrates plate and screw fixation. (j) Panorex one year after reconstruction demonstrates costochondral rib grafts with miniplate fixation.

Pediatric Facial Fractures

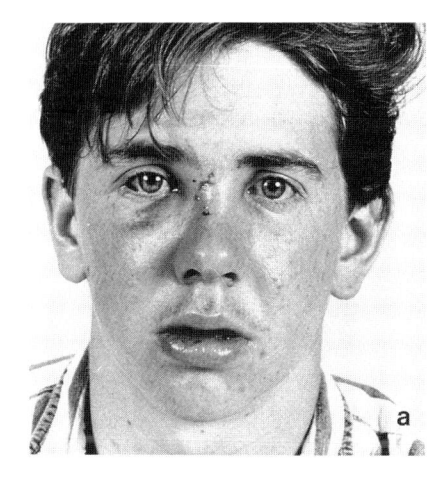

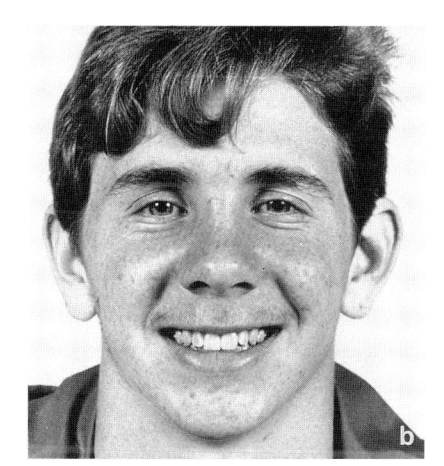

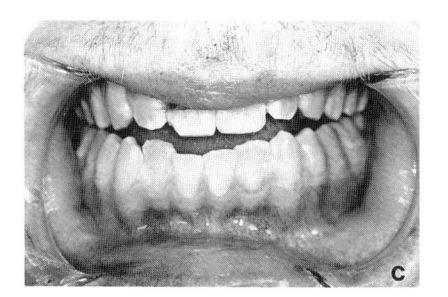

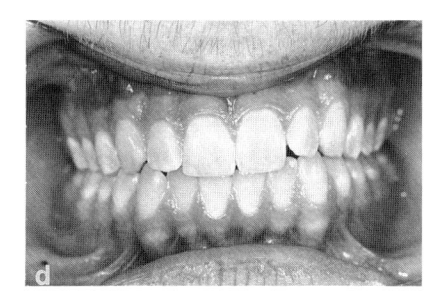

Figure 32.7 This 14-year-old boy sustained combined Le Fort I and II fractures with bilateral orbital floor blowout fractures when he was kicked in the face. (a) Frontal view before repair. (b) Frontal view six months after repair. (c) Occlusal view before repair. (d) Occlusal view six months after repair. (e) CT scan demonstrates nasofrontal bone separation and comminuted medial orbital walls. (f) CT scan demonstrates fractures through anterior and posterior maxillary walls. (g) Three-dimensional CT scan reformations demonstrate Le Fort II fracture with frontonasal separation, and locations of the infraorbital rim and maxillary fractures. (h) Postoperative CT scan shows reduction of the midface fractures. (i) Postoperative plain radiographs demonstrate the location of miniplate and screw fixation.

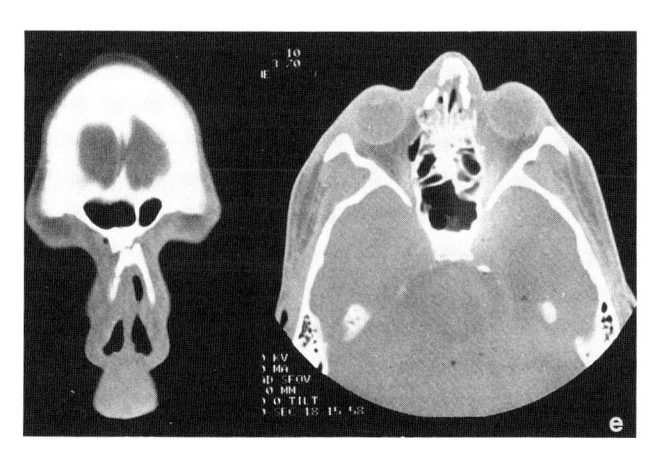

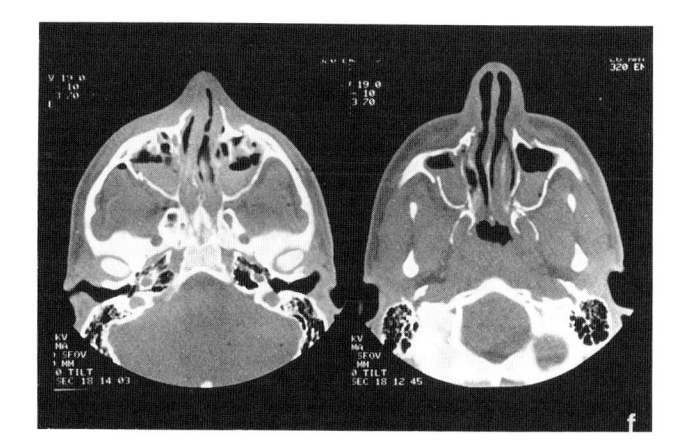

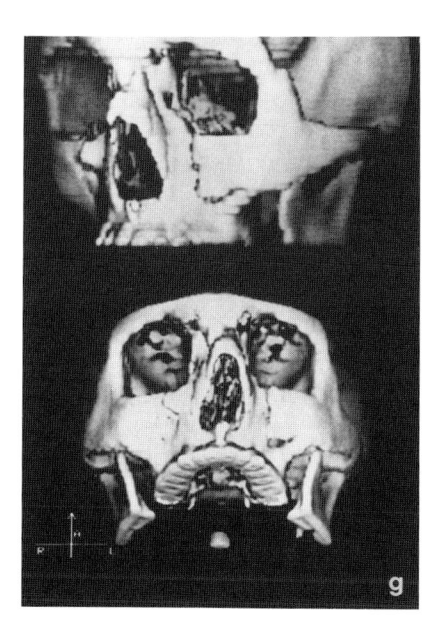

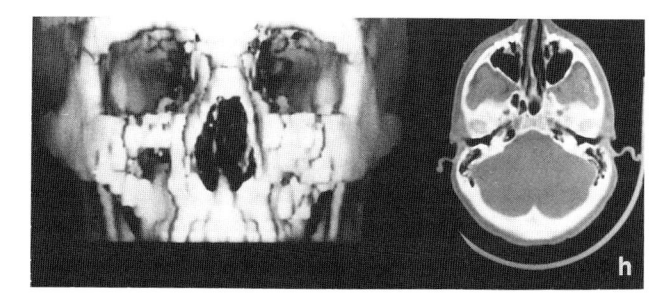

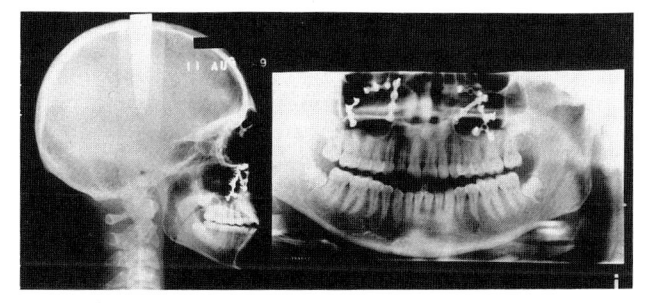

illary sinus into the orbits and autogenous split cranial bone grafts were placed to re-establish orbital volume. He was maintained on a mechanical soft diet with limited physical activity for six weeks.

Critique

The need for complete reduction and then immobilization of this fracture is not disputed. The fact that miniplate and screw fixation can be used effectively with early return of function, as in this case, demonstrates the benefits of this fixation technique even in children and young adults.

After arch bars are placed, along with reduction of any associated dentoalveolar fractures, soft-tissue dissection for exposure of all fractures is completed. Fracture disimpaction and reduction is then accomplished, and the pre-injury occlusion is established and maintained with MMF.

If major bony gaps are present at the vertical pillars (zygomatic buttresses or puriform apertures) and cannot be managed with bone plates alone, then autogenous bone grafts are used. In this case, bone miniplates were placed for stabilization across the zygomatic buttresses, piriform apertures, and infraorbital rims, and autogenous bone grafts were used for the orbital floor blowouts. The orbital floor bone graft is simply placed on the existing circumferential bony shelf. The inset bone graft may then be fixed with a microplate or left to rest in the subperiosteal pocket. Bone microplates probably would have provided adequate stability for fracture fixation at the infraorbital rims without the postoperative difficulty of palpable bone plates being left below the thin-skinned lower eyelids. Although lower-eyelid incisions were used for exposure of the orbital floor, subciliary or subconjunctival incisions probably would have sufficed and would have been cosmetically more acceptable.

Case 6

A seven-year-old boy sustained a naso-fronto-ethmoid fracture in an airplane crash when his forehead and nasal bridge hit the plane's dashboard (see Figure 32.8). This resulted in gross orbital hypertelorism, or increased width between the medial orbital walls. The midfrontal bone was depressed and the nasal bones were crushed, causing a saddle nose deformity. The supraorbital ridge on the left side was also badly comminuted and displaced with a blowin fracture of the orbital roof. The posterior frontal sinus walls were intact. His facial lacerations were sutured, he was stabilized systemically, and then he was transferred to HSC for definitive craniofacial fracture treatment.

At operation, he underwent a coronal incision for exposure of all fractures. The fractures were first reduced and then fixed stably with the application of miniplates and screws across the frontal, orbital, and nasal bone regions. The medial canthi were believed to be adequately repositioned on their bony fragments, which were also reduced and fixed.

His recovery was uneventful, and he was discharged on the fifth postoperative day in the care of his parents. Later a CT scan revealed good reconstitution of the nasal, frontal, and orbital bones. His vision has remained normal. His facial growth has remained on schedule.

Critique

The best time to reconstruct a telescoping nasofronto-ethmoid fracture, for both children and adults, is at the time of injury, before malunion formation. Once a malunion, with its crush orbital hypertelorism deformity, has formed in this region, it is virtually impossible to re-establish a normal nasal and orbital form.

The exposure provided through a coronal incision is almost always required to manage this injury adequately. In this case, we initially attempted to visualize the anatomy by way of the exposure provided by traumatic lacerations through the region around the left eyebrow. However, poor visualization prevented the exposure of all fractures out to normal anatomy. Rather than extending the lacerations into an open-sky-type incision, the coronal incision was selected.

At operation, time was wasted attempting to piece together the multiple eggshell-fractured naso-fronto-ethmoid components, which recollapsed before our eyes because of the poor stabilization afforded by direct wires alone. When two miniplates were placed over the nasofrontal region, the fractured components easily remained in their proper anteroposterior dimension.

This child's fractures healed well and are in good anatomic position. Since the soft-tissue swelling resolved, the miniplates have been palpable, although they are not visible; and this may present a problem if the boy eventually requires spectacles. Our current preference is to use micro bone plates because they provide adequate strength while limiting bulk.

Figure 32.8 This seven-year-old boy sustained a naso-fronto-ethmoid fracture in an airplane crash. The supraorbital ridge on the left was comminuted and displaced with a blowin fracture of the orbital roof. (a) Frontal view before fracture reduction. (b) Frontal view six months after fracture reduction. (c) Oblique view before fracture reduction. (d) Oblique view six months after fracture reduction. (e) This CT scan shows the collapsed naso-fronto-ethmoid and left supraorbital ridge regions before fracture reduction. (f) This three-dimensional CT scan shows the fractures before and after reduction and fixation. (g) This three-dimensional CT scan shows the fractures before and after reduction and fixation. (h) Two-dimensional axial CT scan through midorbits shows the fractures before and after reduction and fixation. The medial orbital rim displacement has been corrected.

Pediatric Facial Fractures

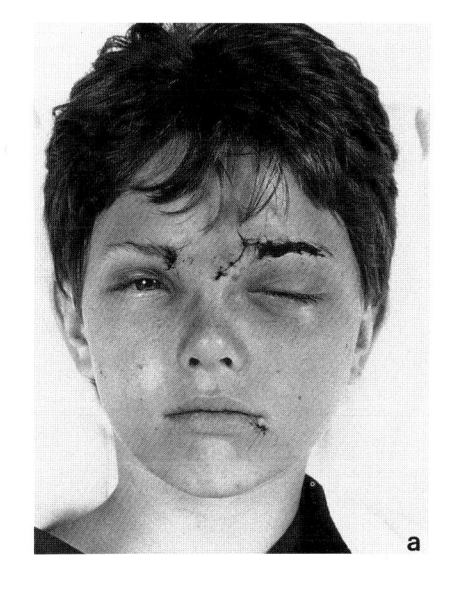

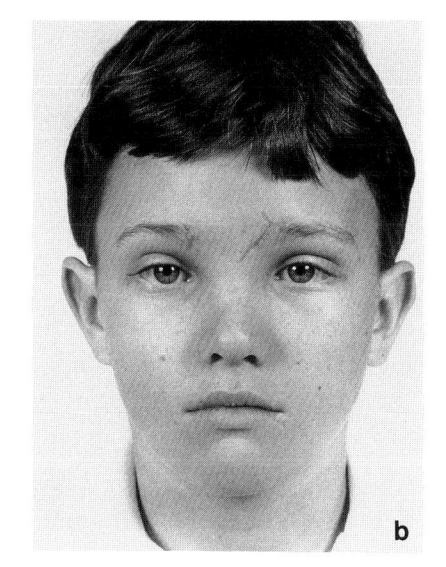

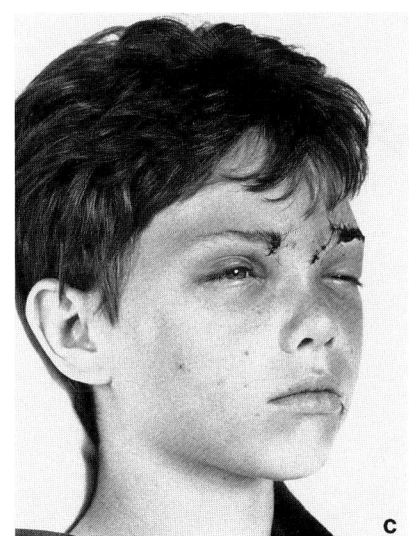

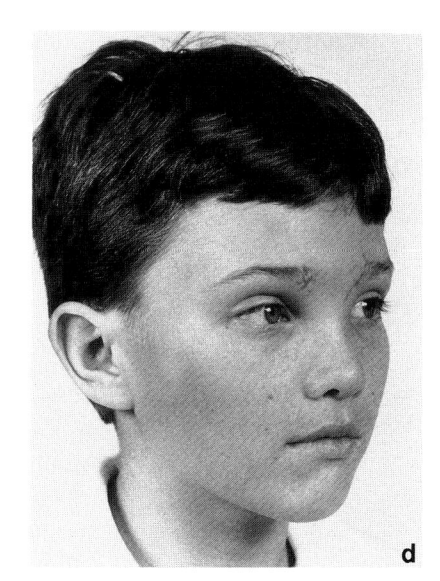

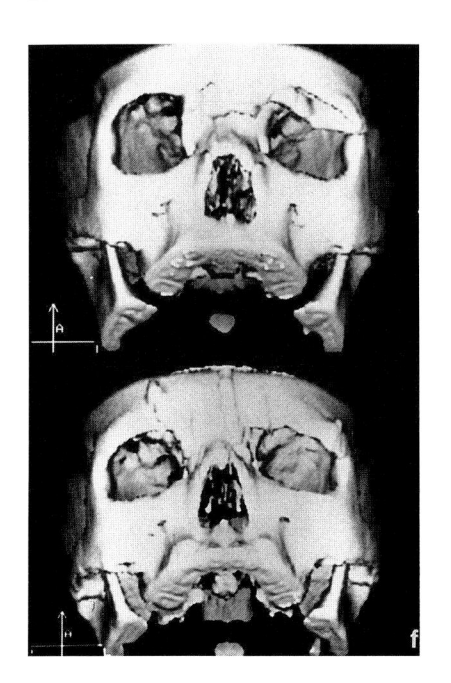

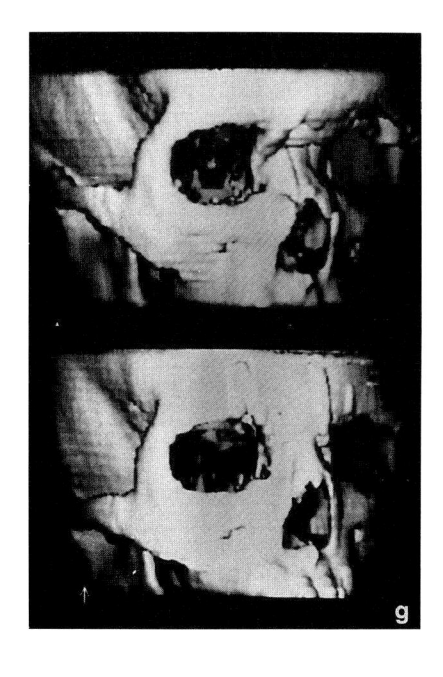

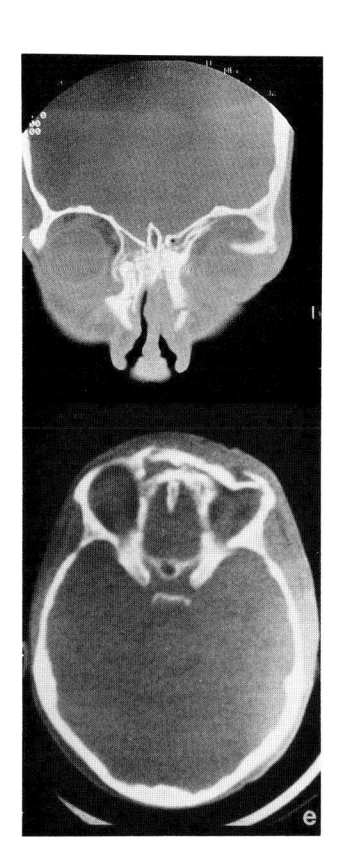

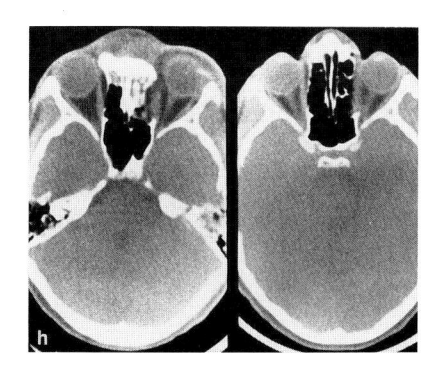

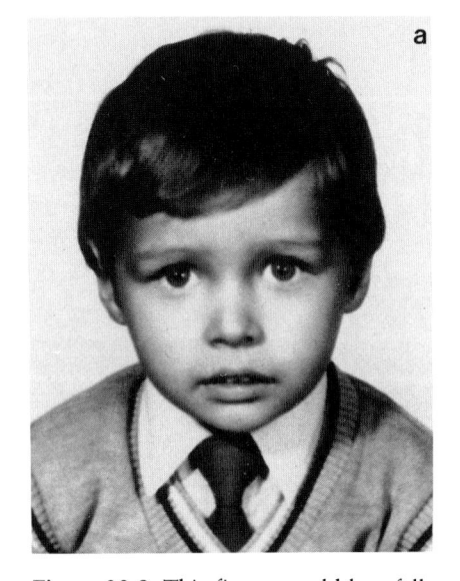

Figure 32.9 This five-year-old boy fell and hit the bridge of his nose on a hard table top resulting in a severe saddle nose deformity. (a) Frontal view just before injury. (b) Frontal view three years after injury. (c) Frontal view six months after nasal reconstruction. (d) Oblique view three years after injury. (e) Oblique view six months after nasal reconstruction. (f) Lateral view three years after injury. (g) Lateral view six months after nasal reconstruction. (h) Worm's eye view three years after injury. (i) Worm's eye view six months after nasal reconstruction. (j) View of nasal dorsum through coronal incision. (k) Crafted full-thickness cranial bone grafts are shown before inset for nasal reconstruction. Stabilization is achieved with microplates and screws. (l) The outer table cranial graft is harvested from the left occipitoparietal region and inset over the full-thickness right occipitoparietal defect. Stabilization is achieved with multiple microplates and screws. (m) This view of the nasal dorsum shows the full-thickness cranial bone grafts stabilized with microplate and screw fixation. (n) Plain radiographs of the nose show fracture before and after reconstruction with cranial bone graft. (o) This three-dimensional CT scan shows fractures before and after reconstruction with cranial bone graft.

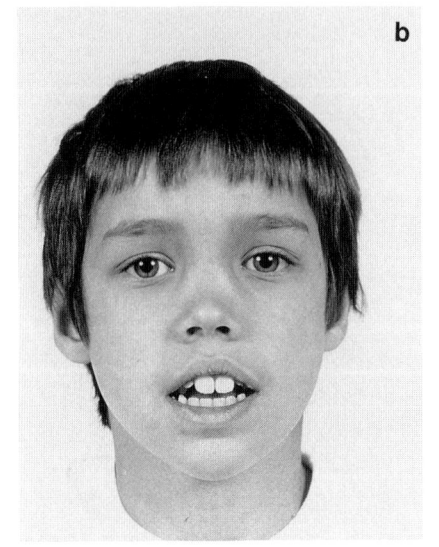

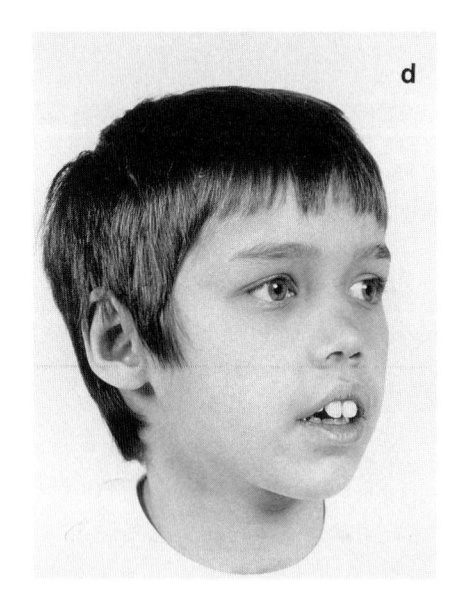

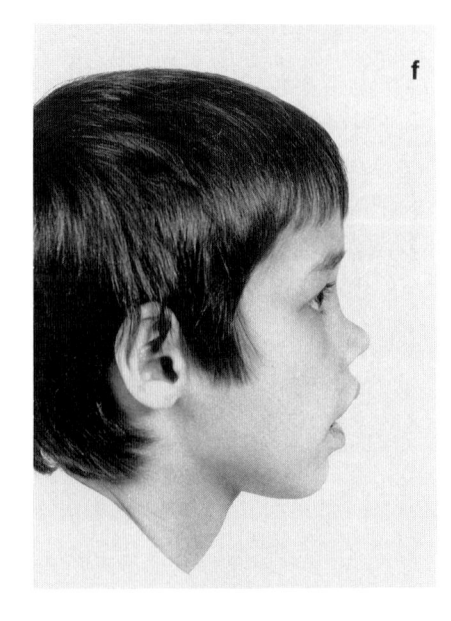

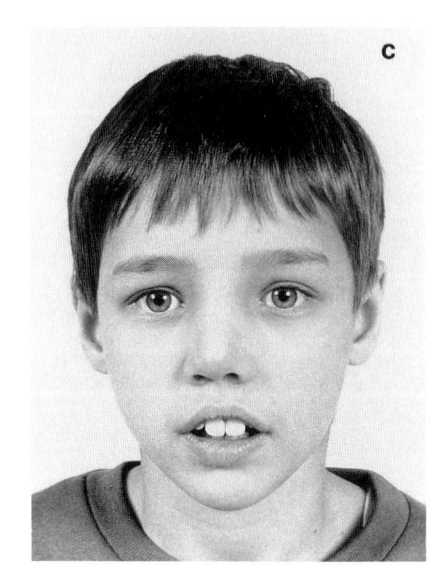

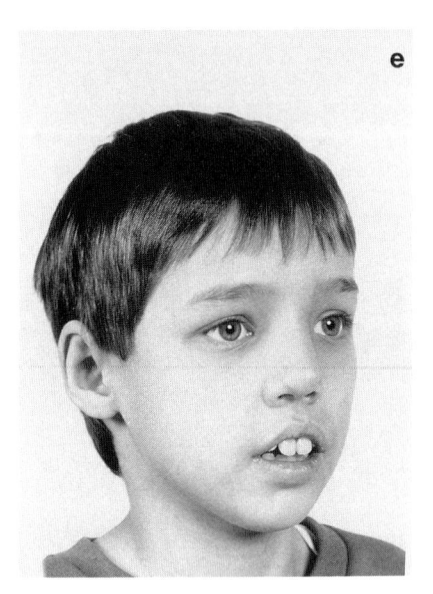

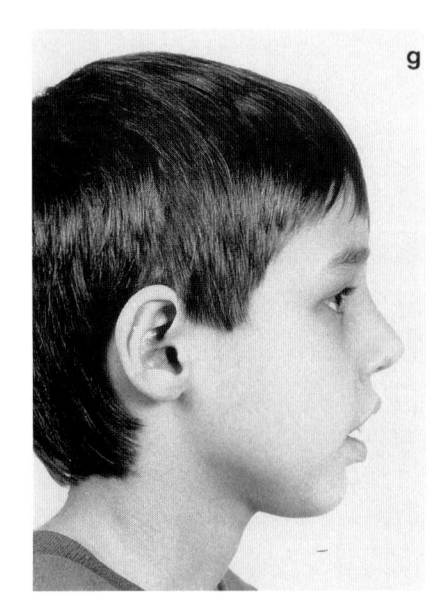

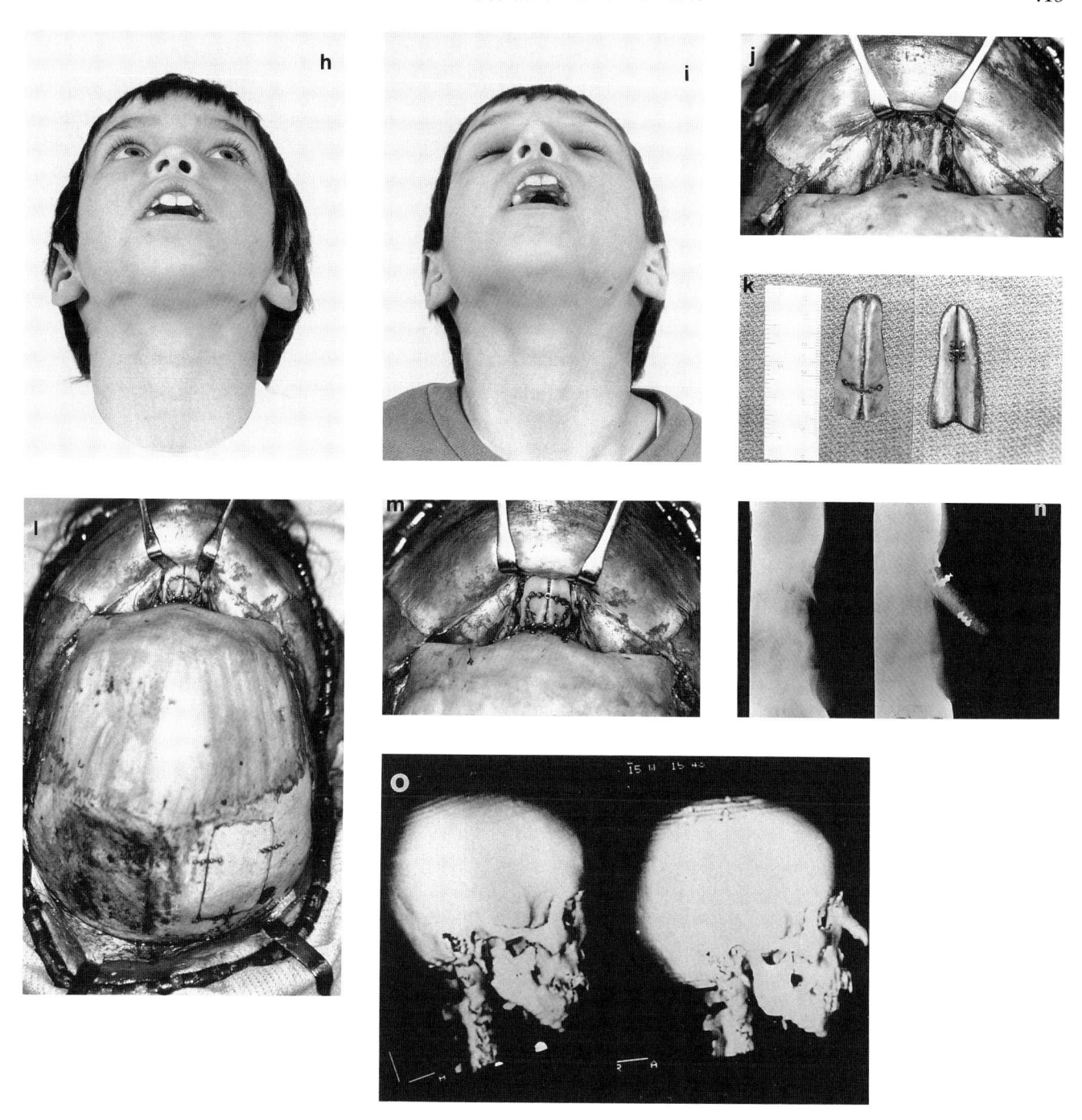

Once bone has healed the bone plates may be removed without concern and perhaps should be removed to prevent distortion of growth. Further experimental and clinical study will be required to clarify this issue. Because his naso-fronto-ethmoid injury occurred early in development, he will be at high risk for a resulting flat dorsum of the nose, which may later require augmentation. No external splinting is required for bony support, but I prefer to place a plaster splint (as in elective rhinoplasty) or steri-tapes to limit swelling of soft tissue in the immediate postoperative period.

Case 7

At age five, this boy fell from a sofa and hit the bridge of his nose on a hard tabletop (see Figure 32.9). There was swelling and nasal bleeding, but no treatment was given and the injury healed. Over the next three months, he developed a marked saddle nose deformity accompanied by difficult nasal breathing.

He was referred for evaluation and treatment at age eight. Examination at the time showed severe flattening over the dorsum of the nose, deviation of the nasal septum, and blockage of the air passage through his nasal cavity.

An axial and coronal CT scan of the craniofacial skeleton confirmed that the nasal skeleton was depressed and the root of the nose was flattened and showed an obtuse nasofrontal angle. The nasal cartilages were also flattened. The anterior third of the nasal septum was deviated.

A psychosocial consultation was obtained because the boy was severely teased and ostracized by his peers both at school and in his neighborhood.

To improve his nasal breathing and encourage better self-esteem, nasal reconstruction was undertaken. Dissection proceeded down to the root of the nose through a coronal incision. Full-thickness cranial bone was harvested from the right parietal region of his skull; from this, two full-thickness cranial grafts were further crafted and joined together with micro bone plates and screws before they were inset. After the grafts were inserted through the coronal incision, they were further stabilized at the nasofrontal angle with several micro bone plates. Split cranial grafts were harvested from the left parietal skull region to reconstruct the full-thickness cranial bone defect over the right parietal region. Stabilization was with micro bone plates.

The patient was discharged from the hospital and permitted limited physical activity for two months. He has now returned to all activities appropriate for his age but is encouraged to avoid trauma to his nose.

Critique

Saddle nose deformities of this severity after direct nasal trauma are rare. Although delaying reconstruction until skeletal maturity may reduce the need for revision surgery, the psychosocial concerns in this case took precedence.

The use of autogenous bone graft for reconstruction, especially when total nasal skeletal reconstruction is required, is my preference. Membranous cranial bone grafts are less likely to resorb, especially when used with plate and screw internal fixation techniques. However, when split, they are often too thin and can be difficult to contour. Full-thickness cranial bone grafts were used in this case to achieve nasal augmentation. Stabilization with micro bone plates limits the visibility or palpability of internal fixation while allowing the theoretical advantage of primary bone healing and limited resorption.

Case 8

While skiing, this 10-year-old boy ran into a post (see Figure 32.10). He sustained right cranio-orbital comminuted fractures accompanied by an underlying brain contusion, dural lacerations, and a cerebrospinal fluid leak.

A CT scan confirmed the comminuted depressed frontal fracture, supraorbital ridge fracture, and comminuted blowin fractures of the orbital roof and medial orbital wall.

At operation, a coronal incision was made, the right frontal craniotomy was completed through the frontal bone fractures, the supraorbital ridge fractured fragment was temporarily removed, and the dural lacerations were repaired with a fascia graft. The components of the orbital roof and superior medial orbital wall fractures were debrided and then reconstructed with cranial bone grafts harvested from the right parietal region. The grafts were stabilized with titanium microplates and screws and attached to each other and then to the cranial base to reconstitute the pre-injury intraorbital volume. The supraorbital ridge was replaced and stabilized, and then the fragmented frontal bone fractures were further secured with additional microplates and screws.

Critique

Fractures of the cranial vault and upper orbital area are common in the pediatric population. When they occur in isolation, the neurosurgeon is often tempted to manage these problems alone. When indicated, a team approach, with a neurosurgeon and plastic surgeon working together, can often diminish the need for secondary revisions. The use of stable micro bone plate and screw fixation has been a major advance that has limited the morbidity related to postoperative infection, recurrent cerebrospinal fluid leaks, and limited vision.

Case 9

This 14-year-old girl sustained multiple traumas, including severe open frontal bone fracture with injury to the underlying brain, in a motor vehicle accident (see Figure 32.11). She required a series of cerebral and cranial bone debridements. She recovered from her cerebral injuries but was left with a very large frontotemporoparietal skull bone defect, which compromised her life style—leaving her unable to participate in any physical activity—and resulted in an aesthetically displeasing appearance, which caused her to shave her hair and wear a wig.

At operation, a formal craniotomy was performed through a coronal incision and full-thickness cranial bone was harvested from the right temporoparietal region. The harvested bone was split into multiple units, and then both the recipient and donor sites were pieced together with split cranial grafts. All grafted areas were stabilized with miniplate and screw fixation.

Critique

In most circumstances even large cranial bone defects can be reconstituted with autogenous cranial bone grafts and stabilization by plate and screw internal fixation. When the defects are large and the thickness of

Pediatric Facial Fractures

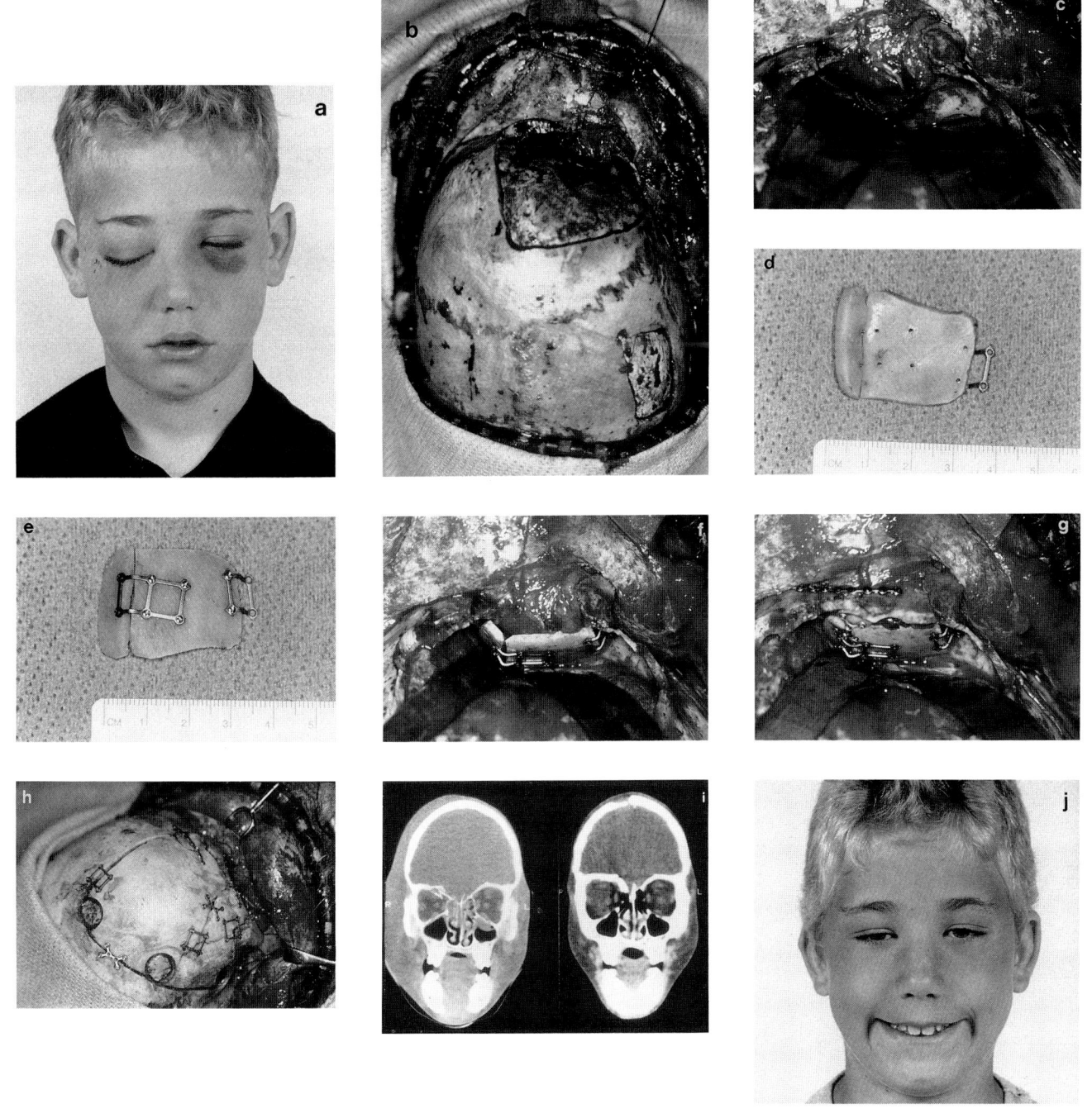

Figure 32.10 This 10-year-old boy sustained right cranio-orbital trauma in a winter skiing accident. His facial fractures included comminuted right frontal bone, associated supraorbital ridge fracture, and comminuted blowin fractures of the orbital roof and superior medial wall. (a) Frontal view five days after injury (before surgery). (b) The cranial vault is seen through the coronal incision. The orbital roof defect is visualized. Cranial bone has been harvested from the right parietal region for orbital reconstruction. (c) This close view of the orbital roof defect shows repair of the dural lacerations. (d) Cranial bone graft is crafted and stabilized with titanium microplates and screws for reconstruction of the orbital roof and medial wall. Inferior view. (e) Superior view. (f) The orbital roof cranial bone reconstruction is stabilized with microplates and screws. (g) The supraorbital ridge fracture is reduced and stabilized. (h) The comminuted frontal bone fracture and craniotomy are stabilized with multiple titanium microplates and screws. (i) Two-dimensional CT scan shows the orbital roof blowin fracture and postsurgical reconstruction. (j) Frontal view of patient just six weeks after reconstruction indicates that normal vision has been restored.

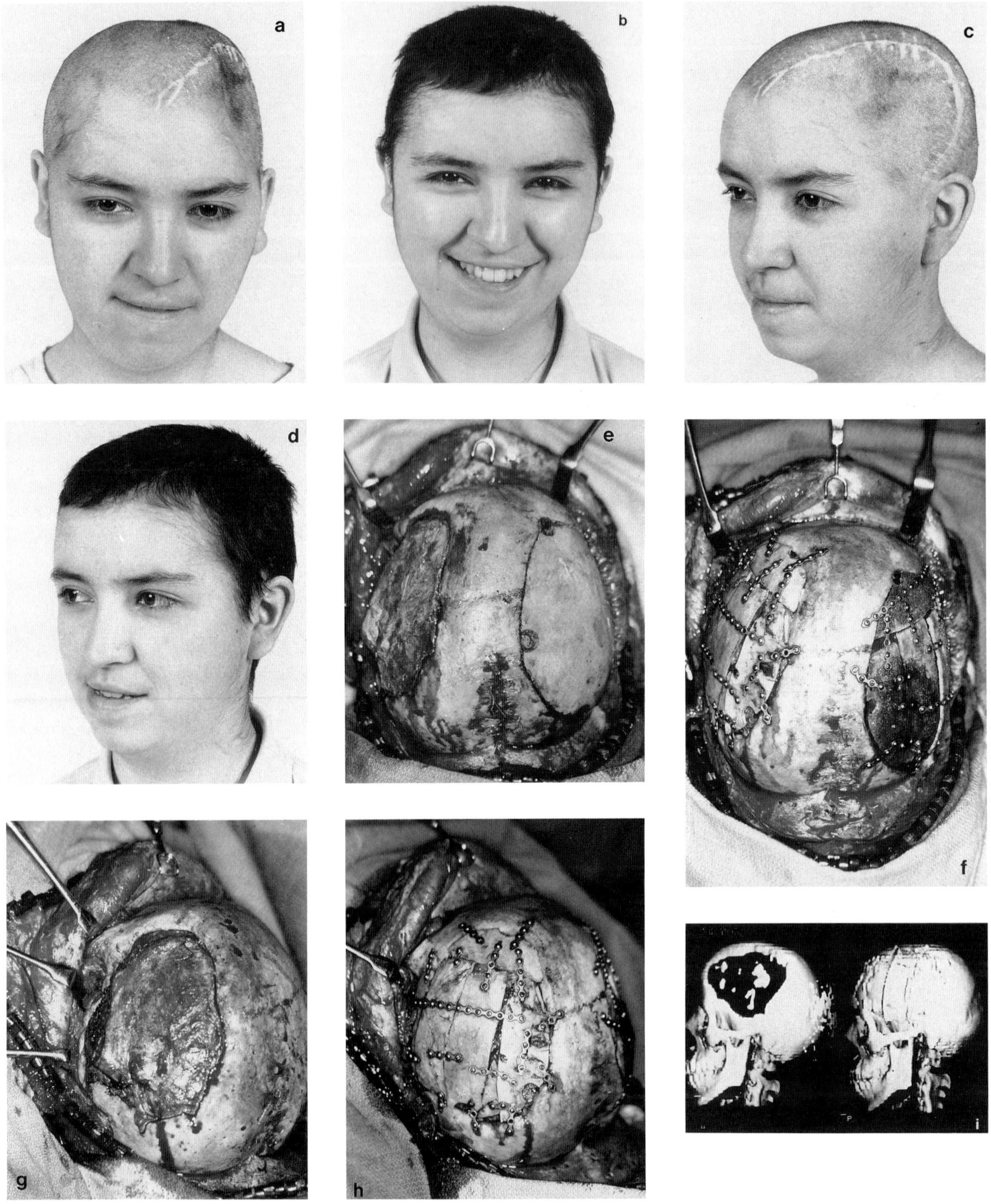
a
b
c
d
e
f
g
h
i

Figure 32.11 In this 14-year-old girl, an initial left cranial vault fracture resulted in a large frontotemporoparietal skull bone defect. (a) Frontal view before reconstruction. (b) Frontal view after reconstruction. (c) Left oblique view before reconstruction. (d) Left oblique view after reconstruction. (e) Bird's eye view of exposed skull through coronal incision shows the large skull defect on the left side and the right craniotomy for harvesting cranial bone for cranioplasty. (f) Bird's eye view of skull shows the cranial bone graft cranioplasty stabilized with multiple titanium miniplates and screws. (g) Left oblique view of cranial bone defect before reconstruction. (h) Left oblique view of skull after reconstruction. (i) Three-dimensional CT scan demonstrate large skull bone defect before reconstruction and method of repair.

the remaining cranial bone is in question, I find it most expedient and safe to harvest full-thickness cranial grafts through a formal craniotomy in conjunction with a neurosurgeon and then to split the units into inner and outer table at the bench. This technique wastes the least cranial bone, limits the chance of accidental injury to the brain, and can be faster when large amounts of cranial bone grafts are required.

I have found that, in addition to decreasing operating time, the miniplates and screws used to stabilize the bone grafts placed for reconstruction when compared to inter-fragmentary wires more predictably ensure bony union between fragments rather than a less desirable fibrous union. With the addition of plate and screw fixation of the cranial bone graft cranioplasty, special protection of the skull is not needed postoperatively.

These multiple miniplates are not visible in the hair-bearing scalp, but they are frequently palpable. We currently prefer to use microplates more routinely to overcome this problem.

SUMMARY

The pattern of craniomaxillofacial fractures in children is different from that in adults, and the differences must be recognized if appropriate treatment is to be provided. Whenever possible, the pediatric trauma patient should be evaluated, treated, and monitored at a pediatric hospital by a surgeon who is familiar with and primarily devoted to the management of pediatric patients. Facial fractures in children may go unrecognized as a result of incomplete communication with the patient, inadequate radiographic examination in the fussy child, or late presentation of the patient by the family.

The more stable forms of fracture fixation currently available have truly revolutionized the treatment of pediatric facial fractures. This does not mean that all pediatric facial fractures will require plate and screw fixation, in fact. However, fixation of fractures with miniplates and microplates and screws may overcome the need for tracheostomy in the multiply-traumatized patient, decrease the incidence of TMJ ankylosis when multiple jaw fractures are present, limit the incidence of infection and malunion in difficult fixation cases, and allow for improved oral hygiene and patient comfort during fracture healing. When knowledge of the locations of the tooth buds enables appropriate placement of plates and screws, injury to the developing or erupted teeth should not be greater than that in the adult.

Plate and screw fixation in the growing jaw will solve many problems in selected facial fracture cases, and less rigid fixation will be required than is usual in adults. The use of heavy reconstructive plates or fracture plates is therefore rarely indicated because miniplates or microplates are more appropriate. Self-tapping screws are preferred; they are placed unicortically or bicortically as indicated. The concept of bone compression (that is, compression plating) to allow for primary bone healing of a fracture is well known. This form of bone healing is not required for the re-establishment and maintenance of pre-injury anatomy for the pediatric patient with facial fracture. For jaw fractures, noncompression plating combined with arch bar placement (tension band concept) coupled with a soft diet and limited physical activity, rather than extended MMF, is usually sufficient.

With the use of noncorroding metals (titanium or Vitallium), removal of plates and screws is no longer a necessity. Once fracture healing is complete, the devices may be removed, although I usually leave them in place and continue to monitor the patient. The concern for growth retardation or distortion is ever present, but it is not known whether this concern is justified. A second operation, with subperiosteal dissection in the growing jaw, may also increase scarring and retard growth. More basic science study and clinical research will be required to resolve this issue.

Late sequelae of pediatric fractures are common, even when appropriate and prompt treatment is instituted. The effects of the trauma event, as well as of the surgical intervention, on growth and development must be considered (Ousterhout 1987).

Long-term follow-up by appropriate practitioners is mandatory to monitor facial growth and development. Intervention at selected intervals may minimize the overall growth distortion and in this way maximize the overall functional, psychological, and aesthetic results for the patient and family.

Acknowledgment

The author thanks Elizabeth Lang and the staff of Medical Publications, The Hospital for Sick Children, for editorial assistance in preparing this chapter.

REFERENCES

Adekeye EO: Pediatric fractures of the facial skeleton: A survey of 85 cases from Kaduna, Nigeria. J Oral Surg 38:355–358, 1980.

Anderson MF, Alling CC: Subcondylar fractures in young dogs. Oral Surg Oral Med Oral Pathol 19:263–268, 1965.

Andreasen JO, Ravn JJ: The effect of traumatic injuries to primary teeth on their permanent successors. II. A clinical and radiographic follow-up study of 213 teeth. Scand J Dent Res 79:284–294, 1971.

Bales CR, Randal P, Lehr HB: Fractures of the facial bones in children. J Trauma 12:56–66, 1972.

Bergland O, Borchgrevink H: The role of the nasal septum in midfacial growth in man elucidated by the maxillary development in certain types of facial clefts: A preliminary report. Scand J Plast Reconstr Surg 8:42–48, 1974.

Bernstein L: Maxillofacial injuries in children. Otolaryngol Clin North Am 2:397, 1974.

Boyne PJ: Osseous repair and mandibular growth after subcondylar fractures. J Oral Surg 25:300–309, 1967.

Bridges CP, Ryan RF, Longenecker CG, Vincent RW: Tracheostomy in children: A twenty-year study at Charity Hospital in New Orleans. Plast Reconstr Surg 37:117–120, 1966.

Campbell RL, Moore RF: Fractured condyle in a 3-month-old infant. Oral Surg 40:45–47, 1975.

Chalmers J: Fractures involving the mandibular condyle: A post-treatment survey of 120 cases. J Oral Surg 5:45–73, 1947.

Coccaro PJ: Restitution of mandibular form after condylar injury in infancy (a 7-year study of a child). Am J Orthod 55:32–49, 1969.

Crysdale WS, Kohli-Dang N, Mullins GC, et al: Airway management in craniofacial surgery: Experience in 542 patients. J Otolaryngol 16:207–215, 1987.

Fortunato MA, Fielding AF, Guernsey LH: Facial bone fractures in children. Oral Surg 53:225–230, 1982.

Freif MG, Baden E: Management of fractures in children. J Oral Surg 12:129–139, 1954.

Gelbier S: Injured anterior teeth in children. A preliminary discussion. Br Dent J 123:331–335, 1967.

Gilhuus-Moe O (ed): Fractures of the Mandibular Condyle in the Growth Period. Stockholm, Scandinavian University Books, 1969.

Graham GG, Peltier JR: The management of mandibular fractures in children. J Oral Surg 18:416–423, 1960.

Hall RK: Injuries of the face and jaws in children. Int J Oral Surg 1:65–75, 1972.

Hall RK: Facial trauma in children. Aust Dent J 19:336–345, 1974.

Harvold EP: New treatment principles for mandibular malformations. In Transactions of the Third International Orthodontic Congress. St. Louis, Mosby, 148–154, 1975.

Jones KM, Bauer BS, Pensler JM: Treatment of mandibular fractures in children. Ann Plast Surg 23:280–283, 1989.

Kaban LB, Mulliken JB, Murray JE: Facial fractures in children: An analysis of 122 fractures in 109 patients. Plast Reconstr Surg 59:15–20, 1977.

Kaplan SL, Mark HI: Bilateral fractures of the mandibular condyles and fracture of the symphysis menti in an 18-month-old child. Two year preliminary report with a plea for conservative treatment. Oral Surg 15:136–147, 1962.

Khosla M, Boren W: Mandibular fractures in children and their management. J Oral Surg 29:116, 1971.

Kissoon N, Dreyer J, Walia M: Pediatric trauma: Differences in pathophysiology, injury patterns and treatment compared with adult trauma. Can Med Assoc J 142:27–34, 1990.

Leake D, Doykos J III, Habal MB, Murray JE: Long-term follow-up of fractures of the mandibular condyle in children. Plast Reconstr Surg 47:127–131, 1971.

Lehman JA Jr, Saddawi ND: Fractures of the mandible in children. J Trauma 16:773–777, 1976.

Lu M: Reimplantation of avulsed anterior teeth in patients with jaw fractures. Plast Reconstr Surg 51:377–383, 1973.

MacLennan WD: Injuries involving the teeth and jaws in young children. Arch Dis Child 32:492–494, 1957.

MacLennan WD, Simpson W: Treatment of fractured mandibular condylar processes in children. Br J Plast Surg 18:423–427, 1965.

Manson PN: Skull and midface injuries. In Plastic Surgery in Infancy and Childhood. 3rd ed. Mustarde JC, Jackson IT (eds). New York, Churchill Livingston, 317–334, 1988.

Manson PN, Clifford CM, Su CT, Iliff NT, Morgan R: Mechanisms of global support and posttraumatic enophthalmos: I. The anatomy of the ligament sling and its relation to intramuscular cone orbital fat. Plast Reconstr Surg 77:193–202, 1986.

McCoy FJ, Chandler RA, Crow ML: Facial fractures in children. Plast Reconstr Surg 37:209–215, 1966.

Messinger A, Radkowski MA, Greenwald MJ, Pensler JM: Orbital roof fractures in the pediatric population. Plast Reconstr Surg 84:213–218, 1989.

Moos K, El-Attar A: Mandible and dental injuries. In Plastic Surgery in Infancy and Childhood. 3rd ed. Mustarde JC, Jackson IT (eds). New York, Churchill Livingstone, 345–364, 1988.

Morgan WC: Pediatric mandibular fractures. Oral Surg 40:320–326, 1975.

Moss ML, Bromberg BE, Song IC, Eisenman G: The passive role of nasal septal cartilage in mid-facial growth. Plast Reconstr Surg 41:536–542, 1968.

Nahum AM: The biomechanics of maxillofacial trauma. Clin Plast Surg 2:59–64, 1975.

Ousterhout DK, Vargervid K: Maxillary hypoplasia secondary to midfacial trauma in childhood. Plast Reconstr Surg 80:491–498, 1987.

Posnick JC, Zimbler AG, Grossman JAI: Normal cutaneous sensibility of the face. Plast Reconstr Surg 86:429–435, 1990.

Proffitt WR, Vig KW, Turvey TA: Early fractures of the mandibular condyles: Frequently and unsuspected cause of growth disturbances. Am J Orthod 78:1–24, 1980.

Rakower W, Protzell A, Rosencrans M: Treatment of displaced condylar fractures in children: Report of cases. J Oral Surg 19:517–521, 1961.

Rowe NL: Mandibular joint lesions in infants and adults. Int Dent J 10:484–495, 1960.

Rowe NL: Fractures of the facial skeleton in children. J Oral Surg 26:505–515, 1968.

Schettler D, Rehrmann A: Long-term results of functional treatment of condylar fractures with the long bridle according to A Rehrmann. J Maxillofac Surg 3:14–22, 1975.

Schultz RC: Facial trauma in children. In Facial Injuries. 3rd ed. Marshall DK (ed). Chicago, Year Book Medical Publishers, 471–491, 1988.

Smith KA, Posnick JC, et al: Facial fractures in the pediatric population: Ten years experience. Proceedings of the 43rd Annual Meeting of the Canadian Society of Plastic Surgeons, 1, June 1989.

Thomson HG, Farmer AW, Lindsay WK: Condylar neck fractures of the mandible in children. Plast Reconstr Surg 34:452–463, 1964.

Waite DE: Pediatric fractures of jaw and facial bones. Pediatrics 51:551–559, 1973.

Walker DG: The mandibular condyle. Fifty cases demonstrating arrest in development. Dent Practitioner (Bristol) 7:160–168, 1957.

Walker RV: Traumatic mandibular condylar fracture dislocations. Effect of growth in the Macaca Rhesus monkey. Am J Surg 100:850–863, 1960.

Winstanley RP: Collapse of the condylar head of the mandible in children and subsequent ankylosis. Br J Oral Surg 16:3, 1978.

Zide MF: Open reduction of mandibular condyle fractures. Indications and technique. Clin Plast Surg 16:69–76, 1989.

Zide MF, Kent JN: Indication for open reduction of mandibular condyle fractures. J Oral Maxillofac Surg 41:89, 1983.

PART III

Clinical Applications

Orthognathic Surgery

CHAPTER 33

Rigid Fixation of the Le Fort I and the Sagittal Split Ramus Osteotomies

William H. Bell

Restoration of normal jaw function or improved function, optimal facial aesthetics, and long-term dental and skeletal stability are essential for successful orthognathic surgery. The key to achieving these objectives is to analyze facial proportions and then to establish and implement aesthetic priorities through the use of cephalometric planning and occlusal studies (Guernsey 1971) to achieve normal function after surgical repositioning of the jaws. The combined surgical–orthodontic approach, combining maxillary, mandibular, and chin surgery, when used in concert will small bone plate osteosynthesis and systematic muscular rehabilitation after surgery, increases treatment efficiency and frequently improves jaw function.

This chapter presents techniques of repositioning and stabilizing the maxilla by the Le Fort I downfracture and the mandible by the surgical split ramus osteotomy (SSRO). Osteotomy design, anatomical considerations, biologic principles, and techniques of sectioning the upper and lower jaws are discussed. Special emphasis is placed on the use of plate and screw fixation techniques.

THE LE FORT I OSTEOTOMY

The Le Fort I downfracture technique affords the surgeon great latitude and safety in correcting maxillary deformities. The ability to reposition the maxilla in all three dimensions of space dramatically increases efficiency of treatment by the surgeon and orthodontist.

Biological Foundation

Successful transposition of the maxillary dento-osseous segments by Le Fort I osteotomy depends on preservation of the vascularity of the segment by proper design of the soft-tissue and bony incisions. The collateral circulation within the maxilla and its enveloping soft tissues and the many vascular anastomoses in the maxilla permit many technical modifications of the Le Fort I osteotomy.

Recent studies have supported our clinical impressions about the nature of the circulation to the maxilla and guided our design of surgical incisions and osteotomies. In a cadaver study You et al. (1990) found that the normal blood supply of the maxilla originates centrifugally from the alveolar medullary arterial system. The mucoperiosteal arterial system also gives many branches that penetrate the cortical bone and supply blood to the maxilla. The multiple sources of blood supply to the maxilla and the abundant vascular communications between the hard and soft tissues is the biological foundation for maintaining dento-osseous viability despite transection of the medullary blood supply after osteotomies.

That the integrity of the descending palatine vessels is not essential to maintain maxillary viability has been shown experimentally. When Le Fort I osteotomies were done in Rhesus monkeys (You 1991a) ligation of the descending palatine vessels only reduced blood flow to the maxilla acutely. Over time, no statistical difference was found in the blood-flow changes or in osseous viability.

In addition to the bone and soft-tissue healing, Le Fort I osteotomy design should provide for the long-term integrity of the teeth and for the development of growing teeth. We have made a preliminary examination of these issues in our patients. Seventeen maxillary third molar teeth from 10 patients whose postsurgical follow-up ranged from 6 months to 78 months (mean, 40 months) were extracted. The long-term biologic effects of Le Fort I osteotomy on the pulp and on the development of teeth were retrospectively evaluated with clinical and standard histologic techniques. Normal teeth from patients who were not operated on were used as controls. Histologic examination revealed an intact pulpal circulation and minimal pathologic changes in the pulpal tissue. Sixty percent of the completely developed teeth in the study showed normal pulpal architecture after surgery. The significance of calcific alterations in the pulp cavity of the other 40% of the completely developed teeth is questionable. These findings require further elucidation.

Clinical and radiographic studies showed that the growing teeth developed normally after surgery. The Le Fort I downfracture procedure had little discernible long-term effect on the pulp and on the development of human third molar teeth. The results of this study parallel biologically the clinically favorable consequences associated with the LeFort I downfracture procedure and support the use of early surgery in adolescents with incompletely developed roots of teeth.

Since our initial description of the downfracture technique for segmentation of the maxilla, we have had experience with more than 2000 Le Fort I osteotomies at our institution. Approximately two thirds of these have been segmental operations. The descending palatine vessels were either intentionally or inadvertently transected in approximately one fourth of these cases without discernible clinical consequences. In all probability, however, the vessels were unknowingly transected in even more cases. A reasonable effort is routinely made to preserve the integrity of these vessels whenever feasible; there is, however, no reluctance to clamp them with a vascular clip or cauterize them to gain accessibility or enhance visualization. Superior or posterior repositioning of the posterior portion of the maxilla are movements in which transection of the vessels may most frequently be indicated in order to visualize and gain access to the junction of the tuberosity and the pterygoid plate and to reposition the maxilla.

There have been relatively few reports of the loss of small or large maxillary dento-osseous segments with Le Fort I osteotomies. Undoubtedly, however, many such cases have gone unreported. A study of the circumstances involved when segments are lost generally reveals that the operating surgeon has violated a basic biologic or surgical principle. Most frequently, the vascular pedicle has not been maintained by proper design of the soft-tissue flap, or circulation to the mobilized segment has not been preserved by way of attached palatal mucoperiosteum. Excessively long and traumatic surgery, imprudent selection of interdental osteotomy sites, and strangulation of the circulation by improperly positioned suspension wires are other causes of compromised wound healing.

Design

Superior, anterior, or posterior maxillary repositioning may result in poor bony interfaces and few abutment areas because bone of the lateral maxillary walls is frequently thin and friable and may not support the use of rigid skeletal fixation. When osteotomies are made in the superior aspect of the lateral maxilla, where bony walls are angular, the margins of the proximal and distal segments may not be juxtaposed. This may cause telescoping of the posterior maxilla into the antrum and long-term osseous instability (see Figure 33.1).

Individualization of the geometric design of the osteotomy, the use of rigid skeletal fixation, and bone grafting in selected cases will avoid most of these problems. The osteotomy design should ideally form a well visualized strong bony base for the use of small bone plates and screws anteriorly and posteriorly. Additionally, it should provide a buttress for the predictable placement of inlaid stabilizing bone grafts. By varying the position and angulation of the lateral maxillary osteotomy, numerous variations of the Le Fort I osteotomy can be designed. In general, these modifications can be divided into three types: (1) traditional Le Fort I (low-level) osteotomy, (2) maxillary step osteotomy, and (3) high Le Fort I osteotomy (see Figure 33.2).

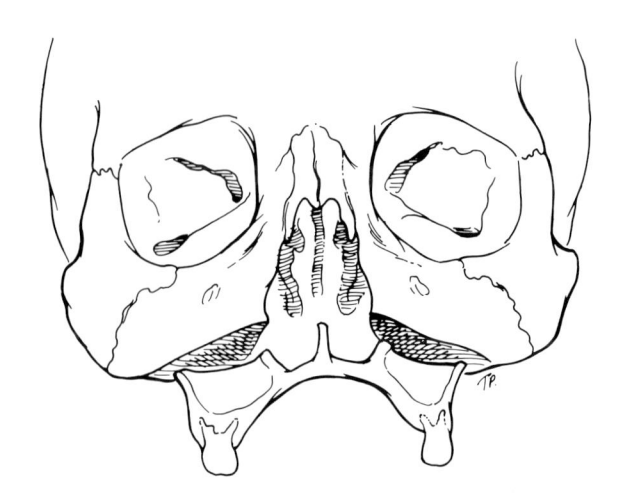

Figure 33.1 When osteotomies are made in the superior aspect of the lateral maxilla, where bony walls are angular, the margins of the proximal and distal segments may not be juxtaposed, allowing telescoping of the posterior maxilla into the maxillary antra and possible osseous instability and difficulty in stabilizing the repositioned maxilla.

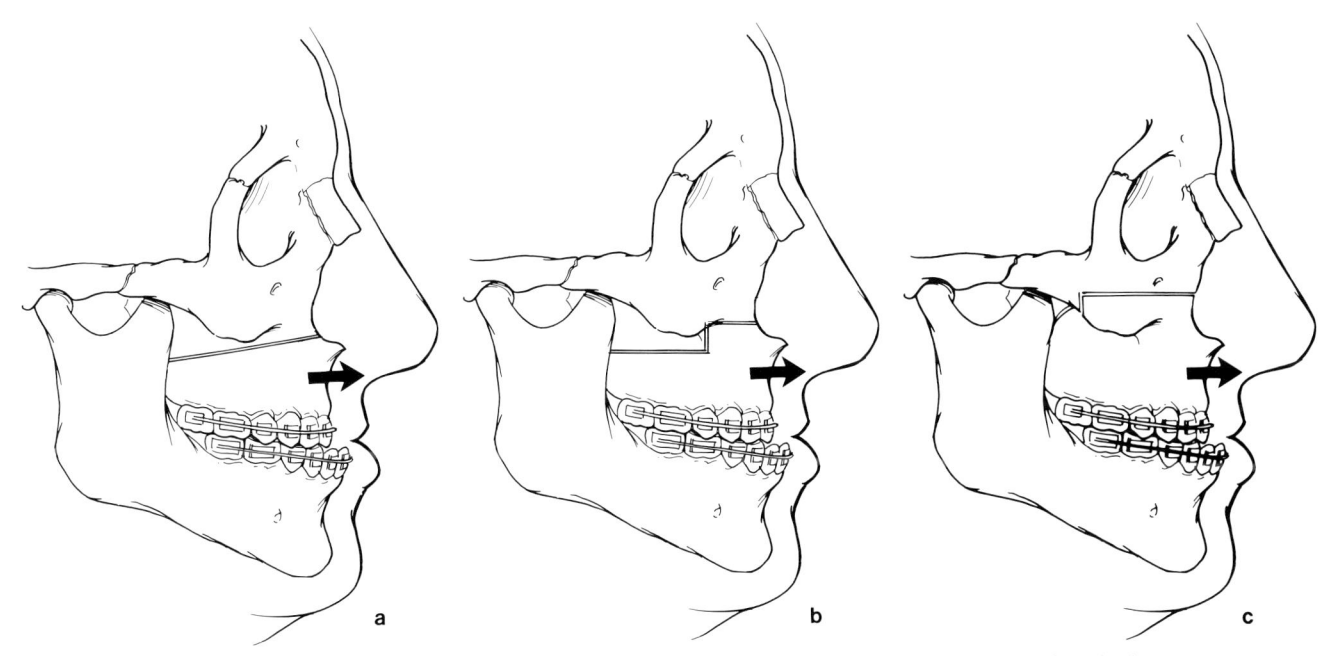

Figure 33.2 Various designs for Le Fort I osteotomy: (a) traditional Le Fort I, (b) step Le Fort I, and (c) high Le Fort I.

Traditional Le Fort I Osteotomy

The traditional Le Fort I (low-level) osteotomy (see Figure 33.2a) places the lateral maxillary osteotomy a safe level above the cuspid and molar roots and extends it to a level just beneath the zygomatic buttress. Because the cuspid root is considerably longer than the molar roots, and because of the low position of the zygomatic buttress, the traditional Le Fort I is by necessity inclined anteroposteriorly. This anterior–posterior inclination combined with anterior maxillary repositioning can lead to significant reduction in upper incisor show, which must be taken into account in preoperative planning.

If one is not aware of this ramping effect when designing maxillary osteotomies, unpredicted changes in vertical dimension can arise, compromising aesthetics. It is possible to take advantage of this ramping effect with the traditional LeFort I osteotomy, where superior and anterior repositioning of the maxilla is desirable. It is important to note that because of the inclination of the lateral maxillary osteotomy combined with the anterior repositioning, the amount of osectomy is always less than the magnitude of superior repositioning. It is for this reason that careful cephalometric planning and accurate surgery are necessary to prevent unpredictable changes in the vertical positions of the incisors.

The traditional low-level Le Fort I osteotomy is indicated when a small (5-millimeter) anterior movement with good bony interfaces is anticipated following maxillary advancement (frequently combined with superior–inferior maxillary repositioning). Advantages and indications for the traditional Le Fort I osteotomy design include (1) speed, (2) general familiarity with osteotomy design, (3) simplicity, (4) facility to reposition the maxilla superiorly and posteriorly, and (5) ease of segmentation. In addition, the traditional Le Fort I osteotomy may be combined with Le Fort III osteotomy in selected cases. Disadvantages include (1) possible telescoping of repositioned segments, (2) difficulty obtaining sufficient bone for application of screw and/or plate osteosynthesis in individual cases with aberrant anatomy (for example, exceedingly thin anterior maxillary walls), (3) difficulty positioning corticocancellous bone grafts in the pterygopalatine region, (4) potential for unpredictable changes in vertical maxillary position, and (5) relatively poor augmentation of malar, infraorbital, and paranasal areas. The traditional Le Fort I osteotomy may not be feasible at an early age because of developing tooth beds contiguous to the planned line of bone sectioning.

Maxillary Step Osteotomy

In an effort to improve the predictability and accuracy of maxillary advancement surgery and to eliminate the incline or ramping effects seen with the traditional Le Fort I osteotomy, the maxillary step osteotomy was designed (Bennett 1985) (see Figure 33.2b). In this technique, the lateral maxillary osteotomy is made parallel to the Frankfort horizontal. This places the osteotomy higher into the zygomatic buttress, where a vertical step is made. A horizontal osteotomy is then continued posteriorly to the pterygoid plates, parallel to the anterior horizontal osteotomy (see Figure 33.2b). It is important to keep the anterior and posterior osteotomies parallel to minimize interferences during maxillary repositioning. This osteotomy design enables easy anterior and superior maxillary repositioning by way of an ostectomy along the lateral maxillary walls.

The design of this osteotomy is dependent on accurate cephalometric prediction studies. The apices of the cuspid and molar roots are first identified. Utilizing the cephalometric prediction tracing, a line is scribed from low on the piriform rim, superior to the cuspid apex, to the zygomatic buttress parallel to the Frankfort horizontal. At the time of surgery, this bone cut is sequentially extended posteriorly until the thick portion of the zygomatic buttress is sectioned. Careful assessment of bone thickness in the planned vertical osteotomy site in the zygomatic maxillary buttress may be helpful in designing and positioning the osteotomy in denser bone. A vertical step is then extended inferiorly. The inferior extent of this vertical step, together with the horizontal osteotomy extending posterior to the pterygoid plates, must be sufficiently superior to avoid injury to the molar roots. It is important that the anterior and posterior horizontal osteotomies remain parallel to avoid interferences during anterior repositioning of the maxilla. Once the osteotomy has been designed on the prediction tracing, the vertical distance from the cuspid and molar occlusal surfaces is recorded. These measurements are transferred to the lateral maxillary wall at the time of surgery by placing reference marks at the predetermined level above the cuspid adjacent to the piriform aperture and above the molars at the zygomatic buttress. Once the osteotomy design has been transferred to the patient, the LeFort I downfracture is accomplished in the routine manner. With the cephalometric prediction studies used as a guide, the lateral osteotomy is initiated at the piriform rim and extended posteriorly until the thick bone of the zygomatic buttress is sectioned. In this manner, a sufficient quantity of bone is assured for the application of screw and plate osteosynthesis.

Advantages and indications for this osteotomy design include (1) pure anteroposterior maxillary repositioning where a vertical change at the incisor is undesirable, (2) vertical osteotomy at the zygomatic buttress provides a well visualized place for corticocancellous bone graft placement and superior augmentation of the paranasal area. Disadvantages include (1) technical difficulty, (2) requires accurate cephalometric prediction studies for predictable results, and (3) insufficient bone along the lateral maxillary wall or zygomaticomaxillary buttress may preclude application of screw and/or plate osteosynthesis.

The Le Fort I downsliding technique is a variation of the maxillary step osteotomy (Bennett 1985, Reyneke 1985). Patients with a combination of vertical and anteroposterior deficiency are ideal candidates for this osteotomy design. In these individuals, the surgical treatment plan would include maxillary advancement combined with corticocancellous bone grafting to increase the vertical dimension. Instead of the traditional low-level Le Fort I osteotomy, the downsliding osteotomy is designed to provide an inclined plane that allows for vertical lengthening as the maxilla is advanced. The proper angulation and position of the lateral maxillary osteotomy is determined from careful preoperative cephalometric prediction studies.

Indication for the sliding Le Fort I osteotomy design is limited to patients with combined vertical and anteroposterior maxillary deficiency where the required advancement is equal to or greater than the required vertical increase. Advantages of this technique include (1) increased stability, and (2) less corticocancellous bone graft is required. This procedure is technically more difficult and provides less augmentation of the paranasal area.

High Le Fort I Osteotomy

The difficulties encountered with the previous techniques in placing screws and plates along the thin lateral maxillary wall can be circumvented by modifying the design of the Le Fort I osteotomy to extend the lateral maxillary osteotomy high into the zygomatic root (see Figure 33.2c). Such a modification provides for excellent bony interfaces following maxillary repositioning as well as the necessary bone for the application of bone screw and/or plate osteosynthesis.

The position and angulation of the high Le Fort I osteotomy is based upon a correlated clinical examination, aesthetic treatment objective, cephalometric planning studies, and model surgery. The lateral maxillary osteotomy extends from the piriform aperture at a level just beneath the infraorbital foramen posteriorly into the dense bone of the zygoma, 6 to 8 millimeters or more above the inferior aspect of the zygoma. The degree of penetration of the zygoma and the posterior extension of the lateral maxillary osteotomy is dependent upon the pneumatization of the maxillary antrum, the position of the posterior maxillary wall, the planned surgical movement, and the aesthetic treatment objectives. Due to the high level of the maxillary osteotomy, soft-tissue projection of the infraorbital malar and paranasal regions will increase significantly. The need for augmentation in these regions (i.e., infraorbital, paranasal, zygomatic) must be determined by a meticulous clinical facial aesthetic analysis. If the soft-tissue contour in these regions is deemed adequate, then a different osteotomy design must be chosen to meet the aesthetic treatment objectives. Fixation for this osteotomy design is accomplished with positional screws in the zygomatic root combined with miniplates or screw osteosynthesis and interpositional bone grafts at the piriform aperture. Augmentation of the malar bones and the infraorbital and paranasal areas is frequently accomplished with alloplastics or corticocancellous bone grafts. Refinements in the contours of the advanced maxilla are made with a combination of avitene and hydroxyapatite.

The integrity of the nasolacrimal system is at risk with the high Le Fort I osteotomy, as evidenced by the reports of transient or permanent epiphora after this procedure (Freihofer 1990, Keller 1990). Our cadaver studies (You 1991b) showed that when the osteotomy is made just beneath the infraorbital foramen and extends to the pyriform rim at the level of the attachment of the inferior turbinate, the nasolacrimal duct within or its bony canal will usually not be jeopardized.

The meatal portion of the nasolacrimal duct is its extension into the inferior nasal meatus as it exits the bony canal. There is large variability in the length of the meatal portion. Because the high Le Fort I osteotomy is frequently made above the level of the ostium of the nasolacrimal duct, we emphasize the importance of elevating the lateral nasal mucoperiosteum, which contains the meatal portion of the nasolacrimal duct, up to the base of the inferior turbinate to protect the meatal portion from injury when the osteotomy is made.

To date no such problems have been observed in our series of patients who have had high Le Fort I osteotomies for correction of dentofacial deformities. If clinicians understand the regional anatomy well, position the osteotomies of the lateral nasal wall precisely, and protect the meatal portion of the nasolacrimal duct carefully, the danger of permanent injury to nasolacrimal structures is in all likelihood very low.

Indications for this osteotomy design in addition to maxillary anteroposterior deficiency include those patients who require augmentation of the zygomatic, infraorbital, and/or paranasal regions. Potential advantages of the modified high Le Fort I osteotomy include (1) enhanced stability with screw and plate osteosynthesis; (2) versatility of osteotomy design, enabling both vertical and anteroposterior maxillary skeletal deformities to be corrected; (3) extension of the lateral maxillary osteotomy high into the zygomatic root, allowing for augmentation of the zygomatic, infraorbital, and paranasal regions; (4) reduction of telescoping of posterior segments following maxillary repositioning; (5) reduction of injury to tooth root apices following screw placement; and (6) avoidance of possible damage to developing tooth buds, enabling maxillary surgery to be performed at an early age. Experience with this technique has demonstrated the following disadvantages: (1) increased operating time; (2) technical difficulty; (3) potential for fracture of the zygoma; (4) undesirable changes in vertical dimension can result if position and angulation of the lateral maxillary osteotomy is not carefully determined from cephalometric prediction tracings and model surgery; (5) asymmetric maxillary movements can produce undesirable soft-tissue changes;

and (6) posterior and superior repositioning of the maxilla is technically difficult and problematic.

Exposure of the Osteotomy Site

Successful transposition of the maxillary dentoosseous segments by Le Fort I osteotomy depends on preservation of viability of the segment by proper design of the soft-tissue and bony incisions. The collateral circulation within the maxilla and enveloping soft tissues, and the vascular connections in the maxilla, permit many technical modifications of the Le Fort I osteotomy.

A horizontal incision is made in the maxillary vestibule superior to the mucogingival junction, extending from the first molar region of one side to a similar area on the contralateral side. At the zygomatic buttress the mucoperiosteal incision is made high in the vestibule, where the soft tissue is relatively thick and extensible. Anteriorly, the incision is made more inferiorly—3 or 4 millimeters above the mucogingival line—to minimize disruption of some of the muscles of facial expression attached to the upper lip.

To maintain maximum circulation to the maxillary bone and teeth, the inferior mucoperiosteal tissues are elevated just enough to allow visualization and palpation of the bone encasing the apices of the teeth and to facilitate interdental osteotomies. Therefore, a maximum buccolabial and palatal pedicle to the mobilized segments is maintained.

The margins of the superior flap are raised to expose the infraorbital nerve and the maxilla immediately lateral and medial to the nerve (see Figure 33.3). Dis-

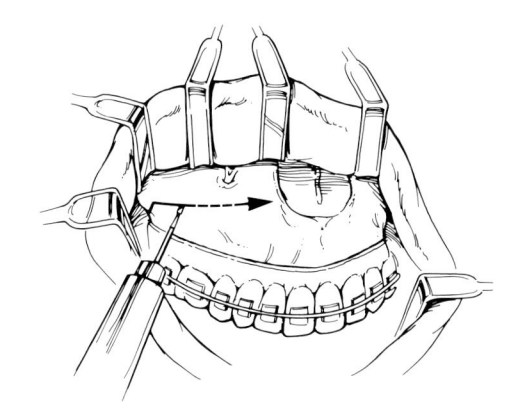

Figure 33.3 The margins of the superior flap are raised to expose the infraorbital nerve and the maxilla immediately lateral and medial to the nerve, the root of the zygoma, the inferior aspect of the zygoma, the anterior nasal floor, the piriform aperture, and the pterygomaxillary junction. Anterior and posterior vertical reference lines and planned lateral maxillary osteotomies are etched into the lateral maxilla at the desired level with a fissure bur.

section is carried anteriorly to facilitate reflection of the nasal mucoperiosteum from the lateral and inferior aspects of the piriform rim and the anterior nasal floor. The mucoperiosteum is detached from the nasal floor, the base of the nasal septum, and the lateral nasal walls. Tunneling subperiosteally to the pterygomaxillary junction enables visualization of the posterolateral portion of the maxilla. With the tip of a curved right-angle retractor positioned at the junction, the mucoperiosteal reflection is extended over the inferior aspect of the zygoma. After the masseter muscle is released to gain access and exposure to the inferior-medial aspect of the zygoma, a cottonoid pack is placed to retract the inferior contents of the infratemporal fossa away from the osteotomy sites.

Osteotomy Design

Vertical reference lines are inscribed into the lateral aspect of the piriform aperture at the zygomaticomaxillary buttress perpendicular to the occlusal plane. On the basis of measurements made from the cephalometric prediction studies and transferred to the bone with calipers, the proposed osteotomies are inscribed into the lateral maxilla with a fissure bur (see Figure 33.3). The inferior bone cut is positioned at a safe level above the apex of the maxillary canine.

Position and angulation of the osteotomies is based upon a correlated clinical examination, cephalometric planning studies, and model surgery. Accurate transfer of cephalometric information is facilitated by the geometric design of the osteotomy made through the lateral maxilla and the root of the zygoma. Osteotomies are designed and positioned to improve stability of the proximal and distal segments by maximum interfacing of the bony margins. Anteriorly, the osteotomy is designed so that the largest possible bony interface can be created while the bone cut is positioned at a safe distance above the tooth apices in the thicker part of the maxilla. The lateral maxillary osteotomy courses from the piriform aperture posteriorly into the denser bone of the root of the zygoma, 5 millimeters or more above the inferior aspect of the zygoma. The osteotomy design must also be consistent with the aesthetic objectives of the planned surgery.

When osteotomies or ostectomies are made in the thick roots of the zygomas, the margins of the proximal and distal segments are consistently juxtaposed after surgery. The posterior portion of the maxilla is sectioned with a fissure bur to determine sequentially the relative thickness of the zygomatic maxillary buttress and to provide a stable index and reference for subsequent sectioning of the lateral maxilla. The degree of penetration of the root of the zygoma and the posterior extension of the lateral maxillary osteotomy will vary according to the degree of pneumatization of the antrum and the position of the posterior wall of the antrum. When trial sectioning of the maxilla and zygomaticomaxillary buttress reveals relatively thick bone, the maxillary step osteotomy may be used and is technically easier (Bennett, 1985). If the posterior portion of the lateral maxilla and the zygomaticomaxillary buttress are very thin, great care and meticulous technique are exercised to avoid fracturing the root of the zygoma. Even if this should occur, as it has in two patients, the fractured free segment can be repositioned as planned and stabilized to the distal segment with an interosseous wire, a circumzygomatic wire, or a bone plate.

Sectioning the Maxilla

The major portion of the lateral maxilla is sectioned from the contralateral side with a reciprocating saw blade; the osteotomy is then extended anteriorly to the lateral piriform rim. With a periosteal elevator or a small malleable retractor passed subperiosteally medial to the lateral nasal wall to protect the nasal mucoperiosteum, the anterior aspect of the lateral nasal wall is sectioned with the reciprocating saw blade (see Figure 33.4).

The horizontal osteotomy is extended posteriorly into the dense root of the zygoma to a point 5 or 6 millimeters above the inferior aspect of the body of the zygoma and 4 to 6 millimeters distal to the zygomaticomaxillary suture line (Lemke and Della Rocca, 1990; Van Sickels, Jeter, and Aragon, 1985). For the step osteotomy, a vertical through-and-through osteotomy is made with a reciprocating or oscillating saw blade to the inferior and deep aspect of the zygoma. With the contents of the infratemporal fossa reflected, the osteotomy is directed inferiorly and medially at a 45-degree angle to the pterygomaxillary junction (see Figure 33.5). Because the bone in this area is generally relatively thin, the osteotomy can usually be made with a finely ta-

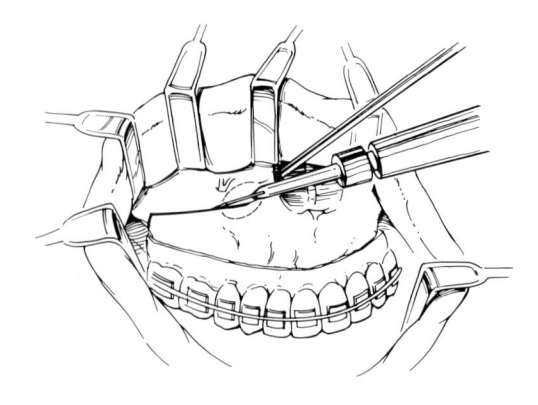

Figure 33.4 The major portion of the lateral maxilla is sectioned from the contralateral side with a reciprocating saw blade.

pered, curved osteotome. When the bone is thick, however, the posterior vertical osteotomies are made with an oscillating or reciprocating saw blade. Finally, the maxilla is separated from the pterygoid process by malleting an osteotome directed medially and anteriorly into the pterygomaxillary suture.

The midportion of the medial antral wall is sequentially sectioned with a fissure bur and a finely tapered osteotome positioned between the margins of the lateral maxillary ostectomy. Sectioning of the medial antral wall is terminated at least 1 centimeter short of the perpendicular plate of the palatine bone to avoid transecting the descending palatine vessels. The thin antral wall contiguous to the vessels generally fractures when the maxilla is downfractured.

A nasal septal osteotome positioned parallel to the hard palate is malleted toward a finger positioned on the posterior nasal spine to separate the base of the posterior bony nasal septum from the maxilla. Gradually increasing inferior pressure on the anterior aspect of the maxilla facilitates visualization of the nasal surface of the maxilla and lateral nasal walls. While the midface structures are stabilized by the assistant, the surgeon uses both hands to hinge the maxilla inferiorly and posteriorly. The assistant simultaneously detaches the remaining mucoperiosteum from the nasal floor and horizontal plane of the palatine bone to facilitate downfracturing.

The posterior part of the maxilla is separated from its remaining bony attachments by forward pressure of a periosteal elevator or similar instrument against the thick and strong posterior aspect of the horizontal plate of the palatine bone to achieve mobility and movement of the maxilla to the contralateral side (see Figure 33.6). A similar procedure is accomplished on the opposite side.

With the maxilla in the downfractured position, bone interferences in any area can be readily identified and removed under direct visualization. Reduction of the height of the lateral nasal walls is accomplished with rongeurs. Meticulous and sequential reduction of the posterior aspect of the lateral nasal wall and alveolopalatal junction in the area opposite the second and third molars is accomplished with rongeurs and burs. Finally, osteotomes, burs, and/or Kerrison forceps may be used carefully to expose the descending palatine vessels (see Figure 33.7). After the overlying bone has been excised, an effort is made to preserve the integrity of these vessels whenever feasible. When the planned posterior and superior movements are problematic, the vessels can be sharply transected or cauterized after vascular clips have been placed. With large retractors positioned, the posterior maxillary tuberosity can be removed to facilitate posterior maxillary repositioning.

The height of the vomer is reduced an amount proportional to the planned superior movement of the maxilla. A mid-sagittal groove is made in the superior aspect of the maxilla to accommodate the nasal septum and to prevent its lateral displacement. Submucous resection of the cartilaginous nasal septum is accomplished to facilitate superior movement of the repositioned maxilla and to prevent buckling of the septum. The mucoperichondrium enveloping the inferior aspect of the cartilagenous septum is incised and detached bilaterally from the inferior-lateral aspect of the septum. The height of the cartilage is reduced an amount proportional to the superior movement of the maxilla. The maxilla can now be rotated upward into the planned

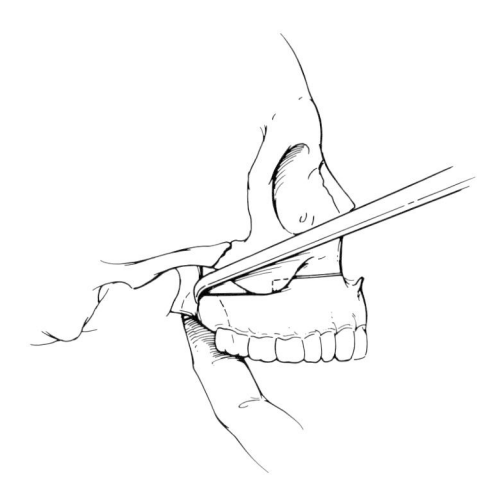

Figure 33.5 Bone is sectioned with a sharp, curved osteotome, which is directed inferiorly and medially at a 45-degree angle to the pterygomaxillary junction.

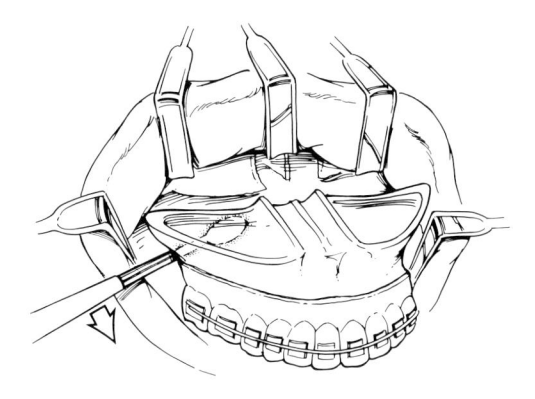

Figure 33.6 The mobilized maxilla has been hinged inferiorly on an axis that passes through the condylar heads. The mucoperiosteum has been detached and separated from the nasal surface of the maxilla and the horizontal plate of palatine bone to facilitate downfracturing. The posterior part of the maxilla is separated from its remaining bony attachments by forward pressure of a periosteal elevator or similar instrument against the thick posterior aspect of the horizontal plate of the palatine bone to achieve mobility.

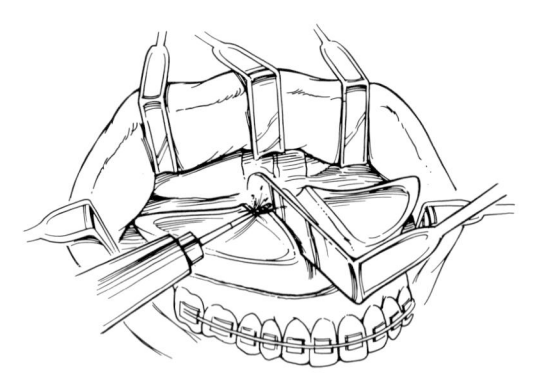

Figure 33.7 With the maxilla downfractured, the vertical dimension of the posterior aspect of the lateral nasal wall and alveolopalatal junction in the area opposite the second and third molars is carefully reduced with a No. 701 fissure bur to expose the descending palatine vessel. Retractors are positioned to protect the contiguous soft tissues and to enhance accessibility and visualization; the typical vertical bony prominence of these structures lies lateral to the descending palatine vessel.

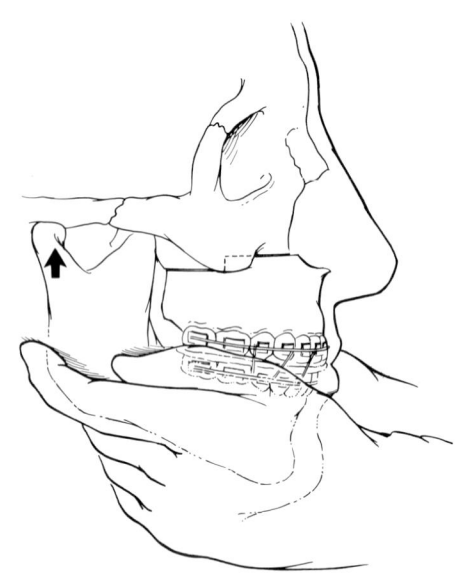

Figure 33.8 After the interocclusal splint is precisely ligated to the maxilla, the mandibular teeth are indexed into the splint; MMF is accomplished with wire ligatures between vertical lugs attached to the arch wire. With the condyles held upward and forward against the posterior slopes of the articular eminences, the maxillary-mandibular complex is repeatedly rotated closed to the desired vertical position.

relationship without buckling the septum. The mucosal margins are then closed with catgut sutures.

After the maxilla is completely mobilized, the interocclusal splint is precisely ligated to the maxilla. The mandibular teeth are indexed into the splint, and maxillomandibular fixation (MMF) is accomplished with wire ligatures between the vertical lugs attached to the arch wire. The maxillary-mandibular complex is moved as a unit through the mandibular arc of rotation so that the areas of bone contact can be visualized as the maxilla is positioned upward and forward. Bone is removed from the posterior margins until the mobilized segment can be passively seated in the desired vertical position and the margins of the lateral maxillary osteotomies are juxtaposed. With the condyles held upward and forward against the posterior slopes of the articular eminences, the maxillary-mandibular complex is repeatedly rotated closed to the desired vertical position (see Figure 33.8). Finally, the maxilla is stabilized in the planned position by appropriate bone plate osteosynthesis.

Stabilization with Rigid Fixation

Through the use of many different combinations of biocompatible and corrosion-resistant bone plates and screws for stabilization, the Le Fort I downfracture is even more versatile than previously used methods (Beals 1987, Drommer 1981, Harle 1980, Harsha 1986, Horster 1980, Luhr 1968, 1979, Rosen 1986, Steinhauser 1982, Van Sickels 1985). The drastic shortening of the period of MMF from 6 to 12 weeks to only a few days or, more commonly, the total elimination of MMF, is one of the principal advantages of the mini bone plate technique. Therefore, it is possible to open the mouth in the always potentially critical period after extubation without the danger of displacing the segments. Because airway problems are avoided, there is, generally speaking, no need to keep the patient in an intensive care unit for the first postoperative night. The opening of the mouth, moreover, facilitates oral hygiene, prevents temporomandibular joint hypomobility, and minimizes the progression of pre-existing periodontal disease, which might occur during prolonged MMF. Rigid fixation shortens the hospital stay (Rosen 1986) and indeed the entire period of morbidity following Le Fort I osteotomies. Further, the ability to open the mouth after surgery has a profound comforting effect on the patient.

Whenever feasible, four plates are placed anteriorly and posteriorly where relatively thick cortical bone is present. With the application of rigid fixation in Le Fort I osteotomies, the need for bone grafting has decreased (Horster 1980). This is another advantage of miniplate fixation. Despite the improved stability of these techniques, however, bone grafting across the osteotomy sites and bone gaps may be essential to facilitate bone healing. For instance, bone grafting is generally necessary in selected cases when the vertical dimension of the maxilla and midface is to be increased and in cleft palate patients with severe atrophy on the affected side.

The main disadvantage of bone plates is the inability to adjust the appliance once it has been placed. Also, the method may take longer than wire osteosynthesis when the surgeon is not familiar with this technique. However, once the individual has gained some experience and routinely works with experienced assistants, there is little time difference between the two methods. This is particularly true in cases of major maxillary advancements, inferior repositioning of the maxilla, and segmentation of the maxilla (where interosseous wire fixation is difficult). Interosseous wires are effective when tension forces can be applied—in one direction only—whereas plates can stabilize segments in all three dimensions.

Miniplates are available in different designs and varying lengths. The two eccentric holes on either side of the bony gaps on the straight, curved, or T plates are designed to provide compression (Luhr 1968, 1979). Because this mechanism is rarely indicated in the clinical practice of orthognathic surgery, these miniplates are usually applied in a noncompressive mode. Minifixation plates, which were specifically designed for orthognathic surgery, do not have eccentric holes, and therefore the potential for bone movement while screws are tightened is avoided. A bone plate of proper length and shape should routinely provide two holes for screws in the stable segment and two holes for fixing the repositioned segment. Because of their small size and thinness, miniplates are versatile and may be adapted to almost any variety of contoured bone surfaces. The specific application and configuration of the small bone plates will depend on the bone contour and the varieties of bony steps that result from segmenting the maxilla. Usually, the plate requires some amount of bending and trial fitting to adapt to the underlying bone.

Selection of the appropriate length and contouring of the plate for implantation is facilitated by the use of very thin and malleable templates. A template is custom fitted and adapted to the individual contour of the maxilla across the osteotomy site with light digital pressure. A similar type and size of bone plate is then formed with bending forceps so that it will duplicate the shape and configuration of the template. Now the plate is formed with the bending instruments until it lies passively across the osteotomy side and is flat against the bone surfaces. If the plate does not contact the underlying bone, the movable, repositioned dentoalveolar segment of the maxilla will be displaced when the screw is tightened. The resultant torquing may create a malocclusion.

Once contoured to lay passively against all bone surfaces, the plate is held in position with plate-holding forceps and secured to both the distal and proximal segments with two screws (see Figure 33.9). Minifixation plates (which do not have any eccentric holes) are preferred for orthognathic surgery since they minimize the risk of segment movement due to horizontal screw movement during the insertion process.

The bone is drilled with a drill bit of 1.5-millimeter diameter. It is important to maintain a speed lower than 1000 revolutions per minute and to irrigate the drill to minimize thermal damage to the bone. Besides bone necrosis, high-speed drilling will cause an undesirable enlargement of the drill hole (the drill bit is turned off center by centrifugal forces). Only a precise 1.5-millimeter diameter drill hole will provide maximum holding power for the self-tapping 2.0 millimeter screw. Because the screw pull-out strength is directly related to bone thickness and screw size, bone screws are more stable when placed in the thickest available bone. A 2-millimeter diameter self-tapping screw 6, 8, or 10 millimeters in length is inserted with a screw-holding clamp and tightened snugly (see Figure 33.9b). Adaptation of the plate to the movable portion of the maxilla is con-

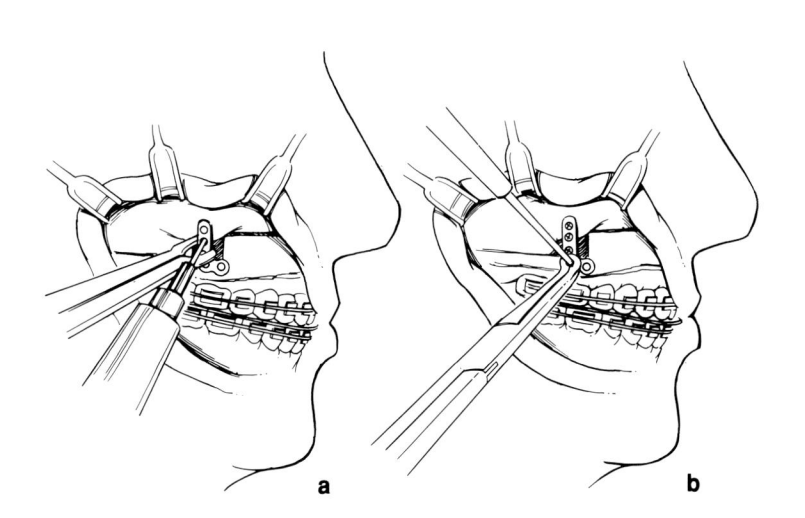

Figure 33.9 (a) A curved bone plate is held in position with plate-holding forceps as bone is drilled with a 1.5-millimeter drill bit. (b) A 2-millimeter diameter self-tapping screw is held in place with a screw-holding clamp and tightened snugly with a Phillips screwdriver. The proximal and distal segments are stabilized with four screws.

firmed. If necessary, the screw can be loosened somewhat and the plate can be rotated to achieve the desired location and the adaptation to the underlying bone. To fix the maxilla in the desired position, a second screw is inserted into the outermost hole of the stable proximal portion of the zygoma and tightened. Osteosynthesis is completed when the third and fourth screws are sequentially placed in the two innermost holes adjacent to the osteotomy site.

Next, the appropriate bone plate is positioned and stabilized to the opposite zygoma. The method of stabilizing the bone plates is based upon individual anatomical and planned positional considerations. Numerous and varied methods are utilized. Final stabilization of the repositioned maxilla is achieved with two additional bone plates, trial-fitted passively and secured to the piriform rim areas. Depending on the individual anatomical situation, four-hole, slightly curved, T-, or L-shaped plates are utilized. Typical means of stabilization of the variations of the Le Fort I osteotomy design are presented in Figure 33.10.

Fixation of the traditional Le Fort I osteotomy following maxillary advancement with superior repositioning can be achieved with piriform miniplates combined with posterior miniplates in the zygomatic buttress region or with zygomatic suspension wires secured to the buccal tube on the maxillary first molar. The lack of sufficient bone thickness along the lateral and anterior maxillary walls frequently encountered in the hypoplastic maxilla may preclude the use of screw and/or plate osteosynthesis. Occasionally, planned telescoping of the lateral maxillary walls following superior repositioning enables positional screws to be placed in the anterior. Additional stability to resist posterior relapse can be achieved by "sandwiching" corticocancellous bone grafts between the telescoped maxillary segments with positional screws and/or plates. Fixation of the step osteotomy can be achieved with either anterior piriform miniplates combined with posterior zygomatic suspension wires or with miniplates. Fixation of the high Le Fort I osteotomy is accomplished with positional screws in the zygomatic root combined with miniplates or screw osteosynthesis and interpositional bone grafts at the piriform aperture.

By subperiosteal tunneling at the lateral and inferior aspects of the piriform aperture, and with careful retraction and visualization, the surgeon can assess the anatomy of the inferior and lateral piriform rim areas. Here the lateral and medial walls of the maxilla become confluent to form a relatively thick and discernible buttress of bone. Placement of bone screws through both cortices of this thickened bone usually provides a means

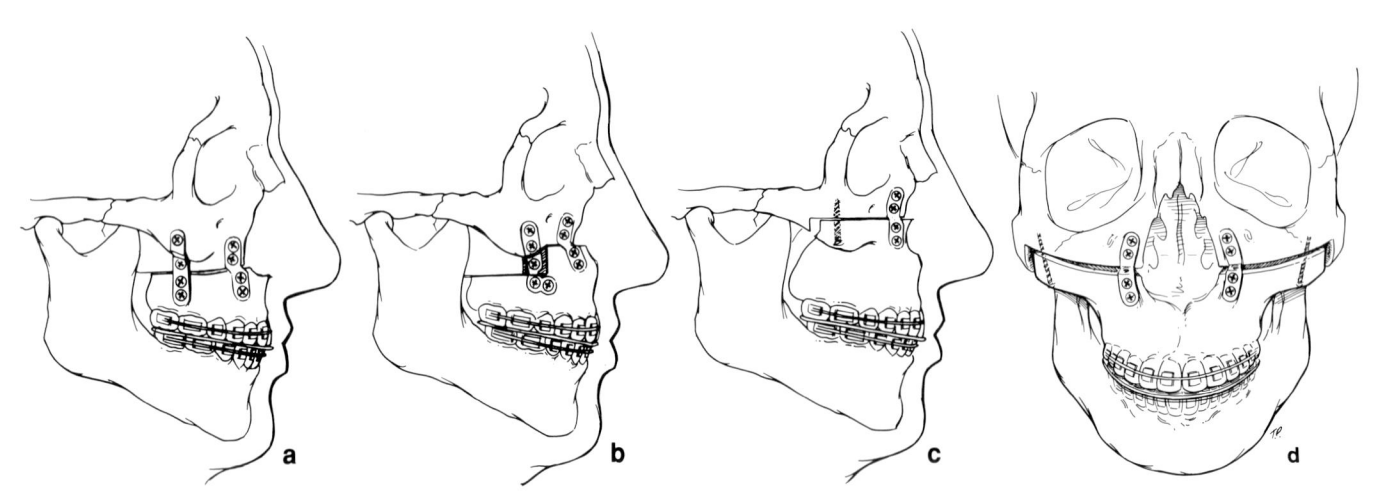

Figure 33.10 Typical means of fixation of the variations of the Le Fort I osteotomy. (a) Fixation of the traditional Le Fort I osteotomy following maxillary advancement with superior repositioning can be achieved with piriform miniplates combined with posterior miniplates in the zygomatic buttress region (shown here) or with zygomatic suspension wires secured to the buccal tube on the maxillary first molar. The lack of sufficient bone thickness along the lateral and anterior maxillary walls frequently encountered in the hypoplastic maxilla may preclude the use of screw and/or plate osteosynthesis. Occasionally, planned telescoping of the lateral maxillary walls following superior repositioning enables positional screws to be placed in the anterior. Additional stability to resist posterior relapse can be achieved by "sandwiching" corticocancellous bone grafts between the telescoped maxillary segments with positional screws and/or plates. (b) Fixation of the maxillary step osteotomy can be achieved with either anterior piriform miniplates combined with posterior miniplates (shown here) or with zygomatic suspension wires. (c) Fixation for the high Le Fort I osteotomy design is accomplished with positional screws in the zygomatic root combined with miniplates or screw osteosynthesis and interpositional bone grafts at the piriform aperture (lateal view). (d) Augmentation of the malar bones and the infraorbital and paranasal areas is frequently accomplished with alloplastics or corticocancellous bone grafts. Implants are frequently used to augment the zygomas and infraorbital areas (A-P view).

of stabilizing a bone plate in the anterior part of the maxilla. The relatively thick inferior aspect of the piriform rim of the repositioned segment consistently provides stable anchorage.

Finally, MMF is released and the stability of the maxilla is confirmed. With superior digital pressure in the angles of the mandible to maintain the proper relationship between condyle and fossa, the mandible is rotated closed into the occlusal splint. The mandible should index passively and precisely into the splint without interferences or condylar shifts. In selected patients, when the maxilla has not been segmented and stable occlusion has been achieved, the occlusal splint may be removed and the patient allowed to function immediately.

The failure to remove adequate bone from the posterior and medial aspects of the repositioned maxilla is probably the single most important cause of apparent "relapse" and anterior "open bite" after surgery. If premature contacts and open bite exist after release of MMF, the rigid fixation is removed and the entire procedure is repeated until the mandible can be rotated passively into the desired relationship.

Segmentation of Maxilla

Presently, about 75% of all patients undergoing orthognathic surgery are treated by the Le Fort I downfracture and various mandibular surgical procedures. Maxillary repositioning is accomplished in approximately two thirds of patients treated by sectioning the maxilla into two, three, or four segments (Bell, 1984). Many technical modifications of this versatile technique are feasible to facilitate simultaneous anterior-posterior, vertical, or horizontal movements of the maxilla. Space closure, arch alignment, leveling, and increased arch length can be accomplished by vertical interdental osteotomies. The design of the osseous and soft-tissue incisions is individualized to maintain the largest possible dento-osseous segment and to preserve the maximum viable soft-tissue pedicle.

Three- and Four-Segment Le Fort I Osteotomies

Interdental osteotomies are frequently made in the canine-lateral incisor interspaces with relatively little risk to the contiguous teeth (see Figure 33.11). The planned changes must be carefully simulated by correlated model surgery and cephalometric planning studies. Segmentation of the anterior maxilla to improve the axial inclination of the anterior teeth and to increase arch length without ostectomy or extractions is the treatment of choice in selected cases. When interdental osteotomies produce large spaces between the teeth, bone grafts or hydroxyapatite may be placed between the margins of the sectioned bone to stabilize and consolidate the segments and obviate periodontal problems. Hydroxyapatite is not used when teeth are to be orthodontically repositioned into an alveolar graft site after surgery. In such cases autogenous particulate marrow is routinely used.

Two-Segment Le Fort I Osteotomy

Increasing the arch length by sectioning the maxilla into two segments by parasagittal palatal osteotomy can facilitate correction of moderately crowded and rotated incisors (see Figure 33.12). Additionally, an ideal Class I canine relationship can be achieved by widening or narrowing the maxilla. The inferior aspect of the expanded maxilla is stabilized with an interocclusal splint; the superior portion may be stabilized adjunctively with a mini bone plate fixed across the interdental osteotomy site. A bone graft or hydroxyapatite (see Chapter 35) may also be placed between the margins of the expanded segments.

When the interocclusal splint is removed, a new arch wire is placed to maintain horizontal stability and to facilitate alignment of the anterior teeth by closure of the interincisal space. If the posterior part of the maxilla is widened significantly, horizontal stability is maintained with a transpalatal arch or acrylic splint. The facility to achieve additional maxillary expansion is another advantage of the transpalatal arch.

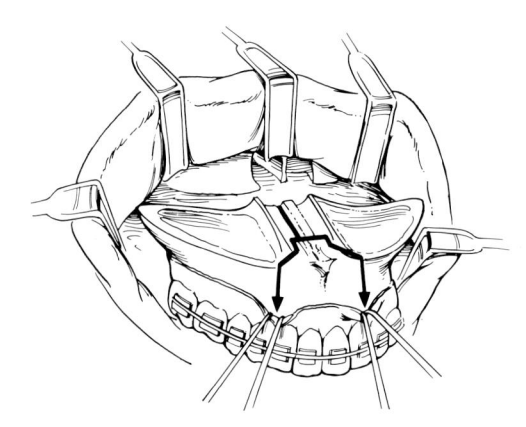

Figure 33.11 Sectioning the maxilla into three segments by Le Fort I osteotomy. In the canine-lateral incisor region there is usually a wider and thicker zone of keratinized gingiva than is normally found in the canine-premolar region, where there is frequently a high frenum attachment and a narrower and thinner band of keratinized gingiva. Consequently, healing of a vertical incision made in this area is usually uncomplicated, and dehiscence of the wound margins is rare. Vertical interdental osteotomies in the lateral incisor-canine interspaces are connected by a U-shaped transpalatal osteotomy distal to the incisive canal; the posterior aspect of the maxilla is sectioned parasagittally.

Figure 33.12 (a) Two-segment Le Fort I osteotomy to increase anterior maxillary arch length. The parasagittal palatal bone is sectioned with a No. 703 fissure bur in the area midway between the midpalatal suture and the junction of the horizontal and vertical parts of the maxilla. (b) Widening the maxilla and increasing anterior arch length by two-segment Le Fort I osteotomy. (c) After the interocclusal splint is removed, a new arch wire is placed to maintain horizontal osseous stability and to facilitate alignment of the anterior teeth by closure of interincisal space.

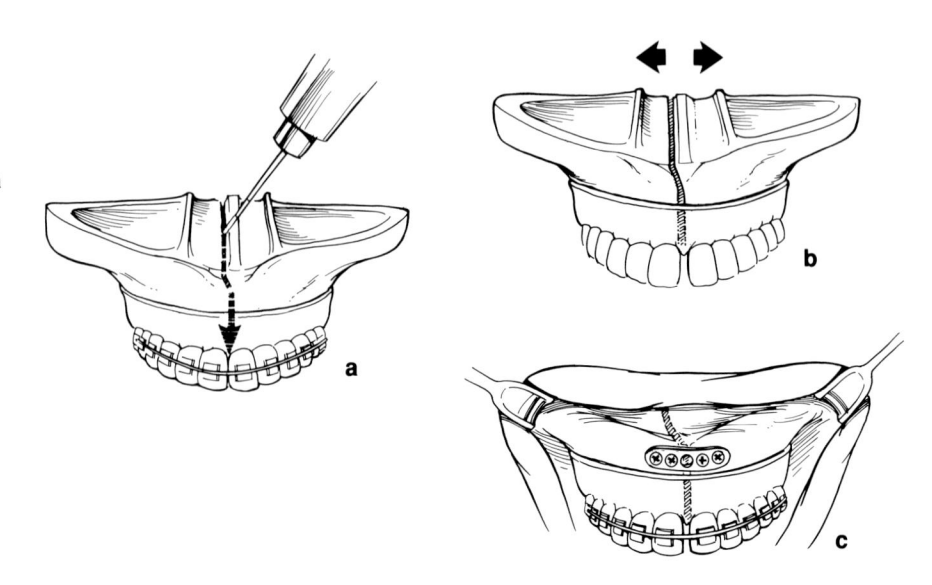

It should be realized that even the placement of very rigid plates beside the piriform aperture and the zygomatic buttress may not prevent transverse relapse of a parasagittally sectioned maxilla. To maintain the desired width, a prefabricated, strong transpalatal arch or splint should be inserted after surgery. The patient should wear this appliance for at least the first four to six months after surgery.

Inferior Repositioning of the Maxilla

The successful use of mini bone plates does not depend on an absolute bony stop. If, for example, an increased vertical or anterior-posterior space between osseous margins is desired, bone plates are initially used to stabilize the maxilla. Then an autogenous bone graft is wedged into the osseous defect.

The stability of the inferiorly repositioned maxilla may be improved by altering the geometric design and position of the lateral maxillary osteotomy so that interfaces between the margins of the segments are favorable. Additionally, rigid skeletal fixation is employed routinely to increase the vertical stability of the inferiorly repositioned maxilla. Anteriorly, the lateral maxillary osteotomy is usually made as low as feasible with a tapered reciprocating saw blade in the thicker part of the maxilla. This osteotomy design maximizes the interface between the maxilla and the interposed bone graft and facilitates miniplate osteosynthesis. In effect, based on clinical and radiographic studies, the anterior maxillary height may usually be increased while an unfavorable increase of the posterior maxillary height is minimized. The repositioned maxilla is stabilized with two anterior and two posterior bone plates. Sequentially, the anterior aspect of the maxilla is fixed in the planned vertical position with a bone plate on either side.

When anteroposterior maxillary deficiency is corrected, stabilization of the anteriorly repositioned maxilla is vital. Vertical osteotomies in the root of the zygoma or zygomatic maxillary buttress provide an excellent site for bone grafting and bone plate osteosynthesis.

Downsliding Technique

When anteroposterior maxillary deficiency is associated with vertical maxillary deficiency, the surgical plan should include maxillary advancement in addition to correction of the vertical discrepancy. In selected cases, both corrections may be achieved by a downward and forward sliding movement of the maxilla. The lateral maxillary osteotomy designs are individualized. The osteotomy is angled so as to provide an inclined plane that will increase the vertical dimension as the maxilla slides forward. The horizontal length from the piriform rim to the lateral aspect of the zygoma is measured on a lateral cephalogram. From this measurement the downward angulation of the osteotomy and position of the vertical step are calculated.

Anteriorly, an angulated cut extends from high on the lateral aspect of the zygoma to low on the anterior piriform rim. Posteriorly, the osteotomy is directed inferiorly and medially at a 45-degree angle to the pterygoid plate. As the maxilla is advanced, bony defects are created at the vertical steps. In selected cases of minimal vertical maxillary deficiency, the lip-to-tooth relationship and anteroposterior deficiency can be corrected solely by the Le Fort I downsliding technique. When vertical maxillary deficiency is more severe, the Le Fort I osteotomy is combined with interpositional bone grafting.

Technical Disadvantages and Complications

Since 1984 the modified Le Fort I downfracture technique described in this chapter has been used frequently but selectively to reposition the maxilla in all three planes of space to achieve excellent skeletal and occlusal stability. Although the procedures are technically more demanding than the traditional Le Fort I osteotomy technique, relatively few problems have been experienced. Segmentation of the posterior part of the maxilla, where the lateral maxillary walls are frequently thin and friable, can produce undesirable fracturing and instability. In two patients, inadvertent fracturing occurred through the zygomaticomaxillary area. In both these patients, the fractured segment was stabilized as a free graft with a bone plate.

Certain positional movements of the maxilla are difficult and potentially problematic: excessive posterior and superior repositioning of the maxilla is technically difficult because more areas of bony contact must be meticulously reduced to facilitate passive adaptation of the margins of the osteotomized segments. Finally, asymmetric movement of the maxilla may produce asymmetric prominence of the zygomas. Such problems are minimized by individualizing the osteotomy design.

SAGITTAL SPLIT RAMUS OSTEOTOMY

The sagittal split ramus osteotomy (SSRO) allows two-dimensional skeletal changes of the mandible. This osteotomy configuration offers a broad area of bone contact for stability and bone healing. It also lends itself to stabilization using rigid fixation techniques. Its most frequent indication is for the treatment of mandibular deficiency alone or in combination with correction of maxillary deformities (see Figure 33.13). The SSRO may also be used to treat situations of mandibular excess when a vertical change and an anteroposterior change are anticipated because it provides better bone contact than may be possible with the intraoral vertical subcondylar procedure.

We believe that the sagittal split osteotomy technique as described below has certain advantages over the Obwegeser–Dal Pont technique (Dal Pont 1961, Trauner 1957a, 1957b). Because the horizontal bone incision of the vertical ramus is much shorter, the surgery is easier to execute. Most of the medial pterygoid and masseter muscle attachment on the segments is retained. Increased blood supply to the proximal segment is enhanced. The previously "blind" aspects of the surgical technique are eliminated, and stripping of the masseteric–pterygoid sling is not necessary. As a result, the proximal segment of the mandible, with most of the masseter and pterygoid muscles attached, maintains the same spatial relationship that existed before surgery. Consequently, there is minimal anatomic or functional change in the muscle and bone relationship of the proximal segment. In addition, nuances in osteotomy design and execution, based on anatomic studies, are intended to minimize the likelihood of damage to the inferior alveolar nerve and to optimize conditions for the application of rigid fixation.

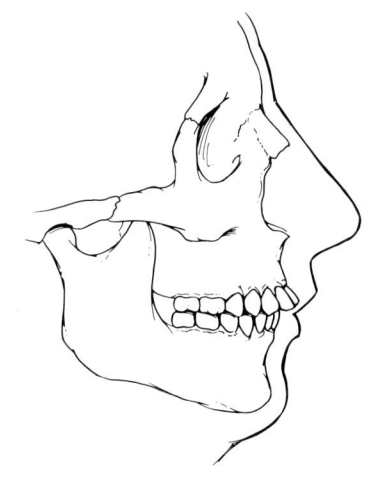

Figure 33.13 Typical dental, skeletal, and facial features of mandibular deficiency are shown with the mandible in centric relation and lips relaxed: The mandible is retropositioned; the lower lip is procumbent and everted; and a Class II malocclusion is present.

This section presents the author's techniques of SSRO and its rigid fixation for the treatment of mandibular deficiency.

Techniques of the Sagittal Split Ramus Osteotomy (SSRO)

Exposure

After the patient is positioned on the operating table and the oropharynx is packed, the mouth is stabilized in an open position with a prop. Adequate lighting for the intraoral sagittal splitting technique is mandatory, and either a fiberoptic system or a headlight is suggested. When hypotensive anesthesia is not used, local anesthesia (such as lidocaine 2%) with a vasoconstrictor (such as epinephrine 1:200,000) is infiltrated along the lateral oblique ridge, along the medial aspect of the vertical ramus, and inferolaterally in the molar region of the mandible. Transection of the buccal artery as it transverses the vertical ramus, herniation of the buccal fat pad into the surgical site, and difficulty in closing the mucosal incision because of inadequate access to the jaws following MMF are problems commonly experienced with the intraoral approach to the

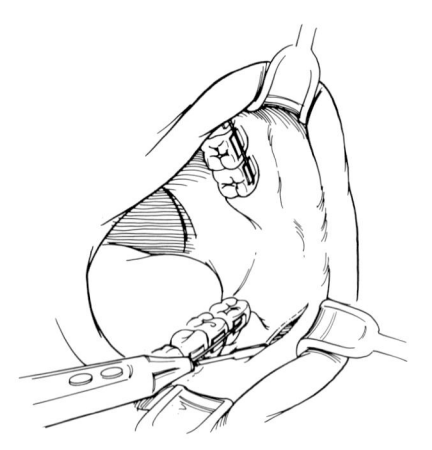

Figure 33.14 The mucosal incision is made in the lateral aspect of the buccal vestibule opposite the second and third molar areas over the external oblique ridge.

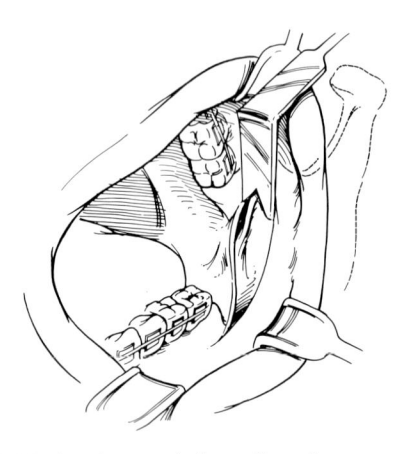

Figure 33.15 An elevator helps reflect the temporalis tendon. The coronoid process is exposed with a V-shaped right-angle notch retractor that is positioned against the anterior and inferior aspect of the coronoid process.

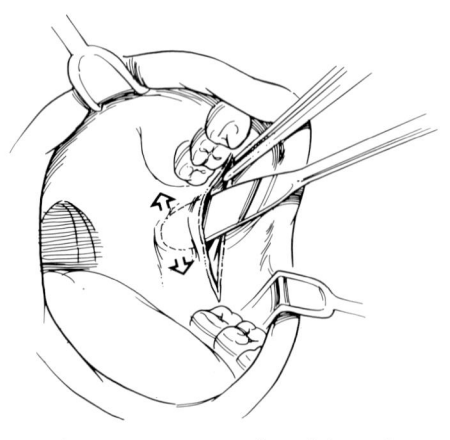

Figure 33.16 The periosteum is reflected from the anterior and medial aspect of the ramus superior to the lingula and carried to a point immediately posterior to the neurovascular bundle. The arrows indicate the area of subperiosteal tunneling.

vertical ramus. Such problems are minimized by using a modified soft-tissue incision in the mucogingival fold, carrying it parallel with the posterior teeth from the area opposite the third molar to the area opposite the first molar (Booth 1976) (see Figure 33.14). After the initial incision through the mucosa, the wound margins are separated to expose the underlying buccinator muscle. Care should be taken to prevent incising the most superior fibers of the buccinator muscle. Leaving the superior fibers intact prevents herniation of the buccal fat pad into the operative field. Any portion of the buccinator muscle that is not incised easily can be retracted superiorly to expose the anterior border of the ramus (see Figure 33.15).

The muscle and periosteum are detached from the underlying bone with a periosteal elevator. Minimal subperiosteal dissection is performed on the lateral aspect of the mandibular ramus to maintain the attachment of the masseter muscle. A subperiosteal dissection is extended inferolaterally to the area of the antegonial notch. Two periosteal elevators are then placed in the superior aspect of the soft-tissue incision to reflect the mucoperiosteum superiorly away from the coronoid process. A V-shaped right-angle notch retractor positioned against the anterior and inferior aspect of the coronoid process is retracted superiorly by the assistant to facilitate the surgeon's stripping off the muscular and tendinous attachments of the temporalis muscle until the coronoid notch is exposed (see Figure 33.15). A relatively small mucobuccal fold incision provides adequate access to the surgical site owing to the extensibility of the soft tissues.

The medial periosteal reflection is extended posteriorly by subperiosteal tunneling to expose the medial surface of the ramus from the anterior border above the lingula and mandibular foramen to a position immediately posterior to the lingula (see Figure 33.16). Care should be exercised to avoid damaging the inferior alveolar nerve, artery, and vein, which will be enclosed in a neurovascular bundle of periosteum (see Figure 33.17). Only the superior aspect of the neurovascular bundle is visualized. The neurovascular bundle generally enters the mandibular foramen inferior to the occlusal plane of the mandibular teeth or at about the midpoint of the ramus superoinferiorly (Bremer 1952). It is commonly believed that the mandibular foramen is at the midpoint of the ramus both anteroposteriorly and superoinferiorly. Rather, the mandibular foramen is located about two-thirds of the distance from the anterior to the posterior border of the ramus (Rajchel 1985, Hayward 1977).

One end of a dental curette is placed in the sigmoid notch for the purpose of orientation. The lingual subperiosteal tunnel facilitates placement of a modified lingual-channel retractor without damaging the lingual flap or neurovascular bundle (see Figure 33.17). The modified retractors can be placed along the lingual aspect of the mandible with minimal soft-tissue reflection. Proper positioning of the retractor provides adequate visualization and accessibility for the lingual osteotomy. Excessive medial retraction is unnecessary; it may stretch the inferior alveolar nerve and also risks laceration or stretching of the nerve and vessels over the sharp edge of the mandibular foramen.

Osteotomy

The cut on the medial aspect of the mandible is normally accomplished first. With the medial channel retractor in place, the medial surface of the mandible can be easily observed (see Figure 33.17). Only rarely is it necessary to reduce the superior extension of the internal oblique ridge with a large, round bur to facilitate visualization of the medial surface of the mandible. A horizontal osteotomy is then made with a Lindemann bur or reciprocating saw (see Figure 33.18) on a plane parallel to the occlusal plane. This horizontal cut is placed at a level immediately above the mandibular foramen and the inferior alveolar neurovascular bundle. The horizontal cut is made at or near the tip of the lingula through the lingual cortex to a depth equivalent to half the medial-lateral thickness of the ramus from the area immediately posterior to the inferior alveolar neurovascular bundle to the anterior border of the mandible.

Clinical experience (Wolford 1987), now substantiated by anatomic studies (Smith 1988), has shown that positioning the medial osteotomy at or near the tip of the lingula places the cut beneath the position of fusion of the buccal and lingual cortical plates. The cancellous bone between the two plates allows a plane in which a favorable surgical fracture can take place.

Multiple small holes are drilled into the cancellous bone along the anterior border of the ramus, medial to the lateral oblique line, to facilitate the sagittal osteotomy. A No. 702 or 703 tapered fissure bur is used to continue the osteotomy along the anterior border of the ascending ramus (see Figure 33.19). The depth of the cut along the anterior border of the ascending ramus should be maintained parallel to the sagittal plane of the ramus. Care should be taken to keep the depth of the cut from impinging on the inferior alveolar nerve canal. The sagittal cut is carried anteriorly and inferiorly to connect with the planned vertical osteotomy at the lateral aspect of the body of the mandible.

At the junction of the first and second molar teeth, the lateral body cut is made perpendicular to the inferior border of the mandible, down to bleeding bone or the marrow-vascular space (see Figure 33.20). The cortex is cut with a reciprocating saw blade.

In order to make the sagittal split occur more easily and to allow the split to occur along the inferior border rather than higher on the lingual side, we carry the lateral vertical osteotomy completely through the

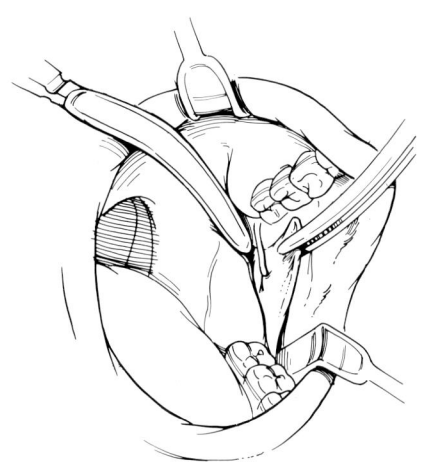

Figure 33.17 The end of the periosteal elevator or Henhan retractor is positioned immediately superior and posterior to the neurovascular bundle to facilitate visualization of the medial surface of the ramus.

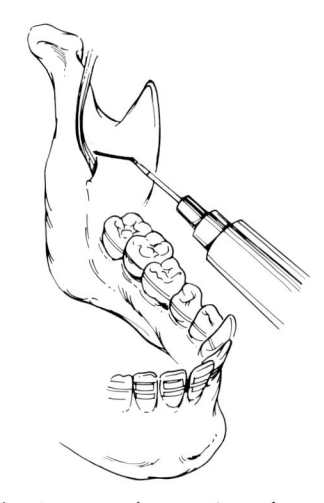

Figure 33.18 A laminectomy bur sections the medial vertical plate. The beveled horizontal medial cut is positioned as close to the lingula as possible. The beveled cut (30 to 35 degrees) is made to minimize irregularities between the proximal and distal segments.

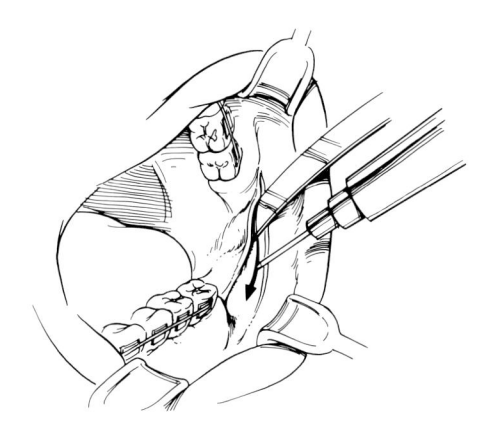

Figure 33.19 The fissure bur continues the cut anteriorly medial to the external oblique ridge.

Figure 33.20 (a) At the junction of the first and second molar teeth, the osteotomy is carried vertically to the inferior border of the mandible. (b) The lateral vertical cut in the first and second molar region is made tangential to the buccal surface of the bone (posterior bevel) to facilitate precise positioning and visualization of the special reciprocating saw blade that is used to section the inferior border of the mandible. (c) The inferior border of the mandible is split by blades that are offset to the left or right side to provide access for cutting on either side of the mandible. The cut is commenced anteriorly adjacent to the vertical buccal osteotomy. The blade (hidden by lingual cortex) is oriented so that the cutting edge is parallel to the inferior border of the mandible as it bisects the buccal-lingual thickness of the cortex. The 5-millimeter height of the blade allows it to penetrate the inferior border cortex without damaging the neurovascular bundle. The reciprocating action of the blade is started at low speed and sunk to the approximate depth before the speed is increased. The blade is then directed posteriorly to the distal aspect of the antegonial notch area. It is next directed immediately lingual so that it will exit through the lingual cortex anterior to the angle of the mandible at the area of the gonial notch. The reciprocating saw's handpiece and blade should be oriented so that the blade will cut maximally up into the bone. The blade is oriented parallel to the inferior border of the mandible and should bisect the buccal-lingual thickness of the inferior border cortex. Once the saw blade has been engaged, the handpiece is rotated superiorly so that the triangular blade can cut most efficiently. The rounded shaft of the inferior aspect of the blade limits the blade from excessive vertical sectioning into the osteotomy area. The inferior border of the mandible cut is started adjacent to the vertical buccal osteotomy.

inferior cortex (Epker 1975, Wolford 1987, 1990). The osteotomy is accomplished with a specially designed reciprocating sawblade. The blade extends vertically up from the inferior border at a maximum cutting depth of 5 millimeters. A recent anatomic study (Rajchel 1985) indicates that the minimum distance from the inferior aspect to the inferior border was just over 5 millimeters, thereby making the inferior sawblade safe when used from the second molar posteriorly.

The osteotomy should be inspected to ensure that the bleeding marrow-vascular space is noted throughout the entire course of the osteotomy. Failure to complete the cortical bone cuts prior to initiating a sagittal split of the mandible may result in an unfavorable fracture. Selection of the junction of the first and second molar teeth as the position of the vertical osteotomy is based on knowledge of the mediolateral position of the canal as it courses through the mandible. A recent study addressing this area showed that the distance from the medial aspect of the buccal cortical plate to the mandibular canal (horizontal medullary bone width) was significantly greater at the distal half of the first molar than at any other area of the posterior body or ramus of the mandible. The mean distance from the mandibular canal to the buccal plate of bone was 4.05 millimeters at the first molar, 3.61 millimeters at the second molar, 1.72 millimeters at the third molar, and 1.97 millimeters immediately anterior to the mandibular foramen. (One standard deviation for each section was 1.1 millimeters) (Rajchel 1985).

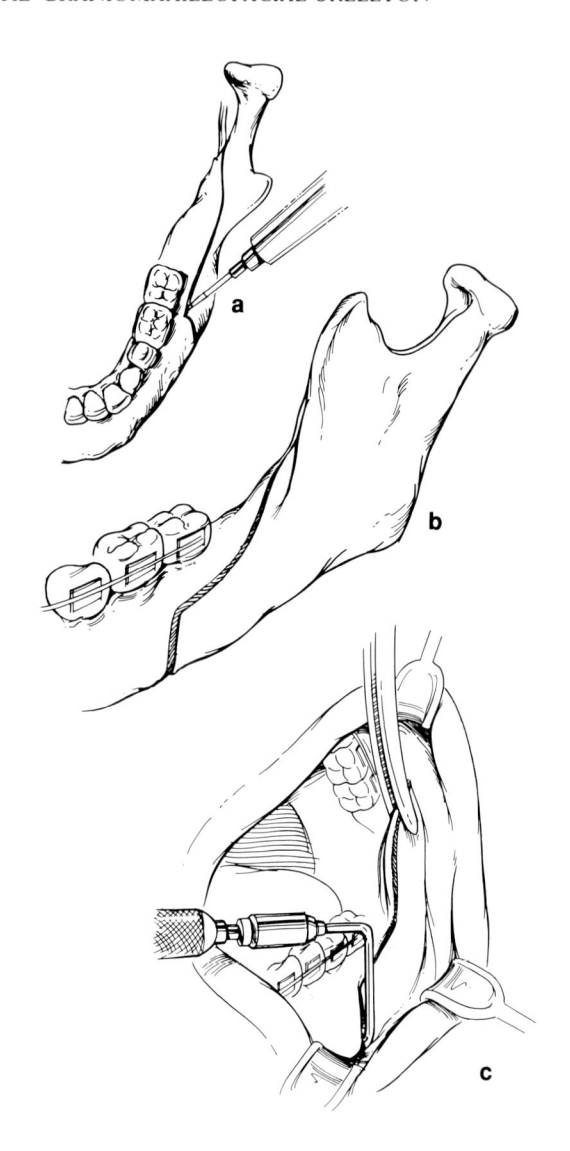

A spatula osteotome with a finely tapered blade is malleted inferiorly with light taps into the sagittal osteotomy site at the junction of the sagittal and vertical osteotomies in the first and second molar regions. The osteotome, directed parallel to the lateral cortex of the ramus, is malleted carefully to section the body of the mandible at the juncture of the buccal cortical plate and the intramedullary bone. The osteotome must not be malleted too deeply to obviate the possibility of transecting the inferior alveolar neurovascular bundle. A second osteotome, similar in size to the first, is malleted into the sagittal osteotomy site slightly posterior to the

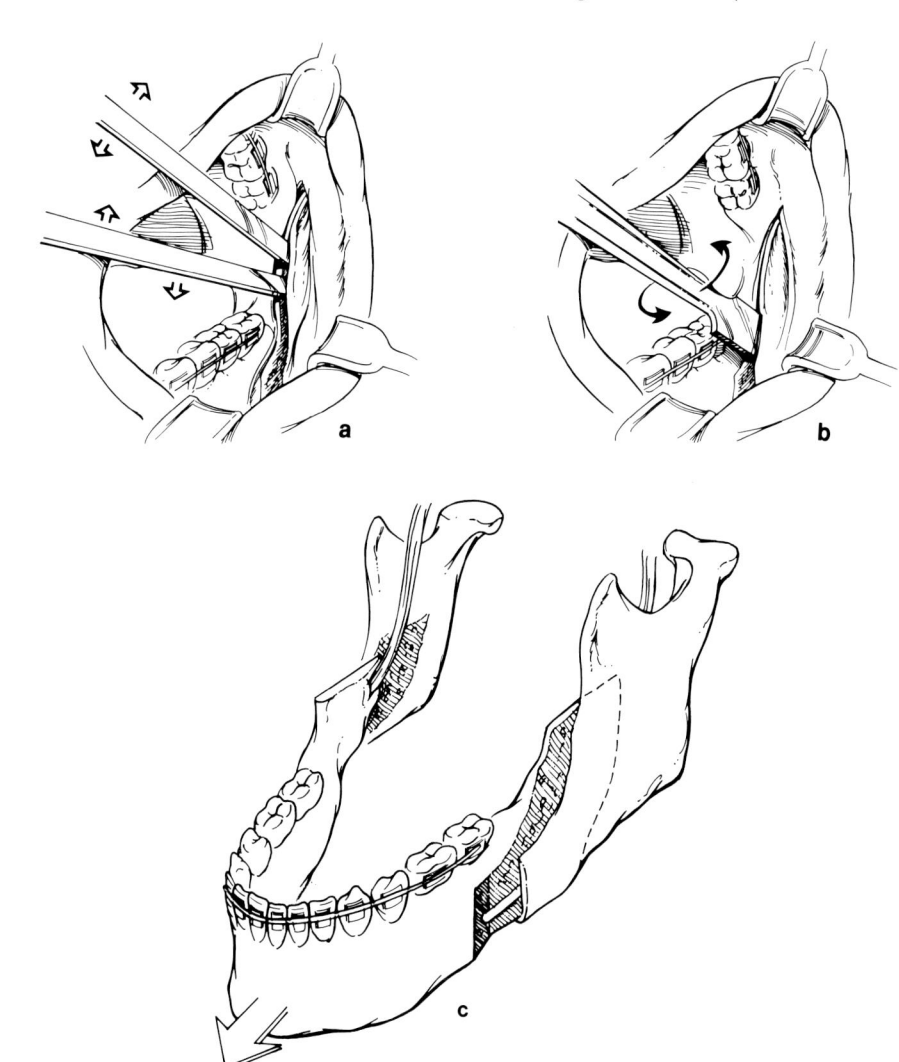

Figure 33.21 (a) Spatula osteotomes are malleted to partially section the body of the mandible. Care is taken to keep the spatula osteotomes directed just subjacent to the cortical plate to prevent damage to the neurovascular bundle. If the mandible splits, care is taken to visualize the course of the neurovascular bundle to make sure that portions of the nerve are not contained in the proximal condylar segment. A curved osteotome is used to partially split the lateral-medial aspect of the ramus. An osteotome is levered against the distal segment to apply force against the inner surface of the proximal segment. An orthopedic osteotome is inserted in the split and twisted to separate the ramus segments. (b) A bileveled osteotome is utilized to pry the mandibular segments apart. Bone anterior to the vertical cut should be used as the principal fulcrum. If separation is not complete, a splitting chisel completes the cut at the inferior border of the mandible. (c) Completeness of separation is verified by grasping the proximal and distal segments and moving them apart in an anterior–posterior direction and inspecting for full separation.

previously placed osteotome. A small, finely tapered, sharp, curved osteotome is malleted between the sectioned bony margins at the inferior border of the body of the mandible at the junction of the incompletely sectioned proximal and distal bone fragments (see Figure 33.21a). The osteotome is carefully malleted parallel to the sagittal plane of the mandibular body to facilitate sectioning of the inferior border of the mandible. The maneuver tends to eliminate the "bad split" caused by incomplete sectioning of the inferior border of the mandible. Next, the osteotome is levered against the lateral aspect of the distal segment so that force is directed laterally against the inner surface of the proximal segment. When there is resistance to separation of the proximal and distal segments, all the bone incisions are carefully re-examined to be certain that the osteotomies have been made completely through the cortical bone into the underlying cancellous bone. Then the levering manipulations against the proximal and distal margins are repeated. In most cases the entire ramus can be split in this manner. If the proximal and distal segments are not split, a thin osteotome is lightly malleted between the sectioned bone margins of the anterior border of the ascending ramus at the juncture of the buccal cortical plate and the intramedullary bone.

After the mandible is split, a larger orthopedic osteotome is then inserted in the anterior aspect of the sagittal osteotomy (see Figure 33.21b). (These large osteotomes are not used when the width of the mandible is small.) The surgeon may use two osteotomes to test the completeness of the osteotomy cut by gently twisting the blades and noting whether the ramus fragments separate. Care should be taken to ensure that the osteotome does not impinge on the inferior alveolar neurovascular bundle as the instrument is directed between the lateral and medial fragments of the ramus. Final splitting is completed by gentle twisting or prying with either one or both osteotomes. As the osteotome separates the medial and lateral fragments of the ramus, the cutting blade of the instrument should be directed against the inner surface of the cortex of the proximal fragment. The contents of the mandibular canal are usually visualized at this time, and care should be taken to ensure that no portions of the contents of the mandibular canal are adhering to the lateral (proximal) fragment. It may be necessary to detach the nerve carefully from the bony trabeculae in the proximal segment. After the neurovascular bundle is exposed and visualized within an incomplete split, the split is completed by malleting a spatula osteotome through the inferior border of the mandible. The residual attachments of the medial pterygoid muscle to the distal segment are detached with a periosteal elevator through the distracted proximal and distal segments. The same procedure is accomplished on the opposite side. When the inferior alveolar neurovascular bundle is entrapped in the mandibular canal in the proximal segment and the planned movement is minimal, it may be unnecessary to expose and detach the nerve from the body trabeculae in the proximal segment. The distal segment may be advanced because the nerve can stretch when the segment is moved only a short distance.

Stabilization with Rigid Fixation

Many studies that have critically evaluated skeletal stability of mandibular advancement using nonrigid fixation have documented a high incidence of significant relapse (Behrman 1972, Guernsey 1971, Lysell 1960, McNeill 1973, Sandor 1984). The rigid fixation of sagittal osteotomies has shown great promise in reduction of relapse as well as having advantages of patient comfort and easy jaw mobilization and return to function (Paulus 1982, Spiessl 1976b, Van Sickels 1985a, 1986). Before rigid fixation of the osteotomized segments, MMF in the planned occlusion is achieved with anterior intermaxillary wires and posterior circummandibular wires. The proximal segment is gently manipulated, positioned, and stabilized with a ramus pusher; extraoral superiorly directed digital pressure at the posterior ramus and simultaneous counter pressure with the ramus pusher at the anterior portion of the ramus produces a net anterosuperior force on the condyle (see Figure 33.22). We prefer the placement of position screws as our means of rigid stabilization. When the transcutaneous approach is used, access to the osteotomy site for screw placement is gained through a stab skin incision 1 to 2 centimeters above the inferior border of the mandible in the area of the gonial notch. Following infiltration of the cheek with local anesthetic, a 4- to 5-millimeter incision is made through the skin only. A pointed trocar is introduced through the lumina of the drill guide and bluntly dissected through the underlying muscle and periosteum to the lateral surface of the ramus. Once the end of the drill guide is exposed intraorally, a self-retaining retractor holds the cheek tissues on the inner side away from the end of the drill guide and stabilizes the guide, allowing improved visualization. The necessary bore holes can be drilled and screws placed through one properly placed skin incision (see Figure 33.23). The tissue protractor clamp is used to stabilize the tissue protector and maintain cheek retraction. A neutral drill guide insert is used in concert with the tissue protector. Drill holes through the proximal and distal segments are made with a slowly rotating 1.5-millimeter drill and a mini pin driver. A continuous flow of saline is maintained at the drill–bone interface. After the neutral guide insert is removed, a screw depth gauge is used to determine the millimetric depth of the screw hole. Position screws maintain passive separation of the proximal and distal bony segments. The screws should perforate the lingual cortex and extend 1 millimeter deeper than the depth of the drill hole to assure bicortical engagement.

The inferior border of the mandible is digitally palpated to simulate the alignment of the inferior border of the mandible, consistent with the cephalometric prediction studies. The proximal and distal segments are stabilized passively in the desired position with a modified bone clamp positioned at the area of maximum bone contact. After the drill hole is made, a 2-millimeter-diameter screw of the required length is seated in the previously drilled screw hole on a screw-holding instrument. A screwdriver is inserted through the trocar to tighten the screw firmly (see Figure 33.24). The pattern of placement for positional screws depends on the osteotomy design and the availability of bone (see Figure 33.25).

Placement of two screws at the upper border and one at the inferior border is preferred for reasons of

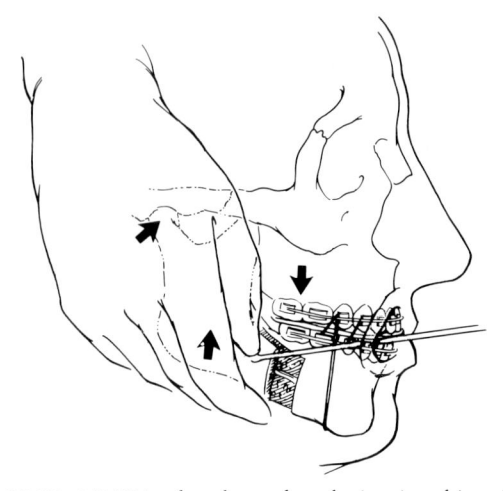

Figure 33.22 MMF in the planned occlusion is achieved with anterior maxillomandibular wires and posterior circummandibular wires. The proximal segment is gently manipulated, positioned, and stabilized with a ramus pusher (wire director); extraoral superiorly directed digital pressure at the posterior ramus and simultaneous counter pressure with the ramus pusher at the anterior portion of the ramus produces a net anterosuperior force on the condyle (arrows).

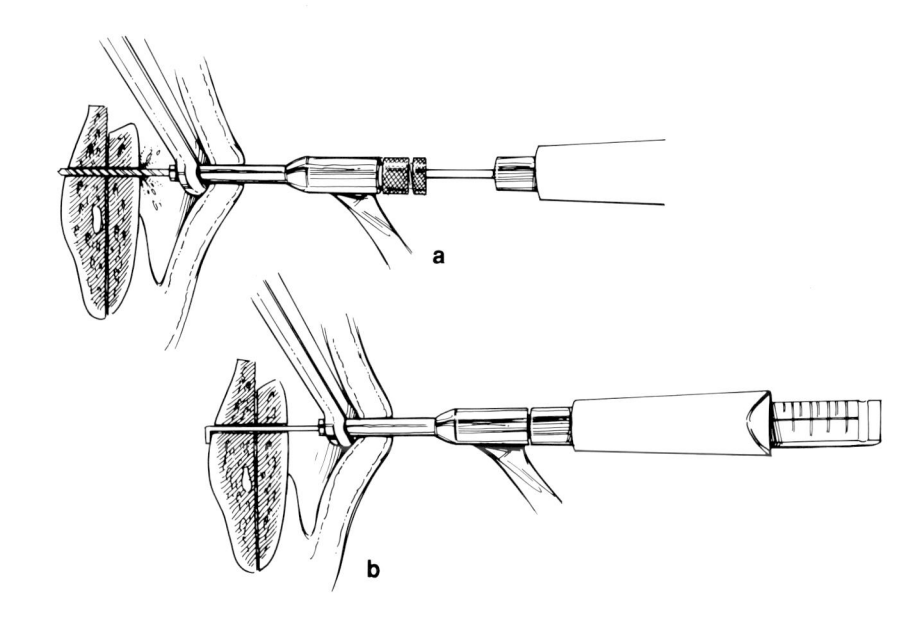

Figure 33.23 (a) The tissue protector clamp is used to stabilize the tissue protector and maintain cheek retraction. A neutral drill guide insert is used in concert with the tissue protector. Drill holes through the proximal and distal segments are made with a slowly rotating 1.5-millimeter drill and a mini pin driver. A continuous flow of saline is maintained at the drill–bone interface. (b) After the neutral guide insert is removed, a screw depth gauge is used to determine the millimetric depth of the screw hole. Position screws maintain passive separation of the proximal and distal bony segments. The screws should perforate the lingual cortex and extend 1 millimeter deeper than the depth of the drill hole to assure bicortical engagement.

access, adequacy of bone stock, and biomechanics. A cadaver study (Smith 1988) showed that both the buccal and lingual cortical plates at the external oblique ridge (superior border) are significantly thicker than those at the inferior border. This increased cortical bone thickness at the superior border is an advantage over the inferior border for the placement of screws. Furthermore, the amount of bone available at the inferior border on the distal segment (lingual cortex) is often compromised because the split frequently occurs high near the mandibular canal (Jonsson 1979). In addition to providing thicker bone for screw purchase, the arrangement of two screws at the superior border and one at the inferior border has theoretical (Speissl 1976a) and experimental (Ardary 1989, Foley 1989) biomechanical advantages. For example, the placement of screws at the superior border would locate the fixation at the tension band (according to the biomechanical model of mandibular fracture (prepared) by Spiessl (Foley 1989) (See also Chapter 14). This would then resist the tendency for postoperative increase in gonial angle and anterior facial height, as well as the tendency for horizontal relapse that was shown to occur after mandibular advancement surgery (Schendel 1980).

Erupted or impacted third molar teeth are extracted 9 to 12 months before surgery. Subsequent healing of the extraction sites minimizes the possibility of a "bad sagittal split" because of the improved contact of the segments and a larger area to place at least two or three screws. Gross interferenes between the proximal and distal segments are removed to facilitate improved apposition of the segments. Splaying of the proximal and distal segments associated with mandibular advancement, asymmetric mandibular movements, and isolated areas of poor contact of the proximal and distal segments may be improved by judicious contouring of the segments. Ideal apposition of the segments is infrequent.

Bicortical screws provide the best osseous stability, but it may not always be possible to place such screws without damaging the underlying teeth. In such cases, miniplates and unicortical screws provide sufficient stabilization of the segments. The plates must be very precisely adapted to the underlying bone to prevent condyle displacement after the screws are tightened. In selected cases, it may be necessary to utilize two plates to achieve the desired stabilization (see Figures 33.26 and 33.27). When rigid fixation methods are utilized, the surgeon must release the MMF after surgery and assess whether the mandible will rotate into the planned position without distraction of the condyle from the fossa. To rotate the mandible into the splint without distracting the condyle, pressure should be applied only beneath the angles, carefully noting initial occlusal contact. If there is positional shifting of the mandibular teeth to achieve a maximum occlusion, the rigid fixation appliances must be removed, MMF must be re-established, and the proximal condylar fragment must be repositioned. Then the rigid fixation appliances are reapplied. It should be possible to rotate the mandible into the planned position repeatedly with minimum effort and without displacement. If an excellent occlusion results and the repositioned segments are stabilized well with rigid fixation appliances, thought can be given to removing the splint and allowing the patient to occlude naturally into a normal Class I occlusion.

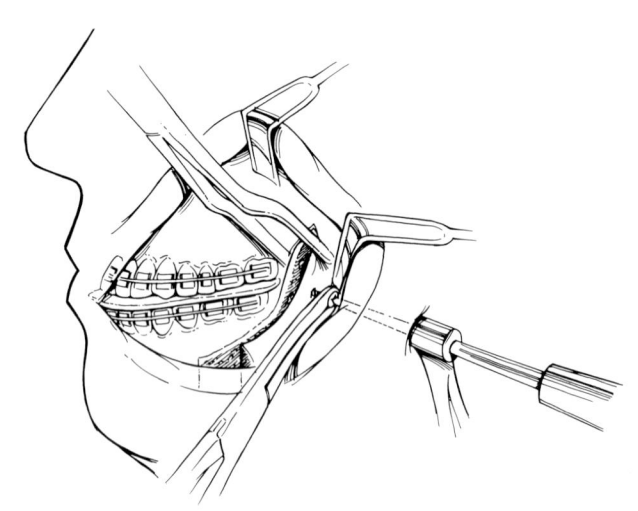

Figure 33.24 The inferior border of the mandible is digitally palpated to simulate the alignment of the inferior border of the mandible, consistent with the cephalometric prediction studies. The proximal and distal segments are stabilized passively in the desired position with a modified bone clamp positioned initially at the area of maximum bone contact. After the drill hole is made, a 2-millimeter-diameter screw of the required length is seated in the previously drilled screw hole on a screw-holding instrument. A Phillips screwdriver is inserted through the trocar to tighten the screw firmly.

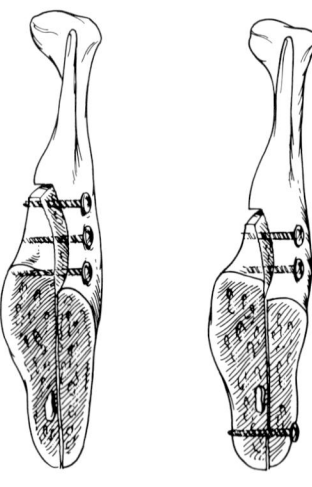

Figure 33.25 The pattern of placement for positional screws depends on the osteotomy design and the availability of bone. On the left, three 2-millimeter-diameter screws are placed through the superior border of the proximal and distal segments. On the right, two 2-millimeter-diameter bicortical screws are placed at the superior border and one or two at the inferior border of the mandible, avoiding the neurovascular canal. This screw placement pattern is usually feasible when the inferior border of the mandible is successfully split. Ideally, the screw at the inferior border of the mandible will transect the cortical portion of the proximal and distal segments.

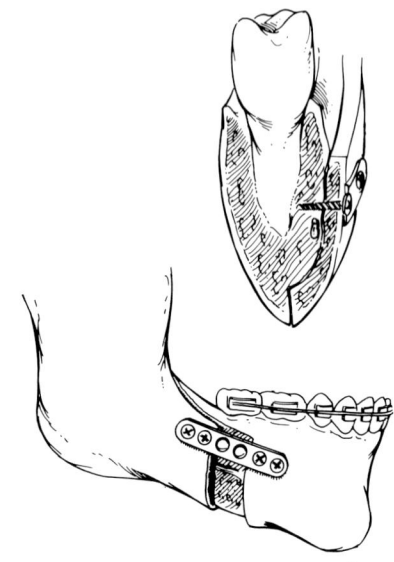

Figure 33.26 Bicortical screws provide good osseous stability, but in selected cases placing such screws without damaging the underlying teeth is impossible. In such cases, unicortical screws used in concert with miniplates usually provide sufficient stabilization of the segments. The plates must be very precisely adapted to the underlying bone to prevent condyle displacement when the screws are tightened. A neutral drill guide is used in concert with a tissue protector to facilitate symmetric drilling of a hole through the outer cortex. An example of such a need is when impacted third molar teeth are removed simultaneously with the sagittal split ramus osteotomy. In selected cases, it may be necessary to use two plates or a larger reconstruction plate to achieve the desired stabilization.

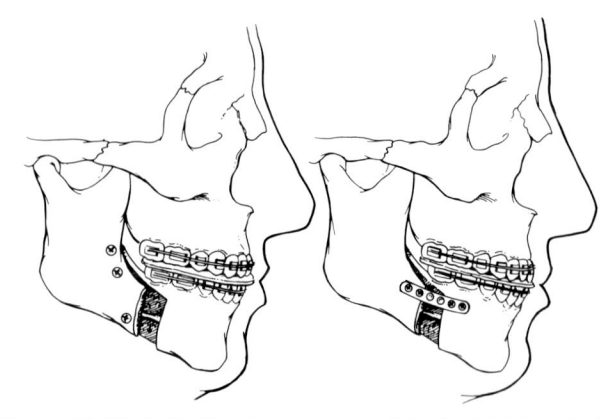

Figure 33.27 (left) Fixation is accomplished with bicortical position screws. (right) Fixation is accomplished with miniplates and unicortical screws.

Neuromuscular Rehabilitation

Following the patient's recovery from surgery, several training elastics are placed to facilitate occlusal and neuromuscular rehabilitation. A day or two after surgery, the occlusion is checked in a clinical environment with good light, suction, and assistance. Laminiographic radiographs of the temporomandibular joints are taken in centric relationship and compared with preoperative radiographs. If the condyle is improperly seated or associated with a shift in centric relationship versus centric occlusion, repositioning of the maxilla and restabilization with rigid skeletal fixation appliances is mandatory.

Light vertical training elastics are placed bilaterally between soldered interproximal lugs attached to maxillary and mandibular orthodontic arch wires in the canine–first-molar interspaces (Bell 1983, Storum 1986). Range-of-motion exercises four or five times per day are usually commenced on the second or third postoperative day. Gentle, assistive, one- or two-handed range-of-motion exercises are usually performed within three to five days after surgery.

Appropriate training elastics are placed during the day and night. Once a stable and desired occlusion has been achieved and the patient has learned habitually to occlude properly, progressively longer periods of daytime use of the mandible without elastics is permitted. The duration of rehabilitation is determined by surgical procedure, patient compliance, individual variability, resultant occlusion, and clinical judgement (Bell 1984). In the absence of a TMJ internal derangement, three to eight weeks of therapeutic exercises is generally adequate to achieve an interincisal opening comparable to the presurgical measurement.

The objectives of occlusal and neuromuscular rehabilitation are to achieve a stable Class I occlusion, adequate interincisal distance, normal protrusive and lateral movements, and functional position of the condyles. Routine monitoring of condylar position is accomplished with open- and closed-mouth laminographic analyses of the temporomandibular joints until translatory movements of the condyles are normalized and the condyles are seated into the glenoid fossae.

CLINICAL EXAMPLES

Case 1

A.S., a 14-year-old student sought treatment to decrease the prominence of her maxillary incisors, improve her smile line, increase the prominence of her chin, and correct her malocclusion (Figure 33.28 a,b,c). Additionally, she was concerned about episodic pain and popping in her right temporomandibular joint. She habitually postured her mandible forward to compensate for her retrognathic mandible and Class II malocclusion, which was associated with vertical maxillary hyperplasia. The results of the clinical assessment implicated the disparity between centric relation and centric occlusion as a possible contributing cause of her mandibular dysfunction (Figure 33.28 m,n,o).

The surgical treatment plan consisted of the following:

1. Two-segment Le Fort I step osteotomy to superiorly reposition the maxilla (7 millimeters in the anterior and 5 millimeters in the posterior), to reduce the interlabial gap and amount of incisor exposure, and to widen the maxilla.
2. Bilateral sagittal split ramus osteotomies to advance the mandible 5 millimeters into a Class I canine and molar relationship.
3. Osteotomy of the inferior border of the mandible with interpositional bone grafting to increase the chin prominence (5 millimeters) and chin height (5 millimeters).
4. Submental lipectomy to reduce submental fat and improve the submental-cervical angle.

Treatment

Complete leveling and alignment of the maxillary arch, without extractions, were accomplished by extruding the premolars and first molars and proclining the maxillary incisors. The mandibular arch was aligned and partially leveled without extractions. After these objectives were accomplished, there was a 6-millimeter overjet and the maxillary and mandibular incisors were in good relationship to their bony bases. The maxillary and mandibular osteotomies and genioplasty were performed simultaneously and the jaws stabilized by rigid skeletal fixation.

Concomitant extraction of impacted mandibular third molars and sagittal split ramus osteotomies required stabilization of the mandible with a five-hole curved Vitallium bone plate. The proximal portions of the ramus segments were fixed and stabilized with 12-millimeter bicortical screws; 8-millimeter unicortical screws were used to stabilize the distal segments to avoid damage to the roots of the molar teeth. Anterior-posterior and vertical facial height proportions were achieved by orthodontic and surgical treatment (Figure 33.28 j,k,l). Occlusal and skeletal stability have been maintained over a six-year postoperative follow-up period (Figure 33.28 s,t,u,v).

Case 2

P.C., a 19-year old Latin American female was referred for treatment of her asymmetric long face (Figure 33.29 a,b,c). She had received many years of orthodontic treatment during adolescence.

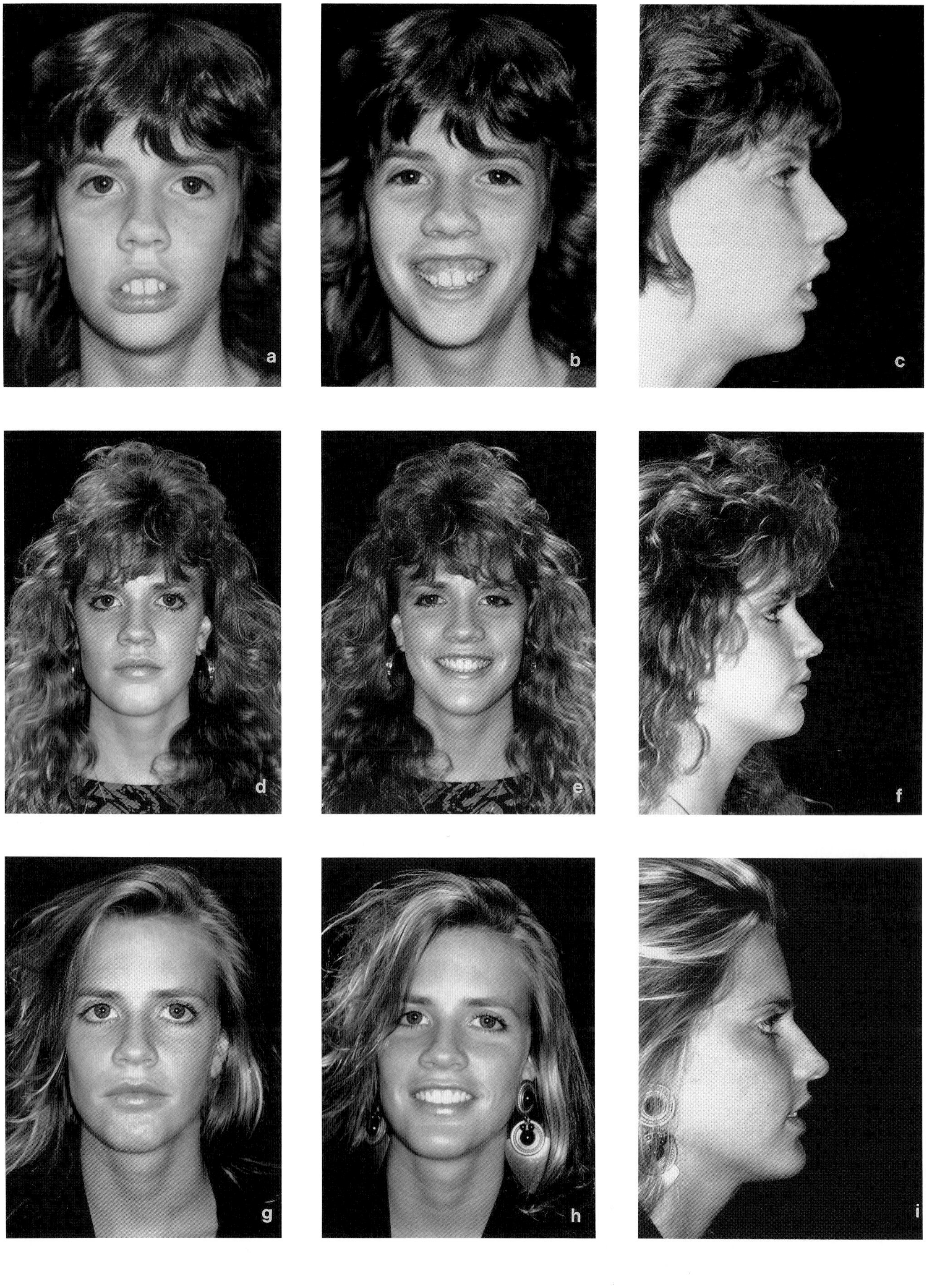
a
b
c
d
e
f
g
h
i

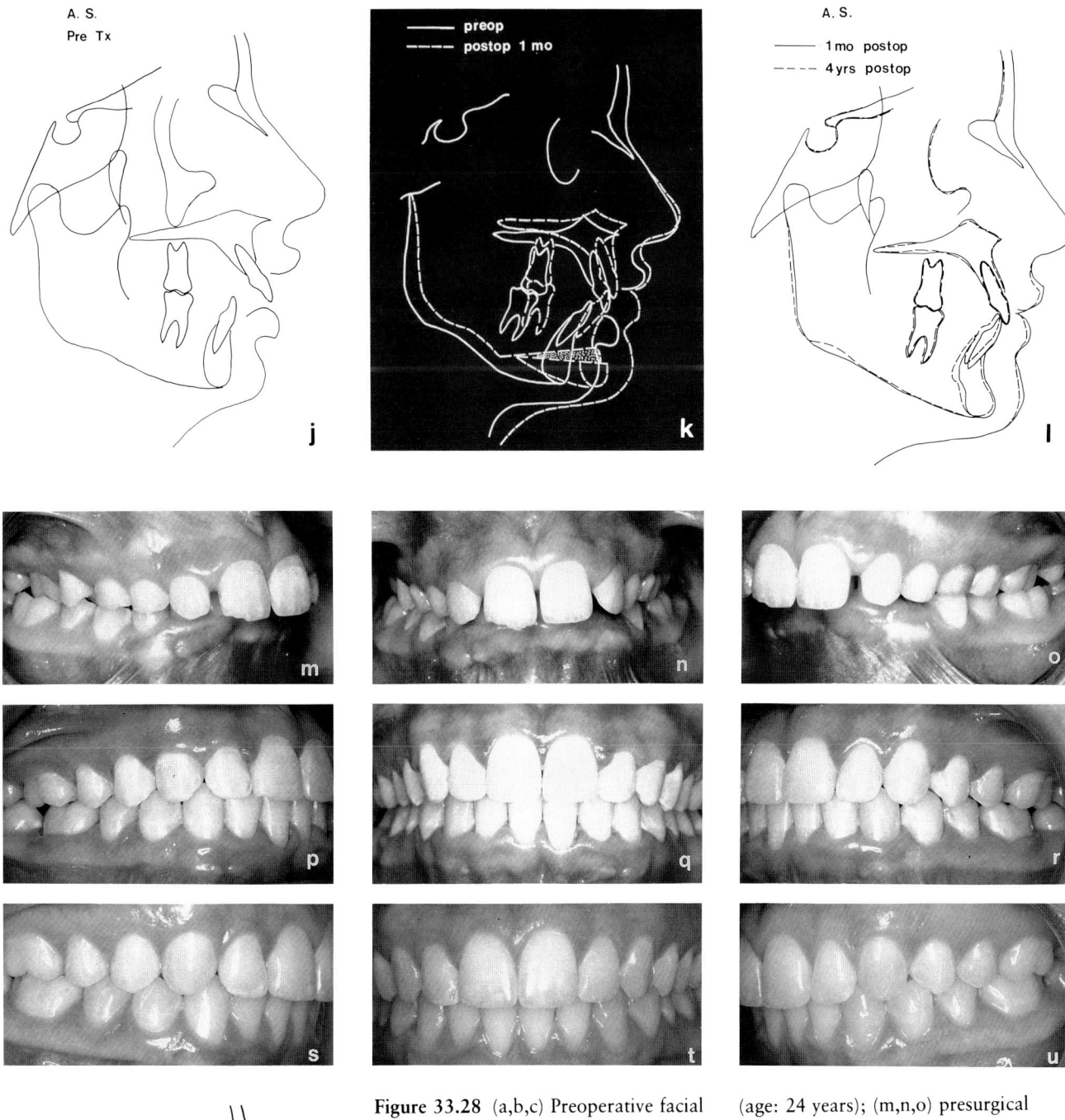

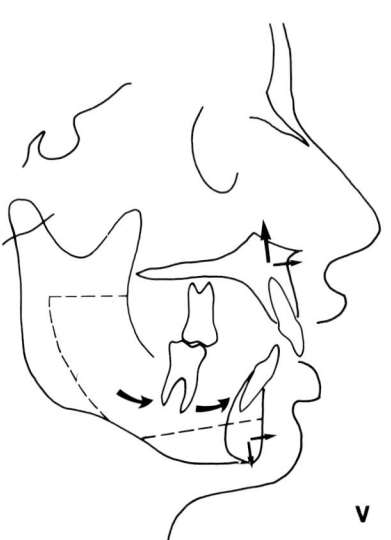

Figure 33.28 (a,b,c) Preoperative facial appearance of 15-year-old patient; (d,e,f) facial appearance two years after orthognathic surgery; (g,h,i) facial appearance six years after orthognathic surgery; (j) pretreatment cephalometric tracing (age 15 years) with mandible in centric relationship and lips in repose; (k) pre- and postorthognathic surgery cephalometric tracings (age: 18 years); (l) skeletal and dental stability indicated by cephalometric tracings before and six years after orthognathic surgery (age: 24 years); (m,n,o) presurgical asymmetric Class II malocclusion; (p,q,r) Class I occlusion after orthognathic surgery and orthodontic treatment; (s,t,u) occlusion six years after surgical-orthodontic treatment; (v) plan of surgery: Le Fort I osteotomy to superiorly and anteriorly reposition maxilla, bilateral sagittal split ramus osteotomies to advance mandible, genioplasty to increase prominence and height of mandible, and suction lipectomy of submental cervical region.

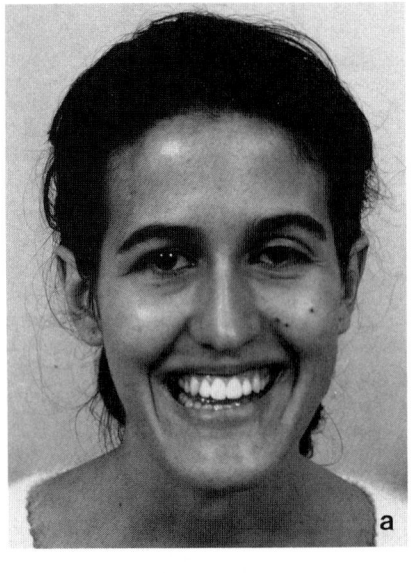

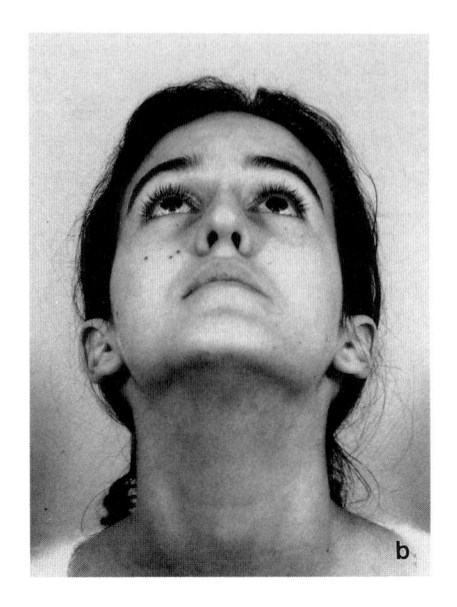

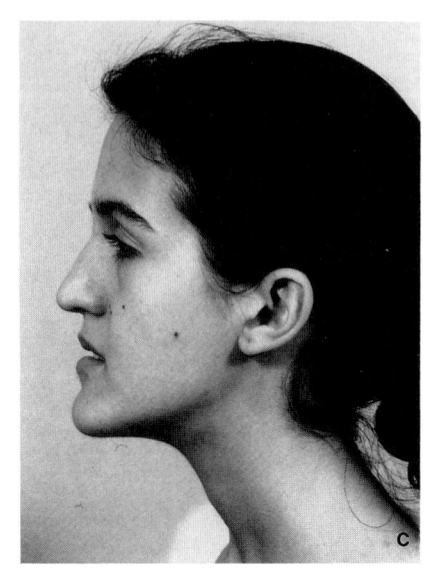

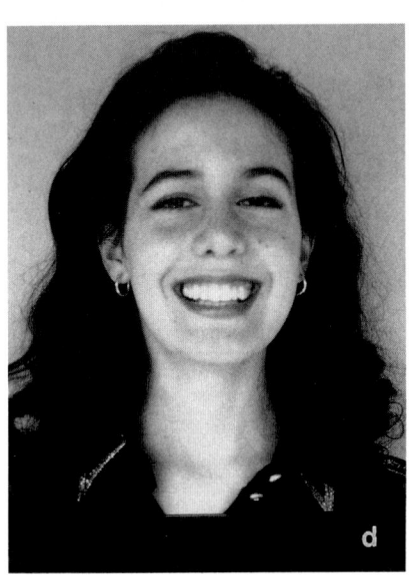

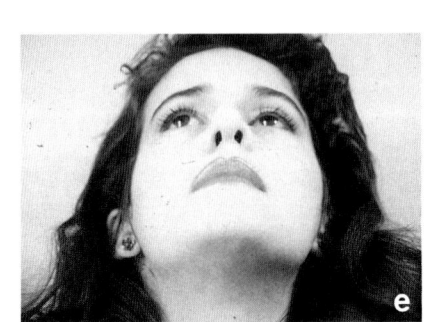

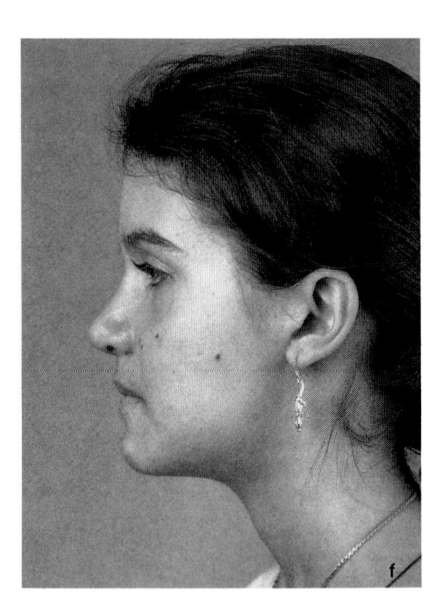

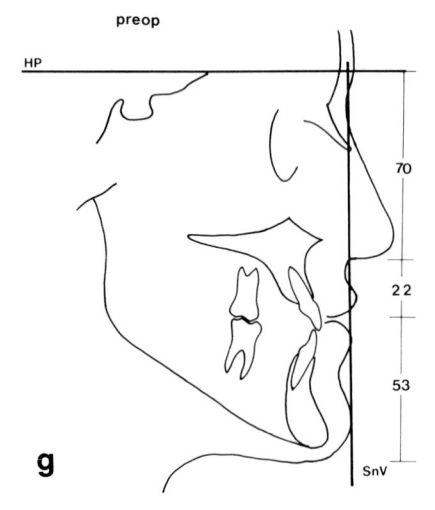

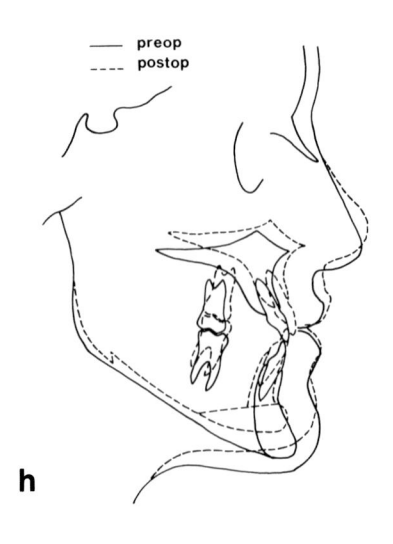

446   RIGID FIXATION OF THE CRANIOMAXILLOFACIAL SKELETON

Figure 33.29 (a,b,c) Preoperative facial appearance of 19-year-old girl with asymmetric long face, relative mandibular excess, and nasal deformity; (d,e,f) facial appearance one year postrhinoplasty and two years postorthognathic surgery; (g) preoperative cephalometric tracing; (h) composite cephalometric tracings before and two years after surgery; (i,j,k) asymmetric Class III malocclusion before surgery;

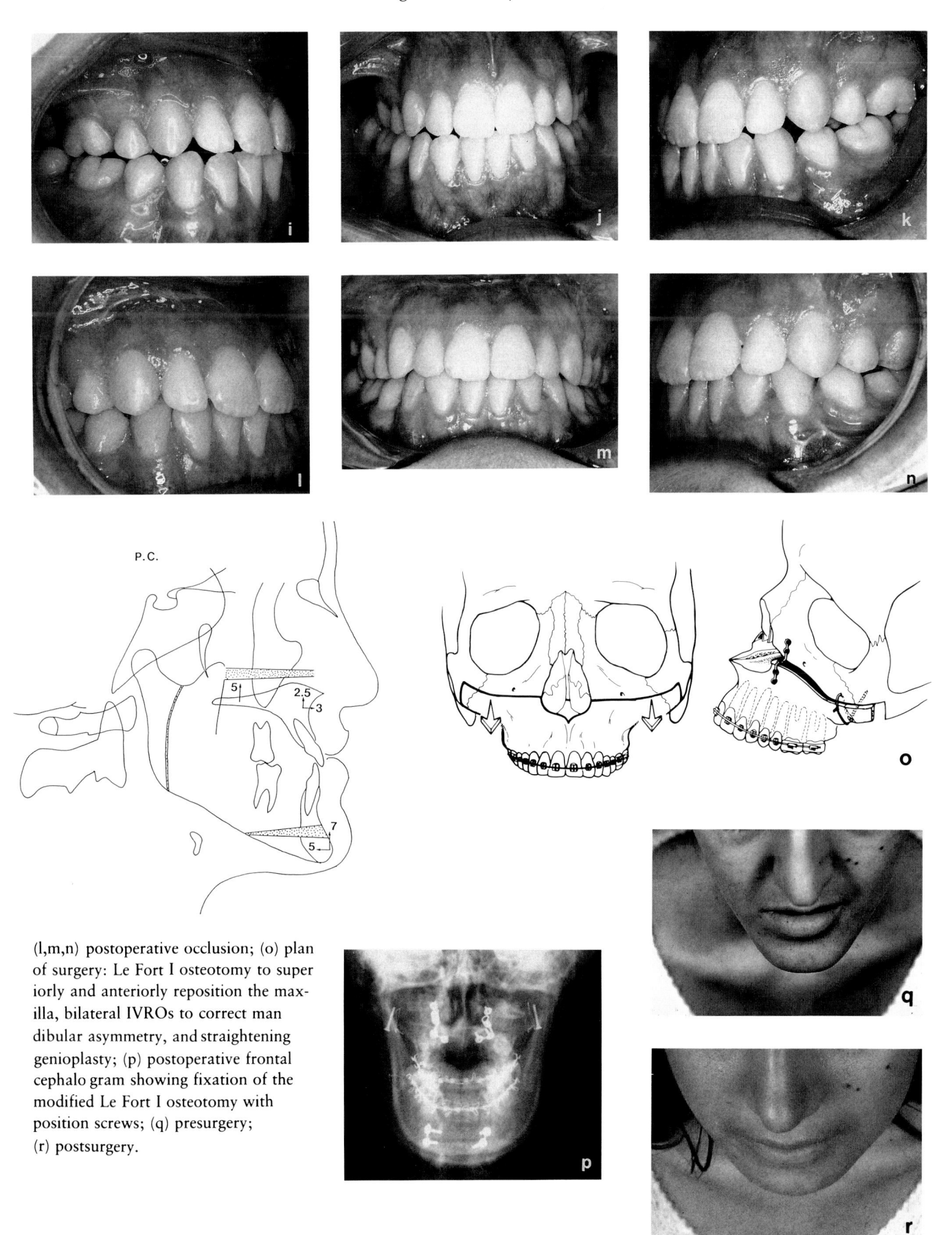

(l,m,n) postoperative occlusion; (o) plan of surgery: Le Fort I osteotomy to superiorly and anteriorly reposition the maxilla, bilateral IVROs to correct mandibular asymmetry, and straightening genioplasty; (p) postoperative frontal cephalogram showing fixation of the modified Le Fort I osteotomy with position screws; (q) presurgery; (r) postsurgery.

Problem List—Aesthetics

The patient exhibited a mildly asymmetrical long face with excessive chin prominence and height. Clinical and cephalometric examination (Figure 33.29 g) showed the typical dentofacial features of asymmetric relative mandibular prognathism with mild vertical maxillary hyperplasia and lip incompetence. Profile analysis revealed an acute nasolabial and nasocolumellar angle, bilateral flattening of the paranasal and malar regions, and excessive chin prominence and height. The nose was narrow and asymmetric because of a bulbous right lateral cartilage. The patient's prominent nasal dorsum and nasolabial disproportion indicated the need for rhinoplasty after orthognathic surgery.*

An asymmetric Class III malocclusion was associated with adequate alignment of the maxillary and mandibular arches. A correlative study of the nasolabial proportions, columella length, nasal prominence, and projection was used adjunctively to construct a new SNV reference line that was calculated to achieve harmony between the nose and upper lip and aid in planning for the anteroposterior soft tissue changes. In view of the fact that a functional occlusion could be achieved, the patient refused additional orthodontic treatment.

Plan of Surgery

Stage I

1. Le Fort I osteotomy to superiorly and anteriorly reposition the maxilla. The maxilla was repositioned anteriorly 6 millimeters by a high-level Le Fort I osteotomy (through the roots of the zygomas and subjacent to the infraorbital foramina) to increase the malar and paranasal prominence and widen the base of the nose. With the maxilla downfractured, a section of nasal cartilage was excised and preserved in a freezer for subsequent nasal tip surgery. This secondary nasal septal surgery was accomplished ten weeks after the definitive orthognathic surgery.
2. Intraoral vertical ramus osteotomies to correct the mandibular asymmetry and achieve the desired Class I occlusion.
3. Reduction of chin height 6 millimeters and chin prominence 4 millimeters by ostectomy of the inferior border of the mandible. Chin was repositioned laterally to achieve chin symmetry.

Stage II Ten weeks postorthognathic surgery, we corrected the nasal asymmetry and residual nasolabial disproportion by open rhinoplasty to narrow the lateral nasal cartilages, increase the nasal tip prominence, and reduce the dorsal nasal prominence.

Follow-up

The maxillary, mandibular, and chin surgery were accomplished simultaneously to shorten the face, increase the malar and paranasal prominence, correct the malocclusion, and widen the nasal ala.

Several months later, rhinoplasty was performed under local anesthesia in an out-patient setting to reduce the dorsal nasal hump, narrow the right lateral cartilage, and rotate the nasal tip with a preserved autogenous cartilaginous nasal strut previously harvested at the time of Le Fort I osteotomy. A Weir procedure was accomplished on the right side where asymmetric widening of the nasal alar base occurred after Le Fort I osteotomy. Balanced anterior-posterior, vertical, and transverse facial proportions were achieved by orthognathic and nasal surgery (Figure 33.29 d,e,f,h). The postoperative Class I occlusion has remained stable and functional over a two-year follow-up period (Figure 33.29 l,m,n).

Sequencing Considerations of Nasal Surgery

In this particular patient, surgery was programmed in two stages to facilitate clinical observation of nasal tip changes resulting from superior and anterior repositioning of the maxilla. Such changes cannot be predicted with certainty despite the fact that in this individual they would usually be calculated to be positive after maxillary surgery.

The nose is evaluated both independently and relative to the upper lip and midface: Based upon the clinical findings, the patient was deemed to have an independent nasal deformity. If the nasolabial angle is acute (downturned nasal tip), forward maxillary movement can be reasonably expected to raise the nasal tip and have a positive aesthetic effect on the nasal and facial proportions. When the nasolabial angle is acute, when the columella appears long in its anterior-posterior dimension, and the upper lip is retrusive, the maxilla can be repositioned anteriorly to alleviate undesirable aesthetics in the midface and nose. A correlated study of the nasal-labial proportions, columella length, and the upper lip drape is used adjunctively in planning anteroposterior maxillary changes and nasal tip changes. It is important to know and understand the limitations of nasal surgery—how much change in the nasal proportions can be reasonably expected to occur with the rhinoplasty done some two to six months after surgical repositioning of the maxilla. The amount of forward maxillary movement will depend on simulated rhinoplasty and the calculated changes that will occur in the nasal tip.

---

*Surgeons: William H. Bell, D.D.S., and Douglas P. Sinn, D.D.S., Dallas, Texas. Orthodontics: Jose Carlos Elgoyhen, D.D.S., Buenos Aires, Argentina.

To place the treatment into proper clinical perspective, the orthognathic and nasal surgery analyses and treatment objectives must be coordinated. The limitations of nasal surgery must be understood and carefully coordinated with the changes that can be reasonably expected with both nasal and orthognathic surgical procedures. The amount of forward maxillary movement depends on simulated rhinoplasty and changes that occur in the nasal tip. Freehand tracings of a "new" upper lip contour are made with cephalometric planning studies aided by constructing a subnasale vertical reference line that is used adjunctively to achieve proportionality between the upper lip and the nose. An overall knowledge of the anticipated soft tissue changes associated with three-dimensional movements of the jaws and teeth is combined with the surgeon's individual artistic sense of facial proportionality and beauty.

Precise predictions of nasal tip changes are not always possible. Even in the best of hands, it may be difficult if not impossible to predict the delicate soft tissue changes associated with maxillary advancement and its effect on abnormal tip position. Successful orthognathic and nasal surgery mandates predictability of soft tissue changes associated with orthognathic surgery.

SUMMARY

Our present-day Le Fort I osteotomy and SSRO techniques are the harvest of yesterday's research. Current clinical results are memorials to the courage, persistence, ingenuity, and research of the surgical pioneers of the Le Fort I downfracture and the SSRO. Recent technical innovations combined with new osteotomy designs, efficient orthodontic treatment, systematic neuromuscular rehabilitation, and rigid skeletal fixation facilitate the achievement of improved jaw function, dental and skeletal stability, and balanced facial proportions.

REFERENCES

Ardary WC, Tracy DJ, Brownridge GW, Urata MM: Comparative evaluation of screw configuration on the stability of the sagittal split osteotomy. Oral Surg Oral Med Oral Pathol 68:125, 1989.

Beals SP, Munro JR: The use of miniplates in craniomaxillofacial surgery. Plast Reconstr Surg 79:33, 1987.

Behrman SJ: Complications of sagittal osteotomy of the mandibular ramus. J Oral Surg 30:554, 1972.

Bell WH, et al: Muscular rehabilitation after orthognathic surgery. Oral Surg Oral Med Oral Pathol 56:229–235, 1983.

Bell WH, et al: Simultaneous repositioning of the maxilla, mandible and chin. In Bell W, Proffit W, White R (eds): Surgical Correction of Dentofacial Deformities, vol 3. Philadelphia, W.B. Saunders Co, 1984.

Bennett MA, Wolford LM: The maxillary step osteotomy and Steinman pin stabilization. J Oral Maxillofac Surg 43:307–311, 1985.

Booth DF: A simplified approach to the sagittal osteotomy. J Oral Surg 34:745, 1976.

Bremer G: Measurements of special significance in connection with anesthesia of the inferior alveolar nerve. Oral Surg Oral Med Oral Pathol 5:966, 1952.

Dal Pont G: Retromolar osteotomy for the correction of prognathism. J Oral Surg 19:42–47, 1961.

Della Rocca RC, Nesi FA, Lisman RD: Anatomy of ocular adnexa and orbit. In Smith BC: Ophthalmic Plastic and Reconstructive Surgery. Vol I, Mosby Company, ST Louis, pp 15–74, 1987.

Drommer R, Luhr HG: The stabilization of osteotomized maxillary segments with Luhr mini-plates in secondary cleft surgery. J Maxillofac Surg 9:166, 1981.

Epker BN: Modifications in the sagittal osteotomy of the mandible. J Oral Surg 35:157–159, 1975.

Foley WL, Frost DE, Paulin WB Jr, Tucker MR: Internal screw fixation: Comparison of placement of pattern and rigidity. J Oral Maxillofac Surg 47:720, 1989.

Freihofer HPM, Brouns JJA: Midfacial movement. Oral and Maxillofac Surg Clin North Am 2:761–773, 1990.

Guernsey LH, DeChamplain RW: Sequellae and complications of the intraoral sagittal osteotomy in the mandibular rami. Oral Surg Oral Med Oral Pathol 22:176, 1971.

Harle W: Le Fort I osteotomy (using mini-plates) for correction of the long face. Int J Oral Surg 9:427, 1980.

Harsha BC, Terry BC: Stabilization of Le Fort I osteotomies utilizing small bone plates. Int J Adult Orthod Orthognath Surg 1:69, 1986.

Hayward J, Richardson ER, Malhotra SK: The mandibular foramen: Its antero-posterior position. Oral Surg Oral Med Oral Pathol 44:837, 1977.

Horster W: Experience with functionally stable plate osteosynthesis after forward displacement of the upper jaw. J Maxillofac Surg 8:176, 1980.

Jonsson E, Svartz K, Welander U: Sagittal split technique I. Immediate postoperative conditions: A radiographic follow-up study. Int J Oral Surg 8:75, 1979.

Keller EE, Sather AH: Quadrangular Le Fort I osteotomy. J Oral Maxillofac Surg 48:2–11, 1990.

Lemke N, Della Rocca RC: Surgery of the Eyelids and Orbit: An Anatomical Approach. Appleton & Lance, Norwalk, pp 96–135, 1990.

Luhr HG: Aur stabilen Osteosynthese bei Unterkieferfrakturen. Dtsch zahnaerztl Z 23:754, 1968.

Luhr HG: Stabile Fixation von Oberkiefer-Mittelgesichtsfrakturen durch Mini-Kompressionsplatten. Dtsch zahnaerztl Z 34:851, 1979.

Lysell G, Nyquist G, Obert T: Positional changes of the teeth and mandibular "fragments" during the immobilization period with cap-splints after treatment for mandibular prognathism by the Babcock-Lindemann method. Acta Odontol Scand 18:293, 1960.

McNeill RW, Hooley JR, Sundberg RJ: Skeletal relapse during intermaxillary fixation. J Oral Surg 1, 31: 212, 1973.

Paulus GW, Steinhauser EW: A comparative study of wire osteosynthesis versus bone screws in the treatment of mandibular prognathism. Oral Surg Oral Med Oral Pathol 54:2, 1982.

Rajchel JL: The medio lateral course of the mandibular canal. Master's Thesis, The University of Michigan. 1985.

Reyneke JP, Mosureik CV: Treatment of maxillary deficiency by a Le Fort I downsliding technique. J Oral Maxillofac Surg 43:914–916, 1985.

Rosen HM: Miniplate fixation of the Le Fort I osteotomies. Discussion by H.G. Luhr. Plastic Reconstr Surg 78:748, 1986.

Sandor GKB, Stoelinga PJW, Tideman H, Leenen RJ: The role of the intraosseous osteosynthesis wire in sagittal split osteotomies for mandibular advancement. J Oral Maxillofac Surg 42:231, 1984.

Schendel SA, Epker PN: Results after mandibular advancement surgery: An analysis of 87 cases. J Oral Surg 38:265, 1980.

Smith BR: The anatomy of the mandible as it relates to the medial ramus osteotomy and rigid fixation of the sagittal split osteotomy. Master's Thesis. Baylor University. 1988.

Spiessl B: Principles of rigid internal fixation in fractures of the lower jaw. In Spiessl, B (ed.): New Concepts in Maxillofacial Bone Surgery, Springer-Verlag, Berlin, p. 21, 1976a.

Spiessl B: Rigid internal fixation after sagittal split osteotomy of the ascending ramus. In Spiessl, B (ed.): New Concepts in Maxillofacial Bone Surgery, Springer-Verlag, Berlin, p 115, 1976b.

Steinhauser EW: Bone screws and plates in orthognathic surgery. Int J Oral Surg 11:209, 1982.

Storum KA, Bell WH: The effect of physical rehabilitation on mandibular function after ramus osteotomies. J Oral Maxillofac Surg 44:94–99, 1986.

Trauner R, Obwegeser H: The surgical correction of mandibular prognathism and retrognathia with consideration of genioplasty. I. Oral Surg Oral Med Oral Pathol 10:677–689, 1957a.

Trauner R, Obwegeser H: The surgical correction of prognathism and retrognathia with consideration of genioplasty. II. Oral Surg Oral Med Oral Pathol 10:787–792, 1957b.

Van Sickels JE, Flanary CM: Stability associated with mandibular advancement treated with rigid osseous fixation. J Oral Maxillofac Surg 43:341, 1985a.

Van Sickels JE, Jeter T, Aragon S: Rigid fixation of maxillary osteotomies: A preliminary report and technique article. Oral Surg Oral Med Oral Pathol 60:262–265, 1985b.

Van Sickels JE, Larsen AJ, Thrash WJ: Relapse after rigid fixation of mandibular advancement. J Oral Maxillofac Surg 44:698, 1986.

Wolford LM, Bennett MA, Rafferty CG: Modification of the mandibular ramus sagittal split osteotomy. Oral Surg Oral Med Oral Pathol 64:146, 1987.

Wolford LM, Davis WM: The mandibular inferior border split: A modification in the sagittal split osteotomy. J Oral Maxillofac Surg 48:92, 1990.

You ZH, Zhang ZK, Zhang XE, Xia JL: The study of vascular communication between jaw bones and their surrounding tissues by SEM of resin casts. West China J Stomatol 8:235–237, 1990.

You ZH, Zhang ZK, Zhang XE: Le Fort I osteotomy with descending palatal artery intact and ligated: A study of blood flow and quantitative histology. Contemp Stomatol. In press. 1991a.

You ZH, Bell WH, Finn RA: Anatomy of nasolacrimal canal and high Le Fort I osteotomy. Presented at the 73rd annual meeting of American Association of Oral and Maxillofacial Surgeon, Chicago, 1991b.

SUGGESTED READING

Bell WH: Modern Practice in Orthognathic and Reconstructive Surgery, Vols. 1, 2 and 3. Philadelphia, W.B. Saunders Co. 1991 and 1992.

CHAPTER 34

Rigid Fixation in Combined Surgery of the Maxilla and Mandible

Joseph G. McCarthy

P. Craig Hobar

Barry H. Grayson

Combined surgery of the maxilla and mandible is indicated when

1. both jaws show evidence of pathology,
2. discrepancies between the two jaws are of such a magnitude that correction of the occlusion with an osteotomy of a single jaw is not technically feasible,
3. the degree of movement of a single jaw results in a suboptimal esthetic result, or
4. single jaw movement is of such a magnitude that relapse is inevitable.

Two-jaw surgery may be applicable in congenital, developmental, and acquired deformities that result in occlusal abnormalities. Other indications include asymmetric skeletal deformities of both the maxilla and mandible, and bimaxillary protrusion. Simultaneous movement of the maxilla and mandible is capable of providing some of the most dramatic changes in maxillofacial surgery; however, the procedure is associated with increased technical difficulty, unique problems with condylar position, increased operative time and blood loss, a higher complication rate, and greater rehabilitative demands. Consequently, careful patient selection and thorough preoperative planning are essential.

A complementary working relationship between the orthodontist and surgeon is critical to efficient planning of two-jaw surgery. The preoperative plan provides a blueprint to allow achievement of ideal occlusion and optimal esthetics. The surgical procedure then becomes an efficient and precise technical means to deliver the desired results.

ANATOMY

The anatomic principles of jaw surgery are identical to those of isolated surgery of the maxilla and mandible and will not be repeated (see Chapter 33). Pertinent anatomic points will be presented in the section on technique.

DIAGNOSIS

As in other types of maxillofacial surgery, a detailed history is essential. Prior orthodontic or surgical therapy should be documented. It is important to discern what the patient considers abnormal or esthetically displeasing. A realistic understanding of the problem and eventual outcome are important requirements on the part of the patient. This is the time when the doctor/patient relationship is formed, and it remains important through the extended period of preoperative orthodontic therapy, hospitalization, and postoperative rehabilitation.

The preoperative analysis should include documentation of the soft tissue and bony characteristics of the face. Nasal, lip, and chin soft-tissue anatomy is intimately related to the underlying bony and dental anatomy and is affected by both pathology and surgical alteration. Both molar and incisal occlusal relationships should be noted.

Skeletal analysis begins with a posteroanterior and lateral cephalogram. Key cephalometric landmarks can be marked and measured after the cephalogram is traced on acetate film. Measurements can be made directly from the acetate tracing or calculated and recorded through several commercially available computer programs. Key landmarks and measurements are illustrated in Figures 34.1–34.5.

Dental models prepared by the orthodontist allow precise evaluation of arch configurations and decisions regarding the need for preoperative orthodontic therapy. Mock surgery on the dental models allows creation of an intermediate occlusal splint, which will be used intraoperatively to position the maxilla in relationship to the existing mandibular configuration (see Figures 34.6 and 34.7). The definitive occlusal splint is then made from the corrected maxilla to allow precise positioning of the mandible (see Figure 34.7).

An in-depth review of presurgical analysis and planning can be obtained from several references (Zide and associates 1981a, 1981b, 1982, Grayson 1989, McCarthy and associates 1990). A representative case study sequence will be presented at the end of the chapter.

TECHNIQUE

General endotracheal anesthesia is administered through a nasotracheal tube fixed to the membranous septum with a large silk suture. In the rare instance that nasotracheal intubation is not possible, a tracheostomy is performed. The patient is monitored with a digital oximeter, an arterial line, a presternal stethoscope, and a rectal temperature probe, and is maintained with two large-bore intravenous lines. Packed red blood cells are available—preferably donated previously by the patient or donated by a member of the family and cross-matched for compatibility (donor specific).

Rigid fixation is the preferred method of fixation in two-jaw surgery. It allows safe extubation in the early postoperative period, improved oral hygiene, better patient tolerance, and early rehabilitation of the temporomandibular joint and muscles of mastication. In rare instances, the quality of the bone is inadequate to achieve reliable rigid fixation, and maxillo-mandibular fixation (MMF) must be used. The quality of the bone is usually inadequate when extenuating circumstances such as previous trauma, irradiation, or tumor resection make rigid fixation of the bone tenuous in the presence of the strong pull of the muscles of mastication. In all instances, the definitive occlusal splint is left attached only to the maxillary teeth. This maneuver allows careful monitoring of the occlusion by the orthodontist. If severe relapse does occur, it is recognized immediately and the teeth can be replaced in MMF. When it is clear

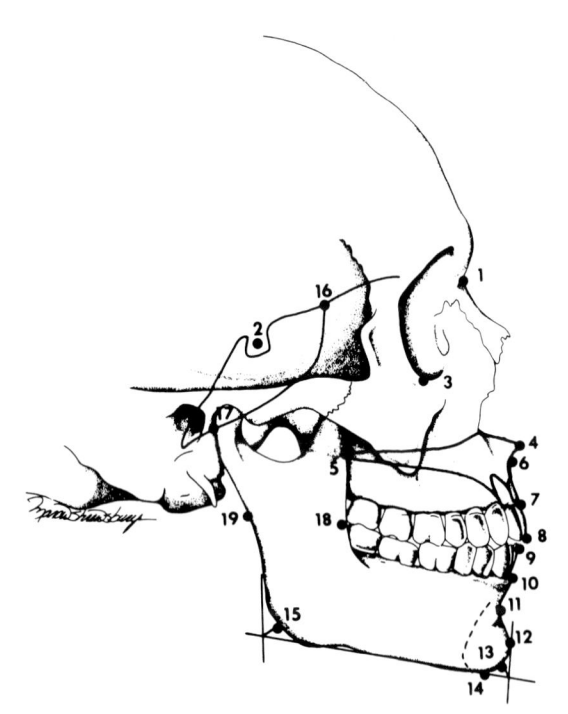

Figure 34.1 Key cephalometric landmarks: 1. nasion, 2. sella, 3. orbitale, 4. anterior nasal spine, 5. posterior nasal spine, 6. point A, 7. supradentale, 8. upper incisal edge, 9. lower incisal edge, 10. infradentale, 11. point B, 12. pogonion, 13. gnathion, 14. menton, 15. gonion, 16. sphenoid-ethmoid intersect, 17. articulare, 18. anterior border of mandible, 19. posterior border of mandible. (Modified from Zide B, Grayson B, McCarthy JG: Cephalometric analysis: Parts I, II, and III. Plast Reconstr Surg 68:816, 1981.)

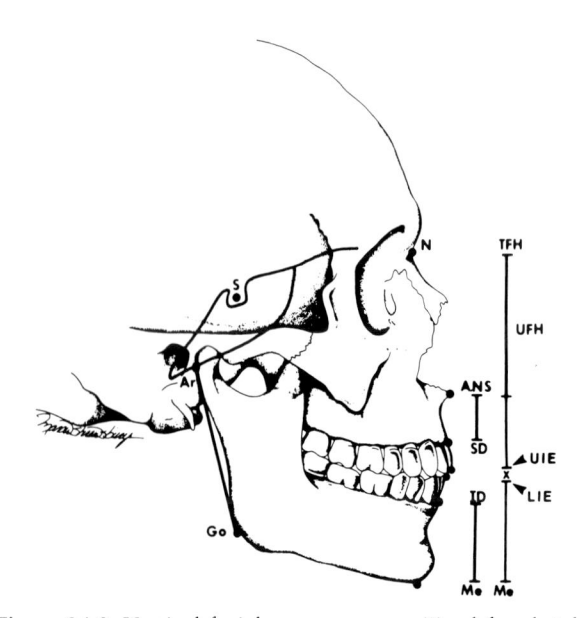

Figure 34.2 Vertical facial measurements. Total face height (TFH, ME to N) may be divided into upper face height (UFH N to ANS) and lower face height (LFH, ANS to Me). Lower face height consists of five components: ANS to SD, ANS to UIE (upper incisal edge), interincisal gap (x), ME to LIE (lower incisal edge), and ME to ID. Posterior lower face height is defined as AR to GO. (Modified from Zide B, Grayson B, McCarthy JG: Cephalometric analysis: Parts I, II, and III. Plast Reconstr Surg 68:816, 1981.)

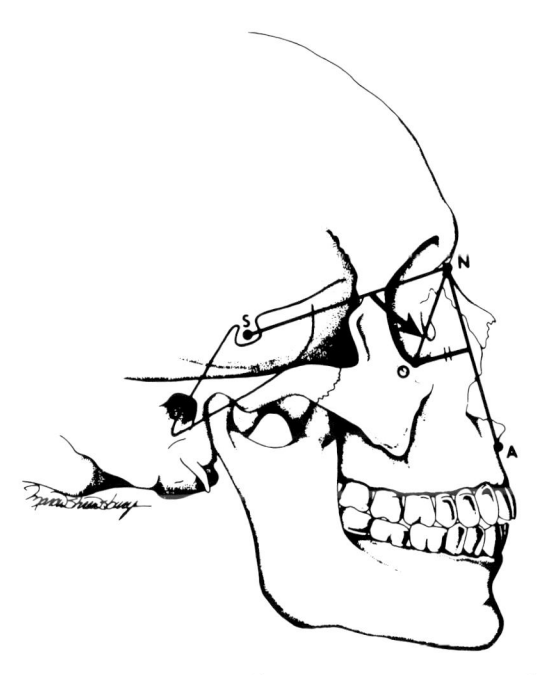

Figure 34.3 Horizontal midface measurements. Hypoplasia of the upper midface is manifest by a reduced angle SNO (arrow). The hypoplasia may be confirmed by measuring the linear distance from orbitale (point O) perpendicular to NA. If SN length deviates from normal, the value of angle SNO will be affected. If point A is retruded or protruded, the distance from O to NA will be affected. (Modified from Zide B, Gayson B, McCarthy JG: Cephalometric analysis: Parts I, II, and III. Plast Reconstr Surg 68:816, 1981.)

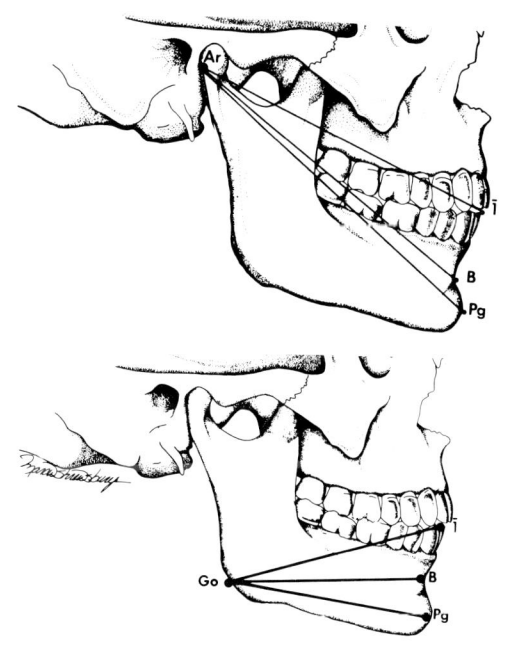

Figure 34.4 Horizontal lower face measurements. Measurements from Ar to anterior points define the overall oblique length of the mandible, including the ramus. Measurements from Go to anterior points define the horizontal length of the body of the mandible. (Modified from Zide B, Grayson B, McCarthy JG: Cephalometric analysis: Parts I, II and III. Plast Reconstr Surg 68:816, 1981.)

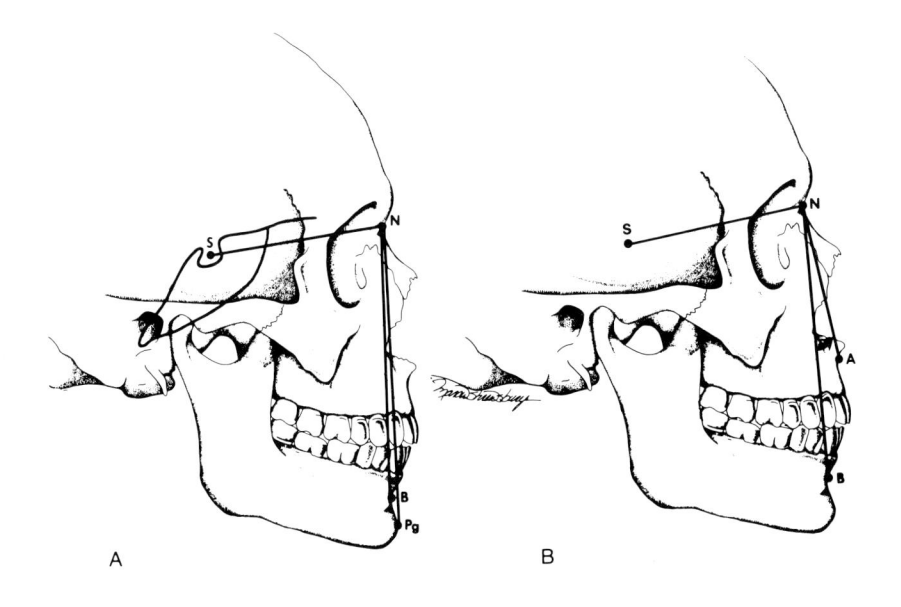

Figure 34.5 Horizontal lower face measurements. (a) SNB defines the position of the mandible relative to the anterior cranial base. SN-Pg describes bony development at the symphysis and assists in determining the requirement for surgery at the symphysis. (b) The anteroposterior position of the mandible relative to the maxilla is described by angle ANB. (Modified from Zide B, Grayson B, McCarthy JG: Cephalometric analysis: Parts I, II and III. Plast Reconstr Surg 68:816, 1981.)

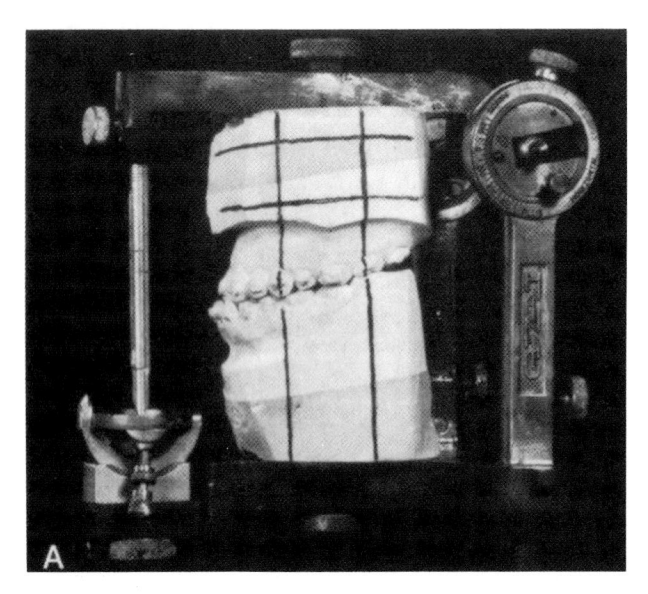

Figure 34.6 (a) Dental study models are mounted on an articulator that simulates the path of mandibular excursions and facilitates presurgical orthodontic planning. (b) The maxillary cast is cut and advanced into the "ideal" occlusion. Markings drawn on the cast bases may be used to measure the amount of advancement needed to achieve the planned occlusal relationships. (From McCarthy JG, Kawamoto HK, Grayson BH, et al: Surgery of the jaws. In Plastic Surgery, McCarthy JG (ed). Philadelphia, Saunders, 1990.)

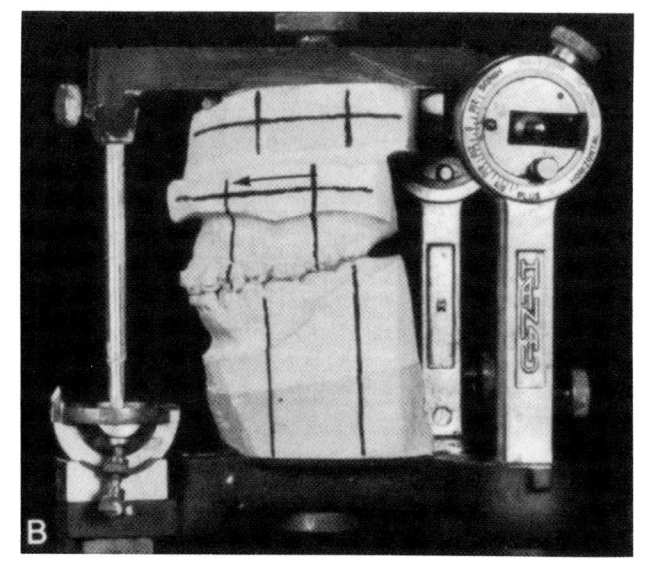

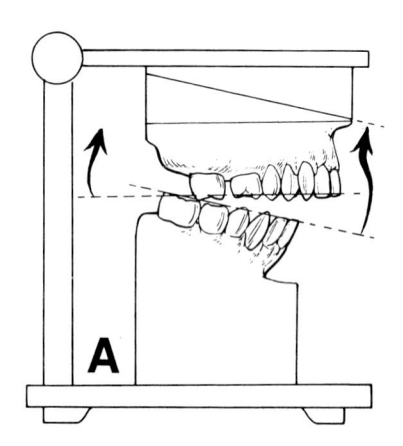

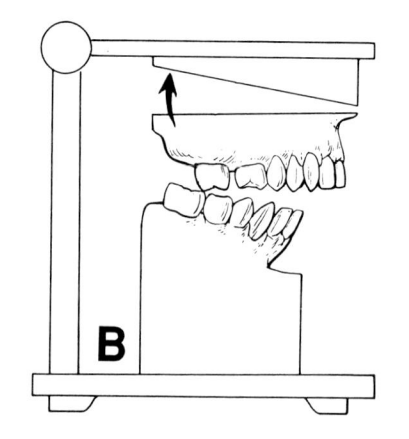

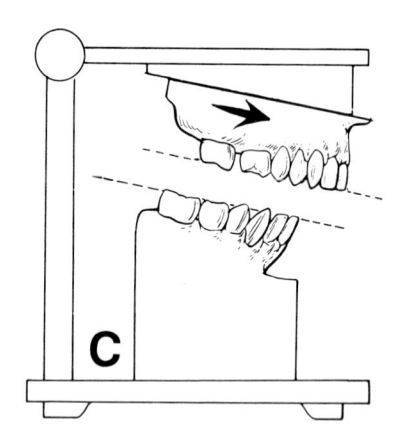

Figure 34.7 (a) Preoperative occlusion is demonstrated on dental models. (b) Projected posterior vertical maxillary impaction. Note the mock surgery (arrow) on the maxillary model. (c) Associated advancement (arrow) of the maxillary cast. (d) The intermediate splint is constructed on a study model simulating posterior impaction and anterior advancement of the maxilla. (e) The final, or definitive, splint is constructed after advancement (arrow) of the mandibular cast. (From McCarthy JG, Kawamoto HK, Grayson BH, et al: Surgery of the jaws. In Plastic Surgery, McCarthy JG (ed). Philadelphia, Saunders, 1990.)

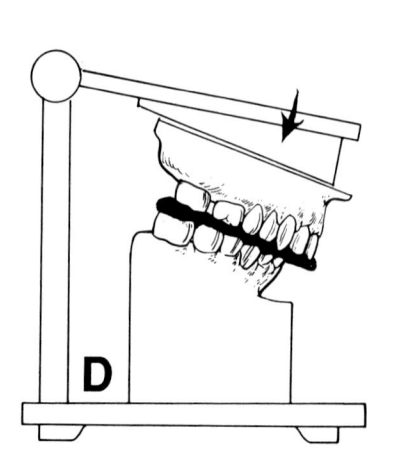

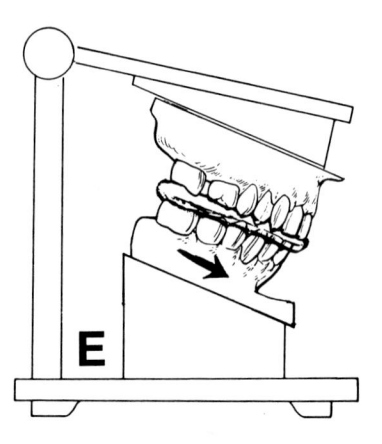

that the occlusion is stable without MMF, the occlusal splint is removed.

Condylar Positioning

A critical factor in assuring a successful outcome of two-jaw surgery is proper seating of the condyles in the temporomandibular joints. The joint is considerably mobile multidimensionally, especially under general anesthesia and the associated muscular relaxation. The maxilla and/or mandible must be rigidly fixed in occlusion with the condyles precisely seated in the glenoid fossae in their centric position. If this is not done, when the MMF is released and the muscular relaxation no longer exists, the condyles will shift into their centric position with a resultant malocclusion of the teeth. Previously, when prolonged postoperative MMF was employed, some remodeling of the condyles was possible; however, if the required remodeling is greater than only a minor accommodation, excessive strain will be placed on the condyles, predisposing to degenerative changes (Ewers 1984, Freihofer 1977, Hadjianghelou 1981). Rigid skeletal fixation techniques and immediate mobilization offer no opportunity for condylar remodeling. Assuring proper condylar seating has thus become more critical.

The simplest, but not necessarily the most precise, method of condylar positioning when rigid fixation is applied to the maxilla is to apply pressure on the condyles in a superior and posterior direction after ensuring they are seated within the fossae. The joints, highly mobile in an inferior and anterior direction, can be dislocated easily when general anesthesia results in muscular relaxation; therefore, this possibility must be guarded against. After completion of rigid skeletal fixation, MMF should be removed, and the excursion of the mandible and occlusal relationships with the maxilla should be carefully noted. If the mandible does not move easily through a complete arc of rotation, and if it does not meet the maxilla in the desired occlusal relationship, the rigid fixation should be removed and repeated until it is correct. As an alternative to this somewhat inexact method, Luhr (1989a) outlined an intraoperative method that utilizes a splint connected to a face bow for control of condylar positioning in maxillary surgery.

When the main body of the mandible is separated from the condylar segments by osteotomies, the method of applying superior and posterior pressure is no longer applicable. The segments are susceptible not only to anterior and inferior dislocation but also to rotation. A reliable method of establishing optimal condylar positioning of the mandible in two-jaw surgery was outlined by Luhr (1989b). An acrylic splint is made preoperatively with the condyles in centric occlusion. Referred to as the *condylar positioning splint,* (CPS), it is independent of the intermediate and definitive occlusal splints. If there is any question as to the patient's ability to position the teeth in centric occlusion, a panorex is taken at the precise time of splint impression to document and assure proper condylar seating.

At the beginning of the procedure, the (CPS) is placed and the teeth are wired to the splint—a maneuver that effectively places the condyles in the centric position. Intraoral buccovestibular incisions are made to expose both the maxilla and the ramus of the mandible in the subperiosteal plane. The proposed sites of the maxillary and mandibular osteotomies are selected and scored with a side-cutting bur. An L-shaped plate is placed bilaterally from the ramus of the mandible to the zygomatic buttress. Mandibular fixation is performed on the condylar segment at a distance from the osteotomy, and the maxillary fixation is above the planned site of the Le Fort I osteotomy (see Figure 34.8). This technique allows precise anatomic association of the condylar segments of the mandible to the stationary portion of the maxilla with the condyles optimally seated in the temporomandibular joint. A centric relationship is established which should not change with osteotomy and surgical movement of the segments. The plate can be removed, but the position is secured by the marks of the screw holes. The majority of mandibular movements can be achieved with bilateral sagittal split (ramisection) osteotomies; however, if an osteotomy other than a sagittal split is performed, it is important to adjust the placement of the mandibulozygomatic plate to assure control of the condylar segment.

Osteotomies

The osteotomies necessary to achieve the sagittal split of the mandibular rami are performed first, because they are technically easier prior to fixation of the teeth in the intermediate splint. The completion of the osteotomies and actual splitting of the rami are not performed because integrity of the mandible is essential for positioning of the maxillary segment with the intermediate splint.

The maxillary osteotomy is then performed completely. Multiple variations allow precise movement of the maxilla in several planes (advancement, retrodisplacement, superior repositioning, inferior repositioning, or rotation). The intermediate splint fabricated by mock surgery on the dental models allows precise control of the anteroposterior, transverse, and rotational movements. The vertical height of the maxilla, however, can vary as the mandible rotates and thus must be controlled intraoperatively by the surgeon. The precise change in the vertical height of the bony maxilla can be determined by scoring the bone transversely above and below the proposed osteotomy. A second measurement is also performed from an ink mark placed on the medial canthus to the superior aspect of the ipsilateral in-

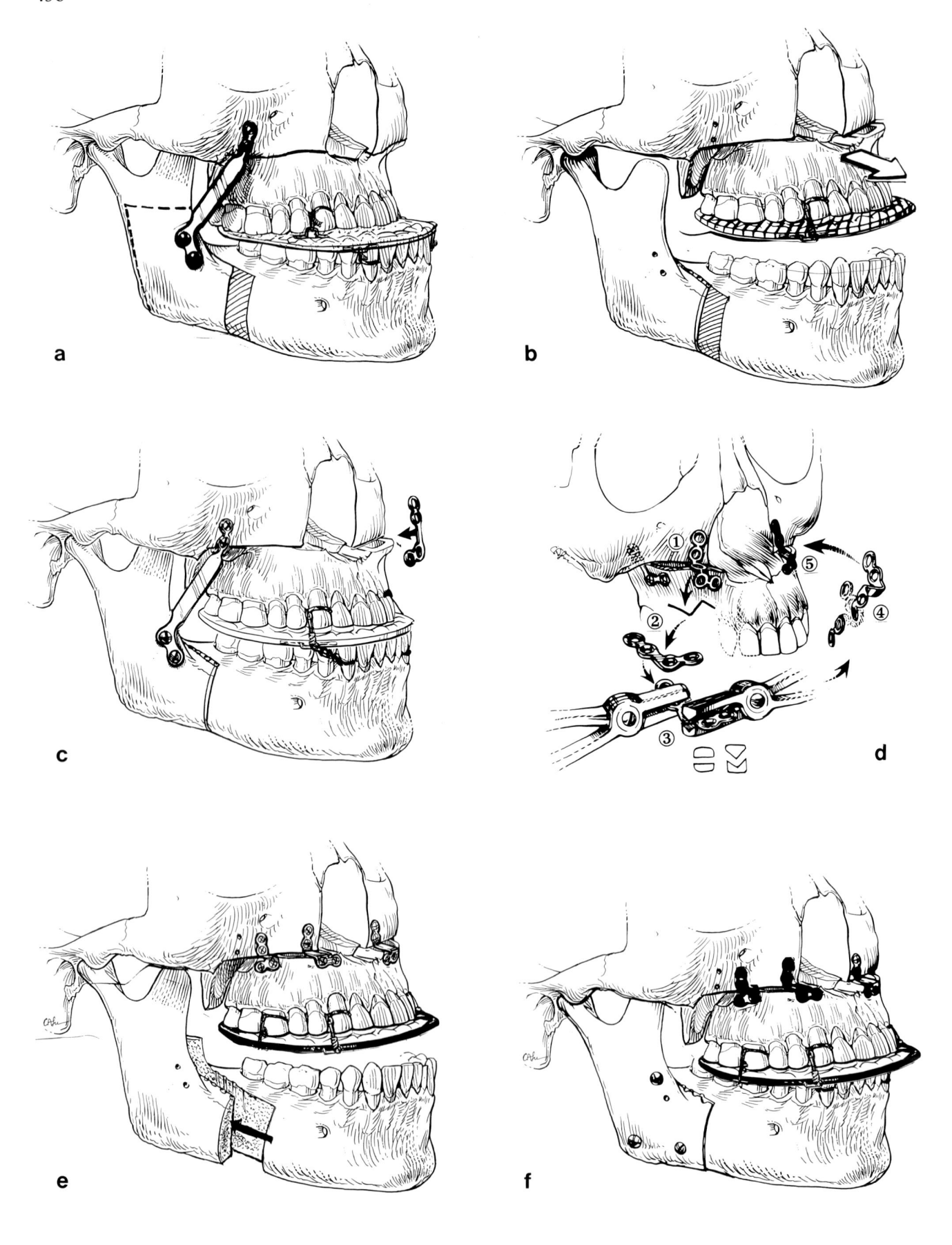

456 Rigid Fixation of the Craniomaxillofacial Skeleton

Figure 34.8 (a) A special mandibulozygomatic positioning plate is used to bridge the distance between the mandibular ascending ramus and the zygoma. The plate holes are countersunk on both sides. The same type of plate may be used on the left and right sides of the patient. One end of the plate is fragmented to facilitate the contouring of the plate until it fits passively to the bone. (This type of plate may also be used with the positioning technique in mandibular sagittal split osteotomies.) If it is too long, it may be shortened by simply cutting off the outer two links with a wire cutter. The positioning plate serves as a surgical instrument and may be used repeatedly. Note the outlines of the mandibular and maxillary osteotomies. The ascending ramus is connected with the root of the zygoma at the beginning of the procedure. The anterior pair of screws must be placed well above the planned Le Fort I osteotomy line. It is presumed that the application of the positioning plate is performed when the position of the condyles is exactly in centric relation, which must be assured by a CPS and MMF. (b) Before the osteotomies are performed, the positioning plate (as well as MMF) must be temporarily removed, leaving the four screw holes on each side as reliable skeletal reference points for reinsertion of the plate and screws. The direction of advancement of the Le Fort I segment is shown. The intermediate splint is in position, and the mandibular osteotomy is almost completed. (c) Miniplates are used to fix the Le Fort I segment. The intermediate splint is secured with MMF. The mandibulozygomatic positioning plate can be reapplied to confirm proper condyle seating. (d) The miniplates are contoured to secure the Le Fort I segment. (e) The definitive splint has been applied, and the mandible will be recessed. Note the rigid fixation of the maxilla and the previously drilled holes associated with the mandibulozygomatic positioning plate. (f) Lag screws are inserted after drill holes are made through a percutaneous trocar. The inferior alveolar nerve must be avoided. This is done before the MMF of the definitive splint is released.

cisor dentogingival junction (Kawamoto 1989). The ink mark may actually be more precise than the bone scores because the external appearance of the relationship between lip and incisor is the ultimate aesthetic goal in impaction or distraction osteotomies of the maxilla. Impaction requires precise removal of a predetermined segment of the maxilla through parallel osteotomies or through a single osteotomy and graduated removal of bone until an optimal relationship of medial canthus to incisor is achieved. Overimpaction should be avoided because it may cause upper lip camouflage of the maxillary incisors and an unappealing short face. Vertical elongation of the maxilla is achieved by a single osteotomy and distraction of the superior and inferior segments. Any resultant bone gap exceeding 3 millimeters is grafted with split calvarial bone or hydroxyapatite.

Rigid Fixation

Rigid skeletal fixation is achieved with the upper and lower jaw secured in the intermediate splint and the condyles properly positioned by exerting superior and posterior pressure or by the face bow method of Luhr (1989a). Optimal fixation is achieved with four plates placed in the vertical maxillary buttresses (right and left nasomaxillary buttresses, right and left zygomaxillary buttresses) (see Figure 34.8c). The ideal sites for screw fixation are limited to these buttresses because the remainder of the maxilla is composed of the thin cortical bone overlying the maxillary sinus. It is usually preferable to use the four-hole 90° or 120° angled 2-inch plates to allow placement of the vertical limb firmly to the maxillary buttresses and placement of the transverse limb across the inferior maxillary segment above the apices of the teeth. It is essential to plan osteotomies and fixation to allow screw placement in the buttresses and in that position of the dentoalveolar segment superior to the roots of the teeth.

After fixation of the Le Fort I segments, the intermediate splint is removed and the mandibular osteotomy is resumed and completed. The numerous variations on the osteotomies of the mandibular ramus are beyond the scope of this discussion. If the anatomy of the ramus is adequate, a sagittal split is the preferred osteotomy because it provides maximal bone-to-bone contact and allows rigid screw fixation, albeit at the risk of damage to the inferior alveolar nerve. Prior to fixation, the mandibulozygomatic (condylar fixation) plate is replaced and fixed; the previously placed screw holes are used (see Figure 34.8a). This maneuver precisely seats the condyles in the center of the temporomandibular joints. The maxilla and mandible are then wired into the definitive splint. The sagittal split of the ramus is fixed with screws (see Figure 34.8f). No attempt should be made to tighten this fixation excessively because this will predispose to compression of the inferior alveolar nerve between the bone segments and will place undesired forces on the mobile condylar segment after the condylar fixation plate is removed. For these reasons, the use of lag screws and compression plates is avoided.

If the configuration or bone stock of the ramus is inadequate for performance of a sagittal split, a vertical osteotomy of the ramus, positioned posterior to the lingula and inferior alveolar nerve, is performed. In mandibular advancement, this results in a bone gap. Bone gaps exceeding 3 millimeters are filled with either split calvarial bone or hydroxyapatite. When bone grafting is necessary, exposure is facilitated by a submandibular or Risdon incision. Fixation is achieved with plates and screws.

The MMF is removed, as is the zygomaticomandibular plate. The definitive splint is left attached to the maxillary segment for the reasons previously given. This allows safe postoperative management of the airway without the need for prolonged intubation or intensive nursing care. The patient is prescribed liquids on the first postoperative day and is quickly advanced to a soft diet. Interdental rubber bands ease postoperative discomfort and allow smoother transition to acceptance of the new occlusal relationships. The patient is followed carefully, and if any change in the occlusal relationships is seen, the patient is placed in stronger rubber bands or even MMF. When the occlusal relationship is stable, the splint is removed from the maxilla.

COMPLICATIONS

Complications for two-jaw surgery are the same as those for single-jaw surgery of the maxilla or mandible. They include skeletal relapse, hemorrhage, infection, condylar displacement, and secondary changes in sensation of the lower lip.

LONG TERM FOLLOW-UP

The effects of rigid fixation on stability of combined surgical movements of maxilla and mandible are still being investigated. Welch (1989), in a review of the literature of the past 33 years concerning postoperative stability following orthognathic surgery, came to the following conclusion: Maxillary superior repositioning tends to be a stable procedure, whereas maxillary inferior repositioning tends to be unstable with movement occurring in variable and unpredictable directions; maxillary advancement tends to be stable, whereas mandibular advancement tends to be less stable; mandibular setback is perhaps the most stable procedure, possibly making this the only procedure in which rigid fixation is not necessary; and a cleft palate deformity makes a Le Fort I procedure as unstable as it is in patients with vertical maxillary deficiency. Studies are conflicting as to whether simultaneous surgery of the maxilla and mandible increases skeletal instability as compared to single-jaw surgery (Le Banc 1982, Quejada 1987, Luyx 1985).

CASE STUDY

K.C. is a 36-year-old female whose chief complaints included lip incompetency and the appearance of a long face. Clinical examination found 4 to 5 millimeters of incisal show at rest, a 3-millimeter interlabial gap at rest, and approximately 4 millimeters of gingival show on smiling. Projection of the chin was deficient (see Figure 34.9). Intraoral examination found a class I molar occlusion on the right and a class II on the left with a 7-millimeter overjet. Presurgical cephalometric evaluation found a mild midface vertical maxillary excess (ANS to Superdentale) and deficient mandibular body length (Go to Pg). In addition, the mandibular body appears retropositioned with respect to the cranial base (SN) (see Figure 34.10).

The surgical plan involved a vertical maxillary impaction (3 millimeters anteriorly and posteriorly), bilateral sagittal split of the ramus with advancement of 5 millimeters, and a horizontal osteotomy of the mandible (genioplasty) with advancement of 5 millimeters.

Preoperative impressions of the teeth were made for the construction of an occlusal splint. An intermediate splint was constructed with the maxilla reposi-

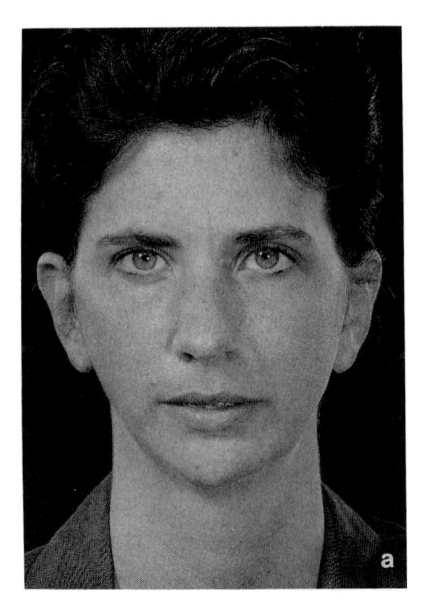

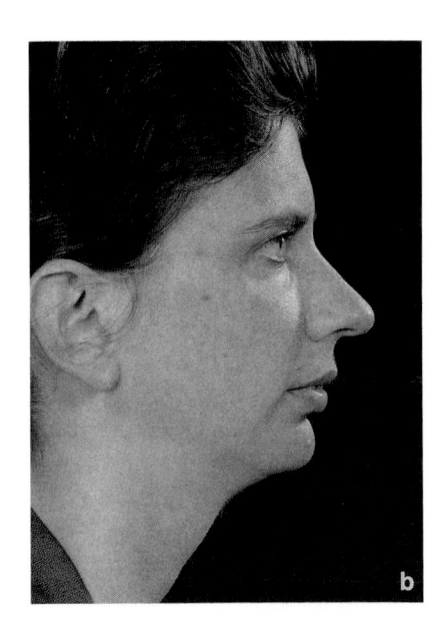

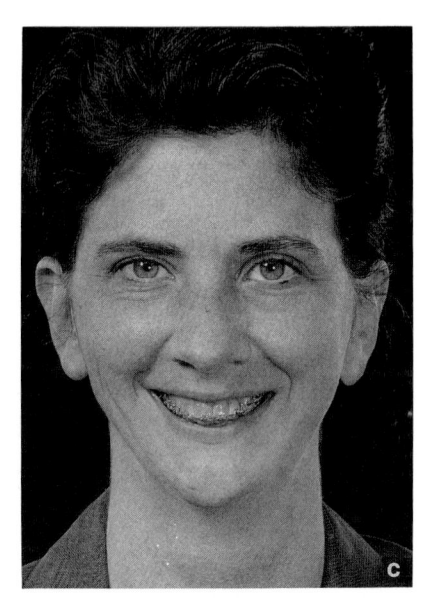

Figure 34.9 This 36-year-old female has a long face, inadequate chin projection, incisal show at rest and interlabial gap: (a) full face view, (b) oblique profile and (c) smiling view.

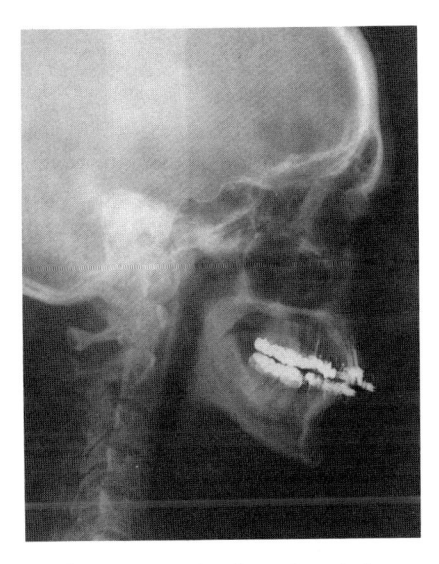

Figure 34.10 This preoperative lateral cephalogram documents midface vertical maxillary excess and deficient mandibular body length. The mandibular body is also retrodisplaced. Note the overjet.

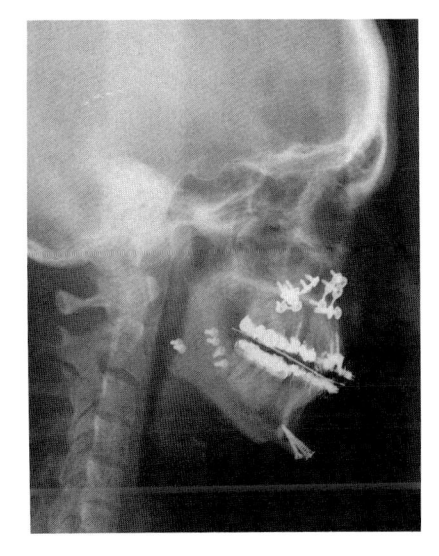

Figure 34.11 Postoperative lateral cephalogram shows miniplate fixation of the Le Fort I segment and lag screw fixation of the mandibular rami. Note the screw fixation of the genioplasty fragment.

tioned 3 millimeters superiorly. The splint was inserted intraoperatively, after the Le Fort I osteotomy was performed but prior to completion of the mandibular osteotomies (see Figure 34.8). This allowed for repositioning of the maxillary osteotomy segment in relation to the "unoperated mandible." Rigid skeletal fixation of the Le Fort I osteotomy was achieved. The intermediate splint was removed, and the mandibular osteotomy was completed. A definitive splint was inserted to reposition the mandible forward (5 millimeters). Rigid skeletal fixation (three screws on each side) was placed to secure the ramus osteotomy. The patient was removed from MMF intraoperatively.

Postoperatively the patient was placed on a soft diet for eight weeks, at the end of which time the maxillary splint was removed. Examination of the occlusion revealed 1 to 2 millimeters overjet and 1 to 2 millimeters overbite (see Figure 34.11). She shows decreased facial convexity, improved chin projection, and lip competency at rest (see Figure 34.12).

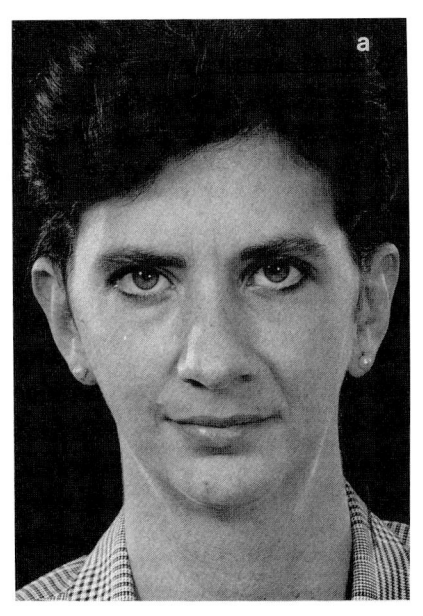

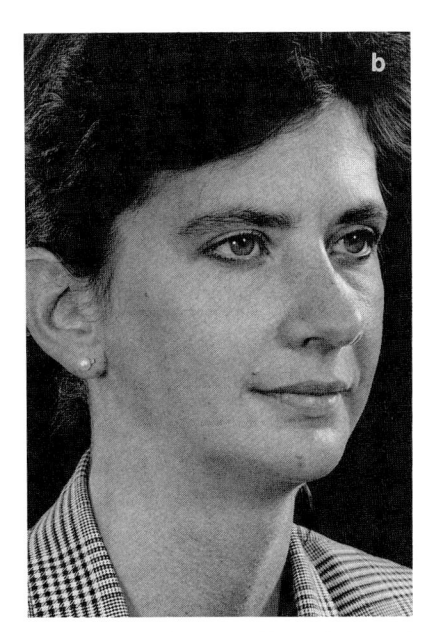

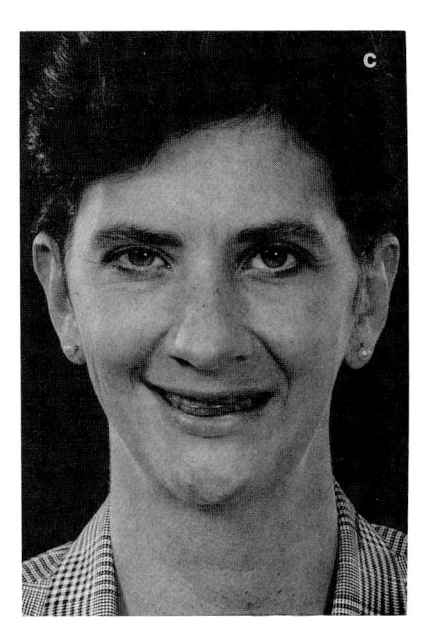

Figure 34.12 Postoperative views: (a) full face view, (b) oblique profile and (c) smiling view.

BIBLIOGRAPHY

Ewers R: Die tempromanubularen Strukturne Ewashsener und die Reaktion auf opertive Verlagerugen. Eine Tierexperimentelle Sutdie an ausgewachsenen Cercopithecus-aethiopsAffen. Z Stomatol 81: 73, 1984.

Freihofer HP: Modellversuch zur lageveranderung des Kieferkipfchens nach sagittaler Spltung des Unterkiefers. Shweiz Mschr Zahnheilk, 87:12, 1977.

Grayson BH: Cephalometric analysis for the surgeon. Clin Plast Surg 16:4, 1989.

Hadjianghelou O: Zurcher Erfahrungen mit der Zugschraubenosteosynthese bei der sagittalen Spaltung des Ramus. Ortschr kiefer-Gesichts Chir 26: 94, 1981.

Kawamoto HJ: Simplification of the Le Fort I osteotomy. Clin Plast Surg 16:4, 777, 1989.

La Banc JP, Turvey T, Epker BN: Results following simultaneous mobilization of the maxilla and mandible for the correction of dentofacial deformities: Analysis of 100 consecutive patients. Oral Surg Oral Med Oral Pathol 54:607, 1982.

Lindorf HH, Steinhauser EW: Correction of jaw deformities involving simultaneous osteotomy of the mandible and maxilla. J Maxillofac Surg 6:239, 1978.

Luhr HG, Kubein-Meesenburg D: Rigid skeletal fixation in maxillary osteotomies: Intraoperative control of condylar position. Clin Plast Surg 16:157, 1989a.

Luhr HG: The significance of condylar position using rigid fixation in orthognathic surgery. Clin Plast Surg 16:1, 147, 1989b.

Luyx NH, Ward-Booth RP: The stability of Le Fort I advancement osteotomies using bone plates without bone grafts. J Maxillofac Surg 13:250, 1985.

McCarthy JG, Kawamoto HK, Grayson BH, et al: Surgery of the Jaws. In Plastic Surgery, McCarthy JG (ed). Philadelphia, Saunders, 1990.

Moser K, Freihofer HPM: Long-term experience with simultaneous movement of the upper and lower jaw. J Maxillofac Surg 8:271, 1980.

Quejada JG, Bell WH, Kawamura H, et al: Skeletal stability after inferior maxillary repositioning. Int J Adult Orthod Orthogn Surg 2:67, 1987.

Turvey TA: Simultaneous mobilization of the maxilla and mandible: Surgical technique and results. J Oral Maxillofac Surg 40:96, 1982.

Welch TB: Stability in the correction of dentofacial deformities: A comprehensive review. J Maxillofac Surg 47:1142, 1989.

Zide BM, Grayson B, McCarthy JG: Cephalometric analysis: Part I. Plast Reconstr Surg 68:816, 1981a.

Zide BM, Grayson B, McCarthy JG: Cephalometric analysis for upper and lower midface surgery: Part II. Plast Reconstr Surg 68:816, 1981b.

Zide BM, Grayson B, McCarthy JG: Cephalometric analysis for mandibular surgery: Part III. Plast Reconstr Surg 69:155, 1982.

CHAPTER 35

Rigid Fixation and Bone Substitutes in Orthognathic Surgery: Stable Expansion of the Facial Skeleton

Harvey M. Rosen

Despite the increasing use of rigid fixation in elective facial osteotomies, skeletal relapse remains a problem. This is particularly true in extensive maxillary advancements (especially in cleft patients with lip or palate), transverse maxillary expansions, and inferior maxillary repositioning procedures. In the performance of these skeletal expansion procedures, the restrictive forces of soft tissue in combination with large osteotomy gaps create an environment in which repositioned dentoosseous segments inexorably drift toward their preoperative position. Rigid fixation must not be considered a panacea that will prevent this phenomenon.

Although bone grafting of osteotomy gaps in combination with rigid fixation may minimize this potential for relapse, it certainly does not eliminate it. Data supporting this statement are available for cleft maxillary advancements and for maxillary inferior repositioning procedures. One can only extrapolate these data when considering the relapse potential of extensive noncleft maxillary advancements and extensive transverse maxillary expansions.

In an effort to eliminate osseous instability associated with maxillary skeletal expansive procedures, porous, block hydroxyapatite, a nonresorbable bone graft substitute, has been used in selected patients in combination with rigid fixation. This has been done since June 1986 at Pennsylvania Hospital. In this chapter we describe that experience.

PATIENT SELECTION

The clinical material was derived from 52 nonconsecutive patients who underwent elective maxillary osteotomies. Patients were considered appropriate candidates for implantation of block hydroxyapatite only if autogenous bone would have been harvested for interpositional placement into an osteotomy gap had the hydroxyapatite not been available; that is, the implant material was used in lieu of interpositional bone grafts only. Accordingly, operative indications include

1. all patients undergoing inferior maxillary repositioning unaccompanied by significant advancement (10),
2. all maxillary advancements in patients with no cleft of 8 millimeters or greater (21),
3. all maxillary advancements in patients with cleft lip or palate (6), and
4. all transverse maxillary expansions of 5 millimeters or greater (15).

This accounted for 117 implanted anatomic areas. The distribution of these areas were as follows: 74 in the anterolateral maxillary wall, 20 in the lateral nasal wall and 23 in the nasal floor.

ANATOMY AND TECHNIQUE

In all maxillary advancements, a vertical step osteotomy is used at the zygomatic maxillary buttress. This osteotomy provides an accessible area of thick cortical bone in which to wedge the implant block (see Figure 35.1). Alternatively, a larger rectangular block may be placed in the step that extends anteriorly along the entire anterolateral maxillary osteotomy gap (see Figure 35.2).

Sagittal palatal osteotomies to expand the maxillary arch transversely are performed off the midline through the right or left nasal floor. Blocks are then

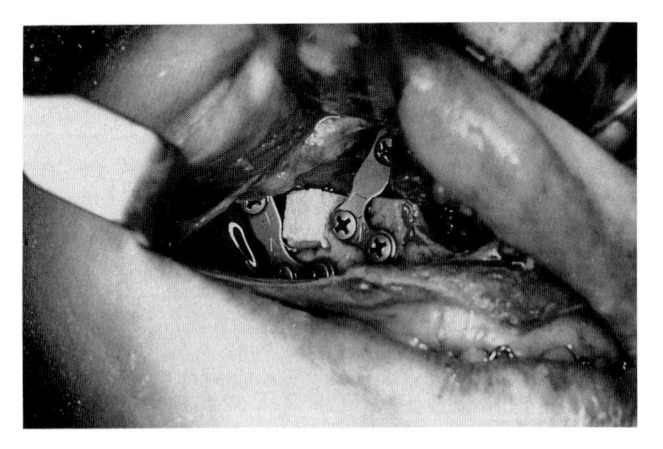

Figure 35.1 This Le Fort I osteotomy is to produce maxillary advancement of 8 millimeters. Hydroxyapatite blocks are placed in the step osteotomy made in the thick cortical bone of the zygomatic maxillary buttress.

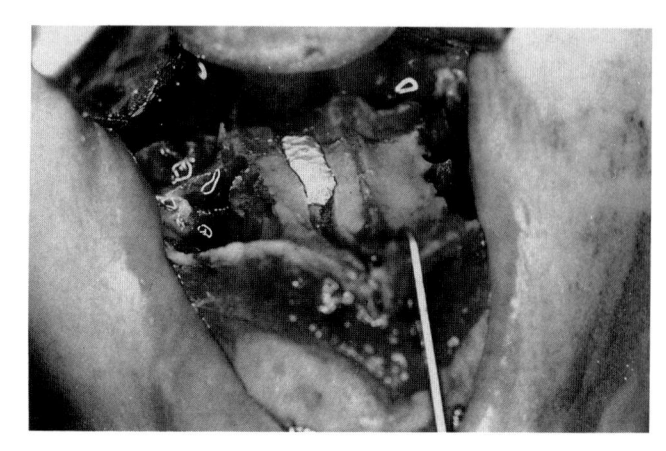

Figure 35.3 This two-piece Le Fort I osteotomy is to produce a 6.5-mm transverse expansion at the region of the first molar. Note the parasagittal palatal osteotomy through the right nasal floor. Hydroxyapatite blocks are placed in the palatal osteotomy gap to maintain transverse expansion.

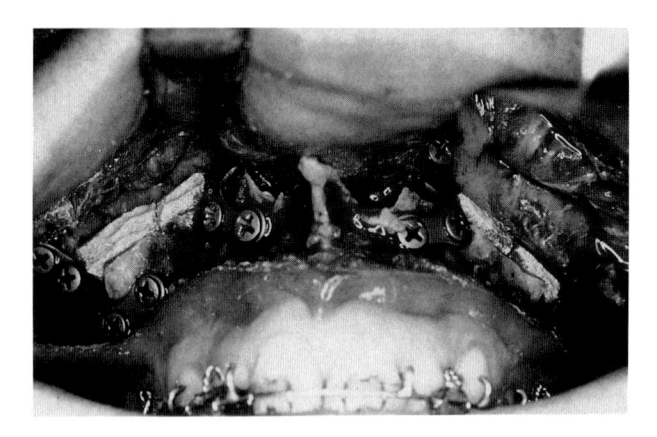

Figure 35.2 This Le Fort I osteotomy is to produce maxillary advancement of 11 millimeters. Hydroxyapatite blocks extend from the step osteotomy anteriorly along the entire anterolateral osteotomy gap.

placed in the osteotomy gap to help maintain the transverse expansion (see Figure 35.3). This parasagittal location is characterized by thinner bone and thicker palatal mucosa than the palatal midline. Thick mucosa is less prone to perforate, minimizing the chance of chronic exposure of the implant to the oral cavity. Similarly, inadvertent tears in the nasal mucosal floor should be repaired to avoid chronic exposure of the implants to the nasal cavity. These considerations with regard to soft tissue will minimize the complication rate associated with the use of hydroxyapatite blocks in this location.

Le Fort I osteotomies to reposition the maxilla inferiorly must be performed high on the lateral nasal wall because the apices of the tooth roots are well superior to the nasal floor in patients with a vertical maxillary deficiency. Performing these osteotomies high on the lateral nasal wall will also provide enough room to place bone plates and screws above the root apices. Once the maxilla is down fractured, implant blocks are placed along the lateral nasal walls; pyriform aperture plates are then applied. The remainder of the anterolateral osteotomy gap is then implanted with hydroxyapatite, followed by application of the zygomatic buttress bone plates. This is the only instance in orthognatic surgery in which compression is used in order to hold the implant blocks tightly in place (see Figure 35.4).

RESULTS

Patients were followed up from 6 to 34 months; the mean was 14.6 months. The complication rate attributed to the use of the implants was 2%. The single complication was a dislodged implant block in the nasal floor, which presented as a movable submucosal nasal mass. Its removal was required.

Despite the fact that all implants were either adjacent to an open maxillary sinus or in the nasal floor, no infections occurred. All patients were treated with prophylactic systemic antibiotics and decongestants for one week.

The stability achieved by the combined use of rigid fixation and porous blocks of hydroxyapatite has been excellent. All sagittal advancements of the maxilla in those patients without a cleft have demonstrated complete stability throughout the period of follow up. Inferior maxillary repositioning procedures have also demonstrated a remarkable stability. The range of in-

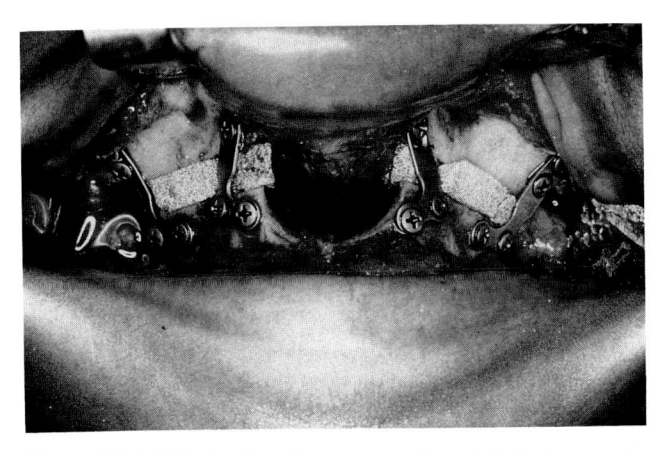

Figure 35.4 This Le Fort I osteotomy is to inferiorly reposition the maxilla 6 millimeters anteriorly. Hydroxyapatite blocks are placed in the lateral nasal wall and anterolateral maxillary osteotomy gaps. Compression plating is used to help hold the blocks in position.

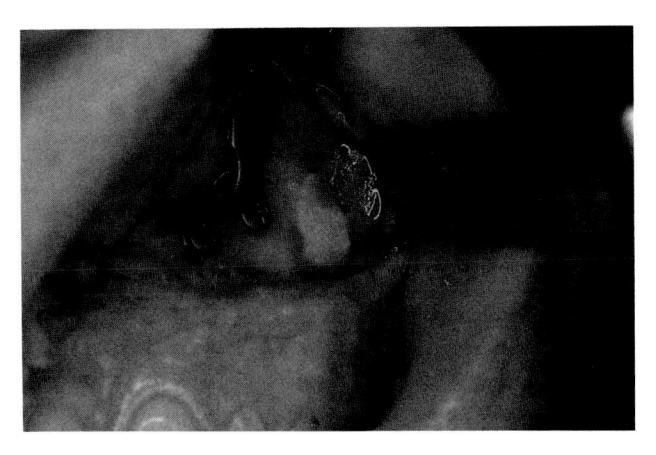

Figure 35.5 An implanted hydroxyapatite block is shown 13 months after placement in a zygomatic buttress osteotomy gap. Note the distinct interfaces between implant and bone and punctate bleeding from the cut surface of the implant.

ferior maxillary movements ranged from 5 to 8 mm, with a mean of 6.5 millimeters. At the time of follow up all maxillae were within ±0.5 millimeters of their immediate postoperative positions. This is well within the margin of error for cephalometric tracing techniques.

Postoperative instability has been noted in 2 of the 15 patients who underwent transverse maxillary expansions. Two patients, who underwent transverse expansions of 8 millimeters and 9 millimeters, were noted to undergo transverse relapse following their active phase of postoperative orthodontics at three and five months, respectively.

Gross and Histologic Findings

Ten of these 52 patients later consented to open biopsy of the implant material and bone/implant interface. The time from implantation to biopsy ranged from 3 to 15.2 months, with a mean of 12.6 months. A total of 23 biopsy specimens were obtained. Specimens were harvested from the zygomatic buttress (18) following maxillary advancements and inferior repositionings, and from the piriform buttress (5) following inferior repositionings.

At the time of biopsy, the implant remained clearly distinguishable from bone; distinct bone/implant interfaces were seen. Implants, whose preimplantation color was white, appeared slightly pink and bled in a punctuate fashion when cut with a contour bur (see Figure 35.5). Specimens remained undecalcified and were thick-sectioned with a low-speed diamond saw and stained with modified Villanueva-Goldner trichrome stain.

Twenty-one of 23 specimens had healed by forming an osseous union with no fibrous tissue between implant and bone (see Color Plate 19). No resorptive or remodeling activity (osteoclasts or Howships lacunae) could be seen in the bone immediately adjacent to the implant. Two specimens had healed by forming a fibrous union. In all biopsies that had healed with a direct osseous union, bone ingrowth was observed in the pores of the implant material. The extent of bone ingrowth was highly variable and independent of the time from implantation, the anatomic site implanted, and the surface area of the bone/implant interface. A consistent healing process involving the presence of osteoid tissue, calcified bone, and fibrovascular tissue within the implant pores was observed in all specimens with bone ingrowth (see Color Plates 20 and 21). Because no osteoclasts could be seen in association with the presence of osteoid tissue, a reasonable conclusion is that ongoing net bone production is taking place. Unfortunately, serial implant biopsies from the same patient would be needed to document this theory.

Radiographic Findings

Following implantation of hydroxyapatite blocks, 8 patients have been followed radiographically for 24 to 32 months. Standard lateral cephalometric x rays best visualized blocks placed in the anterolateral maxillary wall and lateral nasal wall. Panorex films were accompanied by too much distortion to afford good visualization.

It was found that implants remain virtually unchanged in their radiographic appearance. The density of the blocks and their marginal discreteness were identical to their immediate postoperative appearance (see Figure 35.6).

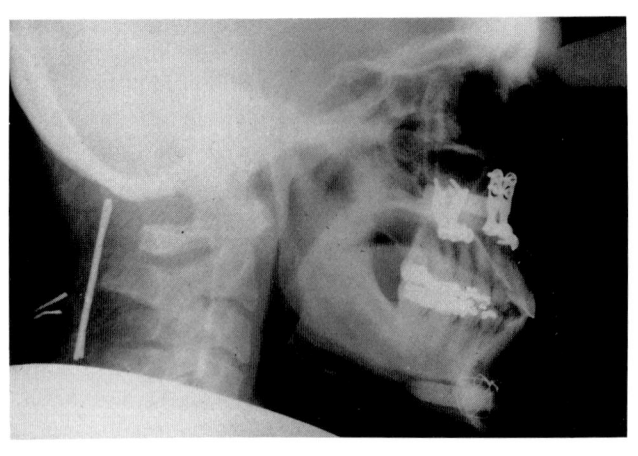

Figure 35.6 This lateral cephalometric x ray was taken 26 months after vertical lengthening of the maxilla with hydroxyapatite blocks along the lateral nasal and anterolateral maxillary walls. The implant blocks remained well defined with unchanged radiodensity (the chin has also been vertically elongated with hydroxyapatite implant blocks).

DISCUSSION

Surgical repositioning of the maxilla frequently creates large osteotomy gaps. As the magnitude of osseous repositioning increases, bone contact decreases and osseous gaps enlarge.

Although the necessity for grafting bone gaps has decreased with the increasing use of rigid plate and screw fixation, it should again be emphasized that rigid fixation may not reliably prevent relapse in the presence of minimal bone contact, large bone gaps, and restrictive soft-tissue forces. Such is the case following extensive maxillary advancements, transverse expansions, and inferior maxillary repositioning procedures. Under such conditions osseous relapse can be shown to occur in the early postoperative period despite tight screw placement and unchanged plate contour. The explanation for this relapse, which may be similar to bone drift as described by Enlow, is not dissimilar to the mechanics involved in orthodontic movement of teeth.

In this environment interpositional bone grafting becomes necessary to promote stability of repositioned dento-osseous segments. Unfortunately, bone grafting in conjunction with rigid fixation has not eliminated this potential for relapse because of the marked tendency of autogenous bone to undergo early postoperative resorption. Resorption of a bone graft arises as a result of pressure generated from soft-tissue restrictive forces in extensive advancements and, presumably, in transverse expansions. It also is caused by masticatory forces generated both during and after maxillomandibular fixation (MMF) following inferior maxillary repositioning.

Accordingly, the concept of using nonresorbable substitutes for bone grafts for interpositional use has much appeal. Such a bone graft substitute would ideally have the following biomechanical characteristics:

1. structural rigidity,
2. promotion of rapid tissue incorporation and direct osseous healing,
3. minimal loss of volume, and
4. a low complication rate associated with its use.

Early data suggest that porous hydroxyapatite blocks possess these properties.

The implant blocks are derived from specific marine corals that have a completely interconnected porous nature. The pore size ranges from 190 to 230 μm. The $CaCO_3$ skeleton is converted by the manufacturer (Interpore International, Irvine, California) to $CaPO_4H_2O$. This mineral matrix is, therefore, architecturally and chemically similar to the inorganic component of human cortical bone. Accordingly, this porous structure provides a suitable scaffold for rapid ingrowth of fibrovascular tissue and bone. This healing process has been repeatedly demonstrated in experimental and clinical settings. This material clearly has no intrinsic osteoinductive properties. When placed in soft tissue and/or when implant blocks heal with a fibrous union (as in two specimens in our patient series) no bone ingrowth takes place. The material must be in direct contact with bone; that is, it is osteoconductive only.

Dry implant blocks are extremely brittle but gain strength as tissue incorporation proceeds. The compressive strength of the ingrown implant far exceeds masticatory forces. The torsional strength of the ingrown implant has been estimated to be 60% to 70% of human cortical bone.

Loss of volume of the implant has been minimal, estimated as less than 2% within two years. This helps explain the unchanged radiographic appearance of the implant blocks seen in our patient series.

Stress shielding of adjacent host bone is not a significant consideration because the elastic modulus of ingrown, porous hydroxyapatite has been shown to be similar to that of human bone. As seen in our histologic studies, no evidence of resorption or remodeling of host bone adjacent to the implant has been observed. Apparently the intimate bonding of host bone to implant transfers stress directly to the bone adjacent to the implant.

These biomechanical properties of porous, block hydroxyapatite favor its use as an interpositional bone graft substitute in orthognathic surgery for obliteration of osteotomy gaps. Rigid fixation of maxillary osteotomies should be used in conjunction with this implant material. This will allow tissue ingrowth to take place so that the implant will achieve adequate compressive

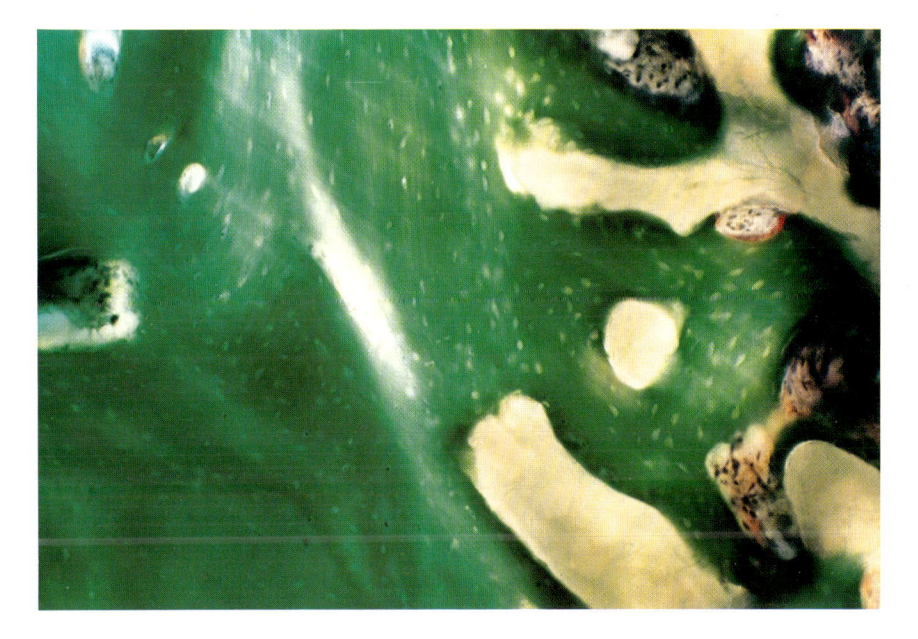

Color Plate 19 Direct osseous union between bone (green) and hydroxyapatite implant (unstained material) is shown. No resorptive or remodeling activity of adjacent host bone takes place. This biopsy was retrieved 11 months following implantation. Modified Villanueva Goldner trichrome stain was used.

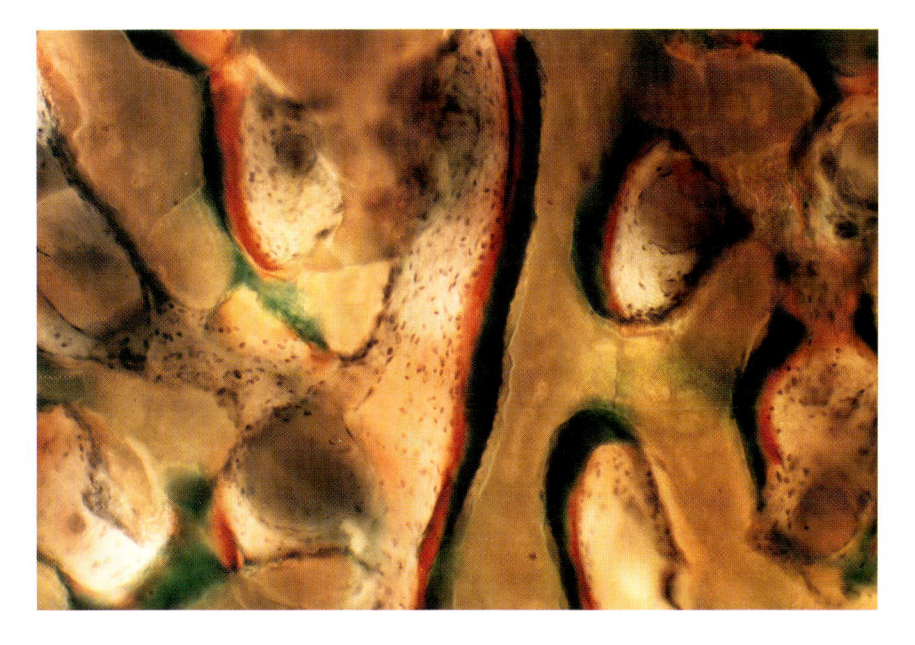

Color Plate 20 Typical healing process within pores of an implant is characterized by deposition of calcified bone adjacent to the implant wall (green), osteoid tissue adjacent to bone (orange), and fibrovascular tissue filling the central portion of the implant pore. Modified Villanueva Goldner trichrome stain was used.

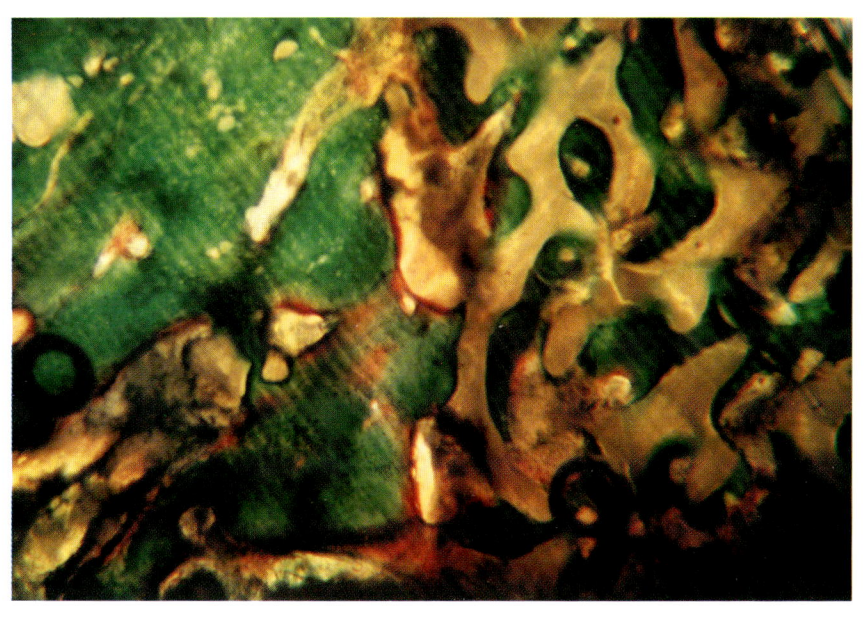

Color Plate 21 More advanced healing is shown in a 14-month specimen. Note that the pores are filled with calcified bone and a small amount of osteoid tissue. Modified Villanueva Goldner trichrome stain was used.

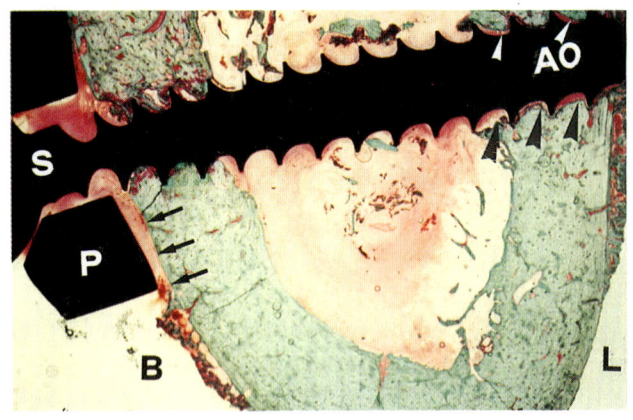

Color Plate 22 After 3 months the ASIF screws nearest to the resection borders reveal the reactions mentioned. Arrows indicate resorption underneath the plate. Soft-tissue interposition along the thread (arrowheads) is most evident at the apical part. (B = buccal, L = lingual aspect of the dog mandible, S = 100s screwhead in the hole of the plate.) (See Figure 49.9.)

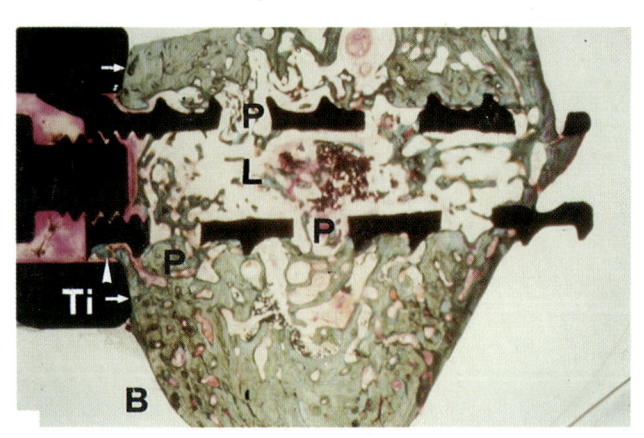

Color Plate 23 Human histological results were obtained after defect bridging and full exposure to functional loads. THORP screw nearest to the resection border is shown after defect bridging for 26 months and irradiation with 7000 rads. Bone has grown into the lumen (L) and perforations (P), anchorage is optimal, and bone–thread contact is direct. Bone apposition between the head of the screw and plate (arrows) is shown. There is no bone resorption underneath the plate, indicating transmission of physiological stress.

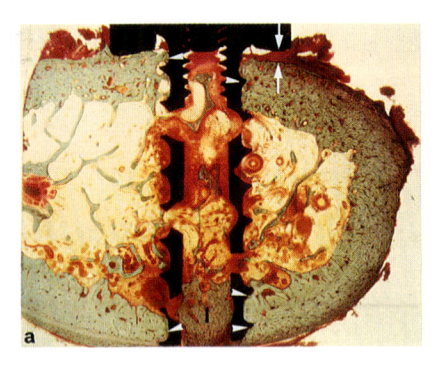

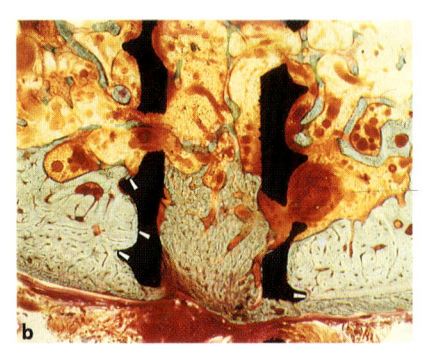

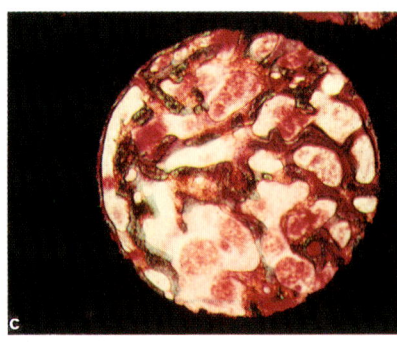

Color Plate 24 The experimental series of Figure 49.10 is shown with a THORP plate fixed by only two screws bridging the contralateral mandibular defect. (a) Optimal stability of the hollow screw with direct bone contact is seen along the thread (arrowheads). There is no bone resorption underneath the plate, although one side was not intraoperatively adapted to the bone (arrows). (I = ingrowth of bone tissue into the lumen.) (b) A view of the apical end of the screw of Color Plate 23(a) at higher magnification confirms the perfect anchorage of the THORP system, in contrast to the ASIF system. (c) A rare section of a side perforation shows one of the screws examined after only four weeks implantation time. In spite of the short interval, bone tissue has already been appositioned.

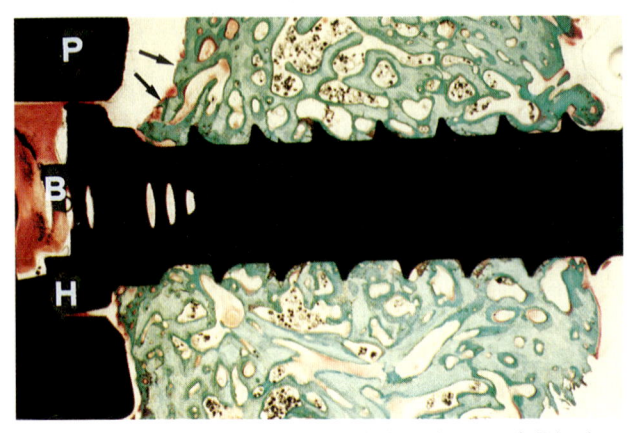

Color Plate 25 Human histological slice shows a full-body screw one year after reconstruction. Irradiation was with 4200 rads. Although intraoperative optimal plate adaptation was impossible (arrows), the rigid fixation of the head (H) to the plate (P) by the expansion bolt (B) was stable.

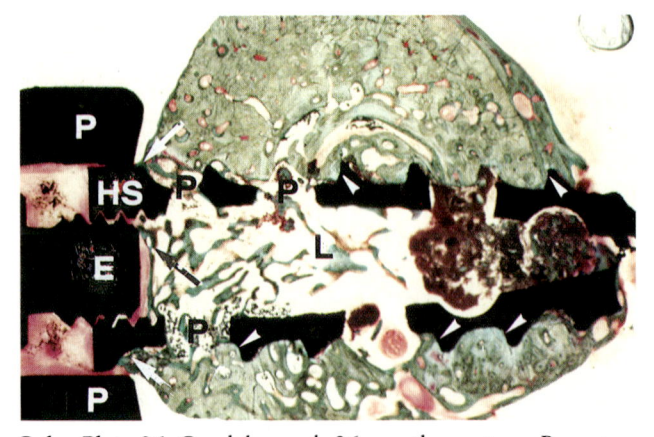

Color Plate 26 Condylar neck 26 months post op. Bone apposition (arrows) is seen up to the head (HS); between the screw head and plate (arrowheads). New bone formation appears in the screw lumen (L) up to the expansion bolt (E) through the perforations (P) (fuchsia, green light × 14).

strength before it is subjected to masticatory loads. These masticatory forces can be generated with chewing or during MMF. Rigid fixation obviates MMF, and patients are placed on soft diets for six weeks.

The high compressive strength of the implant coupled with its low rate of resorption and lack of host bone remodeling help to explain the tremendous osseous stability seen in this patient series. Relapse of transverse maxillary expansions in two patients most likely represents medial rotation of the hemimaxillary segments, the point of rotation of which was at the implanted osteotomy site. Transverse medial movement of the palatal shelves themselves is extremely unlikely.

The low rate of complication associated with the implant for interpositional use in orthognathic surgery is primarily attributed to secure coverage of soft tissues. The previously mentioned considerations with regard to soft tissues will help to minimize exposure of the implant. The absence of infected implants or sinusitis when hydroxyapatite is placed adjacent to an open maxillary sinus has been a consistent finding in our experience and that of others. This probably relates to the prophylactic use of antibiotics, the rapid vascularization of the implant block, and the forgiving nature of the maxillary sinus.

A word of caution should be offered concerning the extent to which one can stably and safely advance and/or transversely expand the maxilla. Despite the use of rigid fixation in combination with block hydroxyapatite, one must not exceed the physiologic limits of the tethered palatal mucosa to perfuse the repositioned osseous segments. In addition, a tight upper lip in a patient with cleft lip or palate may orthodontically retract the maxillary incisors following an extensive maxillary advancement. This action may masquerade as a skeletal relapse. The technology of rigid fixation and nonresorbable bone graft substitutes should not lull the surgeon into performing a nonphysiologic operative procedure.

On the other hand, one should take advantage of the tremendous stability afforded by this technique. No longer is the excuse of instability valid when aesthetic considerations demand maxillary advancement. This technique is as reliable as mandibular setback, which was considered to be its more stable counterpart. Similarly, when there is lack of facial height with lack of incisal show, inferior repositioning of the maxilla should be performed without undue concern about superior relapse. Fear of overlengthening the maxilla with subsequent impingement on freeway space does not appear to be a significant concern. This is probably more applicable in the patient who needs prosthetic dentistry than in the patient with a natural dentition. Finally, transverse expansion of the maxilla in order to achieve proper occlusion should be performed surgically rather than depending on orthodontic expansion of the maxillary arch, which in most cases will prolong treatment and lead to unstable results.

Facial skeletal expansion in all planes can be executed in a stable and predictable fashion. When considerations of aesthetics and occlusion dictate expansive vectors of osseous movement, appropriate surgical treatment planning must follow.

BIBLIOGRAPHY

Bell WH, Scheiderman GB: Correction of vertical maxillary deficiency: Stability and soft tissue changes. J Oral Surg 39:666–670, 1981.

Holmes RE, Wardrop RW, Wolford LM: Hydroxyapatite as a bone graft substitute in orthognathic surgery: Histologic and histometric findings. J Oral Maxillofac Surg 46:661–671, 1988.

Persson G, Hellern S, Nord PG: Bone plates for stabilizing Le Fort I osteotomies. J Maxillofac Surg 14:69–73, 1986.

Posnick JC, Ewing M, Ross RB: Skeletal stability after Le Fort I maxillary advancement in patients with unilateral cleft lip and palate. Plast Surg Forum 11:77–79, 1988. (Abstr.)

Rosen HM: Miniplate fixation of Le Fort I osteotomies. Plast Reconstr Surg 78:748–754, 1986.

Rosen HM: Porous, block hydroxyapatite as an interpositional bone graft substitute in orthognathic surgery. Plast Reconstr Surg 83:985–990, 1989.

Rosen HM: Definitive surgical correction of vertical maxillary deficiency. Plast Reconstr Surg 85:215–221, 1990.

White E, Shors EC: Biomaterial aspects of Interpore 200™ porous hydroxyapatite. Dent Clin North Am 30:49–67, 1986.

Wolford LM, Wardrop RW, Hartog JM: Coralline porous hydroxyapatite as a bone graft substitute in orthognathic surgery. J Oral Maxillofac Surg 45:1034–1042, 1987.

CHAPTER 36

The Role of Plate and Screw Fixation in the Treatment of Cleft Lip and Palate Jaw Deformities

Jeffrey C. Posnick
Mark P. Ewing

The satisfactory management of cleft lip and palate presents considerable challenge for reconstructive surgeons. It requires the close cooperation of many specialists, who must concentrate not only on their area of expertise but also on pooling their talents to meet the overall needs of each patient.

The first step is thorough assessment of the patient. In the case of patients with repaired clefts, skeletal dysplasia (jaw deformity), and malocclusion, assessment must include evaluation of breathing pattern, speech and language function, occlusion, facial soft- and hard-tissue aesthetics, and psychosocial status. Although the patient may request correction of a lip scar deformity and nasal distortion or correction of poor speech caused by a congenital deformity and previous surgical procedures, a true correction may necessitate the establishment of a normal bony architecture. In such cases, simple soft-tissue camouflage is not appropriate.

The central problem for most cleft patients who have skeletal dysplasia and malocclusion is maxillary hypoplasia, which is caused by the original birth defect and previous surgical interventions.

This is often complicated by the presence of residual oronasal fistula, a cleft-dental gap in the region of the congenitally missing lateral incisor tooth and an alveolar bony defect with residual mobility of the maxillary segments. In these patients, skeletal reconstruction must begin with the Le Fort I maxillary osteotomy in one or more segments. This procedure was developed in Europe over 100 years ago. In 1867, Cheever performed a unilateral Le Fort I osteotomy to remove a nasopharyngeal tumor. In 1935, Wassmund performed an osteotomy of the maxilla using the fracture lines that had been described by Rene Le Fort in 1901 in a patient with an open-bite deformity (Freihofer 1977).

In 1942, Schuchardt performed the first separate Le Fort I osteotomy at the pterygoid plates. Gillies and Rowe in 1954 described the mobilization of collapsed maxillary segments in patients with clefts, and Obwegeser (1955) showed that the down-fractured maxilla could be moved in any direction either as a unit or in segments. In experiments in dogs, Bell (1973) demonstrated revascularization in bone healing with this procedure. Well-planned and meticulously executed orthognathic surgery can clean up many of the residual clefting problems that the adolescent may present with.

The use of internal miniplate, microplate and screw fixation techniques has allowed for more predictable, immediate, and long-term results (Posnick and Ewing, 1990) and has reduced the early morbidity associated with surgical procedures involving the jaw (Luhr 1979).

DIAGNOSIS AND TREATMENT PLANNING

Facial Aesthetics

A basic appreciation of facial aesthetics and a thorough, systematic approach to the analysis of facial deformities are prerequisites for planning strategy as well as for correcting jaw deformities. Facial proportions, facial symmetry, and the relationship of the maxillary anterior teeth to the upper lip—both smiling and in repose—must also be considered (Bell 1980). A combination of cephalometric analysis, anthropometric surface measurements, and computerized tomography (CT) techniques can supplement, but not replace, a thorough clinical examination by an experienced surgeon.

Since antiquity, man has sought the elusive embodiment of beauty in the human face. However, concepts of facial beauty vary and do not always conform to reality. For many centuries, the nine classical Greek canons for facial proportion, which were frequently depicted by Renaissance artists, provided the accepted standard; however, Farkas (1985) found significant differences between the actual proportions of vertical and horizontal anthropometric measurement in Caucasian faces and the relationships dictated by the canons. Ricketts (1982) suggested that the golden mean could be applied to the human face. However, it has long been known that absolute symmetry is uninteresting and even monotonous (Farkas 1987).

Numerous cephalometric systems have been devised to evaluate the relationships among the cranium, facial bones, and dental structures. Each system has attempted to obtain information about the relationships of jaw to jaw, cranial base to jaw, and tooth to jaw.

The relationship between the upper lip and the maxillary anterior teeth must be considered in both smile and repose when a patient with a jaw deformity is assessed. Ideally, with the upper lip at rest, about 2 to 3 mm of the vertical height of the central incisor tooth is visible. With a broad smile, 1 to 2 mm of the vertical height of the gingiva shows above the central incisor crowns.

In patients with clefts and maxillary hypoplasia, the teeth and gingiva often do not show below the upper lip, causing an edentulous appearance. On the other hand, some patients with bilateral cleft lip and palate may have an elongated premaxilla that exposes an excessive amount of tooth and gingiva. A congenital cleft lip that has undergone surgical repair and multiple revisions may deviate considerably from the norm; the dynamic range of the upper lip may be drastically reduced, and the middle portion of the bilateral cleft lip is often immobile. In such patients, planning jaw surgery may necessitate compromise; for overall aesthetic improvement, the upper jaw may have to be placed so that tooth exposure is slightly excessive with the lip at rest and gingival exposure is slightly inadequate with the lip in a broad smile. Ideally, the dental midlines and the midline of the chin should match the facial midline.

Attempts should be made to predict the response of soft tissue to orthognathic surgery. The ratio of soft-to-hard tissue change rarely approaches a one-to-one relationship (Bell 1981). Ratio tables have been generated that permit relatively accurate prediction of results (Bell 1981). However, the response of soft tissue to movement of bone in the scarred and tethered cleft lip differs from that of the normal lip.

ANALYSIS OF OCCLUSION

Analysis of occlusion is essential in planning jaw surgery. However, before this is done, alginate dental impressions should be obtained, cast in stone, and mounted on an articulator with a face-bow transfer. To achieve maximum correction of occlusal plain canting, open-bite deformity, cross bites, and dental gaps and to position the dental midlines on the facial midline, orthodontic techniques must be combined with jaw surgery. By completing mock surgery on dental models preoperatively, the surgeon and orthodontist can plan to the millimeter the anterior-posterior, horizontal, and vertical maxillary and mandibular changes required to achieve optimum facial aesthetics and occlusion.

Intraoperatively, judging facial aesthetics and lip-to-tooth relationships is difficult. The surgeon must therefore rely heavily on his or her preoperative judgment of the desired aesthetics and on the precise measurements calculated with the orthodontist during the model surgery phase. A cut-as-you-go approach in orthognathic surgery is rarely advised. Greater accuracy is achieved by using a prefabricated acrylic interocclusal final splint in one-jaw surgery and by adding an intermediate splint in combined maxillary and mandibular, or two-jaw, surgery.

RESIDUAL DEFORMITIES

Unilateral Cleft Lip and Palate: Residual Deformities

The residual clefting deformities that an adolescent with UCLP presents with will vary, but may include: a degree of maxillary hypoplasia resulting in a concave midface profile, Class III malocclusion and negative overjet. Despite a general preference for fistula closure in the mixed dentition, residual oronasal fistula may be present. Previous attempts at fistula closure may have ended in failure, or this problem may have been neglected earlier in life. Residual bony defects of the alveolus, palate and floor of the nose with an inferiorly displaced nasal sill may also be present. A cleft-dental gap in the region of the congenitally-absent lateral incisor tooth at the cleft site is a common finding. The chin may be vertically long and retrognathic. This is due to a mouthbreathing habit. Mandibular dysplasia may be present with canting of the occlusal plane, resulting in a facial asymmetry.

Bilateral Cleft Lip and Palate: Residual Deformities

The BCLP adolescent may have residual clefting deformities which vary from the other cleft types and include: maxillary dysplasia, the premaxilla may be either vertically long or short and is often horizontally retruded. The lateral segments may be constricted and hypoplastic with Class III malocclusion. Despite a general preference for fistula closure and bone grafting in mixed dentition, residual oronasal fistula may be present. Previous attempts at fistula closure may have ended in failure and other patients may have been neglected. In these cases, the premaxilla will be mobile. Cleft-dental gaps, resulting from the congenital absence of the lateral incisor teeth are frequent findings and unless successful bone grafting and fistula closure was accomplished in the mixed dentition residual bony defects, through the alveolus, floor of the nose and palate will be present. Chin dysplasia with increased vertical length and retrogenia occurs but mandibular dysplasia, due to is true mandibular prognathism is rare. Mandibular asymmetries with occlusal canting may occur.

Isolated Cleft Palate: Residual Deformities

A degree of maxillary dysplasia may be present and when it is, it often follows one of two patterns. A frequent finding is horizontal maxillary retrusion with a minor degree of vertical hypoplasia. Another common pattern is vertical maxillary excess with a minor degree of horizontal retrusion. Residual oronasal fistula may be present, either at the incisal foramen region or within the soft palate and associated with residual bony defects in the hard palate. Chin dysplasia will generally present as increased vertical length with retrogenia. Mandibular dysplasia may be in the form of mandibular retrognathism if part of the Pierre Robin sequence. Where present, this tends to mask the degree of maxillary hypoplasia.

SURGICAL TECHNIQUES

Maxillary Surgical Techniques

The maxillary surgical techniques required for correction of the residual clefting deformities seen in adolescence are unique. They depend on the patient's presenting residual clefting problems which is a reflection of their cleft type (i.e., BCLP, UCLP, and ICP), previous surgery and growth potential. In the past, authors have developed various modifications of the Le Fort osteotomy and attempts to correct these residual problems and minimize morbidity (Braun, 1982, Garrison, 1987, Tessier, 1984, Tideman, 1980, James, 1985, Poole, 1986, West, 1990, and Westbrook, 1983). The senior author has further modified the maxillary Le Fort I osteotomy to conform to the cleft type (e.g., BCLP, UCLP and LCP) and residual clefting deformities that the adolescent presents with, allowing for safe one-stage correction (Posnick J.C., 1991, Posnick J.C., Dagys A.P., 1991, Posnick J.C., 1991) (see Figures 36.4 and 36.7).

With the use of miniplate and screw internal fixation, the cleft maxilla, once dysimpacted and advanced, can be securely stabilized. The maximum horizontal advancement I have achieved in the cleft patient is 27 millimeters. The miniplates are placed vertically across the osteotomy and secured; one plate is placed at each zygomatic buttress region, and one plate is placed at each nasal piriform aperture region. In the UCLP patient I also place a microplate and screws horizontally across the cleft site to give added stability. Internal fixation techniques ensure reliable placement of osteotomy segments and may diminish postoperative skeletal relapse (Beals 1987, Drommer 1981, Harsha 1986, Horster 1980, Luhr 1979, Rosen 1986, Posnick and Ewing 1990). With stable internal fixation, the jaws may be left unwired for postoperative airway management with little concern for immediate relapse of skeletal segment position.

Postoperative relapse may occur despite the best planning and the use of current surgical techniques, including internal bone miniplate and screw fixation (Posnick and Ewing 1990). This is especially true in the patient with cleft lip and palate who has a scarred hypoplastic maxilla requiring a Le Fort I osteotomy. It is hoped that the tendency to relapse is decreased by the use of both maxillo-mandibular fixation (MMF) and miniplate and screw fixation techniques in the postoperative period. Interposition autogenous iliac bone grafts are placed at osteotomy gaps, including between the zygomatic buttress and the nasal aperture regions. In addition, all cleft defects are filled with cancellous bone graft. The placement of bone graft may be a major factor in preventing relapse (Araujo 1978, Tessier 1984). Wiring a prefabricated interocclusal splint to the orthodontic brackets on the upper teeth adds stability to the segmented maxilla.

After the ideal occlusion is achieved intraoperatively and after the MMF is released to check the bite, the jaws are often left unwired to permit extubation in the operating room and rapid postoperative recovery. This will depend on the specific airway protocol at a particular hospital. In the majority of cleft patients, it remains my preference to place MMF either in the operating room or before the patient is discharged from the hospital in attempts to further limit skeletal relapse.

Mandible Surgery

Surgical repositioning of the mandible is not usually required in cleft patients, with the exception of those with Pierre Robin syndrome and in cases of associated mandibular prognathism or facial asymmetry. Overall functional and aesthetic needs determine whether simultaneous mandibular repositioning is indicated. Camouflage procedures consisting of mandibular setback to obviate the need for maxillary surgery should be avoided in most circumstances.

When mandibular repositioning is required, I prefer to use a sagittal split osteotomy technique, which gives a more physiological correction and allows better bone-to-bone contact of segments. To achieve stabilization, I usually use three bicortical screws placed through a transbuccal trocar system at each osteotomy site. One or two are placed along the lateral oblique ridge and then one or two close to the inferior border. Great care is taken to avoid injury to either the inferior alveolar neurovascular bundle or the dentition. Other surgeons prefer the placement of bone plates (Beals 1987,

Drommer 1981, Harsha 1986, Horster 1980, Luhr 1979, Rosen 1986). In any case, the basic principle is to ensure that the condyles are well seated in their glenoid fossa before osteotomy stabilization.

Residual malocclusions can occur after mandibular osteotomy stabilized with internal fixation devices such as miniplates, bicortical screws, or lag screws. These difficulties have led to the development of intricate techniques to maintain the preoperative position of the condyle in the glenoid fossa (Reuther, personal communication 1986, Luhr 1989). Osteotomies can then be completed and the mandible repositioned and stabilized with bone miniplates or screws. Whether the additional time, dissection, and manipulation required ultimately limit postoperative malocclusion remains to be seen.

The transbuccal trocar system is extremely useful for stabilizing the mandibular segments with bone miniplates or bicortical screws while limiting the external incisions required. The recent introduction of right-angle drills and screwdrivers may allow intraoral exposure as required for plate and screw fixation of the mandible, thereby circumventing the need for the trocar system, which involves small but definite 4-millimeter facial incisions.

Chin Surgery

Patients with clefts often have vertically long and retrognathic chins. An intraoral vertical reduction and horizontal advancement genioplasty can be safely completed with minimal morbidity if basic principles are adhered to. The mucosa is incised to the depth of the vestibule to ensure an adequate mucosal wound edge at closure. This limits the incidence of wound dehiscence and prevents postoperative problems with the attached gingiva. The blood supply to the chin should be meticulously maintained through soft-tissue attachment along the inferior and lingual aspects of the bone flap.

The inferior borders of the mandible are exposed through subperiosteal dissection. Dissection superior to the mental nerve should be avoided to prevent excessive traction and accidental avulsion of the neurovascular (mental nerve) bundle. When performing a horizontal osteotomy, the surgeon should leave at least 2 millimeters (and ideally 4 millimeters) of bone below the mental foramina to avoid lacerating the nerve in the mandibular canal.

Satisfactory chin stabilization is often achieved by placing three transosseous direct stainless steel wires. My personal preference is the placement of two microplates secured with microscrews. However, when significant chin advancement is required, and a scarred or deficient skin bed are present, two well placed miniplates are preferred. The importance of adequate stabilization cannot be overemphasized.

The posterior extent of the chin osteotomy must be carefully selected to avoid bony discrepancies. The greater the vertical reduction, the more posteriorly the osteotomy should be extended to avoid a visible postoperative step-off on either side of the junction of the chin and the mandibular body. If a step-off is present, it should be reduced intraoperatively by bone burring with a rotary drill. Major spontaneous remodeling of the bony step-off should not be expected postoperatively.

CASE REPORTS

A spectrum of clefting types and presenting deformities demonstrate the range of problems that benefit from cleft-orthognathic surgery.

Case 1: Unilateral Cleft Lip and Palate

This 17-year-old girl was born with complete left cleft lip and palate (see Figure 36.1). She underwent soft-tissue repairs in infancy and early childhood.

She developed maxillary hypoplasia with a class III malocclusion. She was congenitally missing the lateral incisor tooth at the cleft site. The cleft dental gap had been successfully closed through the orthodontic treatment initiated in the mixed dentition.

Preoperative othodontic treatment was followed by a standard maxillary Le Fort I osteotomy with horizontal advancement. Stabilization was achieved with titanium miniplates and screws, iliac bone graft, prefabricated acrylic splint, and MMF.

Postoperative orthodontic detailing of occlusion continued for a six-month interval, and she was then placed in orthodontic retainers.

Case 2: Unilateral Cleft Lip and Palate

This 28-year-old woman was born with a complete cleft of the right primary and secondary palate (see Figure 36.2). By history she had undergone 16 previous cleft lip procedures while living in Hong Kong, including cleft lip and palate repairs, as well as a superiorly based pharyngeal flap for velopharyngeal incompetence and an attempted Le Fort I osteotomy.

On our initial assessment, she was found to have multiple residual problems that included a hypoplastic maxilla with residual oronasal fistula, residual bony defects, a scarred and tethered pharyngeal flap resulting in borderline velopharyngeal competence, mandibular prognathism, and a vertically long chin. She had congenital absence of the left maxillary central and lateral incisors and canine tooth, resulting in a large cleft dental gap.

She underwent preoperative orthodontic treatment to align each arch. Following this, she underwent a maxillary Le Fort I osteotomy in two segments with advancement, simultaneous closure of the residual oronasal fistulas, iliac bone grafting to alveolar and palatal bony defects, bilateral sagittal split osteotomies of

470   RIGID FIXATION OF THE CRANIOMAXILLOFACIAL SKELETON

Figure 36.1 This 17-year-old girl was born with a unilateral cleft lip and palate. She developed a maxillary hypoplasia and a class III malocclusion and required a maxillary Le Fort I osteotomy with horizontal advancement. (a) Preoperative frontal view. (b) Postoperative frontal view. (c) Preoperative frontal view with smile. (d) Postoperative frontal view with smile. (e) Preoperative profile view. (f) Postoperative profile view. (g) Preoperative occlusal view. (h) Postoperative occlusal view. (i) Articulated dental models ready for model surgery. (j) The maxilla advanced and ready for splint construction. (k) Preoperative radiographs. (l) Postoperative radiographs.

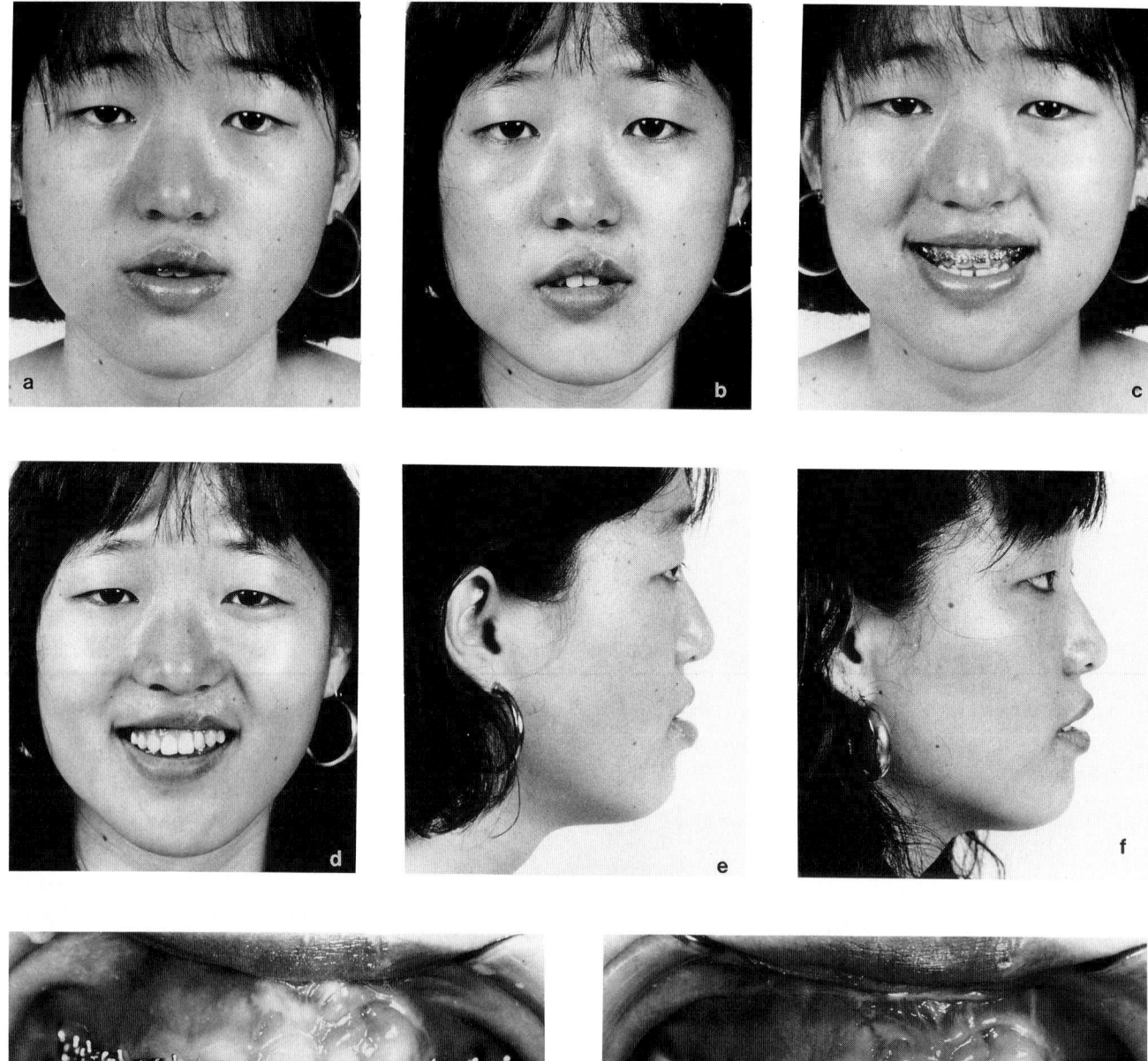

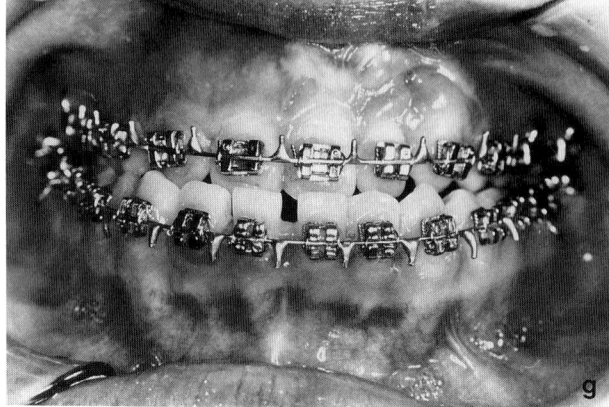

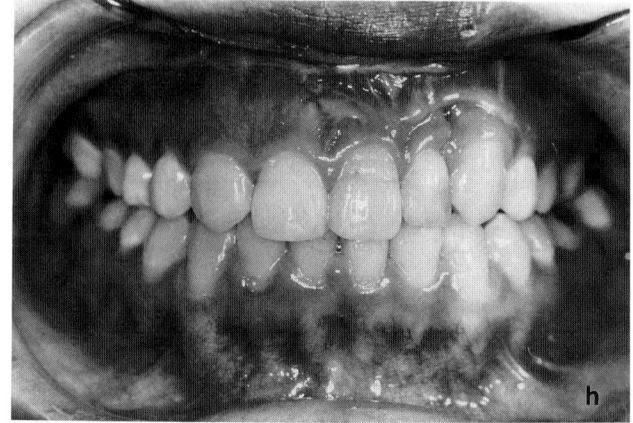

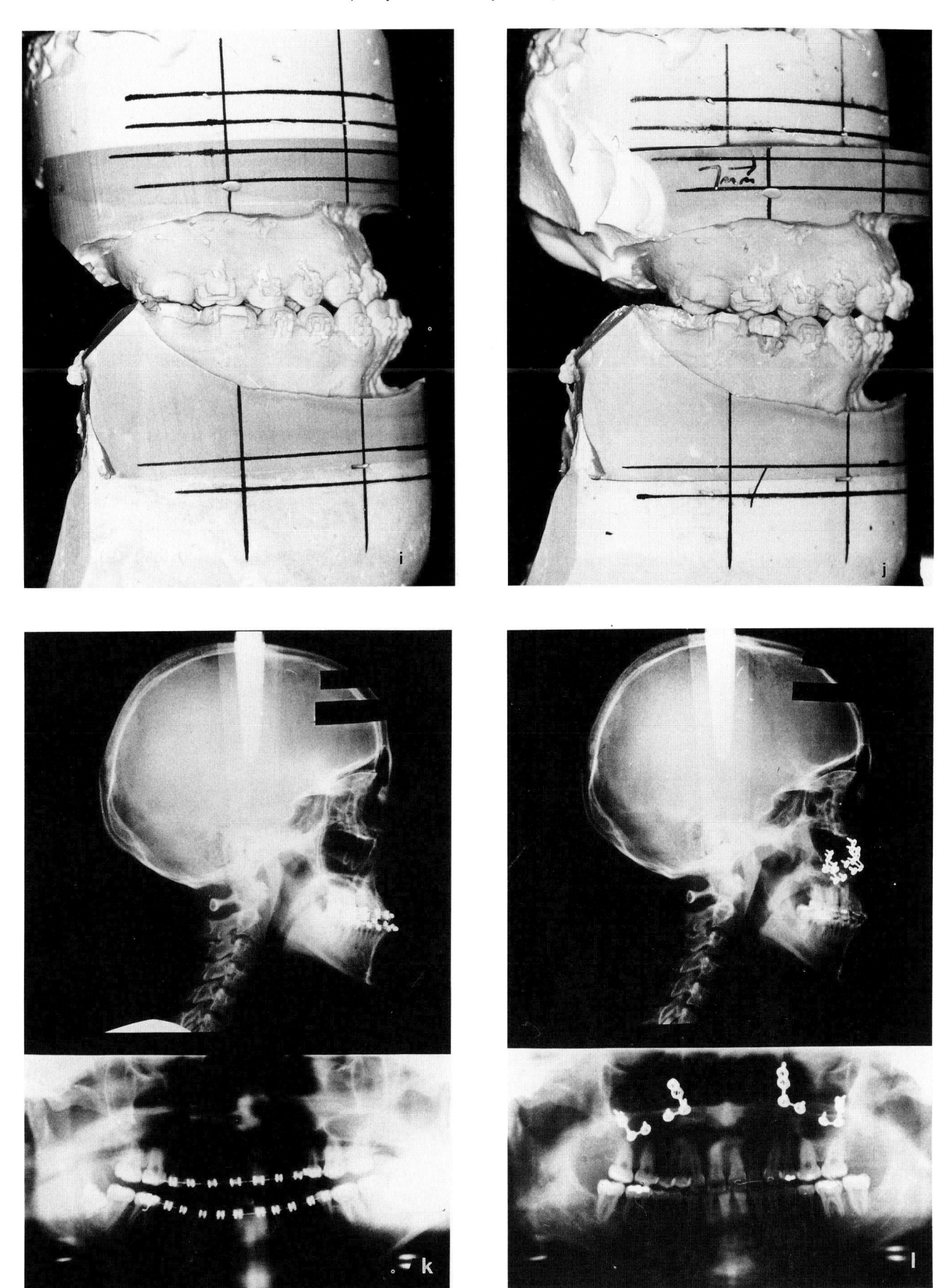

Cleft Lip and Palate Jaw Deformities

Figure 36.2 This 28-year-old woman had a repaired unilateral cleft lip and palate with residual deformities requiring Le Fort I osteotomy in two segments, closure of oronasal fistula, iliac bone grafting, bilateral sagittal split osteotomies of the mandible, and genioplasty. (a) Preoperative frontal view with smile. (b) Postoperative frontal view with smile. (c) Preoperative profile view. (d) Postoperative profile view. (e) Preoperative occlusal view. (f) Postoperative occlusal view. (g) Articulated dental models ready for model surgery. (h) Maxilla advanced and ready for intermediate splint construction. (i) The mandible set back and ready for final splint construction. (j) The transbuccal trocar system in place. (k) Screwdriver through transbuccal trocar system at sagittal split site. (l) The bony chin exposed for a vertical reduction and advancement genioplasty. (m) Genioplasty completed and stabilized with titanium miniplates and screws. (n) Preoperative and postoperative lateral cephalometric radiographs.

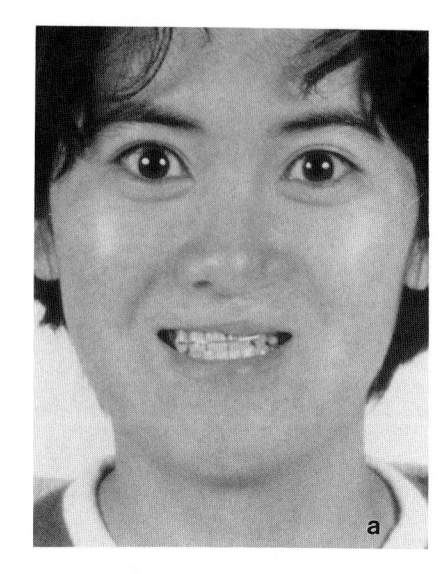

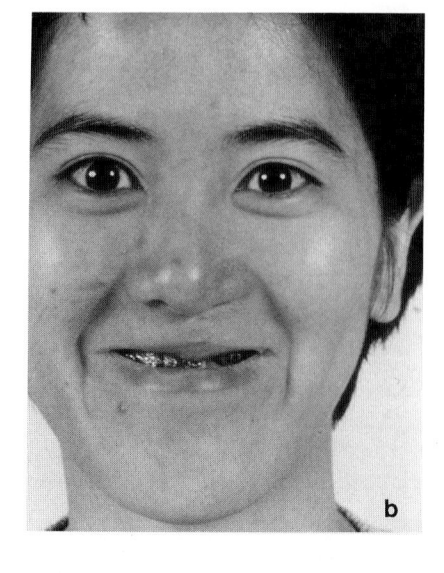

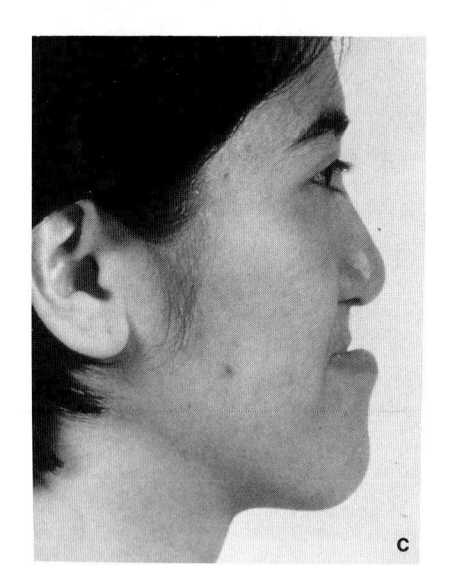

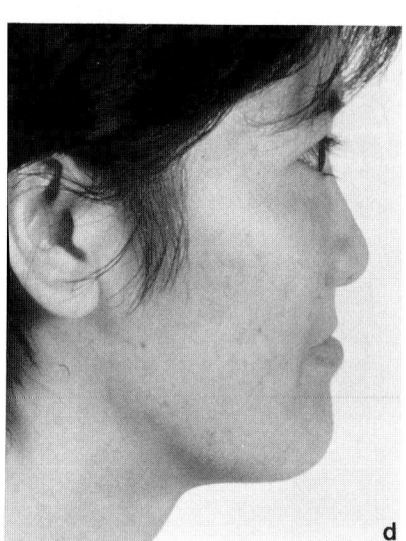

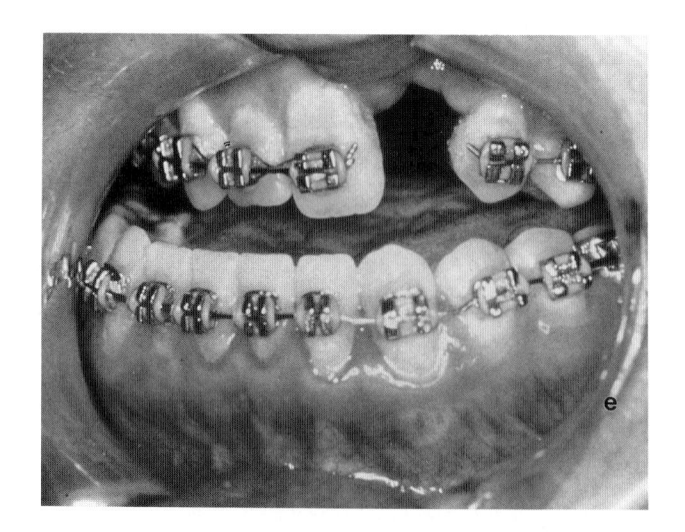

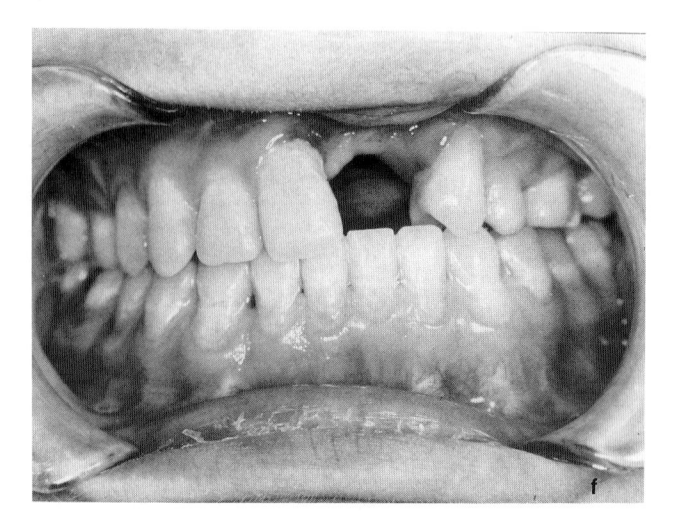

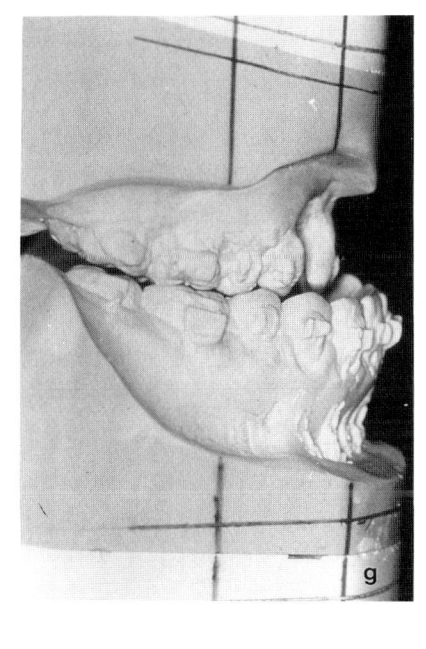

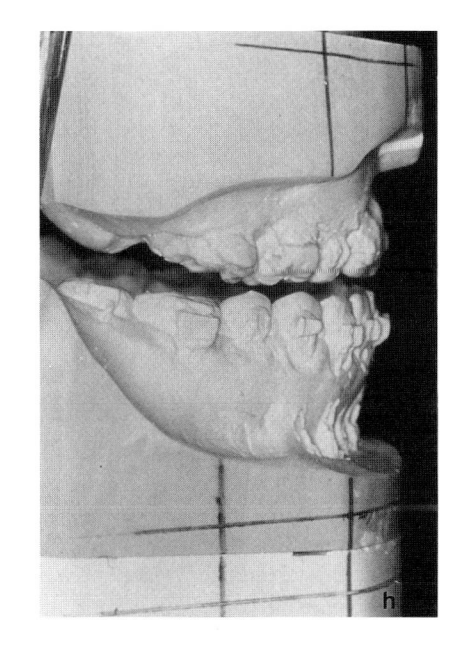

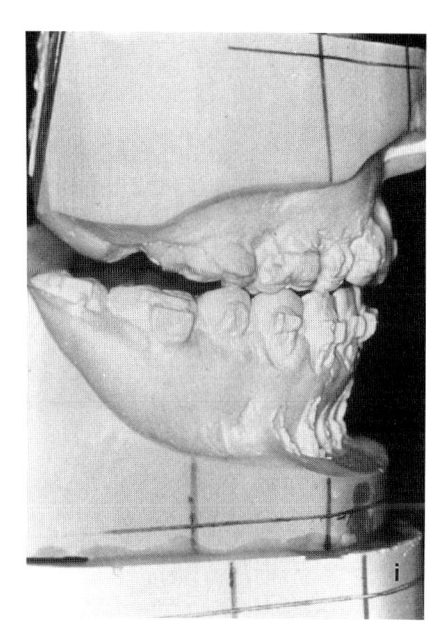

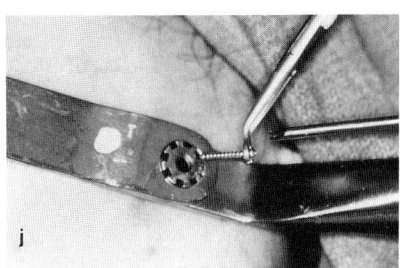

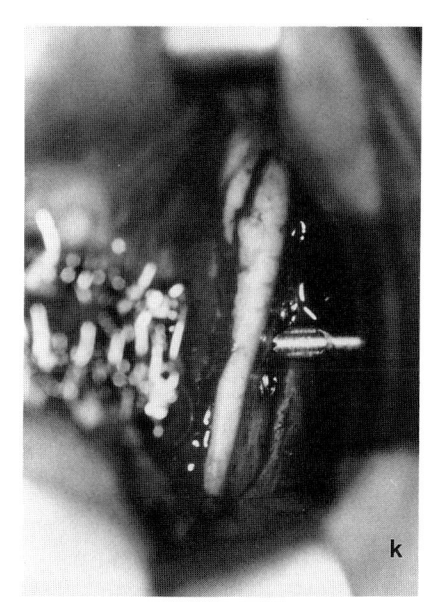

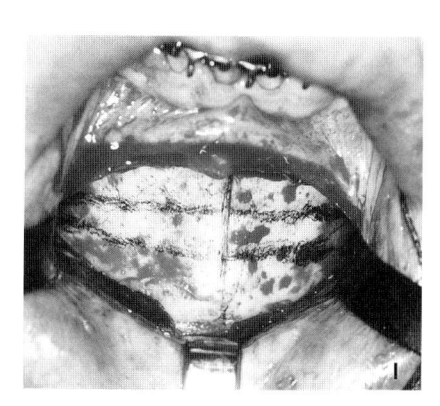

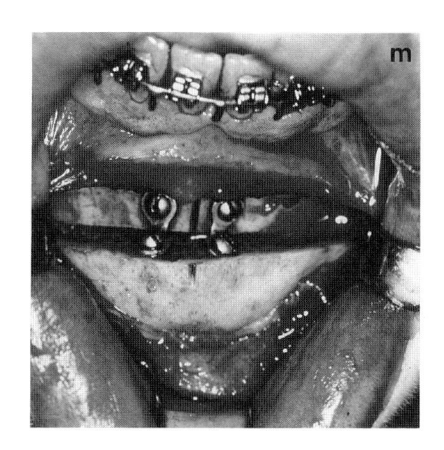

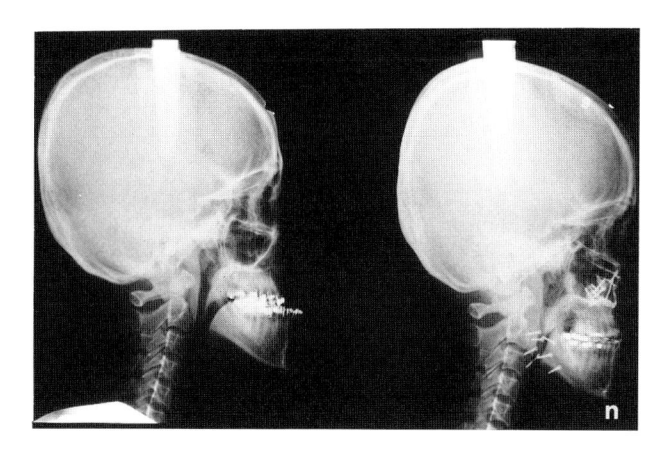

Cleft Lip and Palate Jaw Deformities

the mandible with setback, and a vertical reduction and advancement genioplasty. Stabilization was achieved with a combination of titanium miniplates and screws in the maxilla and bicortical screws in the mandible, as well as a prefabricated acrylic splint and MMF.

Postoperatively, she continued her orthodontic treatment and required a revision of her superiorly based pharyngeal flap to improve her velopharyngeal closure pattern. Now that the orthodontic work is completed, she is ready for prosthetic restoration of missing maxillary teeth.

Case 3: Unilateral Cleft Lip and Palate

This patient (see Figure 36.3) was born with a complete cleft of the left lip and palate. He had undergone lip closure at 4 years of age, followed by a cleft palate repair with push-back flaps at age 6. Cleft lip revision and a pharyngoplasty were performed at age 15.

His residual problems included a cleft-dental gap with a poorly formed, palatally displaced, rudimentary lateral incisor tooth at the cleft site, a perialveolar oronasal fistula, an anterior open bite, a Class III malocclusion, and a vertically long and retrognathic chin. At age 16, the patient received orthodontic brackets to level and align the teeth on each maxillary segment and the mandible in preparation for orthognathic surgery carried out 1 year later.

He underwent a modified Le Fort I osteotomy in two segments with differential repositioning to close the gap and the oronasal fistula and to correct the anterior open bite and Class III malocclusion. A vertical reduction and advancement genioplasty was also performed.

He is shown 1 year after surgery with improved function and appearance and without the need for prosthetic rehabilitation.

Case 4: Bilateral Cleft Lip and Palate

A Caucasian boy with complete BCLP underwent bilateral lip repair at 3 months of age, which was followed by cleft palate repair at 18 months with bilateral push-back flaps. He underwent lip-scar revision at the age of 2 years, followed by columella lengthening at 3 years, 11 months of age. Brackets were placed at the age of 13 for what was felt to be his final orthodontic treatment to align the teeth on each segment.

At the age of 16, the patient was referred for surgical consideration of his mobile premaxilla and closure of his oronasal fistula with the thought that fixed bridgework would replace the missing lateral incisors. Examination revealed a mobile premaxilla, congenitally missing maxillary lateral incisor teeth with cleft-dental gaps, labial and palatal residual oronasal fistulae, and a vertically long and retrognathic chin.

Cleft-orthognathic surgery was carried out at the age of 17 (see Figure 36.5). The modified maxillary Le Fort I osteotomy was completed to reposition the lateral segments differentially for closure of the cleft-dental gaps and oronasal fistula, to stabilize the premaxillary segment, and to improve periodontal support to the teeth adjacent to each cleft. A vertical reduction and horizontal advancement genioplasty was also completed to improve his lip closure and appearance.

He is shown 2 years after surgery and after successful management of these problems; he has a more attractive smile and does not require prosthetic rehabilitation. His poor oral hygiene continues to cause a generalized gingivitis.

Case 5: Bilateral Cleft Lip and Palate

This patient with BCLP underwent bilateral lip repair at 3 months of age, followed by cleft palate repair at 18 months with bilateral push-back flaps (see Figure 36.6). He had lip-scar revision at age 2, followed by columella lengthening at age 4. At 13 years of age, brackets were placed for what was believed to be his final orthodontic treatment to align the teeth in each segment.

At age 16, the patient was referred for surgical correction of his mobile premaxilla and oronasal fistula closure with the thought that fixed bridgework would replace the missing lateral incisors. Examination revealed a mobile and hypoplastic premaxilla, congenitally missing maxillary lateral incisors with cleft-dental gaps, labial and palatal residual oronasal fistulas, and a vertically long and retrognathic chin.

At age 17, he underwent a modified maxillary Le Fort I osteotomy to reposition the lateral segments differentially for closure of the cleft-dental gaps and oronasal fistulas, to stabilize the premaxillary segment, and to improve periodontal support for the teeth adjacent to each cleft (see Figure 36.7). A vertical reduction and horizontal advancement genioplasty was also completed to improve his lip closure and appearance.

He is shown 2 years after surgery with successful management of these problems and a more attractive smile, without the need for prosthetic rehabilitation.

Case 6: Isolated Cleft Palate

This 23-year-old woman was born with an isolated cleft palate (see Figure 36.8). She underwent repair of the cleft palate at 18 months of age and a superiorly based pharyngeal flap at age 12 to correct velopharyngeal incompetence.

She presented to me with maxillary hypoplasia, class III malocclusion, and velopharyngeal incompetence. Following preoperative orthodontic treatment, she underwent a maxillary Le Fort I osteotomy with hori-

Cleft Lip and Palate Jaw Deformities

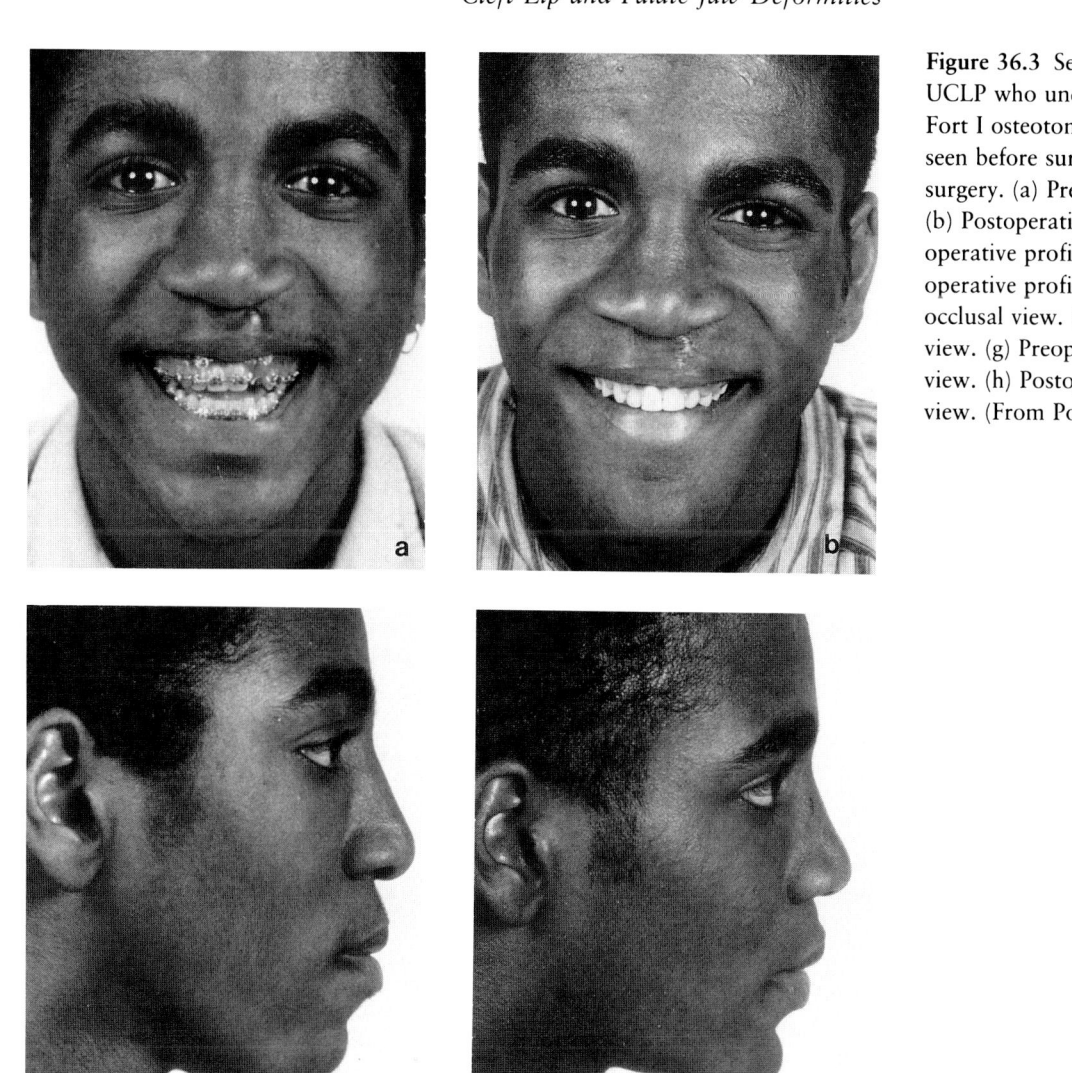

Figure 36.3 Seventeen-year-old with UCLP who underwent a modified Le Fort I osteotomy in two segments is seen before surgery and 1 year after surgery. (a) Preoperative frontal view. (b) Postoperative frontal view. (c) Preoperative profile view. (d) Postoperative profile view. (e) Preoperative occlusal view. (f) Postoperative occlusal view. (g) Preoperative lateral occlusal view. (h) Postoperative lateral occlusal view. (From Posnick 1991b.)

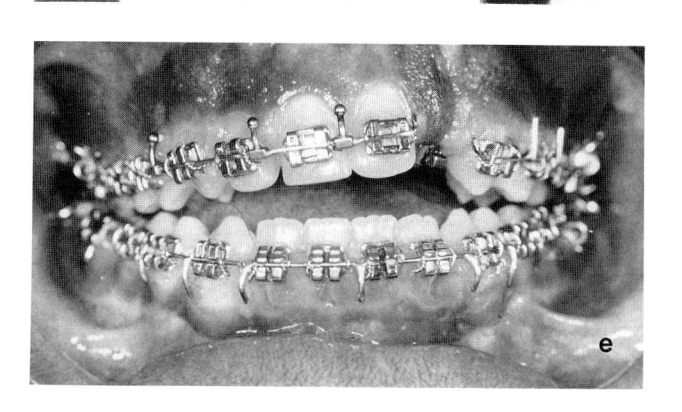

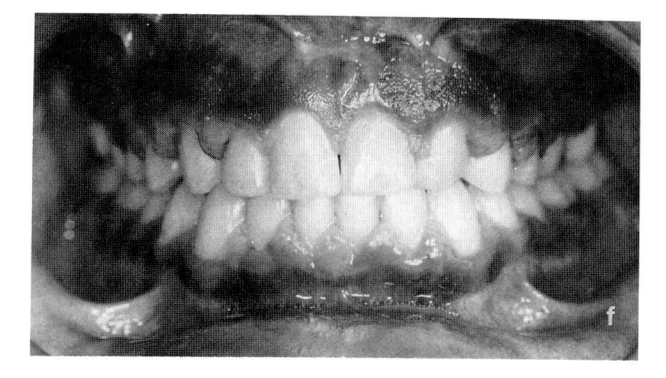

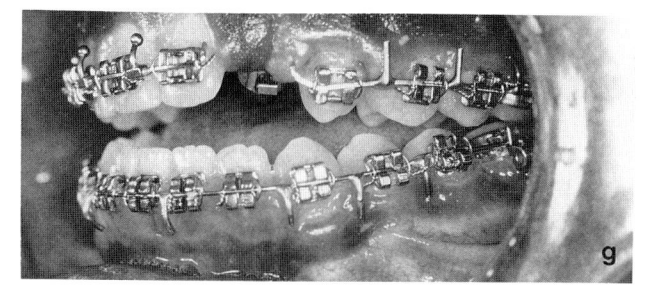

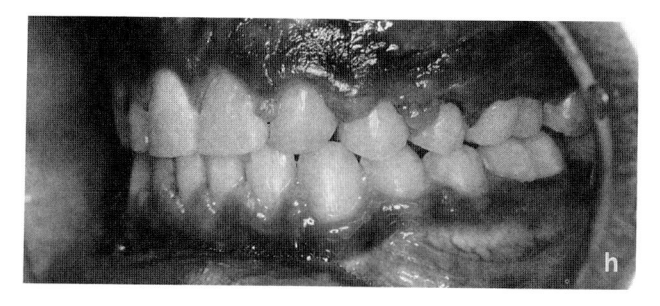

Figure 36.4 Illustrations of modified Le Fort I osteotomy in two segments. (a) Frontal view of bony skeleton before and just after fixation of Le Fort I osteotomy in two segments. The inferior turbinates have been reduced, and a submucous resection of the deviated nasal septum has been performed. Iliac cancellous bone graft has been placed along the nasal floor. (b) Lateral view of maxillofacial skeleton before and just after fixation of modified Le Fort I osteotomy. (c) Illustration of direct incisions for completion of osteotomies and fistula closure. (d) Illustration of down-fractured Le Fort I in two segments after submucous resection of the septum, reduction of inferior turbinate through the nasal mucosa opening, followed by watertight nasal-side closure. (e) Illustration indicating oral-side wound closure on both labial and palatal aspects after differential segmental repositioning. (f) Palatal view of bony segments before and after repositioning. (From Posnick [in press]).

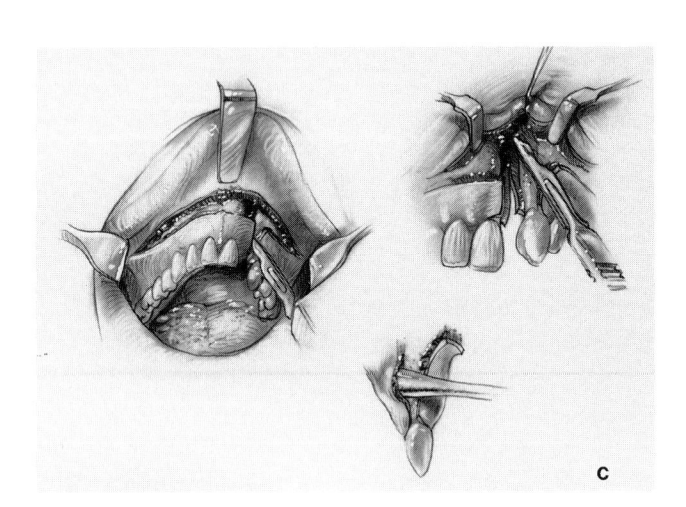

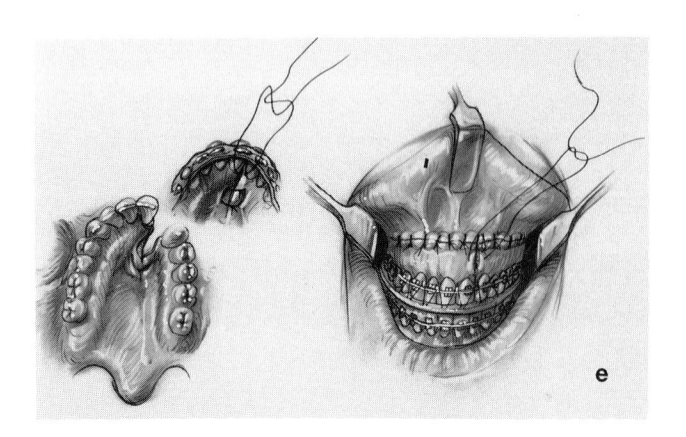

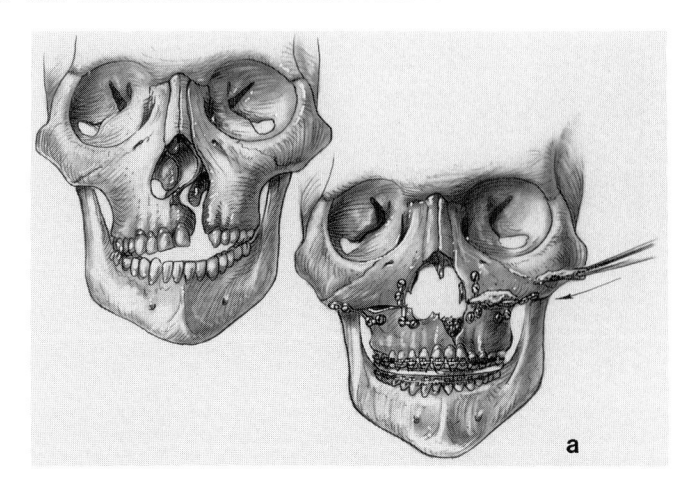

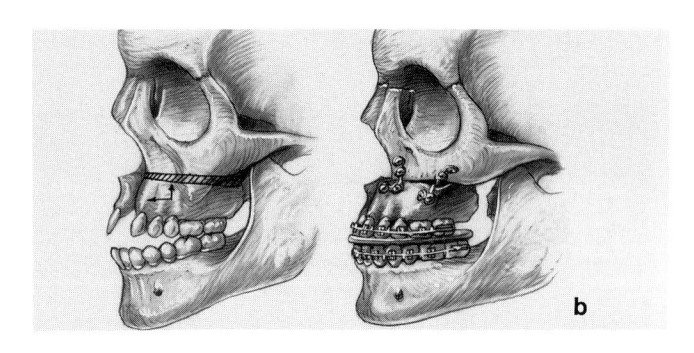

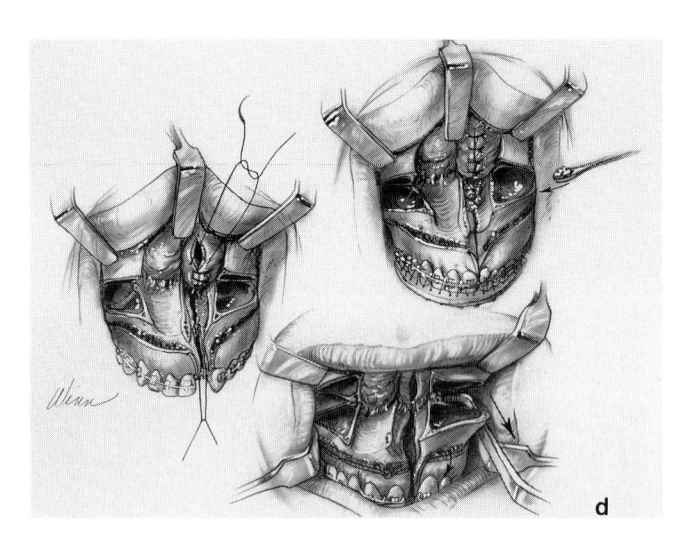

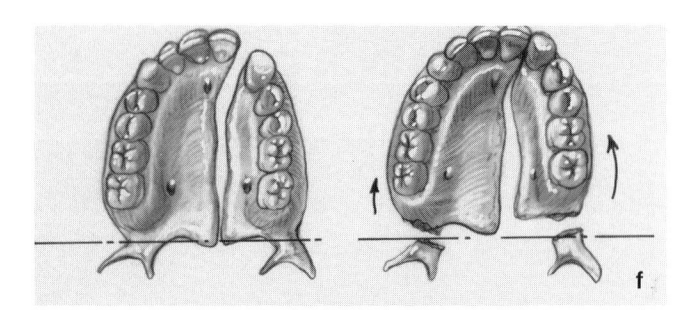

Cleft Lip and Palate Jaw Deformities

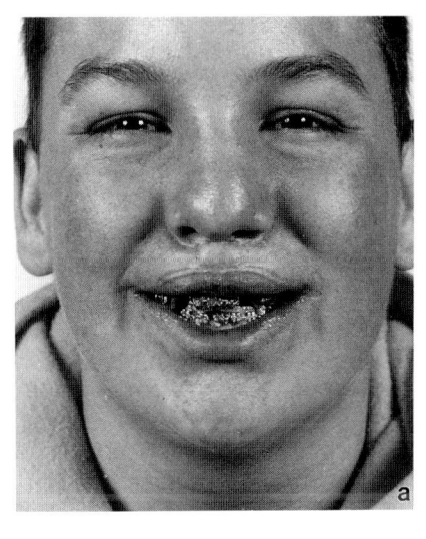

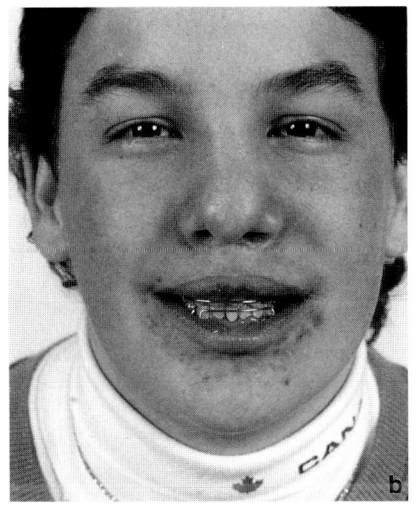

Figure 36.5 Seventeen-year-old with bilateral cleft lip and palate who underwent a modified Le Fort I osteotomy in two segments with premaxilla remaining intact. He is shown before surgery and 2 years later. (a) Preoperative frontal view, (b) postoperative frontal view, (c) preoperative profile view, (d) postoperative profile view, (e) preoperative occlusal view, (f) postoperative occlusal view, (g) preoperative palatal view, (h) postoperative palatal view. (From Posnick and Dagys 199.)

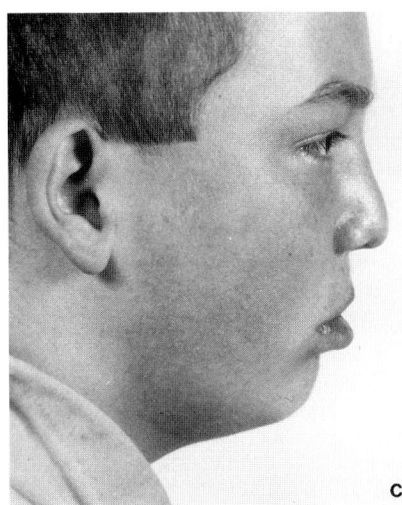

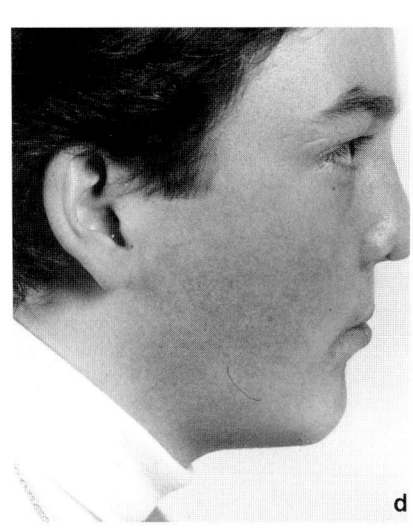

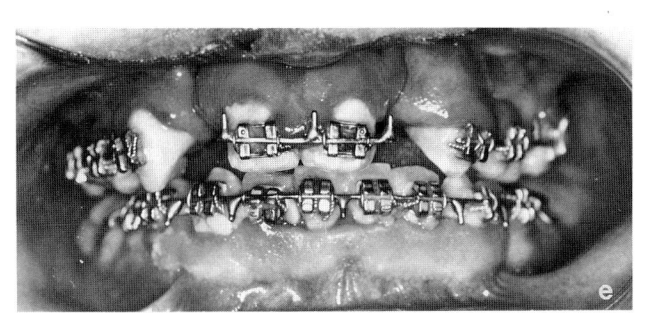

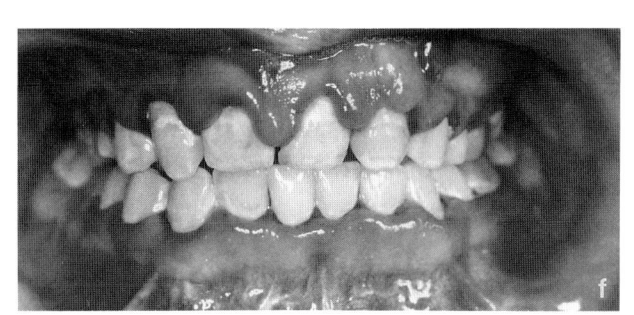

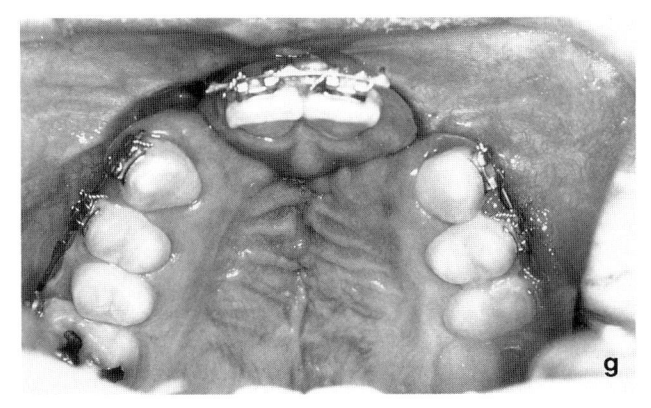

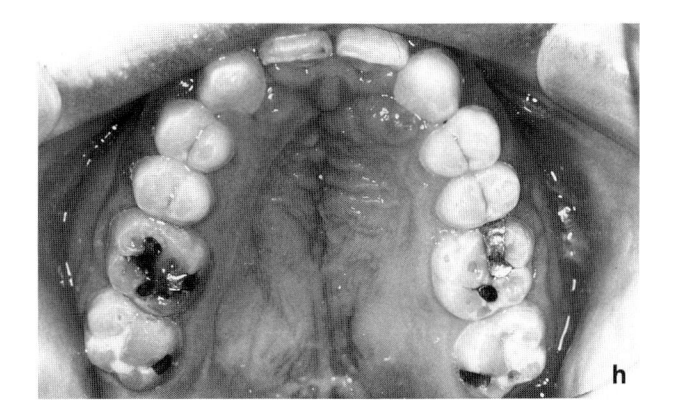

Figure 36.6 A 17-year-old with BCLP who underwent a modified Le Fort I osteotomy in two segments with the premaxilla remaining intact. He is shown before surgery and 2 years later. (a) Preoperative frontal view. (b) Postoperative frontal view. (c) Preoperative profile view. (d) Postoperative profile view. Fron Posnick JC and Dagys AP: Orthognathic surgery in the bilateral cleft patient, Philadelphia, WB Saunders, 1991. (e) Preoperative occlusal view. (f) Postoperative occlusal view. (g) Preoperative palatal view. (h) Postoperative palatal view. (From Posnick 1991b.)

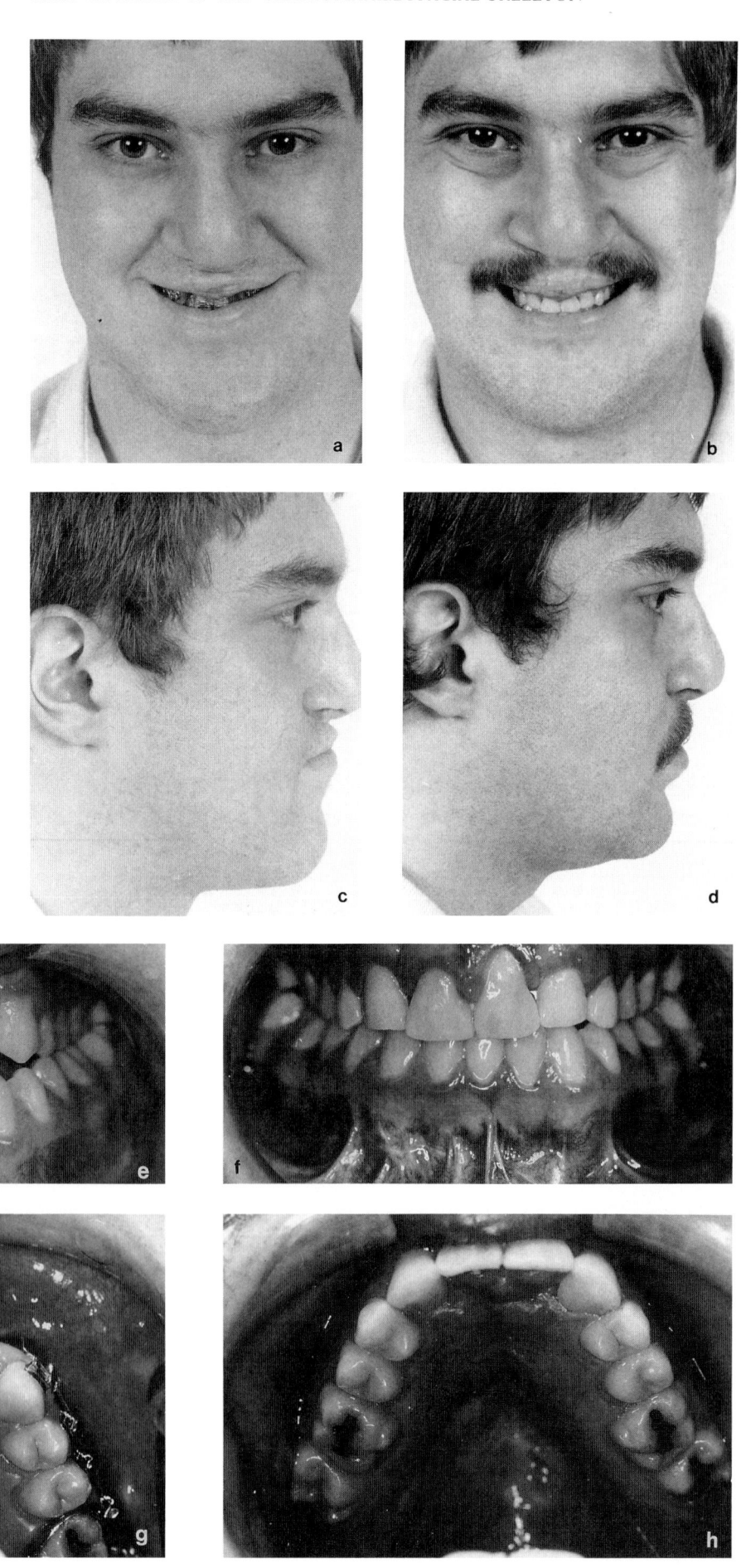

Cleft Lip and Palate Jaw Deformities 479

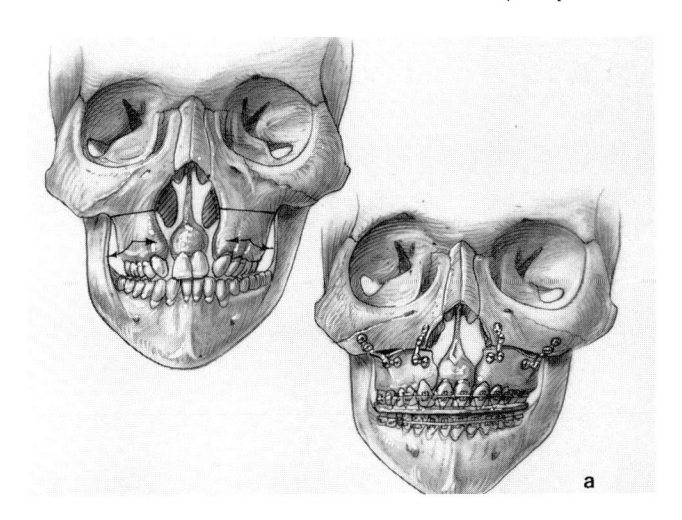

Figure 36.7 Illustrations of modified Le Fort I osteotomy in two or three segments. (a) Illustration of the BCLP patient before and after lateral segmental osteotomies and repositioning. (b) Illustrations before and after three-part maxillary osteotomies with repositioning of the segments. (d) Illustration of down-fractured lateral segments demonstrating exposure for nasal-side closure of oronasal fistula and additional view of oral mucosa incisions. (e) Illustration of premaxillary osteotomy from palate side using either a chisel, rongeur, or reciprocating saw. (f) Illustration demonstrating oral wounds sutured at the end of procedure. (g) Palatal view of bony segments before and after repositioning for closure of cleft-dental gaps. (From Posnick 1991b.)

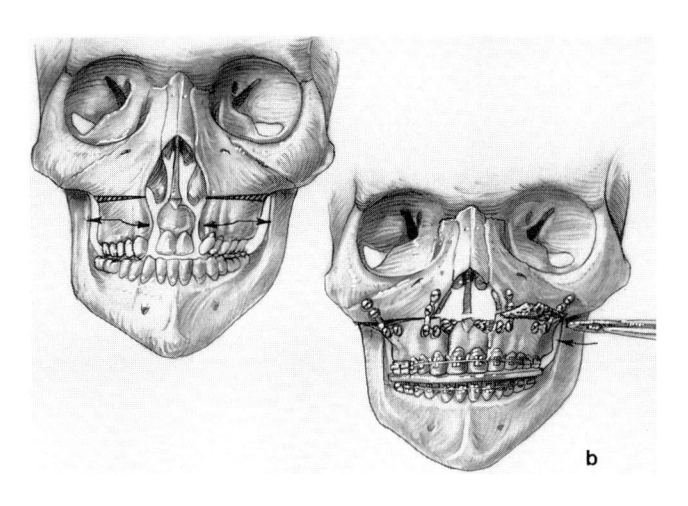

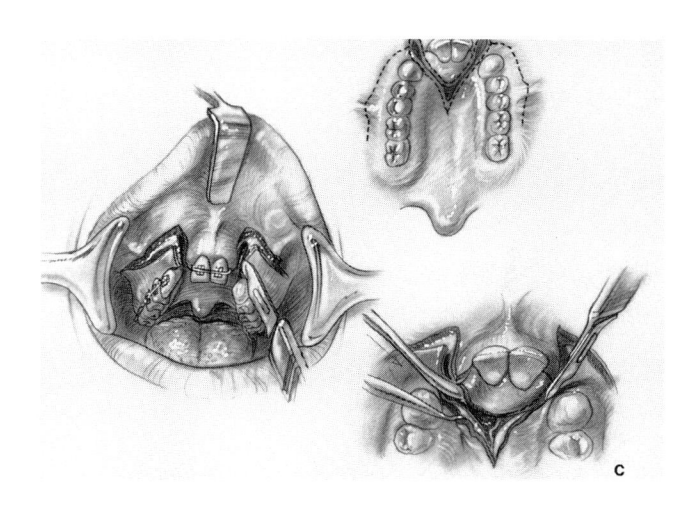

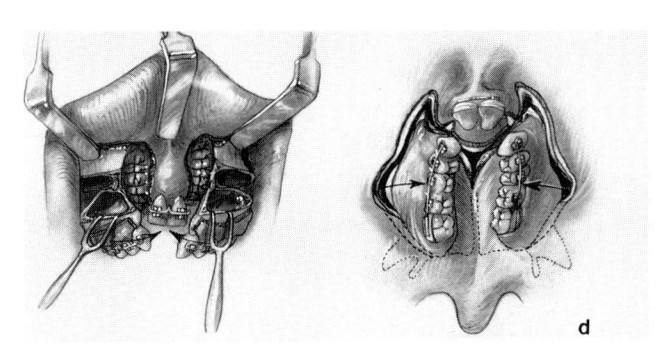

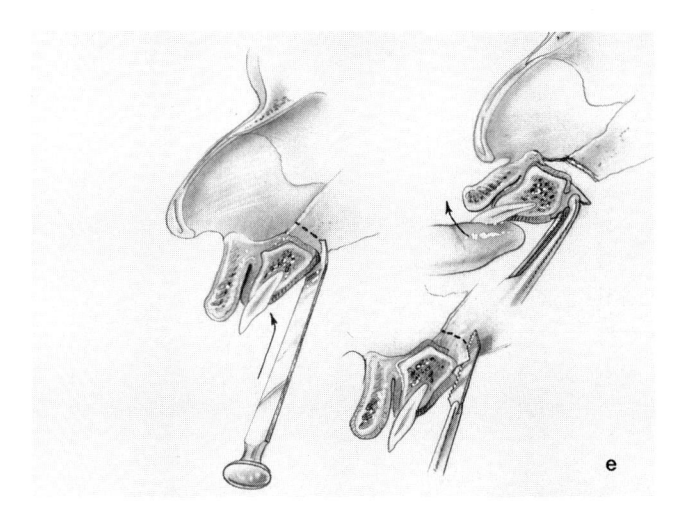

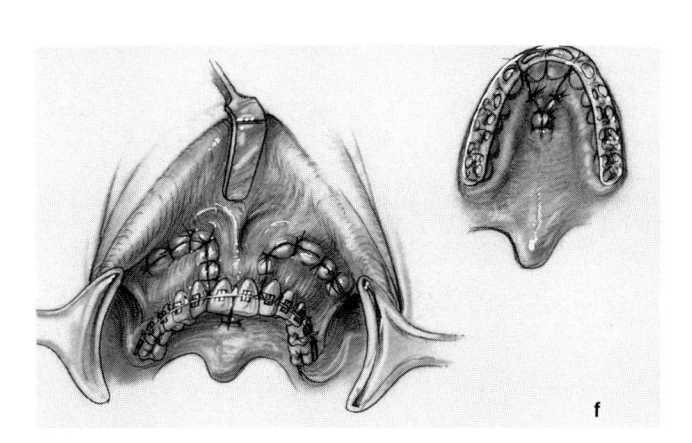

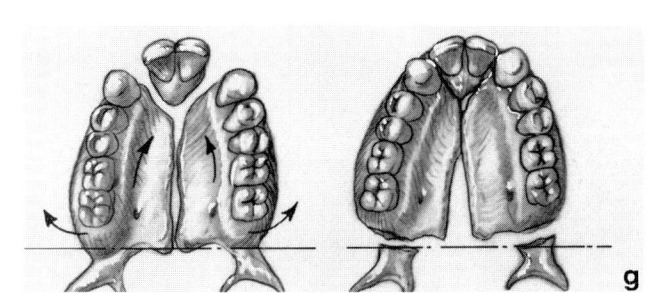

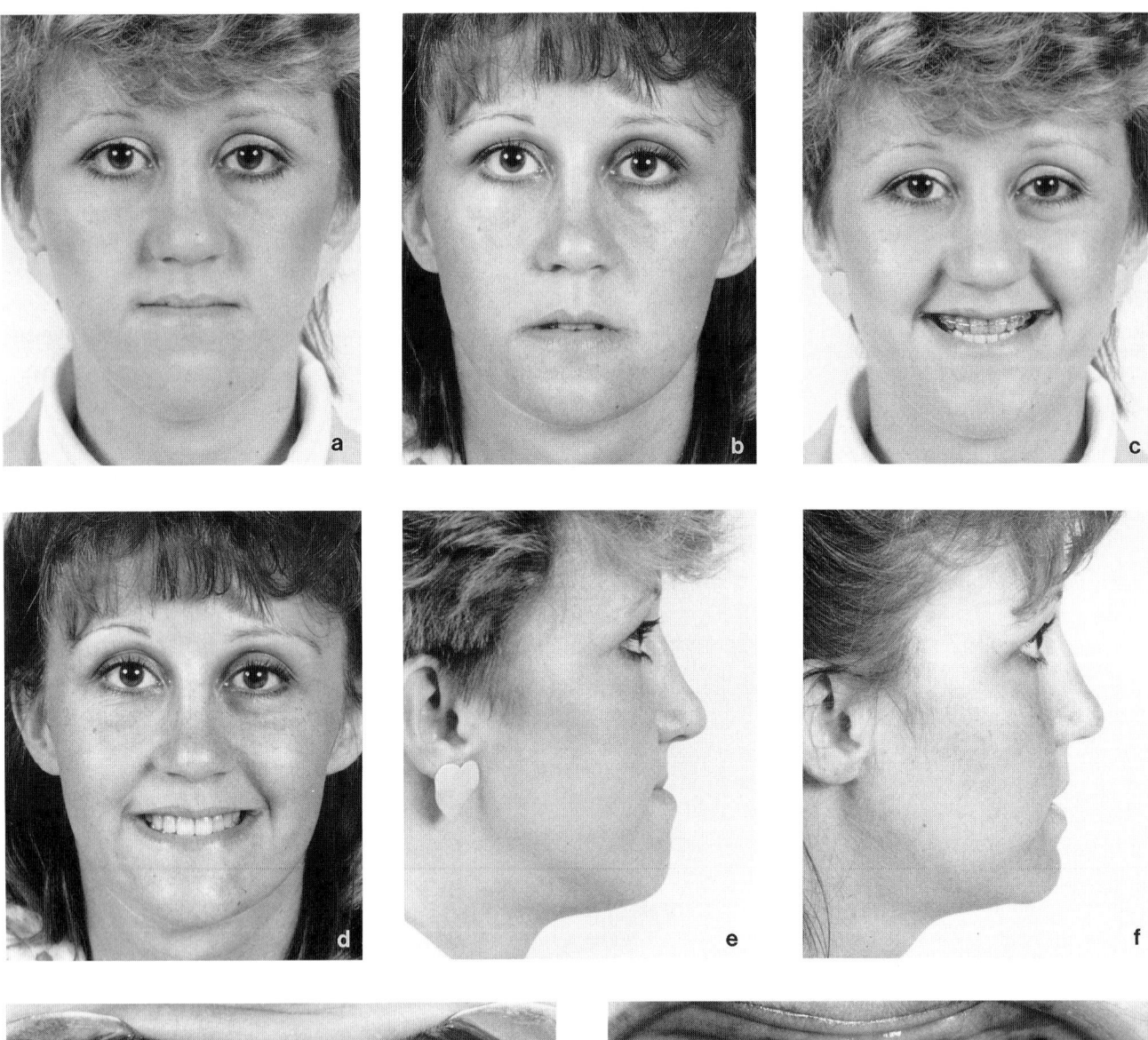

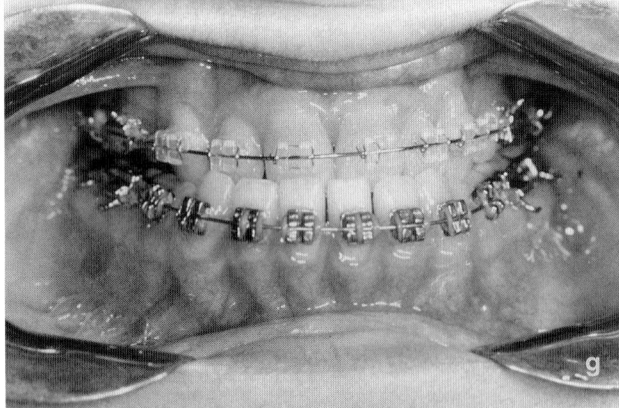

Figure 36.8 This 23-year-old woman was born with isolated cleft palate. She underwent a maxillary Le Fort I osteotomy with horizontal advancement and a vertical reduction and horizontal advancement genioplasty. (a) Preoperative frontal view in repose. (b) Postoperative frontal view in repose. (c) Preoperative frontal view with smile. (d) Postoperative frontal view with smile. (e) Preoperative profile. (f) Postoperative profile. (g) Preoperative occlusal view. (h) Postoperative occlusal view. (i) Articulated dental model ready for model surgery. (j) The maxilla advanced and ready for splint reconstruction on articulator. (k) Intraoperative view of Le Fort I osteotomy stabilized with titanium miniplates and screws. (l) Intraoperative view of vertically reduced and horizontally advanced genioplasty stabilized with three direct transosseous wires. (m) Preoperative lateral cephalometric radiograph. (n) Postoperative lateral cephalometric radiograph. (From Posnick [in press].)

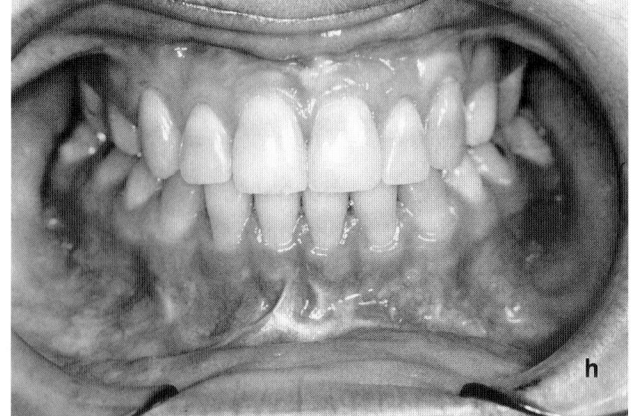

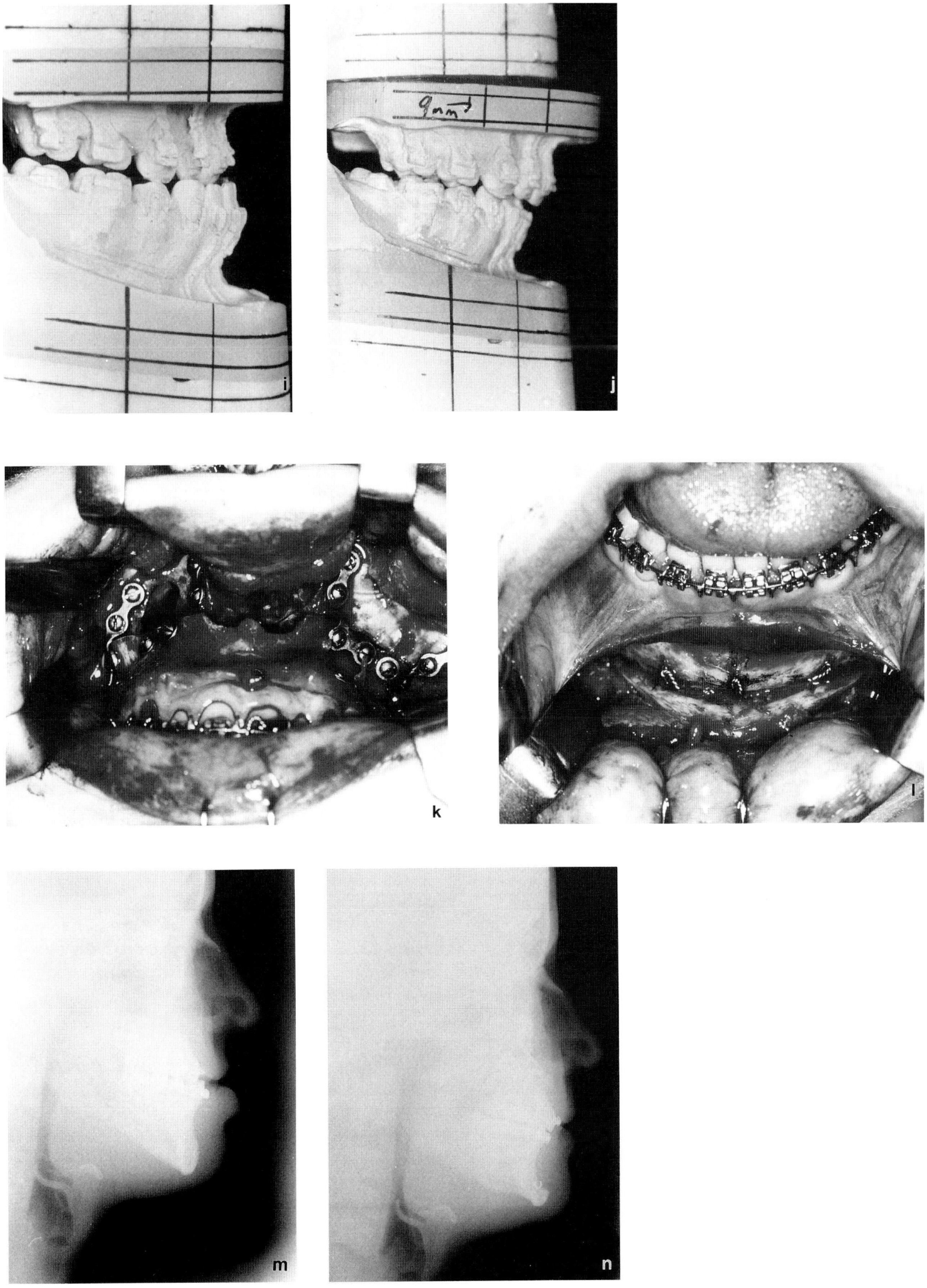
i
j
k
l
m
n

zontal advancement, posterior intrusion, and anterior (vertical) extrusion. Titanium miniplates and screws were used for stabilization in combination with a prefabricated occlusal splint, iliac bone graft and MMF. She also underwent a horizontal advancement genioplasty.

Postoperatively, she required a revision of her superiorly based pharyngeal flap for the management of velopharyngeal incompetence.

COMPLICATIONS

Apart from the problems associated with general anesthesia and perioperative airway compromise, perhaps the most devastating complication of jaw surgery is the loss of bone segments and teeth secondary to avascular necrosis. With traditional described techniques, the risks are greatest after Le Fort I segmental osteotomies in patients with bilateral clefts (Freihofer 1977); however, when careful surgical technique is used as described these complications should be extremely rare (Posnick 1991).

Residual malocclusion may arise, it can often be traced to poor planning, difficulties with execution of the operation, unpredictable skeletal or dental relapse, or limited compliance of the patient. However, patients of even the most skilled surgeons and orthodontists may experience postoperative malocclusion necessitating a second surgical procedure. The need for reoperation can be minimized through correct diagnosis, meticulous preoperative orthodontic treatment and surgical technique tailored to match the presenting deformities. The surgical technique includes aggressive soft-tissue dissection, planned overcorrection in anticipation of relapse, mini- and microplate and screw, internal fixation techniques, autogenous bone grafting, postoperative MMF, and class III elastics (when indicated).

When either a ramus osteotomy or a genioplasty of the mandible is performed, the inferior alveolar-mental nerve, which runs directly through the mandible, may be bruised, producing temporary paresthesia; or it may be lacerated, producing a permanent loss of sensation. Permanent sensory loss in the region of the lower lip and chin is seen in at least 10% of patients (Nishioka 1987, Walter 1979). Injury to the infraorbital nerve leading to sensory loss in the upper lip area may occur after a maxillary Le Fort I osteotomy but is rarely permanent. In general, poor objective documentation of changes in neurosensibility after osteotomies makes the true incidence of permanent sensory loss and resulting disability difficult to judge (Posnick 1990).

The premaxillary segment in the BCLP patient may have residual mobility after maxillary surgery. Although its true incidence is not known, the mobility can be minimized through meticulous three-layer fistula closure techniques, autogenous cancellous bone grafting, and miniplate and screw internal fixation combined with a prefabricated acrylic splint wiring to the maxillary teeth for eight weeks postoperatively. Recurrent oronasal fistulas and nonunion of the maxillary segments are rare occurrences in patients with unilateral clefts.

LONG-TERM RESULTS

Skeletal Stability after Le Fort I Maxillary Advancement in Patients with Clefts

Recently we (Posnick and Ewing 1990) studied the long-term skeletal outcome in UCLP patients who had undergone maxillary Le Fort I osteotomies. The charts of 30 adults and adolescents unergoing jaw surgery between 1974–1986 were reviewed retrospectively. These patients, who were judged to be skeletally mature, had unilateral cleft lip and palate and underwent Le Fort I advancement. The purpose of the study was to determine the amount and timing of relapse, correlation between advancement and relapse, effect of performing multiple jaw procedures, outcome with different types of bone graft, effect of a pharyngeal flap in place at the time of osteotomy, and the advantages of various methods of internal fixation. Tracings of preoperative and serial postoperative lateral cephalograms (immediately after surgery and six to eight weeks, one year, and two years after) were digitized to calculate horizontal (see Table 36.1) and vertical (see Table 36.2) changes in the maxilla.

No significant differences in outcome were seen between patients who had maxillary surgery alone and those who had simultaneous operations on both jaws. Nor did the outcomes vary significantly with the type of autogenous bone graft used (hip versus rib) or the segmentalization of the Le Fort I osteotomy.

The mean effective advancement was greater immediately and two years after surgery in patients who did not have a pharyngeal flap in place before the operation (see Table 36.3). Advancement was also greater immediately and two years after surgery in the group who underwent miniplate fixation than in patients with direct-wire fixation (see Table 36.4). Significant relapse is likely to occur between the operation and the initial, or immediate, cephalometric examination (two to seven days after the operation) in patients with direct-wire fixation. However, in those with miniplate fixation, early relapse is probably prevented and the bone is more likely to heal in the preferred position. This theory could be tested if it were possible to take a cephalometric radiograph in the operating room immediately after jaw stabilization.

During the first year the patients continued to show skeletal relapse, but there was no change either vertically or horizontally after that time (see Tables 36.1 and 36.2). It was interesting to find that there was no significant correlation between the amount of horizontal advancement (see Figure 36.9) or vertical displacement (see Figure 36.10) and the amount of relapse.

Table 36.1 Le Fort I osteotomy in unilateral cleft patients: horizontal advancement and relapse

Time after Operation	Effective Advancement (mm) Mean	SD	Min.	Max.	Mean Relapse from Previous Position (mm)
1 week	6.7	2.6	1.7	12.2	Unknown
6 weeks	5.7	2.5			1.0
1 year	4.9	2.6			0.8
2 years	4.8	2.6	1.0	10.7	0.1

(From Posnick and Ewing 1990.)

Table 36.2 Le Fort I osteotomy in unilateral cleft patients: vertical displacement and relapse

Time after Operation	Downward Displacement (mm) Mean	SD	Min.	Max.	Mean Relapse from Previous Position (mm)
1 week	2.6	3.0	−3.4	8.6	Unknown
6 weeks	1.4	2.7			1.2
1 year	1.2	2.5			0.2
2 years	1.2	2.5	−2.9	7.0	0.0

(From Posnick and Ewing 1990.)

Table 36.3 Le Fort I osteotomy in unilateral cleft patients: effects of pharyngoplasty on horizontal advancement and relapse

Pharyngoplasty in Place	Time after Operation	Effective Advancement (mm) Mean	SD	Mean Relapse from Previous Position (mm)
No (N = 24)	1 week	7.4	2.5	
	1 year	5.2	2.6	2.2 mm
Yes (N = 6)	1 week	5.5	3.0	
	1 year	3.6	2.5	1.9 mm

(From Posnick and Ewing 1990.)

Table 36.4 Le Fort I osteotomy in unilateral cleft patients: comparison of horizontal advancement and relapse between patients with direct-wire and miniplate fixation

Fixation	Time after Operation	Effective Advancement (mm) Mean	SD	Mean Relapse from Previous Position (mm)
Direct wire (N = 25)	1 week	6.5	2.7	
	1 year	4.6	2.7	1.9 mm
Miniplate (N = 5)	1 week	8.0	1.7	
	1 year	6.4	2.2	1.6 mm

(From Posnick and Ewing 1990.)

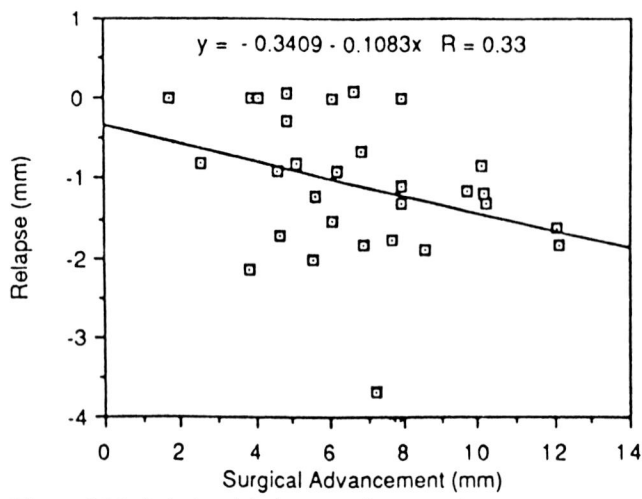

Figure 36.9 Relationship between horizontal surgical advancement and relapse after one year. (From Posnick and Ewing 1990.)

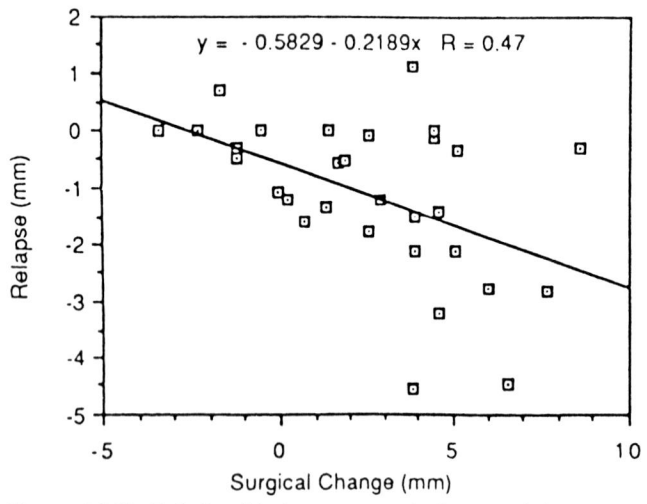

Figure 36.10 Relationship between vertical surgical displacement and relapse after one year. (From Posnick and Ewing 1990.)

SUMMARY

Over the past five years I have performed maxillary Le Fort I osteotomies on approximately 100 patients with repaired clefts. When the concepts and techniques described have been used, the most gratifying results of orthognathic surgery have frequently been in patients with the worst preoperative situation: bilateral clefts with collapsed hypoplastic lateral maxillary segments, mobile premaxilla, large residual oronasal fistulas, alveolar bony cleft defects, bilateral congenital (lateral incisor) dental gaps, and a vertically long and retrognathic chin. The use of internal fixation with bone miniplates and screws in cleft jaw surgery has become an integral part of the overall surgical plan. However, it has not supplanted the simultaneous use of autogenous bone grafts, prefabricated splints, MMF, and planned overcorrection to reduce the functional and aesthetic effects of skeletal relapse and to maximize the end result. Precise diagnosis, careful planning of combined surgical and orthodontic treatment, and meticulous technique make possible the resolution of these multiple residual clefting problems at one operation.

Acknowledgment

The author wishes to acknowledge and thank Dr. A. Dagys, Dr. R.B. Ross, Dr. M. Taylor, Dr. D. Engel, Dr. B. Tompson, and Dr. N. Shapera from the Division of Orthodontics, The Hospital for Sick Children, for their assistance with the surgical planning and orthodontic treatment of the patients presented. Without their collective and individual guidance, this work would not have been possible.

The author thanks Elizabeth Lang and the staff of Medical Publications, The Hospital for Sick Children for editorial assistance in preparing this chapter.

REFERENCES

Araujo A, Schendel SA, Woford LM, Epker BN: Total maxillary advancement with and without bone grafting. J Oral Surg 36:849–858, 1978.

Beals SP, Munro IR: The use of miniplates in craniomaxillofacial surgery. Plast Reconstr Surg 79:33–38, 1987.

Bell WH. Biological basis for maxillary osteotomies. Am J Phys Anthropol 38:279–289, 1973.

Bell WH, Proffit WR, White RP: Surgical correction of dentofacial deformities. vol 1 and 2. Philadelphia, Saunders, 1980.

Bell WH, Scheideman GB: Correction of vertical maxillary deficiency: Stability and soft tissue changes. J Oral Surg 39:666–670, 1981.

Braun TW, Stotereanos GC: Long term results with maxillary advancement in cleft palate patients in oral and maxillofacial surgery. Proceedings from the 8th International Conference on Maxillofacial Surgery 1982, p 265.

Drommer R, Luhr HG: The stabilization of osteotomized maxillary segments with Luhr mini-plates in secondary cleft surgery. J Maxillofac Surg 9:166–169, 1981.

Farkas LG, Hreczko TA, Kolar JC, Munro IR: Vertical and horizontal proportions of the face in young adult North American Caucasians: Revision of neoclassical canons. Plast Reconstr Surg 75:328–338, 1985.

Farkas LG, Kolar JC: Anthropometrics and art in the aesthetics of women's faces. Clin Plast Surg 14:599–616, 1987.

Freihofer HP Jr. Results of osteotomies of the facial skeleton in adolescence. J Maxillofac Surg 5:267–297, 1977.

Garrison BT, Lapp TH, Bussard DA: The stability of Le Fort I maxillary osteotomies in patients with simultaneous alveolar cleft bone grafts. J Oral Maxillofac Surg 45:761–766, 1987.

Harsha BC, Terry BC: Stabilization of Le Fort I osteotomies utilizing small bone plates. Int J Adult Orthodon Orthognath Surg 1:69–77, 1986.

Horster W: Experience with functionally stable plate osteosynthesis after forward displacement of the upper jaw. J Maxillofac Surg 8:176–181, 1980.

James DR and Brook K: Maxillary hypoplasia in patients with cleft lip and palate deformity—the alternative surgical approach.

Luhr HG. Zur stabilen Osteosynthese bei Unterkiefertfrakturen. Deutsch Zahnaerztl Z 23:754, 1968.

Luhr HG: Stabile Fixation von Oberkiefer-Mittelgesichtsfrakturen durch Mini-Kompressionsplatten. Dtsch Zahnaerztl Z 34:851, 1979.

Luhr HG. The significance of condylar position using rigid fixation in orthognathic surgery. Clin Plast Surg 16:147, 1989.

Nishioka GJ, Zysset MK, Van Sickels JE: Neurosensory disturbance with rigid fixation of the bilateral sagittal split osteotomy. J Oral Maxillofac Surg 45:20–26, 1987.

Obwegeser H: In Zur Operationstechnik bei der Progenie und anderen Unterkieferanomalien. Trauner R, Obwegeser H. Deutsch Zahn-, Mund- u Kieferheik 23:1, 1955.

Poole MD, Robinson PP, and Nunn ME: Maxillary advancement in cleft lip and palate patients, J Maxillofac Surg 14:123–127, 1986.

Posnick JC, Ewing MP: Skeletal stability after Le Fort I maxillary advancement in patients with unilateral cleft lip and palate. Plast Reconstr Surg 85:706–710, 1990.

Posnick JC, Grossman JAI, Zimber AG: Normal cutaneous sensibility of the face. Plast Reconstr Surg 86:429–433, 1990.

Posnick JC: Discussion: Orthognathic surgery in cleft patients treated by early bone grafting. Plastic and reconstructive surgery 87(5):840–842, May 1991a.

Posnick JC, Dagys AP: Chapter: Orthognathic surgery in the bilateral cleft patient: An integrated surgical and orthodontic approach. Oral and Maxillofacial Surgery Clinics of North America, (Hudson JW eds) W.B. Saunders Co., 693–710, Vol. 3, No. 3, August 1991.

Posnick JC: Chapter: Orthognathic surgery in the cleft patient. Instructional courses, plastic surgery education foundation and C.V. Mosby Co. (Russel, RC eds), 1991b.

Posnick JC: Chapter: Secondary skeletal deformities in cleft patients. Mastery of surgery: plastic and reconstructive surgery (Cohen, Mimes eds), Little, Brown and Co. 1992 (in press).

Ricketts RM: Divine proportion in facial esthetics. Clin Plast Surg 9:401–422, 1982.

Rosen HM: Miniplate fixation of Le Fort I osteotomies. Plast Reconstr Surg 78:748–755, 1986.

Tessier P, Tulasne JF: Secondary repair of cleft lip deformity. Clin Plast Surg 11:747–760, 1984.

Tideman H, Stoelinga P, Gallia L: Le Fort I advancement with segmental palatal osteotomies in patients with cleft palates. J Oral Surg 38:196–199, 1980.

Walter JM Jr, Gegg JM: Analysis of postsurgical neurologic alteration in the trigeminal nerve. J Oral Surg 37:410–414, 1979.

West A: Orthognathic surgery, Oral Maxillofac Surg Clin North Am 2(4):761, 1990.

Westbrook MT Jr, West RA, and McNeil RW: Simultaneous maxillary advancement and closure of bilateral alveolar clefts and oronasal fistulas, J Oral Maxillofac Surg 41:257, 1983.

CHAPTER 37

The Use of Rigid Fixation for Cleft Lip and Palate

David S. Precious

Rigid fixation, when used in the management of deformities that result from both the presence and treatment of labiomaxillopalatine clefts, can enhance stability and predictability of results. However, the clinician should be acutely aware that bony relapse of the operated parts, both maxilla and mandible, in spite of rigid fixation, remains a significant problem.

Many aspects of pathologic facial disequilibrium in patients with clefts are due to inadequate and inaccurate primary muscle surgery of both the lip and the palate. Further confusion arises when these imbalances are magnified and modified by subsequent facial growth, the quality of which depends to a great extent on the degree to which either "normal" function or dysfunction is present during the growing years. The surgeon must understand the anatomy of the primary faults, the shortcomings of the primary operations, the effects of these shortcomings on subsequent facial growth, and, finally, the highly variable nature of secondary deformities associated with labiomaxillopalatine clefts.

ANATOMY

In the normal case the anterior muscles of the face form three rings (see Figure 37.1):

- a superior, or nasolabial, ring that consists of the transverse nasal muscles and the levator muscles of the upper lip and nose,
- a middle, or labial, ring formed by the orbicularis oris muscles of the upper and lower lips, and
- a lower, or labiomental, ring formed by the mentalis muscles and the depressor muscles of the lower lip.

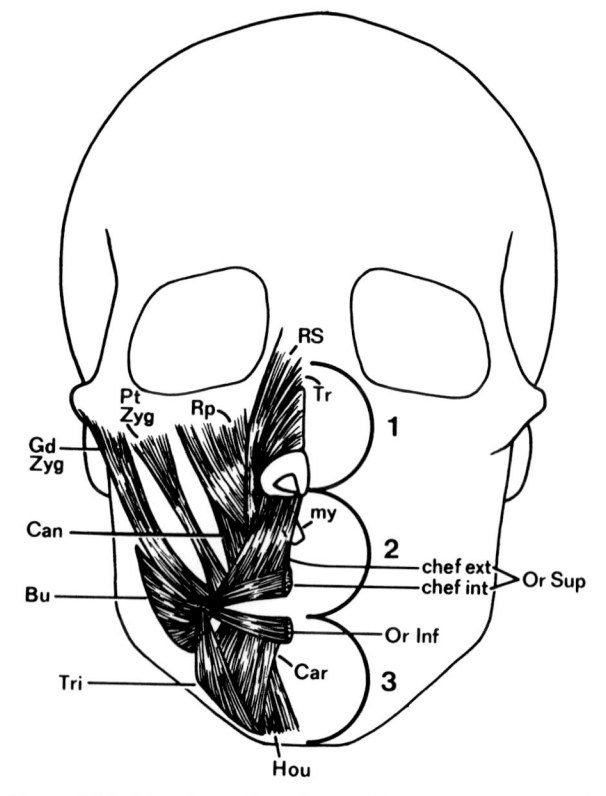

Figure 37.1 The three rings formed by the anterior muscles of the face: (1) the superior, or nasolabial, ring; (2) the middle, or labial, ring; and (3) the lower, or labiomental, ring.

The transverse nasal muscle is the most important functional element in the superior ring because it surrounds the nasal orifice and has two important functions, nostril constriction and support of its corresponding half of the upper lip. The latter function is particularly related to support of the external head of the orbicularis oris muscle, which in turn supports the labial commissure. The nasal septum, on both sides of which symmetrical muscles are normally inserted, remains in the midline. The median interincisive suture, the septopremaxillary ligament, and the median ligament of the upper lip also remain in the midline.

In patients with total unilateral labiomaxillopalatine clefts, the muscles on the cleft side remain lateral to the defect and are therefore deprived of the nasal septum as a point of anchorage. This situation favors posterior positioning and medial rotation of the anterior part of the minor segment. The uncleft side is often referred to in error as the normal side. The muscles on the uncleft side that do insert on the nasal septum drag it into the noncleft nostril and to a lesser degree into the anterior portion of the minor segment, the median interincisive suture, and the two incisive processes. The premaxilla is less developed than normal on the cleft side because of the periosteal discontinuity and the resultant absence of normal muscular periosteal stimulation. The uncleft side is also abnormal, and it is underdeveloped by an amount equal to the degree to which the interincisive suture is bent to this side. The alar cartilage on the cleft side is unsupported and displaced lateroinferiorly, as is the bony pyriform aperture itself. Although the nasal cartilaginous deformities can be considerable, true hypoplasia of the alar cartilages is rare except in cases such as holoprosencephaly. The nasal bones are deviated to the uncleft side, but on the cleft side the poorly supported nasal capsule induces an internal rotation of the ascending anterior maxillary pillar, which in turn causes lateral displacement of the medial canthus. This lateral displacement gives the appearance of unilateral hypertelorism when in fact frequently only telecanthus is present.

All of these imbalances are exaggerated when a complete velopalatine cleft accompanies the labiomaxillary cleft. This exaggeration is caused by the distortions in the premaxillary-vomerine suture and in the function of the vomer with the palatal shelf on the cleft side, where a membranous suture is found. The sutured soft palate and fibromucosa of the hard palate in the classic repair establish a transverse narrowing of the palate, which alters vertical growth of the hard palate and the maxilla. Growth also appears to be altered in the anteroinferior portion of the maxilla, which, when coupled with the vertical problem, leads to a malpositioned, retruded, anterior maxillary dental arch.

The general scheme of things as outlined above can serve as a basis to evaluate, to a greater or lesser degree, both incomplete and bilateral clefts. In the bilateral case, however, one must appreciate that the premaxilla is longer than normal because of excessive stimulation of the premaxillary-vomerine suture; because of the presence of the lower lip—which pushes from below and behind the maxillary alveolar process—because of the absence of the muscular sling of the upper lip; and, finally, because of the active role of the nasal septum as it grows downward and forward.

Given this abnormal anatomy and its attendant dysfunction coupled with the fact that primary surgery is rarely perfect from a functional point of view, it is clear that by the time the patient has reached adolescence (frequently having had orthodontic treatment and teeth extracted) the clinician needs a method that will permit the development of an accurate objective assessment of the abnormalities with which the patient now presents. These abnormalities include muscular, dental, cutaneous, and bony problems, each of which requires attention in the treatment plan in order to achieve the optimum functional and aesthetic result.

DIAGNOSIS

Clinical Examination

Rigid fixation techniques are applicable, in cleft lip and palate deformities, to adolescent and adult patients who require some form of orthognathic surgery and/or bone grafting. It is extremely important to recognize that the presence of vestibular oral-nasal fistula (ONF) is clinical proof of deficiency in the muscular elements of the floor and in the lateral aspect of the nose. Muscular dysfunction is present when there is vestibular ONF, deviation of the nasal septum to the uncleft side, and inability of the patient to project the upper lip symmetrically (see Figure 37.2).

Correction of muscular dysfunction of the nose and upper lip is based on the establishment of balance among the anterior nasal spine of the maxilla, the cartilaginous nasal septum, the nasolabial and labiomental muscles, the teeth, the maxilla, and the mandible. All of these structures can be assessed, to a greater or lesser degree, in a cephalic context by the use of the architectural and structural craniofacial analysis of Delaire (1978).

Cephalometric Analysis

Cephalometric analysis is composed of two distinct phases. The lines of craniofacial balance, which allow us to view objectively and quantify the variations between the patient being examined and the "normal" in the patient's peer group, represent the architectural analysis. Direct study of the cephalometric radiograph of the osseous structures, taking note of the structures, dimensions, degree of ossification, trabeculation, and cortication (external contour), and study of neighboring

Figure 37.2 The three principal clinical features of muscular dysfunction: (a) vestibular oral-nasal fistula, (b) deviation of the nasal septum to the uncleft side, and (c) inability to project the upper lip symmetrically.

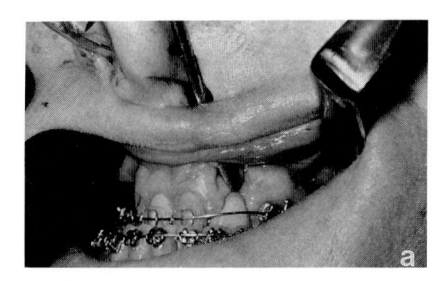

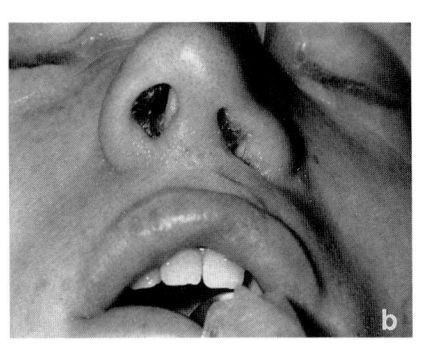

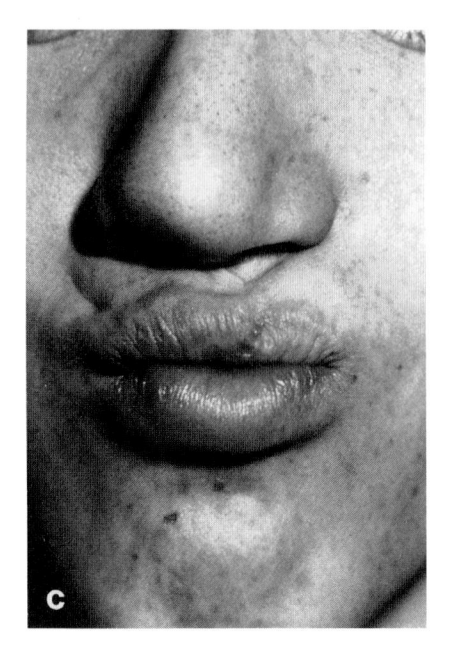

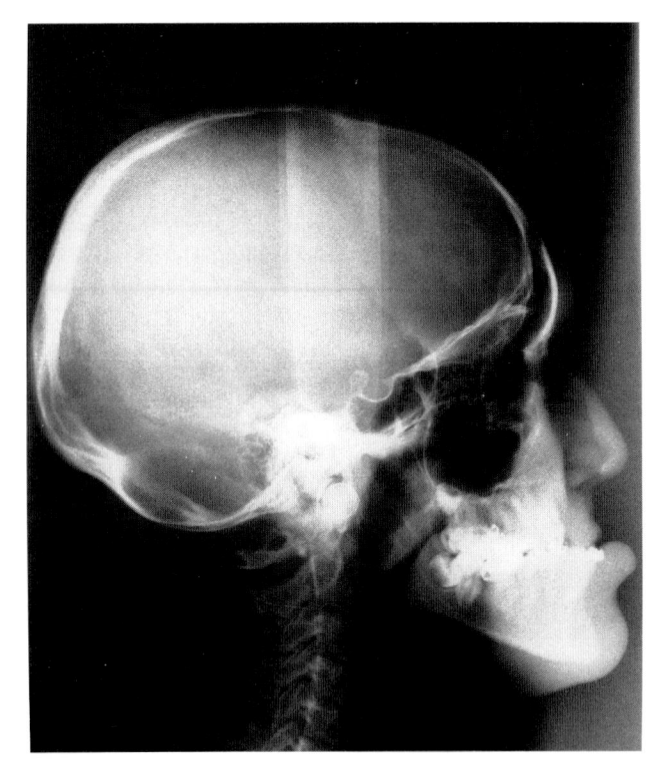

Figure 37.3 This lateral craniofacial cephalometric radiograph is suitable for analysis.

soft tissues (both superficial and deep), represents the structural analysis.

Architectural Analysis

Architectural analysis requires a lateral cephalometric radiograph of high quality, showing clearly the hard and soft tissues of the whole head and neck. It should be taken with the patient staring into infinity, the mandible closed in centric relation, and the lips in repose (see Figure 37.3). The analysis consists of a cranial portion, a facial portion, and two lines of dental orientation.

Cranial Analysis Three reference points must first be identified: point M (see Figure 37.4), situated at the junction of the frontonasal and nasomaxillary sutures; point CT (see Figure 37.5), the temporal condylar point, situated on the posteroinferior border of the radiographic outline of the articular eminence; and point Clp (see Figure 37.6), situated at the apex of the posterior clinoid process, behind the sella turcica.

To trace the four cranial lines one begins with C1 (see Figure 37.7), the craniofacial baseline that joins points M and CT. Line C1 extends posteriorly until it meets line Oi, its perpendicular, which is drawn tangent to the external outline of the occipital bone. Line C1 should pass in the immediate vicinity of the top of the pterygomaxillary fissure and the center of the mandibular condyle. "Ideally" the posterior border of the mandibular condyle (Cp) should be situated exactly halfway along line C1 (that is, 50% of the distance from M to Oi, at the point Cp). Thus the distance Cp to Oi, the craniospinal area, is normally equal to the distance Cp to M, the craniofacial area.

The Use of Rigid Fixation 489

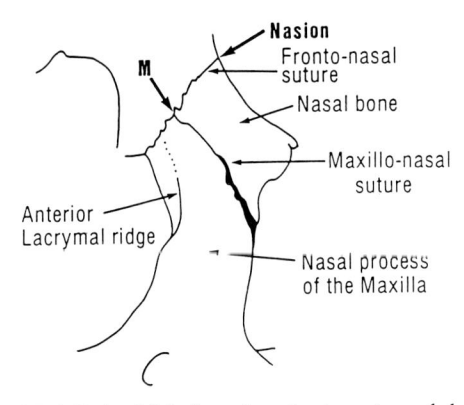

Figure 37.4 Point M is found at the junction of the fronto-nasal and nasomaxillary sutures.

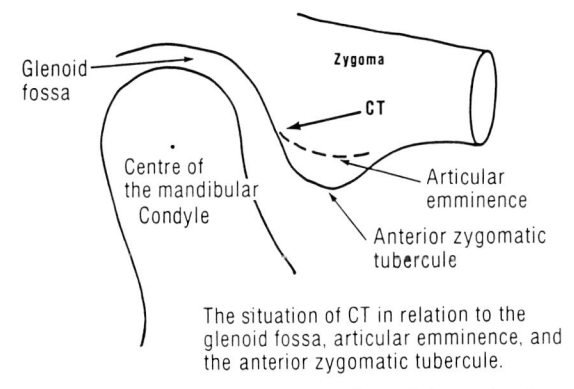

Figure 37.5 Point CT, the temporal-condylar point, is shown.

The cranial height, line C2, is traced perpendicular to C1 at its center (the center of C1 ideally is coincident with Cp, although this is not always the case). If the point Cp is in front of the midpoint of line C1, this indicates a shortening of the craniofacial area, which often has a tendency toward a class III skeletal pattern. Conversely, if point Cp is behind this midpoint, this indicates an elongation of the craniofacial area and tendency to a class II skeletal pattern. Line C2 intersects the calvaria at point Sc (the cranial summit).

The superior line of the cranial base, C3, is drawn from M to Clp (the apex of the clinoid process) and extended posteriorly until it intersects the external surface of the occipital bone of Op. Point Op is normally the most posterior extremity of the occipital bulbosity. Normally line C3 passes just over and parallel to the cribiform plate, then close to the upper lip of the optic chiasmal groove, and then by the anterior clinoid process.

The basilar slope, line C4, is drawn by connecting point Clp to a point at a tangent to the posterosuperior edge of the apex of the odontoid process (Od). Normally C4 is tangent to the dorsum of the sella turcica, to the cerebral surface of the basioccipital bone, and to the basion. It should pass very close to the posterosuperior surface of the mandibular condyle. When it does not, one must suspect an error of centric relation during the taking of the radiograph, thus initiating a verification check of the position of the condyle in its fossa.

Cranial analysis also calls for the measurement of the following angles:

- C1/C3, the anterior cranial base angle, is normally between 20° and 22°. A greater angle favors a class III skeletal pattern, and a smaller angle favors a class II skeletal pattern.
- C3/C4, the sphenoidal angle, is normally between 115° and 120°. A greater angle favors a class II skeletal pattern, and a smaller angle favors a class III skeletal pattern.

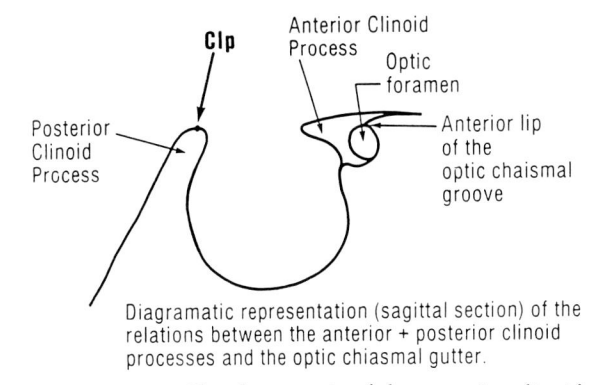

Figure 37.6 Point Clp, the summit of the posterior clinoid process, is shown.

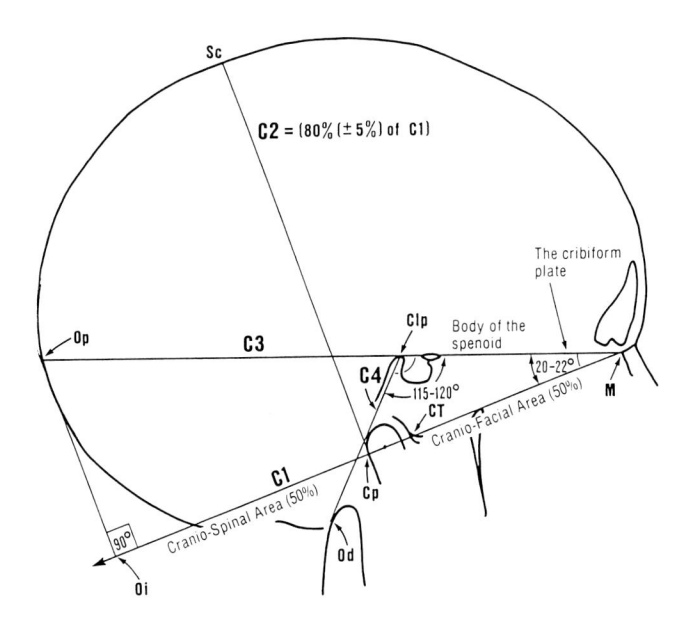

Figure 37.7 The cranial analysis begins with a tracing of the four cranial lines.

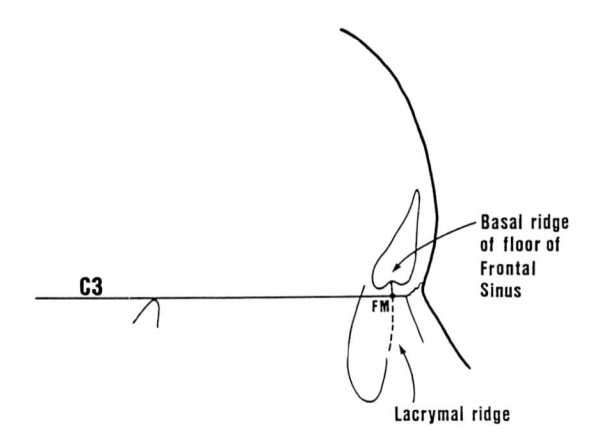

Point FM

Figure 37.8 The relationship of point FM to the lacrymal ridge, line C3, and the basal ridge of the floor of the frontal sinus, is shown.

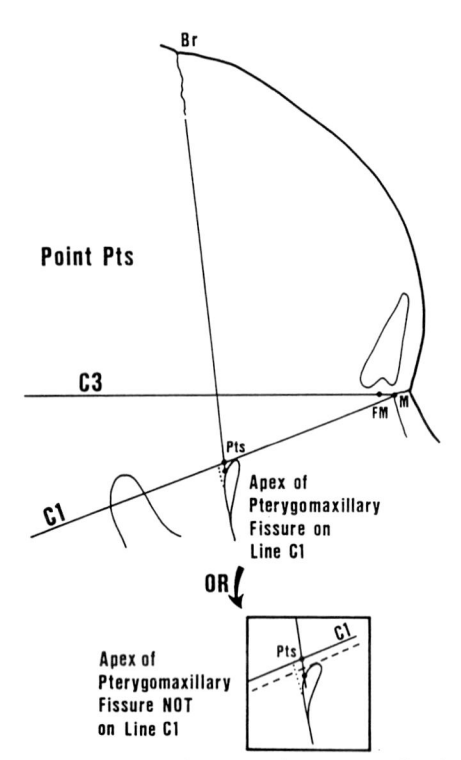

Point Pts

Figure 37.9 Points Br and Pts are shown. Usually the apex of the pterygomaxillary fissure just touches line C1.

Facial Analysis Facial analysis consists of drawing eight craniofacial lines, CF1 through CF8. Lines CF1 through CF3 permit analysis of the anteroposterior balance of the facial skeleton with respect to the cranium and cervical column. Lines CF4 through CF8 permit analysis of the vertical relationships. Three points must be located before tracing these lines: the frontomaxillary point (FM), the bregma (Br), and the superior pterygoid point (Pts).

Point FM (see Figure 37.8), the frontomaxillary point, anatomically corresponds to the middle of the upper border of the ascending nasal process of the maxilla and its sutural articulation with the frontal bone. Point FM can be found by continuing the upward extension of the lacrimal ridge to the frontomaxillary suture. These anatomic specifications may aid in exact siting of point FM on the teleradiograph: It lies upon line C3; it resides at the center of the bony opacity created by the superior extremity of the ascending nasal process of the maxilla (which spans the distance between point M and the lacrimal groove); and it can be located directly below the ridge of reinforcement that forms a part of the base of the frontal sinus.

Point Br (see Figure 37.9), the bregma, is situated at the upper extremity of the coronal suture (frontoparietal). This point is generally easy to find in the young (except in cases of premature craniostenosis), but in the adult the suture may be completely closed. In this case, the surgeon must be aided by the existence of a small depression in the external cortical plate, just behind what used to be the sutural bevel.

Point Pts (see Figure 37.9), the superior pterygoid point, is found where the superior outline of the pterygomaxillary fissure forms a tangent to line C1.

Anteroposterior Relationships The anterior line of craniofacial balance, line CF1, passes through point FM (see Figure 37.10). Angle C3/CF1 differs, depending on the age and sex of the subject. In children, the angle is always about 85°. After pubescent growth is complete, the angle is about 85° in females and about 90° in males. Line CF1 extends upward to its intersection with the external frontal cortical bone and downward to pass below the bony menton.

The middle line of craniofacial balance, line CF2, links points Br and Pts and extends down to intersect with the inferior border of the mandible, the pterygomandibular point (Ptm).

The posterior line of craniofacial balance, line CF3, is parallel to line CF2 and passes through point Cp. Its upper extremity stops at the point of intersection with the external cortical plate of the calvaria. It extends below the mandibular angle.

Normally, irrespective of the value of angle C3/CF1, CF1 passes through the frontal sinus, FM, and the anterior borders of the nasopalatine canal (point NP) (in children, here line C1 passes through the cuspal tip of the developing permanent canine tooth, which may superimpose upon NP). Line CF1 then passes through the hypomochlion (the point of union of the apical third and the coronal two-thirds of the root length of the nonresorbed deciduous canine, or the permanent canine after complete eruption), the distal slope of the occlusal edge of the crown of the upper canine (a small distance in front of the distal contact point), the apex of the lower central incisor, and finally through the menton (point Me) (see Figure 37.11).

The presence of a dentofacial dysmorphosis can modify these relationships. In cleft patients point NP commonly does not coincide with line CF1. In this case, a new line FM–NP is extended to the inferior border of the mandible. The situation of the various points of reference with respect to these craniofacial lines gives the following information: the degree of anteroposterior displacement between the maxilla and mandible, both in relation to the "ideal," and in relation to one another; the degree of maxillary prognathia or retrognathia; the degree of mandibular prognathia or retrognathia; the retroposition or mesioposition of the maxillary canine tooth; the degree of mesioversion or distoversion of the maxillary canine tooth; and the mesioposition or retroposition of the lower central incisor, which is generally associated with a corresponding proclination or retroclination of the lower anterior segment.

Thus, the line CF1 and the line extended from FM to NP have already revealed a large amount of information on their own. Nevertheless, one should interpret these results as a function of each particular case. Indeed, in some "normal" subjects the angle of orientation of line CF1 has a greater or lesser value than average. Thus, some male adults can have an angle $C_3/CF_1 = 85°$ (instead of 90°) as large as 95°. By the same token, some females can have an angle equal to or greater than 90°. Nevertheless, for every case, the subject is well balanced only if all the reference points are well aligned.

Line CF2 (see Figure 37.12) normally runs downward from point Br, passes through point Pts, and passes closely alongside the anteroinferior border of the pterygoid plate. As it continues, line CF2 follows closely the anterior border of the ramus and eventually intersects the inferior border of the body of the mandible at point Ptm. Point Ptm is normally situated close to the middle of the segment defined by the mental symphysis and the posterior extremity of the mandibular angle. Dentofacial dysmorphoses exhibit a forward or backward tilting of the anterior border of the pterygoid plate, a forward or backward tilting of the anterior border of the mandibular ramus, and a positioning too far forward or backward of the point Ptm in relation to the middle of the mandible (see Figure 37.13).

Line CF3 (see Figure 37.14) normally is tangent to the posterior surface of the mandibular condyle (point Cp) and also is tangent to the posterior border of the

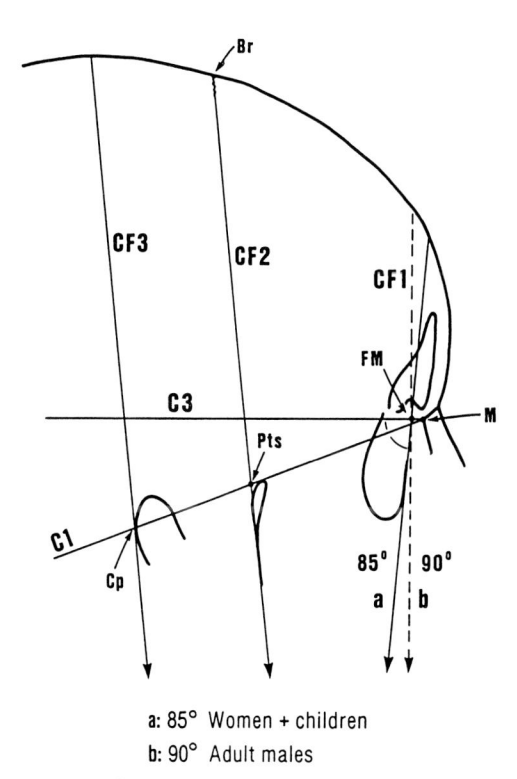

a: 85° Women + children
b: 90° Adult males

Figure 37.10 The relationships of lines CF1, CF2, and CF3 are shown.

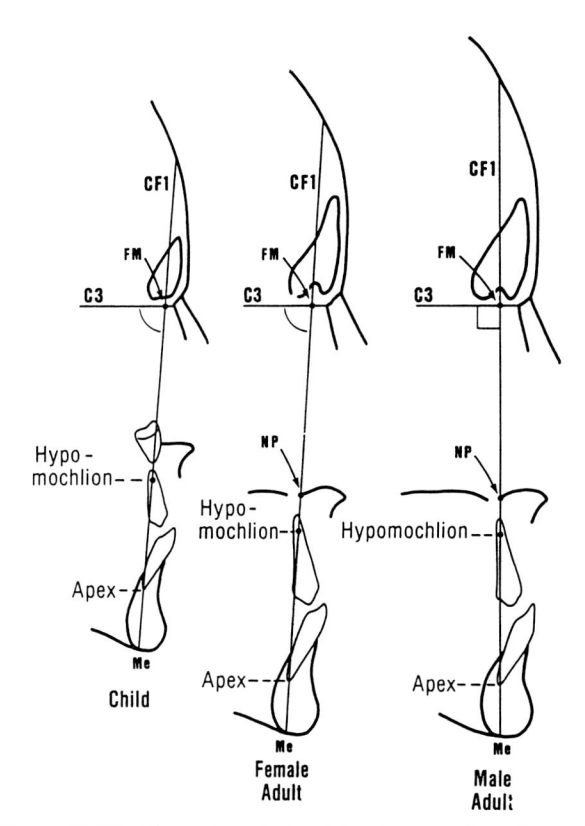

Figure 37.11 The strict relationship of anatomic points with line CF1 when facial balance is present is shown.

Figure 37.12 The relationships of line CF2 to the cranium, the maxilla, and the mandible are shown.

Figure 37.13 Maxillary and mandibular imbalances of class II and class III skeletal patterns are shown in relation to line CF2.

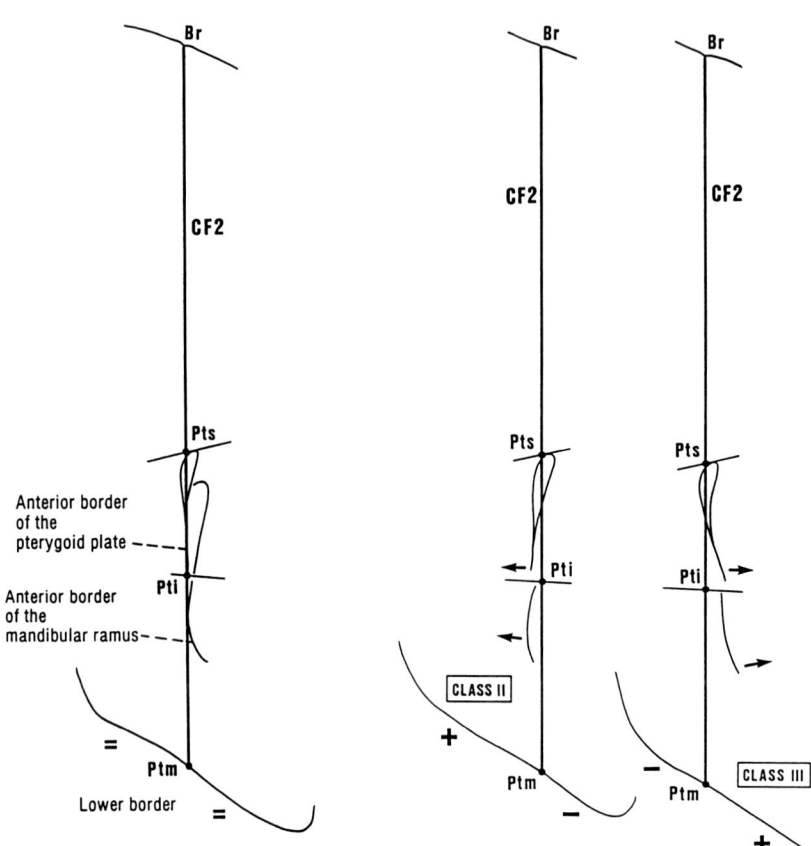

Figure 37.14 Normal relationship of line CF3 to the posterior border of the mandibular ramus is shown.

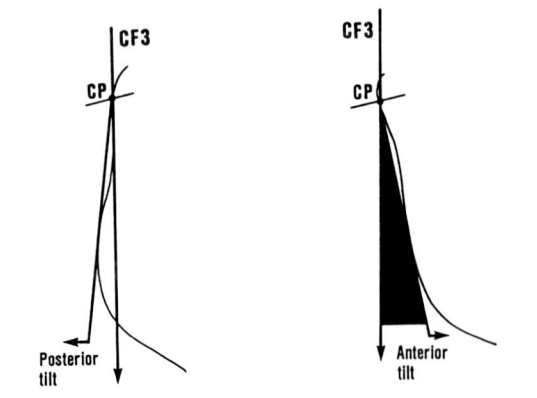

Figure 37.15 Posterior and anterior rotation of the ramus can be demonstrated with line CF3.

ramus, above the mandibular angle. Between these two points of tangency the posterior border of the ramus is slightly concave. As it continues downward, CF3 normally passes in front of the anterior curvature of the atlas. Dentofacial dysmorphoses often exhibit an anterior or posterior tilting of the mandibular rami (see Figure 37.15). The tracing of lines CF1, CF2, and CF3 divides the craniofacial area of line C1 into two segments: line M–Pts, called the maxillary area; and line Pts–Cp, called the mandibular area. The length and proportions of the craniofacial, craniospinal, maxillary, and mandibular areas objectively relate to certain predispositions of the cranial base to facial dysmorphosis. A reduction in the craniofacial area predisposes to class II skeletal pattern, and an increase in the craniofacial area predisposes to class III skeletal pattern. A reduction in the maxillary area leads to a shortening of the maxilla, and an increase in the maxillary area leads to a lengthening. A reduction in the mandibular area favors mandibular excess, and an increase in the mandibular area leads to a mandibular deficiency (see Figure 37.16).

The Use of Rigid Fixation 493

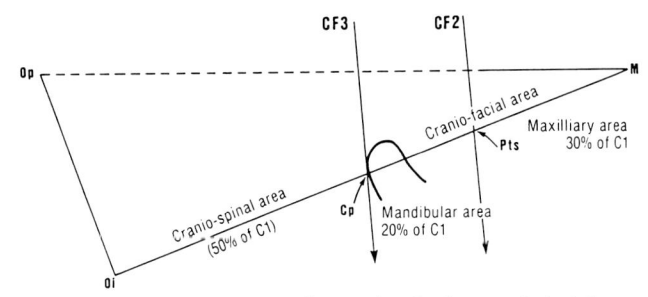

Figure 37.16 Lines CF2 and CF3 divide the craniofacial area into mandibular and maxillary fields. The relationship of these fields or areas deviates from the norm when craniofacial deformity is present.

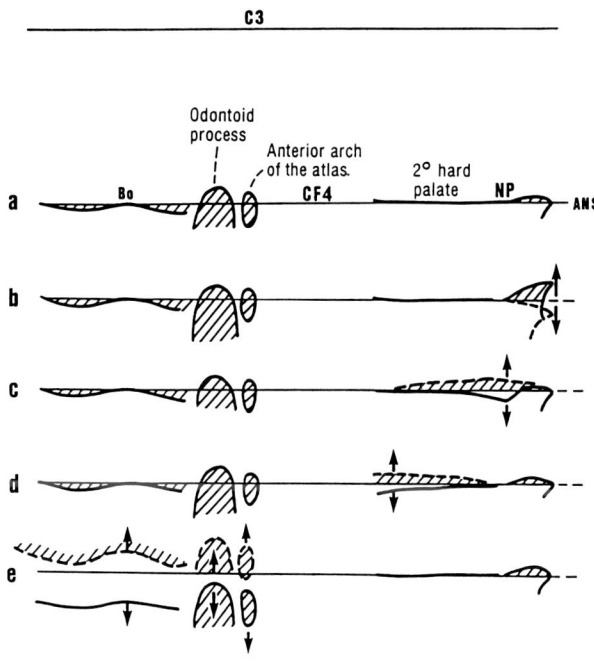

The tracing of CF4 when one or more points of reference are non-aligned. (parallel to C3)

Figure 37.17 The vertical relationships of cranial, spinal, and maxillary structures are illustrated.

Vertical Relationships Lines CF4 through CF8 permit vertical analysis of craniofacial balance. The craniopalatal line, line CF4, is traced parallel to line C3 from the summit of the anterior nasal spine (ANS) to just below the lowest point of convexity of the squamous occipital bone (Om). Line CF4 normally passes anteroposteriorly through NP (the upper anterior border of the nasopalatine canal) and the craniocervical articulation (represented by the anterior arch of the atlas, the tip of the odontoid process, and the occipital condyles). The level of the craniocervical articulation varies with age. Line CF4 subsequently lightly slices or forms a tangent to the squamous occipital bone (see Figure 37.17). Along its course, line CF4 cuts line CF2 at the inferior pterygoid point (Pti). This point should be confused neither with the posterior nasal spine nor with the inferior extremity of the pterygomaxillary fissure. In children, line CF4 normally passes through the apex of the odontoid, slightly above the anterior arch of the atlas, and through the Bolton point, Bo (found at the occipital retrocondylar notch). In adults, line CF4 passes at a lower level, often passing by the upper half of the odontoid process (below the dens) and by point Od before arriving at point Bo. Moreover, depending on the degree of tilt of the head, noting the relative vertical positions of Bo and the anterior arch of the atlas, with respect both to one another and to the apex of the odontoid process, may be useful. When the parallel to line C3 beginning at ANS does not pass through the other points mentioned, the surgeon, suspecting the position of ANS to be abnormal and of no use in relation to the analysis, must employ another method of tracing. By convention, we draw line CF4 so that it passes through the maximum of the other points of reference; that is, so that it passes through NP, the 2° hard palate, the apex of the odontoid, and Bo. Nevertheless, in some cases no parallel drawn to line C3 will pass through at least two of the reference points. This situation indicates an important vertical craniofacial imbalance having, in particular, incongruency between the upper face (and nasal complex) and the occipitomandibular area. The position of line CF4 should be adapted to the particular situation. It can be represented by a band demarcated by two lines, one passing by ANS and the other passing by the most reliable of the occipitocervical points, that is, either the apex of the odontoid or point Bo. If this representation is used, the other lines of craniofacial balance (CF5 through CF8) (see Figure 37.18) will each be represented by a band. Alternatively, they can be represented by a line that takes the "average" of the points, if point ANS can be well located at a predictable, reasonable level. Point ANS can be located by using line CF8 as a point of reference.

The line of theoretical facial height, line CF5, is drawn perpendicular to line CF4 (and thus also to line CF3) and through point ANS (see Figure 37.18). Above point ANS, the line halts directly opposite (point Na), at the projection of Na (point Na'). Below point ANS, the line halts at the projection at the level of the "theoretical" menton (point Me'). The relative lengths of these two segments of line CF5 are determined by the rule that the distance of point ANS to point Me' is 55% of the total length of line CF5. Therefore the length of the segment from point ANS to point Na' is 45% of the total anterior facial height (from point Na to point Me). In practice the position of Met is simply calculated

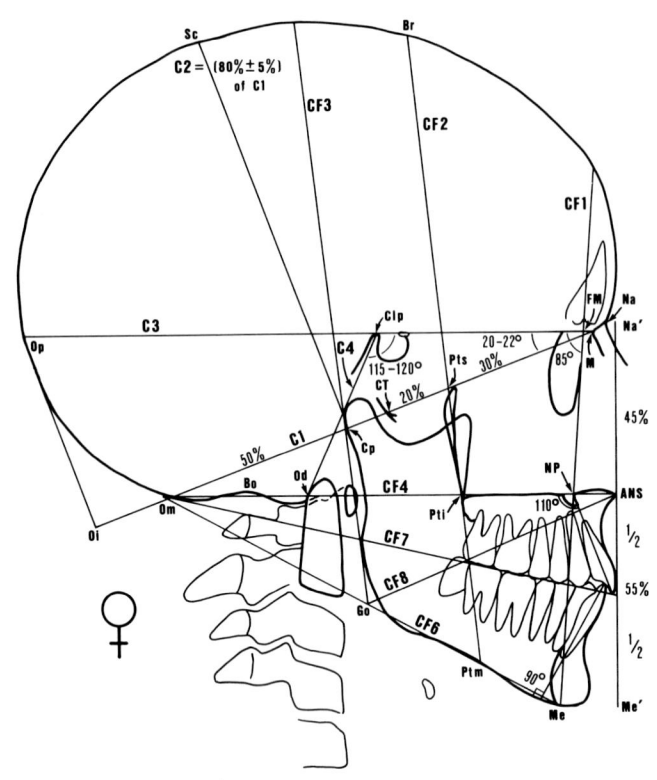

Figure 37.18 Architectural craniofacial analysis of Delaire. Note that the upper face constitutes 45% of the total facial height.

by doubling the distance of Na' to ANS and adding 1/9 to it. Once the theoretical level of the osseous mental point has been defined, the "ideal" situation for the point Me is easily obtained. It is situated at the intersection of line CF1 and the parallel to CF4 drawn through Me'. This situation may vary in the anteroposterior plane depending upon the orientation of CF1 and according to age, sex, and facial type. Where the line CF4 has been replaced by a band CF4, one must draw two points Me' and Me'' that delineate a band of theoretical mental height. The osseous mental point of the patient under analysis usually is situated between the two extremities Me' and Me'', because its position is subject to constraints generated at the same time from the facial, cervical, and lingual musculature. Point Na' is usually 1 to 3 mm in front of point Na. Line CF5 is tangent to the buccal faces of the upper central incisors. Maxillary retrusion or premaxillary hypoplasia can place point Na more posterior (the converse is also true). If line CF5 is not tangent to the buccal face of the upper central incisor a palatal or vestibulo version of these teeth is implied.

The craniomandibular line, line CF6, drawn from Me, runs tangent to the base of the squamous occipital bone, and ends at its union with line CF4 at point Om (see Figure 37.18). Normally CF6 follows closely the inferior border of the mandible from Me to the antegonial notch. As it continues, it just touches the inferior extremity of the mandibular angle, then crosses CF3 at the gonion point (point Go). In most people, point Me coincides with point Me' and point Om is closely positioned to the external cortical plate of the squamous occipital bone.

The cranio-occlusal line, line CF7, joins point Om to the midpoint of that portion of line CF5 that extends from point ANS to point Me'. Thus line CF7 does not exactly bisect the angle CF4 Om CF6, but it comes close to doing so (see Figure 37.18). Normally, line CF7 is tangent to the occlusal surfaces of the deciduous molars and the first permanent molars. Anteriorly, line CF7 passes in close proximity to the incisal edge of the upper central incisor after passing slightly below the incisal edge of the lower incisor. In dentofacial dysmorphoses, the situation and orientation of the occlusal plane is often very different due to a higher or lower posterior occlusal level and an increased or decreased overbite or anterior open bite.

The line of anteroposterior, vertical facial balance, line CF8, is normally drawn parallel to line C1 through point ANS. When the anterior nasal spine is well placed, line CF8 passes exactly through Go at the intersection of CF3 and CF6. The anterior nasal spine can be abnormally high or low, or too far forward or backward. In other respects the craniofacial area can be excessively long or short. Any of these abnormalities can move CF3, and thus the position of Go, forward or backward. Hence, the tracing of line CF8 should often be interpreted as a function of the information already provided by the other lines of craniofacial balance. This line is nevertheless very useful for objective visualization of the vertical shortening of maxillary depth as well as of any anomaly in the position of point ANS. Line CF8 is of great service in placing the points Go and Om when point ANS is well placed and occipital anomalies are present.

The Dental Analysis Despite its simplicity, dental analysis gives a good idea of the relationship of the dental arches to their bony bases, and also reveals the orientation of the anterior teeth (upper and lower incisors and upper canines). Line CF1 normally passes through the hypomochlion of the maxillary canine tooth, the distal sloping edge of the occlusal surface of the maxillary canine, and the apex of the mandibular central incisor. Line CF4 passes 3 to 4 mm above the apices of the upper first permanent molars. Line CF5 is tangential to the buccal face of the upper central incisors. Line CF7 is tangential to the occlusal plane of the deciduous molars and the first permanent molars. Three specific dental lines are also traced. First, the line of the long axis (incisal tip to root apex) of the maxillary central incisor, which normally creates an angle of 110° to line CF4, passes through NP in the normal subject. Sec-

The Use of Rigid Fixation   495

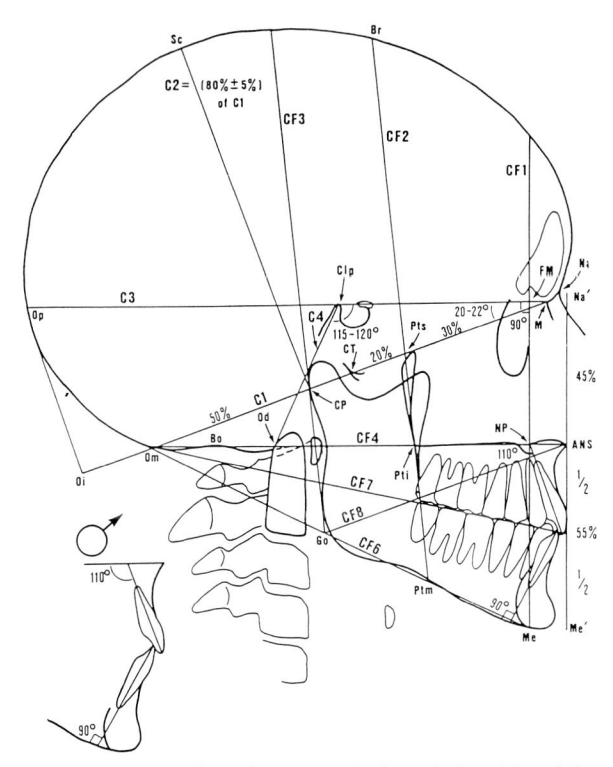

Figure 37.19 Dental analysis reveals the relationship of the dental arches to their bony bases and indicates the orientation of the anterior teeth.

ond, the line of the long axis of the upper canine normally creates an angle of 105° with line CF4. Third, the lower incisal line, which joins the incisal tip and apex, is normally perpendicular to the lower border of the mandible (see Figure 37.19). These dental lines disclose not only either linguoversion or buccoversion of the teeth but also either propositioning or retropositioning of their associated alveolar bone.

The Structural Study

The architectural analysis should be enhanced systematically by a structural study, which is a direct study of a lateral skull cephalometric radiograph. This study encompasses the examination of the state of various elements of the cranial, facial, and cervical skeleton and all the visible soft tissues. The structural study gives valuable information about the functional influences to which the skeleton is subject; about its characteristics of ossification, which may or may not enter into the classification of a syndrome; and about the functions of the craniofacial musculature.

SURGERY

Patients who suffer from the sequellae of both a labiomaxillopalatine cleft and a primary surgery have several common surgical requirements. These are functional genioplasty, maxillary osteotomy, which is frequently combined with alveolar bone graft, and total revision of the nasolabial musculature (not only to reorient these muscles but also to repair the vestibular oral-nasal fistula).

Functional Genioplasty

Functional genioplasty begins with the patient under controlled hypotensive general anesthesia, which is maintained via a cuffed oral-endotracheal tube. Lidocaine 1% with 1/100,000 is routinely used for infiltration hemostasis in the soft tissues overlying the anterior mandibular region. A vertical reference incision is made just through mucosa to aid accurate closure of soft tissue at completion of the operation. An intraoral incision is made in the unattached mucosa from the left first molar to the right first molar. The anterior aspect of the mandible is exposed by carefully elevating the soft tissues in the subperiosteal plane, such that the integrity of periosteum and muscle is maintained. The mental foramina are identified from a superoposterior approach before the dissection is inferiorly extended. The mental nerves are identified while the inferior border of the mandible is dissected free of its periosteal-muscle attachments well posterior to the mental foramina (see Figure 37.20). Lateral and midline vertical reference lines are scored on the facial surface of the mandible with a fine fissure bur. A thin malleable retractor is then placed at the inferior border of one side of the mandible. The osteotomy outlines are scored on the labial cortex of the mandible, after which they are completed with a reciprocating saw. A similar maneuver is carried out on the opposite side. The tenon thus created has vertical dimensions equal to the amount of vertical correction determined during the architectural analysis. With the inferior mandibular segment retracted inferiorly, two wedges of bone are removed to complete the tenon (see Figure 37.21). These bony wedges are useful for grafting the maxilla because their

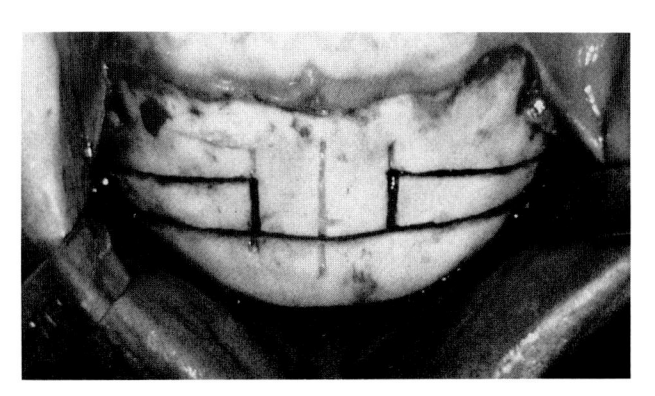

Figure 37.20 The facial surface of the mandible is exposed posterior to the mental foramina.

embryonic origin is similar to that of the maxilla and they are conveniently shaped. A mortise is now cut from the lingual cortex of the inferior mandibular segment, leaving intact bone between the labial cortex and the anterior wall of the mortise. This intact bone is equal to the desired amount of chin advancement (see Figure 37.22). The mortise of the inferior mandibular segment is now placed on the tenon of the superior mandibular segment, thus affecting a precise superoanterior reposition of the chin. This relationship can be stabilized with a plate and screws, with screws alone, or with double-strand stainless steel surgical wires (see Figure 37.23). The clinician must be aware that there is a well documented pattern of bony resorption/apposition following chin advancement surgery. This pattern should be taken into account when the method of fixation is decided. The soft-tissue reconstruction is delayed until maxillary surgery is completed.

Incisions

For unilateral deformities, the functional approach of Delaire is taken to identify the appropriate landmarks on which the incision design is based. The nasal domes are marked, followed by identification of the base of the columella on the uncleft side. A parallelogram is then constructed in order to identify the desired position of the columellar base on the cleft side. An incision line is extended from this point to the scar. An incision line is next drawn from the alar base on the cleft side to the cleft scar at the point where the incision line from the columellar base meets the cleft scar. An incision line is drawn superiorly across the nostril sill into the base of the nose. The actual vertical lip incisions are determined to some extent by the primary surgical scar. In any case the principle is such that position of the summit of the cupid's bow on the cleft side is

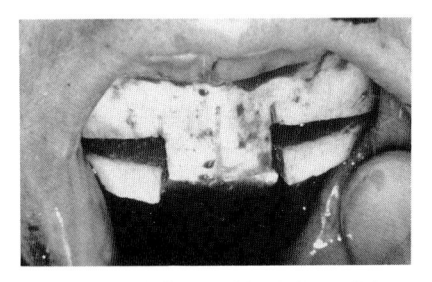

Figure 37.21 Surgical creation of the tenon is illustrated. The vertical arms of the tenon correspond to the amount of planned vertical reduction.

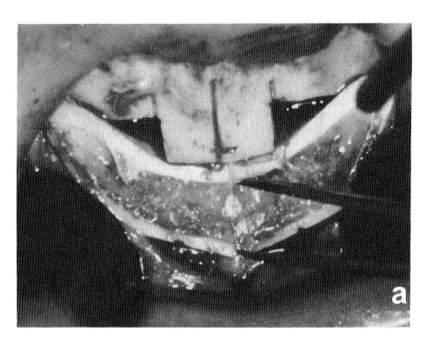

Figure 37.22 (a) Measurements are taken to determine the size of the mortise. (b) The mortise is cut in the lingual aspect of the inferior segment.

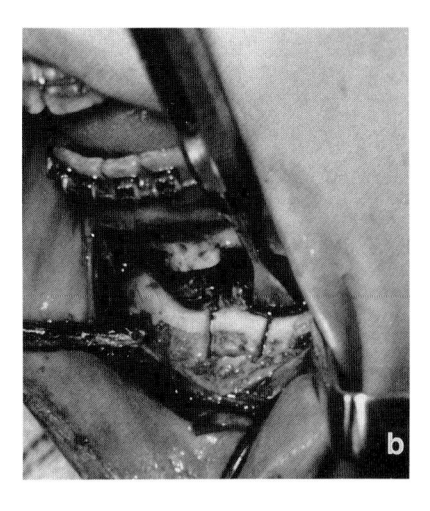

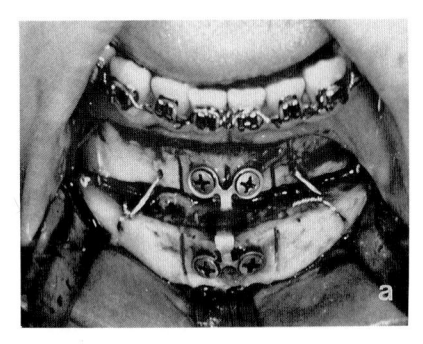

Figure 37.23 Fixation can be accomplished with (a) plate and screws, (b) screws alone, or (c) double-strand stainless steel wires.

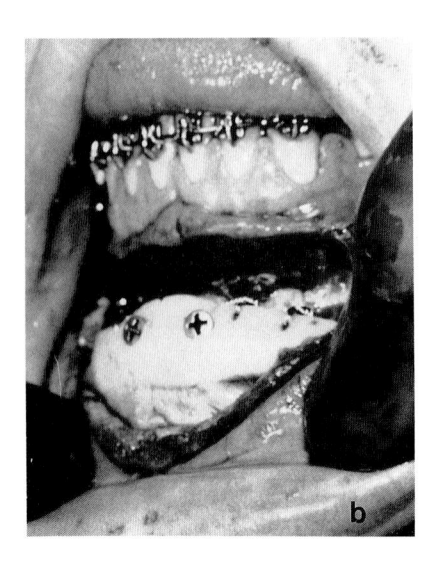

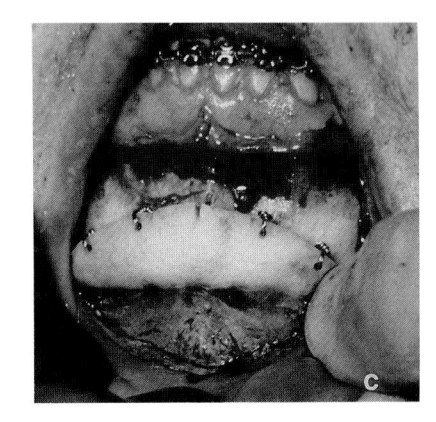

vertically and laterally equidistant from the midline relative to the uncleft side. In order to achieve this symmetry, excision of a small portion of cutaneous tissue on the cleft side is sometimes necessary. The incision line continues over the vermilion border and into the mouth, so that the maxillary labial frenum is always left on the uncleft side of the incision (see Figure 37.24). Once the incision lines have been drawn, the actual cutaneous incisions are completed prior to the infiltration of local anesthesia with 1/100,000 epinephrine since this infiltration distorts the cutaneous landmarks. When a vestibular oral-nasal fistula is present, the incision that divides the lip should become continuous with the fistula to facilitate accurate reconstruction of the floor of the nose and nasolabial musculature.

Maxillary Osteotomy

The maxillary osteotomy of preference is usually the Le Fort I type, but the clinician should be aware of the applicability of the modified Le Fort III or maxillomalar osteotomy when there is deficiency in the anterior projection of the malar aspect of the face. The approach to the maxilla for the Le Fort I osteotomy is similar to that described by Bell (1975) with several modifications. The horizontal incision is kept very low so that only a few millimeters of unattached mucosa remain on the inferior segment. This modification, when combined with very wide subperiosteal exposure—particularly on the cleft side—allows for maximum advancement of soft tissue toward the midline. We invariably use a superior step in the zygomatic region of the maxilla (see Figure 37.25) in order to enhance the accuracy of intraoral spatial orientation, to provide solid bone for application of rigid fixation devices, and to maximize contact of the bony fragments (Precious 1989). We do not use a chisel to separate the maxilla from the pterygoid plates for reasons that have been previously discussed. The maxilla is then oriented to the mandible by way of an intermaxillary occlusal splint, which is initially ligated to the maxillary arch. Contoured miniplates are most frequently used to fix the maxilla in its planned position (see Figure 37.26). In addition maxillo-mandibular wire skeletal fixation is used to supplement dental fixation. This wire is left in place for approximately six weeks. Concomitant mandibular surgery, which is occasionally necessary, can be performed more easily if an armored oral endotracheal tube exits the mouth on the uncleft side via the buccal space from behind the occlusal splint.

Reconstruction of Nasolabial Muscles

Three important muscles and muscle groups must be reconstructed in order to achieve symmetry and good function of the upper lip. First, the lateral nasal muscle

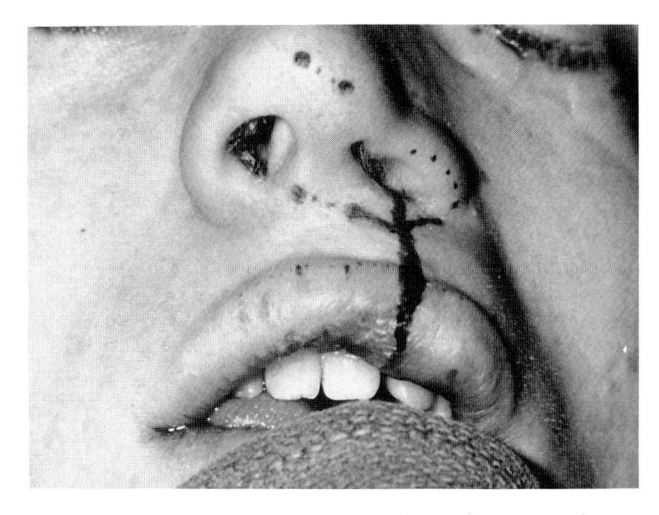

Figure 37.24 Planned incisions are shown for a secondary functional cheilorhinoplasty.

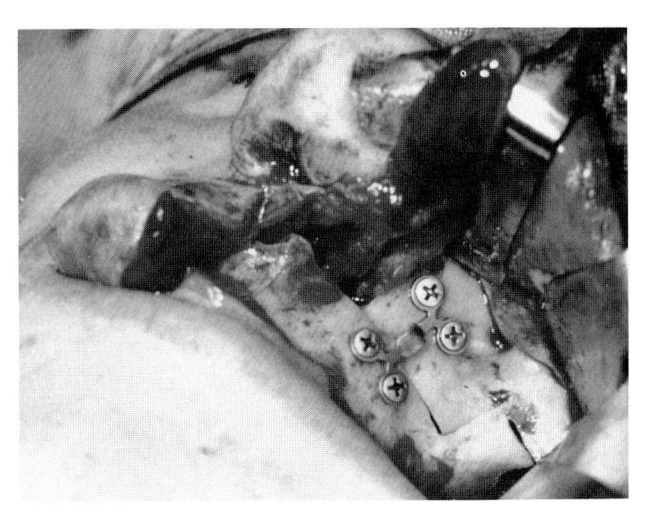

Figure 37.25 The superior step design of the Le Fort I osteotomy improves bony contact when the inferior segment is advanced.

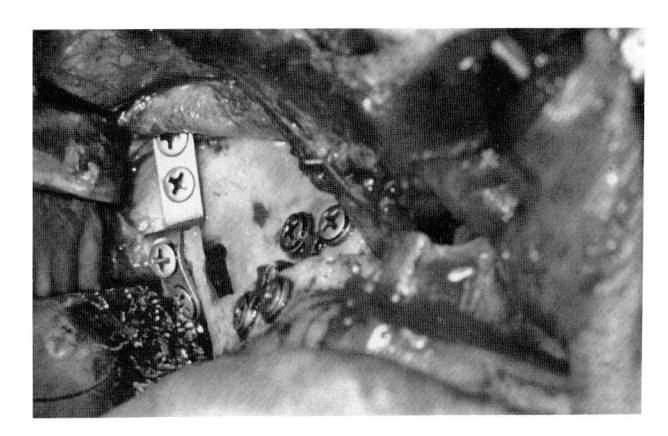

Figure 37.26 Careful contouring of the miniplates improves the accuracy of the fixation.

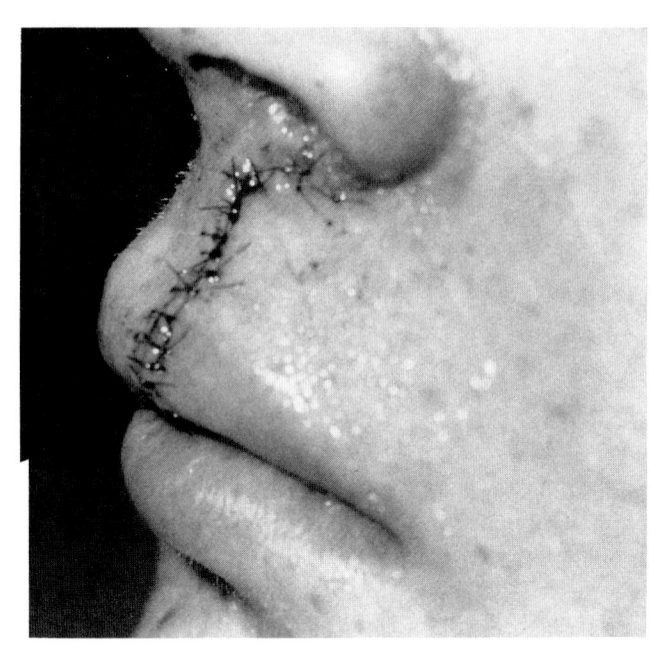

Figure 37.27 Posture of the lip is shown two days postsurgery.

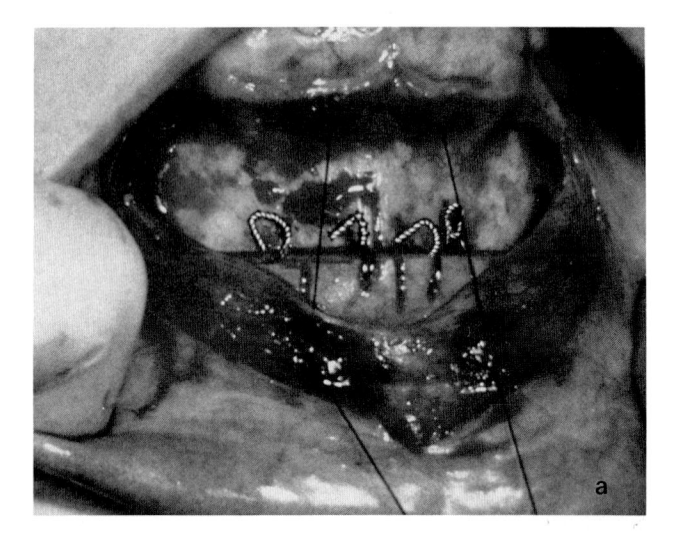

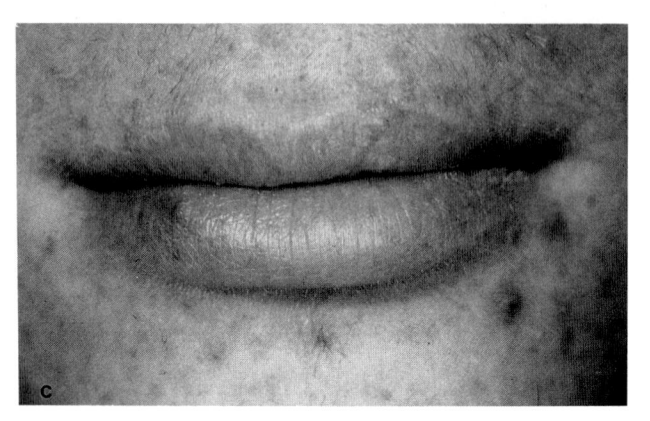

must be identified and sutured, with nonresorbable material, to the base of the cartilaginous nasal septum near the anterior nasal spine. Second, the levator muscles of the lip must be identified and sutured to the nasal septum anterior to the position chosen for the lateral nasal muscle. Finally, the pyramidal portion of the orbicularis oris muscle must be identified and sutured to the most anterior portion of the nasal septum. The upper lip can be thought of as a circus tent with the central pole being the anterior nasal spine and septum. If this reconstruction is carried out meticuluosly, good eversion and protrusion of the lip should be possible after surgery (see Figure 37.27).

The mentalis muscles must also be reconstructed with nonresorbable sutures to assure improved lower-lip function, which in itself has a beneficial effect on upper-lip function (see Figure 37.28).

SUMMARY

In the management of secondary deformities associated with labiomaxillopalatine clefts, the use of rigid fixation can aid immensely in both accuracy and stability. Careful clinical examination will usually reveal deviation of the nasal septum to the uncleft side, nasolabial and labiomental muscular dysfunction, maxil-

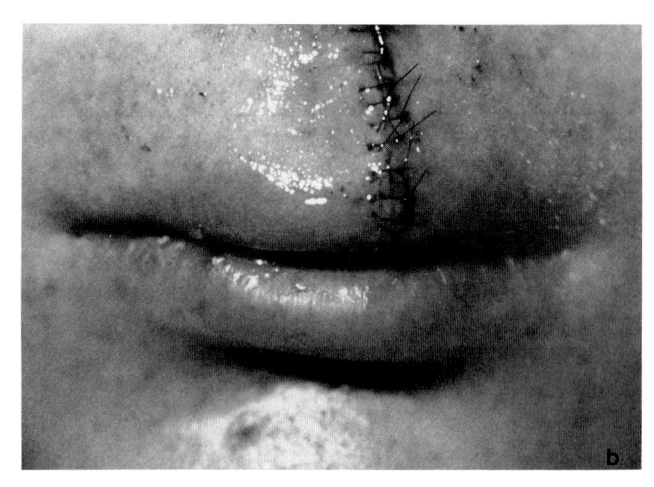

Figure 37.28 (a) Suturing the divided mentalis muscles in order to restore muscular function. (b) Relationship of upper and lower lips two days postsurgery. (c) Same patient two years after surgery.

lary deficiency, and vertical mandibular excess. Accurate planning of movement of both hard and soft tissue can be enhanced with the use of the architectural craniofacial analysis of Delaire. Accurate muscular reconstruction can be accomplished only on a good skeletal base. In order to achieve optimum aesthetic results, the clinician should adopt the functional approach to the correction of both primary and secondary cleft deformities.

REFERENCES

Bell W: Le Fort I osteotomy for correction of maxillary deformities. J Oral Surg 33:412, 1975.

Delaire J: Theoretical principles and technique of functional closure of the lip and nasal aperture. J Maxillofac Surg 78:93, 1977.

Delaire J: L'analyse architectural et structural craniofaciale (de profil); principes theorique quelques examples d'emploi en chirurgie maxillofaciale. Rev Stomatol 79:1, 1978.

Delaire J, Precious D: Influence of the nasal septum on maxillary growth in patients with congenital labiomaxillary cleft. Cl Pal J 23:270, 1986.

Precious D, Delaire J: Correction of anterior mandibular vertical excess: The functional genioplasty. Oral Surg Oral Med Oral Path 59:229, 1985.

Precious D, Ricard D, Morrison A: Pterygomaxillary separation without the use of osteotome: 426 cases. 71st Annual meeting of the American Association of Oral and Maxillofacial Surgeons. San Francisco, Calif., 1989.

CHAPTER 38

Orthodontic Considerations and Rigid Fixation

James L. Ackerman

Harvey M. Rosen

The introduction of plates and screws as a method of achieving rigid fixation in orthognathic surgery has dramatically improved the efficacy of these procedures. In spite of this advance, the use of rigid fixation is not universally accepted by surgeons and orthodontists. This is primarily because this fixation method is, as its name states, rigid, and therefore unforgiving. Subsequent to rigid fixation, little, if any, opportunity arises for the treating orthodontist to manipulate repositioned dento-osseous segments by means of elastic traction in the postoperative period. As a result, any significant improvement in the occlusion achieved at the time of surgery will require postsurgical movement of teeth. If a skeletally based malocclusion remains following surgery, correction through movement of the teeth will prolong total treatment time, may aesthetically compromise the final result, and will most likely be unstable. The surgeon therefore must be capable of consistently producing the planned occlusal relationships at the time of surgery. If the surgeon cannot do this, the use of rigid fixation should be abandoned in favor of the more forgiving and less exacting fixation method of wire osteosynthesis with maxillo-mandibular fixation (MMF).

From the patient's point of view, however, the elimination of MMF in the postoperative period has remarkably enhanced the recovery experience and has made surgical correction of dentofacial deformities much more acceptable. In the past, the specter of six to eight weeks of postsurgical MMF has been the single greatest stumbling block for patient acceptance of combined orthodontic/surgical correction of dentofacial deformity.

With the introduction of rigid fixation, surgeons and orthodontists have had to modify and refine their traditional procedures to accommodate this technique's inherent lack of forgiveness. It has always been important for the surgeon and orthodontist to work closely in the planning and treatment of the orthognathic surgical patient. The use of rigid fixation made the coordination of orthodontics and surgery even more important. Our goal in this chapter is not to provide a definitive text on all aspects of orthodontics with regard to treating the orthognathic surgical patient. Our purpose is to point out the ways in which these techniques have had to be modified due to the introduction of rigid fixation.

PREOPERATIVE CONSIDERATIONS

The key to treatment planning in orthognathic surgery, regardless of whether or not one utilizes rigid fixation, is in establishing a correct diagnosis. This determination is made primarily on the basis of physical findings and the assessment of facial form. The various diagnostic aids, such as cephalometric and panoramic radiographs, facial photographs, study models, and other measurements, are extremely helpful in confirming the preliminary diagnosis, which is based on the physical examination. In spite of the many diagnostic tools available today, including the newer imaging techniques as well as computerized simulation approaches, astute treatment planning still comes down to clinical judgment.

Knowledge of the patient's prior orthodontic treatment, if any, is essential. If unstable tooth movement has been previously accomplished, relapse is likely following the period of active postoperative orthodontics. Unstable tooth movement includes attempted closure of skeletal open bite, excessive transverse expansion of the maxillary arch, and anterior dental compensations to camouflage a class II or III malocclusion. These unfavorable dental compensations should be eliminated preoperatively in order to minimize the possibility of dental relapse in the postoperative period.

In patients with malocclusions severe enough to warrant orthognathic surgery and who have not had prior orthodontic therapy, spontaneous adaptive changes in the positions of the teeth often mask the underlying jaw disproportion. These adaptive changes are referred to as *spontaneous dental compensations* (see Figure 38.1). In this situation, the maxillary and mandibular teeth rarely fit together nicely when the surgeon attempts to simulate the most optimal occlusion with the "hand-held" dental casts. One or more teeth can be removed from the plaster casts and reset in wax to simulate the outcome of the presurgical orthodontic movement of the teeth. The surgeon also can judiciously grind small areas on the occlusal surfaces of the plaster teeth to simulate the result of adjusting the occlusion by the selective grinding of enamel. This diagnostic set-up indicates the extent of the orthodontic movement of teeth that will be required in conjunction with the orthognathic surgery.

The placement of orthodontic appliances serves two functions. The first is to achieve the changes in tooth position that were simulated on the diagnostic set-up and to remove any dental compensations that had spontaneously arisen or that had taken place due to prior orthodontic treatment. The dental arches must be coordinated to allow for proper interdigitation of the opposing teeth while maintaining the proper axial inclination in their supporting basal bone.

There are two schools of thought as to how much orthodontic tooth movement should be accomplished prior to surgery and how much should remain for the postsurgical phase of treatment. Prior to the use of rigid fixation, an interocclusal wafer or splint was routinely used to index the teeth for the duration of MMF. Because the teeth did not have to interdigitate well during this period, many orthodontists thought that performing a great deal of presurgical orthodontics held little merit and left much of the tooth movement to be accomplished postsurgically. In other words, the surgery was used to change the underlying skeletal pattern, and once the skeleton was normalized, the patient was treated like any other orthodontic patient.

This approach has always presented a major disadvantage. Upon completion of surgery, the patient would like to have the orthodontic appliances removed as soon as possible after healing. Telling the patient that the occlusion will be compromised if the orthodontic appliances are removed too soon is often not compelling. This patient management problem can be solved by accomplishing most of the required orthodontics presurgically. In addition, with the advent of rigid fixation and the elimination of MMF in the immediate postoperative period, patients can immediately function into their planned occlusion. With the exception of those patients who require segmental Le Fort I maxillary osteotomies, the use of final surgical splints can be entirely eliminated provided that the bulk of the necessary orthodontic tooth movement has been accomplished presurgically. In those patients who have had minimal presurgical orthodontic tooth movement, immediate mandibular function in the postoperative period becomes problematic. For example, the postoperative patient who has temporarily lost proprioception and does not have a stable, well interdigitating occlusion will frequently shift the mandible into an eccentric position to establish what he or she perceives to be the best occlusal fit. The surgeon's effort to achieve a reproducible, physiologic relationship between the condyle and the glenoid fossa is now lost. Therefore, if the patient is to function in the immediate postoperative period when only minimal presurgical orthodontics have been accomplished, a final surgical splint must be used. This obviates one of the advantages of using rigid fixation, that is, the ability of the treating orthodontist to apply maxillo-mandibular elastics in the early postoperative period in order to resume finishing postsurgical orthodontic tooth movement. When a patient wears a final surgical splint, this possibility is eliminated. The orthodontist must then wait until the splint is removed before resuming the postsurgical phase of orthodontic treatment.

For all these reasons, completing as much of the orthodontic treatment as possible during the presurgical phase of treatment is beneficial. If tooth extraction is not necessary as part of the orthodontic treatment, accomplishing presurgical orthodontic tooth movement takes from six to nine months. Thus, with an additional

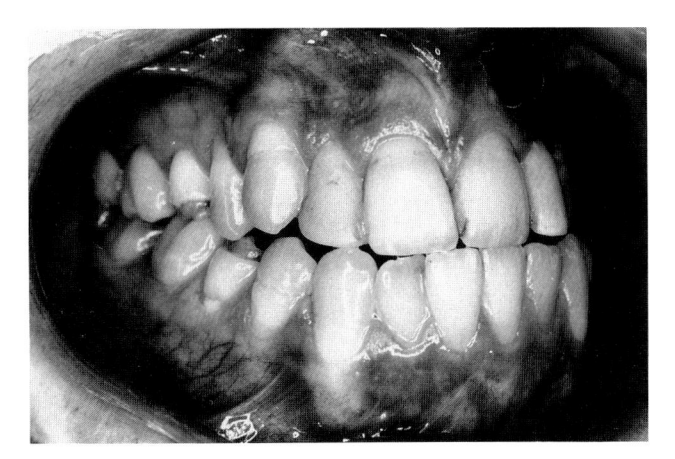

Figure 38.1 Spontaneous dental compensations are shown in a patient with a class III malocclusion. Notice the lingual inclination of the anterior mandibular teeth in an effort to minimize skeletal disproportion. This should be eliminated by presurgical orthodontic treatment.

two months for postsurgical orthodontic treatment, most patients requiring a combination of orthodontics and orthognathic surgery can be treated in less than a year.

As previously mentioned, when leveling and aligning the teeth orthodontically, it is important not to tip teeth that later will be repositioned surgically in a more bodily fashion. Minimizing intrusion or extrusion of teeth orthodontically is also important, because these tooth movements can relapse quickly in the postoperative period and can jeopardize an otherwise good surgical result. Attempted orthodontic transverse expansion by buccally tipping the posterior teeth is also ill advised, because this is likely to relapse following the active phase of postoperative orthodontics.

The second function of orthodontic appliances is to serve as points of attachment for the MMF that is required intraoperatively. Almost any kind of orthodontic appliance can be used for this purpose. Use of orthodontic bands for the molar teeth and bonded attachments on the remaining teeth is usually prudent. Because many, if not most, patients are adults, using ceramic brackets for the anterior teeth makes the orthodontic aspect of treatment more acceptable. In general, a bracket slot size of 0.022 by 0.028 appears to work best. Because MMF is used only intraoperatively, the surgical hooks can be placed on undersized, 0.018 by 0.025 stainless-steel rectangular wires without much concern that the wire won't be rigid enough or that there will be an unfavorable torsion placed on the wire (see Figure 38.2). In maxillary segmental cases, 0.021 by 0.025 posterior segmental wires should be used to avoid rotation of the wire.

After these final surgical wires are placed, a two-week interval is allowed to accommodate any additional movement of teeth. Final impressions are then taken, and the dental casts are mounted on a semi-adjustable anatomic articulator; a face-bow transfer is used to mount the maxillary cast. The mandibular model is then mounted relative to the maxillary cast with the use of either a wax or silicone bite that is taken with the mandible in centric relation, that is, when the condyles are as close as possible to the physiologic center of the glenoid fossa. A final lateral cephalometric radiograph must be taken with the mandible in this position. This is particularly important in Class II and mandibular asymmetry cases, in which case the patient may be posturing forward or to one side without knowing it. If the surgeon is unable to determine whether the patient is functionally shifting the mandible, an interocclusal wafer of acrylic is interposed between the maxillary and mandibular teeth, eliminating the interferences of occlusion. This disarticulation of the teeth allows the musculature to dictate the best physiologic position of the mandible.

After the final models are mounted on a semi-anatomic articulator, the model surgery is performed.

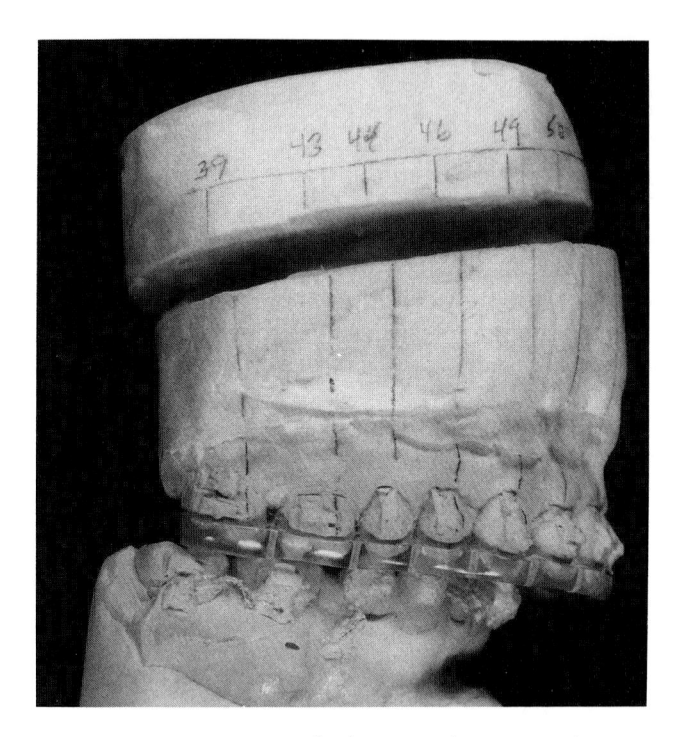

Figure 38.2 Customary orthodontic appliances are shown used in conjunction with rigid fixation. Brackets with slot size of 0.022 by 0.028 are directly bonded to all teeth except molars, which are banded. A stainless steel continuous arch wire of 0.018 by 0.025 is fitted in slots. Surgical hooks (either crimped or soldered) are attached to the arch wire.

The most important role that this serves is to allow fabrication of an intermediate splint (see Figure 38.3) if double-jaw surgery is to be performed or a final surgical splint (see Figure 38.4) if maxillary segmentation is planned. Double-jaw surgery is always performed with intermediate splints in order to position the maxilla correctly in the sagittal plane. Vertical hash marks scored on the lateral maxillary walls at the time of surgery are, at best, inaccurate. In addition, the occlusal plane is less likely to tilt, either sagittally or transversely, with an intermediate splint.

Double-jaw surgery, which includes multiple segmentation of the maxilla, requires fabrication of a composite splint (see Figure 38.5). This obviates removal of the maxillary splint once the maxillary dento-osseous segments have been mobilized and repositioned. One must realize that rigid fixation offers the least resistance to relapse in transversely expanded maxillary segments. Splint removal once these segments have been plated is, therefore, ill advised.

The necessity for a final surgical splint depends on two factors. The first is whether the maxilla has been segmentalized (see Figure 38.4). If maxillary segmentation has been carried out, a maxillary splint into which the mandible functions is mandatory. The second factor

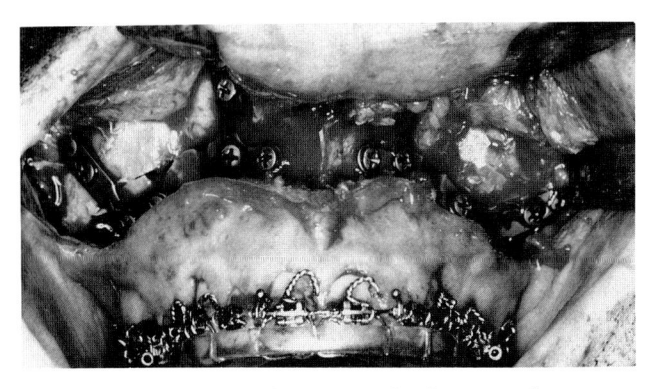

Figure 38.3 An intermediate surgical splint is used to position the maxilla accurately in the sagittal plane without risk of transverse or sagittal tilting. The mandible has yet to be surgically advanced into class I occlusion.

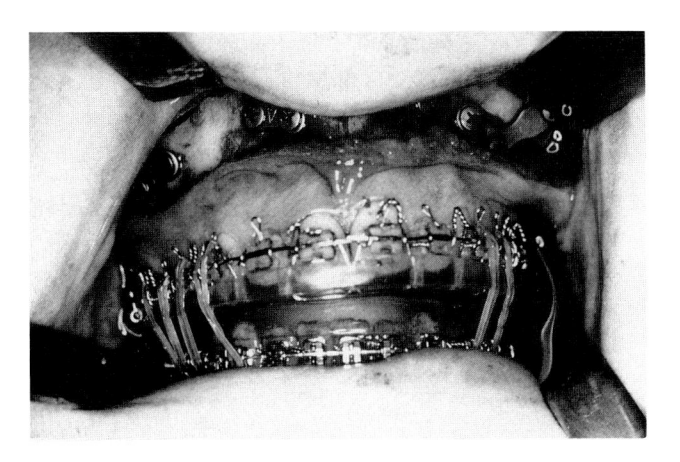

Figure 38.4 A final surgical splint is used for four-piece maxillary segmentation. Each dento-osseous segment is wired into the splint by using the most mesial and distal tooth in each segment.

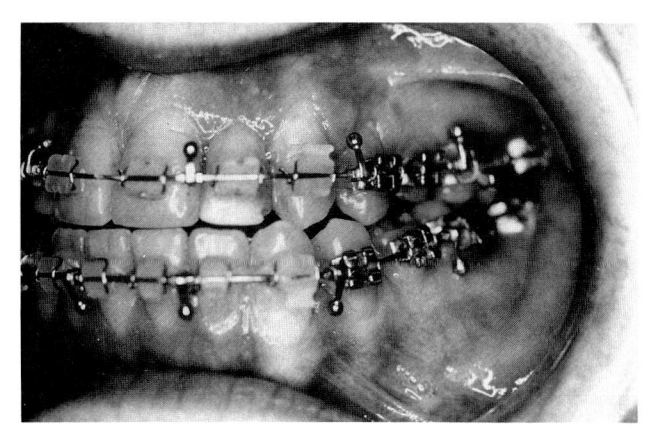

Figure 38.5 A composite surgical splint (intraoperative view) is composed of a fixed maxillary splint, already wired to the maxilla, and an intermediate splint that indexes into the maxillary splint to position the maxilla accurately in the sagittal plane. Once the mandible is mobilized, its teeth will index into the maxillary splint to dictate the sagittal position of the mandible.

is the extent to which presurgical orthodontics has been accomplished. If the patient has a stable occlusion into which he or she can reproducibly bite without interference or functional shifting of the mandible, a final surgical splint is not necessary.

INTRAOPERATIVE CONSIDERATIONS

The single most important intraoperative step for the successful use of rigid fixation is the release of MMF once the jaws have been rigidly immobilized. This presents the surgeon with a unique opportunity to help ascertain whether the mandibular condyles were correctly positioned at the time of segment fixation. On release of MMF, if the mandible does not occlude properly with the maxillary dentition or surgical splint, rigid fixation must be dismantled, the previous surgical steps must be repeated, and new drill holes must be used. Once the planned surgical occlusion has been achieved, the operation is terminated. No MMF, either wires or elastics, is in place at the end of the procedure.

POSTOPERATIVE CONSIDERATIONS

Within the first 24 hours following surgery, the following determination must be made: Is the anatomic relationship between condyle and glenoid fossa established at the time of surgery the correct physiologic relationship for the patient? On the first postoperative day, the patient is asked to occlude. If the patient functions comfortably and reproducibly into proper occlusion without mandibular translation, one can assume that the condylar position established at surgery is correct. Baseline lateral and P-A cephalograms are then obtained. If the patient is unable to occlude properly (usually represented as areas of open bite), condylar distraction must have existed at the time rigid fixation was accomplished. Under this circumstance the patient should undergo reoperation as soon as the problem is discovered. This situation, when it arises, follows a Le Fort I intrusive procedure and is caused by inadequate posterior maxillary ostectomy. A somewhat nebulous situation exists when the patient can properly occlude but minor degrees of mandibular translation (either laterally or forward) must take place to accomplish this. Under this circumstance, the patient is asked to occlude fully while transcranial radiographic exposures of the temporomandibular joints are obtained. Reoperation is indicated if the condyle is distracted. If the condyle is well seated, the patient is placed in light training elastics

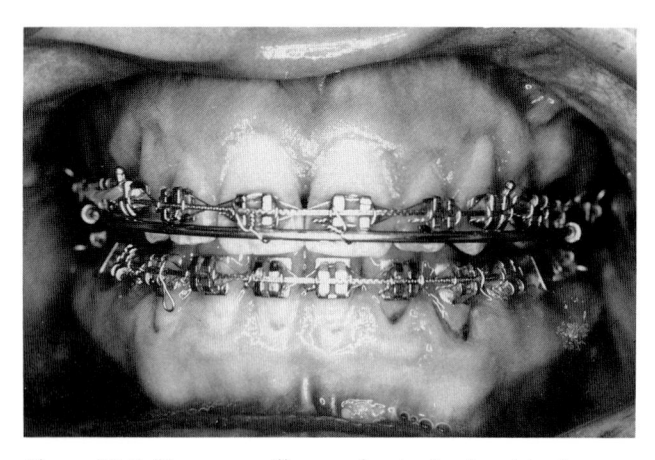

Figure 38.6 Heavy maxillary arch wire is placed in the headgear tubes and ligated to the tooth brackets to help stabilize transverse expansion after the splint is removed.

to guide the mandible into proper occlusion. Baseline lateral and P-A cephalograms are then obtained.

Prior to the use of rigid fixation, when MMF was required for six to eight weeks, the condylar distraction may not have been discovered until the patient was completely healed. Such patients had the terrible inconvenience, as well as psychological trauma, of having to be readmitted to the hospital for further surgery at that late date. Although reoperation using rigid fixation is required in approximately 5% of patients, these patients are saved this disappointment so long after initial surgery.

Surgical splints used in multiple segment Le Fort I procedures are generally left in place for four to five weeks. If significant transverse expansion has been surgically accomplished, the patient is seen by the orthodontist the day the splint is removed. At this time a heavy arch wire is ligated to the orthodontic brackets to help stabilize the transverse expansion (see Figure 38.6). Remember, rigid fixation offers the least resistance to skeletal relapse in the transverse plane. In those patients who do not undergo maxillary segmentation and therefore do not have final surgical splints wired into place, the orthodontic arch wires with surgical hooks can usually be removed within 10 to 14 days postsurgically. Plain, rectangular nickel-titanium arch wires, which are less rigid, can be placed and the finishing stages of the orthodontic tooth movement can commence.

CONCLUSIONS

In this chapter we have discussed some orthodontic considerations in treating patients undergoing orthognathic surgery with rigid fixation techniques. Both the surgeon and the orthodontist must work together closely to plan treatment of patients. Their techniques must be refined sufficiently to achieve results that are within the narrow tolerances dictated by the inability to obtain orthopedic change postsurgically. Ideal occlusion is rarely, if ever, achieved immediately postsurgically, and it is through the short course of postsurgical orthodontic treatment that optimal occlusion is established. The surgeon is compelled to deliver to the orthodontist a postsurgical malocclusion that can be corrected by minor orthodontic movement of teeth in a relatively short period. The comfortable interdigitation of the teeth must coincide physiologically with the centered condylar positions within the glenoid fossa.

Orthognathic surgery today, although based on scientific principles, remains a clinical art. Diagnosis still relies on clinical judgment, and the outcome of treatment relies on the imagination and skill of the surgeon and orthodontist.

BIBLIOGRAPHY

Epker BN, Fish LC: Dentofacial deformities: Integrated orthodontic and surgical correction. St. Louis, Mosby, 1986.

Fish LC, Epker BN: Prevention of relapse in surgical-orthodontic treatment: Mandibular procedures. J Clin Orthod 20:826–841, 1985.

Fish LC, Epker BN: Prevention of relapse in surgical-orthodontic treatment: Maxillary procedures. J Clin Orthod 21:33–47, 1987.

Proffit WR, Epker BN: Treatment planning for dentofacial deformities. In Surgical Correction of Dentofacial Deformities. Bell WH, Proffit WR, White RP (eds). Philadelphia, Saunders, pp 155–200, 1980.

Rosen HM: Miniplate fixation of Le Fort I osteotomies. Plast Reconstr Surg 78:748–754, 1986.

PART III

Clinical Applications
Congenital Craniofacial Deformities

CHAPTER 39

Stability of Skeletal Fixation in Congenital Craniofacial Surgery

Jean-Francois Tulasne

Paul Tessier

In the treatment of craniofacial malformations, osteotomies, mobilization and fixation of bone segments are the three usual steps taken to provide balance to the skeleton. Onlay and inlay grafts are frequently used alone or in combination with osteotomies.

Stability of the fragments, essential for bone healing, depends on the direction and degree of displacement and the type of fixation. The displacement dictates the design of the osteotomy; whenever possible, a self-retention device is incorporated. Bone grafts are often necessary both to fill the gaps and to help stabilize the fragments. Large areas of contact between the fragments guarantees fast consolidation. Rigid fixation can be helpful in preventing mobility and creating even compression between the fragments which allows primary bone healing (Reitzik 1983).

For almost 20 years, rigid fixation has proven to be extremely useful in the treatment of facial fractures. More recently, it has been given good results in the treatment of dentofacial deformities. However, wire fixation is still widely used in both maxillofacial and craniofacial surgery. Reasons for using wire instead of miniplates and screws are

- satisfactory results with wire fixation,
- reluctance to use a new system,
- possibility of adverse effects on adjacent structures (temporomandibular joint, teeth, nerves),
- increased operating time, and
- higher cost of rigid fixation systems.

Having used miniplates and screws in orthognathic surgery for several years, we believe that rigid fixation represents major progress in bone surgery. Therefore we have abandoned wire fixation in the treatment of patients with dentofacial deformities. Does rigid fixation offer such advantages for craniofacial surgery?

Although the use of miniplates and screws is the method of choice to stabilize bone segments, in some cases their use is not an absolute necessity, and stable fixation can be achieved much more simply with a few wires. Moreover, wires will remain useful for orienting fragments before stabilization.

GENERAL RULES

Stabilization of Bone Grafts

Inlay grafts usually maintain their position without fixation when they are cut to the proper size. Self-retention osteotomies can be made by burring either the recipient site or the graft to improve stability (see Figure 39.1). Onlay grafts are often unstable and always benefit from fixation. Rigid fixation with screws is the pro-

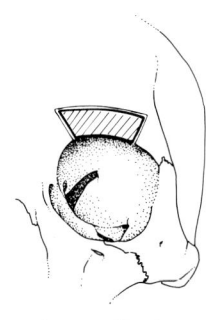

Figure 39.1 Inlay grafts usually do not require any type of fixation, particularly if a self-retention device is incorporated.

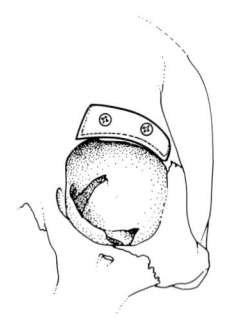

Figure 39.2 Onlay grafts are best stabilized with one or two screws.

Table 39.1 Comparison of successive steps following osteotomy and mobilization of the bone fragment in orthognathic and craniofacial surgery. The role of wire is far from negligible.

	Positioning according to	Temporary fixation	Definitive fixation (stabilization)
Orthognathic	Precise reference points	Wires (MMF)	Plates and screws
Craniofacial	Surgical experience more than calculation	Wires	Wires, or plates and screws

cedure of choice, as it combines compression with stability (see Figure 39.2).

Stabilization of Bone Segments

Four steps are involved in the repositioning of bone fragments. These steps, in order, are osteotomy, mobilization, positioning the fragment, and stabilization. The osteotomy is the minor part of the operation. Mobilization must be complete and can be difficult to obtain in some cases. Stabilization is essential for bone healing and is usually done without difficulty, not requiring a great deal of surgical experience. The crucial step is positioning the fragment (see Table 39.1).

In orthognathic surgery, the main reference for positioning the fragments is the dental occlusion. In trauma cases, the fracture lines are the guides for anatomic reduction. In craniofacial malformations, the ideal position of the bone fragment is not determined by precise criteria and therefore rarely is found immediately. According to her or his experience, the surgeon will make one or several trials before determining the best position. For each position a temporary fixation is necessary. This temporary fixation is best achieved with wires. By loosening some wires and tightening others, the surgeon can move the bone fragment until the ideal position is found. At this time, definitive and firm stabilization is accomplished with miniplates, screws, or additional wires, according to the case.

In general,

- wires are sufficient to maintain fragments in apposition;
- rigid miniplates are very helpful when the fragments are comminuted; a plate must be used to maintain gaps between fragments;
- screws are indicated when fragments overlap;
- rigid miniplates are useful to maintain straightening or bending of a bone segment (see Figure 39.3).

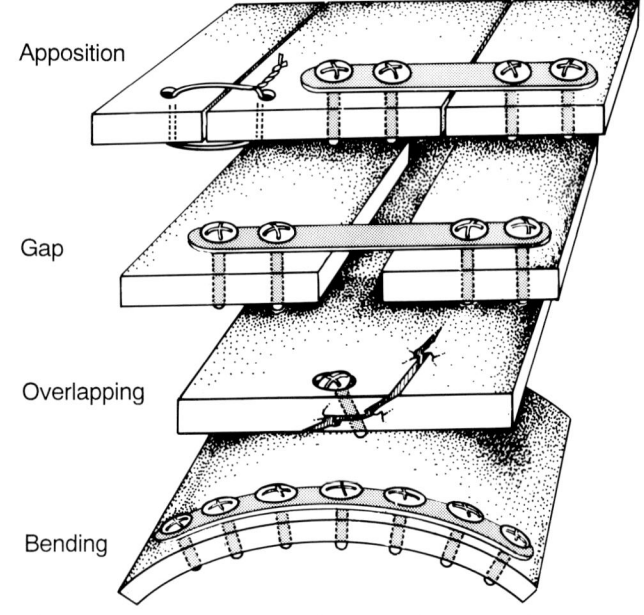

Figure 39.3 Various types of osteosynthesis are shown according to the position of the bone segments.

STABILIZATION ACCORDING TO THE DEFORMITY

Craniosynostosis

Surgery in infancy is performed primarily to release the stenosed sutures of the skull. The deformed parts of the cranial vault are mobilized, reshaped, and repositioned. They are not firmly stabilized but rather left "floating" to respond to the pressure of the growing brain (Marchac 1979). Therefore, the bone segments are fixated with wires or even with polyglycolic sutures.

In older children, a long miniplate helps to keep the reshaped fragment in the ideal anatomic position. Also, in some cases miniplates can stabilize a fronto-orbital advancement more simply and more rapidly than wires do.

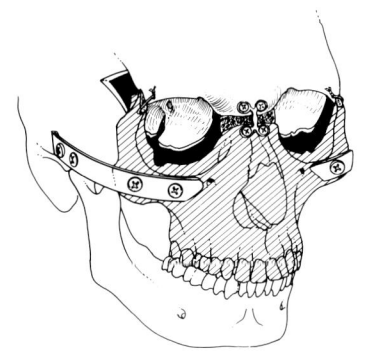

Figure 39.4 The midface can be perfectly stabilized with miniplates at the frontonasal junction and by screws fixating the temporozygomatic cranial grafts to the cranial vault and to the face.

Craniofaciostenosis

A midfacial advancement can be stabilized by a self-retaining type of osteotomy (Tessier V) and maxillomandibular fixation (MMF). Bone grafts that fill the gaps between the cranium and face provide increased support to the midfacial fragment. Rigid fixation at the zygomatic level reduces the duration of, or even avoids, MMF (see Figure 39.4).

A frontofacial monobloc advancement which results in a large continuous gap between the cranium and the face may be stabilized with bone grafts. Stable advancement is more easily obtainable with miniplates (Muhlbauer 1983).

Orbital Hypertelorism

Following the orbital osteotomies the orbits are brought together by tightening one or two interosseous wires. The supraorbital ridges are then anchored to the frontal bar with two additional wires. The position is checked and the wires are tightened to achieve the ideal position and stable fixation (see Figure 39.5). Additional stabilization with miniplates is not needed unless the lateral orbital walls must be bent posteriorly. The stability of results following wire fixation in orbital hypertelorism surgery has been confirmed by study over 25 years (Tessier 1989).

Hemifacial Microsomia

The treatment of hemifacial microsomia is essentially surgery of the jaws to correct facial asymmetry. Rigid fixation is therefore routinely used as in orthognathic surgery (see Figure 39.6). In severe cases with a missing ramus, a costochondral graft is secured to the body of the mandible with two or three screws. Screws are also used to stabilize cranial grafts in the other

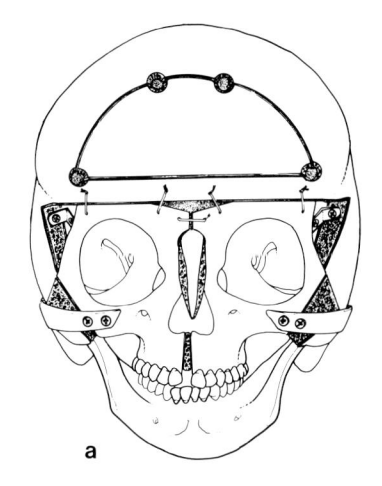

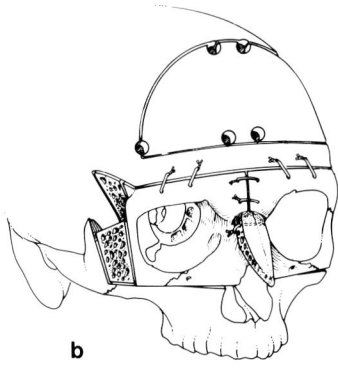

Figure 39.5 The correction of orbital hypertelorism is done by medial translocation of either (a) the two hemifaces or (b) the orbital cavities alone, which is best achieved with wires bringing the orbits together. Additional wires between the supraorbital ridges and the frontal bar are sufficient for a complete stabilization. A miniplate can be helpful laterally to maintain bending of the two segments.

underdeveloped areas: the mandible, the zygoma, and the parietal region (Munro 1989).

Treacher Collins Syndrome

The radical midfacial rotation for treatment of Treacher Collins syndrome, developed by Tessier (1989), consists of a Le Fort II osteotomy, mandibular lengthening, and reconstruction of the orbital region with cranial bone graft. Stability at the frontonasal angle is provided by two interosseous wires. The key point for sagittal stability and further consolidation is the bone graft interposed between the temporal bone and the maxilla (see Figure 39.7). Fixation with screws or miniplates simplifies both positioning and stabilization of the grafts (see Figure 39.8).

On the mandible, miniplate fixation can provide enough stability to avoid or minimize MMF (see Figure 39.9).

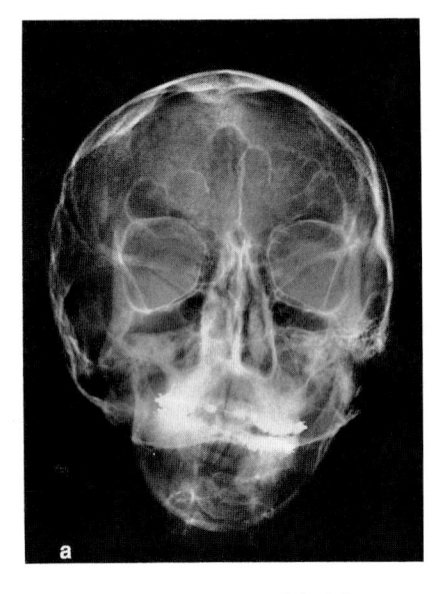

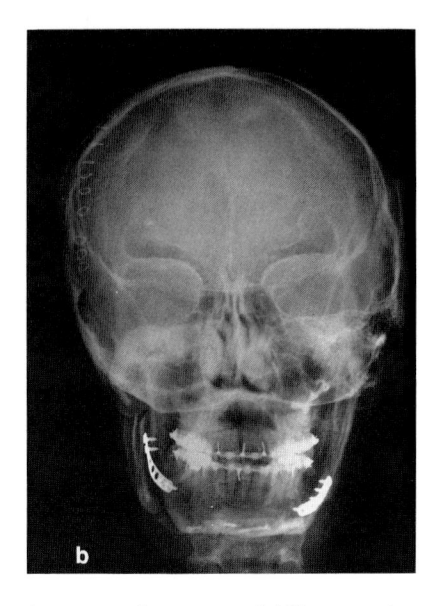

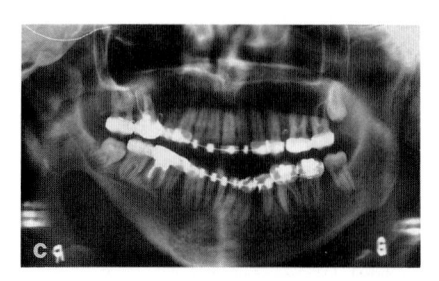

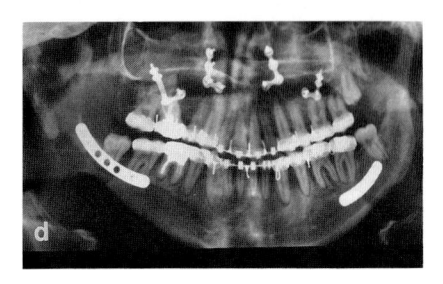

Figure 39.6 Correction of facial asymmetry in a case of hemifacial microsomia is shown. Stabilization of the maxilla and mandible was achieved with miniplates, without MMF. (a) Preoperative posterior-anterior radiograph, (b) postoperative posterior-anterior radiograph, (c) preoperative panorex, (d) postoperative panorex.

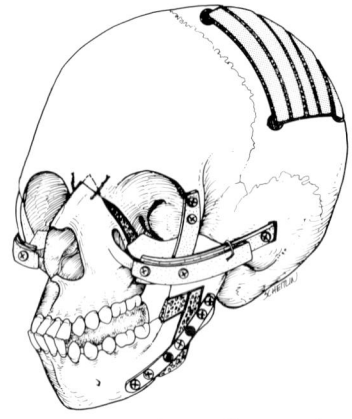

Figure 39.7 Treacher Collins syndrome treated by combined rotation of the midfacial segment and mandibular lengthening. Total reconstruction of the zygomatic arches, malar bones, and orbits with cranial grafts is shown.

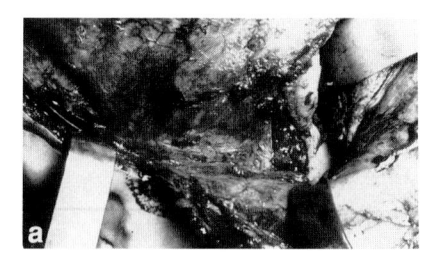

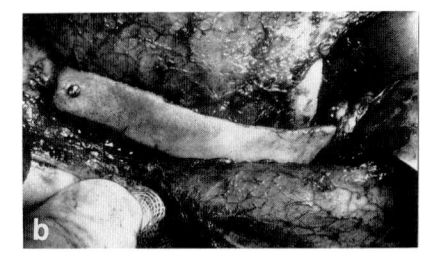

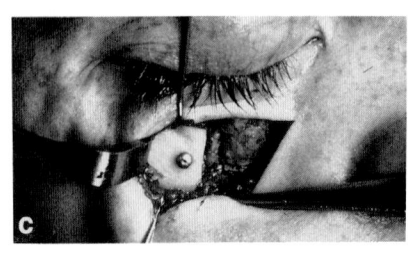

Figure 39.8 (a, b, c) Total reconstruction of the zygomatic arch is achieved with a cranial graft stabilized by screws in the temporal and infraorbital areas.

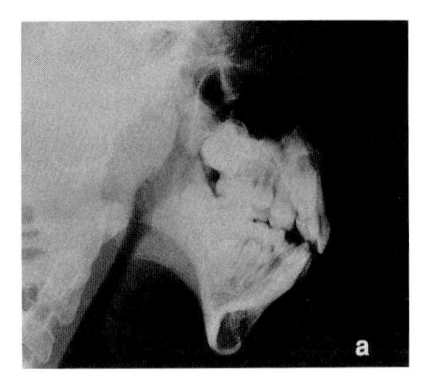

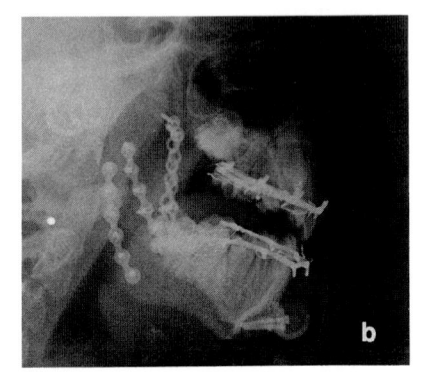

Figure 39.9 (a, b) Stabilization of the mandible with miniplates is accomplished following a bilateral V-shaped osteotomy of the ramus and advancement of the mandibular body. The genioplasty was stabilized with two screws.

CONCLUSION

Although less revolutionary than their role in orthognathic surgery, rigid fixation techniques are a major advance in the treatment of congenital craniofacial deformities. However, interfragmentary wiring is a technique that should not be abandoned. For example, it provides an excellent means of temporary fixation when there is a doubt about the ideal position of the bone fragments. In many cases, the combination of interfragmentary wiring and miniplate fixation represents the most straightforward and rapid way to achieve a stable result.

BIBLIOGRAPHY

Marchac D, Renier D: Le front flottant, traitement précoce des faciocraniosténoses. Ann Chir Plast 24: 121–126, 1979.

Muhlbauer W, Anderl H, Marchac D: Complete frontofacial advancement in infants with craniofacial dysostosis. Transactions of the 8th International Congress of Plastic Surgery, Montreal, pp 318–320, 1983.

Munro IR: Rigid fixation and facial asymmetry. Clin Plast Surg 16:1, 187–194, 1989.

Reitzik M: Cortex-to-cortex healing after mandibular osteotomy. J Oral Maxillofac Surg 41:658–663, 1983.

Tessier P, Tulasne JF: Stability in correction of hypertelorism and Treacher Collins syndrome. Clin Plast Surg 16:1, 195–204, 1989.

CHAPTER 40

The Role of Plate and Screw Fixation in the Treatment of Craniofacial Malformations

Jeffrey C. Posnick

The notorious trench warfare of World War I resulted in thousands of combined soft- and hard-tissue facial injuries that required urgent treatment. The names of two doctors in particular stand our for their work during this period, Dr. Varaztad Kazanjian and Sir Harold Gillies. During and after World War I, and again during World War II, these men laid the foundation for the specialty we now call maxillofacial surgery. The level of their success in repairing traumatic injuries to the face brought hope to people with congenital facial anomalies.

After World War II, Sir Harold Gillies saw increasing number of patients with previously untreated congenital craniofacial malformations. He applied the knowledge he had gained in treating war injuries to these problems, and in 1950 (Gillies 1950) he reported an encouraging experience involving total midface advancement for Crouzon syndrome. Later, however, to the great discouragement of Sir Harold, the patient's face relapsed to its preoperative status.

In 1967, after many years of work in the field, Dr. Paul Tessier described a new approach to the management of Crouzon syndrome and Apert syndrome (Tessier 1967). His landmark presentation and publication were the beginning of modern craniofacial surgery. To overcome the problems encountered by Gillies, Tessier developed a new basic surgical approach which included new osteotomy locations and the use of autogenous bone grafts. He also applied an external fixation device to maintain bony stability. The following year, Dr. Joe Murray from Boston Children's Hospital published his experience with the Tessier midface advancement for Crouzon syndrome (Murray 1968). He also used an external fixation device for osteotomy stabilization.

During this same period, Hans Luhr, a young maxillofacial surgeon who was still training in Hamburg, Germany, learned of the benefits of internal fixation (bone plates) for extremity fracture healing. In 1968, he proposed that miniature bone plates could be constructed and used as compression plates for mandibular fracture fixation (Luhr 1968). Despite Dr. Luhr's enthusiasm, his concepts of internal fixation for the craniofacial skeleton did not take hold. Many innovative craniofacial osteotomies were developed by Tessier, Ortiz-Monasterio, and others (Ortiz-Monasterio 1978, Tessier 1967, 1971, van der Meulen 1983). These brilliant techniques became less favored because they were associated with major infections (that is brain abscess, meningitis, osteomyelitis) (Israele 1989). It was not until Luhr's concepts of improved osteotomy and bone graft fixation in craniofacial surgery were further developed that the next giant leap in craniofacial surgery could occur.

Now, with the liberal use of mini- and microplate and screw internal fixation techniques, several of the excellent early osteotomies have resurfaced and can be performed in combination with stable miniplate and screw fixation techniques (Muhlbauer 1987, Posnick 1991). When designed, executed, and stabilized well, these combining cranial vault and total midface osteotomies carried out through an intra-cranial approach can often simultaneously solve the problems of diminished intracranial volume, shallow hyperteloric orbits, and deficient midface. When these osteotomies are combined with bone plate and screw fixation and autogenous cranial bone grafting, their associated morbidity rate is acceptably low. However, important questions arise. Should bone plates be used in the growing child? Will the placement of a bone plate inhibit or distort further bone growth? Because no answers are yet available, those of us who use bone plates in growing patients must follow the growth and development of these patients closely and make appropriate clinical observations.

The following cases illustrate how internal bone plate and screw fixation can be used in the surgical management of craniofacial malformations.

CASE REPORTS

Case 1: Crouzon Syndrome

Procedure: Total Cranial Vault Reshaping and Monobloc Osteotomy with Advancement

A 12-year-old Nicaraguan boy presented with unrepaired Crouzon syndrome (see Figure 40.1). He has above average intelligence and a good sense of humor. His only previous surgery was the placement of two ventriculoperitoneal shunts.

Physical examination and computed tomography (CT) scan revealed severe oxycephaly, shallow orbits, bulging eyes, and total midface deficiency. He had mild optic atrophy and corneal abrasions from chronic exposure keratitis.

At operation he underwent total cranial vault craniotomy and reshaping and monobloc (orbits and midface) osteotomy with anterior repositioning. Surgical exposure was through a coronal incision only, and it was not necessary to complete a tracheostomy. The orbits were brought forward 18 millimeters at the level of the supraorbital ridge. Fixation was achieved with multiple titanium miniplates placed at the level of the cranial vault, orbits, nose, and zygomas. Postoperatively, his course was uneventful; he was discharged on the tenth day after surgery and returned home to Nicaragua two months later.

Critique

The use of stable plate and screw fixation techniques allowed for the careful and cautious use of a combined intracranial and extracranial approach to the problems of total midface deficiency, exorbitism, exophthalmus, and cranial vault dysplasia. The combined cranial vault and midface osteotomies and reshapings could be predictably carried out with minimal morbidity and rapid recovery.

This form of stable fixation made unnecessary maintenance of a separate supraorbital bar component to preserve spacial relations and to provide a point for adequate fixation, as initially described by Ortiz-Monasterio (1978). Although this patient's jaws did not have to be wired together postoperatively, it was necessary to apply Erich arch bars to both jaws and to obtain maxillo-mandibular fixation (MMF) by using a prefabricated acrylic splint to achieve the jaw relationship at the occlusal level.

Case 2: Apert Syndrome

Procedure: Total Cranial Vault Reshaping and Facial Bipartition Osteotomy with Reshaping and Advancement

This 5-year-old girl was born with Apert syndrome (see Figure 40.2). She underwent suture release and forehead reshaping in infancy. She presented with a tall, flat, wide forehead; shallow orbits with bulging eyes; orbital hypertelorism; and total midface deficiency.

At operation through a coronal incision, she underwent a facial bipartition osteotomy with three-dimensional repositioning of the two halves of the face to correct her orbital hypertelorism, shallow orbits, and midface deficiency. In addition, the cranial vault was totally reshaped. Stabilization was achieved with cranial bone grafts, multiple titanium miniplates, and MMF. A tracheostomy was not needed. Her recovery was uneventful, and she was discharged on the sixteenth postoperative day.

As part of her staged reconstruction, she will require a maxillary Le Fort I osteotomy and genioplasty in combination with orthodontics. These procedures will be performed when the skeleton matures (at age 14 to 16).

Critique

The use of multiple miniplates and screws allowed stable placement of the midface halves of the facial bipartition osteotomy. Because of the opening created from the nose through the anterior cranial base, which is always present at the end of this surgical procedure, it is important that the osteotomy units and placed bone grafts be stably fixed to allow for early healing. This limits the chance of infection, which can be a devastating complication of this operation. When a significant anteroposterior advancement (15 millimeters) is desired, it is virtually impossible to achieve a watertight seal of the anterior cranial fossa from the nasal cavity. Some surgeons prefer to inset a pericranial flap for a layered closure. I advise caution in this regard, because the pericranial flap elevated, especially in a repeat coronal incision, may be a random pattern flap. Turning the flap down 180° and then reconstructing the bony framework allows the flap to pass through only a small bony window, also diminishing the potential blood supply through this tunnel. This may lead to an ischemic flap within an area of dead space that already carries contaminants from the sinus and nasal passage. This is the worst possible scenario that would increase the likelihood of infection. Partial closure of the anterior cra-

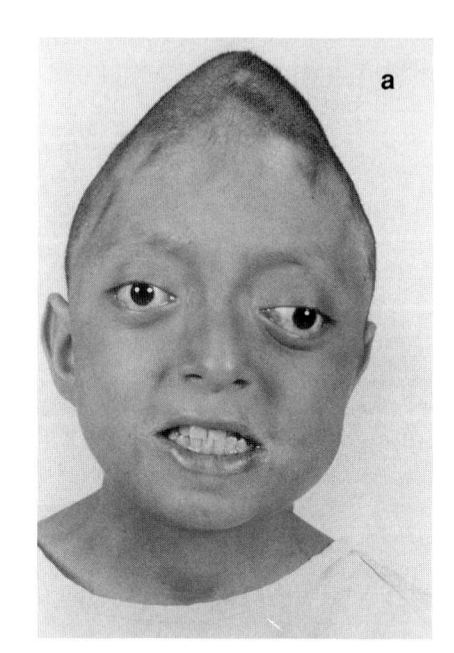

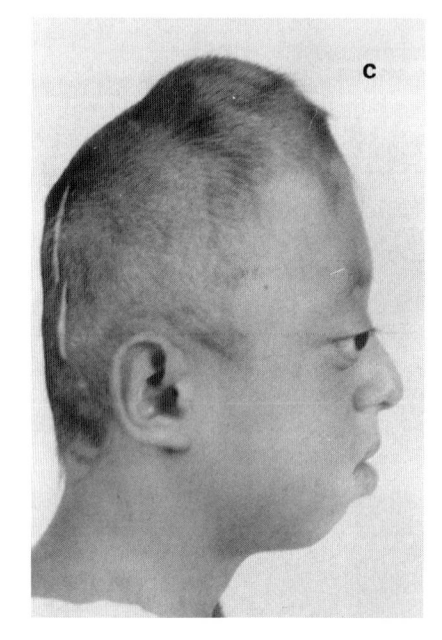

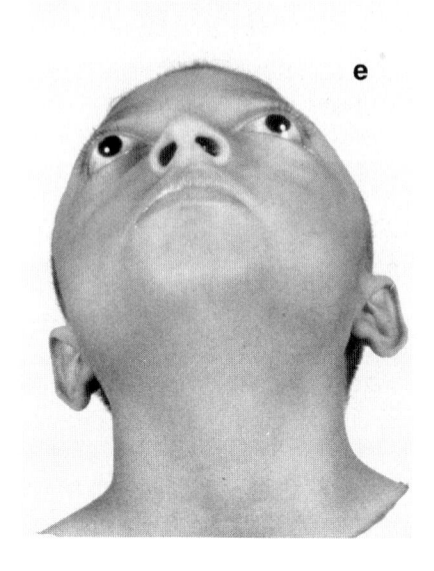

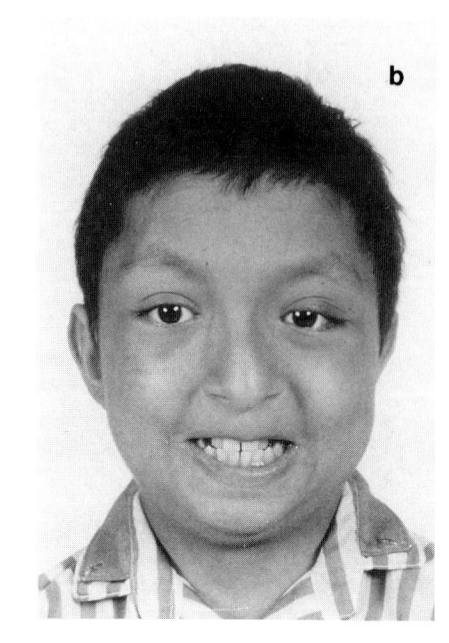

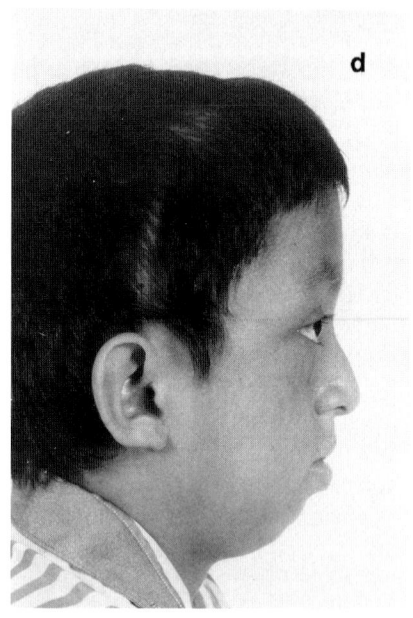

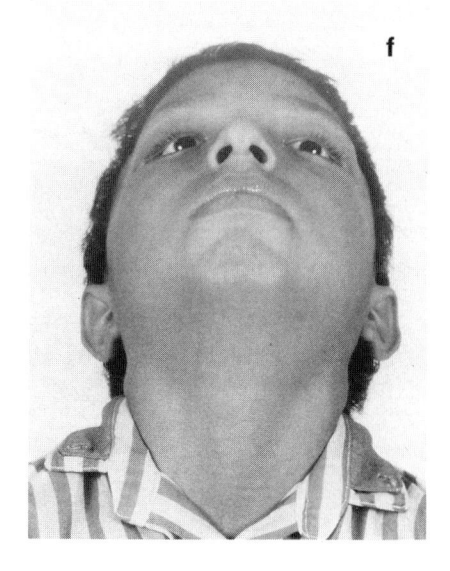

Figure 40.1 This 12-year-old boy with unrepaired Crouzon syndrome underwent total cranial vault and monobloc osteotomies with reshaping and advancement. (a) Preoperative frontal view. (b) Postoperative frontal view. (c) Preoperative lateral view. (d) Postoperative lateral view. (e) Preoperative worm's eye view. (f) Postoperative worm's eye view. (g) The extent of eyeball proptosis is demonstrated with hemostats touching orbital rims. (h) Illustrations show this patient's craniofacial morphology, osteotomies, and fixation technique. (i) Intraoperative lateral view shows cranial vault and orbital bony morphology before osteotomies. (j) Intraoperative lateral view shows cranial vault and orbital bony anatomy after osteotomies, cranial bone grafting, and titanium bone plate and screw fixation. (k) Intraoperative bird's eye view shows the cranial vault before osteotomies. (l) Intraoperative bird's eye view shows the cranial vault after total cranial vault reshaping with cranial bone grafting and titanium bone plate and screw fixation. (m) Three-dimensional CT scans show the reformations. The lateral view is shown before and after osteotomies. (From Posnick 1991.)

Craniofacial Malformations

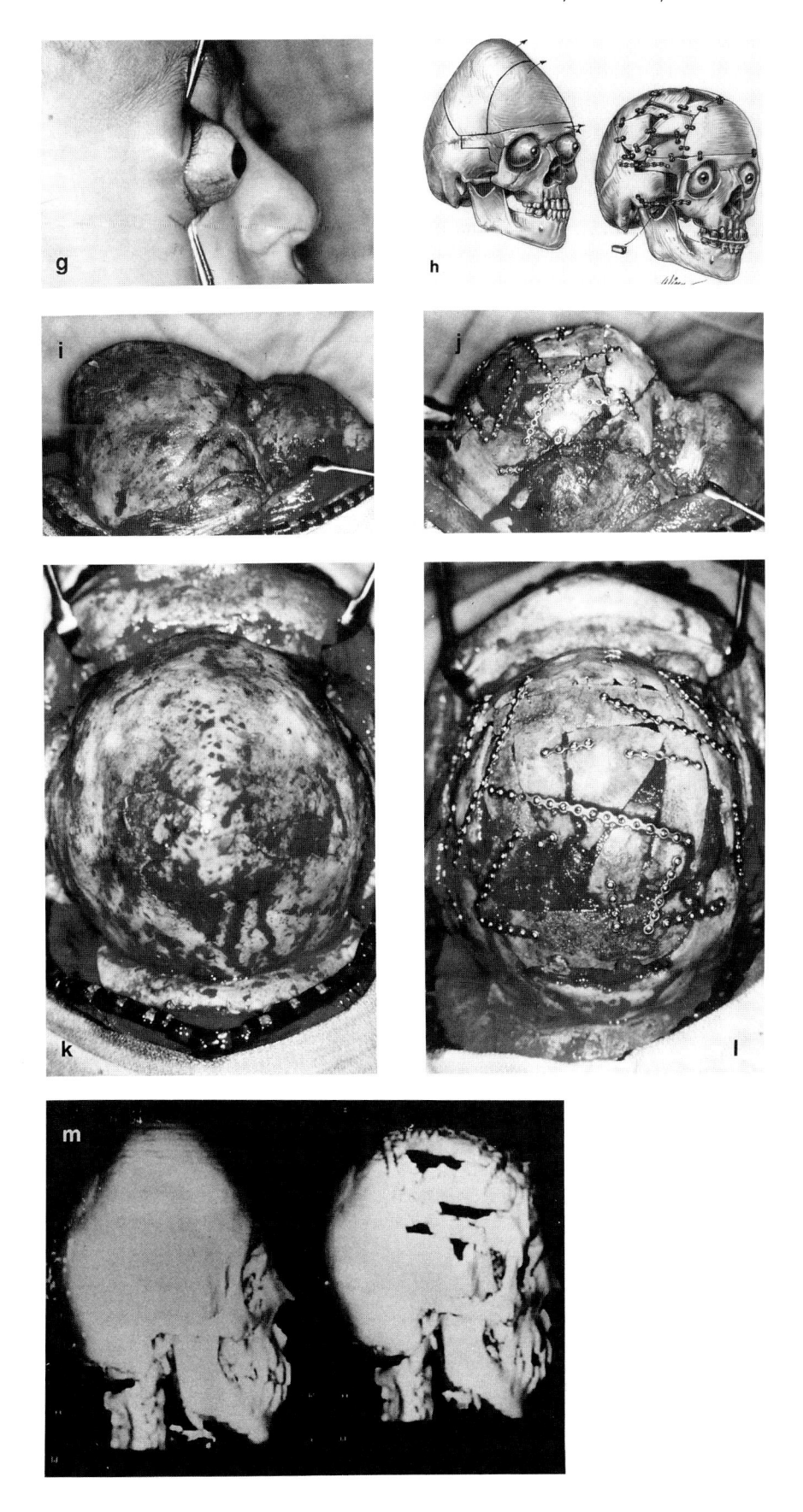

515

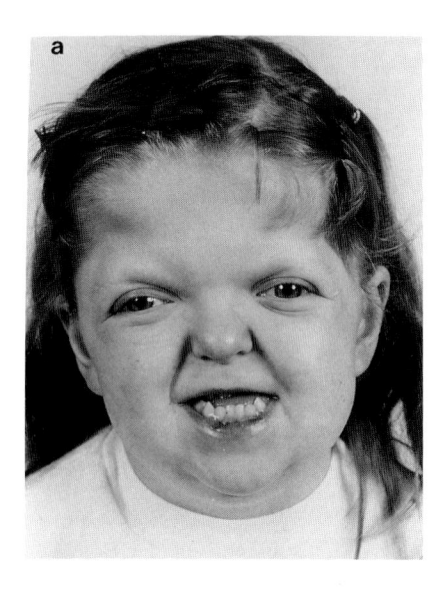

Figure 40.2 This 5-year-old girl with Apert syndrome underwent cranial vault and monobloc bipartition osteotomies with reshaping and anterior repositioning. (a) Preoperative frontal view. (b) Postoperative frontal view at one year. (c) Preoperative lateral view. (d) Postoperative lateral view at one year. (e) Postoperative oblique view at one year. (f) Illustrations demonstrate her bony anatomy before and after cranial vault and monobloc bipartition osteotomies with reshaping. (g) Intraoperative lateral view shows the cranial vault, orbits, and zygomatic arches after osteotomies stabilized with cranial bone grafts and multiple miniplates and screw fixation. (h) Preoperative and postoperative axial-sliced CT scans through midorbits demonstrate the improvement in orbital hypertelorism and orbital depth with diminished eyeball proptosis. (i) Three-dimensional CT scans show oblique view before and after reconstruction.

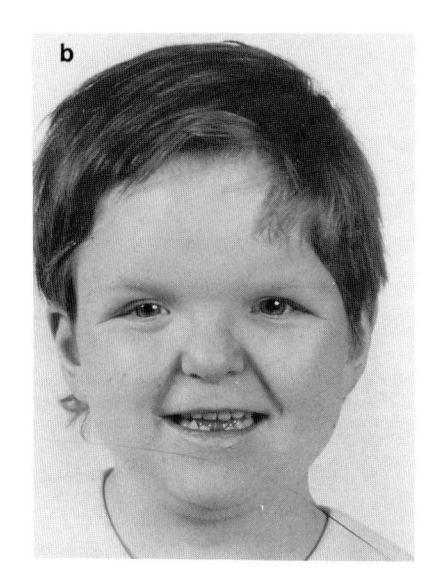

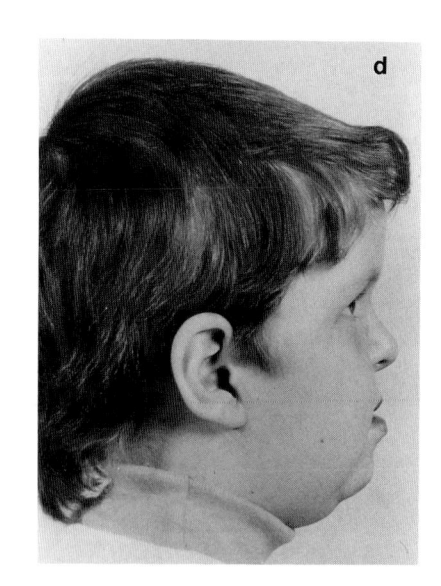

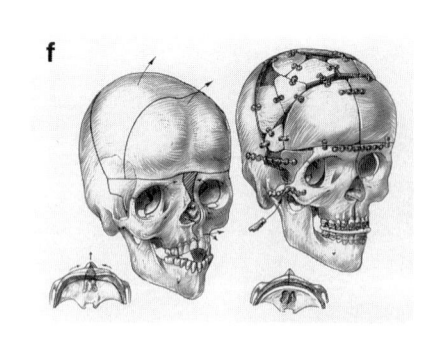

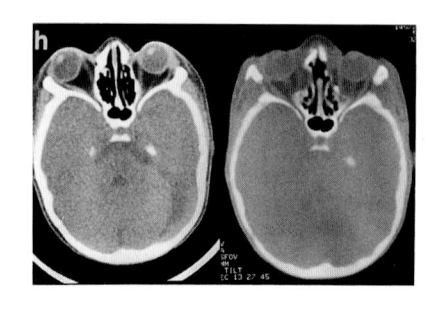

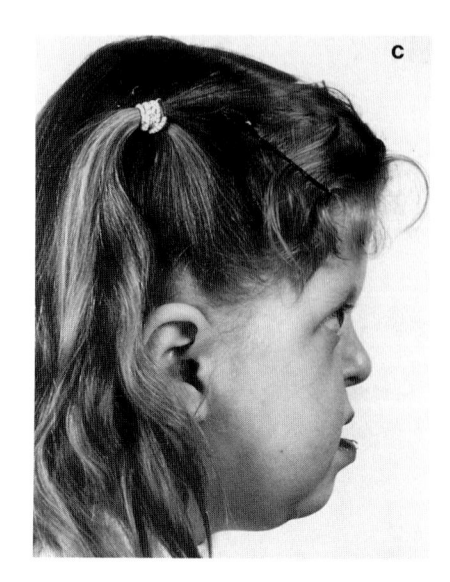

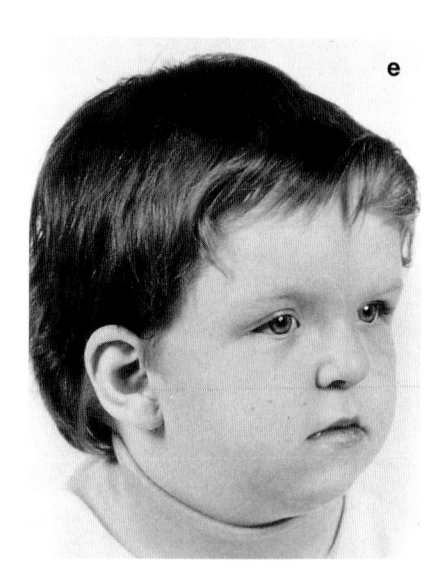

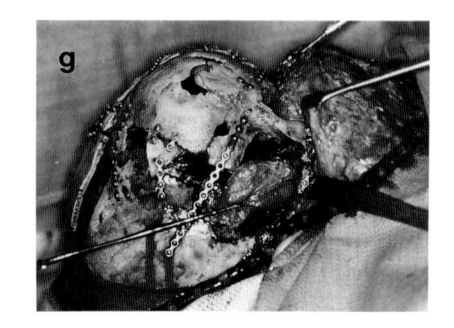

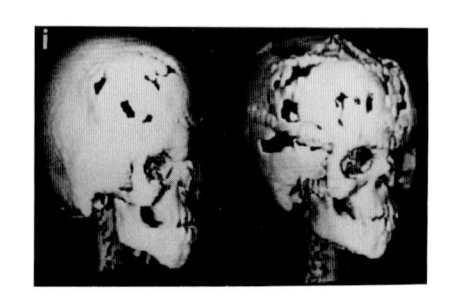

nial base can be achieved with bone grafts. Initially this space in the anterior cranial fossa is filled with air and blood. The brain then expands into the increased intracranial volume. The critical regions in which to gain bony stability are at the occlusal level, zygomatic arches, and tenon extension of the supraorbital ridges, as well as throughout the cranial vault.

Case 3: Midline Cranio-orbital Cleft with Orbital Hypertelorism

Procedure: Anterior Cranial Vault and Facial Bipartition Osteotomy with Reshaping and Repositioning

This child, born with Tessier 0- and 14-midline craniofacial clefts (Tessier 1972; Tessier et al. 1973), underwent repair of the soft-tissue midline cleft of the lip, nasal skin, and palate (see Figure 40.3). She was referred to me and, after full assessment by the craniofacial team, underwent a facial bipartition osteotomy through an intra-cranial approach at 5 years of age. At operation, the two halves of her face were repositioned medially to correct her facial hypertelorism, bringing her left and right nasal bones back into the midline. The palate arch width was widened, and excess midline nasal skin was excised.

Stabilization was accomplished with cranial bone grafts and multiple titanium miniplates and screws for stable fixation. A tracheostomy was not required. Healing was uneventful, and the patient was discharged from the hospital two weeks postoperatively.

Later in adolescence, she will require further bony augmentation of the dorsum of her nose. She will also require a maxillary Le Fort I osteotomy combined with orthodontics when the skeleton matures (at age 14 to 16).

Critique

The use of plate and screw fixation was a major factor in the success of this patient's surgery. It not only allowed the stable placement of bone osteotomy units at surgery but also gave added stability, minimizing motion and thus encouraging the rapid closure of minor cerebral spinal fluid leaks, which inevitably occur early on through the nose.

By delaying hypertelorism repair until about five years of age, final reconstruction can be achieved at the level of the cranial vault and orbits. Further growth requirements and additional distortion will likely occur in the regions of the nose and jaws.

Case 4: Trigonocephaly

Procedure: Anterior Cranial Vault and Three-quarter Orbital Osteotomies with Reshaping

An 18-month-old boy presented with premature closure of the metopic suture, which had caused a vertical midline ridging of the forehead, flatness and recession to the supraorbital ridges (which were more severe laterally), and a degree of orbital hypotelorism (see Figure 40.4). Overall, these features gave a triangular shape to the anterior cranial vault (Marchac 1978, Whitaker 1977).

At operation, he underwent a coronal incision, through which anterior cranial vault and three-quarter orbital osteotomies with reshaping were carried out via an intracranial approach. The orbital units, which were badly misshapen, required three-dimensional reshaping. In addition, the orbits were separated in the midline to correct his hypotelorism. A bone miniplate was helpful in stabilizing the orbital units in the midline, and direct wires were used in many locations to stabilize weakened areas in the orbital rims. The total orbital units were re-inset, and the anterior cranial vault was reconstructed. Healing was uneventful, and the skin sutures were removed on the tenth postoperative day.

Critique

Although I use miniplates sparingly in infants, they can reduce operative time and improve the overall esthetic result. The theoretical concern that bone miniplates may inhibit or distort further growth of the bone on which they sit is legitimate but not proven. I currently use micro bone plates and screws in infants when stable fixation is indicated. My initial impression is that these small bone plates do not further inhibit growth in the abnormal bony situations where they are placed.

Case 5: Crouzon Syndrome

Procedure: Le Fort III Osteotomy with Advancement

This 16-year-old girl presented with a mild form of total midface hypoplasia resulting in shallow orbits, bulging eyes, increased scleral show, flat midface, and decreased gingival and tooth show (see Figure 40.5). At operation, she underwent an extracranial Le Fort III osteotomy with advancement through a coronal incision. Stabilization was achieved with split cranial bone grafts and titanium miniplate and screw internal fixation. A tracheostomy was not required.

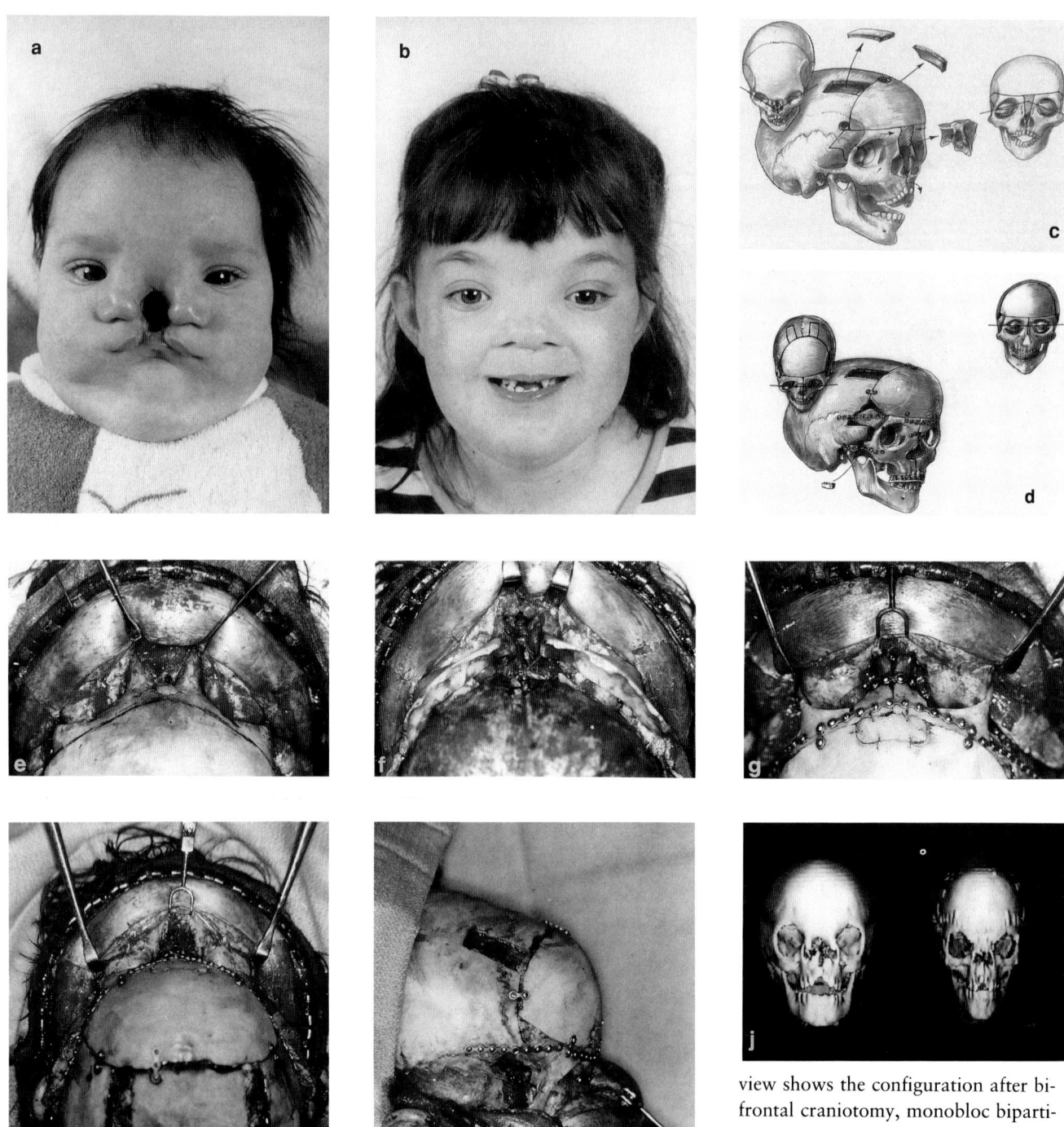

Figure 40.3 This 5-year-old girl, born with a severe cranio-orbital facial midline cleft, underwent a monobloc bipartition osteotomy with medial repositioning. (a) Preoperative frontal view in early infancy. (b) Postoperative full-face frontal view after repair. (c) Illustration shows the preoperative craniofacial morphology and proposed osteotomies. (d) Illustration shows the craniofacial morphology after osteotomies and repositioning. (e) Intraoperative close-up view shows the anterior cranial vault and upper orbital and nasal bony anatomy through the coronal incision. (f) The same intraoperative view shows the configuration after bifrontal craniotomy, monobloc bipartition osteotomy, and osteotomy of excessive midline orbital and nasal bone. (g) The same intraoperative view shows the situation after medial repositioning of the facial halves. Stabilization is achieved with multiple titanium bone plates and screws. (h) Intraoperative bird's eye view shows the cranial vault after osteotomy stabilization. (i) Intraoperative lateral view shows the cranial vault and orbits after osteotomy stabilization. (j) Three-dimensional CT scans show frontal views before and after reconstruction.

Craniofacial Malformations 519

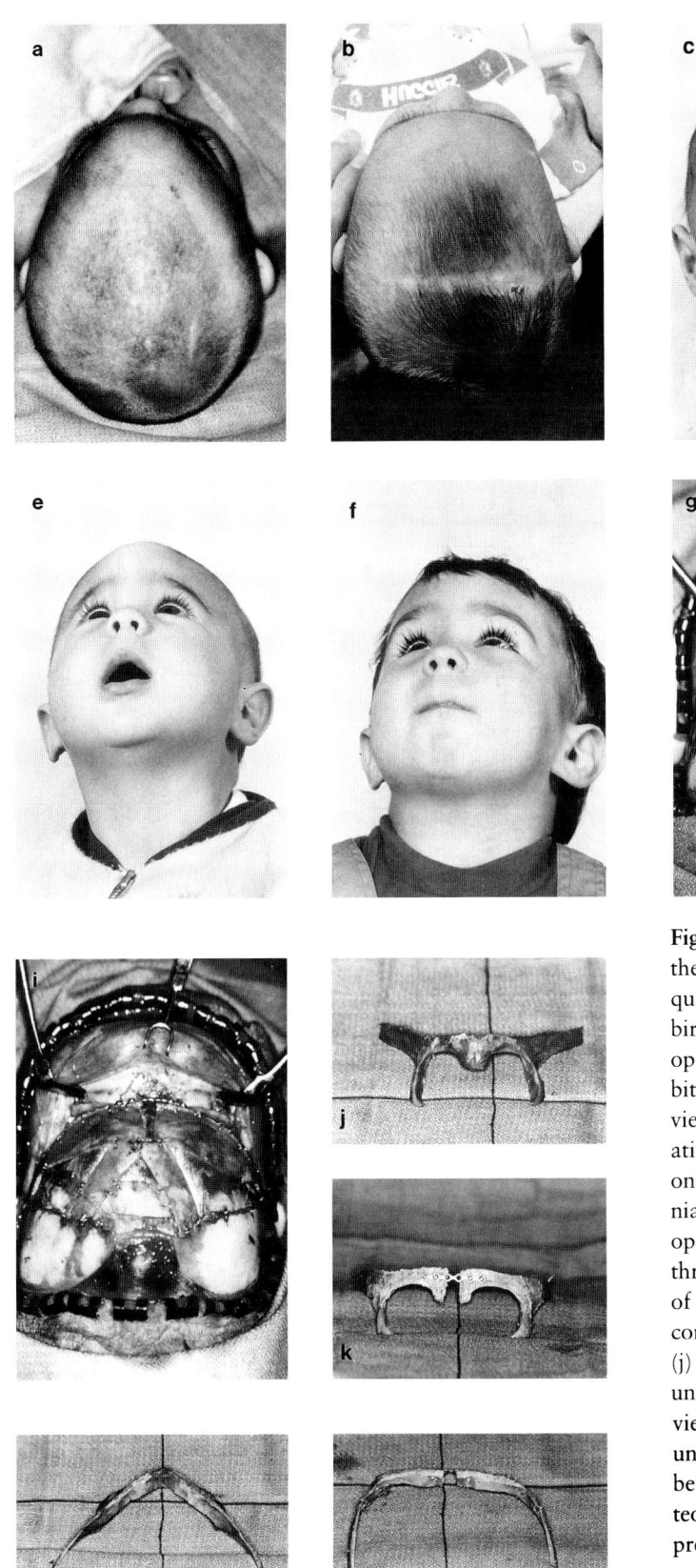

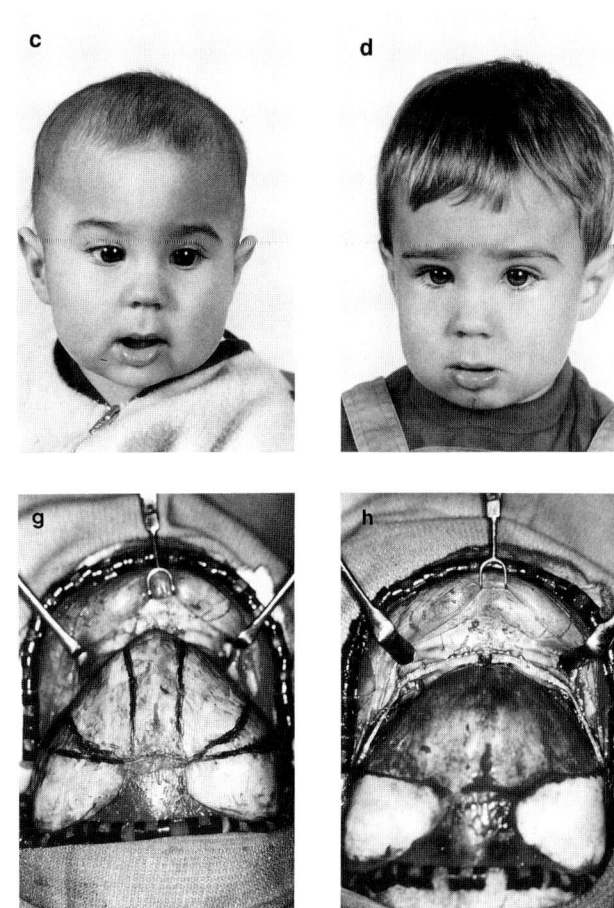

Figure 40.4 This 18-month-old boy's premature closure of the metopic suture required anterior cranial vault and three-quarter orbital osteotomies with reshaping. (a) Preoperative bird's eye view demonstrates trigonocephaly. (b) Early postoperative bird's eye view demonstrates normalization of orbital and cranial vault morphology. (c) Preoperative frontal view. (d) Postoperative frontal view at one year. (e) Preoperative worm's eye view. (f) Postoperative worm's eye view at one year. (g) Intraoperative bird's eye view shows the cranial vault through the coronal incision. (h) The same intraoperative view shows the situation after craniotomy, and three-quarter osteotomies with reshaping and then re-inset of orbital unit. (i) The same intraoperative view shows the configuration after additional reshaping of the cranial vault. (j) Front view shows the three-quarter orbital osteotomy units with tenon extensions before reshaping. (k) The same view shows the configuration after reshaping of the orbital unit. (l) Bird's eye view shows the orbital osteotomy units before reshaping. (m) Bird's eye view shows the orbital osteotomy units after reshaping. (From Posnick et al. [in press].)

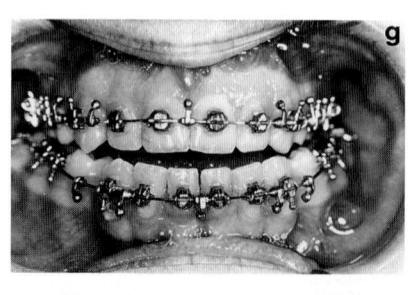

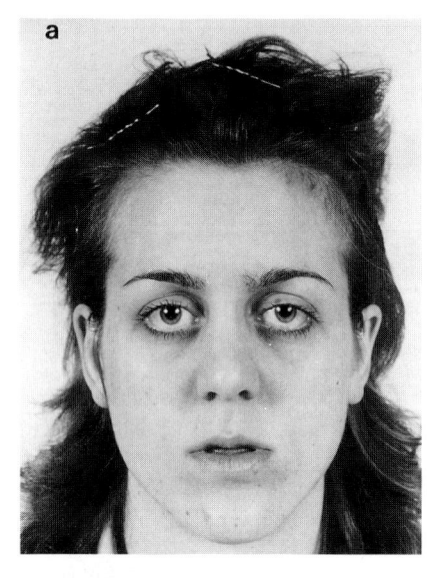

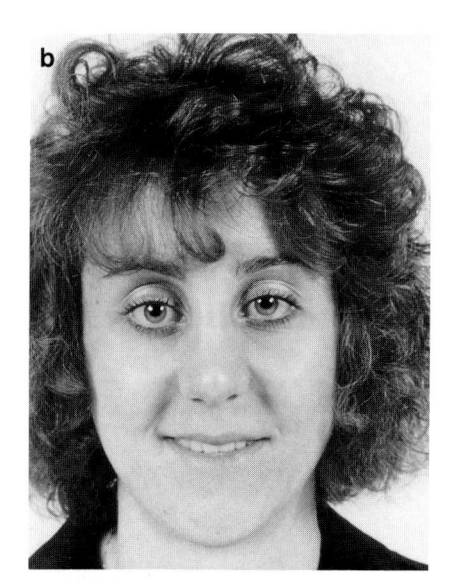

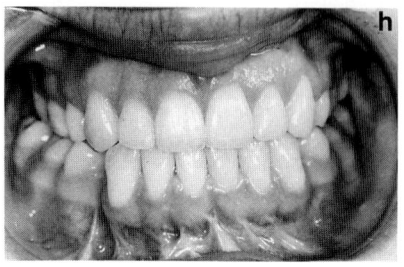

Figure 40.5 This 16-year-old girl with mild form of Crouzon syndrome underwent an extracranial Le Fort III osteotomy with advancement. (a) Frontal view before osteotomy. (b) Frontal view one year after Le Fort III osteotomy. (c) Profile before osteotomy. (d) Profile one year after Le Fort III osteotomy. (e) Worm's eye view before osteotomy. (f) Worm's eye view one year after Le Fort III osteotomy. (g) Occlusal view before osteotomy. (h) Occlusal view one year after Le Fort III osteotomy. (i) Intraoperative view shows the zygomatic complex after osteotomies. The view is through the coronal incision. (j) The same intraoperative view shows stabilization with titanium bone plates and screws. (k) Intraoperative bird's eye view shows the cranial vault and orbits through the coronal incision. Stabilization of the Le Fort III osteotomy is accomplished with bone plates and screws. Split cranial grafts have been harvested from the left parietal region and interposed in the nasofrontal region and zygomatic arches.

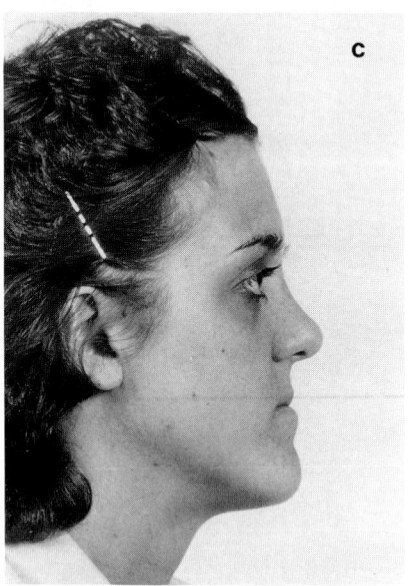

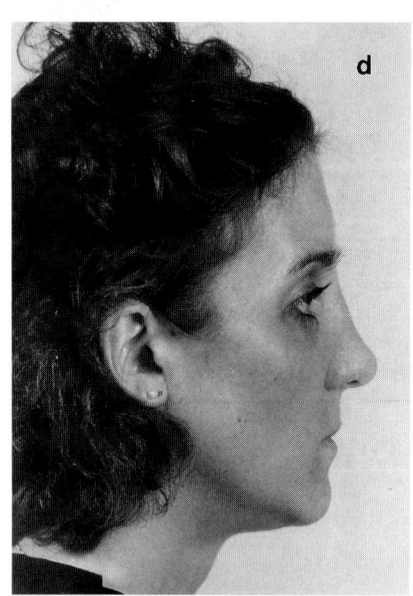

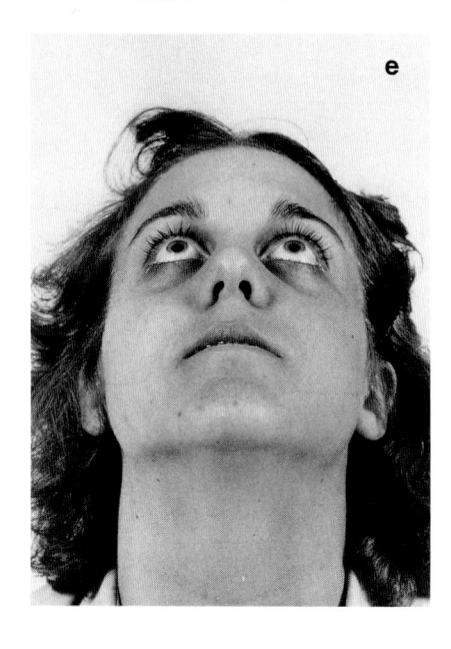

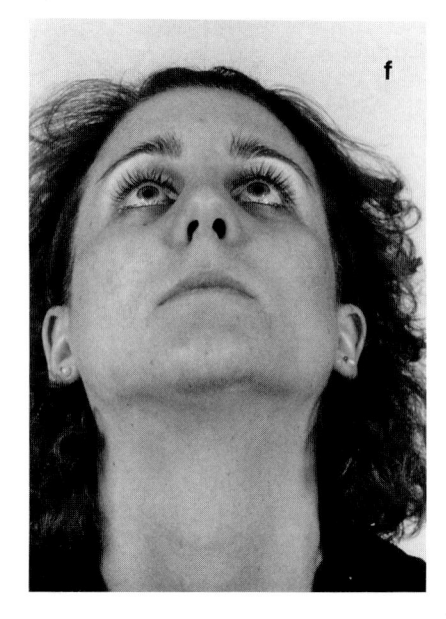

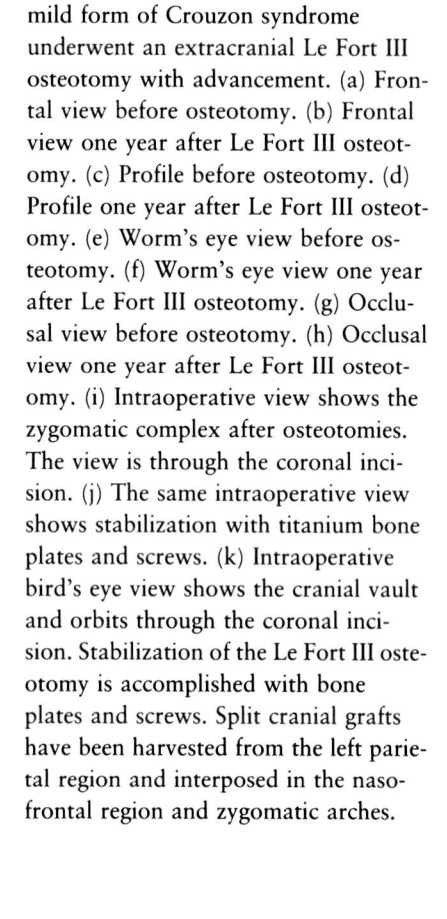

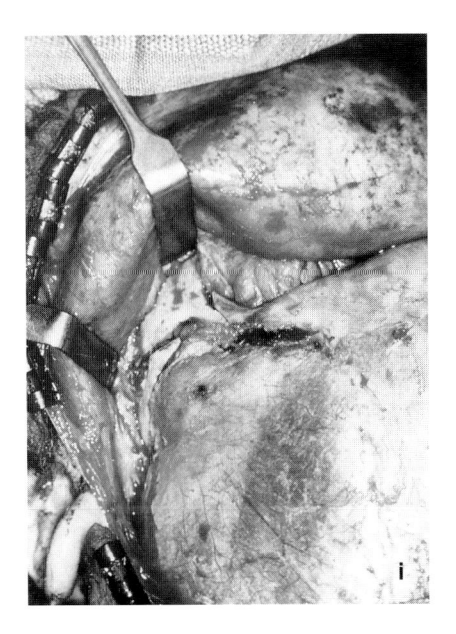

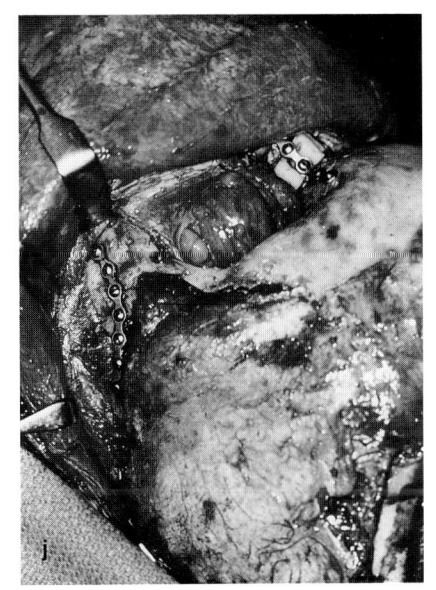

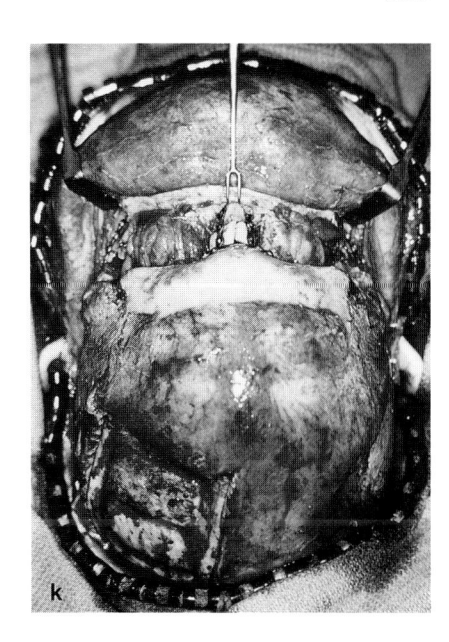

Critique

In the right situation, the Le Fort III osteotomy can give a good aesthetic result. However, one must keep in mind the aesthetic problems that may arise from this procedure: elongation of the nose and step-offs in the lateral orbital rims. Difficulties with enophthalmus can arise if the midface is advanced too much in the attempt to accommodate for occlusion. The use of plate and screw internal fixation and cranial bone grafts have allowed the Le Fort III osteotomy to become a routine procedure in certain situations.

Case 6: Treacher Collins Syndrome

Procedure: Total Zygomatic Reconstruction with Full Thickness Cranial Grafts

This 5½-year-old boy was born with Treacher Collins syndrome (Tulasne and Tessier 1986) (see Figure 40.6). He had small, cupped ears and required bone-conductive hearing aids. His orbits were dystopic, and his zygomas were hypoplastic with bilateral clefting through the arches. The palate was constricted, and the proximal mandibles were hypoplastic with decreased posterior facial height but with functioning condyles. There was an anterior open-bite deformity and a vertically long and retrognathic chin. The soft tissues of the lower eyelids and cheeks were deficient because of colobomas. The lateral canthi were downwardly displaced.

Dissection through a coronal incision exposed the cranial vault, orbits, anterior maxilla, and zygomas. Templates were fashioned for the hypoplastic zygomas and then taken to the posterior cranium, where full-thickness cranial bone grafts were harvested for bilateral zygomatic reconstruction. Stabilization was with bicortical screws to the fronto-zygomatic suture region, to the anterior maxilla, and to the posterior temporal bone as required. Each lateral canthus was then identified and raised to the newly located fronto-zygomatic suture region.

Healing was uneventful, and he was discharged on the tenth postoperative day.

Critique

This patient is now seven years old. His CT scan confirms improved bony morphology achieved and then maintained in the zygomatic regions. However, residual soft-tissue deficiency of the lower eyelids, temporalis muscles, fat pads, and cheek skin remains and limits his overall esthetic improvements.

Although a degree of bony resorption is likely, it can be limited by use of stable bone graft fixation techniques. Because I do not believe that the placed bone grafts grow, even after bone graft take, I postpone cheekbone reconstruction until an age when I can craft and place cheekbone units that are close to adult size. This requires waiting until the patient is five to seven years old.

He will require maxillary, mandibular, and chin osteotomies in combination with orthodontic treatment when his facial bones reach maturity.

Case 7: Brachycephaly (Bilateral Coronal Synostosis)

Procedure: Anterior Cranial Vault and Three-quarter Orbital Osteotomies with Reshaping and Advancement

This infant was born with a flat forehead (see Figure 40.7). Examination revealed a symmetrical forehead that was flat and wide (brachycephaly). The supraorbital ridges were recessed, and bony ridges were palp-

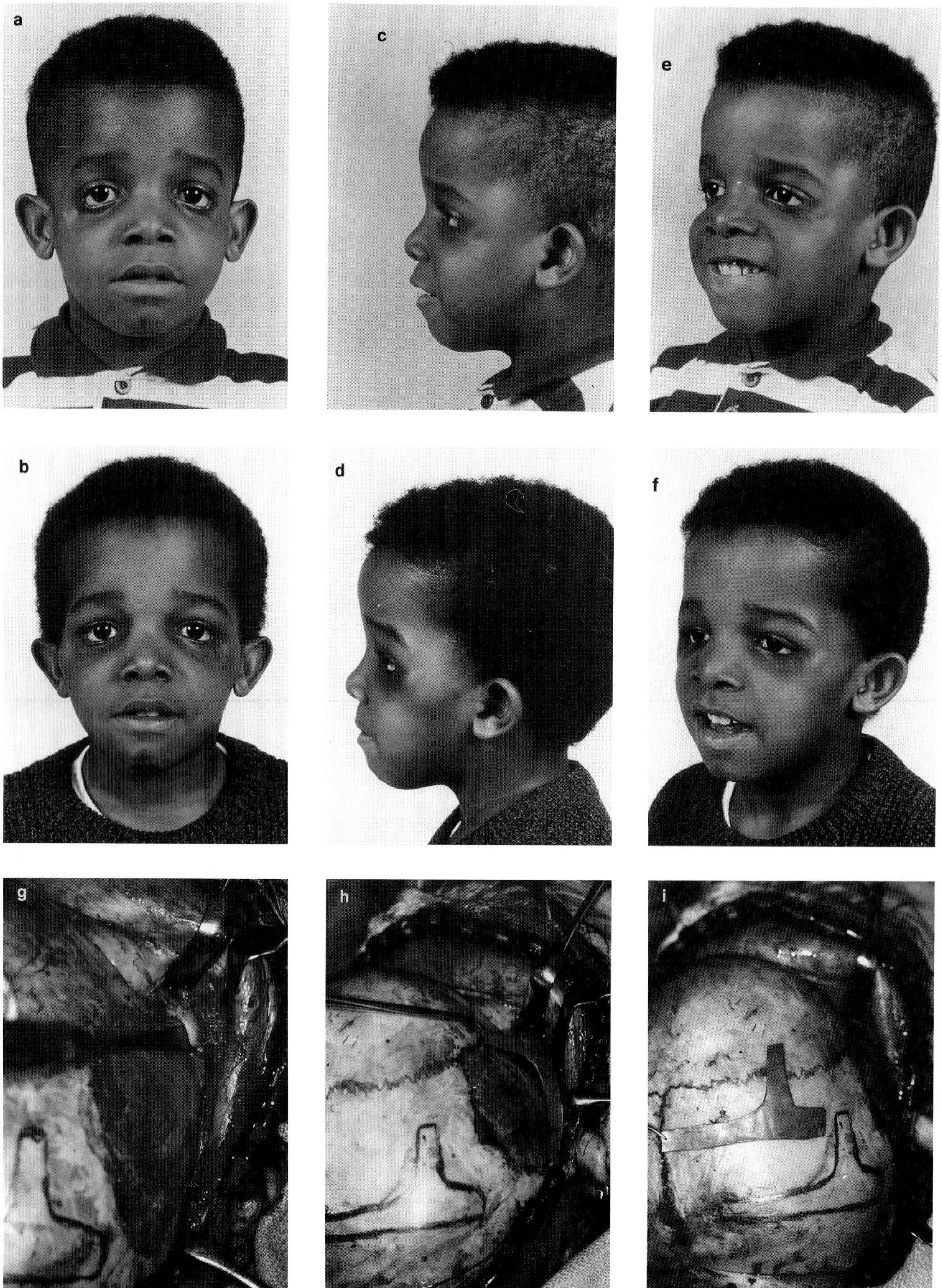
a
c
e
b
d
f
g
h
i

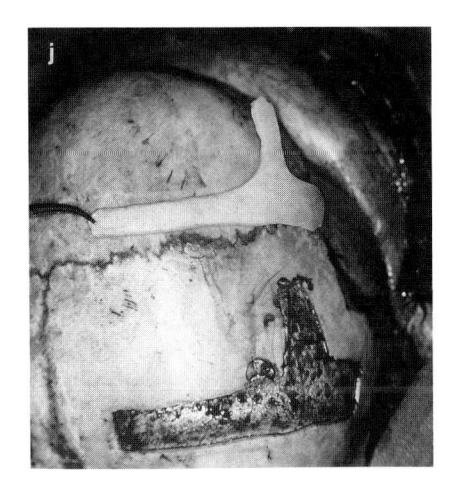

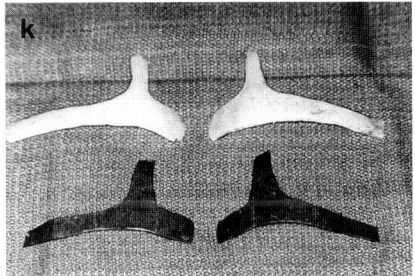

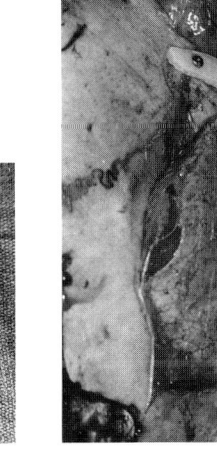

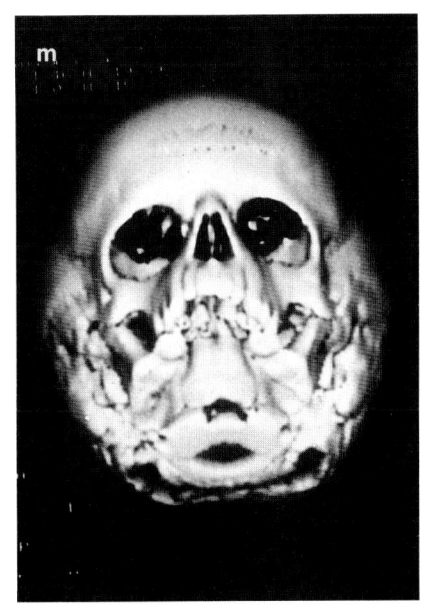

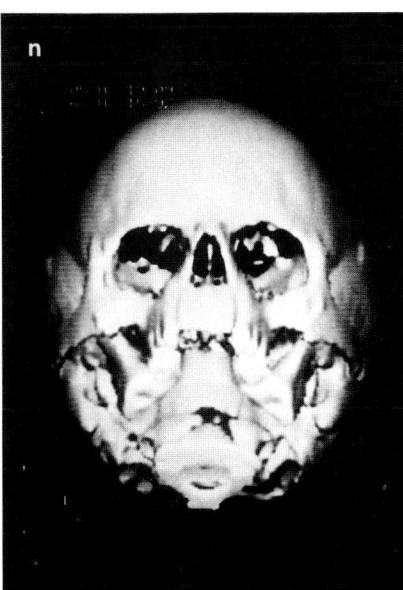

Figure 40.6 This 5½-year-old boy, born with Treacher Collins syndrome, underwent full-thickness cranial bone graft reconstruction of the zygomatic bone through a coronal incision. (a) Frontal view before reconstruction. (b) Frontal view after bilateral zygomatic reconstruction. (c) Profile before reconstruction. (d) Profile after zygomatic reconstruction. (e) Oblique view before reconstruction. (f) Oblique view after zygomatic reconstruction. (g) Intraoperative view shows the cleft zygomatic arch. (h) A metal template is constructed to match the bony requirements of the recipient site. (i) The template taken to the occipitoparietal skull region is specifically selected for correct curvature. (j) A craniotomy is performed to harvest the bone graft for reconstruction. (k) Both cheekbones and templates are shown. (l) The reconstructed cheekbone is inset and stabilized with titanium bicortical screws. (m) Three-dimensional CT scan shows the reformations before reconstruction. (n) Three-dimensional CT scan shows the reformations after reconstruction.

Figure 40.7 This one-year-old infant's unrepaired bicoronal synostosis required suture release, and anterior cranial vault and three-quarter orbital osteotomies with reshaping and advancement. (a) Oblique view before surgery. (b) Oblique view after reconstruction. (c) Profile view before surgery. (d) Profile view after reconstruction. (e) Intraoperative lateral view shows the orbits and cranial vault after reshaping and micro bone plate fixation. (f) Close-up of anterior cranial vault demonstrates the micro bone plate fixation to the supraorbital ridge. (g) Three-dimensional CT scan reformations show the craniofacial skeleton in oblique views taken before and after reconstruction. (h) Three-dimensional CT scan reformations show of the cranial base before and after reconstruction and demonstrate the increased depth of the anterior cranial base.

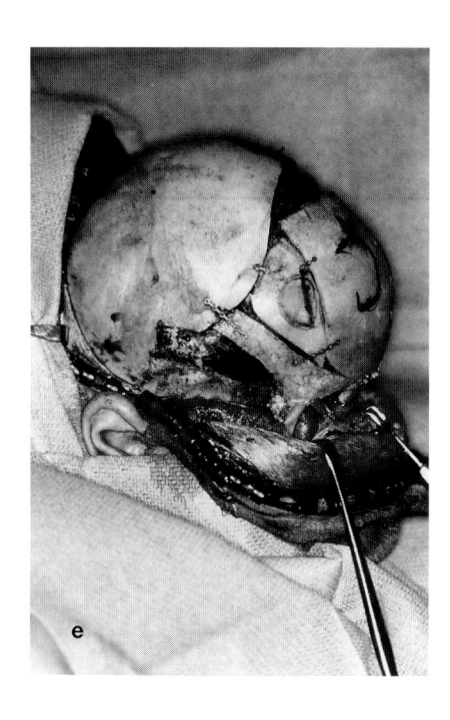

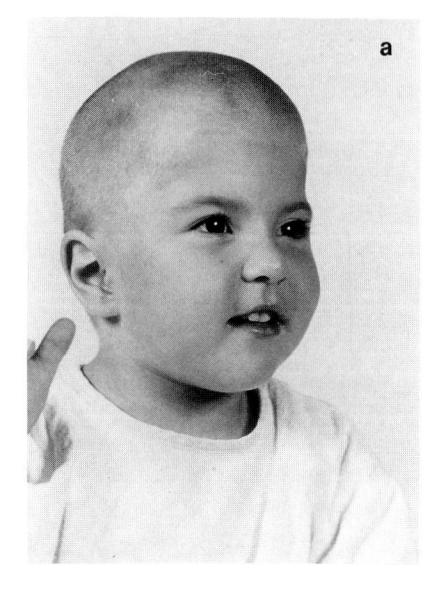

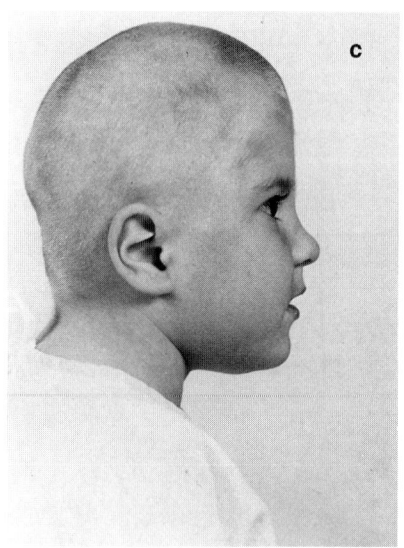

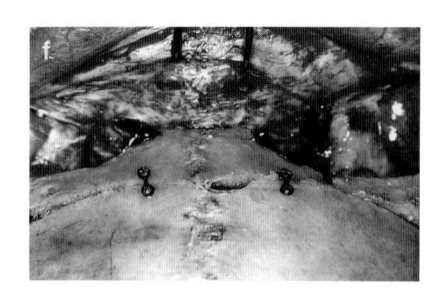

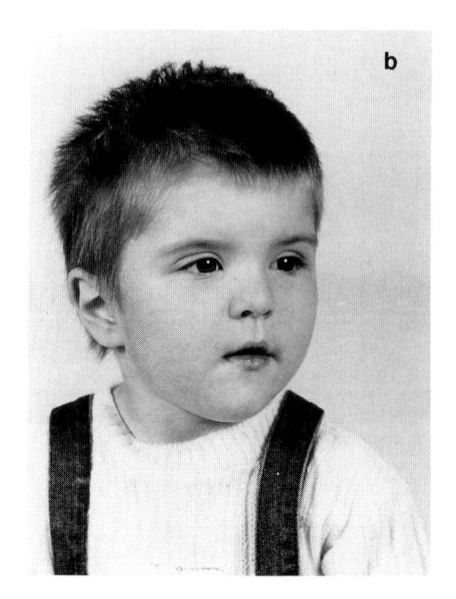

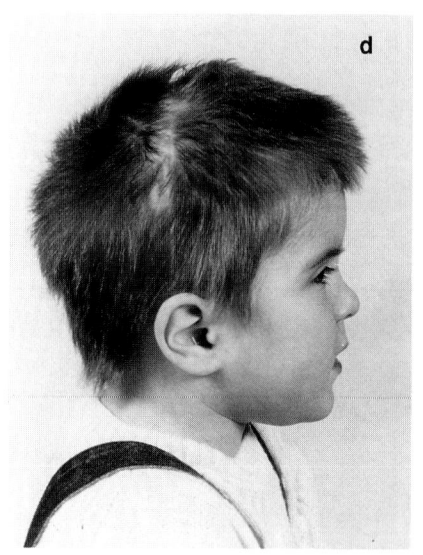

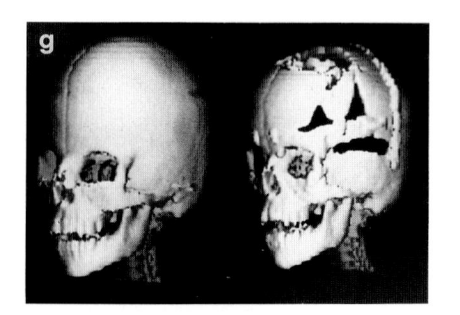

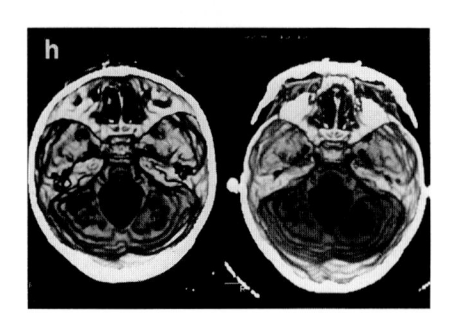

able over the coronal suture regions. A CT scan of the craniofacial skeleton revealed bilateral coronal suture synostosis with resulting short and wide anterior cranial base, shallow orbits, and bulging eyes.

At operation, through a coronal incision, the cranial vault and orbits were exposed in the subperiosteal plane. A bifrontal craniotomy was completed with retraction of the frontal and temporal lobes of the brain. Three-quarter orbital osteotomies with tenon extensions were completed. The orbital units were reshaped and then replaced into the operative field in an advanced position to increase the depth of the anterior cranial base and increase the intra-cranial volume. Stabilization was achieved with micro bone plates and screws. The anterior cranial vault was further sectioned and then replaced to establish a normal forehead configuration. Additional micro bone plates and screws were used for stabilization.

Critique

Marchac and Renier (1982) have pointed out that as many as 42% of children with more than one prematurely closed cranial vault suture will develop significantly increased intracranial pressure. For this reason, suture release and simultaneous cranial vault and orbital reshaping are mandatory to increase intracranial volume during the rapid brain-growth phase.

The selective use of micro bone plates and screws can help to establish the more exact cranio-orbital morphology desired, to maintain the advancement forehead and orbital position achieved once the scalp flaps are sutured, and to decrease operative time. Further study is required to evaluate their routine use in small children.

DISCUSSION

The use of bone miniplate and microplate and screw internal fixation in treating craniofacial malformations has literally revolutionized pediatric craniofacial surgery. The individual cases selected for discussion here illustrate some of the major concepts, controversies, and indications involved.

The chief advantages of this form of osteotomy and bone graft fixation include the ease of three-dimensional shaping of the osteotomies and bone graft units, the ability of the placed osteotomy units to withstand the natural deforming forces (that is, scar tissue, congenitally inadequate soft-tissue drape, muscles of mastication, postural molding, and wound contracture), and the primary or early secondary bone healing. In addition, the incidence of infection may be greatly diminished, early and late skeletal relapse may be diminished, and there should be less overall bone graft resorption.

The disadvantages of stable internal plate and screw fixation for osteotomies and bone grafts include the need for specialized instrumentation and necessity for the surgeon and operating-room team to develop new technical skills. The question of leaving implanted foreign material, which may cause an allergic reaction or lead to late exposure or extrusion, is always a concern with any implanted device. Some of these risks appear to be reduced by the use of either titanium or Vitallium metal. Once postoperative swelling has resolved and perhaps some bone graft resorption has occurred, palpable or visible plates and screws can present an aesthetic problem. Should this occur, a secondary operation to remove them can be done on an outpatient basis and is frequently combined with other necessary minor revision surgery. The ever-increasing innovations to internal bone plate and screw fixation, such as microplate systems, and our ability to select cases that are amenable to low-profile screws and plates when miniplates are required are making this problem much less common than it was several years ago. The question of whether bone plates and screws interfere with progressive growth of the craniofacial skeleton is unresolved and demands additional experimental and prospective clinical study (Enlow 1982).

The basic principles of bony surgery should always be kept in mind. They include appropriate osteotomies, stable immobilization, adequate fixation, and remobilization of the jaws at the appropriate time for the bones involved. In the developing face, the timing and staging of reconstruction is of critical importance.

SUMMARY

A radical surgical approach to the management of craniofacial malformation is often required. The osteotomies and bone grafting procedures carried out must be timed and sequenced according to the patient's overall staged reconstructive plan. An understanding of differential cranial and facial bony growth patterns is essential to maximize the functional and aesthetic results, to minimize the need to repeat surgery in the same region, and to limit retardation of further bony growth potential in the regions operated on. The appropriate use of bone miniplate and microplate and screw internal fixation for osteotomy and bone graft stabilization has revolutionized the surgical management of craniofacial malformations.

Acknowledgment

The author thanks Elizabeth Lang and the staff of Medical Publications, The Hospital for Sick Children, Toronto, for editorial assistance in the preparation of this chapter.

REFERENCES

Enlow DH: Handbook of Facial Growth. Second edition. Philadelphia, Saunders, 1982.

Gillies H, Harrison SH: Operative correction by osteotomy of recessed malar maxillary compound in a case of oxycephaly. Br J Plast Surg 3:123–127, 1950.

Israele V, Siegel JD: Infectious complications of craniofacial surgery in children. Rev Infect Dis 11:9–15, 1989.

Luhr HG: Zur stabilen Osteosynthese bei Unterkierferfrakturen. Deutsch Zahnaerztl Z 23:754, 1968.

Marchac D: Radical forehead remodeling for craniostenosis. Plast Reconstr Surg 61:823–835, 1978.

Marchac D, Renier D (eds): Craniofacial Surgery for Craniosynostosis. Boston, Little, Brown, 1982.

Muhlbauer W, Anderl H: Use of miniplates in craniofacial surgery. Proceedings of the 1st International Congress of the International Society of Craniomaxillofacial Surgeons. Berlin, Springer-Verlag, pp 334–337, 1987.

Murray JE, Swanson LT: Mid-face osteotomy and advancement for craniosynostosis. Plast Reconstr Surg 41:299–306, 1968.

Ortiz-Monasterio F, Fuente del Campo A, Carillo A: Advancement of the orbits and the midface in one piece, combined with frontal repositioning, for the correction of Crouzon's deformities. Plast Reconstr Surg 61:507–516, 1978.

Posnick JC: Ch: Craniofacial Dysostosis: Staging of reconstruction and management of the midface deformity. Neurosurgical Clinics of N. America. Pershing J (ed). Philadelphia, Saunders Vol. 2: No. 3:683–702, 1991.

Posnick JC et al.: Indirect intracranial volume measurements using CT scans: Clinical applications for Craniosynostosis. Plast Reconstr Surg [in press].

Tessier P: Osteotomies totales de la face. Syndrome de Crouzon, syndrome d'Apert: Oxycephalies, scaphocephalies, turricephalies. Ann Chir Plast 12:273–286, 1967.

Tessier P: The definitive plastic surgical treatment of the severe facial deformities of craniofacial dysostosis: Crouzon's and Apert's Syndromes. Plast Reconstr Surg 48:419–442, 1971.

Tessier P: Orbital hypertelorism: I. Successive surgical attempts. Materials and methods. Causes and mechanisms. Scand J Plast Reconstr Surg 6:135–155, 1972.

Tessier P, Guiot G, Derome P: Orbital hypertelorism: II. Definite treatment of orbital hypertelorism (OR.H.) by craniofacial or by extracranial osteotomies. Scand J Plast Reconstr Surg 7:39–58, 1973.

Tulasne JF, Tessier PL: Results of the Tessier integral procedure for correction of Treacher Collins syndrome. Cleft Palate J (Suppl) 23:40–49, 1986.

van der Meulen JCH, Vaandrager JM: Surgery related to the correction of hypertelorism. Plast Reconstr Surg 71:6–17, 1983.

Whitaker LA, Schut L, Kerr LP: Early surgery for isolated craniofacial dysostosis. Improvement and possible prevention of increasing deformity. Plast Reconstr Surg 60:575–581, 1977.

CHAPTER 41

Variations in Osteotomy Design to Facilitate Rigid Fixation in Craniofacial Surgery

Craig R. Dufresne

Craniomaxillofacial surgery is a new field that has evolved as a result of advances in technology, engineering, and medical science. New techniques have been applied to the treatment of massive trauma to the head and neck region, reconstruction following cancer ablation, and the treatment and reconstruction of severe birth defects.

Rigid fixation technology has been accepted rapidly for the reconstructive treatment of craniosynostosis syndromes, facial clefting syndromes, and other types of craniofacial anomalies. Craniofacial malformations are relatively rare conditions that exist in a multitude of patterns and varying degrees of severity. Over 250 craniofacial syndromes have been identified, and an additional 25 to 50 new syndromes are described every year. The literature gives various estimates of the incidence of simple craniosynostosis. The range varies from 0.4/1000 births to 1.6/1000 births (Dufresne 1987).

Since the first use of rigid internal fixation by Hansmann in 1886, several advances have been made in the technology, applications, and use of these materials for the treatment of fractures and congenital reconstructions (Luhr 1985a, 1986, 1987a, 1987b, 1990). Advances in the technology of biomaterials and biocompatibility have resulted in a greater number of product designs and smaller and stronger prosthetic devices, all to deliver a better and more stable reconstruction (Luhr 1987b, 1990). The results have led to greater freedom of design and greater variability of craniomaxillofacial osteotomies to correct the more complex problems encountered clinically (Dufresne 1989).

The use of wires for stabilization of bone flaps in craniofacial surgery has been extensive and universal. The problems usually encountered have been cutting through the thin bone in young infants, breakage, loosening, and stretching. The passage of wires in a retrograde fashion through complex osteotomies and the undersurface of bone flaps often can be quite challenging, frustrating, and sometimes disruptive to the bone flaps for even the best surgeons. Once in place, the delicate framework has to be watched carefully in the hope that shifting, resorption, and collapse are minimal (Converse 1977, Dufresne 1989).

The experience gained by the treatment of facial fractures has shown that the exact repositioning of the bony fragments and rigid interfragmentary fixation with plates and screws offers the best reconstructive results.

The objective in neurocranial reconstruction is the creation of normal shapes and contours which can resist soft tissue deforming forces. This is made possible by rigid fixation techniques. In reconstruction of the maxillofacial skeleton and mandible, plates and screws allow immediate active and pain-free mobilization of the maxilla and mandible without jeopardizing the healing process of the bony skeleton. Advances in rigid fixation technology have led to systems with lower profiles and greater flexibility, which allow greater variation in osteotomy design and techniques as they are applied to craniofacial reconstruction.

RECONSTRUCTION OF THE UPPER CRANIOFACIAL REGION

The goal of craniomaxillofacial surgery is restoration of symmetry, balance of proportions, and normal contours to the cranial and facial skeleton. The human skull, as it has evolved, has tended to brachycephaly (Carlson 1971). The surgeon attempts to find the anomalous anatomy and then to restore shape and aesthetics to as close to the norm as possible. This can also include correction of asymmetrical cranial disorders; expansion of the cranium in microcephalic disorders; cranial reduction, as in hydrocephalus; or correction of widened or elongated cranium (Dufresne 1989).

Most reconstructive modalities for surgery of the craniomaxillofacial skeleton today involve the use of rigid fixation techniques. These techniques enable the surgeon to achieve a more stable and controllable reconstruction, and their use expedites the healing process (Beals 1987, Champy 1982, Drommer 1981, Dufresne 1989, Harle 1980, Jackson 1978, Luhr 1986, 1987a, 1988, 1990, Michelet 1973, Muhlbauer 1987a, 1987b, 1987c).

Congenital disorders such as craniosynostosis are often treated in infancy when the skeleton is quite malleable. Rigid fixation plates have been used successfully to advance frontal bone flaps and supraorbital ridges, and their stability is maintained as the children grow. Also, asymmetrical and symmetrical upper cranial defects can be modified to the desired contours and maintained by the plating (see Figure 41.1).

Previously, complicated interlocking segments and osteotomies had to be designed in a "master carpenter's" fashion to allow wire fixation of the bony struts for stabilization of the advanced flaps and bone fragments (Converse 1977). Too often shifting of fragments due to poor fixation detracted from the end result. The ability to recontour the supraorbital ridge, frontal bone, or other areas of the craniofacial skeleton with plates and screws has enabled the surgeon to achieve a much more stable and predictable reconstruction. This usually can be executed more quickly and easily than the previous techniques employing wire osteosynthesis, which require the design of complex interlocking fragments or flaps.

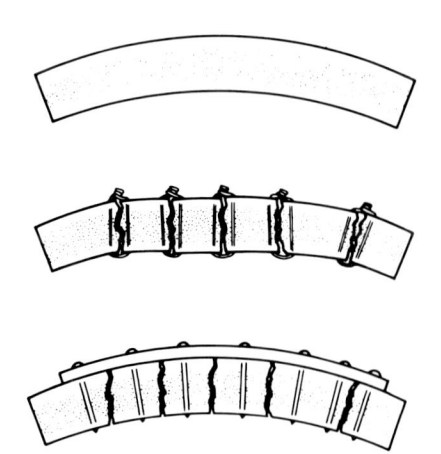

Figure 41.1 Unlike wire osteosynthesis, plate and screw stabilization can maintain bone fragments in complex three-dimensional arrangements.

The most common form of craniosynostosis is the premature closure of the sagittal suture, which causes a narrow, elongated configuration of the neurocranium. This is referred to as *scaphocephaly* or *dolichocephaly* (see Figure 41.2a). A premature (intrauterine) closure of the metopic suture leads to a "keel" deformity of the frontal bone accompanied by some constriction of the temporal areas and hypotelorism. This is referred to as *trigonocephaly* (see Figure 41.2b). The premature closure of the hemicoronal suture leads to an asymmetrical frontal and upper cranial deformity that is referred to as *plagiocephaly* (see Figure 41.2c). The closure of the bilateral coronal suture results in *oxycephaly* or *turricephaly*. This type of deformity is often seen in Crouzon's disease and Apert syndrome (Converse 1977, Dufresne 1987, Whitaker 1980).

The severity of the resultant deformity is directly proportional to the area, the extent, and the sutures involved. The range of the facial deformation can be minimal, as in scaphocephaly; greater, as in trigonocephaly; or quite severe, as in kleeblattschädel syndrome and craniofacial dysostosis, in which multiple sutures are involved (Converse 1977, Dufresne 1987, Enlow 1975, Muhlbauer 1987a, Whitaker 1980).

In unilateral coronal synostosis, the frontal bone is asymmetrical; it is flattened on the affected side and bossed on the contralateral side. The deformities can extend down to the cranial base; when they do, the orbital positions are deformed as well as the supraorbital ridge and the frontal bone. The orbital deformities are often the most disturbing aesthetic aspect of the anomaly. The correction of the plagiocephaly deformity proceeds with first defining the pathology and areas of abnormal contour and development. Osteotomies are then designed that will restore symmetry to the frontal area and supraorbital ridges (Beals 1987, Converse 1977, Dufresne 1989, McNamara 1982, Michelet 1973, Muhlbauer 1987a, 1987b, 1987c, Muhling 1987, Munro 1987, Salyer 1990, Whitaker 1980).

The osteotomies proceed through the area of craniosynostosis and down into the temporal fossa. The release of the fused suture should be as complete as possible, and the risks of an extended release into the region of the cranial base should be weighed. The frontal bone is then elevated off the dura in either a single or two-piece bone flap. Next the supraorbital bar is removed from the fronto-zygomatic sutures, through the orbital roofs and the nasofrontal suture. In most cases the bar is then contoured and secured to the intact lateral cranial vault. The rest of the frontal bone reconstruction is then carried out. At times the frontal halves are rotated and exchanged to achieve the best contours (see Figure 41.3). The previously synostosed coronal suture area is opened during the surgery and is allowed to remain open in order to allow for subsequent symmetrical brain growth and development. Rigid fixation techniques are used to secure bone flaps and grafts to

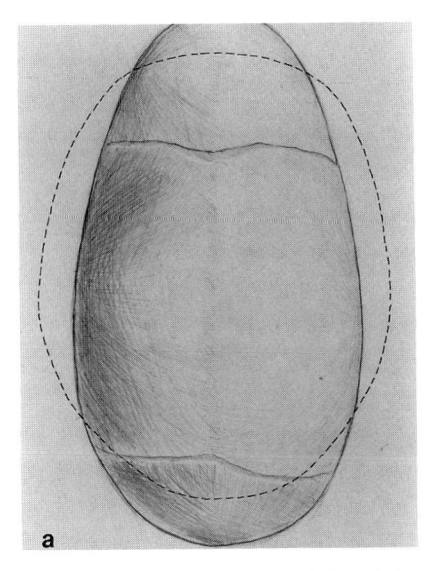

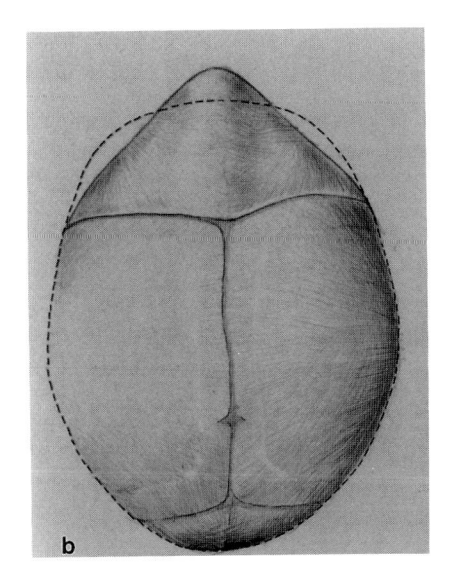

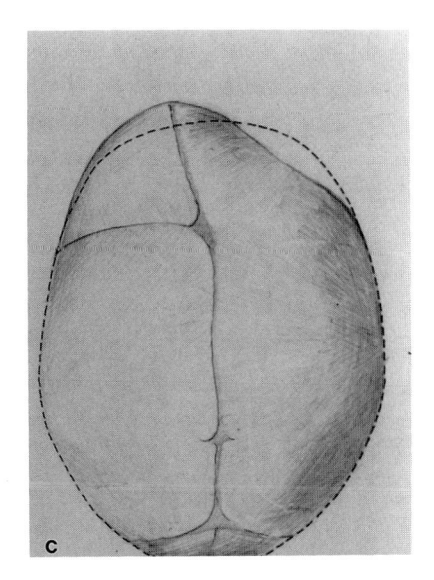

Figure 41.2 Craniosynostosis involving single cranial sutures can lead to profound changes in the shape of the upper cranial area of the craniofacial skeleton. The dashed lines represent the "normal" contours. (a) Scaphocephaly is caused by a premature closure of the sagittal suture and a narrowing and elongation of the skull. (b) Trigonocephaly is caused by premature closure of the metopic suture that imparts a "keel" shape to the anterior frontal bone and narrows the temporal regions and intraorbital distances. (c) Unilateral coronal synostosis leads to a plagiocephaly deformity. This results in a foreshortening of the affected side and often a contralateral bossing of the frontal bone.

allow rapid healing and maintenance of the desired contour and symmetry.

Modified reconstruction and fixation occasionally are required, particularly in young children or in areas where soft-tissue coverage is thin or poor. The use of intracranial plates has been found effective in such cases. This still allows for the creation of new contours as well as for advancement of bone flaps and grafts (see Figures 41.4 and 41.5). In infants, because of their thin, delicate tissues, use of even the smallest wires, plates, or screws can be readily apparent. With the use of intracranial frontal bone fixation, however, palpation of the plates and screws is minimal. This technique involves initially placing the fixation plate intracranially at the point of fixation to the anterior frontal bone or lateral orbital region. The plate is contoured into an "S" shaped configuration that then exits through a bone gap or area of advancement. This will then allow the flaps that are to be secured to the temporal fossa region under the temporalis muscle to be fixed to the region of the cra-

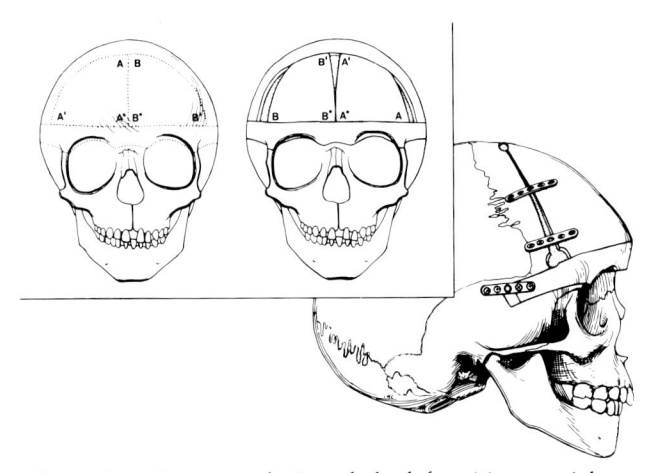

Figure 41.3 In severe plagiocephaly deformities, cranial bone flaps can be advanced or exchanged to achieve the desired contours. They can then be rigidly fixed into position without the need for the interlocking pieces or struts that are needed for wire fixation.

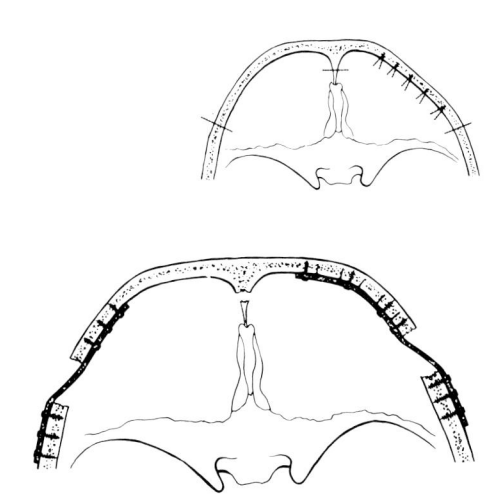

Figure 41.4 Bilateral frontal bone advancement and asymmetrical contouring can be carried out to create the desired morphology by the use of intracranial rigid fixation plates.

Figure 41.5 (a) The desired expansion and contour of the frontal flap can be achieved with precisely contacted intracranial plates. (b) The frontal flap is then secured to the cranial base to which other frontal flaps are fastened.

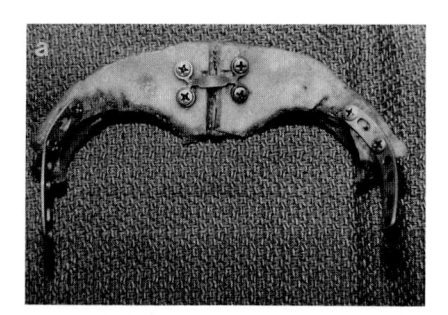

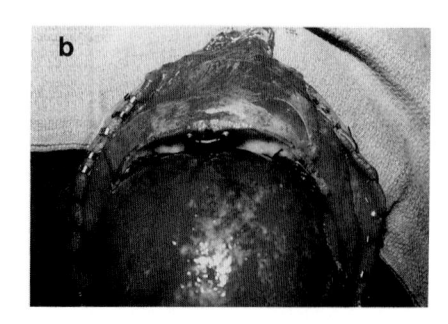

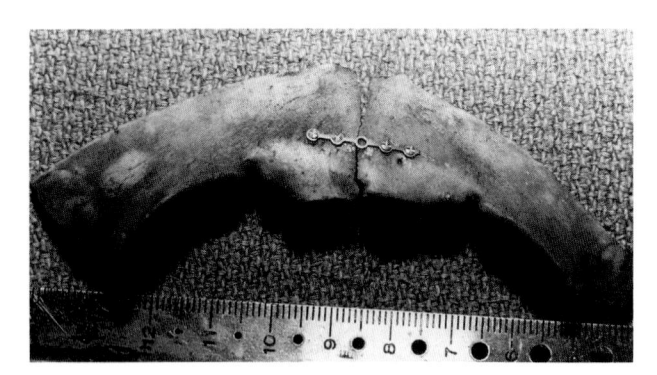

Figure 41.6 The variety of microplate designs is demonstrated. A miniplate is placed in the upper left corner for size comparison.

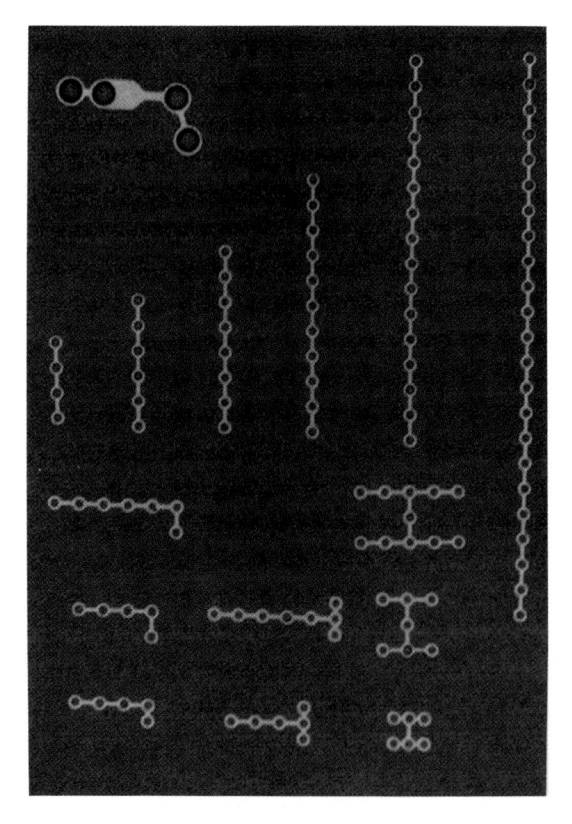

Figure 41.7 The reduced scale of the microplating system allows its external placement for recontouring the frontal bone in a growing infant.

nium that is stable. When the temporalis muscle is to be transposed, the fixation plate offers an ideal support "beam" from which to suspend it. Screw tips noted through the frontal bone or palpable, if any, can be burred down flush to the surface of the flap. In a very thin skull, the brain is protected by the use of cranial or split rib grafts interposed between the hardware and the soft tissues or brain. Recently developed microplating systems make visibility or palpability of the implants unusual (see Figures 41.6 and 41.7).

In surgery on very young patients and infants, only the smallest number of plates is used to achieve rigid fixation of the bone flaps and grafts. The critical areas of fixation are the temporal areas and between the supraorbital bar and frontal bone flaps (see Figure 41.8). This approach has resulted in reproducible and predictable reconstructive methods that have allowed acceptable aesthetic results with minimal complications.

Posterior craniosynostosis can present with significant deformities when unilateral or bilateral lambdoidal synostosis is involved. The approach is similar to those used to correct the deformities resulting from the other prematurely synostosed cranial sutures. The affected sutures are released, and normal contours are created in the abnormal areas of the cranium (see Figures 41.9 and 41.10). The goal is the normal brachycephalic configuration of the neurocranium. In patients less than three years of age, and particularly in those less than a year old, the surgical reconstruction should take into account the considerable amount of brain growth and subsequent skull remodeling which remains. The posterior cranium has to be approached carefully because of the delicate cerebral structures present and the major vascular structures located at the occiput. Surgery in this area is reserved for only severe deformities.

Trigonocephaly and scaphocephaly present with greater deformity and the potential for the operation's causing neurological sequellae is greater because a larger portion of the cranium or a larger number of cranial sutures are involved. The metopic suture, the first cranial suture to close, normally does so just before birth. Premature closure of the metopic suture leads to the frontal bone "keel" and in severe cases can also lead to hypotelorism. Correction is designed to open the con-

Variations in Osteotomy 531

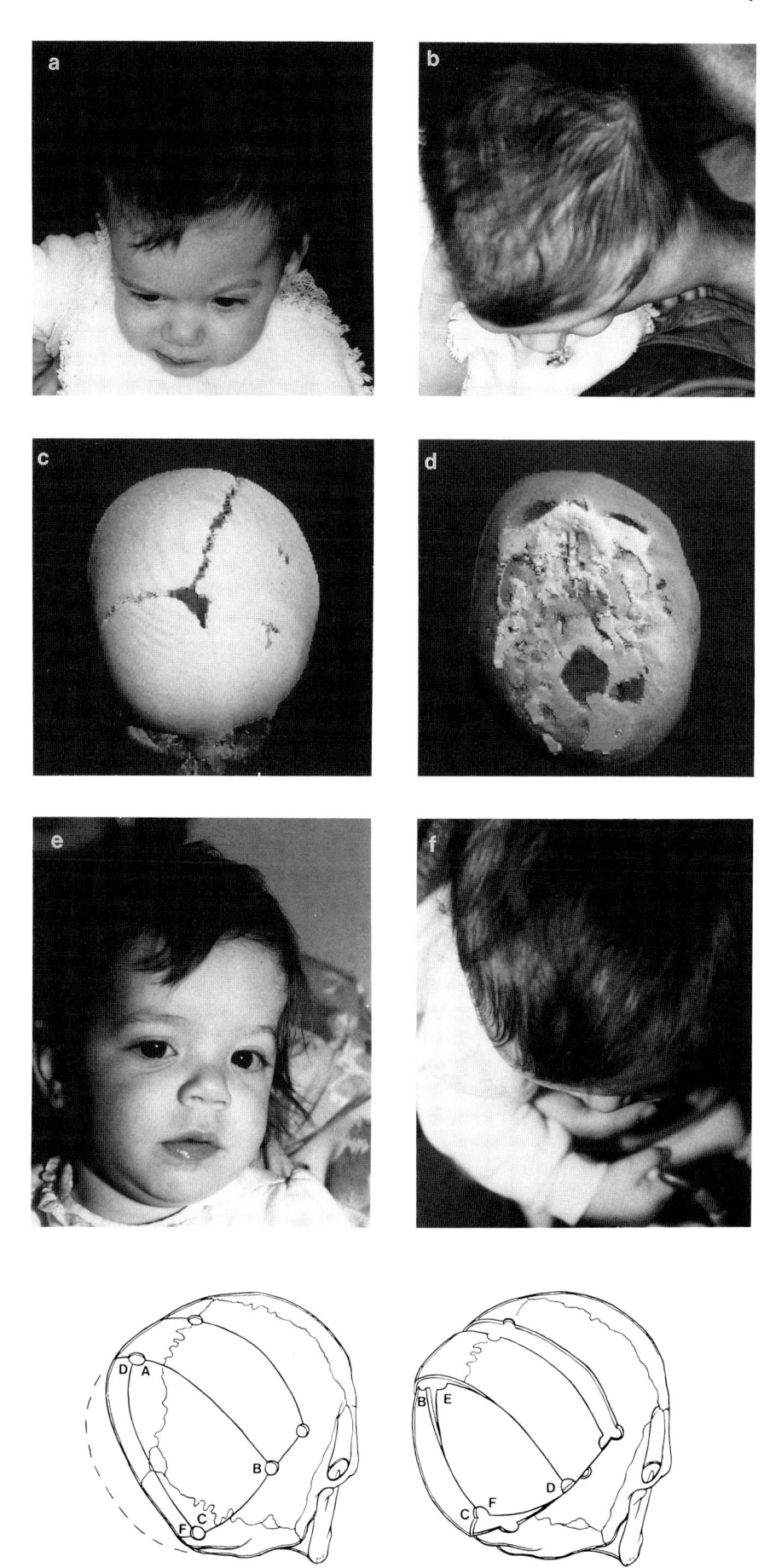

Figure 41.8 (a) This six-month-old patient demonstrates a plagiocephaly deformity secondary to a unilateral coronal craniosynostosis modified frontal view. (b) Overhead view. (c) Three-dimensional CT scans demonstrate the left unilateral coronal synostosis and resultant upper cranial deformity. Overhead view. (d) Worm's eye view. (e) The patient, 1½ years after surgery, shows maintenance of good symmetry and contour. Frontal view. (f) Overhead view.

Figure 41.9 Cranial expansion can be achieved with great stability in any dimension. Open areas are left in young children to allow for brain growth. Here the posterior cranium is expanded and remodeled with the use of multiple bone flaps; their position is maintained with plate screws. The goal is to expand the neurocranium to achieve a more brachycephalic configuration.

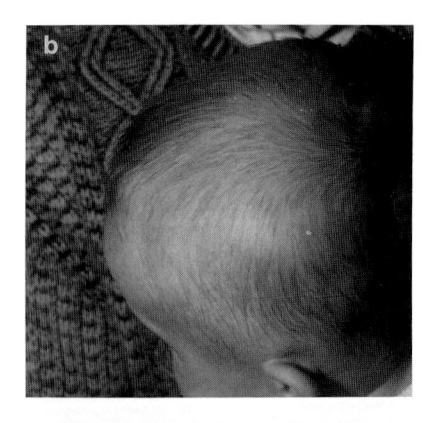

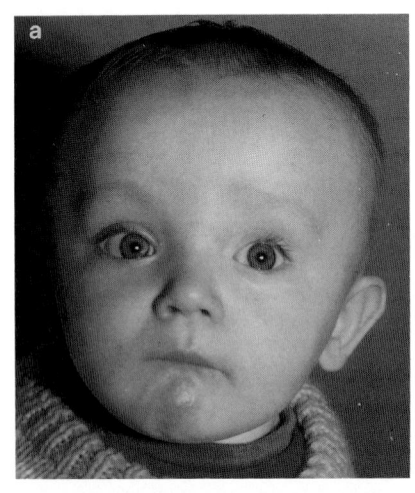

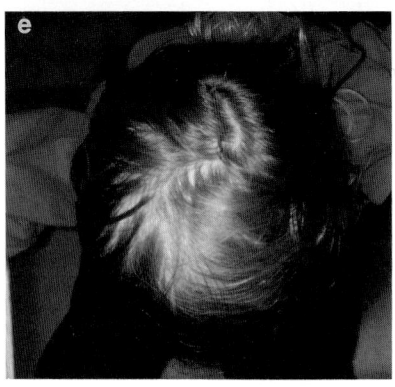

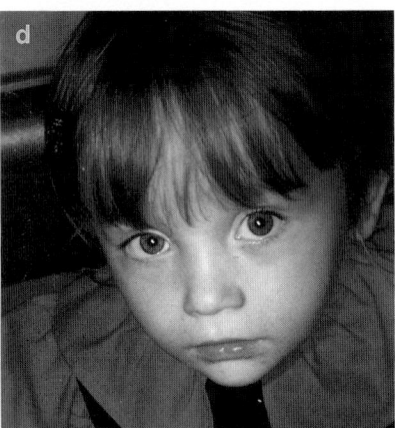

532   RIGID FIXATION OF THE CRANIOMAXILLOFACIAL SKELETON

Figure 41.10 (a) This young patient had bilateral lambdoidal synostosis with severe posterior flattening, foreshortening, and widening of the cranium. Osteotomy design was similar to that shown in Figure 41.9. Anterior view. (b) Posterior oblique view. (c) Posterior view. (d) Postoperative views show the expansion with better contouring. The ears are released of constriction so that further growth can take place. Anterior view. (e) Overhead view. (f) Lateral view.

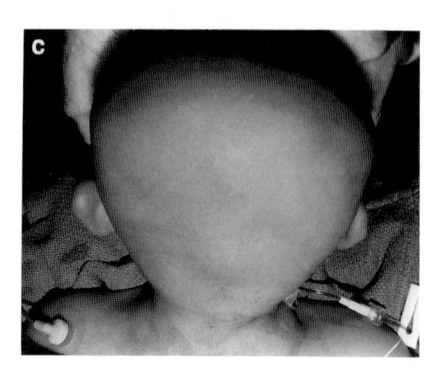

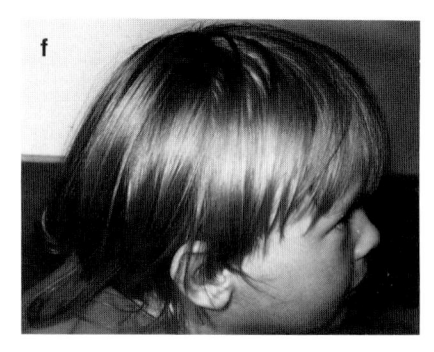

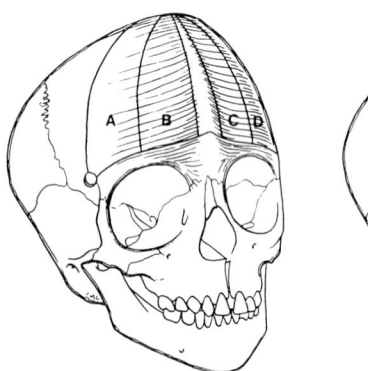

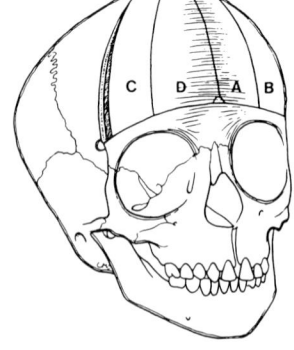

Figure 41.11 In this trigonocephaly deformity, multiple osteotomies of the frontal bone can be performed, and the segments can be reassembled to achieve the desired result. Their position is maintained by long fixation plates or miniplates.

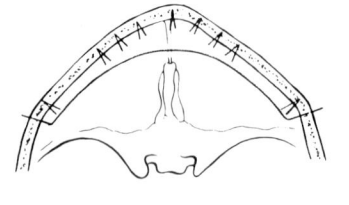

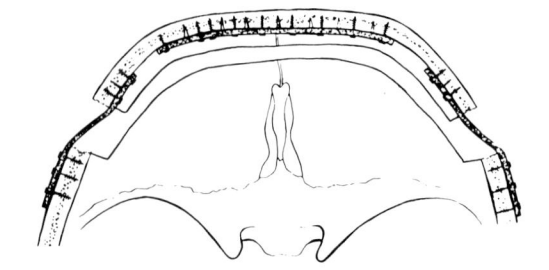

Figure 41.12 Intracranial plating maintains the advancement and contours of the frontal bar in the trigonocephaly deformity. Extracranial plating can also be used.

stricted frontal bone that extends into both temporal fossa and to expand the entire frontal area (see Figures 41.11 and 41.12). This process also includes remodeling the nasal root to correct the keel and, to give the best results, may require correcting the hypotelorism (Converse 1977, Dufresne 1989, McCarthy 1978, Michelet 1973, Muhlbauer 1987a, 1987b, 1987c). Rigid fixation techniques maintain the desired contours and hold bone flaps in place. This can be accomplished readily by either intracranial or extracranial plates and screws. The new microfixation devices offer the best results in the treatment of infants and the very young. The upper neurocranial skeleton is nearly complete at age three, so that expansion can be used with little disturbance to future growth (see Figure 41.13) (Converse 1977, Enlow 1975, McCarthy 1978, McNamara 1982).

Correction of the more severe scaphocephalic deformities requires more extensive surgery. Reconstruction requires anterior to posterior removal and remodeling of the neurocranium. The goals are total release of the upper neurocranium; expansion of the lateral cranium; and, at times, foreshortening of the elongated skull (see Figure 41.14) (Converse 1977, Dufresne 1989, Whitaker 1980). The principles of reconstruction are the same as those described for the less severe skull vault deformities. Rigid fixation is used to stabilize multiple bone flaps, thus enabling dramatic expansion of the cranial vault. The use of multiple bone flaps and rigid fixation allows for greater freedom of design and postoperative stability. With a decreased tendency for positional relapse, revisional surgery is less likely.

Plate and screw fixation is used at the frontotemporal areas and at the occiput for stability of the bone flaps. The middle portion of the cranium, or any other area that is required, is purposely left open to allow further expansion and remodeling of the skull as the brain continues to grow. This often causes decompression of the brain, particularly when clinical signs of increased intracranial pressure are present. Patients may demonstrate improved neurological functioning and motor skills, less headaches and visual disturbances, and improved behavior and sense of well being (Converse 1977, Dufresne 1989, Shilli 1981).

Large cranial bone flaps occasionally must be switched to restore normal contour and appearance. This technique often is the best way to restore a smooth "aesthetic unit" reconstruction, particularly in those patients who have had ablative surgery, who have frontal bone deformity or oxycephaly (see Figure 41.15). This technique allows for rapid and symmetric restoration of certain cranial deformities (see Figure 41.16). The microplate is the implant of choice in the young patient. When properly positioned, it allows for growth and development of the brain and skull.

When severe asymmetric cranial deformities are present in very young infants, rigid fixation techniques can often provide a normal contour and symmetry to the area and allow rapid healing (see Figure 41.17). If extensive plating is required during the reconstruction, then removal of plates is considered after enough time is allowed for healing (three to four months). Because of the thin soft-tissue covering over the devices, in an active child it is sometimes necessary to remove these plates to prevent repeated trauma and exposure of the devices. The techniques of rigid fixation, however, allow the surgery greater freedom during the reconstruction and a more stable fixation that allows the bone to heal in the desired design and configurations.

BONE GRAFTING AND LARGE MESH PLATES

Rigidly fixed bone grafts demonstrate less resorption than unfixed grafts (Phillips 1990). Rigidly fixed split calvarial grafts, which are ideally suited for reconstruction of large defects of the anterior neurocranium, demonstrate the least amount of resorption when compared to grafts harvested from other sites (Phillips 1990). The posterior temporal or parietal bones can be assessed for the proper curvature, contour, and size; and then a full-thickness graft can be taken. The calvarial graft can then be split between the inner and outer tables, and the final details of the design can then be carried out. Once placed in position, the calvarial graft can be rigidly fixed. More often, multiple grafts or flaps can be taken for the reconstruction and then can be contoured to achieve the proper or desired curvature. Long reconstruction plates are, therefore, used to help link all these grafts to achieve the best results.

Follow-up evaluation of patients with calvarial grafts have shown good maintenance of cranial contour. The inner table of the calvarial bone graft is elevated to the level of the surface of the cranium and then secured in position. This has led to minimal problems with healing of the donor site. The stable and close contact of the graft to the margins of the cranial defect accelerate early vascular ingrowth into the area.

Small defects between the grafts or craniotomy bur holes need not always be grafted or filled with a bone substitute (that is, hydroxyapatite blocks) if plates cover the defect. Here plates, wire mesh, or "micromesh" can be used to prevent collapse of the soft tissue into the bony defects and to prevent unsightly pulsatile defects.

Larger defects can be reconstructed with multiple mesh plates that are secured together, or, in areas of large convolutions, custom-tailored plates can be used. With the marriage of space age technology, computer aided graphics, design, and construction, templates or prostheses that fit exactly can be created. These have been helpful in the reconstruction of large, complex defects: A short operation yields very good results (see Figure 41.18) (Morgan 1987). Titanium plates are often used because of their excellent biocompatibility. Bone

Figure 41.13 (a) This patient demonstrates the typical trigonocephaly deformity with constriction of the naso-orbital region. Frontal view. (b) Worm's eye view. (c) Three-dimensional CT scans can be helpful in demonstrating the areas of abnormality to help plan the operative procedure. Frontal view. (d) Overhead view. (e) Intraoperative view of the disarticulated frontal bone and supraorbital rims reflects the abnormal contours demonstrated in the CT scans. (f) Intraoperative view shows restoration of the normal contours and definition by microplate fixation. Note the expansion and multiple scoring of the frontal bone flaps, performed to achieve the desired affect. (g) Appearance of the patient six months postoperatively demonstrates good symmetry and contour. Frontal view. (h) Overhead view.

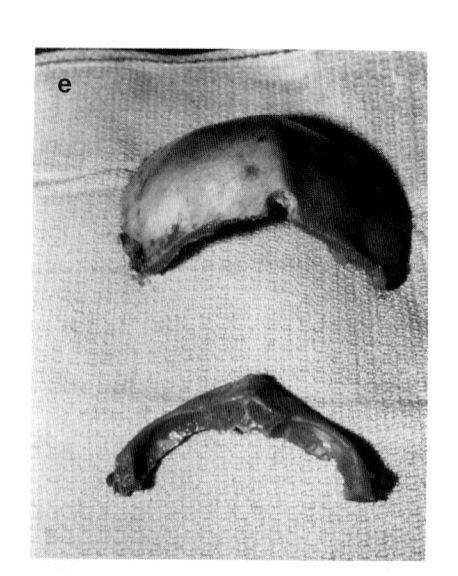

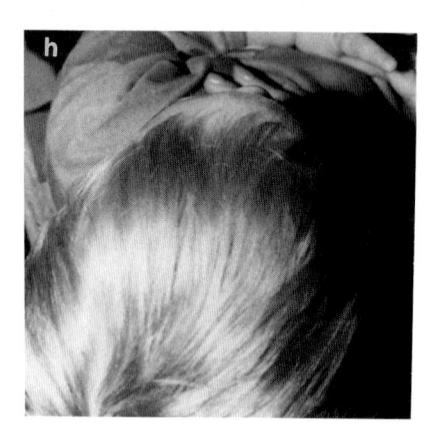

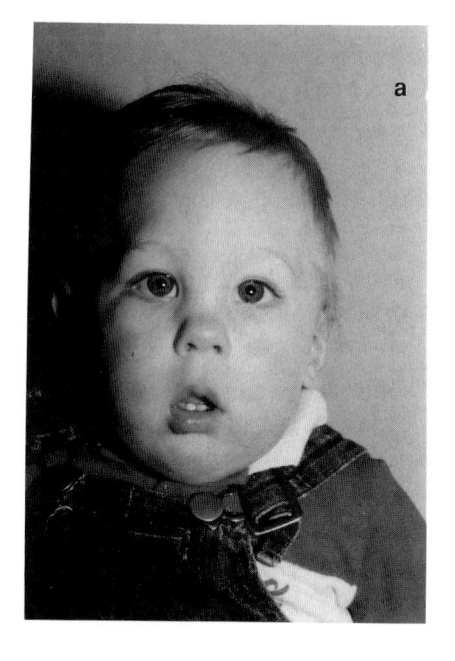

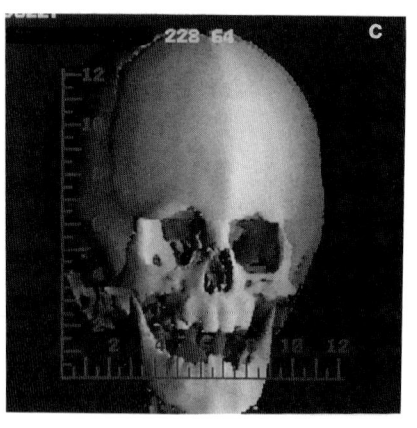

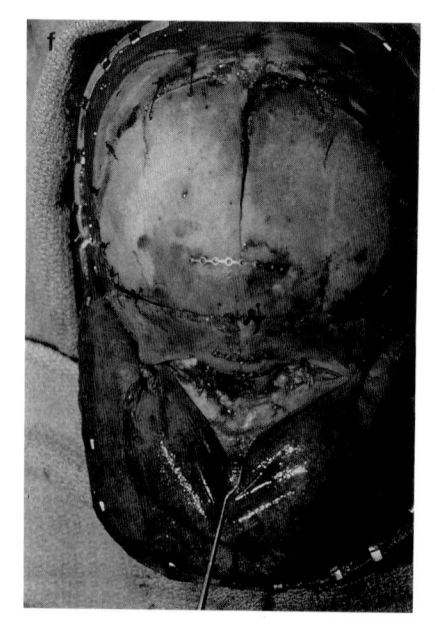

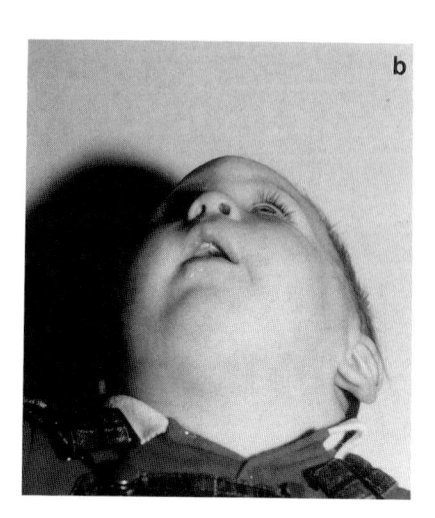

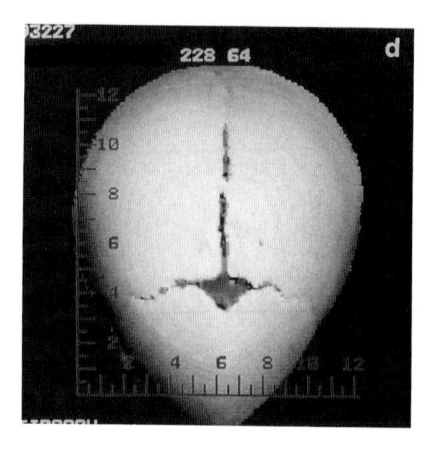

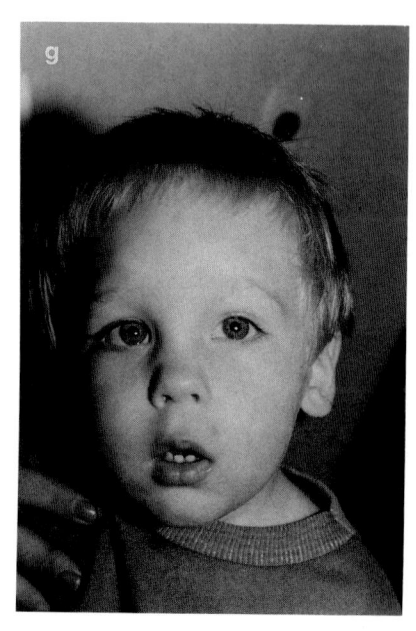

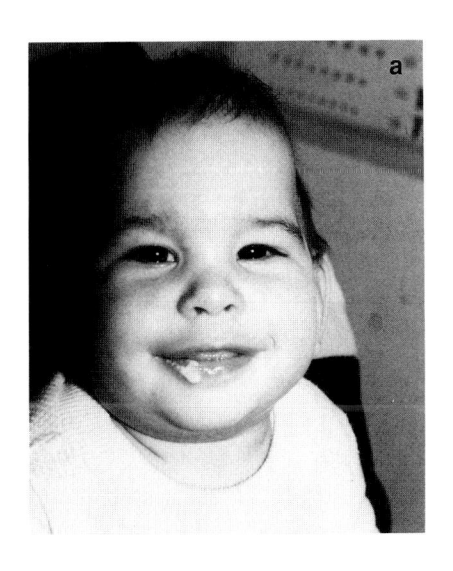

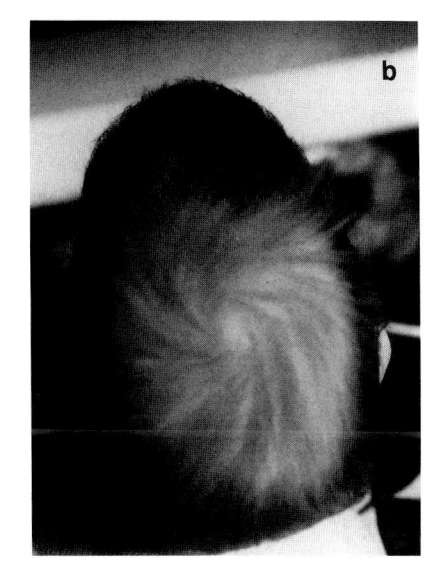

Figure 41.14 (a) Preoperative views show a six-month-old child with severe scaphocephaly and mild signs of developmental delays. The operative plan called for total upper cranial expansion after release of the posterior craniosynostosis. Frontal view. (b) Overhead view. (c) Three-dimensional CT scans reveal lateral cranial constriction and elongation of the anterior and posterior portions of the skull. Frontal view. (d) Overhead view. (e) Lateral view. (f) Intraoperative view shows the degree of expansion of the upper cranial vault and the number of bone flaps used. (g) The patient is shown nearly two years after surgery. Neurologically, he is improved and has reached normal developmental milestones. Frontal view. (h) Overhead view.

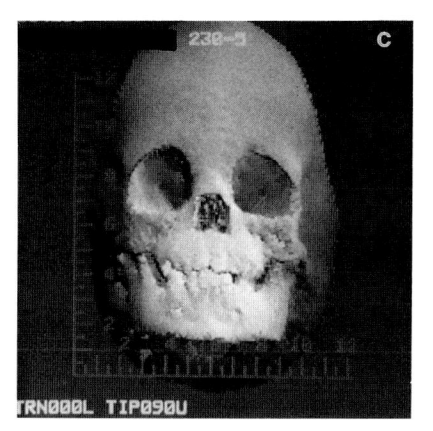

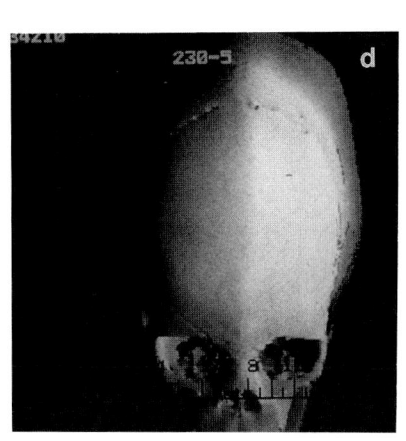

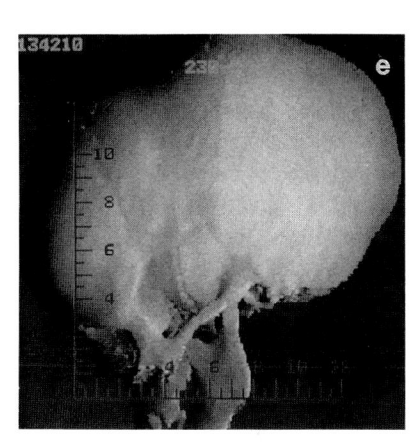

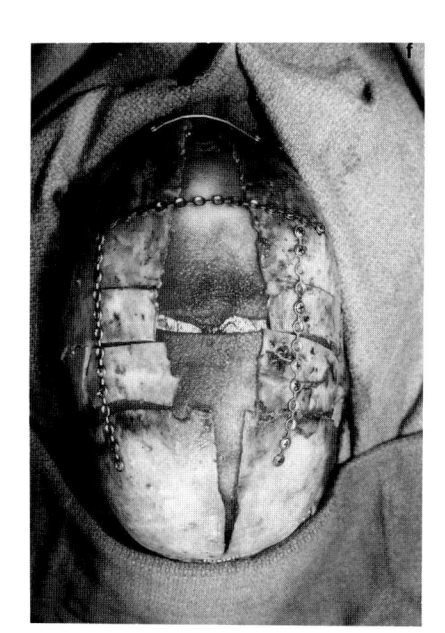

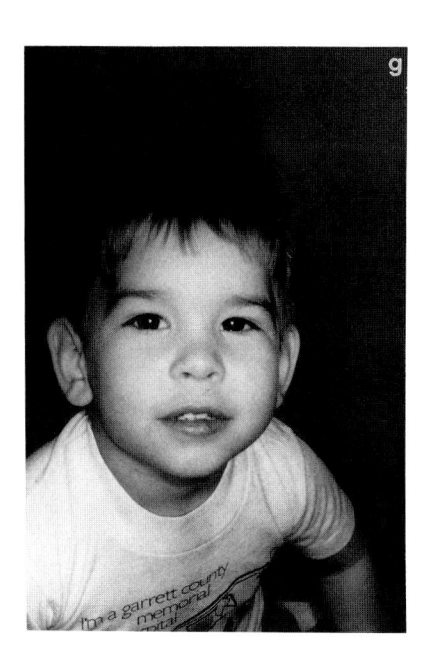

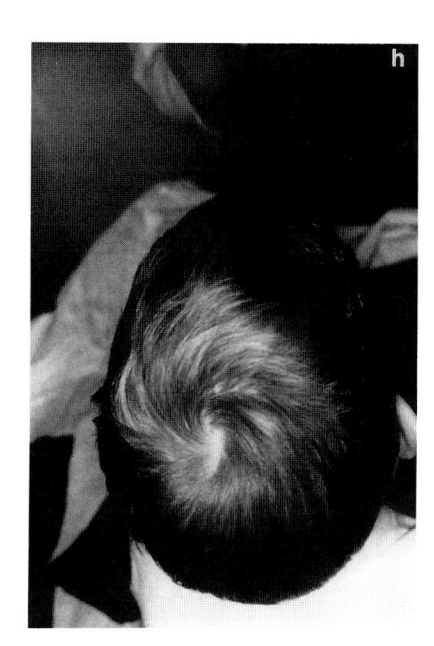

Figure 41.15 Creative osteotomies can be used to obtain the desired curvatures of the bone flaps from other parts of the cranium. The exchange allows for better contouring and improved aesthetic results.

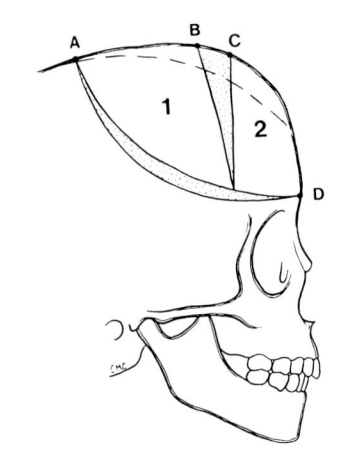

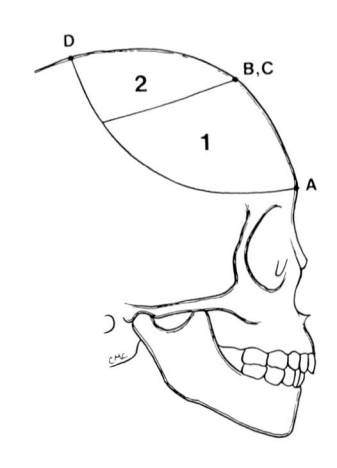

Figure 41.16 (a) This patient had secondary craniosynostosis following placement of a ventriculo-peritoneal shunt. The cranium, which became long and constricted anteriorly, prevented further expansion of the brain. The operative plan was to exchange the middle cranium with the anterior cranium and to allow for overall expansion. Preoperative lateral view. (b) Preoperative overhead view. (c) Three-dimensional scans reveal the areas of abnormal contour and constriction. Overhead view. (d) Sagittal view. (e) The patient is shown one year after flap exchange and reconstruction of the upper cranium. Oblique view. (f) Overhead view.

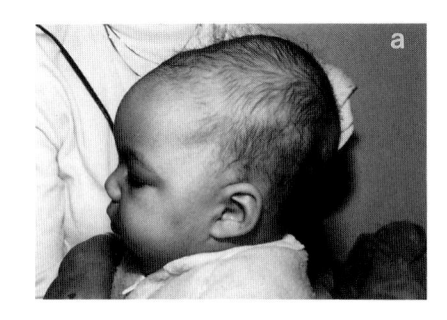

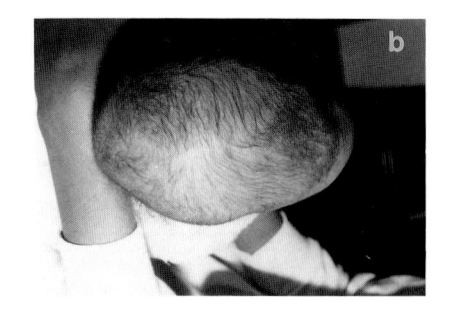

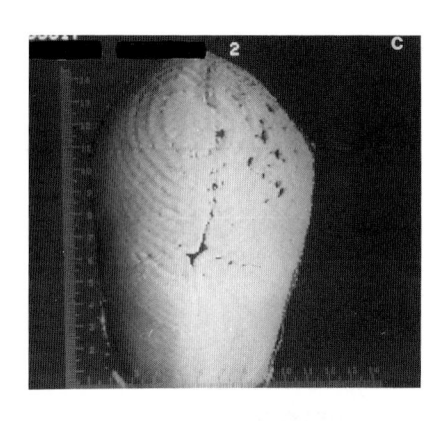

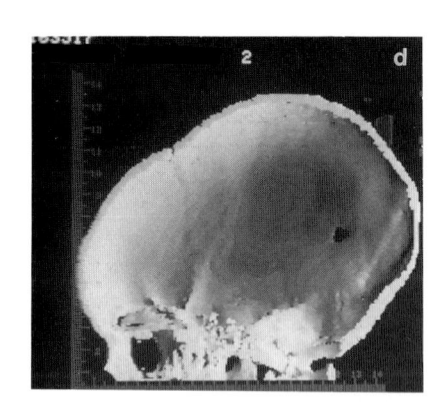

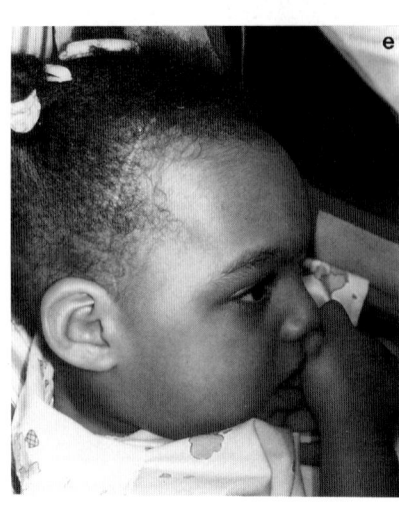

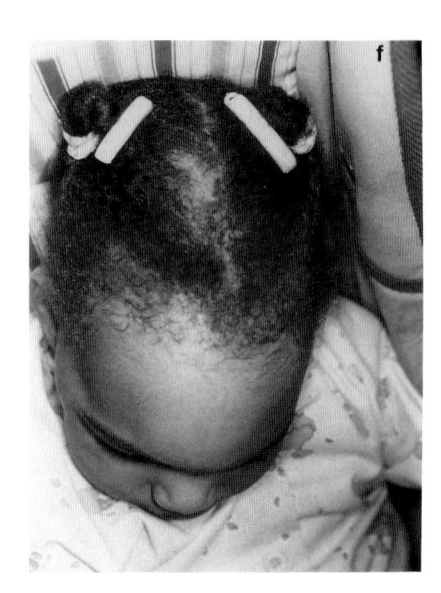

Variations in Osteotomy

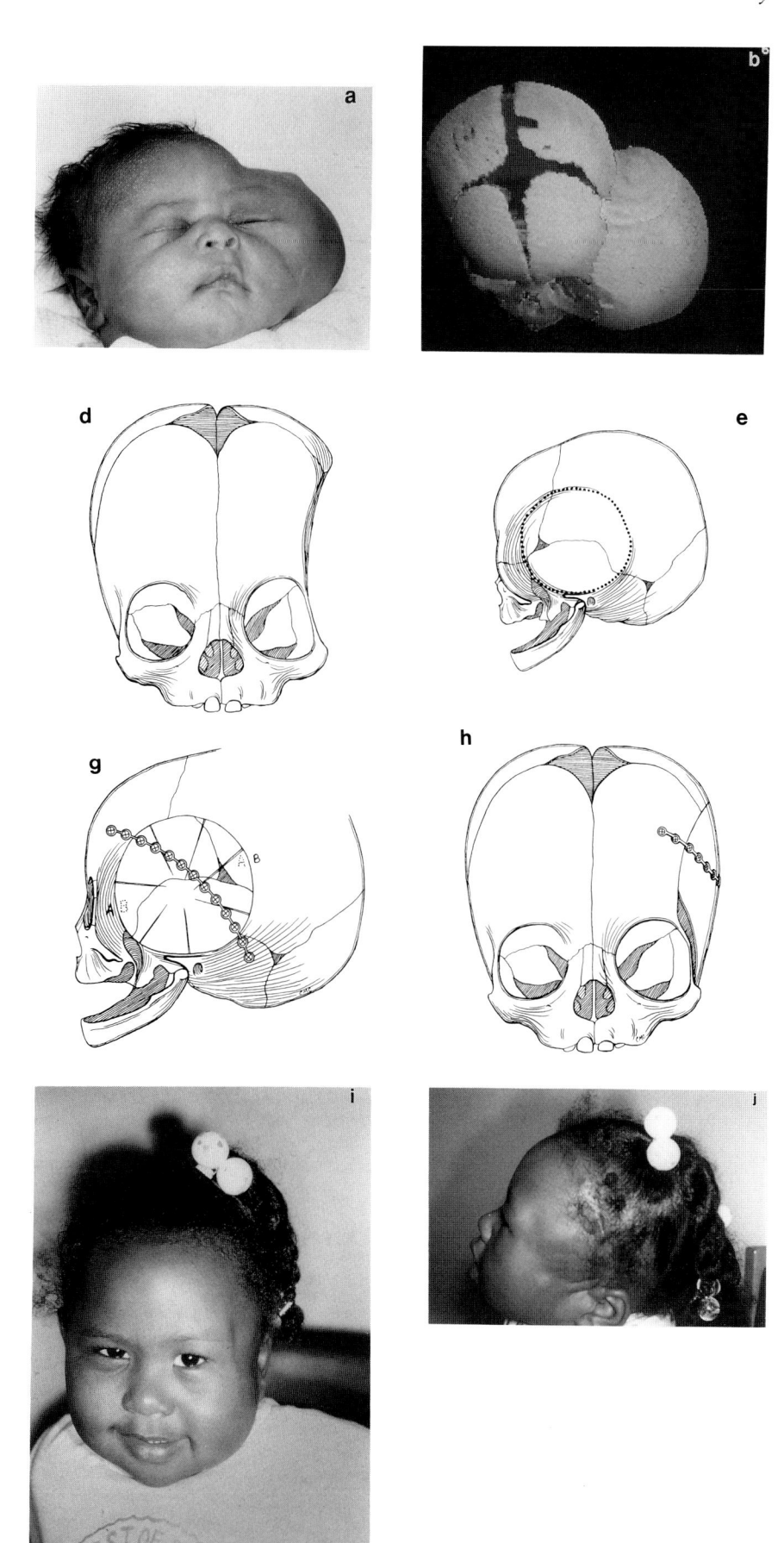

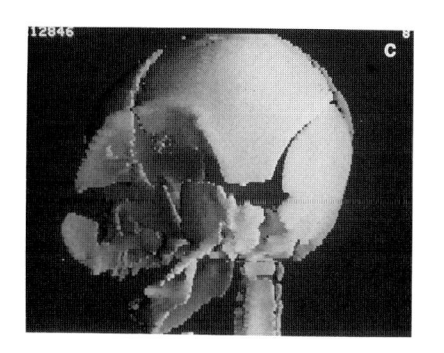

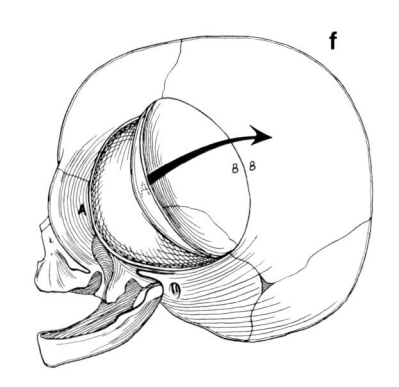

Figure 41.17 (a) Frontal view shows a one-week-old infant with an extensive lateral meningocele that has caused significant distortion of the facial architecture. (b) Overhead three-dimensional CT scans reveal the distortion of the bony structures resulting from the meningocele. (c) A view of the lateral skull shows the meningocele subtracted electronically from the area to reveal the underlying structures. (d) The operative procedure was begun at age three months. The lateral meningocele was resected, and the deformed cranial area was reversed and secured in its new position with a single reconstruction plate. The plate was removed in three months, after bone healing was complete. The lateral orbital wall and the zygomatic arch was greenstick fractured in order to restore a more normal contour and to allow for postoperative remodeling after the pressure from the meningocele was removed. The planned osteotomy is shown. (e) The cranial segment is reversed and replaced. (f) The miniplate is shown in position. (g) The frontal view shows the preosteotomy. (h) A frontal view postosteotomy and fixation. (i) Postoperative appearance is shown two years after surgery. Frontal view. (j) Lateral view.

paste or cancellous bone can be applied to the surface where multiple fenestrations are present. This allows better tissue ingrowth and vascularity, which prevent late infection or extrusion (Morgan 1987).

When the defects are not complex enough to require computer generated contours, then straight mesh plates, after being linked in sequential order, can be used to cover the defect (see Figure 41.19). In order further to camouflage the matrix of the large mesh plates, an additional coverage such as Marlex mesh (C.R. Bard, Inc., Billerica, MA) is sometimes required to prevent the visible detection of the plate after the edema recedes.

Mesh plates have also been useful in the treatment of congenital clefting disorders or to bridge bony gaps (see Figure 41.20). The mesh plates can act as a scaffold

Figure 41.18 Processing of CT data allows for the custom fabrication of models or templates used for reconstructing large skull defects. (a) Oblique view of a three-dimensional scan shows large cranial defect. (b) A computer-generated template is shown. (c) A custom titanium plate is constructed to repair the defect. (d) Intraoperative view shows the plate inset into the defect. (e) The patient is seen eight months after surgery. Frontal view. (f) Lateral view. (g) Posterior view.

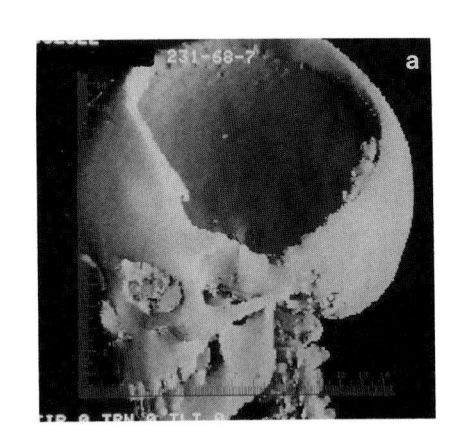

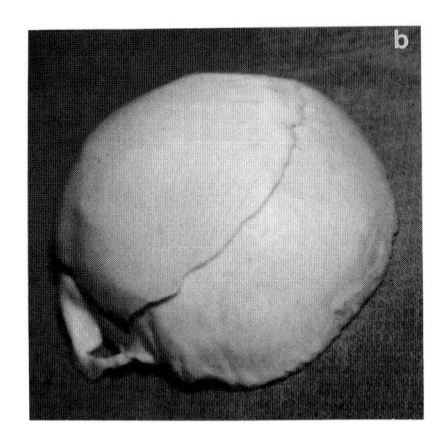

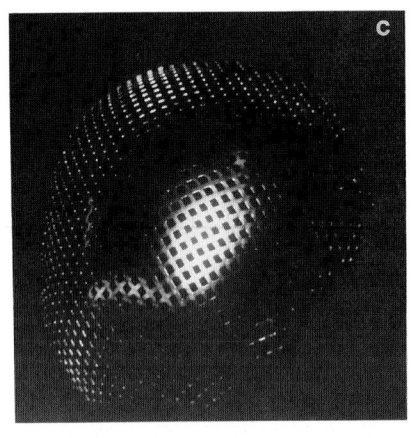

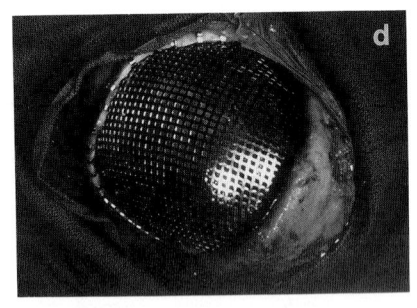

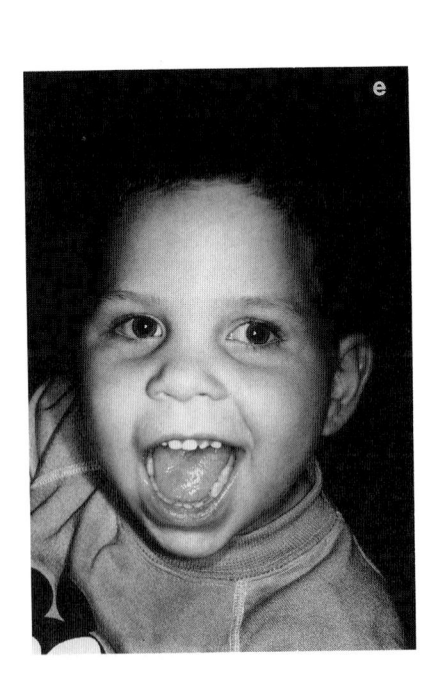

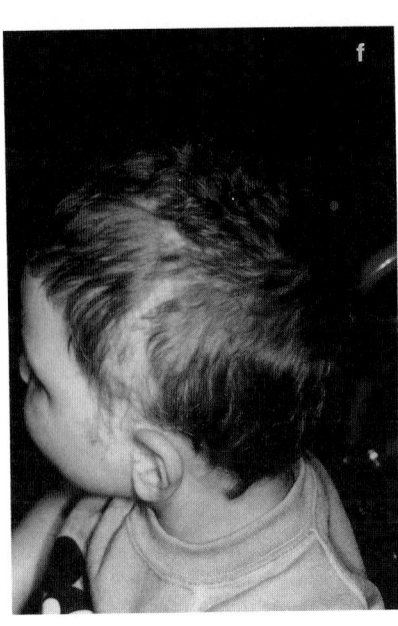

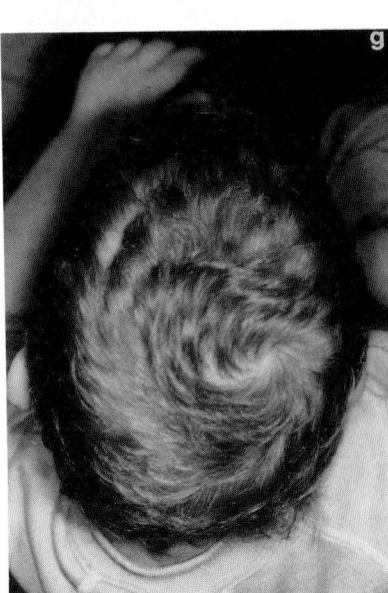

for attachment of additional bone grafts as well as for support of the soft tissue.

MIDFACIAL AND MAXILLARY RECONSTRUCTION

Rigid fixation in upper and midfacial reconstruction has been found to be quite useful and has broadened the surgeon's ability to create more stable and more aesthetic reconstructions. The reconstructive techniques applied to the correction of craniosynostosis deformities involving the neurocranium are also applied to the correction of facial clefting syndromes and miscellaneous craniofacial dysmorphic syndromes involving the facial structures. Reconstruction involves providing balance, symmetry, and normal facial proportions and angles.

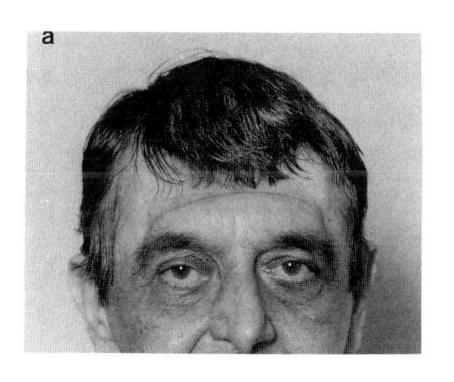

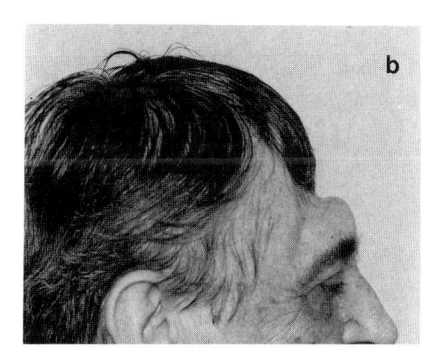

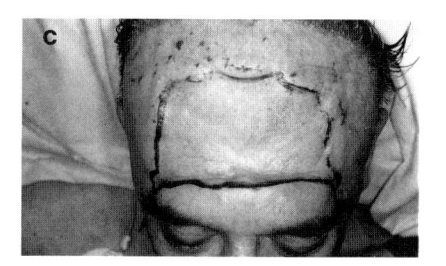

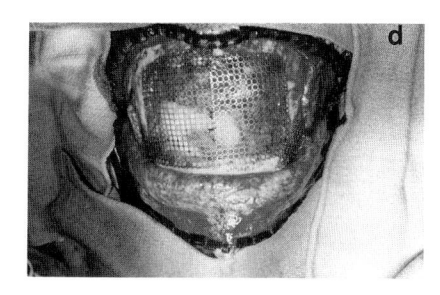

Figure 41.19 The use of micromesh is helpful in areas where defects are not complex. This allows a rapid intraoperative reconstruction with a stable result. This patient demonstrates the loss of the frontal bone flap following an infection. (a) Frontal view. (b) Lateral view. (c) The outline of the defect demonstrates its extent. (d) Two 6 × 8 cm micromesh plates were placed side by side and secured with microscrews to reconstruct the defect. (e) Marlex mesh is used to add support to the soft tissues so that the fenestrated design of the plates will not show through the skin. (f) The patient is shown four months after surgery. A smooth contour is achieved that maintains support of the soft tissue and results in an aesthetically acceptable result. Frontal view. (g) Lateral view.

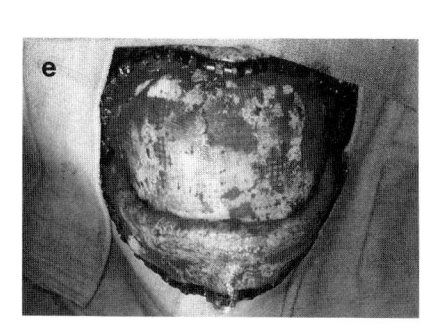

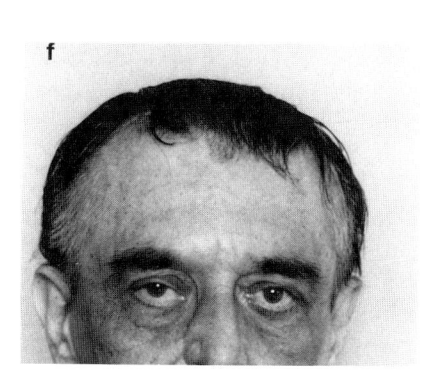

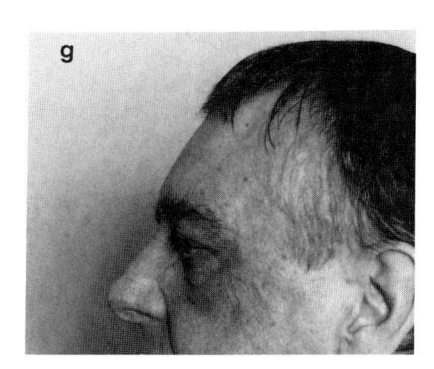

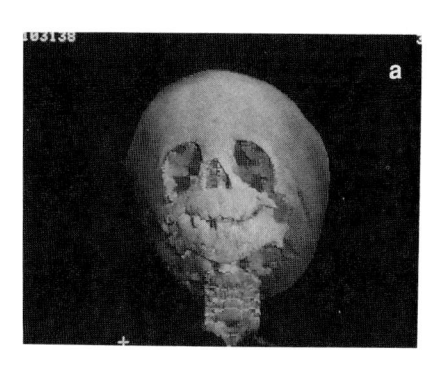

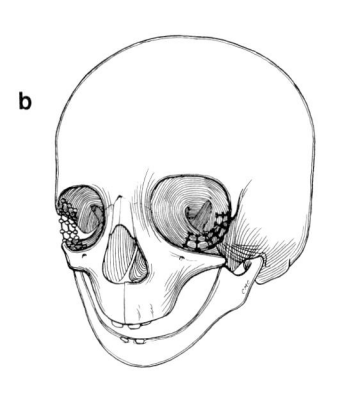

Figure 41.20 (a) In some areas where bone is missing, plating sheet can help create a scaffold for placement of additional grafts for support of additional reconstruction materials. For example, a plating sheet can be used to bridge the bony clefts in this patient, who has Treacher Collins syndrome. Preoperative frontal CT view. (b) Artist's depiction shows mesh bridging the orbital clefts.

(Converse 1977, Dufresne 1989, Luhr 1987b, McNamara 1982, Michelet 1973, Morgan 1987, Muhlbauer 1987a).

Due to the presence of the maxillary sinuses and areas of thin bone, the maxilla is often fractured with traumatic blows to the region. In the case of elective surgery the maxilla is often osteotomized in these areas. Long plates can be used to link the upper cranial base or cranium to the maxilla to establish midface height. These plates are most often placed along the maxillary buttresses in order to produce enough stability to withstand the normal forces of mastication (Kellman 1987, Luhr 1985a, 1985b, 1986, 1987a, 1990). Correction of long or short face syndrome, as well as more complicated rotations, asymmetric advancement, and impaction—as found in hemifacial microsomia patients—can be readily accomplished in a similar manner (Beals 1987, Converse 1977, Munro 1987).

In adult patients, multiple large rigid fixation devices can be used to secure the osteotomies or grafts in the desired position, and these devices can be left in place with little consequence. However, in young children and infants the reconstruction presents more complex problems. The restoration of normal anatomy and contour has to be balanced against the risk of later disturbance of growth potential of various regions. The neurocranial remodeling can be extrapolated or "overcorrected" with relative accuracy because growth is essentially completed by age three (Converse 1977, Enlow 1975). In the facial area, growth can continue up to age 16 in females and over 18 in males (Enlow 1975). Rigid fixation devices are used for only a short while (three to four months) to allow for osteosynthesis, after which they are removed. If left in an area of protracted growth, these devices constrict the full potential of a given region. Careful follow-up and monitoring are needed of children who have required rigid fixation devices, particularly in the facial skeleton.

Facial clefting syndromes can involve the mandible, maxilla, zygoma, orbits, and neurocranium. Reconstruction proceeds as outlined previously, but is often done in stages for the best results. The problems are handled by first reconstructing the skeletal framework of the neurocranium and then dealing with the associated soft-tissue defects of the midface and orbits. Later, the skeletal osteotomies will have to be carried out in the midface in order to "normalize" the facial features as the patient grows (Beals 1987, Carlson 1971, Champy 1982, Converse 1977, Dufresne 1989, Marchac 1978, McNamara 1982, Michelet 1973, Morgan 1987, Muhlbauer 1987a, 1987b).

Hypertelorism reconstruction is a useful example to demonstrate the combination of upper and midfacial reconstruction. Hypertelorism is often the result of a midfacial clefting syndrome. In Tessier's classification, it is referred to as a 0–14 cleft. It will often lead to deformities of the frontal bone, orbits, nose, and maxilla (Converse 1977, Dufresne 1987). Some of the best results are accomplished when the children are about to enter school, when growth is more complete and less subsequent changes are to be expected. Very young patients with severe anomalies can be reconstructed early; however, growth from the maxillofacial region will often have to be corrected or adjusted a number of times as the child continues to grow (see Figure 41.21). Reconstruction is concentrated around the naso-orbital region, with a transposition of the orbits and a combined reconstruction of the nose and maxilla. In very young patients, who have their secondary dentition still high in the upper maxilla, high maxillary osteotomies can be carried out in order to preserve these structures. Here, the osteotomies are carried through only the fronto-zygomatic sutures and medial orbital walls. The globes are transposed and grafts are placed against the orbital wall in order to maintain more medial globe position (see Figure 41.22). In cases such as lateral orbital clefting syndromes, vertical dystopia, and Treacher Collins syndrome—where some lateral orbital skeleton is actually missing—mesh plating has been useful in restoring continuity of the bony tissue. Additional bone grafts can be placed on the mesh plates that act as scaffolding. Plates or screws can also be used to incorporate the medial canthoplasty portion of the procedure to a stable area in the facial skeleton as well as to offer additional support for the reconstruction.

In cases of congenital clefts, bone grafts can be applied to areas where bridging is needed to establish proper width and occlusion. In cases where a class III malocclusion is present, as in some craniosynostosis syndromes or cleft patients, often a two-piece or three-piece Le Fort I maxillary osteotomy has to be carried out. In some patients, expansion of the maxilla is carried out with a split of the midline and intradental as well as upper maxillary fixation. In these instances, stability and fewer incidences of relapse can be brought about by rigid fixation. Immediate mobilization of the mandible without the need for maxillo-mandibular fixation (MMF) has helped to reduce facial edema and discomfort, temporomandibular joint (TMJ) stiffness, and the length of the hospital stay.

Congenital maxillary hypoplasia as seen in Crouzon's disease and Binder's syndrome can easily be treated with Le Fort III/Le Fort I maxillary osteotomies, or, in the latter syndrome, with segmented maxillary osteotomies (see Figure 41.23); or with modified Le Fort I or Le Fort II osteotomies (see Figures 41.24 and 41.25). In these cases, postoperative (MMF) can be avoided. Patients are more accepting of this, and they are better able to maintain oral hygiene. There is less edema and less discomfort without the use of MMF. Cost effectiveness is manifested by minimal need for ICU beds and shortened hospital stay.

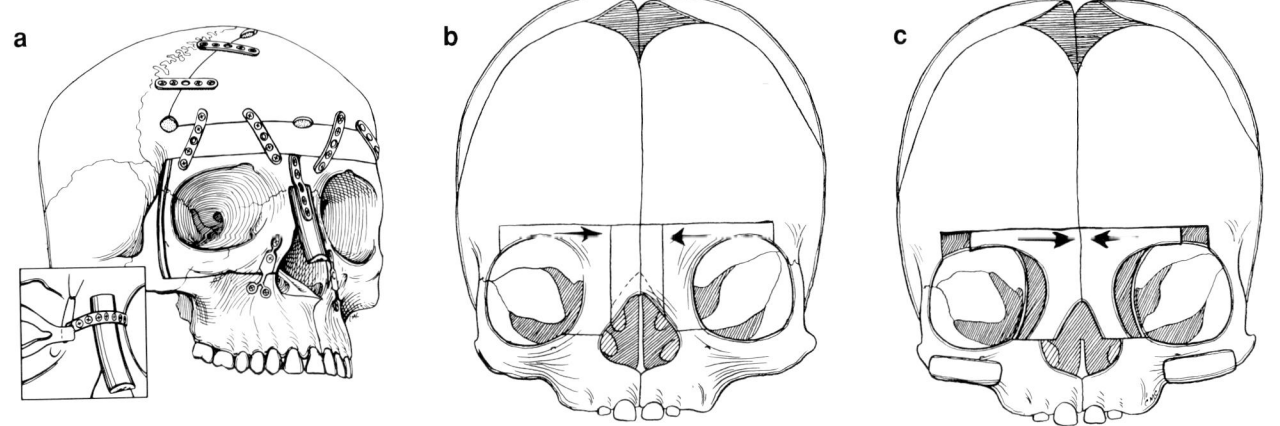

Figure 41.21 (a) Hypertelorism corrections can be quite complicated. Fixation devices may incorporate the medial canthoplasties (inset) and nasal grafts. This results in more predictable and stable reconstructions. (b) In young infants, because of the proximity of the permanent dentition, limited osteotomies are carried out in order to reduce the interorbital tissue. Bone grafts are required at the lateral orbital walls to maintain the globes in the new position. The design of the osteotomy is shown. (c) The medial orbits are shown transposed.

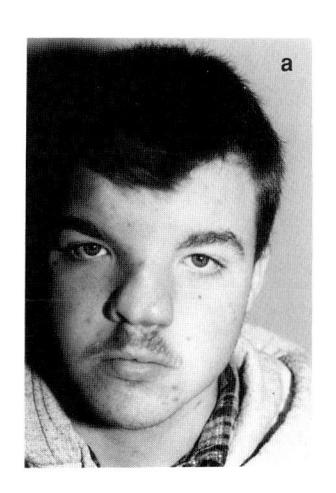

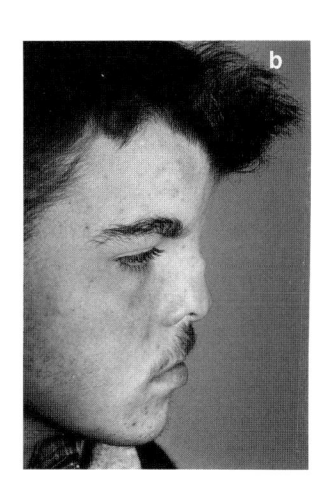

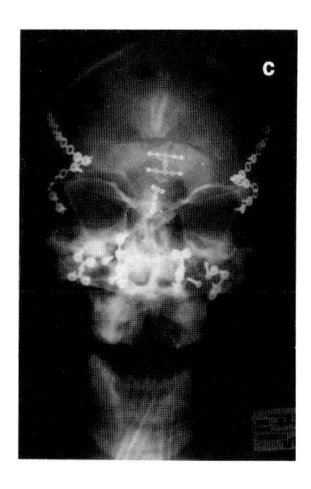

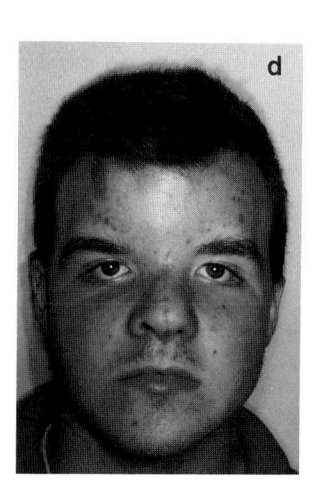

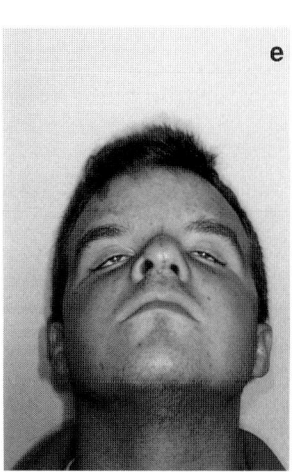

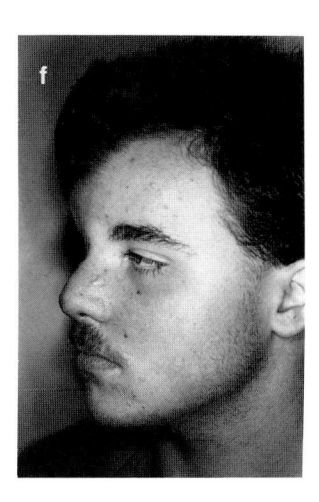

Figure 41.22 (a) This patient reveals a midline clefting syndrome (Tessier 0–14 facial cleft) that has resulted in class II hypertelorism (40-millimeter intercanthal distance). The midface, maxilla, nasal structures, and periorbital structures are affected. Frontal view. (b) Lateral view. (c) Postoperative x ray reveals the fixation of the frontal bone flaps, orbital bone flaps, and the nasal and maxillary bone grafts. (d) The patient is shown three months after surgery. A more balanced and normal facial architecture is seen. Frontal view. (e) Worm's eye view. (f) Oblique view.

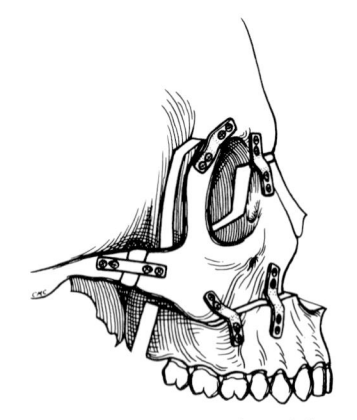

Figure 41.23 The use of rigid fixation has allowed segmentation of maxillary osteotomies accompanied by better security and less chance of relapse. This figure demonstrates a combination of Le Fort I and III osteotomies to allow for a single-stage reconstruction of a severe midface retrusion.

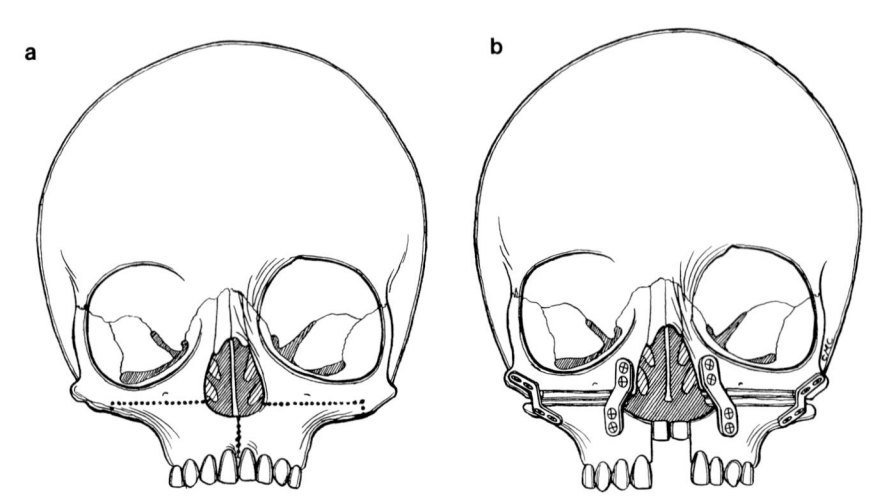

Figure 41.24 In young patients, maxillary osteotomies can be achieved above the permanent dentition. This figure demonstrates the midpalatal split and advancement of the lower maxilla. (a) Proposed osteotomies. (b) After mobilization and fixation.

MANDIBULAR RECONSTRUCTION

Standard mandibular reconstruction often uses lag screws for rigid fixation of advancement or retrusion of congenital mandibular occlusion problems (Prein 1987, Rahn 1987). More aesthetic osteotomies can be made quite stable when combined with such procedures as sliding genioplasties. Here reduction, advancement, and/or augmentation add to the quality of the result because of the surgeon's ability to reconstruct rigidly this portion of the mandible. Segmental osteotomies, which offer better stability and more predictable outcome, can also be easily performed (see Figure 41.26).

SUMMARY

The application of rigid fixation devices has expanded the craniomaxillofacial surgeon's armamentarium and allows her or him greater versatility of osteotomy design and fixation. Further studies are in

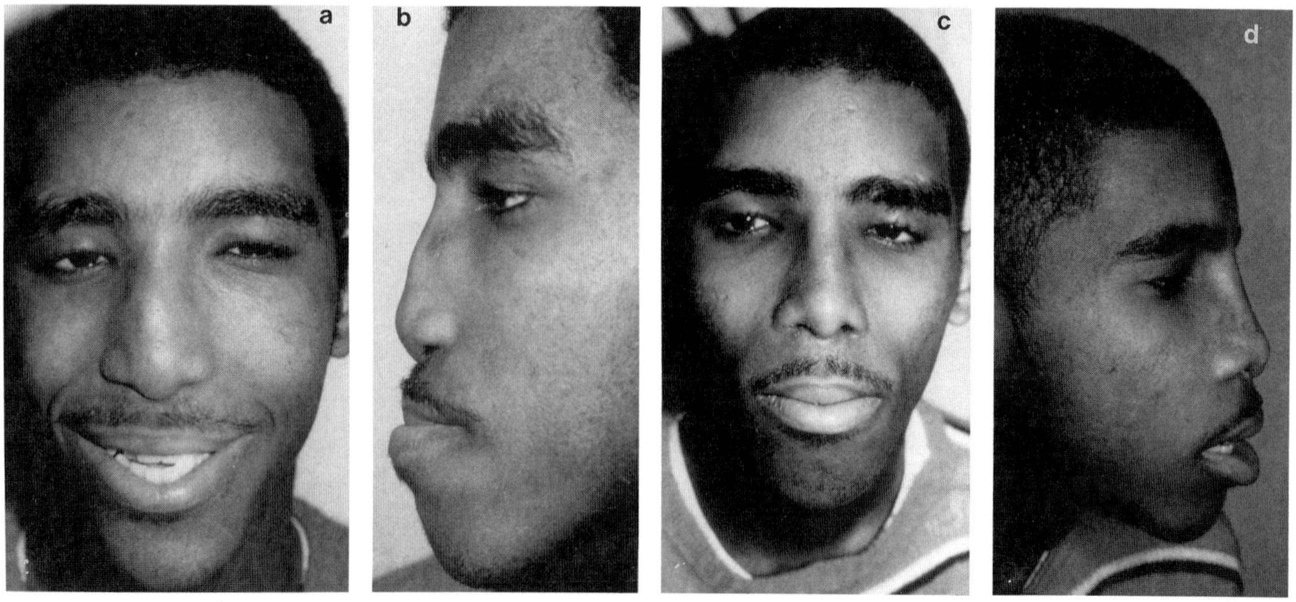

Figure 41.25 This patient demonstrated lower maxillary/nasal dysplasia. A midsegmental maxillary advancement was performed with concomitant nasal reconstruction to improve breathing. (a) Preoperative frontal view. (b) Preoperative lateral view. (c) Postoperative frontal view. (d) Postoperative lateral view.

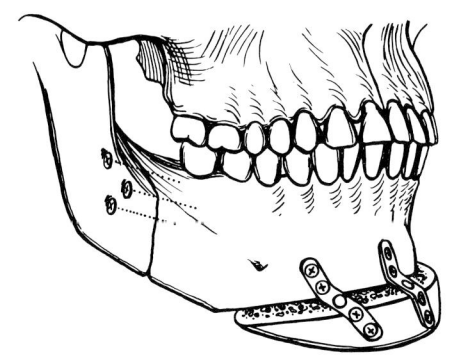

Figure 41.26 Multiple segmental mandibular osteotomies offer better stability when performed with rigid fixation. This figure demonstrates a sagittal split with an advancement genioplasty. The genioplasty segment can also be split, expanded, or reduced in size.

progress to determine the best devices and materials to allow for the most ideal reconstruction. Surgeons want to minimize the degree of disturbance of growth as a result of the application of these rigid fixation devices, and they want to be able to guide the specific pattern of healing and growth in the young craniofacial skeleton. Preliminary studies have shown that the bone is dynamic and "liquid" enough to allow the driving forces of the developing cerebral tissues to remodel and recontour the bone tissue into a normal configuration and contour. Problems with relapse and resorption appear greatly reduced for both bone grafts and flaps following the use of rigid fixation techniques. As the biomaterials industry continues to perfect their devices, and as surgeons continue to be creative in their application of these materials and devices, the future appears to be a very exciting one for craniomaxillofacial surgery.

REFERENCES

Beals SP, Munro IR: The use of miniplates in craniomaxillofacial surgery. Plast Reconstr Surg 79:33–38, 1987.

Carlson DS: Temporal variation in prehistoric Nubian crania. Am J Phys Anthropol 34:191–204, 1971.

Champy M: Treatment of a concave face. Ann Clin Plast 161:27–35, 1982.

Converse JM, McCarthy JG, Wood-Smith D, Coccaro PJ: Principles of craniofacial surgery. In Reconstructive Plastic Surgery. Converse J (ed). Philadelphia, Saunders, vol 4. pp 2427–2492, 1977.

Drommer R, Luhr HG: The stabilization of osteotomized maxillary segments with Luhr miniplates in secondary cleft surgery. J Maxillofac Surg 9:139–198, 1981.

Dufresne C: Rigid fixation: Variations in osteotomy design and technique. Clin Plast Surg 16:165–175, 1989.

Dufresne C, Jelks G: Classification of craniofacial malformations. In Ophthalmic Plastic and Reconstructive Surgery. vol 2. Smith B (ed). St. Louis, Mosby, pp 1185–1207, 1987.

Enlow DH: Handbook of Facial Growth. Philadelphia, Saunders, 1975.

Harle F: Le Fort I osteotomy (using miniplates) for correction of the long face. Int J Oral Surg 9:427–430, 1980.

Horster W: Experience with functionally stable plate osteosynthesis after forward displacement of the upper jaw. J Maxillofac Surg 8:176–181, 1980.

Jackson IT: Transposition cranioplasty to restore forehead contour in craniofacial deformities. J Plast Surg 31:127–130, 1978.

Kellman RM, Schilli W: Plate fixation of fractures of the mid and upper face. Otolaryngol Clin North Am 20:441–456, 1987.

Kruger E, Krumholz K: Results of bone grafting after rigid fixation. J Oral Maxillofac Surg 42:491–496, 1984.

Luhr HG: Basic research, surgical technique and results of fracture treatment with the Luhr mandibular-compression-screw system (MCS-System). In Oral and Maxillofacial Surgery: Proceedings from the 8th International Conference on Oral and Maxillofacial Surgery, Hjorting-Hansen E. Chicago, Quintessence, pp 124–132, 1985a.

Luhr HG, Drommer R, Holscher U, Schauer HW: Comparative studies between the extraoral and intraoral approach in compression osteosynthesis of mandible fractures. In Oral and Maxillofacial Surgery: Proceedings from the 8th International Conference on Oral and Maxillofacial Surgery, Hjorting-Hansen E. Chicago, Quintessence, pp 133–137, 1985b.

Luhr HG: Midface fractures involving the orbit and blow-out fractures. In Oral and Maxillofacial Traumatology. vol 2. Kruger E, Shilli W, Worthington P (eds). Chicago, Quintessence, pp 197–222, 1986.

Luhr HG: Vitallium Luhr systems for reconstructive surgery for the facial skeleton. Otolaryngol Clin North Am 20:573–606, 1987a.

Luhr HG: Rigid facial skeletal fixation: past, present, and future. Presented at the Kazanjian Lecture to the American Society of Maxillofacial Surgeons, Atlanta, Ga. November, 1987b.

Luhr HG: A microsystem for cranio-maxillofacial skeletal fixation. J Cranio-Max Fac Surg 16:312–414, 1988.

Luhr HG: Indications for use of a microsystem for internal fixation in craniofacial surgery. J Craniofac Surg 1:35–52, 1990.

Marchac D: Radical forehead remodeling for craniostenosis. Plast Reconstr Surg 61:823–835, 1978.

McCarthy JG, Coccaro PJ, Epstein F, Converse JM: Early skeletal release in the infant with craniofacial synostosis. Plast Reconstr Surg 62:335–346, 1978.

McNamara JA, Carlov DS, Ribbens KA: The effect of surgical intervention on craniofacial growth. 1982.

Michelet FX, Deymes J, and Dessus B: Osteosynthesis with miniaturized screwed plates in maxillofacial surgery. J Maxillofac Surg 1:79, 1973.

Morgan F: Personal communication, 1987.

Muhlbauer W, Anderl H: Use of miniplates in craniofacial surgery. In Craniofacial Surgery. Proceedings of the 1st International Society of Cranio-maxillo-facial surgery. Marchac D (ed). Berlin, Springer-Verlag, pp 334–337, 1987a.

Muhlbauer W, Anderl H, Heckt P, Ramatschi P, Vertesy E: Early facial advancement in craniofacial stenosis. In Craniofacial Surgery. Proceedings of the 1st International Society of Cranio-maxillo-facial surgery. Marchac D (ed). Berlin, Springer-Verlag, pp 123–129, 1987b.

Muhlbauer W, Anderl H, Ramatschi P, et al: Radical treatment of craniofacial anomalies in infancy and the use of miniplates in craniofacial surgery. Clin Plast Surg 14: 101–111, 1987c.

Muhling J, Reuther J, Sorensen N: Therapy for severe craniostenosis. In Craniofacial Surgery. Proceedings of the 1st International Society of Cranio-maxillo-facial surgery. Marchac D (ed). Berlin, Springer-Verlag, pp 88–90, 1987.

Munro I: The use of miniplates in cranio-maxillo-facial surgery. In Craniofacial Surgery. Proceedings of the 1st International Society of Cranio-maxillo-facial surgery. Marchac D (ed). Berlin, Springer-Verlag, pp 338–340, 1987.

Nand R: Effect of maxillary osteotomy on subsequent craniofacial growth in adolescent monkeys. Am J Orthod 83:391–407, 1983.

Ortiz-Monasterio F, Fuente del Campo A, Carillo A: Advancement of the orbits and the midface in one piece, combined with frontal repositioning for the correction of Crouzon's deformity. Plast Reconstr Surg 61:507–516, 1978.

Paulus GW: A comparative study of wire osteosynthesis versus screws in the treatment of mandibular prognathism. Oral Surg 54:2–6, 1982.

Phillips JH, Rahn BA: Fixation effects on membranous and endochondral bone graft revascularization and bone deposition. Plast Reconstr Surg 85:891–897, 1990.

Prein J, Kellman RM: Rigid internal fixation of mandibular fractures: Basics of AO technique. Otolaryngol Clin North Am 20:559–572, 1987.

Rahn BA: Direct and indirect bone healing after operative fracture treatment. Otolaryngol Clin North Am 20:425–440, 1987.

Raveh J, Vuillemin T: The subcranial-supraorbital and temporal approach for tumor resection. J Craniofac Surg 1:53–59, 1990.

Rittersma J, van der Veld RGM, van Gool AV, Kopperdraarier J: Stable fragment fixation in orthognathic surgery: Review of 30 cases. J Oral Surg 39:671–675, 1981.

Rosen HM: Miniplate fixation of Le Fort I osteotomies. Plast Reconstr Surg 78:748–755, 1986.

Salyer KE, Hall JD: Bandeau: The focal point of frontocranial remodeling. J Craniofac Surg 1:18–31, 1990.

Schatzker J, Sanderson R, Murnaghan JP: The holding power of orthopedic screws, in vivo. Clin Orthop 108:115–126, 1975.

Schilli W, Evers R, Niederdellmann H: Bone fixation with screws and plates in the maxillofacial region. Int J Oral Surg 10 (Suppl. 1):329–332, 1981.

Schmoker R: The eccentric dynamic compression plate: An experimental study as to its contribution to the functionally stable internal fixation of fractures of the lower jaw. AO Bulletin 1–36, April, 1976.

Schmoker R, Van Allman T, Tschop HM: Application of functionally stable fixation in maxillofacial surgery secondary to ASIF principles. J Oral Maxillofac Surg 40:457–461, 1982.

Schmoker RR: Mandibular reconstruction using a special plate: Animal experiments and clinical application. J Maxillofac Surg 11:99–148, 1983.

Steinhausser EW: Bone screws and plates in orthognathic surgery. Int J Oral Surg 11:209–223, 1982.

Vangsness CT, Carter D, Frankel VH: In vitro evaluation of the loosening characteristics of self-tapped and non-self tapped cortical bone screws. Clin Orthop 157:279–290, 1981.

Whitaker LA, Broennle A, Kerr L, Herlich A: Improvements in craniofacial reconstruction: Methods evolved in 235 consecutive patients. Plast Reconstr Surg 65:561–573, 1980.

Wong L, Dufresne C, Richtsmeir JT, Manson PN: The effect of rigid fixation on growth of the neurocranium. Plast Reconstr Surg 88:395–403. October, 1989.

Worthington P, Champy M: Monocortical miniplate osteosynthesis. Otolaryngol Clin North Am 20: 607–615, 1987.

CHAPTER 42

Rigid Fixation of Le Fort III Osteotomies

Joseph G. McCarthy
P. Craig Hobar
Barry H. Grayson

The first Le Fort III osteotomy was reported by Gillies and Harrison in 1950, eight years after it was actually performed (Gillies 1950). Tessier popularized the procedure and wrote extensively on the technical aspects as well as the clinical applications (Tessier 1967, 1971a, 1971b). Several others (Murray 1968, Jabaley 1969, Ortiz-Monasterio 1978, Obwegeser 1969) also contributed to the early development of the operation. The procedure is now commonly performed in many craniofacial centers for the treatment of craniofacial synostosis—for example, Apert syndrome and Crouzon's disease—and other types of midface hypoplasia or retrusion.

The continuing development of pediatric anesthesia, including thermoregulation, oxygen saturation monitoring, and hypotensive techniques, has made the Le Fort III osteotomy a safe procedure with low mortality (less than 1%). Concomitant with improvements in anesthesia has come experience with the Le Fort III osteotomy as performed on younger patients. McCarthy (1984) and Bachmayer (1986) and associates independently demonstrated the safety of the procedure and the absence of adverse developmental effects in young children. The procedure is now frequently performed in children as young as three years of age in some craniofacial centers. A significant recent advance has been the use of rigid skeletal fixation, which in most cases obviates the need for prolonged maxillomandibular fixation (MMF) and tracheotomy.

ANATOMY

In its classic form, the Le Fort III osteotomy produces separation of the entire facial mass (nose, maxilla, and zygomas) from the base of the cranium to allow movement of the face independent of the cranium and mandible (see Figure 42.1). The operation may be performed either through an extracranial (subcranial) or combined intracranial/extracranial approach; the former is preferred unless recontouring of forehead, orbit, or brow is also required.

Advancement of the facial mass relative to the cranium accomplishes several goals:

1. It improves the appearance of the individual with midface hypoplasia by establishing a balance among the key projecting components of the cranium, midface, zygomas, and mandible;
2. It reduces exorbitism by increasing orbital volume; and
3. It corrects the associated class III malocclusion.

DIAGNOSIS

Evaluation of the patient begins with careful inquiry into the patient's perception of his or her deformity. The history should also detail previous surgical procedures and othodontic therapy. Physical examination should pay particular attention to the degree of exorbitism, position of the brows and contour of the frontal bone, position of the inferior orbital rims, projection or retroposition of the cheekbones and pyriform aperture areas, length and projection of the nose, occlusal status, and quality of the overlying soft tissue.

Life-size frontal and lateral photographs aid in preoperative analysis. Cephalograms are essential in defining the skeletal abnormalities and in projecting surgical movements. Dental study models are used to

Figure 42.1 Anatomy of Le Fort III advancement osteotomy. (a) Skeletal pathology of midface hypoplasia with malocclusion and anterior crossbite is shown. (b) The mobilized segment includes the nasomaxillary complex and associated zygomas. Note the anteroinferior (arrow) translation of the segment.

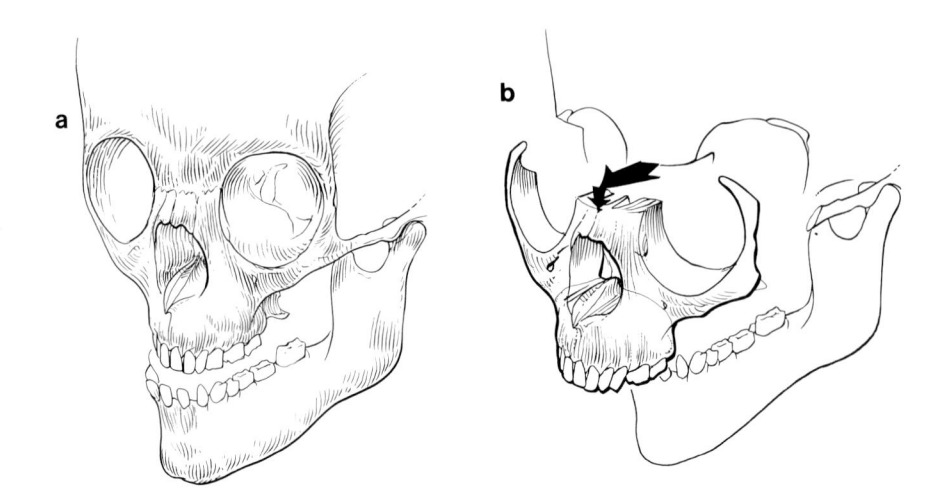

evaluate arch relationships and to plan preoperative orthodontic therapy.

Single-Segment Osteotomy

The classic midface deformity associated with craniofacial synostosis is characterized by (usually symmetric) retropositioning or underdevelopment of the maxilla, zygomatic complexes, and nose. The typical facies includes varying degrees of exorbitism; retruded midface; and a shortened, underprojecting nose. A class III malocclusion is characteristic (see Figure 42.2).

Cephalometric radiographs are taken using standard techniques, and the lateral cephalogram is traced to distinguish bony landmarks. Details of cephalometric analysis are beyond the scope of this chapter, but a summary of important steps pertinent to the Le Fort III osteotomy follows. The analysis is divided into *vertical facial, horizontal midfacial, horizontal lower facial,* and *dental* measurements (Grayson 1989). The patient's results are compared to normative data, controlling for age, sex, and size of the patient. In the patient with midfacial hypoplasia, the usual findings are a marked deficiency of the horizontal midface measurements combined with a variable degree of decreased midface height.

Presurgical orthodontic evaluation is necessary to ensure proper arch relationship for optimal occlusion after movement of the midface complex. Orthodontic therapy (for example, changing incisor inclination, transverse maxillary expansion) may be necessary for six to twelve months before the operation.

Mock surgery on dental study models is undertaken to prepare an interocclusal splint (wafer) that can be used intraoperatively to ascertain the proper position of the maxillary segment relative to the mandibular dentition. The dental study models are mounted on a three-dimensional articulator, and the mock osteotomies are performed on the maxillary segment to produce forward advancement and inferior displacement.

Figure 42.2 This patient has craniofacial synostosis (Crouzon syndrome) characterized by retrusion of the nose and inferior orbital rims, zygoma, and maxilla. (a) Preoperative appearance. (b) Postoperative appearance after Le Fort III advancement and genioplasty. (From McCarthy JG, Epstein FJ, Wood-Smith D: Craniosynostosis. In Plastic Surgery, McCarthy JG (ed). Philadelphia, Saunders, 1990.)

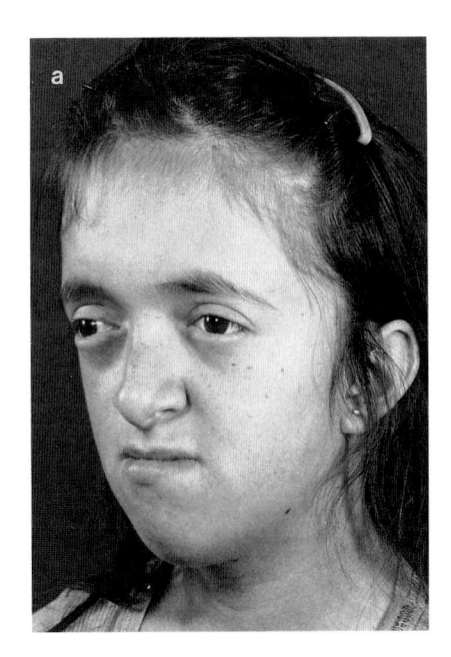

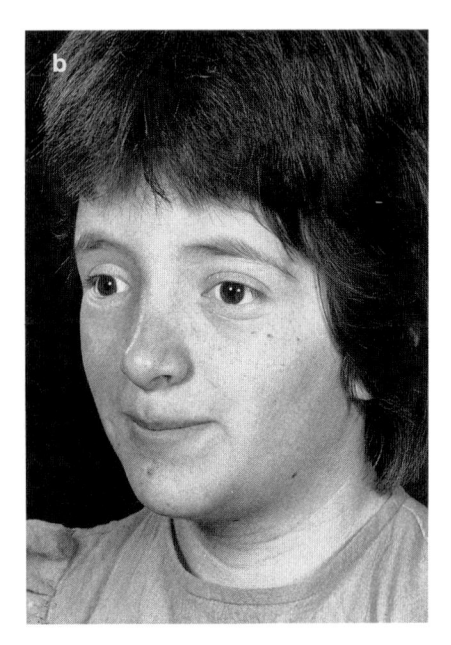

The amount of forward advancement is determined by optimal occlusion and facial appearance. The horizontal midfacial cephalometric landmarks of a representative normal population aid in planning the advancement but should not take precedence over movements dictated by the patient's unique facial morphology and dental occlusion. The soft-tissue attachments to the mobilized segments can limit the degree of advancement that can be accomplished, but 12 to 18 mm of advancement at the incisor level is usually possible.

Inferior displacement (rotation to close an open bite) is limited by the esthetic effects of the corresponding nasal lengthening. In adults, downward rotation is terminated when the desired nasal length is obtained and any remaining open bite is corrected by a separate Le Fort I osteotomy. Closure of a large open bite using a Le Fort III procedure alone can result in an excessively long nose. If a Le Fort I osteotomy is planned in combination with the Le Fort III, two occlusal splints are fabricated, an *intermediate* one and a *definitive* one (see Chapter 34). The intermediate splint retains a calculated amount of open bite to prevent excessive nasal lengthening from inferior displacement of the maxilla after the Le Fort III osteotomy. A Le Fort I osteotomy is then performed, and the ideal occlusion is achieved with the definitive splint, thus preventing undesired nasal lengthening.

In a child, a Le Fort I osteotomy is inadvisable because of the position of the unerupted maxillary teeth, and a residual open bite is preferable to excessive nasal lengthening. The splint is constructed to permit a residual open bite and, if vertical maxillary growth and orthodontic therapy have not corrected the problem by adolescence, a Le Fort I or segmental maxillary osteotomy is done at that time.

Multiple-Segment Osteotomy

At times the various subunits of the midface (nose, maxilla, and zygomas) will not be optimally positioned if moved forward en masse, and differential movements are preferred. This technique requires either staging of the procedure, with secondary movement of one or more of the subunits, or multiple osteotomies that allow movement of the nose, maxilla, and zygomas as separate units, with positioning guided by multiple intermediate splints (Cutting 1991).

TECHNIQUE

General anesthesia is induced via a nasotracheal tube secured with a silk suture through the membranous septum. A minimum of two intravenous lines are inserted, one of which must be sufficiently large to administer packed red blood cells in an unimpeded fashion. The patient is monitored with an arterial line, a transcutaneous oxygen saturation monitor, a rectally placed temperature probe, and a presternal stethoscope. Monitoring devices are purposely kept away from the facial area to avoid interference with the surgical procedure.

A bicoronal scalp incision is made well posterior to the hairline, extending from the root of the helix on one side to the root of the opposite helix. The flap is elevated in a subperiosteal plane centrally and at a level superficial to the deep temporal fascia laterally. Elevation is carried well onto the root of the nose and into the orbit circumferentially in a plane deep to the periorbita. The temporalis muscle is reflected from the fossa to expose the lateral orbital wall. The portion of the temporalis fascia inserting on the zygomatic arch is incised to allow access to the arch; care is taken to remain deep to the frontal branch of the facial nerve. Anterior to the desired osteotomy site, the zygomatic arch is cleared of periosteal and masseter muscle attachments. The lacrimal sac is reflected from the groove in a posterior to anterior direction. The nasolacrimal duct and attachments of the medial canthal ligaments are preserved. The orbital floor is approached through the bicoronal incision and exposed from a lateral to medial direction. Eyelid incisions are optional but can usually be avoided. A sufficient amount of the orbital perimeter is exposed for the osteotomies to be made at least 10 millimeters behind the orbital rim, but caution should be exercised because the orbital depth is markedly reduced in patients with craniofacial synostosis.

Before the osteotomies are begun, hypotensive anesthesia is instituted to minimize blood loss. With a mechanical saw, osteotomies are made in full-thickness fashion through the superolateral aspect of the orbital rim (1), lateral orbital wall (2), and zygomatic arch (3) (see Figure 42.3). A rim of bone is preserved posteriorly in the lateral orbital wall to allow fixation of the bone

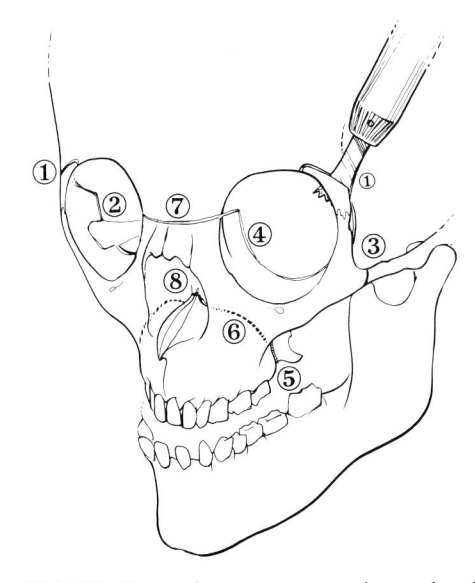

Figure 42.3 The lines of osteotomy are shown for the Le Fort III advancement.

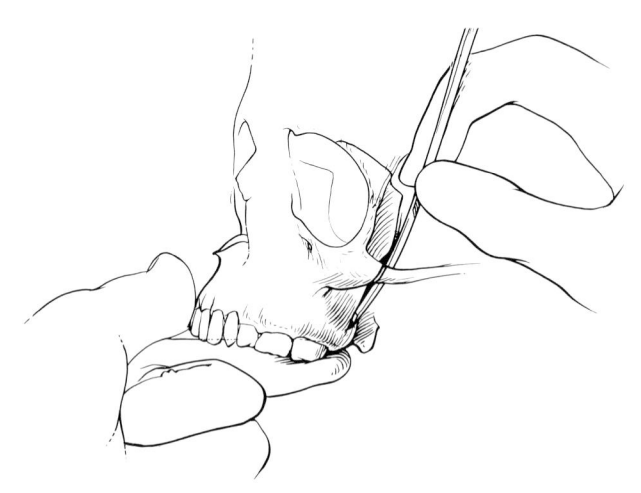

Figure 42.4 Pterygomaxillary dysjunction is demonstrated. The osteotome is placed in the pterygomaxillary fissure via the temporal fossa. The operator's finger placed on the occlusal surface of the maxillary molars ensures accurate placement of the osteotome.

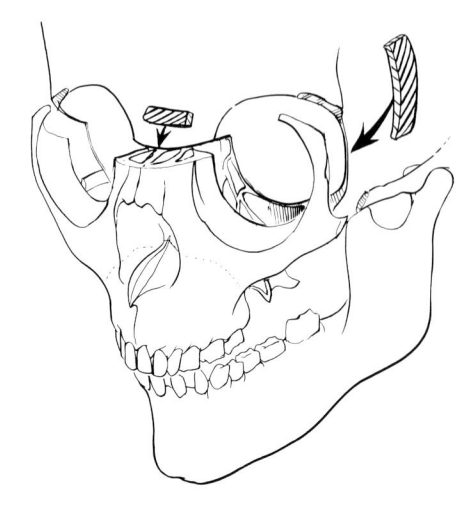

Figure 42.5 Autogenous bone grafts are placed in the defects at the nasofrontal junction and lateral orbital walls. Grafts are not routinely placed in the voids at the zygomatic arches or pterygomaxillary fissures.

grafts. The osteotomies through the orbital floor and medial orbital wall are made with a fine osteotome at least 10 millimeters behind the rim and directed toward the inferior orbital fissure (Tessier 1971a). Pterygomaxillary dysjunction is achieved with a curved osteotome that is inserted through the bicoronal incision and temporal fossa (Murray 1968). The operator's finger is placed behind the alveolar ridge to assure that the osteotome is accurately placed between the maxillary tuberosity and the pterygoid plates, that is, the most avascular plane (see Figure 42.4). Alternatively, the pterygomaxillary dysjunction can be performed through separate buccovestibular (intraoral) incisions.

Intact bone remains only at the root of the nose and between the inferolateral portion of the orbital osteotomy and the pterygomaxillary dysjunction. An osteotome (see Figure 42.3) is inserted through the temporal fossa to the inferolateral portion of the orbital osteotomy and directed toward a finger placed in the mouth at the pterygomaxillary junction (Jabaley 1969). To prevent troublesome bleeding, all soft tissue must be removed from the intervening segment. The osteotomy at the root of the nose is completed last because bleeding from the nasal mucosa is brisk until the facial mass has been completely mobilized (Ortiz-Monasterio 1978). Finally, the septum is transected in a superoanterior to inferoposterior direction with Mayo scissors or a handheld osteotome gently driven by a mallet (Obwegeser 1969). A finger placed around the soft palate and into the nasopharynx prevents injury to the nasotracheal tube and nasogastric tube, if present.

The facial mass is mobilized with Rowe-Killey forceps and/or disimpaction forceps (Tessier) placed posterior to the maxillary tuberosities. Provided all osteotomies are complete and the masseter attachments of the mobilized portion of the zygoma have been elevated, this maneuver should proceed easily.

The previously prepared splint is introduced and wired to the upper teeth by way of either preplaced Guron locks (in adults) or wires suspended from drill holes in the piriform aperture, inferior orbital rims, and/or zygoma (in children). The mobilized segment is then positioned correctly by fitting the lower segment of the splint into the mandibular teeth without displacing the condyles. The previously calculated desired nasal length will determine whether the open-bite deformity will be completely corrected or merely reduced.

After the maxillary segment is stabilized in precise occlusion by use of the splint, permanent stabilization is accomplished with bone grafts and plate fixation. Autogenous bone is the graft material of choice to fill the surgically created defects in the nasofrontal junction, lateral orbital rims, zygomatic arch, and pterygomaxillary space (see Figure 42.5). The preferred donor site is the parietal skull, where split calvarium can be harvested easily through the bicoronal incision. In a young child the calvarium is not reliably developed, and bone is obtained from either the ribs or the ilium. Rigid fixation is established at the nasofrontal junction, lateral orital rims, and zygomatic arches (see Figure 42.6). Vitallium plates are chosen because of their strength when subjected to multiangled configurations and low profile. A T-shaped plate is used at the nasofrontal junction (a microplate should be used in the child with thin overlying skin); C or T-shaped plates are used on the temporal fossa side of the lateral orbital rims; and straight or curved plates are used at the zygomatic arches. Bone grafts are placed in the intervening segments and secured to the Vitallium plates with either wires or screws. After fixation is secure, the maxillo-mandibular wires are removed. Any intraoral incisions are closed with interrupted 3-0 chromic catgut sutures; the reflected temporalis muscles are returned to the temporal fossae (over the miniplates) with sutures; and the scalp is reap-

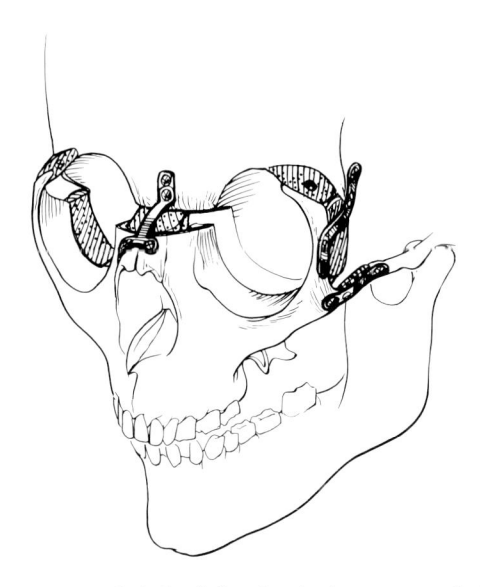

Figure 42.6 Rigid skeletal fixation is demonstrated. A T-shaped miniplate is used at the nasofrontal junction, and a straight or slightly curved miniplate is used at the zygomatic arch. Either a curved or T-shaped miniplate is preferred at the lateral orbital wall. It is important that the miniplate be covered by the repositioned temporalis muscle at the completion of the procedure. Note the associated bone grafts, which can be secured with lag screws (as illustrated) or with interosseous wires.

proximated in two layers. The patient, returned to the recovery room with the nasotracheal tube in place, is extubated when fully awake.

COMPLICATIONS

Several studies evaluating large numbers of patients after major craniofacial procedures (Converse 1975; Whitaker 1979; Munro 1985; David 1987; Poole 1988) show relatively consistent findings: (1) Mortality and morbidity are both significantly higher in intracranial than in extracranial procedures, with mortality rates approximating 1%. (2) Infection is the most common complication but is significantly less in extracranial procedures, averaging approximately 3%. (3) Factors that increase the incidence of infection include prolonged operative time, large areas of dead space (as found in an associated frontal bone advancement), excessive blood loss, and wide communication with the nasal cavity or paranasal sinuses—especially when the patient is mechanically ventilated and the pressure gradient favors transmucosal bacterial contamination of the operative area.

Prophylactic intravenous antibiotics should be administered preoperatively and for 24 to 72 hours postoperatively. If there is communication with the nasal cavity and mechanical ventilation is required, the intravenous antibiotics are continued until either the communication has sealed or the patient is breathing without assistance. A pericranial-galeal flap harvested from the bicoronal flap is used to seal the communication between the cranial and nasal cavities when an intracranial approach is used.

Hemorrhage or excessive blood loss is always a possibility when the highly vascular structures of the face are manipulated. Large areas of exposed soft tissue and bone result from mobilization of the craniofacial skeleton. To minimize blood loss, the procedure should be performed under hypotensive anesthesia and all osteotomy sites should be carefully cleared of soft-tissue attachments. Because transfusion is common in Le Fort III mobilization of the face, this need should be discussed preoperatively with the patient and the family and provisions made for autologous and donor-designated blood for transfusion.

Infrequent complications include injury to the lacrimal drainage apparatus, injury to the frontal branch of the facial nerve, and morbidity related to the bone graft donor sites. These can be avoided with attention to technique.

In affected children, because anterior growth of the midface remains below normal, there is a high incidence of class III malocclusion with anticipated growth of the mandible before and during adolescence. This is an expected sequela, rather than a complication, and is treated by a secondary advancement osteotomy of the maxilla.

Injury to the extraocular muscles should not occur, as all intraorbital dissection is performed in a subperiosteal plane. Strabismus or extraocular muscle dysfunction, if present preoperatively, usually persists postoperatively. If a Le Fort III osteotomy is anticipated, corrective surgery should be deferred until at least six months postoperative (Choy 1979).

LONG-TERM FOLLOW-UP

Multiple reports have documented the long-term stability of the mobilized midface or Le Fort III segment; any occlusal disharmonies observed during long-term follow-up can usually be attributed to expected mandibular growth and development (McCarthy 1984, 1990, Kaban 1984, 1986, Hogeman 1974, Tulasne 1986). Consequently, patients undergoing Le Fort III advancement before mandibular development is complete may require a secondary midface advancement.

Likewise, there can be a recurrence of exorbitism, with recession or remodeling of the advanced zygomatic segment (Hogeman 1974, Tulasne 1986). Studies involving a larger number of patients with longer periods of follow-up are required to document these effects on facial esthetics.

The New York and Toronto centers have independently studied the long-term results of Le Fort III advancement on the growing child under seven years of age (McCarthy 1984, 1990, Bachmayer 1986). All these reports noted the safety of the procedure and the remarkable degree of stability of the mobilized midface segment. Although vertical (inferior) growth of the osteotomized midface segment was demonstrated, anterior growth, if any, was minimal. Any malocclusion that developed during the period of follow-up could be attributed to anticipated mandibular development. Consequently, at operation the child should be placed in an exaggerated class II occlusion, and the family should be forewarned of the need for a secondary midface advancement during adolescence.

CASE STUDY

C.T. is a four-year-old boy with Apert syndrome and a cleft of the soft palate. At age six months he underwent a fronto-orbital advancement.

Clinical Examination: At age four he shows mild exorbitism accompanied by inferior orbital rim deficiency and excess scleral show (see Figure 42.7). The nose is reduced in the vertical dimension, and the midface is hypoplastic and concave. The lips are apart at rest, a finding that is a function of mouth breathing and nasal airway obstruction.

Intraoral Examination: He has a class III malocclusion in the deciduous dentition with an anterior crossbite of 4 millimeters and an open bite of 3 millimeters. The palatal vault is high and narrow (see Figure 42.8).

Presurgical Cephalometric Evaluation: horizontal (ANS–PNS) and vertical (ANS–N and Se–PNS) development of the midface is severely deficient. Total face height is reduced as a consequence of the midface vertical deficiency (see Figure 42.9).

Surgical Plan: The surgical plan involved a Le Fort III maxillary advancement of 10 millimeters at the upper incisal edge, 14 millimeters at the anterior nasal spine, and 16 millimeters at the nasion. This translocation resulted in an advancement with mild rotation in an inferior direction at the incisor level. The consequence of this rotation was to lengthen the nose and reduce the open bite.

Preoperative impressions of the teeth were made for the construction of an occlusal splint. The splint was prepared on dental study models with the maxillary teeth advanced into the surgically corrected position. The splint was inserted intraoperatively to achieve the planned advancement and to stabilize the osseous segment while rigid fixation was inserted. Five miniplates

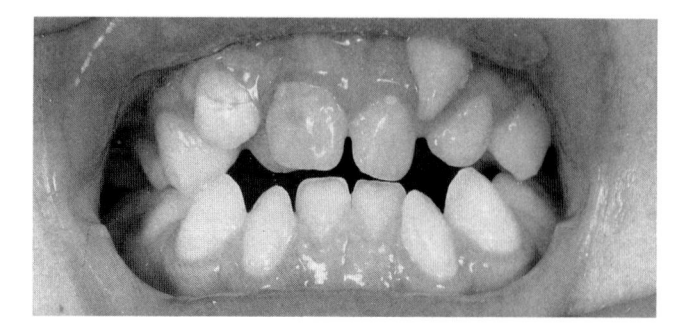

Figure 42.8 Preoperative occlusion.

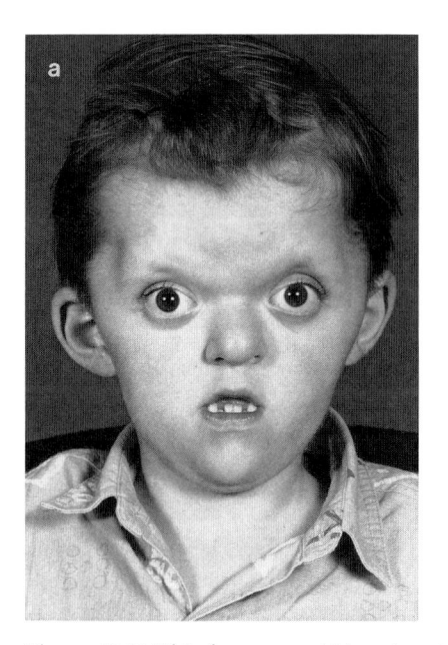

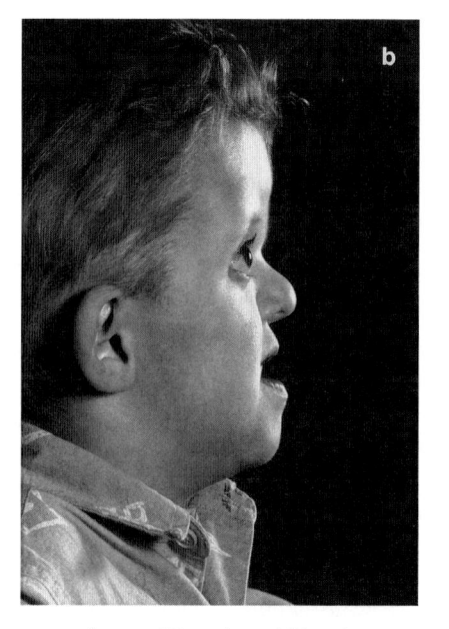

Figure 42.7 This four-year-old boy has Apert syndrome. Note the midface hypoplasia and exorbitism. (a) Frontal view. (b) Profile.

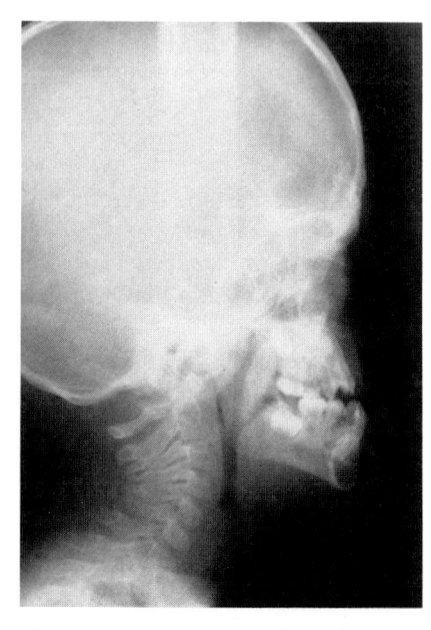

Figure 42.9 Preoperative lateral cephalogram.

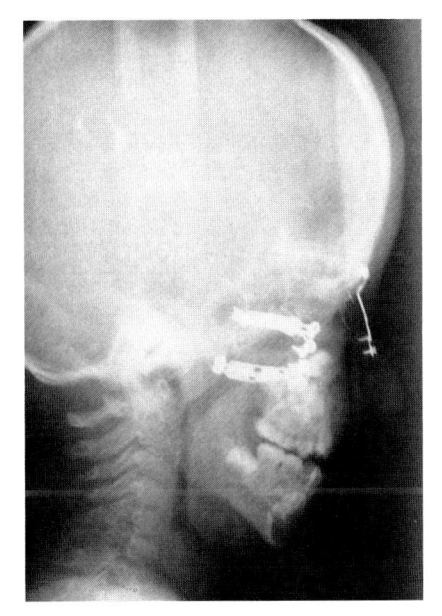

Figure 42.10 Postoperative lateral cephalogram shows the advanced midface segment and miniplates at the nasofrontal junction, temporal fossa, lateral orbital wall (L-shaped) and zygomatic complex (L-shaped).

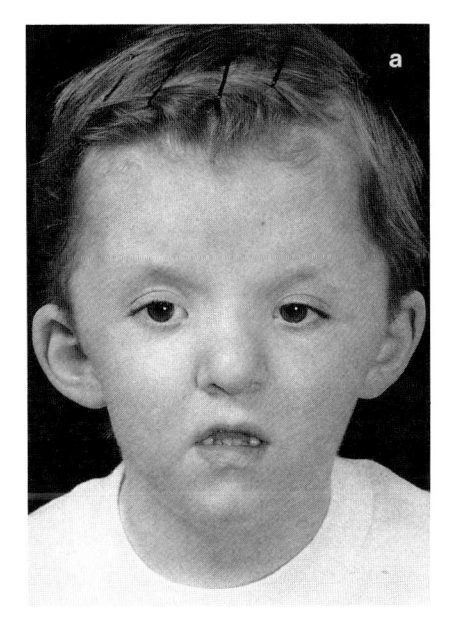

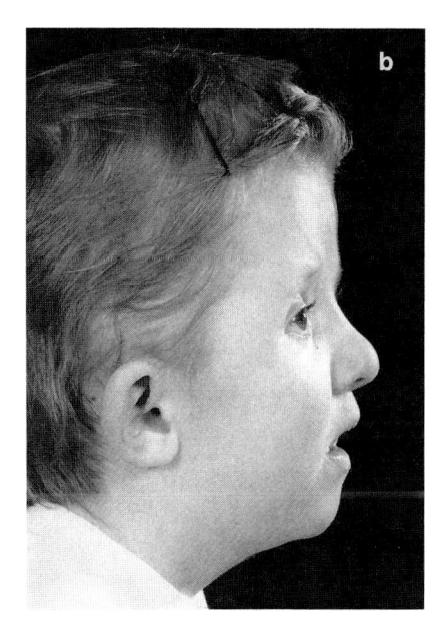

Figure 42.11 Postoperative appearance shows improved midfacial form, lip relationship, and nasal length. The exorbitism has been corrected. (a) Frontal view. (b) Profile.

were used: one at the nasofrontal junction and one each at the left and right temporal fossae and one across each zygomatic arch (see Figure 42.10).

> *Postoperative Course:* The patient was placed on a liquid diet for eight weeks, at the end of which the maxillary splint was removed. Examination of the occlusion revealed an overjet of 3 millimeters with a 2-millimeter open bite. Improved facial convexity and lengthening of the nose were achieved. A functional occlusion was also achieved. The naso-oral airway was opened and the exorbitism was reduced (see Figure 42.11).

REFERENCES

Bachmayer DI, Ross RB, Munro IR: Maxillary growth following Le Fort III advancement surgery in Crouzon, Apert and Pfeiffer syndromes. Am J Orthod Dentofacial Orthod 90:420, 1986.

Choy AE, Margolis S, Breinen GM, McCarthy JG: Analysis of preoperative and postoperative extraocular muscle function in surgical translocation of bony orbits; a preliminary report. In *Symposium on Diagnosis and Treatment of Craniofacial Anomalies.* Converse JM. St. Louis, Mo., Mosby, 1979.

Converse JM, Wood-Smith D, McCarthy JG: Analysis of craniofacial surgery. Plast Reconstr Surg 55:283, 1975.

Cutting CB: Personal communication, 1991.

David DJ, Cooter RD: Craniofacial infection in 10 years of transcranial surgery. Plast Reconstr Surg 80:213, 1987.

Gillies H, Harrison SH: Operative correction by osteotomy of recessed malar maxillary compound in a case of oxycephaly. Br J Plast Surg 2:123, 1950.

Grayson BH: Cephalometric analysis for the surgeon. Clin Plast Surg 16:633, 1989.

Hogeman KE, Willmar K: On Le Fort III osteotomy for Crouzon's disease in children: Report of a four year follow-up in one patient. Scand J Plast Reconstr Surg 8:169, 1974.

Jabaley ME, Edgerton MT: Surgical correction of congenital mid-face retrusion in the presence of mandibular prognathism. Plast Reconstr Surg 44:1, 1969.

Kaban LB, West B, Conover M, et al: Midface position after Le Fort III advancement. Plast Reconstr Surg 73:758, 1984.

Kaban LB, Conover M, Mulliken JB, et al: Midface position after Le Fort III advancement: A long-term follow-up study. Cleft Palate J 23, Suppl: 75, 1986.

McCarthy JG, Grayson B, Bookstein F, Vickery C, Zide B: Le Fort III advancement osteotomy in the growing child. Plast Reconstr Surg 74:343, 1984.

McCarthy JG, LaTrenta GS, Breitbart AS, Grayson BH, Bookstein FL: The Le Fort III advancement osteotomy in the child under seven years of age. Plast Reconstr Surg 86:633, 1990.

Munro IR, Sabatier REC: An analysis of 12 years of craniomaxillofacial surgery in Toronto. Plast Reconstr Surg 75:29, 1985.

Murray JE, Swanson LT: Midface osteotomy and advancement of craniosynostosis. Plast Reconstr Surg 41:299, 1968.

Obwegeser HC: Surgical correction of small or retrodisplaced maxillae: The "dish face" deformity. Plast Reconstr Surg 43:351, 1969.

Ortiz-Monasterio F, Fuente del Campo A, Carrilo A: Advancement of the orbits and midface in one piece, combined with frontal repositioning, for the correction of Crouzon's deformities. Plast Reconstr Surg 61:507, 1978.

Poole MD: Complications in craniofacial surgery. Br J Plast Surg 41:608, 1988.

Tessier P: Osteotomies totales de la face; syndrome de Crouzon; syndrome d'Apert; oxycephalies, scaphocephalies, turricephales. Ann Chir Plast 12:273, 1967.

Tessier P: Total osteotomy of the middle third of the face for faciostenosis or for sequelae of Le Fort III fractures. Plast Reconstr Surg 48:533, 1971a.

Tessier P: The definitive plastic surgical treatment of the severe facial deformities of craniofacial dysostosis. Crouzon's and Apert's diseases. Plast Reconstr Surg 48:419, 1971b.

Tulasne JF, Tessier PL: Long-term results of Le Fort III advancement in Crouzon's syndrome. Cleft Palate J Suppl. 1, 23:102, 1986.

Whitaker LA, Munro IR, Salyer KE: Combined report of problems and complications in 793 craniofacial operations. Plast Reconstr Surg 64:198, 1979.

CHAPTER 43

Rigid Fixation in Block Orbitofacial Advancement and Facial Bipartition Osteotomies

Antonio Fuente del Campo

During the last 15 years, we have been using the block orbitofacial advancement in the majority of our patients with Crouzon's disease. This process simultaneously corrects frontal and midface retrusion. This technique involves the forward projection of the frontal area, orbits, and the middle third of the face in one piece (en bloc). We consider this to be the ideal procedure in patients with Crouzon's disease when the craniostenosis produces an anteroposterior deformity that is generally symmetric and has no vertical alterations.

In patients with Apert syndrome, who in addition may have a rotational component to their orbital midface deformity, the facial bipartition procedure is performed. This process divides the orbital facial complex into two pieces.

Block advancement was accomplished in the frontal area by self-retaining osteotomies and in the midface through the use of bone grafts placed in the pterygomaxillary space. Significant relapse was not seen in the frontal area but was seen in the midface (see Figure 43.1). The use of postoperative maxillo-mandibular fixation (MMF) did not prevent the relapse. The superior and stable results obtained by plate and screw fixation in maxillofacial procedures prompted us to use this

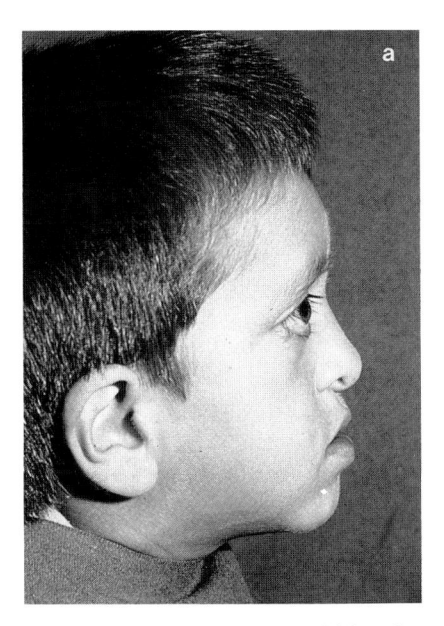

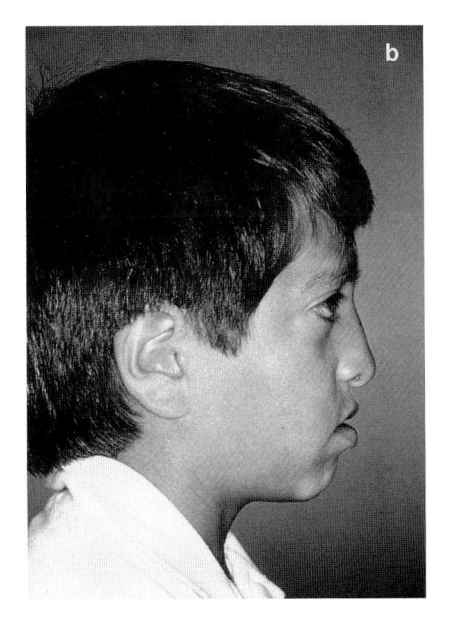

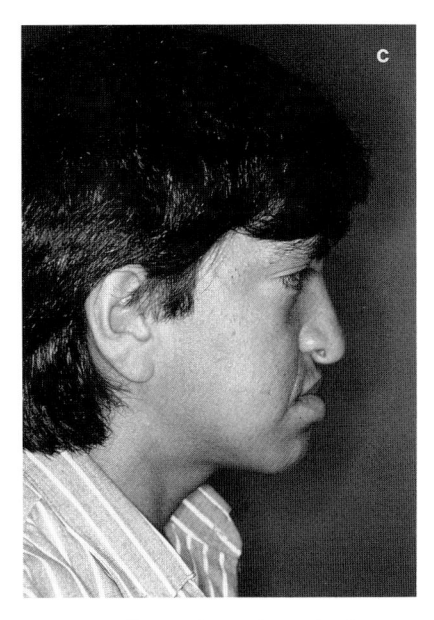

Figure 43.1 (a) This 5-year-old boy has Crouzon syndrome. There is severe exorbitism and maxillary retrusion. (b) Five years after a block advancement, there is some recurrence of the maxillary retrusion. (c) Maxillary relapse is marked 10 years after the procedure, but frontal-orbital advancement remains stable.

technique in block advancement. During the last five years we have used rigid fixation in all cases of Crouzon's disease and Apert syndrome. We feel that its use is particularly important to maintain a satisfactory result in children under four years, in whom a stable occulsion is not present.

SURGICAL PROCEDURE

Craniofacial advancements are performed in two basic procedures: the conventional block advancement described by us in 1978 (see Figure 43.2) for patients with Crouzon's disease, and a block advancement in which the orbital-facial complex is divided into two pieces (facial bipartition) for patients with Apert syndrome.

Exposure

All access is obtained through a bicoronal incision, which begins anteriorly at the top of the ear on each side and extends posteriorly into the parietal area (to avoid having the suture lines over the osteotomies). The scalp flap is dissected in the supraperiosteal plane. The periosteum is incised horizontally 4 centimeters above the supraorbital ridge. The dissection then proceeds in the subperiosteum inferiorly to expose the whole nasal skeleton to the piriform aperture as well as the lateral orbital walls, the malar eminence, and the zygomatic arch. The subperiosteal dissection extends into the orbital cavity. The periorbita are freed from the medial and lateral walls, the floor, and roof to about 1 cm behind the equator of the globe, and the lacrimal apparatus is carefully isolated and preserved. The temporalis muscle is dissected subperiosteally from the temporal fossa in order to expose the external aspect of the lateral orbital wall and the posterior aspect of the zygoma. The dissection is extended inferiorly in a medial direction to the maxillary tuberosity and laterally to the pterygomaxillary junction. This suture is dissected along its length down to the posterior edge of the superior alveolar ridge. No incision in the buccal mucosa is necessary.

Osteotomies

The osteotomies used for block orbitofacial advancement are outlined in Figure 43.2.

The first cut for the frontal craniotomy is made horizontally about 2 centimeters above the superior orbital rim; it extends to the lateral limits of the orbit on each side. It then proceeds at a right angle in a superior direction vertically for about 5 centimeters. The osteotomy again becomes horizontal, directed medially on both sides parallel to the posterior border of the frontal bone. Two quadrangular flaps 2 centimeters in width and 4 centimeters in length extend posteriorly, one on each side of the midline, into the parietal area. These flaps are designed to follow the direction of the planned frontal advancement because they will be used as fixation points to the cranial skeleton. The frontal bone is then removed from the field and wrapped in moist gauze. (It is important to avoid immersing the cranial bones in saline solution while the operation is under way because this will overhydrate the tissues and jeopardize their viability.)

A supraorbital horizontal bar is designed in such a way to allow bone overlap of the lower horizontal osteotomy after frontal advancement. This is accomplished by continuing the lower horizontal osteotomy about 3 to 4 cm into the temporal area and then making a second horizontal osteotomy, parallel to and 1 centimeter below the first, which also extends well beyond the orbital limits into the temporal area. These two parallel osteotomies are joined by a vertical cut that allows the horizontal bar to be removed. The lateral limits of this bar are extended into the temporal area as far as necessary so as to provide bone overlap after frontal advancement. This overlap is necessary for stable fixation.

Figure 43.2 Block frontal facial advancement. (a) Osteotomy sites are shown with dotted lines. The crosshatched frontal area is removed. (b) Fixation is shown after advancement of the frontal and orbital facial segments. The midface advancement is stabilized with the plates and screws. The frontal advancement is stabilized through the self-retaining osteotomies, which are designed so as to maintain bone contact after advancement.

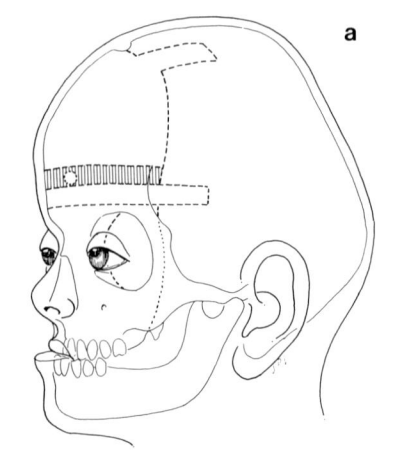

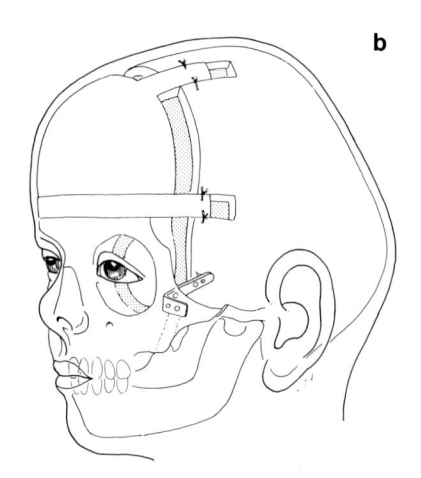

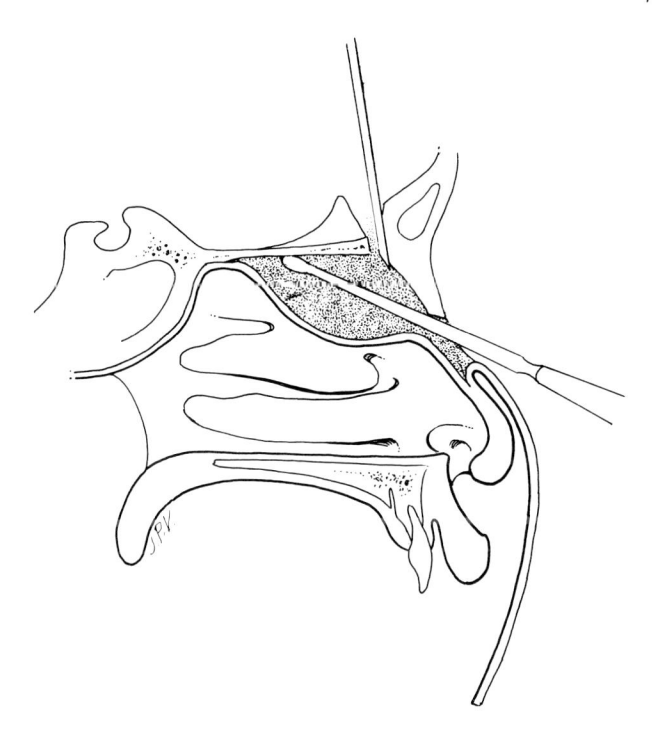

Figure 43.3 The nasal mucosal lining is dissected away from the nasal bones in a subperiosteal plane. The frontal bone is split anterior to the crista galli, and the attachment of the septum to the nasal bone is also separated.

The extradural dissection is then continued intracranially, exposing the anterior cerebral fossa and providing access to the orbital roof. The osteotomies of the orbital roof are made parallel to the supraorbital ridge. They extend medially and then anteriorly to follow the lateral limit of the ethmoid to the crista galli. Inferior retraction of the scalp flap allows the posterior aspect of the nasal bones to be dissected subperiosteally to the level of the angle formed by the vertical and horizontal segments of the frontal bone, thus preserving intact the mucoperiosteal lining of the nose. The angle of the frontal bone is split anteriorly to the crista galli, and the attachment of the septum to the nasal bones is also separated (see Figure 43.3). In this way the integrity of the rhinopharynx is preserved. With the orbital contents properly protected with a malleable retractor, a vertical osteotomy is made through the full thickness of the lateral orbital wall, extending from the lower horizontal osteotomy in the frontal area down to the malar maxillary area and posteriorly to the upper maxillary tuberosity. At the orbital floor the osteotomy is continued medially to the ethmoid area of the medial wall. The zygomatic arch is then cut obliquely to allow bone contact and therefore avoid bone grafts where the orbital facial piece is advanced. The orbital osteotomy is extended inferiorly along the medial orbital wall, passing behind the lacrimal sac to meet the osteotomy of the orbital floor. At this stage the face is attached to the skull only by the pterygomaxillary suture. The frontofacial segment is freed by a vertical osteotomy placed behind one maxillary tuberosity. This may be accomplished either by placing a curved osteotome through the temporal fossa under the zygoma or through a standard transbuccal intraoral approach from below. A Rowe disimpacting forceps is then used to advance the orbital-facial piece to the desired position and expected dental occlusion. The new dental relationship is stabilized interoperatively with intradental wires.

Rigid Fixation

Only two plates, which are placed in the temporal area, are used. The plates are set at 90°, allowing one end to be fixed to the external surface of the temporal bone and the other end behind the malar bone and under the inferior outer angle of the orbits. The plate position provides sufficient stability to avoid the use of bone grafts placed in the pterygomaxillary space to maintain projection of the orbital-facial piece (see Fig-

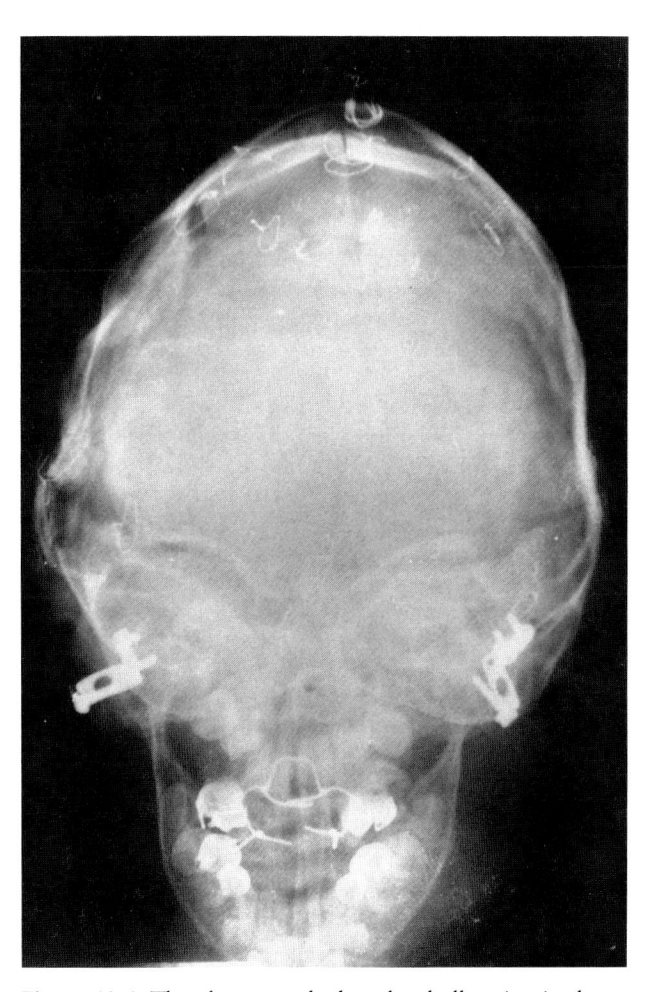

Figure 43.4 The plates attached to the skull maintain the advancement of the orbital facial segment without the need for bone grafts.

Figure 43.5 (a) A periosteal flap is dissected away from the underside of the frontalis muscle and divided in two. (Note the location of the osteotomies in the anterior cranial base.) (b) The periosteal flaps are passed through the gap between the orbits and the supraorbital bar. They are sutured to the meninges of the frontal lobes and then closed in the midline. This bridges the gap in the cranial base created by the orbitofacial advancement and effectively isolates the cranial cavity from the nasal cavity.

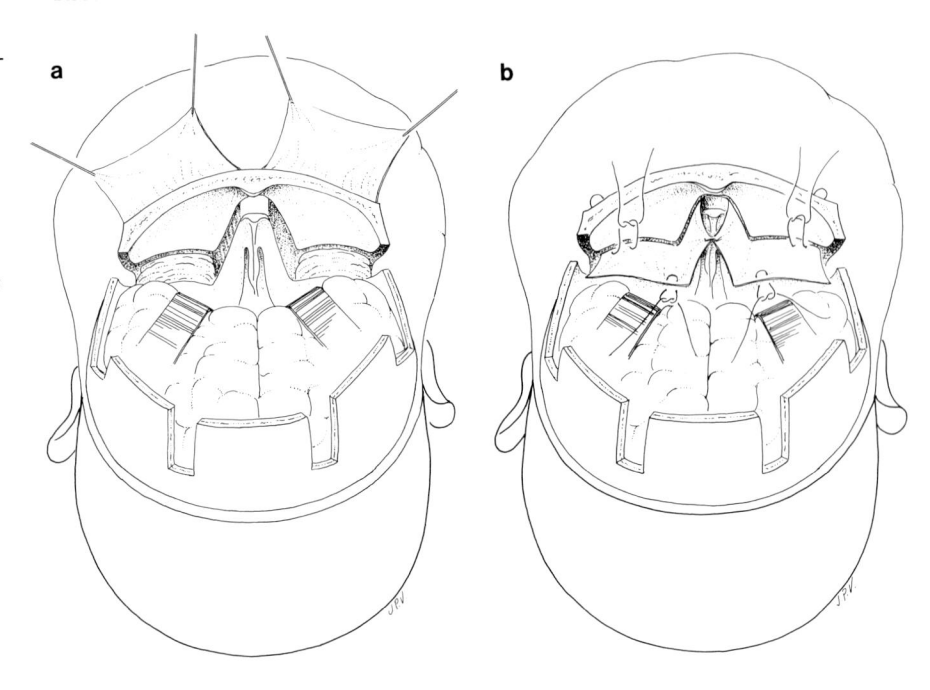

ure 43.4). The horizontal intermediate cranial bar is then replaced in an advanced position that corresponds to the supraorbital ridge, leaving a defect on the temporal end of the horizontal osteotomy. Bone grafts are used only to fill these defects and the gaps created at the lateral walls of the orbits. The gap in the anterior cranial bone is bridged with a periosteal frontal flap based on the supraorbital and supratrochlear circulation. This flap is divided in the midline and passed through the gap between the orbits and supraorbital bar. It is then sutured to the meninges of the frontal lobes and then rejoined in the midline. This technique effectively isolates the cranial cavity from the nasal cavity and also prevents herniation of the brain into the orbits or the nasal cavity. In addition, it prevents adhesions between the meninges and periorbital tissue, which may be a problem in secondary procedures (see Figure 43.5).

Frontal Shortening

Most patients with Crouzon's disease have a vertical, flat, high forehead (see Figure 43.6) whose abnormal configuration is exaggerated where advanced unless its height is simultaneously reduced. This reduction is accomplished by removing a horizontal bone bar at the inferior edge of the bifrontal piece. In this way, reduction of frontal height also decreases the dead space between the bone and the meninges. This decrease in dead space decreases the risk of necrosis and reabsorption of the frontal bone. The removed bone bar provides a source of full-thickness bone grafts to be used where needed. Finally, the frontal bone is fixed to the frontal bar and the parietal area by way of wire osteosynthesis. Before closing, the temporal muscle is rotated anteriorly. Once the procedure is completed, the MMF is released (see Figure 43.7).

APERT SYNDROME

Facial skeletal deformities are much more complex in cases of Apert syndrome. In addition to the anterior–posterior dimensional deformities of Crouzon's disease, Apert syndrome patients have vertical and transverse skeletal abnormalities. These are manifest as excyclotropia of the orbit with orbital hypertelorism, antimongoloid slant of the palpebral fissures; and a significant vertical shortness of the central facial structures that is frequently accompanied by a high, arched palate, a submucous cleft, an anterior open bite, and a very short nose. Block advancement corrects posteroanterior abnormalities but not vertical or the transverse ones (such as hypertelorism). For these patients surgical correction involves a block advancement procedure combined with facial bipartition (see Figure 43.8) as described by Tessier and Van Der Meulen. The procedure is similar to the one described for Crouzon's disease, except that the middle third of the face (orbital facial segment) is divided into two "hemifaces," which are advanced and rotated toward the middle line. The amount of excess bone between both orbits (hypertelorism) is calculated and resected in a triangular shape with a superior base and inferior vertex. The vertex is placed at the level of the anterior nasal spine or the midline at the alveolar ridge, as determined by the necessity to increase the transverse dimension of the maxilla. After the bone in the midline is resected, both "hemifaces" are rotated medially, moving their superior portion to the midline until contact is made. This procedure effectively decreases the interorbital distance levels, the horizontal axes of the orbits, and, in areas, also

Block Orbitofacial Advancement 557

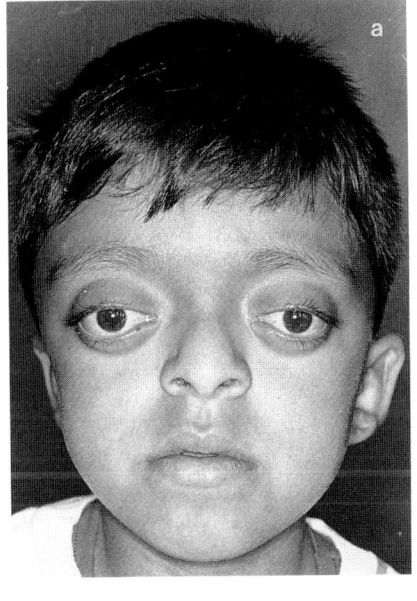

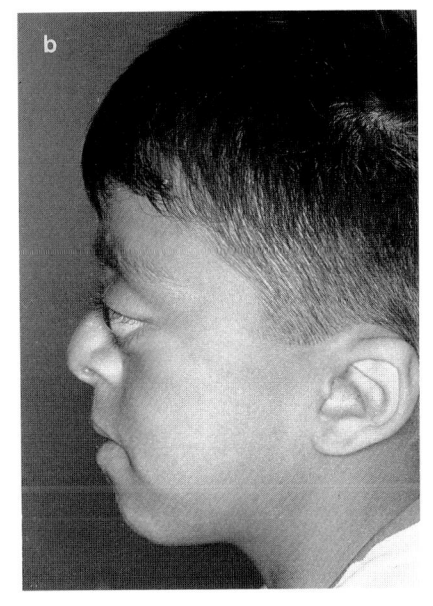

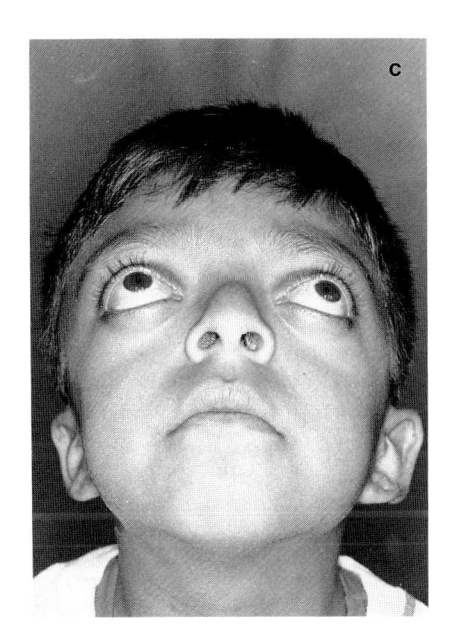

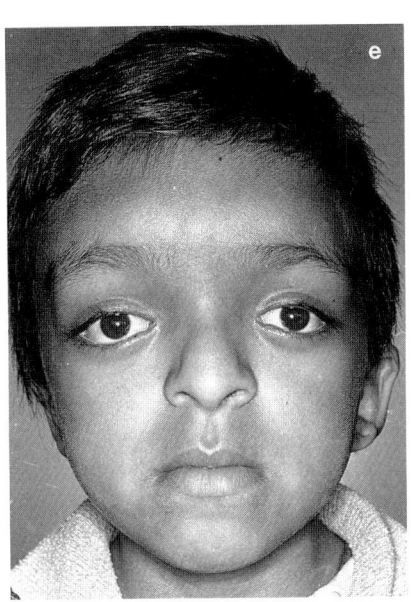

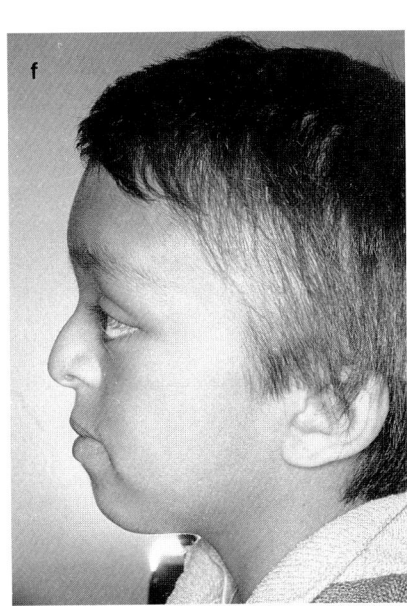

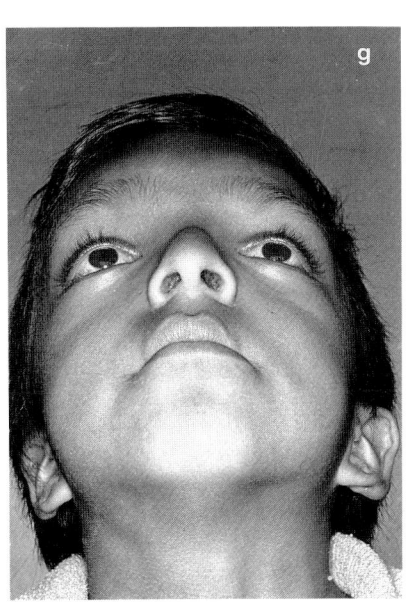

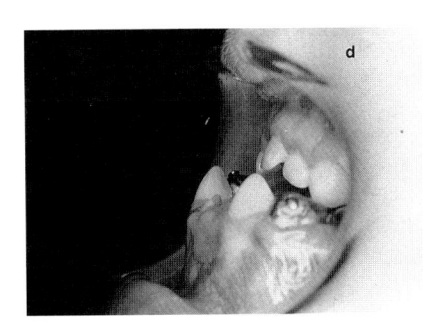

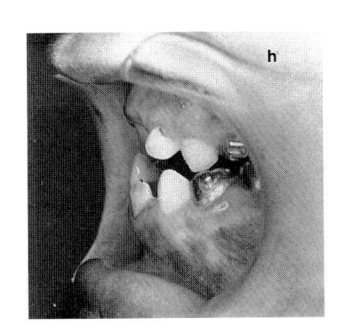

Figure 43.6 This six-year-old boy has Crouzon syndrome. (a) Preoperative frontal view. (b) Preoperative lateral view. (c) Preoperative worm's eye view. (d) Preoperative occlusal view. (e) Fourteen months postoperative frontal view. (f) Postoperative lateral view. (g) Postoperative worm's eye view. (h) Postoperative occlusal view.

Figure 43.7 (a) This five-year-old boy has Crouzon syndrome. (b) Ten months after block advancement, a good proportional relationship is seen.

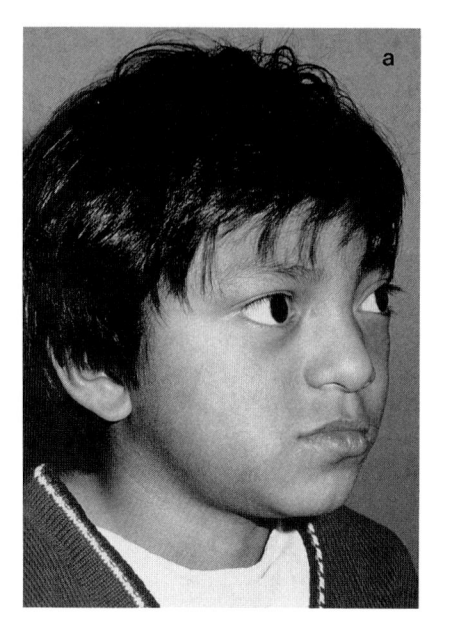

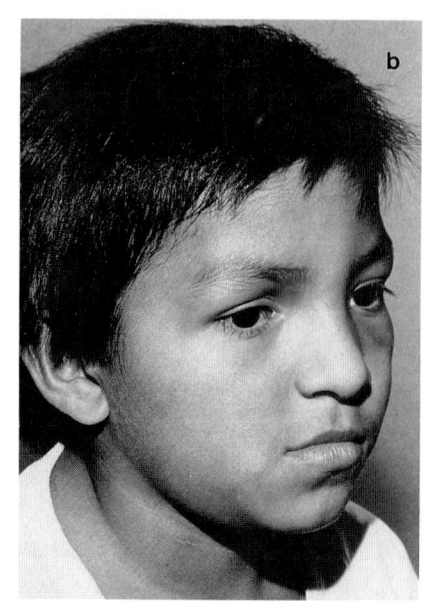

Figure 43.8 The combined block advancement and facial bipartition procedure for Apert syndrome is shown. (a) Frontal and interorbital bone is resected to correct the forehead and the hypertelorism. (b) The two hemifaces are advanced and rotated toward the midline, decreasing the interorbital distance, closing the anterior open bite, and increasing the vertical dimension of the middle third of the face. When there is large bulging of the temporal region, the plates are positioned under pressure with both ends bent at 90°, without using screws.

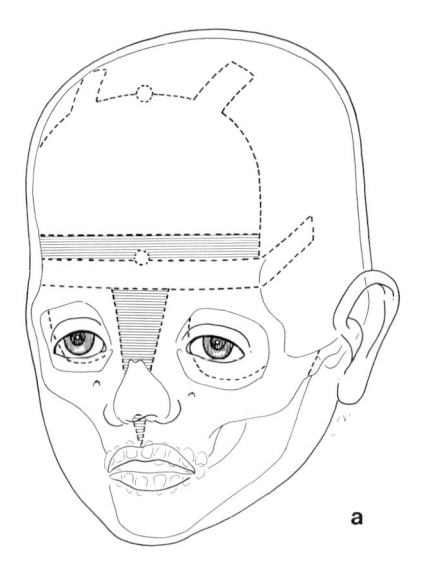

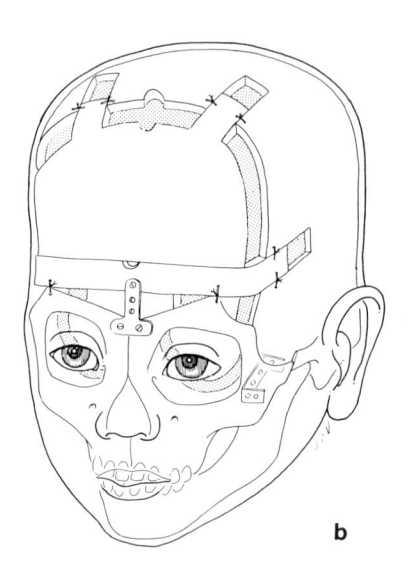

increases the vertical dimension of the middle third of the face. The anterior open bite is also corrected, and the medially rotated hemifacial segments are advanced simultaneously to obtain the best possible occlusion, which is maintained by temporary MMF. Three miniplates are used to fix rigidly all segments of the midface. A plate is placed in each temporal region as in corrections for Crouzon's disease. In cases with large bulging of the temporal regions, the plate is bent 90° at ends and is placed under pressure, without screws, between the outer surface of the temporal bone and the posterior of the latero-inferior angle of the orbit. These plates maintain the facial advancement. To maintain central facial elongation a T plate is positioned with its transverse part joining both orbits and its vertical part fixing them to the horizontal bar (see Figures 43.9 and 43.10). Bicortical bone grafts are placed at the lateral walls of both orbits and in the defects created between the intermediate bar and the superomedial angle of both orbits. The temporary MMF is then removed.

DISCUSSION

Follow-up of these patients in whom rigid fixation was used has been up to three years and six months. In both Crouzon's and Apert cases, results remain stable. In three cases, slight relapse at the occlusal level (2 to 3 mm) was observed. Without rigid fixation, tension exerted by facial muscles and the lack of adequate dental occlusion are known as undesirable factors that compromise the final result and predispose toward relapse. Placing the plates in a diagonal direction and attaching them to the temporal bone completes a pyramidal support of the middle third of the face, which

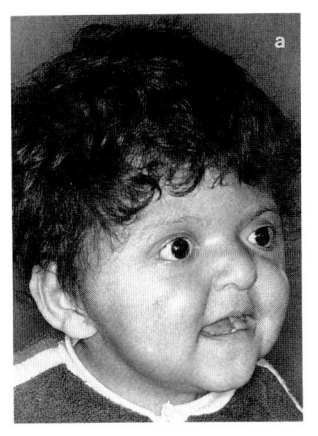

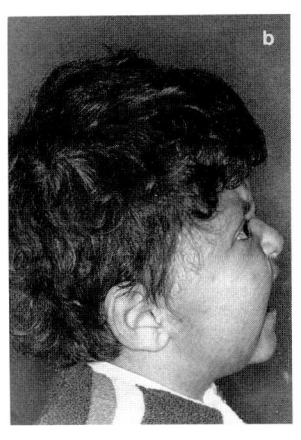

Figure 43.9 This four-year-old boy has Apert syndrome. (a) Preoperative oblique view. (b) Preoperative lateral view. (c) Oblique view two years after a combined block advancement and facial bipartition. (d) Lateral postoperative view. Note the general improvement, particularly the centrofacial elongation.

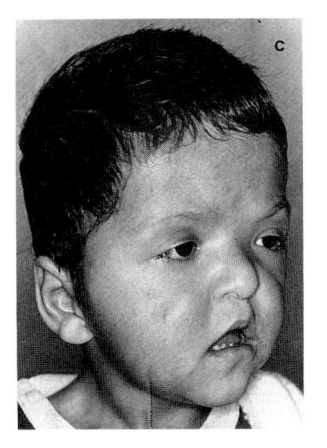

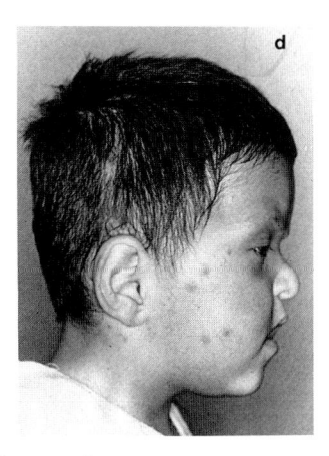

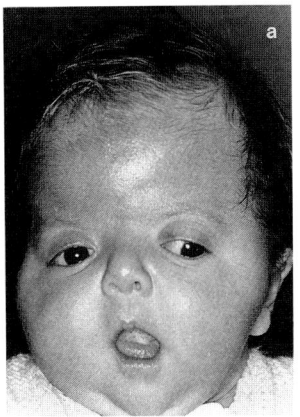

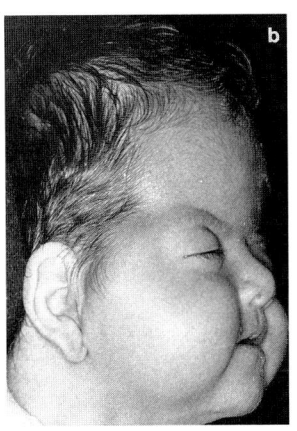

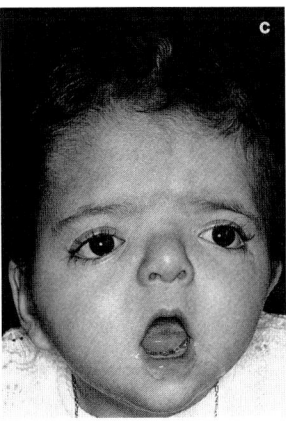

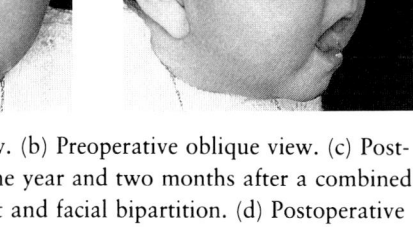

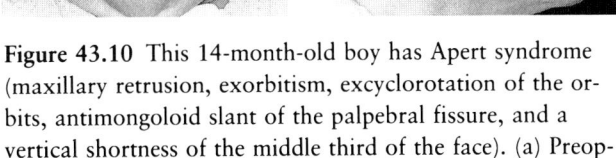

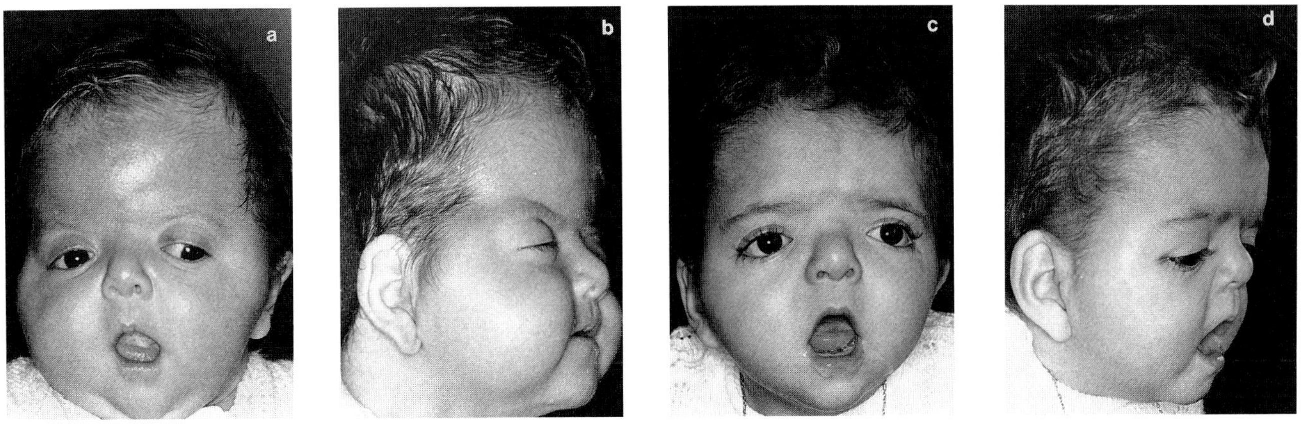

Figure 43.10 This 14-month-old boy has Apert syndrome (maxillary retrusion, exorbitism, excyclorotation of the orbits, antimongoloid slant of the palpebral fissure, and a vertical shortness of the middle third of the face). (a) Preoperative frontal view. (b) Preoperative oblique view. (c) Postoperative result, one year and two months after a combined block advancement and facial bipartition. (d) Postoperative oblique view.

also has an additional point of fixation at the intermediate and frontal fragments, which are solidly fixed to the skull. It is then possible to avoid the muscle tensions that affect the maxilla, causing posterior derotation and relapse at the occlusal level. One of the most discussed points has been the age at which these patients should have operative correction. Previously, we considered an adequate dental occlusion necessary to maintain the advancement at the maxillary level. This would determine whether a block advancement or only a frontal-orbital correction was to be performed. Because the frontal orbital advancement is a partial correction that cannot solve the facial problem but emphasizes the midline disproportion, a second procedure addressing the midface was needed to complete the treatment. None of these patients has had the same satisfactory results as those obtained in patients who have had block advancement. In our experience, the use of plates and screws permits us to do block advancements with stable results in patients of two years of age without postoperative (MMF). Prior to that age, the fronto-zygomatic suture is very fragile and does not provide the required stability without the placement of two additional plates.

Advantages of early surgery are

1. it is technically easier and faster;
2. bones are softer and more malleable;
3. less bleeding occurs;
4. healing is faster, recovery from the surgical trauma is better; and
5. there is less possibility of infection because the paranasal sinuses have not yet developed.

Elimination of MMF reduces the risk of respiratory complications, postoperative time spent in the intensive care unit, the length of the hospital stay, and weight loss. It also prevents loosening of the osteosynthesis by mandibular movements. The effective fixation with plates shortens the time of osteosynthesis and minimizes relapse of the middle third of the face because it does not depend on the occlusion to preserve the advancement. In cases that require postoperative orthodontics, treatment can be started three weeks postprocedure. It is important to mold plates to the surface of the area where they are to be located to avoid antagonistic tensions that could displace them. The plates used in these cases are placed in the fixation, and not the compressive, mode. In the temporal region we use short screws to avoid damage to the dura and meninges. In those cases that show relapse, facial traction masks are soon applied to the upper jaw to achieve a better anteroposterior relationship. In our series of patients we have used block advancement or its variants (with or without rigid fixation) during the last 15 years; infection appeared in five cases (meningitis or osteomyelitis), and this occurred at the beginning of our experience. We have had total loss of the frontal bone flap in four cases and partial loss in eight cases. This was due to aseptic necrosis of the bone; we found no infectious agent. All of these patients were over six years old. In younger patients we have observed thinning of the bone and in some cases partial losses of some small areas. These are important reasons for early surgery and to give special care to the viability of the bone.

BIBLIOGRAPHY

Anderl H, Muhlbauer W, Twerdy K, et al: Frontofacial advancement with bony separation in craniofacial dysostosis. Plast Reconstr Surg 71:303, 1983.

Beals SP, Munro IR: The use of miniplates in craniomaxillofacial surgery. Plast Reconstr Surg 79:33, 1987.

Fuente del Campo A, Ortiz-Monasterio F: Colgajo de Periostio para reconstruir el piso anterior del cráneo en cirugía craneofacial. Cir Plast Iberolatinamer 2:127, 1982.

Fuente del Campo A: Rigid fixation and osteotomy design in frontal orbital advancement osteotomies. Clin Plast Surg 16:205, 1989.

Horster W: Experience with functionally stable plate osteosynthesis after forward displacement of the upper jaw. J Maxillofac Surg 8:176, 1980.

Kaban LB, Conover M, Mulliken JB: Midface position after Le Fort III advancement: A long-term follow-up study. Cleft Palate J (Suppl. 1) 23:69, 1986.

Muhlbauer W: Radical treatment of craniofacial anomalies in infancy and the use of miniplates in craniofacial surgery. Clin Plast Surg 14:101, 1987.

Muhlbauer W, Anderl H, Heeckt P, et al: Early facial advancement in craniofacial stenosis. In Craniofacial Surgery. Marchac D (ed). Berlin, Springer-Verlag, pp 123–129, 1987.

Muhling J, Reuther J, Sorensen N: Therapy of severe craniostenoses. In Craniofacial Surgery. Marchac D (ed). Berlin, Springer-Verlag, pp 88–90, 1987.

Ortiz-Monasterio F, Fuente Del Campo A, Carrillo A: Advancement of the orbits and the midface in one piece, combined with frontal repositioning for the correction of Crouzon's deformities. Plast Reconstr Surg 61:507, 1978.

Ortiz-Monasterio F, Fuente Del Campo A: Refinements on the bloc orbitofacial advancement. In Craniofacial Surgery. Caronni EP (ed). Boston, Little, Brown, pp 263–274, 1985.

Ortiz-Monasterio F, Fuente Del Campo A: Nasal clefts. Ann Plast Surg 18: 377, 1987.

Ousterhout DK: Stability of the maxilla after Le Fort III advancement in craniosynostosis syndromes. Cleft Palate J (Suppl.) 1:91, 1986.

Raposo do Amaral CM: Surgical treatment of orbital hyper- and hypotelorism. In Craniofacial Surgery. Marchac D (ed). Berlin, Springer-Verlag, pp 190–196, 1987.

Steinhauser EW: Bone screws and plates in orthognathic surgery. Int J Oral Surg 11:209, 1982.

Tessier P: Facial bipartition: A concept more than a procedure. In Craniofacial Surgery. Marchac D (ed). Berlin, Springer-Verlag, pp 217–245, 1987a.

Tessier P: The definitive plastic surgical treatment of the severe facial deformities of craniofacial dysostosis: Crouzon's and Apert's diseases. Ann Plast Surg 18:330, 1987b.

Tessier P, Tulasne FJ: Craniofacial Surgery Update. Chicago, Yearbook Medical Publishers, 1986.

Tulasne JF: Long-term results of Le Fort III advancement in Crouzon's syndrome. Cleft Palate J (Suppl.) 1:102, 1986.

Van der Meulen JCH: Surgery of median clefts. In Craniofacial Surgery. Marchac D (ed). Berlin, Springer-Verlag, pp 210–216, 1987.

Van der Meulen JCH, Vaandrager JM: Surgery related to the correction of hypertelorism. Plast Reconstr Surg 71:6, 1983.

Whitaker LA: The craniofacial dysostosis: Guidelines for management of the symmetric and asymmetric deformities. Clin Plast Surg 14:73, 1987.

CHAPTER 44

Advantages of the Subcranial Approach in Craniofacial Surgery

Joram Raveh

Thierry Vuillemin

The term "craniofacial" refers to two separate areas—the cranial-intracranial region and the facial area. These two areas are the domain of different disciplines. Neurosurgeons are responsible for the neurocranium, whereas the facial skeleton is managed by plastic, otolaryngological (head and neck), and oral-maxillofacial surgeons. In our experience, the involvement of various disciplines in the management of traumatic craniofacial injuries (as well as in the correction of congenital anomalies) is disadvantageous. We regard the severe combined fracture pattern of the craniofacial injury as one entity that should be managed by one team. The purpose of this chapter is to highlight the methods developed in our unit which enable an early one-stage surgical procedure. The use of these methods has produced a significant reduction in secondary corrections and morbidity. Two major categories of craniofacial surgery will be described: traumatology and the correction of craniofacial deformities.

CRANIOFACIAL TRAUMATOLOGY

Severe craniofacial injuries often involve the anterior skull base and the parasellar-sphenoidal planes. The comminuted fracture pattern, with major lateral dislocation of the zygomas and the fronto-naso-ethmoidal skeleton, usually results in hypertelorism, flattening of the nasal buttress, and telecanthus. Multiple, extensive dural tears, as well as the compression of the optic nerve, may also complicate these injuries. In our experience, the exposure and definitive management of the frontal skull base is critical in the management of severe craniofacial injuries.

The conventional treatment of the cranial base in severe craniofacial injuries usually involves an intracranial transfrontal approach or a transethmoidal approach. In our opinion, these approaches have the following disadvantages:

1. The management of major intracranial fragment dislocations and multiple dural tears along the frontal area and skull base region performed by the neurosurgical, intracranial, transfrontal approach (Arendall 1983, Bongartz 1981 Gruss 1982, Lieberherr 1985, Loew 1984, Ljunggren 1980, Manson 1986, Meyers 1984, Probst 1986, Strohecker 1984, Westmore 1982) is usually limited to urgent intracranial exploration and local repair. The definite repair of the area of the frontal skull base, including the sellar-sphenoidal planes, makes extensive frontal lobe retraction necessary and represents a major operative procedure for the patient. In many severe cases, brain contusion and edema make this mode of early one-stage management unfeasible. Operative intervention is therefore deferred for 2 or 3 weeks to allow brain contusions and edema to subside (Gruss 1982, Arendall 1983, Loew 1984, Probst 1986, MacGee 1970, Westmore 1982).

   Such delay is a disadvantage for the facial skeletal reconstruction, particularly in the fronto-naso-orbital region. The delayed initial reconstruction is usually inadequate, and secondary surgical corrections and osteotomies are often necessary.

Disadvantages related to the intracranial procedure are (a) a relatively high rate of morbidity, including anosmia, increased brain edema, and protracted hospitalization (Bongartz 1981, Ljunggren 1980, Loew 1984, Probst 1986, MacGee 1970, Rousseaux 1981) and (b) insufficient access to exenterate the ethmoid sinuses, and to reconstruct the frontal sinus and its drainage pathway.

2. The classical, transethmoidal, rhinosurgical approach (Escher 1944, 1960, 1969) for the closure of cerebrospinal fluid (CSF) leaks (Lieberherr 1985, Myers 1984, Westmore 1982, Briant 1987, Calcaterra 1980, 1985, Elies 1982, Park 1983, Samii 1978) provides access only to the midline structures: the frontal sinus, the cribriform plate, and the roofs of the ethmoid and the sellar-sphenoidal planes (see Figure 44.1). This approach does not provide sufficient access to repair multiple or extensive dural tears, particularly if the lesions are dispersed throughout the anterior fossa or when the tears are accompanied by intracranial fragment dislocations. Because this approach provides limited visibility, dural tears may go undetected, which is responsible for a CSF leak recurrent rate of up to 20%, often associated with meningitis.

When tears are allowed to heal by secondary intention the poor quality of the cicatricial tissue in this region is responsible for a permanent risk of delayed CSF leak and meningitis, even after many years (Samii 1978, Calcaterra 1980, 1985, Elies 1982, Westmore 1982, Park 1983, Loew 1984, Myers 1984, Lieberherr 1985, Probst 1986). We strive for a proper surgical closure, even in cases with spontaneous cessation of the CSF leak.

The disadvantages of these procedures prompted us to develop the subcranial technique, which is a modification of the classic transethmoidal ENT procedure. The subcranial technique provides subcranial exposure of the entire anterior fossa, the orbital and ethmoidal roof, and the parasellar sphenoidal planes, thus making it an alternative to the intracranial approach (Raveh 1979, 1981, 1984, 1988a, 1988b).

Treatment Modalities

Nonsurgical Conservative Treatment

No surgical intervention was taken if three conditions existed:

1. no CSF leakage,
2. no pneumocranium, and
3. minimal fracture displacement.

Surgical Treatment

Surgical intervention was taken in cases with manifest CSF rhinorrhea, pneumocranium, and displaced skull base fractures. The absence of CSF leakage and rhinorrhea, particularly in the immediate post-traumatic period may be misleading. Herniation of brain tissue, swelling of the ethmoidal mucosa, and clot formation often obstruct the pathway to the nasal lumen. Presence of this obstruction explains the relatively high rate of latent development of CSF leaks or meningitis (Bongartz 1981, Ljunggren 1980, Arendall 1983, Loew 1984, Probst 1986, Strohecker 1984, Rousseaux 1981,

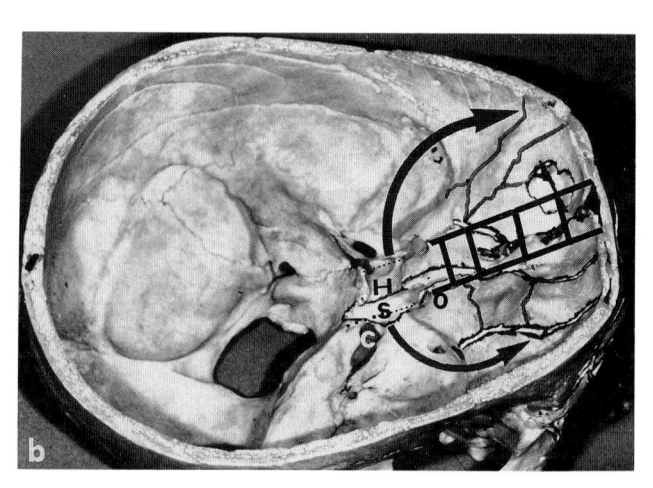

Figure 44.1 Schematic illustration shows the classic transethmoidal ENT approach to the skull base. (a) The classic ENT approach is limited to the frontal sinus and skull base midline structures. (b) Intracranial view shows common skull base fracture patterns. The classic transethmoidal exposure is limited to the midline, skull base, and frontal sinuses (parallel lines). Thus multiple intracranially dislocated fractures dispersed along the fronto-orbital and lateral area (arrows) usually cannot be managed by this approach. (O = optic nerve, H = sella.) Note that the carotid artery (C) is adjacent to the sphenoid (S).

Lewin 1966, Laun 1982, Meirowsky 1981, Paillas 1967, Pia 1979, Raaf 1967). Decisions regarding the neurological condition of the patient and the type and feasibility of the surgical procedure were made in close cooperation with the neurosurgeon, according to the following criteria:

1. Fractures limited to the calvaria without further involvement of the frontal region or skull base were managed by the neurosurgeon;
2. fractures of the frontal cranial vault and all the basal planes of the anterior fossa, including the sellar-sphenoidal region, were managed by our team via the subcranial approach, thus avoiding any frontal lobe retraction; and
3. in cases with vast hemorrhagic brain contusions and damage to the brain tissue, local repair was performed by the neurosurgeon, leaving to the maxillofacial team the subcranial management of the dural tears and skeletal reconstruction of the concomitant fractures of the skull base and orbito-nasal area during the same session.

The radiologic examination included conventional radiographs, tomography, and computerized tomography (CT) scanning. The ophthalmologist evaluates the status of the optic nerve and determines whether decompression is needed.

Clinical Material

From 1978 to 1987, 374 cases with combined midface, frontal, and concomitant skull base fractures were surgically managed. This management included duraplasty and repair of the skull base in a one-stage procedure. Isolated frontobasal or midface fractures are not included in this study. Distributions, and locations of the combined fractures are shown in Tables 44.1 and 44.2.

We consider surgical management and reconstruction of the craniofacial area to be early if it is performed within the first 48 hours. Even severe cases with large multiple dural tears and contusions were managed in a one-stage procedure. Only in cases with an unstable neurological condition, where primary urgent intracranial exploration and limited local repair were necessary, was definite management of the craniofacial fractures postponed.

The Subcranial Approach

In this section, we present the principal surgical and anatomic principles related to the subcranial approach (see Figure 44.2).

Table 44.1 Distribution of midface fractures in relation to 374 concomitant frontobasal fractures

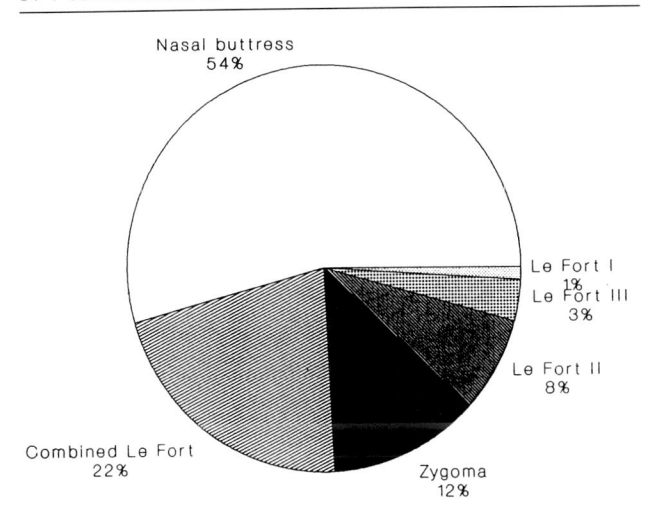

- Nasal buttress 54%
- Le Fort I 1%
- Le Fort III 3%
- Le Fort II 8%
- Zygoma 12%
- Combined Le Fort 22%

Table 44.2 Locations of frontobasal fractures in 374 cases

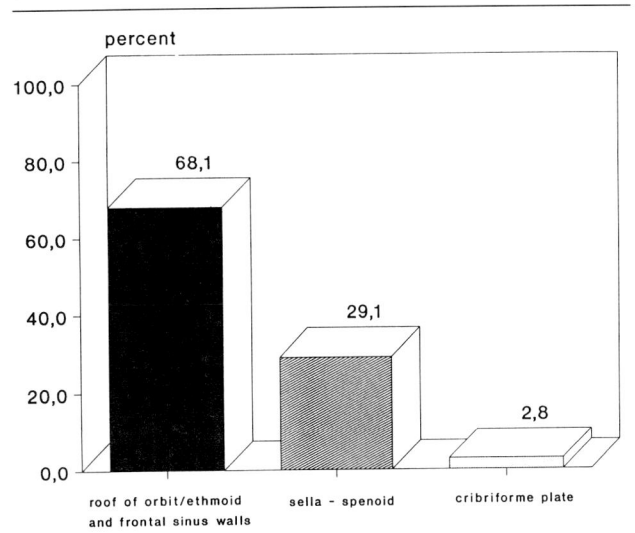

- roof of orbit/ethmoid and frontal sinus walls: 68,1
- sella - spenoid: 29,1
- cribriforme plate: 2,8

Access via the Eyebrow Incision and the Coronal Flap

The eyebrow incision is strictly limited to the eyebrow. If meticulously performed and sutured, it is, in most cases, undetectable. The incision is never extended out of the eyebrow or communicated over the glabella (as is done in the classic ENT procedure) (see Figure 44.3a). In multiple fractures of the frontal cranial vault, and when fragments are dislocated intracranially, a coronal flap is performed (see Figure 44.3b). Both approaches preserve the supraorbital nerve.

Figure 44.2 The subcranial exposure for optimal management of all skull base planes obviates the transfrontal neurosurgical procedure. (a) Broad subcranial exposure including all skull base planes and the fronto-orbito-temporal area, in contrast to the classic transethmoidal ENT procedure, enables adequate repair of vast and multiple dural tears and hemostasis. (b) Subcranial optic nerve decompression is performed by removing the lateral sphenoidal-ethmoidal walls. Expansion of the nerve toward the subcranial compartment underneath the skull base, created after ethmoidectomy, is crucial for functional recovery (arrows).

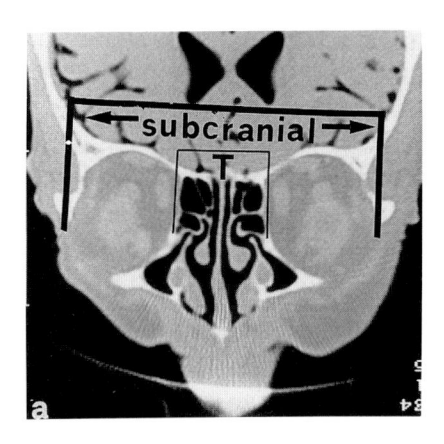

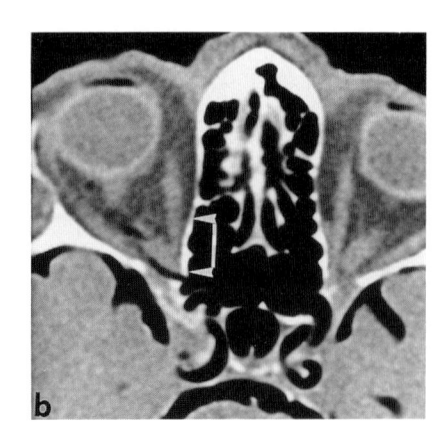

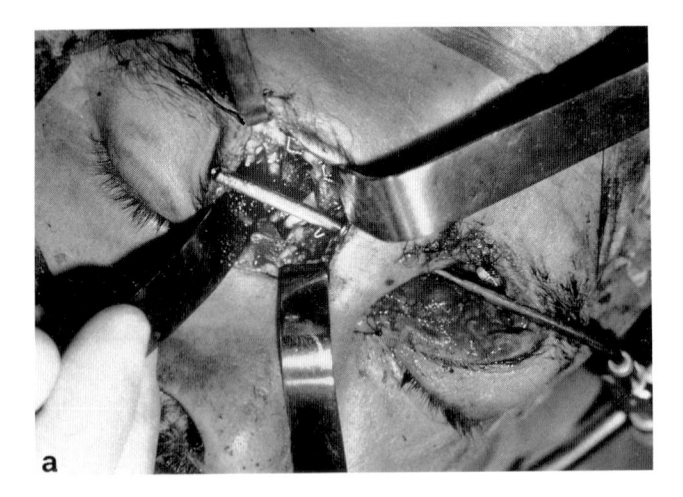

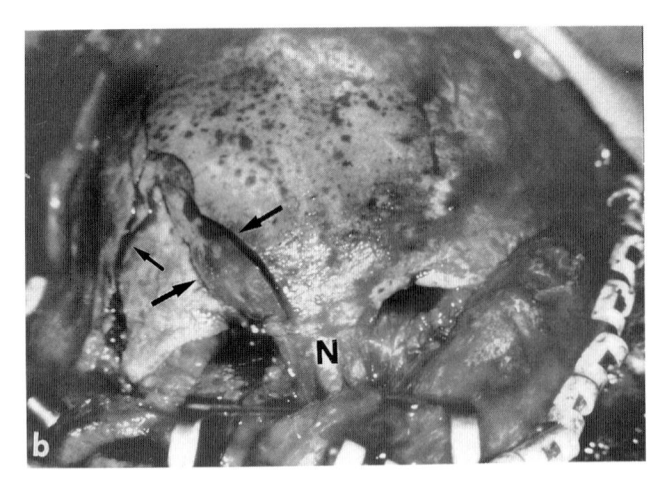

Figure 44.3 Incisions used in the subcranial approach. (a) To avoid unfavorable scars, eyebrow incisions are never extended out of the eyebrow or communicated over the back of the nose. (b) The coronal flap is preferred if major fragment dislocations (arrows) are manifest.

Exposure and Optic Nerve Decompression

Radical exenteration of the ethmoidal cells and exposure of the ethmoidal roof, including the sphenoid, are performed in the same way as in the classic procedure (see Figures 44.1 and 44.2). In contrast to the classic procedure, however, the exposure is then extended over the whole frontal region, including the roof of the orbit up to the apex and the lateral orbital walls (see Figure 44.2). Optic nerve decompression (see Figures 44.4 and 44.5) is performed subcranially by removing part of the orbital wall or, if indicated, the medial wall of the canal (see Figures 44.5 and 44.6). The medial optic nerve canal wall at the upper lateral ethmoidal-sphenoidal conjunction is relatively short. Thus, it is often sufficient to remove the middle section of the medial orbital wall up to the apical end of the nerve canal so as to avoid any development of pressure in the canal itself. Only if fragment dislocation into the canal is manifest is the entire medial canal wall removed (see Figure 44.6). The subcranial compartment, created after the radical ethmoidectomy, enables, in contrast to the conventional intracranial procedure, the expansion of the optic nerve medially. Limiting the resection to the midline of the medial orbital wall, leaving the upper and lower borders intact, is usually sufficient to avoid enophthalmus. If necessary, a lyophilized cartilage layer is interpositioned. The subcranial compartment is drained by means of a Silastic tube inserted into the nasal lumen. This is of utmost importance for the prevention of postoperative development of pressure in the orbital conus; such pressure often leads to an orbital apex syndrome. To visualize and manage all of the dural tears, the various frontal fragments and the major part of the roof of the orbit are temporarily removed (see Figures 44.7 and 44.8).

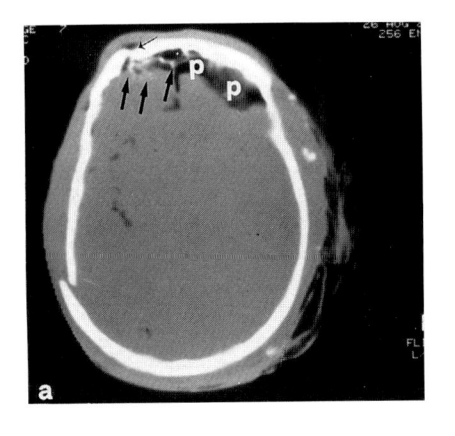

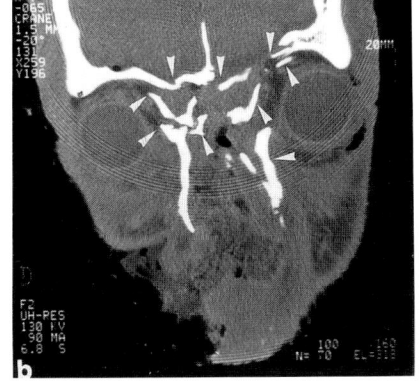

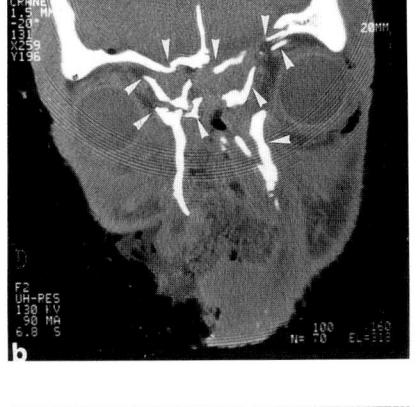

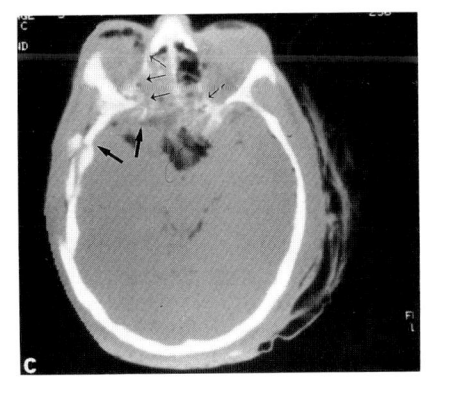

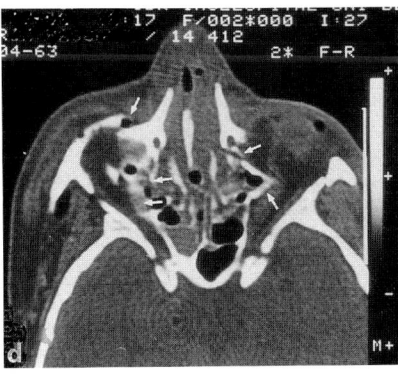

Figure 44.4 Common skull base fracture patterns. (a) Traumatic pressure to the frontal nasal bone often causes fractures (arrows) that are dispersed along the skull base and optic nerve canal and that are accompanied by dural tears. (P = pneumocranium.) (b) Coronal CT of the same patient illustrates the concomitant ethmoidal roof fractures and orbital fragment dislocation toward the optic nerve (arrows). (c and d) Other cases show fronto-ethmoidal skull base fractures (arrows) resulting in optic nerve compression.

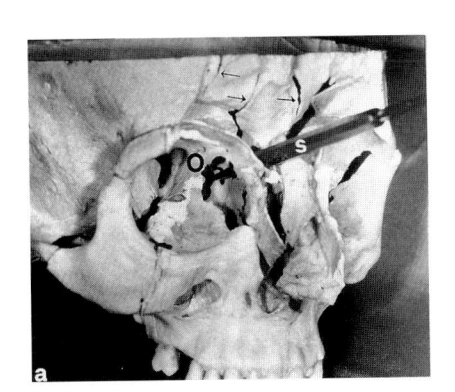

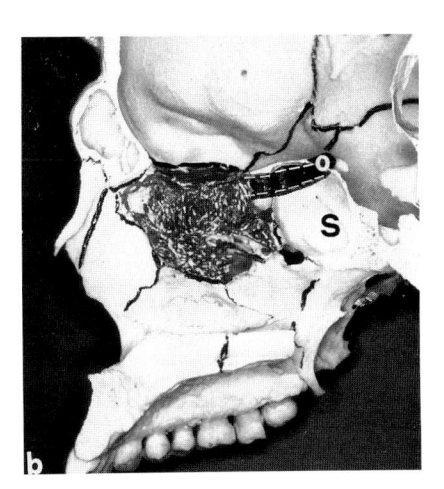

Figure 44.5 Schematic illustrations show skull base fractures and optic nerve decompression. (a) Fragment fractures are present along the posterior frontal sinus walls, fronto-lateral bone, and orbital roof (arrows). Sonde (S) marks the subcranial access for optic nerve decompression. (b) The upper conjunction of the lateral ethmoidal and sphenoidal walls represents the medial wall of the optic nerve canal (dashed line). Removal enables nerve decompression and medial expansion toward the subcranial lumen created after radical ethmoidal cell exenteration.

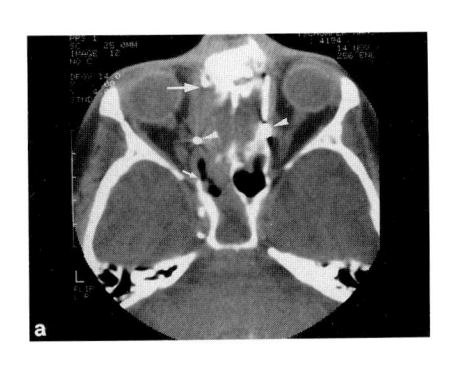

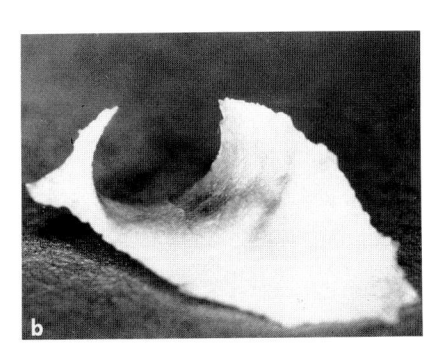

Figure 44.6 (a) Postoperative CT scan. On the right side, the middle part of the medial orbital wall and the optic nerve canal wall (arrows) were removed. Note the ethmoidal artery clips (arrowhead). (b) The removed medial wall of the optic nerve canal is shown.

Figure 44.7 Subcranial technique is illustrated. (a) Major frontotemporal fragment dislocation (arrows) and pneumocranium are present. (b) An eyebrow incision is made, and the fractured frontal bone segment is removed up to the temporal bone (arrows), including the orbital roof. (N = nose, E = eyes, F = closed dural tears with already applied fascia lata layers, S = subcranial and transethmoidal access to the skull base and optic nerve.) (c) The frontal segment (B) and the orbital roof are repositioned. (N = nose.)

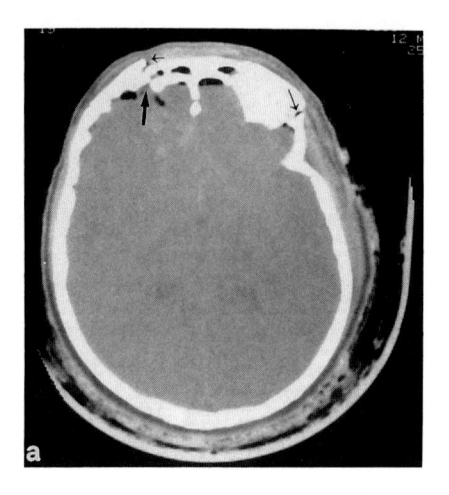

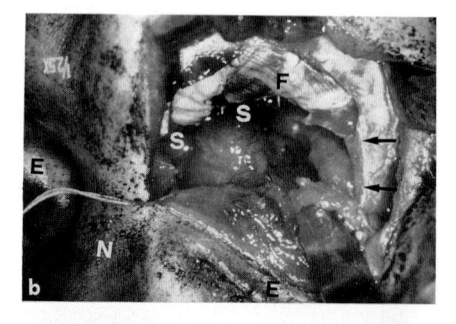

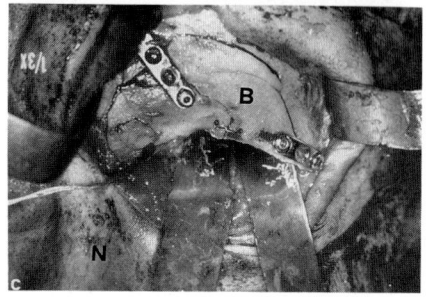

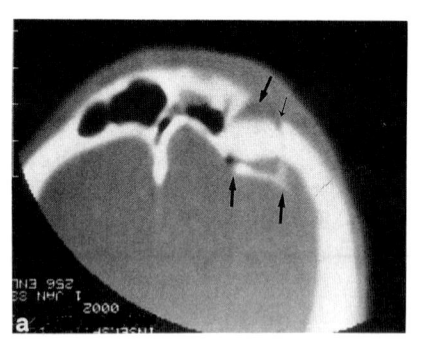

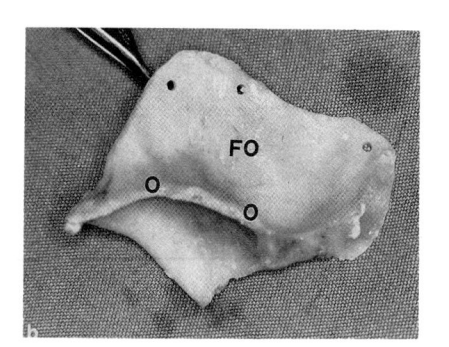

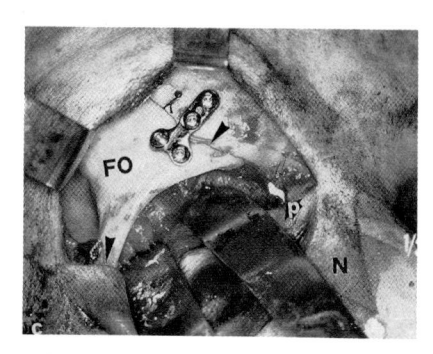

Figure 44.8 (a and b) Pneumocranium and intracranial dislocation of the fronto-lateral (arrows) bone are shown. Removal of the whole segment (FO) including the orbital roof (O) enables exposure and repair of the multiple dural tears including the ethmoidal sphenoidal planes. This procedure obviates the transfrontal approach. (c) The segment is repositioned. (N = nose, P = Portex plastic tube for the drainage of the subcranial compartment and restored frontal sinus into the nasal lumen.)

Dural Repair and Fracture Reduction

The dural tears are sutured and/or covered with a layer of fascia lata and fibrin glue (see Figure 44.7). Even extreme intracranial dislocation of multiple fragments (see Figure 44.9a–e) was managed by the subcranial approach (see Figure 44.9e–i), obviating a transfrontal neurosurgical procedure. In the area of the ethmoidal roof, a second layer of fascia lata is applied that covers the whole underface of the ethmoidal roof, and the sellar and sphenoidal area. This alignment is of utmost importance because it serves as an accessory, watertight barrier to the paranasal spaces. This procedure is performed only after the reduction of concomitant midface or nasal bone fractures (see Figure 44.10). This is because the reduction of the nasal buttress and midface fractures often provokes shifting and displacement of the already partially repositioned fragments of the skull base. In cases with extensive bone loss the defects are bridged with calvarial external table bone grafts.

In our study, the lesions localized to the cribriform plate were very rare (see Table 44.2). We disagree with the opinion of others (Lieberherr 1985) in that we do not dissect the olfactory filaments or expose the underface of the cribriform plate. We do, however, simply remove part of the ethmoidal roof and then explore for dural perforations. With help of the microscope we perform the alignment with fascia lata. Thus iatrogenic, unnecessary damage to the olfactory filaments is avoided.

In comparison to the conventional neurosurgical, transfrontal intracranial procedure, the subcranial ap-

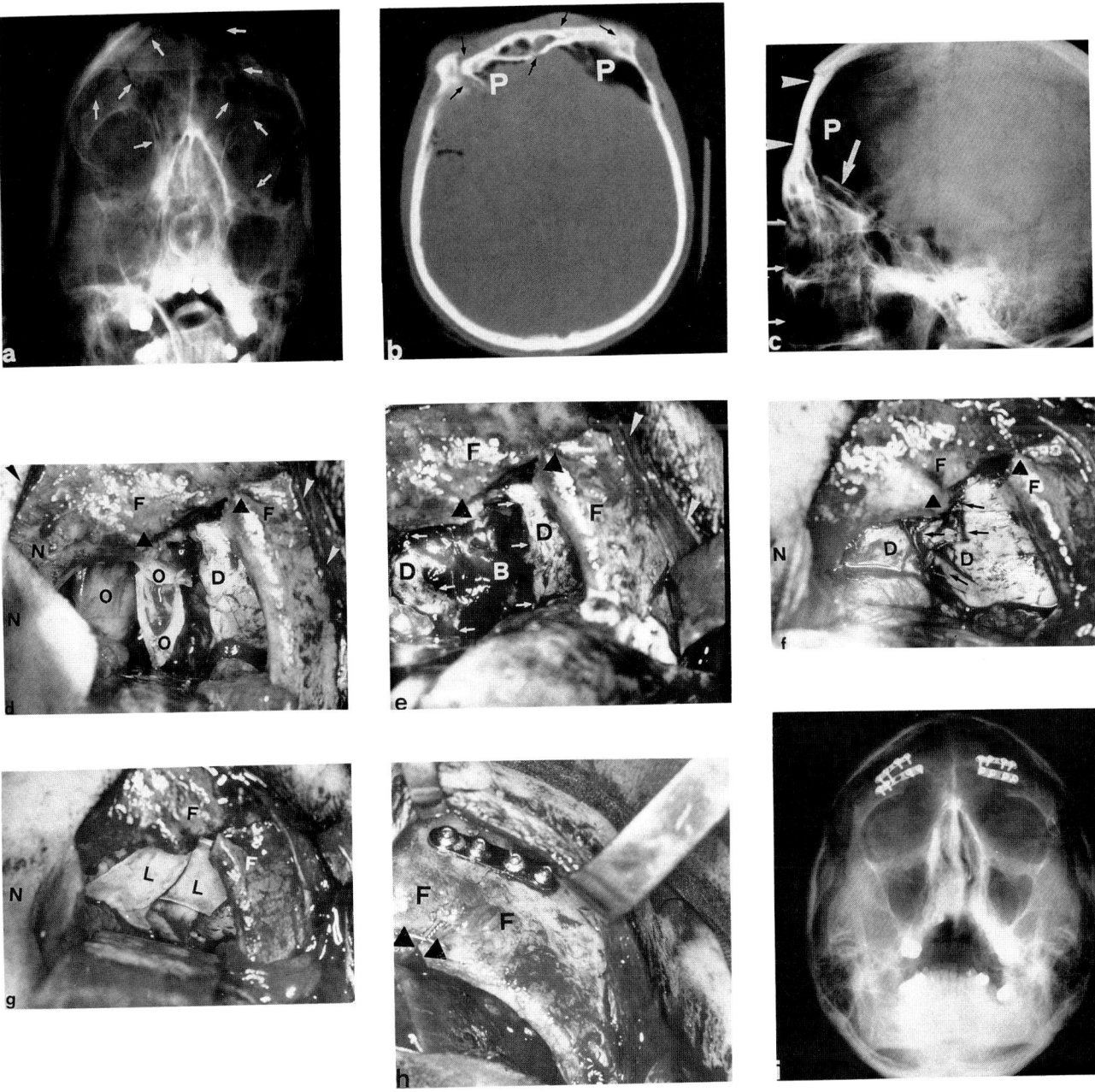

Figure 44.9 (a) Bilateral intracranial fragment dislocation can be seen. (b) This CT illustrates the fractured (arrows), distally dislocated frontal bone and pneumocranium. (c) Lateral radiograph. (P = pneumocranium, arrowheads indicate dislocated frontal bone, arrows indicate intracranially dislocated orbital roof fragments and concomitant skull base involvement.) (d) The situation is shown after removal of intraorbitally prolapsed devitalized brain tissue. (Arrowheads indicate eyebrow incision, triangles indicate dislocated frontal bone (F) segments, O = intracranially penetrating orbital roof fragments, D = dura, N = nose.) (e) F = dislocated (triangles) frontal segments, D = dura after removal of the penetrating orbital roof fragments, B = brain and borders of dura defect (arrows). (f) N = nose, arrows indicate sutured dural defect and repaired ethmoidal and sphenoidal planes. (g) N = nose, L = already applied fascia lata layers. Further layers are aligned along the ethmoidal roof including the sphenoid. (h) Repositioned frontal bone is fixed with the first miniplate. (i) This radiograph shows the frontal bone plating and the zygoma wire ligature osteosynthesis.

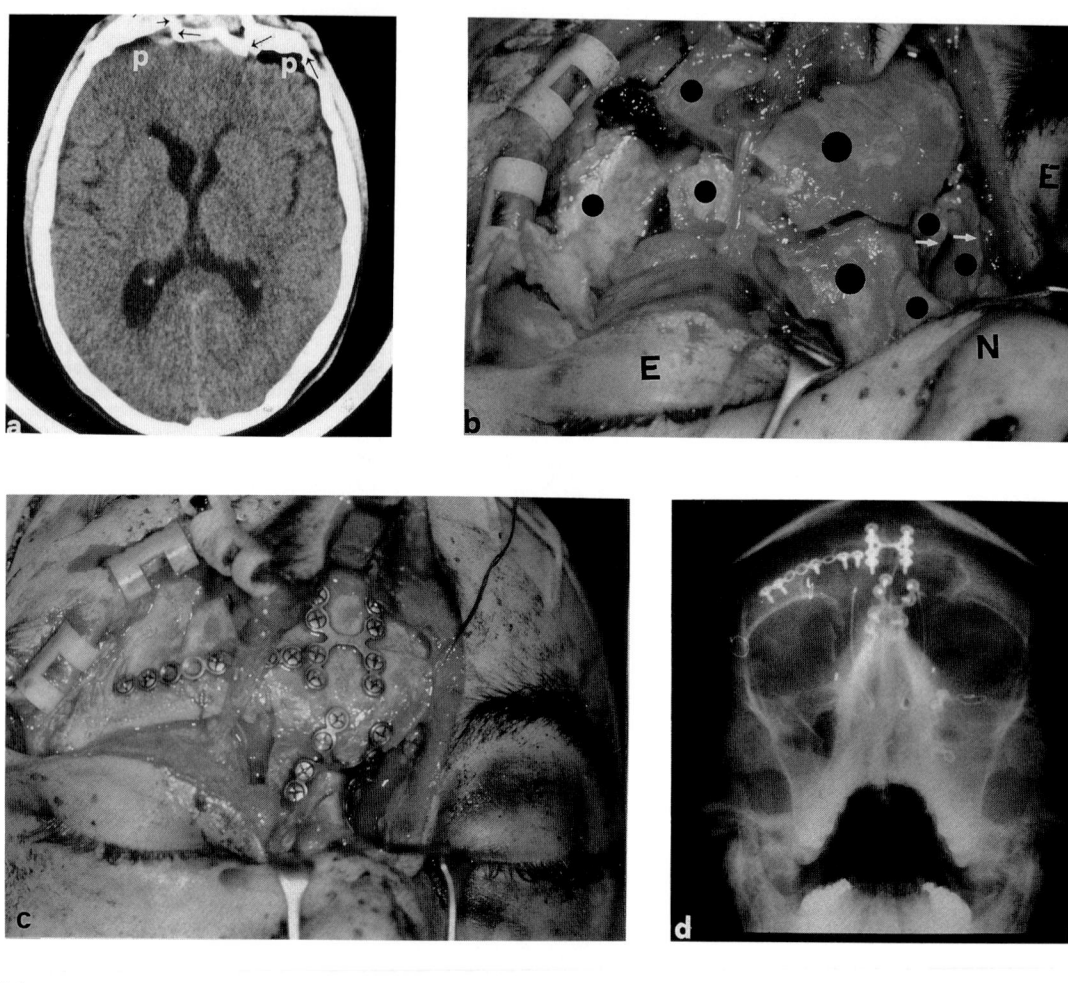

Figure 44.10 Subcranial management of comminuted combined fronto-naso-ethmoidal skull base fractures. (a) CT scan shows pneumocranium (P) and multiple dislocated frontal bone fractures (arrows). (b) Intraoperative view shows subcranial access via the open laceration wound. (E = eye, N = nose.) Multifragmentary and intracranially dislocated fractures of the frontal bone (circles) are shown, as well as the inwardly telescoped and laterally dislocated nasal bone fragments (arrows). Telecanthus is the result. (c) Reduced frontal and nasal bone fragments are shown after subcranial repair and closure of the dural tears along the skull base up to the sphenoid. (Note the miniplates.) (d) Postoperative radiograph. (e and f) Note the patient's scars of traumatic origin.

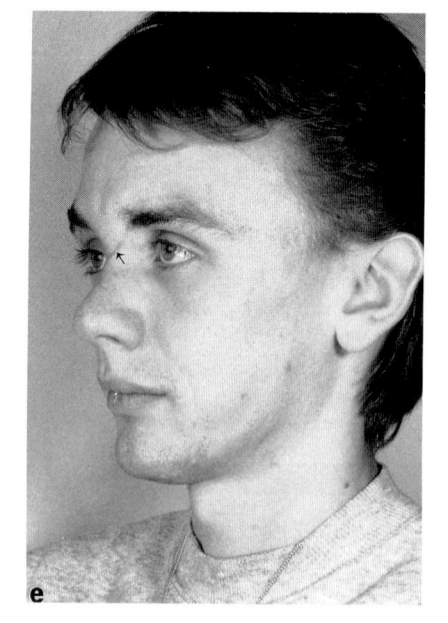

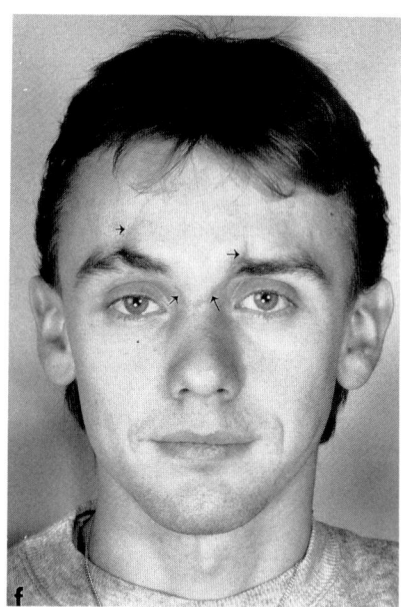

proach practically represents an extracranial management. In an experience, the subcranial approach to the skull base and cranial vault represents the key for early one-stage management and correct reduction of concomitant craniofacial fractures. Each of the following presentations refers to different combined fracture patterns, and illustrates various considerations with regard to combined management.

Case 1: Axial Lateral Midface Dislocation and Concomitant Disruption of the Skull Base Midline Structures

The fracture pattern associated with axial midface dislocation is shown in Figure 44.11.

Apart from the frontal bone fractures, the midface was laterally displaced along with the ethmoidal roof on both sides up to the sella and the cribriform plate, resulting in vast lacerations of the dura, which is extremely adherent to the bone in this area. Copious hemorrhage, brain tissue prolapse into the ethmoidal and orbital region, and CSF rhinorrhea were manifest on this case and are very common with such lesions. The surgeon must be aware that such dislocations may involve the parasellar-sphenoidal planes, including the carotid artery, the sagittal and cavernous sinuses, or the optic nerve and chiasma. Disattachment or lesions of the hypophysis and infundibulum leading to diabetes insipidus were very rare and were manifest in only three of our cases. Utmost caution must be used with regard to these structures so as to avoid iatrogenic damage. The broad exposure and optimal visualization rendered by the subcranial approach are crucial for the success of such surgical procedures. The vast hemorrhagic brain contusion at the frontal-calvaria area (see Figure 44.11a and b) was treated by the neurosurgeon. The further management of the multiple extensive dural tears and the skull lesions, as well as the repositioning of the fragments of the cranial vault, were performed subcranially by our team. An intracranial approach, making frontal lobe retraction necessary, to manage the disrupted frontal skull base planes would have been impossible in this case because of the increased intracranial pressure and cerebral edema. Figure 44.11a–c shows the lateral displacement of the nasal bone and the frontal segment to the left side, along with the intracranial dislocation of the crista galli, the cribriform plate, and the ethmoidal roof. After the subcranial exposure and management of the orbital roofs and the median-paramedian skull base planes and duraplasty (see Figure 44.11d), the fronto-nasal fragments were repositioned and fixed by miniplates (see Figure 44.11e and f). Bone defects are usually bridged by external table grafts or lyophilized cartilage. This patient was mobilized 4 days postoperatively. Figure 44.11(g) shows the patient 10 days postoperatively and Figure 44.11(h), six weeks postoperatively.

Case 2: Intracranial Dislocated Frontal and Basal Skull Base Bone Fragments Including the Orbital Roof, and Major Disto-Caudal Midface Dislocation with Concomitant Orbital Asymmetry

In this case, the impact of the high-velocity trauma, as shown in Figure 44.12 (a and b), has led to lateral displacement of the nasal walls and inward telescoping of the nasal buttress fragments underneath the anterior skull base. Comminution of the ethmoidal cells and manifest nasal CSF leakage are also found. The frontal fragments were intracranially displaced and shifted over the crista galli into the anterior fossa (see Figure 44.12 c and d). The left orbital roof was intracranially dislocated up to the middle cranial fossa. Major caudal and lateral displacement, particularly of the left zygoma and the supraorbital rim, resulted in asymmetry and enlargement of the interorbital distance (see Figure 44.12b). Extensive concomitant dural tears along the skull base up to the sellar sphenoidal region, as well as along the left orbit (see Figure 44.12e) and ethmoid, accompanied by prolapsed devitalized brain tissue, were present. The initial neurosurgical repair was limited to the upper region of the calvaria, through the traumatic skin laceration (see Figure 44.12a and b). The subcranial management of all dural lesions along the frontal skull base planes, including the reconstruction of the cranial vault, was subsequently performed by our team (see Figure 44.12f). With regard to the vast dural tears, brain tissue damage, and edema, an immediate intracranial management of the skull base planes, along with frontal lobe retraction, would have been impossible. Left optic nerve decompression was performed simultaneously. Postoperative development of an orbital Apex syndrome can thus be prevented. Once the frontal fractures were reduced, the correct occlusion was retained by maxillo-mandibular fixation (MMF). The reduction of the orbito-nasal-midface fractures (see Figure 44.12g–i) in correct relation to the already reconstructed frontal area can then be undertaken. The lateral orbital wall and subcranial exposure was performed by the eyebrow incision. Reduction of the infraorbital rim and floor of orbit, even in comminuted fractures, is exclusively performed by the transconjunctival approach. A broad exposure of all the orbital walls up to the apex is essential for correct reduction.

The last step consists of inserting a Portex tube on both sides into the subcranial compartment (the previous ethmoid cell region). The tube protrudes into the nasal cavity, thus maintaining drainage. These tubes are left in situ for six months in order to avoid obstructions of the sinus pathway by granulation tissue. This is essential for the reduction of such complications as mucus retention, empyema, and mucocele. In spite of the severity of the combined fractures, this patient was mobilized and dismissed from the intensive care unit 3 days

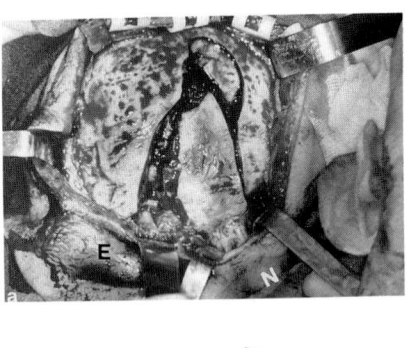

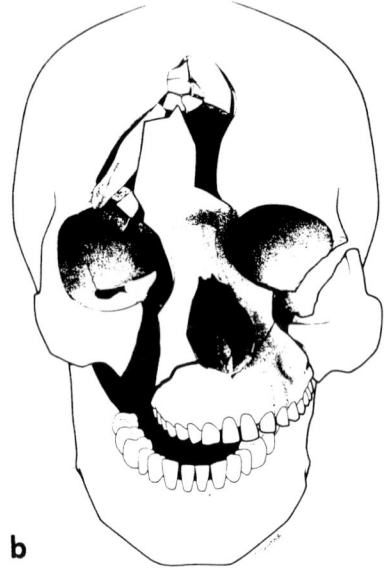

570   Rigid Fixation of the Craniomaxillofacial Skeleton

Figure 44.11 This lateral axial midface dislocation resulted in disruption of the skull base midline planes and concomitant multiple dural tears. (a) Dislocated frontal bone fractures are exposed through the open laceration wound. Axial lateral displacement of the midface and nose (N) are seen. (E = eyes.) (b) Schematic illustration shows the same fractures. (c) Repositioned midface and nasal buttress (N) and partially removed frontal bone fragments are seen. (E = eyes.) (d) The removed frontal bone segments are sutured, and the dural tears (D) are covered with fascia lata (F). (E = eyes, N = nose, S = subcranial approach for the management of the dural tears along the midline planes, sparing the cribriform plate.) (e) Miniplate osteosynthesis of the frontal bone fragments is seen. (E = eyes, N = nose.) (f) Postoperative radiograph. (g) The patient is shown 11 days postoperatively. He was mobilized after 6 days. (h) The patient is shown after two months. Note the scar of traumatic origin.

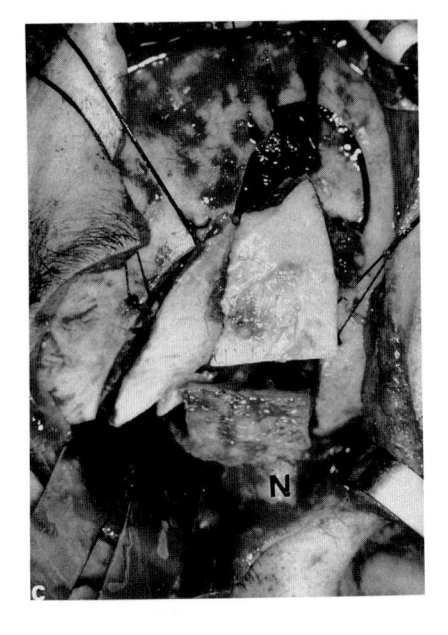

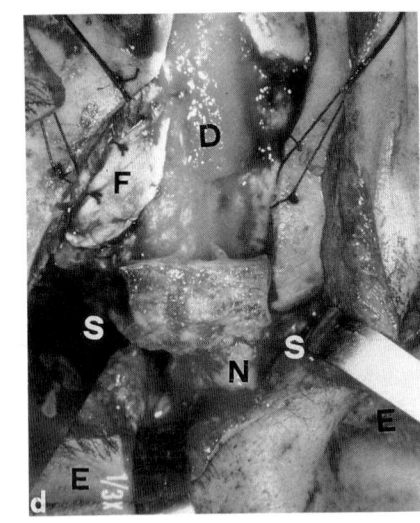

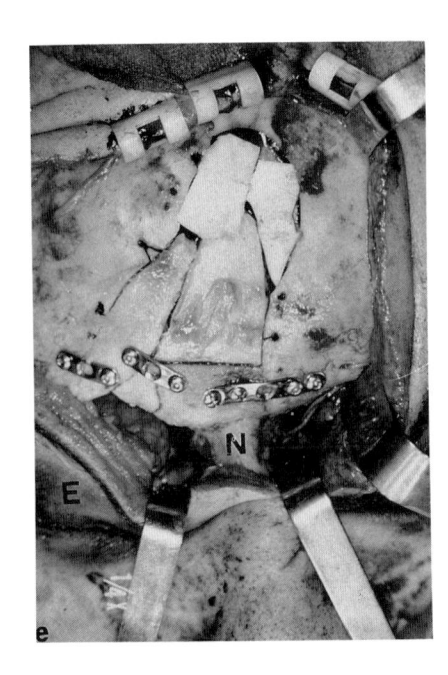

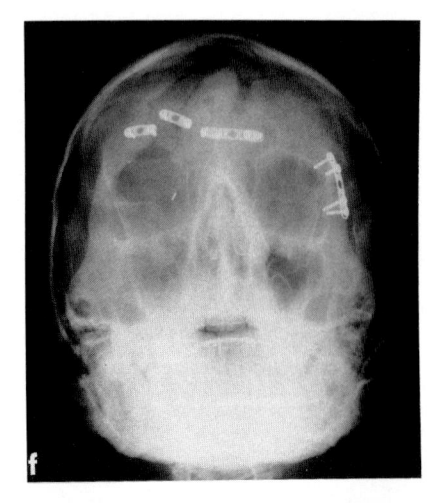

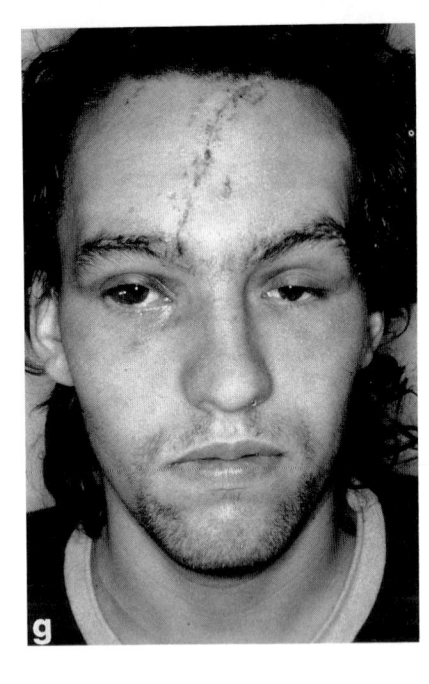

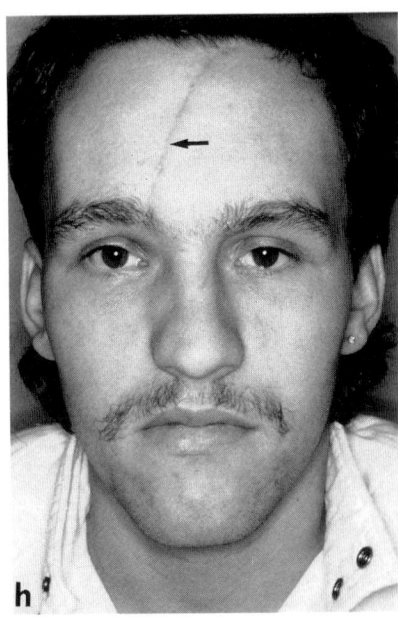

postoperatively; the period of hospitalization was only 12 days. Although this case was managed years ago with only wire ligatures, the results were satisfactory. The functional instability of wire ligatures made necessary immobilization of the jaws by IMF for three to four weeks. This should be considered a disadvantage. For this reason we prefer miniplate osteosynthesis because it enables jaw function.

THE SUBCRANIAL APPROACH FOR THE CORRECTION OF CRANIOFACIAL DEFORMITIES

The conventional methods for the reduction of the interorbital distance in certain craniofacial deformities include:

1. total resection of the midline, including the cribriform plate, the median part of the nasal buttress, and the septum (Murray 1976, Tessier 1967, Derome 1977, Mailard 1982, 1986, Van der Meulen 1983, Lejoyeux 1986);
2. partial preservation of the midline skull base structures (Freihofer 1977, Atkinson 1979, Ortiz-Monasterio 1981, David 1982, Obwegeser 1985, Anderl 1986, Goldin 1986); and
3. paramedian resection, leaving the skeletal midline intact (Converse 1970, Epstein 1975, Benedetti 1979, Munro 1979, 1981, Converse 1981, Pruzansky 1982, Furnas 1982, Jackson 1983, Caronni, 1985).

Common to all these procedures is the fact that the resection of the skull base and the roof of the orbits and the optic nerve decompression are performed by the intracranial transfrontal approach, making necessary the retraction of the frontal lobes and dura. Retraction and resection in this area may result in a higher incidence of consequent brain edema, damage to the olfactory filaments, and protracted hospitalization. The radical exenteration of the ethmoidal and sphenoidal compartment cannot be achieved by this access and the remaining mucosa may lead to the development of mucocele. For these reasons, the subcranial approach through the anterior and posterior walls of the frontal sinus to expose the median-paramedian frontal skull base area has been described (Furnas 1982, Jackson 1983). Proponents of this approach have pointed out that this procedure is time-consuming, and the limited exposure rendered by this access raises the risk of via falsa. Furthermore, significant correction of hypertelorism by the classical, limited transethmoidal access is thought to be impossible (Caronni 1985).

These arguments are fully justified and explain the fact that the transfrontal approach for the osteotomy of the skull base and orbital roof region is still the method of choice, despite the relatively high morbidity rate related to this procedure. The subcranial approach enables exposure and osteotomy of the orbital and ethmoidal roof, as well as the frontal arca, without retraction of the frontal lobes.

Clinical Material

We treated 38 cases surgically, either for fronto-orbital asymmetry and hypertelorism in craniofacial deformites or after inappropriate management of traumatically induced fractures.

Surgical Technique

For the reduction of orbital hypertelorism, we prefer paramedian resection (see Figure 44.13). The ethmoidal orbital roof on both sides, as well as the anterior fossa planes, including the sphenoidal, are broadly exposed by the subcranial approach, just as in the traumatic cases (see Figure 44.13d–f). The radical exenteration of the ethmoidal cells, stripping the mucosa and exposing of the orbital roof up to the apex (including the lateral walls), produces optimal access for subcranial paramedian skull base resection and osteotomy of the roof of the orbits. The optic nerve decompression is also performed by the same route, and the medial wall of the canal is removed. Thus the intracranial approach and retraction of the frontal lobes are unnecessary, the lamina cribrosa is preserved, and damage to the olfactory filaments can be avoided (see Figure 44.13d). A further advantage of this access is the efficient hemostasis of the ethmoidal vessels prior to the paramedian skull base resection.

After the reduction and definitive fixation of the osteotomized segments (see Figure 44.13f and g), the dura is covered with a layer of fascia lata and fibrin glue and with a second layer that lines the paramedian skull base, including the sphenoid. This layer serves as a watertight isolation from the paranasal spaces. This procedure can be performed only if the subcranial exposure has been carried out simultaneously. In order to avoid development of postoperative edema and compression in the apical region of the orbits, which often leads to an orbital apex syndrome, longitudinal incisions are performed in the medial aspect of the periosteum. Thus, periorbital expansion and drainage into the previous ethmoidal compartment is guaranteed. A Silastic tube, which is inserted on both sides underneath the skull base, emerges into the nasal lumen to serve as additional drainage of the subcranial compartment and frontal sinus. This drainage is maintained for six months in order to avoid obliteraton of the drainage pathway by granulation tissue. This case (see Figure 44.13h and i) demonstrates the efficiency of this procedure for the orbital osteotomy and advancement for correction of hypertelorism. In spite of the necessary resection and removal of the bilateral superfluous paramedian frontal ethmoidal roof and nasal bone, as well as the osteotomy

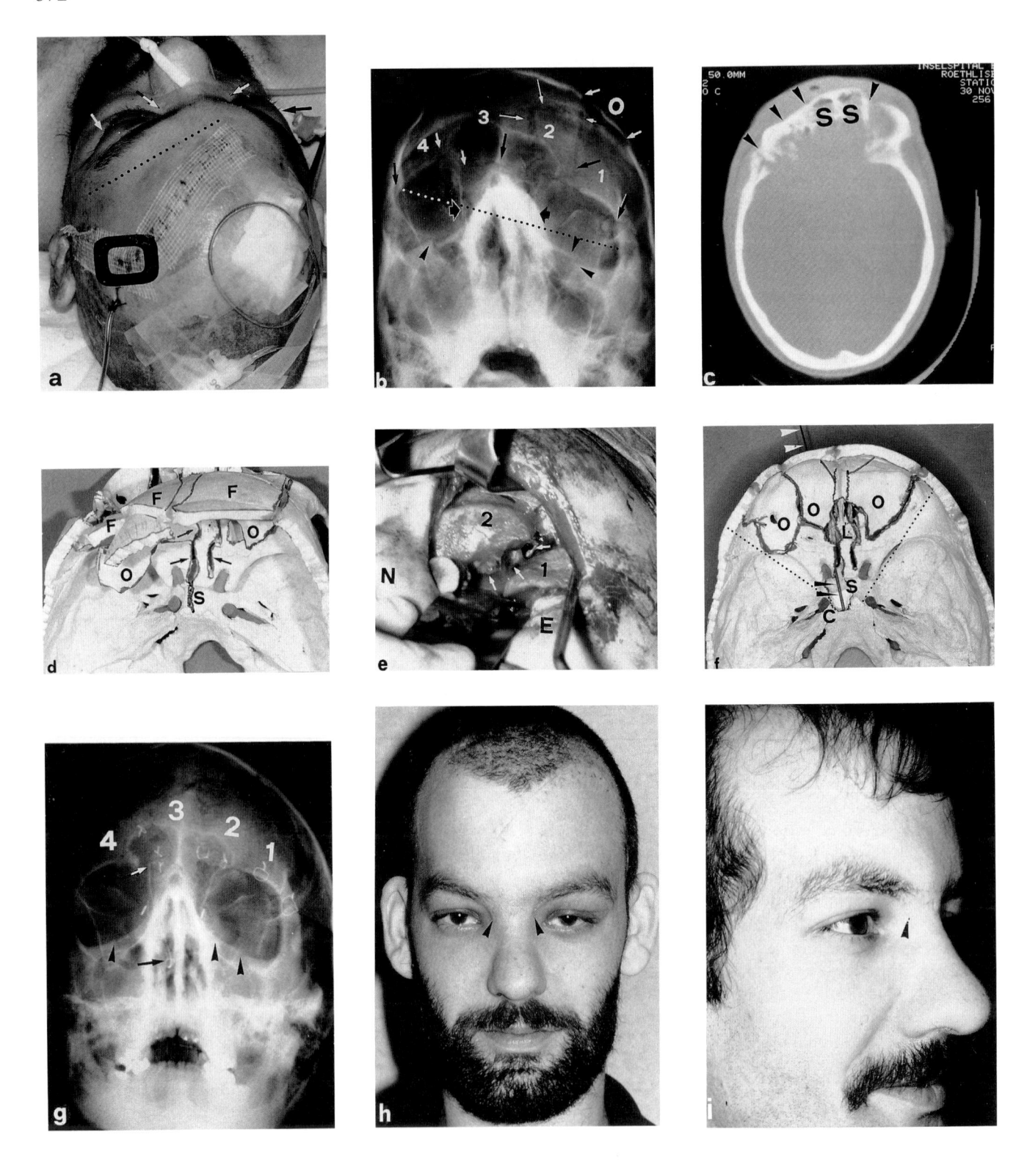

572   Rigid Fixation of the Craniomaxillofacial Skeleton

Figure 44.12 Dislocated multifragmentary fronto-naso-ethmoidal fractures, major dural tears and brain contusion are present in this case, as well as lateral fronto-orbital dislocation, hypertelorism, and concomitant simple midface fractures. (a) Initial neurosurgical local repair was limited to the dislocated calvarial fragment. Note depression of the left frontal bone area (arrows) inward telescoping of the nasal bone, hypertelorism and orbital asymmetry (arrows). (b) Preoperative radiograph. All further lesions were managed subcranially by the maxillofacial surgeon. The displaced frontal fragments are labeled 1–4. (O = site of neurosurgical repair, large arrows indicate lateral displacement of the medial orbital walls and lacrimal crest. Arrowheads indicate Le Fort II, III, and displacement of the infraorbital rim. Dotted line indicates displacement of the orbits and pseudohypertelorism. (c) CT scan shows major intracranial displacement of the multiple frontal fragments (arrowheads). (S = frontal sinus.) (d) Intracranial schematic illustration shows the same fractures. Repair was performed exclusively by the subcranial approach. (F = intracranially displaced fragments, O = major displacement of the orbital roof. Arrows indicate skull base fracture. (e) Intraoperative view shows the subcranial exposure. (E = eyebrow incision on the left, L = upper eyelids, N = dorsum of the nose. 1 and 2 are intracranially displaced fractures corresponding to Figure 44.13b. Arrows indicate dural tears after removal of prolapsed devital brain tissue.) (f) Schematic illustration shows the same skull base planes after frontal bone reduction. The instrument inserted subcranially; arrowheads into the sphenoid (S) indicates the subcranial route for the realignment of the skull base. Note the partially opened sphenoid and the adjacency of the carotid artery (C). (g) Postoperative radiograph shows the frontal bone reduction, corrected interorbital distance, and reduced zygoma fractures (arrowheads). Portex tube drainage (arrows) of the subcranial compartment into the nasal cavity is shown. (h) The patient is shown 17 days postoperatively. Note the slight edema of the upper lids. Incision limited to the left eyebrow. Overextended incision, as on the right, should always be avoided. (i) The patient is shown after one year.

of the orbital roof, no craniotomy was performed (see Figure 44.14f and g). The broad subcranial exposure renders optimal access for optic nerve decompression and necessary osteotomies. Bur holes applied at the paramedian frontal area through both frontal sinus walls, along with the subcranial exposure, enable the paramedian resection along with the preservation of the cribriform plate. Anosmia is avoided by leaving the midline skull base and nasal structures intact.

Three years after unsuccessful reduction of the traumatic fractures, the patient shown in Figure 44.15 was referred with asymmetric displacement of both zygoma and lateral nasal walls. In this case, the subcranial exposure was performed through the eyebrow and the already existing scar over the glabella, obviating a coronal flap. The surgical procedure was performed in the same manner as in the previous case.

Simultaneous Reduction of the Interorbital Distance, Correction of Exophthalmos, and Midface Advancement

In contrast to the already described cases, management of Apert syndrome, as shown in Figure 44.15, requires supplementary orbital and frontal advancement for the reduction of the exophthalmus. Treatment of Apert syndrome also requires midface osteotomy and correction of bone deformity. This case was selected to provide the proof, that despite the osteotomy of the frontal region and cranial vault, the osteotomy and resection can be limited to the paramedian frontal and skull base performed by the subcranial route, without the conventional transfrontal procedure and frontal lobe retraction.

Surgery, although performed in one session, is a major time-consuming procedure. We are of the opinion, however, that a better result can be obtained if the frontal, orbital, and nasal segments, as well as the midface, are simultaneously osteotomized and adjusted. Thus the patient is spared secondary corrections.

In this case, the subcranial exposure of the entire orbitofrontal and skull base area was performed as already described. The orbital and ethmoidal roof osteotomy, as well as that of the frontal region, was performed paramedian to the midline (see Figure 44.15b and c). Even in such cases, the midline structures of the skull base and nose are left undamaged. The optic nerve decompression was performed by the subcranial approach. The entire frontal bone segment (see Figure 44.15b and c) was temporarily removed. Segments of the deformed cranial vault were additionally osteotomized. In contrast to the conventional procedure, however, in none of these surgical stages was frontal lobe retraction performed, thus avoiding any damage to the olfactory filaments. The midface and nasal bone osteotomy was performed subsequently. Any skin incisions to the facial area were avoided.

The osteotomy of the floor of the orbit is always performed by the transconjunctival approach and that of the zygoma by the intraoral access. Visible skin incisions are thus avoided. Resulting defects in the floor of the orbit are bridged by lyophilized cartilage.

After the midface advancement and setting of the correct occlusion, retained by MMF, the orbital segments were advanced, followed by the frontal segment. The cranial vault fragments were exchanged and advanced (see Figure 44.15e and f) so as to achieve an even relief. The fragments were fixed with miniplates.

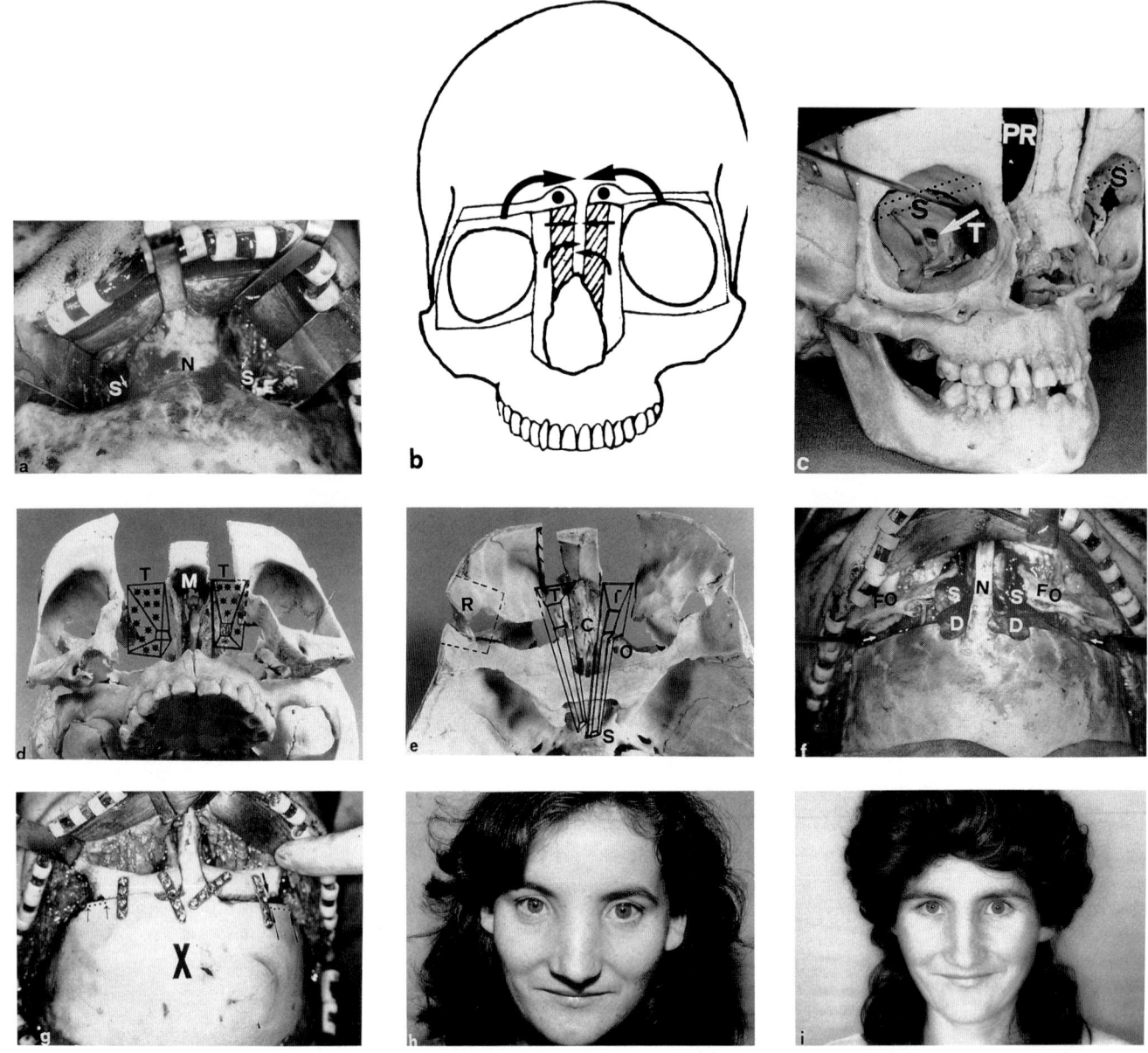

Figure 44.13 The subcranial approach for the correction of craniofacial anomalies obviates the need for craniotomy and transfrontal procedures. (a) Intraoperative view shows the broad nasal bone (N) and wide interorbital distance in Woake's syndrome. (b) Schematic illustration shows the osteotomy and resection. The entire osteotomy is performed via the subcranial-transethmoidal route. The arrows indicate paramedian resection of the lateral nasal walls. The midline structures are preserved. Orbital osteotomy and reduction of the interorbital distance are shown. (c) Prior to the frontonasal paramedian resection (PR) the subcranial (S) and transethmoidal (T) exposure and optic nerve decompression (arrow) are performed. (d) Paramedian resection after radical transethmoidal ethmoidectomy (T) and subcranial exposure preserves the midline structures (M). (e) Intracranial view shows the subcranially performed skull base osteotomy. The cribriform plate is preserved after resection of the ethmoidal roof and osteotomy of the orbital roof are performed by the subcranial and transethmoidal (T) approach. Any retraction of the frontal lobes or dura along the skull base is avoided. Optic nerve decompression (O) is performed via the transethmoidal route. (S = sella, C = cribriform plate.) (f) The patient is shown after paramedian resection. (FO = osteotomized, mobile fronto-orbital segments, D = dura, S = subcranial access for the resection of the ethmoidal and orbital roof, N = spared nasal midline.) (g) The patient is shown after orbital advancement (arrows) and reduction of the hypertelorism. (X = no craniotomy was performed.) (h) The patient is shown preoperatively. (i) The patient is shown postoperatively.

Table 44.3 Complications in 374 frontobasal fractures

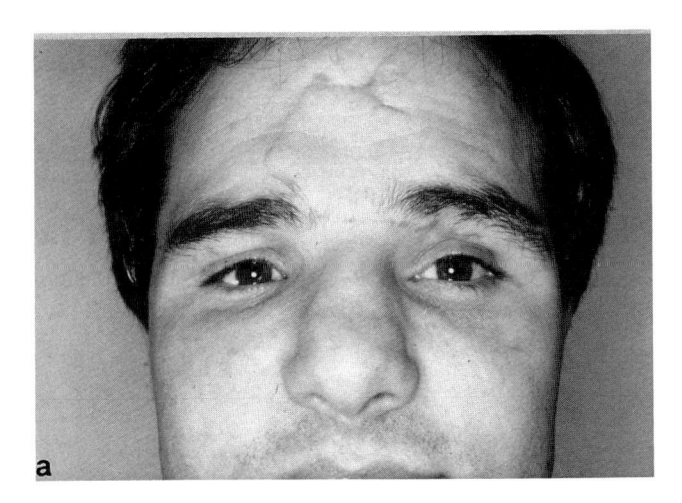

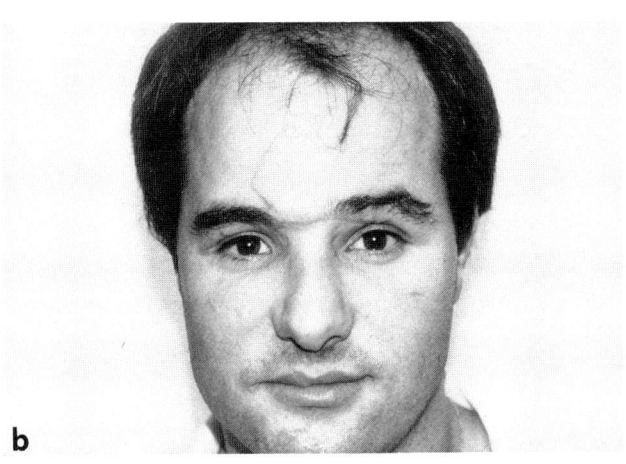

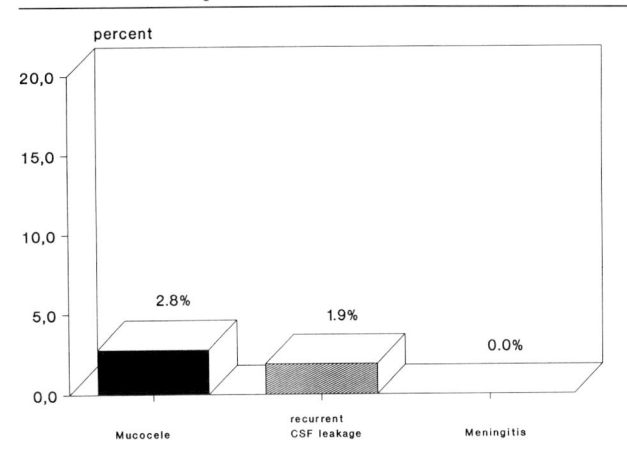

Figure 44.14 (a) This case of orbital asymmetry and hypertelorism of traumatic origin was surgically treated elsewhere three years previously. (b) The patient is shown after surgical correction by the same procedure outlined in Figure 44.13.

The postoperative result is shown in Figure 44.15 (g–j). The patient was discharged 13 days postoperatively, and the follow-up was uneventful.

RESULTS

Evaluation of 374 Surgically Treated Combined Craniofacial Injuries

These cases were kept in close observation and were followed up continuously for five years. After this period the patients were strictly instructed to contact us directly in case of any complications. Close follow-up is possible and particularly effective in Switzerland because of the relatively small territory; thus nearly 95% of patients are compliant. Apart from our team, the following disciplines were involved in the follow-up: neurosurgery; ophthalmology; ENT; and, for the occlusal aspects, the University School of Dental Medicine (Berne, Switzerland). Such continuous evaluation and computerized data collection facilitates evaluation of the postoperative results and obviates the laborous recall of so many patients after many years for a single study.

Our team mainly coordinated the follow-up and the examination of such various procedures performed by the various disciplines as the management of the skull base; orbital, zygoma, and facial asymmetries; vision, nerve, or sinus dysfunction; and occlusion. Such multidisciplinary evaluation is essential to exclude the possibility of any observer bias concerning the statistics and results.

The early surgical management of severe craniofacial injuries, and the fact that the subcranial-extracranial procedure involves less morbidity than the usual neurosurgical intracranial approach, allows reduction of the length of hospitalization. If no other systems were involved, the patients were mobilized after two to three days and discharged after 13.4 days (average).

1. *Recurrent postoperative CSF leaks:* Extension and modification of the classic transethmoidal approach resulted in a marked decrease in recurrent CSF leaks (Raveh 1984) to 1.9% (see Table 44.3). The case evaluations were repeated twice by the neurosurgeons, as well as by an independent physician (general medicine), in order to exclude any errors or missed CSF leaks.
2. *Postoperative meningitis:* None of the cases developed postoperative meningitis (see Table 44.3). The watertight duraplasty, as well as the isolation of the frontal skull base toward the paranasal spaces, proved to be most effective for the prevention of ascending infections.

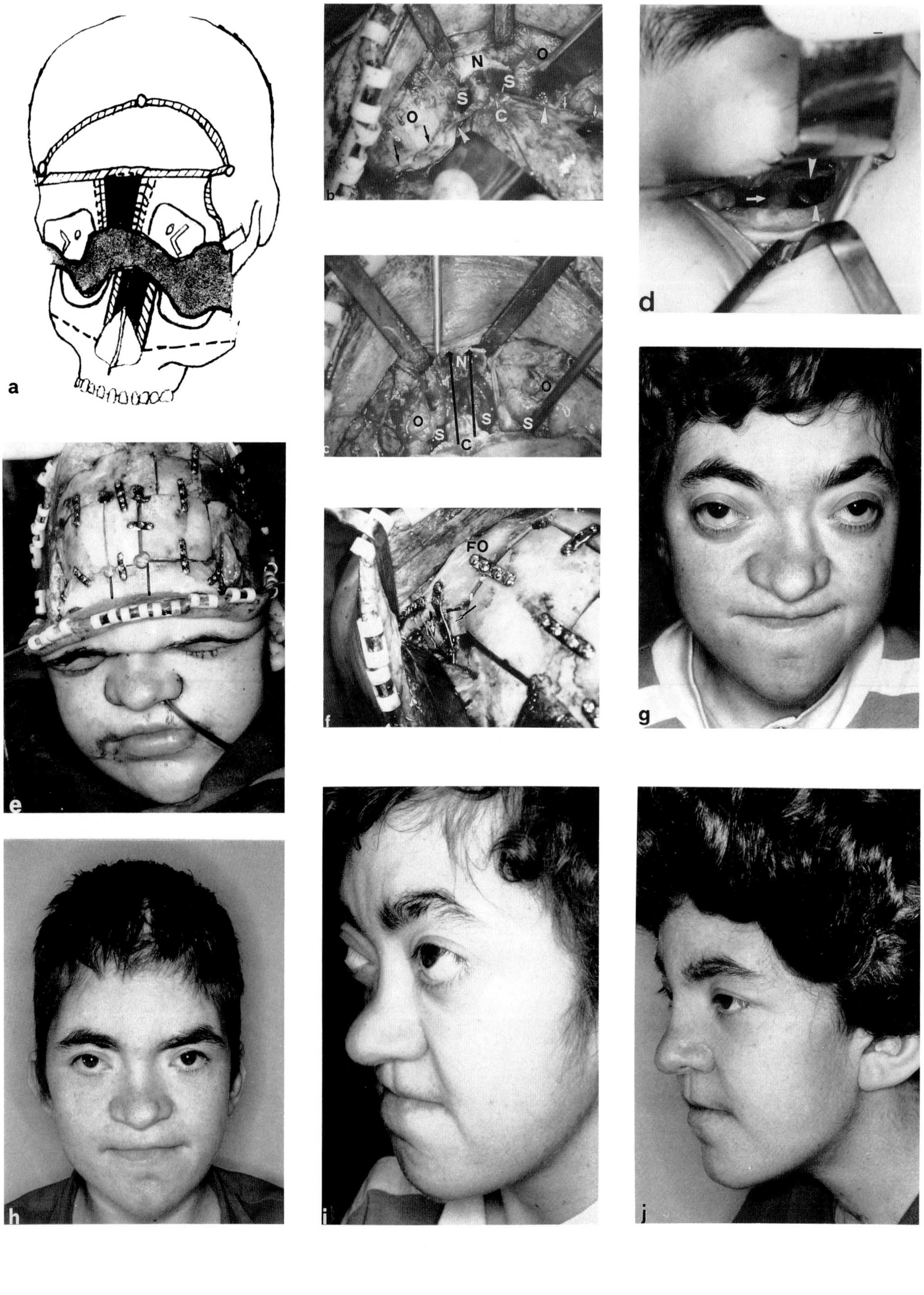
a
N
O
S
S
C
O
b
d
N
O
O
S
S
S
C
c
e
FO
f
g
h
i
j

Figure 44.15 The subcranial approach is shown for the correction of Apert syndrome with simultaneous midface osteotomy. (a) Schematic illustration shows the fronto-orbital and midface osteotomy. Note that the midline structures are spared. (b) Intraoperative view shows subcranial exposure of all the skull base planes. Osteotomy of the orbital (arrows) and ethmoidal roof (arrowheads) and optic nerve decompression by the subcranial approach are shown. The supraorbital and frontal segments are removed. This is done only to enable the advancement. No frontal lobe retraction at any stage is necessary, thus leaving the cribriform plate and olfactory filaments intact. (O = periorbital tissue, C = crista galli, N = osteotomized nasal roof.) (c) The patient is shown after midface advancement is performed. Lines show the degree of advancement. (N = nasal roof, C = crista galli, S = subcranial access, O = orbits.) (d) The transconjunctival approach is shown. Arrowheads indicate the floor of orbit gap with intact infraorbital nerve (arrow) after midface advancement. (e) The patient is shown after midface and consequent fronto-orbital segment advancement and plate osteosynthesis. (f) Lateral view of the advanced (FO) fronto-orbital and calvaria segments. Arrows indicate interpositioned bone grafts. (g) Frontal preoperative view. (h) Frontal postoperative view. (i) Lateral preoperative view. (j) Lateral postoperative view.

Table 44.4 Complications in the reduction of hypertelorism in 168 patients

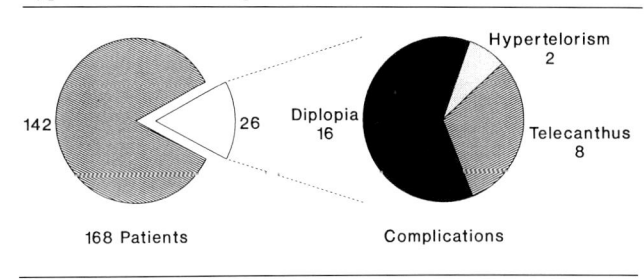

3. *Mucocele:* The exact reconstruction of the anterior and posterior frontal sinus walls and the Portex drainage of both sinuses into the nasal cavity, retained for six months, helped in reducing the incidence of mucocele to a minimum (see Table 44.3).
4. *Anosmia:* Because iatrogenic damage to the fila olfactoria is excluded by the subcranial approach, anosmia was observed only in those patients with direct traumatic lesions of this region. Recovery in those patients has not yet been evaluated.
5. *Interorbital distance, telecanthus, and enophthalmus:* This evaluation included only 168 (45%) of the cases, in which a significant extreme hypertelorism along with consequent naso-orbital wall fractures as well as telecanthus were manifest preoperatively. Such an unfavorable selection is much more significant than including the entire series. The evaluation included the measurements of the interpupillary distance, the corneal light reflex (Hertel ophthalmometer), and the intercanthal distance. We are of the opinion that such measurements are insufficient for determining the success of the operative procedure. The postoperatively measured distance, even if it is within the limits established for the normal population, may represent a significant unaesthetic enlargement for the individual patient when compared to the original intercanthal distance. For this reason, comparison with the patient's previous photographs was included in the evaluation, as well as the opinions of the patient and family members.

   a. *Hypertelorism:* In two cases secondary correction for inadequate reduction of the zygoma complex had to be performed. In no other cases was enlargement of the interorbital distance observed (see Table 44.4).
   b. *Telecanthus:* Eight cases had to be corrected secondarily for postoperative telecanthus (see Table 44.4). In 3, the canthal ligaments were insufficiently adapted; and in the remaining 5 cases, the lateral nasal wall was inadequately reduced. In 15 of the cases, a difference in comparison to the pretraumatic situation was observed, yet the change was so minimal and undisturbing for the patient that a secondary correction was justified.
   c. *Diplopia:* Enophthalmus leading to diplopia was manifest in 16 cases (see Table 44.4). In 7, insufficient reconstruction of the orbital floor made secondary correction necessary. In the remaining cases, conservative treatment by the ophthalmologist was performed. In 10 of these cases, according to the primary surgical report, traumatic lesions and disruption of the periorbital tissue was manifest.
6. *Further statistics:* Complications concerning the midface fractures, such as insufficient reduction of the zygoma, the floor of the orbit, and nasal bone; paranasal sinus dysfunction; occlusional aspects; and bone and cartilage transplant rejection are not the subject of this paper, and statistics regarding them have been deliberately omitted.

Table 44.5 Complications in the subcranial approach for the correction of craniofacial deformities

	Cases	Postoperative CSF Leak	Orbital Apex Syndrome	Mucocele	Secondary Corrections
Apert Syndrome	2	—	1	—	—
Crouzon's Disease	3	—	—	—	—
Woakes Syndrome	1	1	—	—	—
Hemifacial Dysplasia	2	—	—	—	—
Post-traumatic Hypertelorism	11	—	—	—	—
Post-traumatic Fronto-orbital Asymmetry	19	—	—	1	—
Total	38	1	1	1	—

Evaluation of the Surgically Corrected Craniofacial Anomalies

As indicated in Table 44.5, 38 cases were surgically treated. The subcranial exposure was performed in all patients. Hospitalization periods ranged between 11 and 15 days. Most of the patients were mobilized after three to four days. All patients were operated on in a one-stage procedure, and none required secondary corrective surgery.

The only complication occurred in one of the Apert syndrome cases, where an orbital apex syndrome, four days postoperatively, resulted in partial loss of vision in the left eye. We believe this resulted because on this side the incisions to the medial aspect of the periorbital periosteum were omitted, leading to insufficient drainage and expansion of the periorbital tissue into the subcranial lumen. Normal function of the optic nerve was maintained in all remaining cases. Double vision related to the orbital advancement or muscular dysfunction was observed in one case and was corrected by the ophthalmologist.

In one case, as a result of inappropriate alignment of the skull base with fascia lata, CSF leakage limited to the left side developed three days postoperatively. After application of lumbal drainage spontaneous sealing was achieved after five days. In none of the remaining cases was a postoperative CSF leak observed.

None of the patients developed meningitis or postoperative complications, making intensive or special care necessary.

With regard to the subcranial procedure, none of the cases had any diminution of olfactory function and perception postoperatively. In the Woaks syndrome case, the partial pre-existing dysfunction was unchanged postoperatively.

Considering the intraoperative restoration of drainage from the paranasal spaces, it is not surprising that with normal function, complications such as infection, mucus retention, and mucocele were restricted to only one case.

None of the cases developed abberative neurosurgical symptoms or neurological changes, and the morbidity rate was reduced to an absolute minimum.

DISCUSSION

The subcranial exposure and management of the entire frontal and skull base area, including the orbital and ethmoidal roofs, is crucial for performance of the surgical procedures and treatment modalities. In contrast to the transfrontal neurosurgical intracranial approach to the frontal area and skull base planes, the subcranial exposure represents almost an extracranial procedure, because no intracranial manipulation or frontal lobe retraction are performed. In reality the subcranial approach, although it exposes the dura, has nothing in common with the conventional neurosurgical intracranial procedure and is much better. Furthermore, the subcranial approach is the key to an early, one-stage reconstruction of severe craniofacial trauma cases. These severe high-velocity trauma cases (with disruption of the facial skeleton, hypertelorism, concomitant skull base fractures, and multiple dural tears, along with herniation of brain tissue) represent a much greater challenge than craniofacial deformities do if a primary and definite reduction is to be achieved. Correction of the growth in anomaly cases can be managed with well planned osteotomies and transposition of fragments. In contrast, the random pattern of comminuted fractures and the related risks are often unpredictable, in spite of the best radiographs and CT scans. The inwardly telescoped skull base with intracranially dislocated fragments and dysfunction of the orbita; nasal-midface buttresses; and concomitant bleeding emanating from the brain, dural, ethmoidal, and midface vessels represent a greater risk. The surgeon must be well acquainted with the anatomic configuration, so as to avoid iatrogenic injuries to the hypophisis, cavernous and sagittalis sinuses, optic nerve, and via falsa. The exact reduction of the fractures and of the hypertelorism in one session for aesthetic and physiologic restoration is by far the most fascinating field in craniofacial surgery.

The extremely low rate of complications and morbidity in the traumatic cases and the successful early one-stage reconstruction, reducing secondary correction to a minimum, confirm the efficacy of this procedure. The facts that optic nerve decompression by the subcranial technique is more radical than the conventional procedure and that this approach is less traumatic make a significant reduction of the hospitalization period possible. These advantages are also obvious in the treatment of craniofacial deformities.

Aware that in most deformity cases it is not the cribriform plate, but rather the ethmoidal compartment, which is enlarged (Converse 1970, Munro 1979), we always conserve the cribriform plate. The subcranial exposure and radical exenteration of the ethmoidal cells produce optimal visibility for the resection and osteotomy of the ethmoidal and orbital roof. Thus damage to the olfactory filaments can be avoided. Even when the orbital segments have shifted well toward the midline, the subcranial compartment created is broad enough to avoid pressure on the medial aspect of the globe and consequent lateral divergence. From the same transethmoidal access, the entire medial wall of the optic canal can be resected and removed, thus enabling optimal decompression. That the nerve is free to expand toward the midline is of particular significance. In most cases the orbital segments also need to be mobilized in this direction.

A further advantage of this approach is the feasibility of meticulous watertight repair and alignment of the skull base, including the sphenoid, with fascia lata serving as a barrier from the paranasal spaces. Note that in only one of the cases was postoperative CSF leakage observed, in contrast to other (David 1982, Matthews 1979) published reports. In comparison to the usual intracranial approach, the subcranial access is less traumatic and the morbidity rate related to the operation can be considerably reduced.

We are of the opinion that a surgeon, once acquainted with our techniques, will have no doubt as to their tremendous advantages.

Acknowledgment

We are indebted to H. Holzherr for the excellent quality of the schematic drawings and to the editors of the Archives of Otolaryngology—Head & Neck Surgery and European Journal of Cranio-Maxillofacial Surgery for the generous release of published photographs. We are particularly grateful for the excellent secretarial work of A. Zaugg.

REFERENCES

Anderl H, Muehlbauer W, Twerdy K, et al: Craniofaciale Chirurgie. Klin Monatsbl Augenheilkd 181: 331–338, 1986.

Arendall RE, Meirowsky AM: Air sinus wounds: An analysis of 163 consecutive cases incurred in the Korean War, 1950–1952. Neurosurgery 13:377–380, 1983.

Atkinson L, Emmet A, Pabari M: Craniofacial surgery. Med J Aust 1:541–544, 1979.

Benedetti A, Curioni C, Rubini L: Combined maxillofacial and neurological surgery for the correction of the tele-orbitism. J Neurosurg Sci 23:47–52, 1979.

Bongartz EB, Nau HE, Liesegang J: The cerebrospinal fluid fistula: Rhinorrhoea, otorrhoea and orbitorrhoea. Neurosurg Rev 4:195–200, 1981.

Briant TDR, Bird R: Extracranial repair of cerebrospinal fluid fistulae. J Otolaryngol 11:191–197, 1987.

Calcaterra TC: Extracranial surgical repair of cerebrospinal rhinorrhea. Ann Otol Rhinol Laryngol 89:108–116, 1980.

Calcaterra TC: Diagnosis and management of ethmoid cerebrospinal rhinorrhea. Otolaryngol Clin North Am 18:99–105, 1985.

Caronni EP: Craniofacial Surgery. Boston, Toronto, Little, Brown, p 163, 1985.

Converse JM, Ransohoff J, Mathews E, Smith B, Molenaar A: Ocular hypertelorism and pseudohypertelorism. Plast Reconstr Surg 45:1–13, 1970.

Converse JM, McCarthy JG: Orbital hypertelorism. Scand J Plast Reconstr Surg 15:265–276, 1981.

David D, Poswillo D, Simpson D: The craniosynostoses: Causes, natural history and management. Berlin, Heidelberg, New York, Springer, 1982.

Derome PJ, Tessier P: Craniofacial reconstruction in patients with craniofacial malformations: The neurosurgical approach. Clin Neurosurg 24:642–652, 1977.

Elies W: Zum gegenwaertigen Stand der Rhinobasischirurgie. Laryngol Rhinol Otol 61:42–47, 1982.

Epstein FJ, Wood-Smith D, Converse JM, Benjamin MV, Becker HM, Ransohoff J: Radical one-stage correction of craniofacial anomalies. J Neurosurg 42:522–529, 1975.

Escher F: Ein Beitrag aur Versorgung frontobasalen Hirnverletzungen. ORL J Otorhenolaryngol Relat Spec 6:326–332, 1944.

Escher F: Die frontobasalen Schädel-verlet Zungen. Schweiz Med Wochenschr 90: 1451–1458, 1960.

Escher F: Clinical classification and treatment of frontobasal fractures, in *Nobel Symposium: Disorders of the Skull Base Region*, pp 343–352. Alquist and Wiksell, Stockholm, pp 343–352, 1969.

Freihofer HP: Results of osteotomies of the facial skeleton in adolescence. J Maxillofac Surg 5:276–297, 1977.

Furnas DW, DeFeo DR, Kusske JA: Glabellar osteotomy and orbital craniotomies with microscopic control for correction of hypertelorism: A preliminary report of micro-craniofacial surgery in two patients. Plast Reconstr Surg 70:51–63, 1982.

Goldin H, Hockley A, Wake M, Beasley J: Craniofacial surgery. Br J Hosp Med 36:368–373, 1986.

Gruss JS: Fronto-naso-orbital trauma. Clin Plast Surg 9:577–589, 1982.

Jackson IT: The wide world of craniofacial surgery. J Oral Maxillofac Surg 41:103–110, 1983.

Laun A: Traumatic cerebrospinal fluid fistulas in the anterior and middle cranial fossae. Acta Neurochir 6:215–222, 1982.

Lejoyeux E, Tulasne JF, Tessier PL: Maxillary growth following total septal resection in correction of orbital hypertelorism. In Long-Term Results in Craniofacial Surgery. Marsch JL (ed). Burlington, Ontario, Decker, pp 27–39, 1986.

Lewin W: Cerebrospinal fluid rhinorrhea in nonmissile head injuries. Clin Neurosurg 12:237–247, 1966.

Lieberherr U: Zahn Jahre Erfahrung mit der mikrochirurgischen Versorgung fronto-basaler Liquorfisteln. Aktuel Probl ORL 9:48–55, 1985.

Ljunggren K: Liquorrhoea: A review of 66 cases. Acta Neurochir 51:173–186, 1980.

Loew F, Pertuiset B, Chaumier EE, et al: Traumatic spontaneous and postoperative CSF rhinorrhea. Adv Tech Stand Neurosurg 11:169–207, 1984.

MacGee EE, Cauthen JC, Brackett CE: Meningitis following acute traumatic cerebrospinal fluid fistula. J Neurosurg 33:211–316, 1970.

Mailard CF, Montandon D, Berney J: Techniques d'appoint de correction plastique d'hypertélorisme orbitaire. Rev Med Suisse Romande 102:409–415, 1982.

Mailard CF, Montandon D, Goin JL: Die kraniofaziale Chirurgie. Hexagon "Roche" 1:1, 1986.

Manson PN, Crawley WA, Hoopes JE: Frontal cranioplasty: Risk factors and choice of cranial vault reconstructive material. Plast Reconstr Surg 77:888–900, 1986.

Matthews D: Craniofacial surgery: Indications, assessment, and complications. Brit J Plast Surg 32:96–105, 1979.

Meirowsky AM, Caveness WF, Dillon JD, et al: Cerebrospinal fluid fistulas complicating missile wounds of the brain. J Neurosurg 54:44–48, 1981.

Munro IR: Improving results in orbital hypertelorism correction. Ann Plast Surg 2:499–507, 1979.

Munro IR: Craniofacial surgical techniques for aesthetic results in congenital and acute traumatic deformities. Clin Plast Surg 8:303–316, 1981.

Murray JE, Swanson LT, Strand RD, Hricko GM: Reconstructive surgery for major craniofacial deformities. Surg Clin North Am 56:495–512, 1976.

Myers DL, Sataloff RT: Spinal fluid leakage after skull base surgical procedures. Otolaryngol Clin North Am 17:601–617, 1984.

Obwegeser HL, Farmand M: Hypertelorism associated with other facial anomalies. In Craniofacial Surgery. Caronni, EP (ed). Boston, Toronto, Little, Brown, p 166, 1985.

Ortiz-Monasterio F, Fuente-del-Campo A: Nasal correction in hyperteleorbitism. Scan J Plast Reconstr Surg 15:277–286, 1981.

Paillas JE, Pellet W, Demard F: Les fistules ostéméningées de la base du crâne avec écoulement de liquide céphalo-rachidien. J Chir 94:295–303, 1967.

Park JI, Strelzow VV, Friedmann WH: Current management of cerebrospinal fluid rhinorrhea. Laryngoscope 93:1294–1300, 1983.

Pia HW: Schädelhirnverletzungen. Langenbecks Arch Chir 349:247–252, 1979.

Probst C: Neurochirurgische Aspekte bei fronto-basalen Verletzungen mit Liquorfirsteln: Erfahrungen bie 205 operierten Patienten. Aktuel Traumatol 16:43–49, 1986.

Pruzansky S: Craniofacial surgery: The experiment on nature's experiment. Review of three patients operated by Paul Tessier. Eur J of Orthod 4:151–164, 1982.

Raaf J: Post-traumatic cerebrospinal fluid leaks. Arch Surg 95:648–651, 1967.

Raveh J: Schwere Gesichtsschädelverletzungen: Eigene Erfahrungen und Modifikationen. Aktuel Probl ORL 3:145–154, 1979.

Raveh J, Neiger M: Die Wiederherstellung bei schweren Gesichtsschädelverletzungen. Schweiz Monatsschr Zahnmed 91:206–217, 1981.

Raveh J, Redli M, Markwalder TM: Operative management of 194 cases of combined maxillofacial-frontobasal fractures: Principles and surgical modifications. J Oral Maxillofac Surg 42:555–564, 1984.

Raveh J: Kraniofaziale Anomalien: Neue Aspekte chirurgischer Korrekturmethoden. DIA-GM 19:20–37, 1986.

Raveh J, Vuillemin T, Sutter F: Subcranial management of 395 combined frontobasal-midface fractures. Arch Otolaryngol Head Neck Surg 114:1114–1122, 1988a.

Raveh J, Vuillemin T: The surgical one-stage management of combined cranio-maxillo-facial and frontobasal fractures: Advantages of the subcranial approach in 374 cases. J Cranio Maxillofac Surg 16:160–172, 1988b.

Raveh J, Vuillemin T: Advantages of an additional subcranial approach in the correction of craniofacial deformities. J Cranio Maxillofac Surg 16:350–358, 1988c.

Raveh J, Vuillemin T, Lädrach K, Sutter F: Temporomandibular joint ankylosis: Surgical treatment and long-term results. J Oral Maxillofac Surg 47:900–906, 1989.

Rousseaux P, Scherpereel B, Bernhard MH, et al: Fractures de l'étage antérieur: Notre attitude thérapeutique à propos de 1254 cas sur une série de 11,200 traumatismes crâniens. Neurochirurgie 27:15–19, 1981.

Samii M, Draf W: Indikation und Versorgung der frontobasalen Liquorfistel aus HNO-chirurgischer und neurochirurgischer. Sicht Laryngol Rhinol Otol 57:689–697, 1978.

Strohecker J: Zur Akutversorgung offener Frontobasal-Traumen: Primaer- und Spaetergebnisse. Z Unfallchir Versicherungsmed Berufskr 77:21–26, 1984.

Suess W, Corradini C: Bakterielle Meningitiden als Spaetkomplikation persistierender traumatischer Liquorfisteln. Aktuel Traumatol 14:193–194, 1984.

Tessier P, Guiot G, Rougerie J, Delbet JP, Pastorial J: Ostéotomies cranio-naso-orbito-faciales. Hypertélorisme. Ann Chir Plast 12:103–118, 1967.

Van der Meulen JCH, Vaandrager JM: Surgery related to the correction of hypertelorism. Plast Reconstr Surg 71:6–19, 1983.

Westmore GA, Whittam DE: Cerebrospinal fluid rhinorrhoea and its management. Br J Surg 69:489–492, 1982.

Zurbuchen P: Les homogreffons de cartilage lyophilisés. Schweiz Monatsschr Zahnheilk 69:703–804, 1959.

CHAPTER 45

The Use of Rigid Fixation in the Treatment of Facial Asymmetries

Bahman Guyuron

Symmetry is an integral part of pleasing facial aesthetics even though, in reality, most faces have some degree of asymmetry. A disturbance of harmonic symmetry reduces the degree of attractiveness; conversely, the most desirable faces approach 100% bilateral symmetry. The classical concept of facial symmetry was depicted by Leonardo da Vinci and by Albrecht Dürer's drawings of 1507–1508 (Panofsky 1940, 1945). In 1836 Beck (1883) reported unilateral facial hypertrophy as the first medical problem concerning facial asymmetry. It was not until the early twentieth century, with the work of Angle (1907), that more documentation of asymmetric facial deformities received attention. Gruenberg (1912) and Keith (1910) are credited with describing the role of occlusion in facial asymmetry. During the last three decades, advancements in technology such as plain radiology (Forsberg 1984, Berger 1961), computerized axial tomography (CAT) and its three dimensional version (Hemmy 1983, Marsh 1983, Vannier 1984, Cutting 1986), and computer-generated models (Guyuron 1989b) have increased our understanding of asymmetric faces. This increase in understanding has led to proper diagnosis and appropriate surgical planning.

ETIOLOGY AND CLASSIFICATION

The etiology of some rare facial asymmetries might never be clear; however, all facial asymmetries fall into one of two major categories: congenital and acquired (see Table 45.1). A facial asymmetry is congenital if the patient is born with the asymmetry; acquired facial asymmetry develops after birth. A number of conditions encompass an array of congenital facial asymmetries: hemifacial hypertrophy or hyperplasia (Pollock 1985, Sculerati 1985, Adams 1894, Beck 1883, Benson 1963, Bergmen 1973, Bjorklund 1955, Burchfield 1980, Gesell 1921, 1927, Gorlin 1962), hemifacial microsomia (Munro 1987, Poole 1989, Pisarek 1988, Mulliken 1987, Ortiz-Monasterio 1982, Vargervik 1986) craniosynostosis, hemifacial atrophy, and facial clefts (Chierici 1970, Whitaker 1981). The major etiologic factor for acquired facial asymmetry involves a group of asymmetries of idiopathic origin, such as condylar hyperplasia (Reyneke 1979, Mizuno 1988, Rubenstein 1985, Vazirani 1967, Norman 1980, Bruce 1968, Blomquist 1963, Beirne 1980, Kessel 1969), masseteric hypertrophy (Buchner 1979, Roncevic 1986, Hersh 1946), Romberg's disease, torticollis (Keller 1986), acromegaly, and Cauhepe Fieux syndrome (Chateau 1975).

Trauma is another etiology in the development of facial asymmetry. The cause of trauma can be either temporomandibular joint (TMJ) ankylosis (Couly 1980, Vitton 1974) or direct injury of facial bones causing displacement and malunion (see Figure 45.1). A variety of benign processes such as lymphangioma, hemangioma, arteriovenous malformation, neurofibromatosis, fibrous dysplasia, tuberous sclerosis, and Paget disease also result in facial asymmetry (see Table 45.1). Another common etiologic factor for facial asymmetry is irradiation (Guyuron 1983, 1987). According to these studies, high radiation doses result in delayed growth of facial soft tissue and bones. Irradiation doses of 3000 rads or more contribute to the development of asymmetric faces involving the bone. However, soft tissue asymmetry can develop from an irradiation dose as little as 400 rads.

Table 45.1 Etiology of facial asymmetry

Congenital
Facial clefts
Hemifacial microsomia
Craniosynostosis
Hemifacial hypertrophy

Acquired				
Trauma	*Expanding Masses*	*Idiopathic*	*Infections*	*Metabolic*
TMJ ankylosis	Lymphangioma	Condylar hyperplasia	Osteomyelitis	Asymmetric acromegaly
Facial bone fracture with malunion	Hemangioma	Unilateral masseteric hypertrophy	TMJ arthritis	
	Arteriovenous malformation	Romberg's disease		
	Neurofibroma	Torticolis		
	Tuberous sclerosis			
	Paget disease			
	Tumors or cysts			

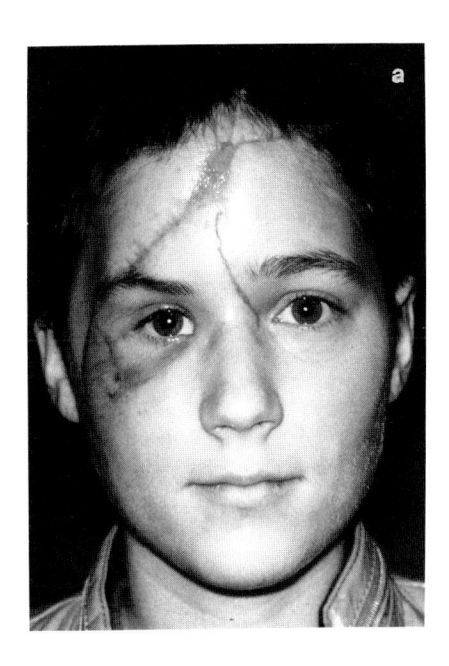

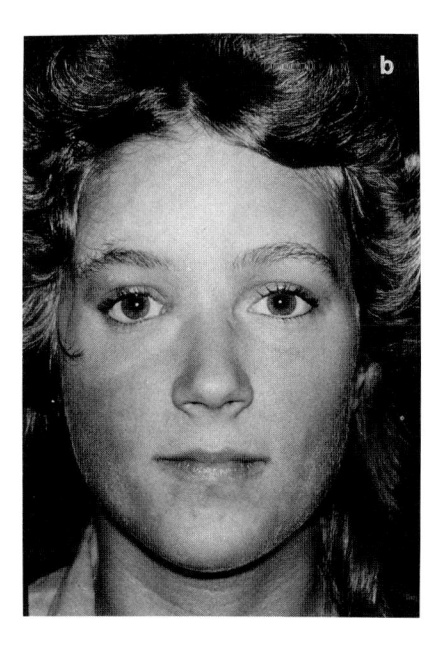

Figure 45.1 (a) A 16-year-old's photograph reveals displaced right orbit due to malunited malar bones. (b) The same patient is shown two years following revision of forehead scars, transposition of right orbit laterally and cephalad, and correction of enophthalmos.

PATIENT ASSESSMENT

A detailed history may assist in differentiating between acquired and congenital facial asymmetry (Smylski 1976). In fact, the history is often the key to proper diagnosis. Physical examination should include a step-by-step, thorough facial evaluation, where the face is divided into three arbitrary, equal portions and each portion is evaluated separately. The first division is from the forehead hairline to the eyebrow level, the second from the eyebrows to the subnasale, and the third from the subnasale to the menton.

The forehead shape, level of eyebrows, eye symmetry, nose, oral commissures, and the chin lineup are examined individually on front view and profile. An overhead and worm's eye view of the patient's face reveals the facial asymmetry more clearly. This becomes especially important in comparing projections of zygomatic arches (Chateau 1975, Benoist and LePesteur 1976). The patient is asked to smile so that the upper lip's relation to the teeth in full smile and in repose can be assessed. The amount of gum show is checked, and the sides are compared. The final step, an important one in assessing facial symmetry, is the placement of a tongue blade in the occlusal plane and the determination of its relationship to the horizontal facial plane and pupil levels. This simple test provides the examiner with important information by clearly revealing horizontal

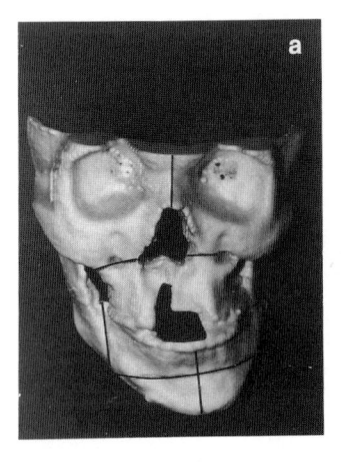

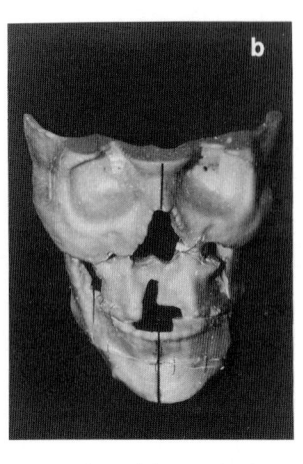

Figure 45.2 (a) This computer-generated model reveals significant asymmetry. (b) Model surgery has been performed. The midline has been aligned, and the movements have been measured and utilized as a surgical blueprint.

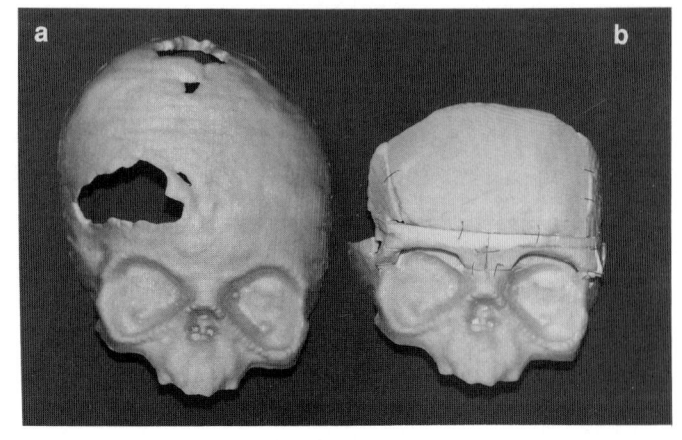

Figure 45.3 (a) This computer-generated skull model shows oxycephaly, cranial asymmetry, and defects in the vertex and the right side of the frontal bone associated with previous surgery. (b) Perfect forehead contour, reduction of forehead height, correction of cranial asymmetry, and forehead advancement are results of model surgery. The movements were measured and recorded, and the segments were utilized as an intraoperative template.

discrepancies, which are a reflection of vertical abnormalities. The fact remains that vertical abnormalities are more visible and aesthetically more significant than horizontal asymmetries. For example, an oral commissure wider on one side than the other will be less noticeable than one that is lower on one side (Munro 1989).

Next, appropriate photographs are taken which include facial front and lateral views, smile, front view slide with or without tongue blade in position, and occlusion. Another important part of the examination is obtaining life-size photographs, which are analyzed via soft tissue cephalometrics (Ginestat 1959, Guyuron 1988). An overlay is used to measure and check the symmetry and to define the pathology. Cephalometric x rays (Nardoux-Sanders 1968) and panorexes will then be obtained. Submental vertex x rays (Forsberg 1984) define the asymmetry of the mandible more precisely. In severe cases, computer-generated models (see Figures 45.2 and 45.3) can be of significant value in defining the deformity and planning the correction (Guyuron 1989b).

INDICATION FOR SURGERY

Even though a majority of the patients presented for surgery are referred because of facial disharmony, a large percentage of these patients suffer from TMJ discomfort; mastication difficulties; digestive complications; and, occasionally, speech abnormalities (Hovinga 1974). Increased interest in facial harmony and awareness of the role of facial proportionality in its attractiveness make it necessary to detect these abnormalities and to correct them appropriately if they are significant enough to disturb the facial balance. TMJ symptoms range from common clicking to complete ankylosis of the joint. Masticatory disturbances are caused by inability to oppose the cusps and grooves of the occlusal surfaces due to crossbite or open bite. Indigestion is caused by ingestion of inadequately masticated food. Furthermore, improper tongue positioning, occlusal abnormalities, and jaw asymmetry may result in speech difficulties. Some patients have expanding tumors, which occasionally can be life-threatening. This, of course, is an absolute medical indication for surgical intervention.

TIMING AND PLANNING OF SURGICAL PROCEDURE

Proper diagnosis is a key to successful planning and management of overall asymmetric facial deformities. The involved portion of the face must also be defined precisely. As stated earlier, the arbitrary divisions of the face are division I, from the vertex to the eyebrow level; division II, from the eyebrow level to the subnasale; and division III, from the subnasale to the mention. If the upper division is involved, a determination is made whether the involvement is soft tissue or, as is more common, the frontal bone and the superior orbital rims. The asymmetric areas in the middle division are normally the orbits, the zygomas, and the nose. The maxilla, the mandible, and the chin compose the usual affected sites in the lower division. Some patients can

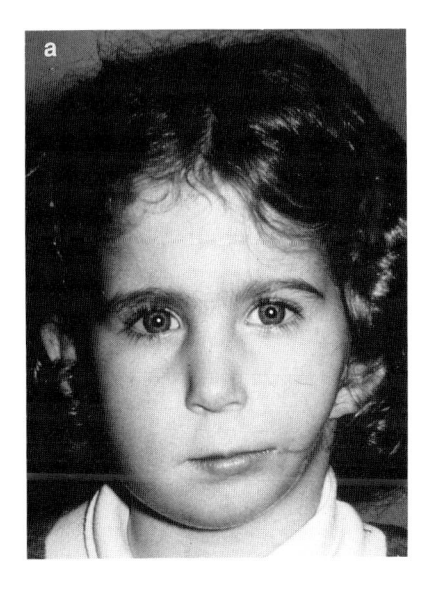

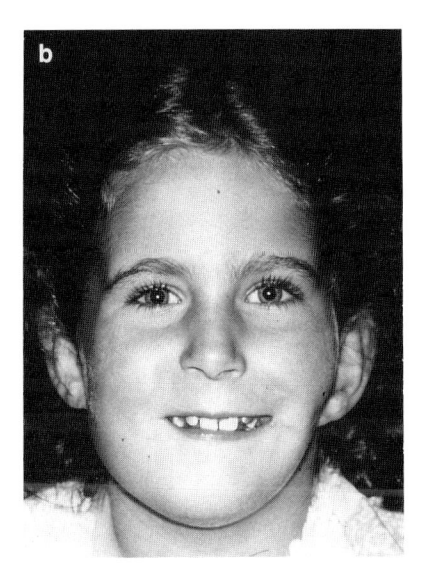

Figure 45.4 (a) This patient, shown before surgery, has left-sided hemifacial microsomia. (b) The same patient is shown three years following a left-side costochondral graft, which provided so much growth that the chin point was displaced toward the patient's right side. The soft-tissue deficiency has not been corrected yet.

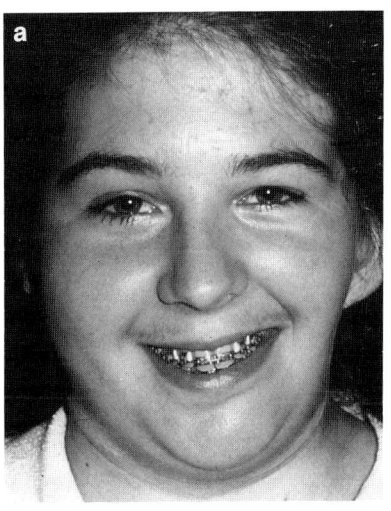

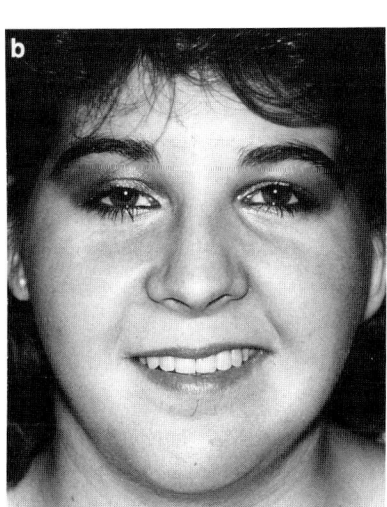

Figure 45.5 (a) Patient with left-sided hemifacial microsomia with a hemifacial microsomia preoperatively and (b) following bimaxillary osteotomy, costochondral graft to the left side, dermis graft for soft-tissue augmentation three years postoperatively.

have asymmetry in a combination of two or three divisions.

The affected tissues must be identified. The pathology can include skin and subcutaneous tissue only (for example, lipodystrophy or Romberg's disease) or a combination of skin muscles in a patient with a radiation-induced deformity if the radiation is given following completion of facial growth. An isolated muscle abnormality may be present, such as unilateral masseteric hypertrophy; or the pathology may be a result of skeletal deformity from unilateral condylar hyperplasia. However, the deformity usually encompasses a combination of these anatomic layers.

The forehead asymmetry is usually the result of either a unilateral coronal synostosis or a bilateral coronal synostosis involving one side more than the other. Under this condition, the preferred time for correction of the deformity is around three months of age, when the bones are firm enough to be advanced in order to correct the forehead asymmetry. If corrected at this time, the deformity often does not affect the orbital growth.

Deformities such as hemifacial microsomia (Kaban 1986) continue to deteriorate with age. Many benign tumors follow the same course. However, some deformities may remain stable and only grow with the patient. Finally, there are rare asymmetries that become less noticeable with age.

Generally, corrections of most bony deformities should be delayed until growth is completed (Souyris 1983), although some authors advocate earlier surgery (Merville 1970, Munro 1987, Ortiz-Monasterio 1982, Vargervik 1986, Kaban 1986). Often, for successful results, treatment must be individualized. I agree with authors who support early treatment of TMJ ankylosis and hemifacial microsomia (Mulliken 1987) (see Figure 45.4). With careful observation, correction of Type I hemifacial microsomia can be delayed until the growth is completed or the deformity becomes more visible (see Figure 45.5).

During surgical planning, definition of midlines can be difficult on patients with major facial asymmetry, particularly when it involves the upper face. If at least one division of the face is in normal position, the symmetry can be achieved by using that division as a reference. If one whole side of the face is asymmetric, then deciding which side is the normal side may be difficult. In such a case, duplicating life-size photographs of each half of the face and placing the reversed halves side by side might be helpful. A decision should be made between the surgeon and the patient, after careful examination of the full-size photograph, as to which side should be corrected. If lower, middle, or upper division on one side is out of proportion, then the task is less challenging because that division can be corrected to match the opposite side. In rare post-trauma cases, all three divisions on both sides are out of position. With the help of a medical artist who uses the patient's old photograph enlarged to life size, the appropriate movements are designed on an overlay. The surgical strategy is then practiced on a computer-generated model, the importance of which in rearrangement of such a distorted anatomy cannot be stressed enough (Guyuron and Ross 1989b).

When an asymmetric single jaw is dealt with following correction of dental compensation by the orthodontist and alignment of the arches, the occlusion is used as a reference to move the abnormal jaw to occlude with the opposite jaw in a normal relationship. If the maxilla is asymmetric, except in trauma cases, often the mandible is involved as well.

When the maxillary vertical repositioning is planned, the best guide is the relation of the upper incisal edge to the upper lip. If the relationship of the upper central incisor to the upper lip is ideal, the maxilla will be lowered on the short side and raised on the long side, pivoting at the midline. This will ensure that the overall maxillary length is not altered. If the upper central incisor show is inadequate, then the short side will be lengthened accordingly to correct the deficiency. If, however, the incisor show is excessive (for example, producing a gummy smile), then the long side is shortened and no change is made on the shorter side. It may be necessary to lengthen or shorten both sides differentially, based on the overall preoperative maxillary excess or deficiency. A mandibular osteotomy is then planned to allow the rotation of the mandible and to re-establish the proper relationship between the upper and lower jaws.

When chin asymmetry is dealt with, the anterior lower facial height is taken into consideration. If the height is ideal, then a segment of bone is removed from the longer half and added to the opposite side (see Figure 45.6). This process will allow rotation of the menton to the resected side. Occasionally, this movement is a slide in a horizontal plain (a transposition rather than a rotation) (see Figures 45.7 and 45.8). If shortening is necessary, then a wedge is resected, based on the long side, and not replaced on the opposite side. This allows reduction in anterior lower facial height at the same time. If the plans include lengthening, the osteotomy is done horizontally, bone graft or hydroxyapatite is added to the short side, and rigid fixation is accomplished.

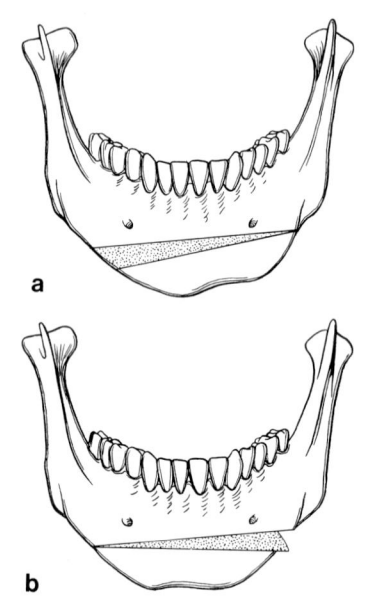

Figure 45.6 An asymmetric caudal mandible due to malposition of the chin. A segment is planned to be removed from the left side and applied to the right side in order to keep the mandibular anterior height stable, yet, correct the asymmetry.

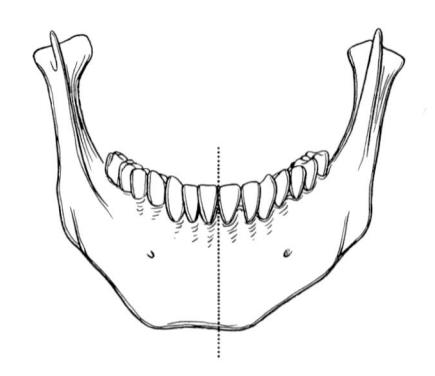

Figure 45.7 Artistic rendering of an asymmetric mandible due to chin deviation to the right side.

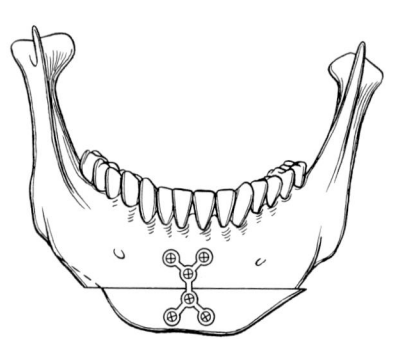

Figure 45.8 Horizontal transposition of the caudal segment following osteotomy and rigid fixation. The irregularities along the mandibular border will be burred down to provide symmetric positioning.

SURGICAL TECHNIQUES

The procedure is done under general anesthesia—except for genioplasty, which possibly can be done as an outpatient procedure under attended local anesthesia (Spear 1987).

For correction of forehead asymmetry due to coronal synostosis, an intracranial approach is used through a bicoronal incision. I strongly suggest the use of a hypotensive anesthesia technique for any major osteotomy involving intracranial procedures or maxillary and mandibular osteotomies. For a simple overlay bone graft to the zygoma, however, normotensive anesthesia is preferred. Furthermore, for the transcranial procedures, the intracranial pressure is reduced by way of a combination of hyperventilation and keeping the intravenous fluid, judged by the urine output, as small as possible. Occasionally, diuresis may be necessary. A forehead skin flap is raised via a bicoronal incision and reflected caudally. The supraorbital, neuro-vascular bundle is freed; this may require a small osteotomy. The periorbita is mobilized circumferentially. Even at an early age, on patients with unilateral coronal synostosis, there usually is compensation on the uninvolved side resulting in frontal bossing; therefore, a bifrontal osteotomy is often necessary (see Figure 45.9). Use of a computer-generated model assures more accuracy and decreases surgical time by enabling proper planning (Guyuron 1989b). A frontal bone flap is removed by the neurosurgeon to allow mobilization of the dura under the frontal bar. The flap is also separated from the anterior fossa to help retraction of the frontal lobes. The osteotomies are made through the orbital roof, lateral orbital wall, and frontal bar. The bar is advanced on the retrusive side and set back on the protruded side, if necessary. A suitable piece of bone is used to rebuild an ideal frontal contour. The remaining bones are then placed back in the sides of the newly constructed frontal bone. I do not believe a free-floating forehead advancement is effective. The bar is fixed by a tongue and groove technique with miniplates and screws. The skin is draped and the wound is irrigated. I prefer to use a conjunctival incision to expose the infraorbital rim if such exposure is necessary. If the condition dictates, the medial canthus is detached and reattached at the completion of the surgery.

For correction of unilateral orbital dystopia, depending on the nature of the asymmetry, the surgical procedure is planned by resecting a segment of the frontal bone cephalad to the orbit. This resection may be necessary on the lateral or medial orbital wall (see Figures 45.10 and 45.11) and on the lateral or caudal portion of the zygoma in order to create a space into which the orbit can be moved (see Figure 45.12). The resected segment from any site is then applied to the defect resultant from transposition of the orbit. The transposed segments are then rigidly fixed in position by thin plates (see Figure 45.13). I use either Würzburg (titanium) or Luhr (Vitallium) plates and screws. Small screws are used for rigid fixation of cranial bone, and screws of larger diameter are used for maxillary/mandibular osteotomies and tension sites. The available screws range from 5 to 15 mm for Würzburg plates (in 2-millimeter increments), and 3, 4, and 6 millimeters for Luhr plates.

In pediatric cases, a newly developed microsystem by Professor Hans Luhr can be used (personal communication). The wound is irrigated copiously with antibiotic solution, and suction drains are placed in position if no persistent communication between the wound and the nasal cavity exists. Otherwise, the drains are connected to an empty intravenous solution bag and left to gravity drainage in order to avoid forced current of bacteria from the nasal cavity into the cranial wound. The forehead flap is draped, and watertight repair is done.

One of the most significant contributions of rigid fixation has been in the area of maxillary and mandib-

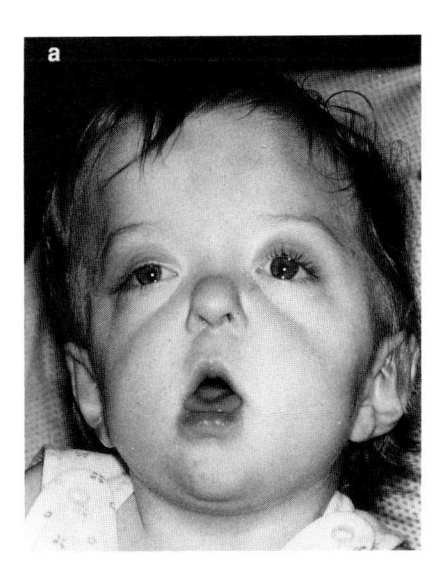

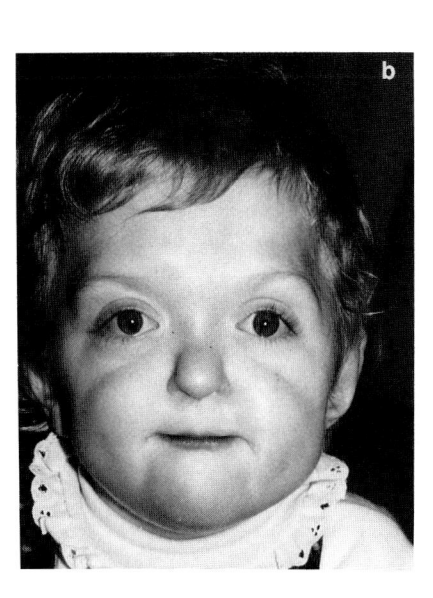

Figure 45.9 (a) Patient with asymmetric coronal synostosis resulting in significant deviation of the skull to the right side before surgery. (b) One year following frontal craniotomy, transpositional bone graft, and transpositional cranioplasty.

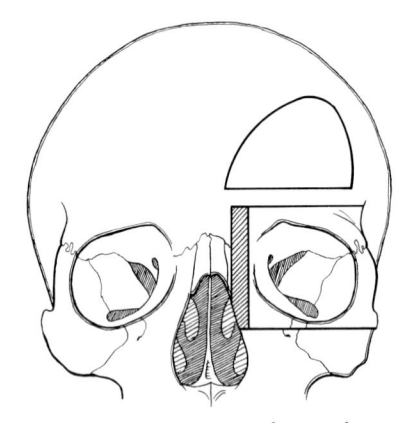

Figure 45.10 Artistic rendering shows the operative approach to horizontal orbital dystopia, which requires resection of the segment of the orbit medially through an intracranial approach by removing a frontal flap.

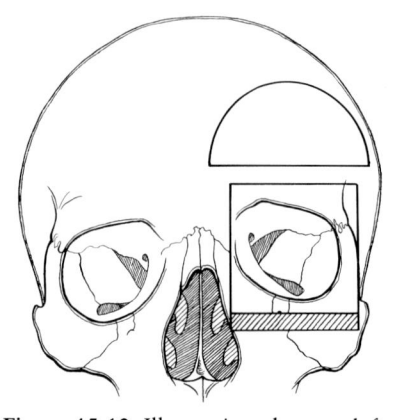

Figure 45.12 Illustration shows a left-sided vertical orbital dystopia and the design of the craniotomy and orbital osteotomy. The line shows the amount of bone that will have to be removed from the zygoma in order to allow the orbit to be lowered vertically.

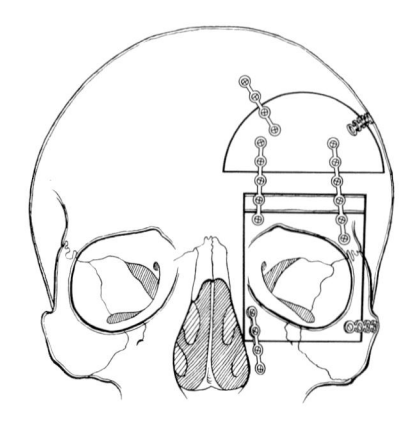

Figure 45.13 Artistic rendering shows a completed correction of vertical orbital dystopia following lowering of the orbit, application of bone graft, and rigid fixation.

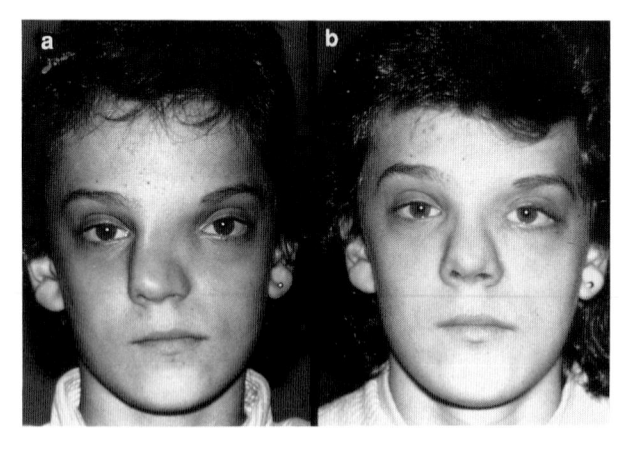

Figure 45.11 (a) This 16-year-old's photograph shows significant left-sided unilateral orbital dystopia and nasal deviation preoperatively. (b) The same patient is shown three years following transcranial correction of orbital dystopia.

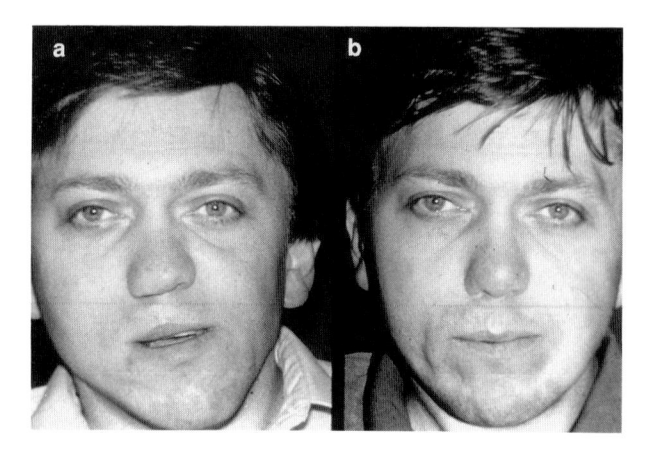

Figure 45.14 (a) Preoperative photograph shows a patient with significant facial asymmetry related to cleft lip/cleft palate. (b) The same patient is shown two years following maxillary and mandibular osteotomy and genioplasty.

ular asymmetry (Munro 1989, Whitaker 1989, Choung 1985, Hall 1984, Brami 1974). However, in order for the rigid fixation to be successful when the occlusion is involved, precise planning and close cooperation with the orthodontist is crucial (see Figures 45.14–45.16).

The procedure is done under general hypotensive anesthesia. The exposure is achieved through an intraoral approach. Seldom in my practice has an external incision for a maxillary or mandibular osteotomy been necessary, except in earlier cases of rigid fixation where a trocar was usually introduced through a small stab incision in the submandibular area to guide the bur. With the use of plates and screws, rather than screws alone, even these small external incisions are avoidable. When a bimaxillary osteotomy is planned, the maxillary surgery is performed first (Guyuron, 1989a). It is very important to have an interim splint fabricated so that the maxilla is guided to a proper position horizontally and vertically. Again, the relationship of the incisal edge to the upper lip is an accurate guide to the length of the maxilla. Furthermore, the degree of gum show and its asymmetry will be used to decide whether the resection will be on only one side (see Figures 45.17 and 45.18) or a resection on one side and bone graft on the opposite side will be required (see Figure 45.19). Occasionally, it is necessary to use bone graft on both sides—more on one side than the other. A rotation along the cephalocaudal axis may also be necessary. All of these movements will have to be planned in advance.

Generally, I use four plates for the maxilla: two at the nasal pyramid level and two at the zygomatic buttress regions. The remaining portions of the maxilla

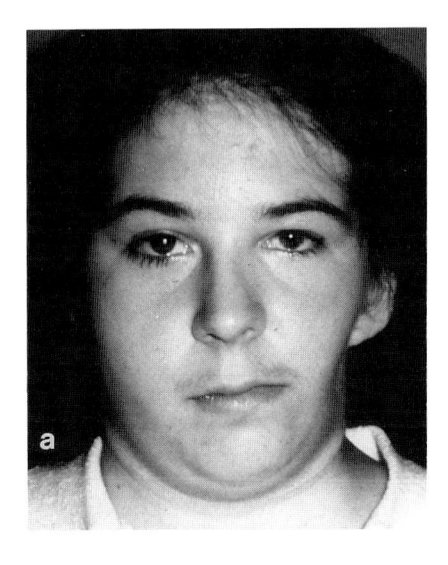

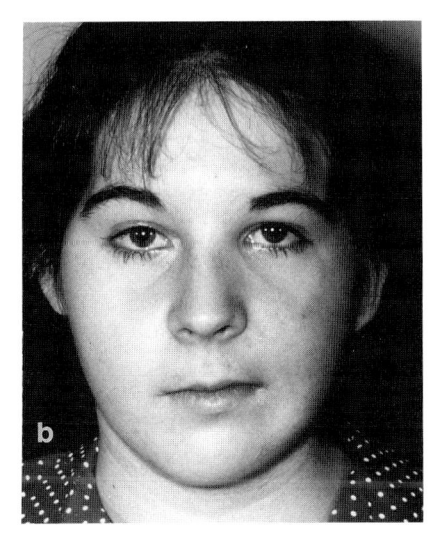

Figure 45.15 (a) This patient has hemifacial microsomia and a combination of soft-tissue and skeletal deficiencies. (b) The same patient is shown five years following maxillary and mandibular osteotomy, bone grafting, reconstruction of left TMJ, and soft-tissue augmentation with fat graft.

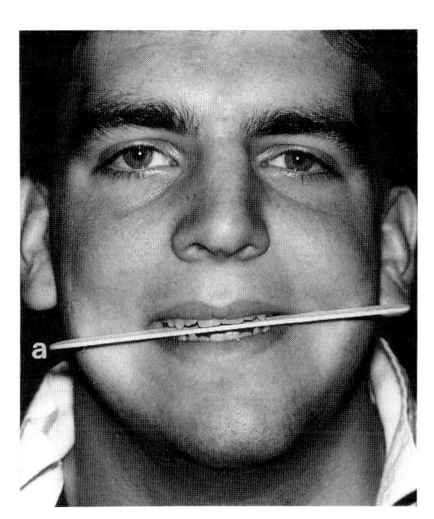

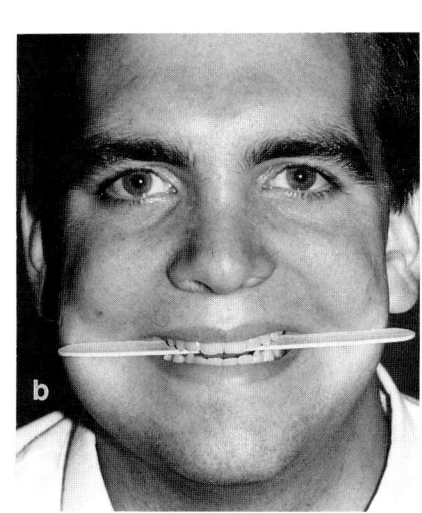

Figure 45.16 (a) Preoperative photograph shows a patient with tongue blade in position to demonstrate the degree of canting of the occlusal plane when the horizontal position of the tongue plate is compared to the imaginary line passing through the pupils. (b) The same view of the patient, one year postoperatively, reveals the corrected plane of occlusion.

either are not accessible or do not contain enough bone for proper fixation. For the anterior maxilla I prefer an L-plate, and for the lateral maxilla an X-plate. Only under unusual conditions, imposed by the maxillary shape, will I deviate from this. With an interim splint in position and temporary maxillo-mandibular wiring, the maxilla is rotated to the desired position and rigid fixation is achieved, while details of rigid fixation principles described in the other chapters of this book are being considered. The wound is irrigated copiously, and the mandibular osteotomy is performed.

I routinely use a sagittal split osteotomy unless a segmental osteotomy is a necessity to achieve proper alignment. Following completion of the osteotomy, the mandible is rotated to position and the ideal occlusion is achieved by way of the second and final splints. Next,

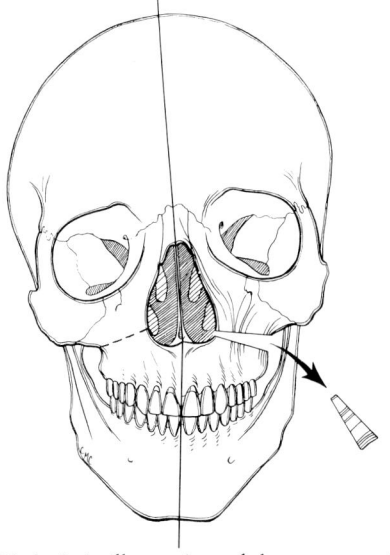

Figure 45.17 Artistic illustration of the asymmetric face shows the rotation of the maxilla and mandible to the right side. The plan was to do a Le Fort I osteotomy to resect a segment from the left side, rotate the maxilla to the left, add bone graft to the right, and use rigid fixation. This bone segment is harvested from the outer table of the skull.

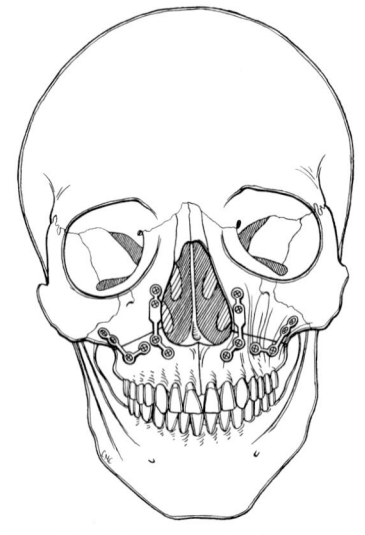

Figure 45.18 By removing bone only from the left side and not adding bone on the right side, one can achieve a symmetric face as long as the incisor show was excessive on the long side.

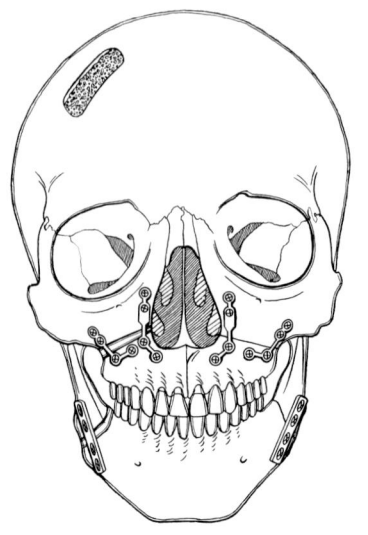

Figure 45.19 Artistic illustration shows a bimaxillary osteotomy for correction of a short, right-sided maxilla following a Le Fort I osteotomy, cranial bone graft, sagittal split mandibular osteotomy, and rigid fixation.

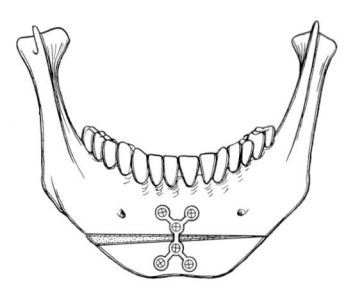

Figure 45.20 The bone graft has been applied to the right side, and rigid fixation has been accomplished with an X plate.

rigid fixation is accomplished between the lateral and medial segments with the condyle being gently positioned by hand in the fossa. Use of monocortical plates for this part of the operation has many advantages. By using this technique, injury to the tooth buds and/or roots is avoidable. Also, minor refinements during the healing period are possible. Furthermore, there is no need for an external incision to guide a bur and screw. Following rigid fixation, the maxillo-mandibular wires are removed. The splint is either extracted or, while in place, used as a precision device to make sure the mandible can be easily rotated in position with no deviation or change in occlusion; this will ensure centric positioning of the condyle. Ideally, temporary maxillo-mandibular wiring is then achieved or elastic bands (to be removed five to seven days later) are applied. The incisions are repaired with 3-0 chromic running locked sutures following copious irrigation of the wound with antibiotic-containing solutions.

If genioplasty is indicated, then the lower labial sulcus incision is made following infiltration with xylocaine containing 1 in 200,000 parts epinephrine. The incision is made on the labial side of the sulcus, leaving enough caudal soft tissue on the gingival side. Next, the periosteum is elevated and the anterior mandible is exposed. Depending on the plan, a horizontal osteotomy (see Figure 45.7) is made, or a wedge is resected with a sagittal saw. The chin is advanced (or rotated), and rigid fixation is achieved with Würzburg chin plates. It is sometimes desirable to create a groove for the plate and screw on the caudal segment. The excess bone along the inferior and lateral borders of the osteotomy is removed with a burr in order to achieve a smooth contour (see Figure 45.8). The wound is irrigated again, and the incision is repaired with 3-0 chromic sutures.

Should bone graft become necessary, split clavarium is the preferred donor material. The bone graft is then prepared and fixed rigidly in position with screws. This can be as an inlay on the chin (see Figure 45.20) or maxillary area (see Figure 45.19), or as an onlay on the zygomatic region.

REFERENCES

Adams SS: A case of hemihypertrophy (giant growth). Arch Pediat 2:901, 1894.

Angle EH: Treatment of Malocclusion of the Teeth. 7th ed. Philadelphia, S.S. White, p 60, 1907.

Beck RT: Med Annalen von Puche H, Chelius and Naegele (1836). Quoted by Ziehl in Virchow's Arch Path Anat, 91, 1883.

Beirne OR, Leake DL: Technetium 99m pyrophosphate uptake in a case of unilateral condylar hyperplasia. J Oral Surg 38:385–386, 1980.

Benoist M, LePesteur J: Considerations sur le bilan preoperatoire des laterognathies mandibulaires, Rev Stomatol 77:96–98, 1976.

Benson PF, Vulliamy DG, Taubman JO: Congenital hemihypertrophy and malignancy. Lancet 1:468, 1963.

Berger H: Problems and promises of basilar view cephalograms. Angle Orthod 31:237–245, 1961.

Bergmen JA: Primary hemifacial hypertrophy. Arch Otolaryngol 97:490, 1973.

Bjorklund SI: Hemihypertrophy and Wilm's tumor. Acta Paediatr 44:286, 1955.

Blomquist K, Hageman KE: Benign unilateral hyperplasia of the mandibular condyle: Report of eight cases. Acta Chir Scand 126:414–426, 1963.

Brami S, Lamarche JP, Souyris F: Treatment of facial asymmetries by one stage maxillary and mandibular bilateral osteotomies. Int J Oral Surg 3:239–242, 1974.

Bruce RA, Hayward JR: Condylar hyperplasia and mandibular asymmetry: A review. J Oral Surg 26:281–290, 1968.

Buchner A, David R, Temkin D: Unilateral enlargement of the masseter muscle. Int J Oral Surg 8:140–144, 1979.

Burchfield D, Escobar V: Familial facial asymmetry (autosomal dominant hemihypertrophy?). Oral Surg 50:321, 1980.

Chateau M: Orthopedie Dento-faciale: Clinique, Diagnostic et Traitement, 5th ed, Paris, Julien Prelat, pp 31–72, 125–143, 150–151, 172, 180, 201, 290, 1975.

Chierici G, Harvold EP, Dawson WJ: Primate experiments on facial asymmetry. J Dent Res 49:847–851, 1970.

Choung PH: Surgical correction of asymmetric mandibular excess. J Korean Dent Assoc 23:1057–1065, 1985.

Couly G: Structure fonctionnelle du Condyle Mandibular Humain en croissance. Rev Stomatol Chir Maxillofac 81:152–163, 1980.

Cutting C, Bookstein FL, Grayson B, et al: Three dimensional computer assisted design of craniofacial surgery procedures: Optimizations and interaction with cephalometrics and CT based models. Plast Reconstr Surg 77:877–887, 1986.

Forsberg CT, Burstone CJ, Hanley KJ: Diagnosis and treatment planning of skeletal asymmetry with the submental-vertical radiograph. Am J Orthod 85:224–237, 1984.

Gesell A: Hemihypertrophy and twinning: Further study of the nature of hemihypertrophy with report of a new case. Arch Neurol Psychiatry 6:400, 1921.

Gesell A: Hemihypertrophy and twinning: Further study of the nature of hemihypertrophy with report of a new study. Am J Med Sci 173:542, 1927.

Ginestet G, Helluy M: Les Etages de la Face. Rev Stomatol 60:506–515, 1959.

Gorlin RJ, Meskin LH: Congenital hemihypertrophy. J Pediatr 61:870, 1962.

Gruenberg J: The symmetroscope: An apparatus for measuring the symmetry or asymmetry of the dental arches. Dent Cosmos 54:490–491, 1912.

Guyuron B, Dagys AP, Munro IR, Ross RB: Effect of irradiation on facial growth: A seven to twenty-five year follow-up. Ann Plast Surg 11:423–427, 1983.

Guyuron B, Munro IR, Dagys AP: Long-term effects of orbital irradiation. Head Neck Surg 10:85–87, 1987.

Guyuron B: Precision rhinoplasty. Part I: The role of life-size photographs and soft-tissue cephalometric analysis. Plast Reconstr Surg 81:489–499, 1988.

Guyuron B: Combined maxillary and mandibular osteotomies. Clin Plast Surg 16:1–7, 1989a.

Guyuron B, Ross RJ: Computer-generated model surgery: An exacting approach to complex craniomaxillofacial disharmonies. J Craniomaxillofac Surg 17:101–104, 1989b.

Hall HD: An improved method for treatment of facial asymmetry secondary to jaw deformity. J Oral Maxillofac Surg 42:673–679, 1984.

Hemmy DC, Davod DJ, Herman GT: Three dimensional reconstruction of craniofacial deformity using computed tomography. Neurosurgery 13:534, 1983.

Hersh JH: Hypertrophy of the masseter muscle. Arch Otolaryngol 43:593, 1946.

Hovinga J, Kraal ER, Roorda LAM: Difficulties in and indications for the treatment of facial asymmetry. Int J Oral Surg 3:234–238, 1974.

Kaban LB, Moses MH, Mulliken JB: Correction of hemifacial microsomia in the growing child: A follow-up study. Cleft Palate J 23:50–52, 1986.

Keith A: Description of a new craniometer and of certain age changes in the anthropoid skull. J Anat Physiol 44:251–270, 1910.

Keller E, Jackson IT, Marsh WR, Triplett WW: Mandibular asymmetry associated with congenital muscular torticollis. Oral Surg Oral Med Oral Pathol 61:216–220, 1986.

Kessel LJ: Condylar hyperplasia: A case report. Br J Oral Surg 7:124–126, 1969.

Marsh JL, Vannier MW: The third dimension in craniofacial surgery. Plast Reconstr Surg 71:759, 1983.

Merville L: Le Traitemente de micromandibulies. Ann Chir Plast 15:298–311, 1970.

Mizuno A, Motegi K: Treatment of an asymmetric mandibular prognathism in an acromegalic patient. J Oral Maxillofac Surg 46:314–320, 1988.

Mulliken JB, Kaban LB: Analysis and treatment of hemifacial microsomia in childhood. Clin Plast Surg 14:91–100, 1987.

Munro IR: Treatment of craniofacial microsomia. Clin Plast Surg 14:177–186, 1987.

Munro IR: Rigid fixation and facial asymmetry. Clin Plast Surg 16:187–194, 1989.

Nardoux-Sanders M: Pour Que la teleradiographie apporte a l'orthopedie dento-faciale des renseignements dans l'espace. Incidence tridimensionnelle, Thesis, Montpellier, 1968.

Norman JE, Painter DM: Hyperplasia of the mandibular condyle. A historical review of important early cases with a presentation and analysis of twelve cases. J Maxillofac Surg 8:161–175, 1980.

Ortiz-Monasterio F: Early mandibular and maxillary osteotomies for the correction of hemifacial microsomia: A preliminary report. Clin Plast Surg 9:509–517, 1982.

Panofsky E: The Codex Huygens and Leonardo da Vinci's Art Theory. London, Warburg Institute, 1940.

Panofsky E: Albrecht Durer. Volume I. London, Oxford University Press, 1945.

Pisarek W: Reconstruction of craniofacial microsomia and hemifacial atrophy with free latissimus dorsi flap. Acta Chir Plast 30:194–201, 1988.

Pollock RA, Newman MH, Burdi AR, Condit DP: Congenital hemifacial hyperplasia: An embryologic hypothesis and case report. Cleft Palate J 53:173–184, 1985.

Poole MD: A composite flap for early treatment of hemifacial microsomia. Br J Plast Surg 42:163–172, 1989.

Reyneke J, Masireol C: Condylar hyperplasia: An alternative method of treatment. J Dent Assoc S Afr 34:335–339, 1979.

Roncevic R: Masseter muscle hypertrophy: Aetiology and therapy. J Maxillofac Surg 14:344–348, 1986.

Rubenstein LK, Campbell RL: Acquired unilateral condylar hyperplasia and facial asymmetry: Report of case. J Dent Child 52:114–120, 1985.

Sculerati N, Jacobs JB: Congenital facial hemihypertrophy: Report of a case with airway compromise. J Cranio Max Fac Surg 8:124–128, 1985.

Smylski PT: Facial asymmetry and the oral surgeon. J Otolaryngol 5:177–183, 1976.

Souyris F, Moncarz V, Rey P: Facial asymmetry of developmental etiology. Oral Surg Oral Med Oral Pathol 56:113–124, 1983.

Spear SL, Mausner ME, Kawamoto HK: Sliding genioplasty as a local anesthetic outpatient procedure: A prospective two-center trial. Plast Reconstr Surg. 80:55–67, 1987.

Vannier MW, Marsh JL, Warrem JO: Three dimensional CT reconstruction images for craniofacial surgery planning and evaluation. Radiology 150:179, 1984.

Vargervik K, Ousterhout DK, Farias M: Factors affecting long-term results in hemifacial microsomia. Cleft Palate J 23:53–68, 1986.

Vazirani SJ, Atterbury RA: Unilateral facial asymmetry: A syndrome. Dent Digest 73:248–251, 1967.

Vitton J: Etude experimentale sur le role du condyle dans la croissance mandibulaire. Rev Stomatol 75:1001–1006, 1974.

Whitaker LA, Schut L, Rosen HM: Congenital craniofacial asymmetry: Early treatment. Scand J Plast Reconstr Surg 15:227–233, 1981.

Whitaker LA: Biological boundaries: A concept in facial skeletal restructuring. Clin Plast Surg 16:1–10, 1989.

PART III

Clinical Applications

Tumors

CHAPTER 46

The Mandibular Reconstruction System (MRS) in Ablative Tumor Surgery

Hans G. Luhr

Juergen Lentrodt

Radical resections of oropharyngeal tumors frequently result in major defects of the mandible. The primary bridging of those defects and the reconstruction of the mandibular arch is desirable in order to prevent a displacement of the resection stumps due to scar traction and uncontrolled muscle pull. A restored mandibular arch prevents facial asymmetry and facilitates speech and masticatory functions. In symphyseal mandibular defects where the suprahyoid muscles and the larynx have lost their suspension, there is always the danger of asphyxia due to the fact that the tongue and the larynx tend to sink backward and downward. This usually requires a tracheostomy—sometimes a life-long tracheostoma. Primary bridging of these anterior mandibular defects and the suspension of the suprahyoid muscles will prevent the need of a tracheostomy and helps the patient with early restoration of speech, swallowing, and masticatory functions.

In order to withstand the remarkable bending forces acting on the resection stumps of the mandible resulting from muscle and scar traction as well as masticatory forces, an alloplastic bridging appliance must provide considerable rigidity. The feasibility of plate and screw fixation to provide this rigidity was first shown by Freeman (1948) and Conley (1951).

Based on experience with plate and screw fixation in fractures and on analysis of the functional requirements of various reconstructive procedures of the mandible the Mandibular Reconstruction System (MRS) was developed (Luhr 1976).

SPECIFICATION OF THE MANDIBULAR RECONSTRUCTION SYSTEM

Plates and screws and the adaptable ramus joint endoprosthesis are made of Vitallium, used for at least 50 years in bone surgery because of its resistance to corrosion and its superior physical properties. The physical properties of Vitallium allow the manufacturing of plates at a thickness of only 1.5 millimeters, thereby reducing the plate's interference with the overlying soft tissues and skin. Plates, screws, drills, templates, and instruments are housed in a sterilizable box with two trays. This box houses the MRS implants as well as plates and templates of the Mandibular Compression Screw (MCS) System. (Lengths and types of screws are the same for both systems; thus they are interchangeable.)

The Screws

The screws are self tapping with a diameter of 2.7 millimeters. The relatively flat conical head is provided with a Phillips slot, which optimizes the transfer of power from screwdriver to screw. Two cutting flutes near the tip of the screw facilitate screw insertion and the cutting of threads into the bone. The standard diameter screws come in lengths of 6, 8, 10, 12, 14, 16, 18, 20, 24, and 28 millimeters. The bone is predrilled by a 2.1-millimeter-diameter surgical drill, which is available in lengths of 15, 20, 30, and 40 millimeters.

If a standard screw is stripped, it can be exchanged for an "emergency screw" with a slightly larger diameter of 3.0 millimeters. This type of screw comes in lengths of 10, 12, and 14 millimeters and can be distinguished easily from a standard screw by its highly polished head.

The screws, drills, and some of the instruments are exactly the same as in the MCS System. Thus they are interchangeable for both systems.

The MRS Plates

Because of the superior physical strength of Vitallium, the thickness of the MRS plates is only 1.5 millimeters. The plate holes are countersunk. Combined with the conical screwheads, this configuration results in a very low screw–plate profile, which minimizes the interference to the soft tissue cover. In addition to the common round holes, all plates are equipped with various eccentric compression holes. This allows the fixation of bone grafts by axial compression. Plates are available in both straight and angle configurations (see Figure 46.1). The straight plates come in lengths of 80, 100, 130, 160, and 190 millimeters. The angle plates are indicated for various reconstructive procedures that affect the mandibular angle area and the ascending ramus. Left and right types of angle plates each come in lengths of 105 millimeters (short), 130 millimeters (medium), 155 millimeters (long), and 193 millimeters (X-long).

MRS-3-D Plates

As a supplement to the common MRS plates, special three-dimensional plates were developed which are equipped with a bending section at the angle (see Figure 46.2). The long plates provide another bending section at the horizontal ramus part. These bending sections allow contouring of the plates in-plane. Thus the angulation of the ramus part of the plate can be varied and contoured to the individual anatomic configuration of the mandible. In-plane contouring is performed with special plate bending pliers. The reconstruction system is supplemented with three-dimensional fragmentation plates (see Figure 46.3) with multiple bending sections that allow simplified three-dimensional plate contouring. This type of plate is mainly indicated in comminuted mandibular fractures and for the fixation of bone grafts in discontinuity defects of the mandible. However, when alloplastic bridging of mandibular defects in ablative tumor surgery is required, the stronger MRS plates should be employed.

The MRS Ramus Joint (Temporomandibular Joint Endoprosthesis)

Based on experience with costochondral grafts, where the proximal part of the cartilage is simply a rounded end, the head of the temporomandibular joint

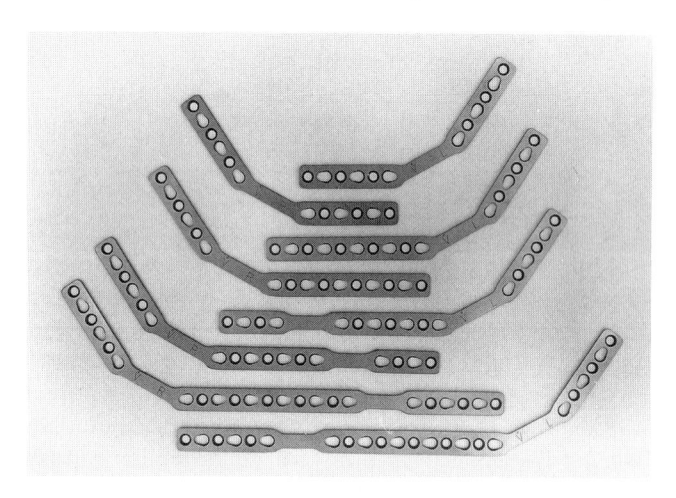

Figure 46.2 Three-dimensional MRS plates with bending sections at the angles are shown. These plates allow in-plane contouring; that is, the angle can be changed when required. The longer plates have an additional bending section at the horizontal part so that they can be contoured at the symphysis area.

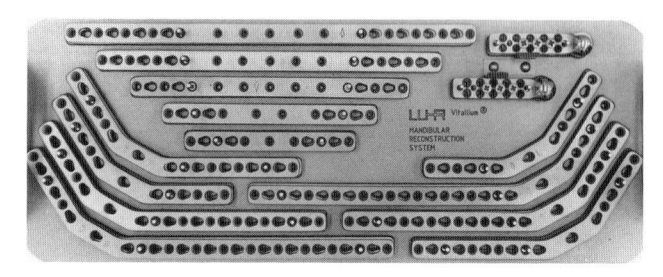

Figure 46.1 Standard MRS plates are shown. All plates are equipped with eccentric compression holes for bone graft fixation by axial compression. The TMJ endoprosthesis appears in the right upper corner.

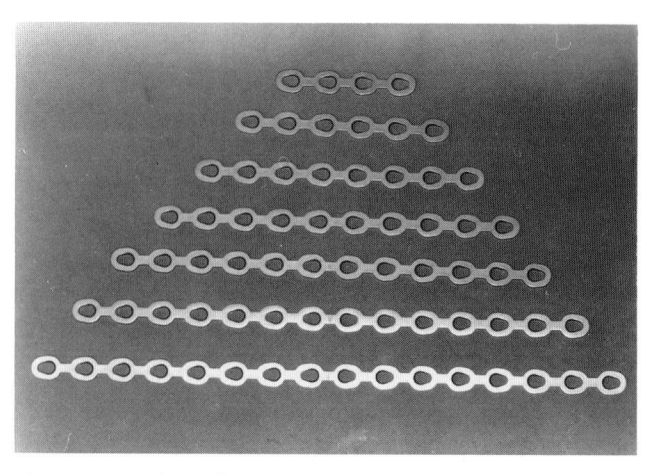

Figure 46.3 Three-dimensional fragmentation plates with multiple bending sections are shown. They are indicated for fixation of bone grafts (and for comminuted mandibular fractures).

(TMJ) endoprosthesis is equipped with a simple, highly polished hemispherical head of 10-millimeter diameter. Because the TMJ is so extremely different biomechanically from the large joints, which have to bear high pressure loads (for example, the hip joint), a special TMJ fossa prosthesis was thought to be unnecessary. As long as the articular fossa itself is not affected, and major parts of the articular disk can be preserved when the condyle is resected in ablative tumor surgery (and this is true in the majority of cases), we see no need for an additional fossa prosthesis. However, when the artificial condyle is inserted, it should be passively seated in the fossa resting on the articular disk, and any pressure should be avoided. We know of no instance of the artificial MRS-condylar head's penetrating the midcranial fossa, and this risk seems to be extremely low.[1]

The TMJ endoprosthesis can be connected to any of the angle plates by means of at least three special screws. The shaft of the endoprosthesis is put beneath the ramus part of the plate. The screws are placed through the plate holes and are inserted into the prethreaded holes of the underlying endoprosthesis (see Figure 46.4). The condylar head can be individually positioned during surgery at different heights (the range of different heights that can be achieved is 20 millimeters).

Instrumentation

The basic instrumentation is identical to the instruments of the MCS System. It consists of screwdrivers (standard and self-retaining), bending pliers for plate contouring, plate- and screw-holding clamps, a protective sleeve for the transbuccal approach, and a depth gauge (see Figure 46.5). Supplementary instruments are bone holding forceps to keep the plate in place while the screw holes are drilled and special bending pliers for in-plane contouring of the three-dimensional MRS plates (see Figure 46.6). Figure 46.7 shows how in-plane contouring is performed when a change of the angle of the plate is required.

INDICATIONS FOR USE OF THE MANDIBULAR RECONSTRUCTION SYSTEM

There are two main indications for use of the MRS. The first group of indications is for alloplastic bridging of mandibular defects in ablative tumor surgery or defects resulting from shotgun blasts. This includes the replacement of the condyle by a TMJ endoprosthesis (see Figure 46.8). The second indication is for rigid fix-

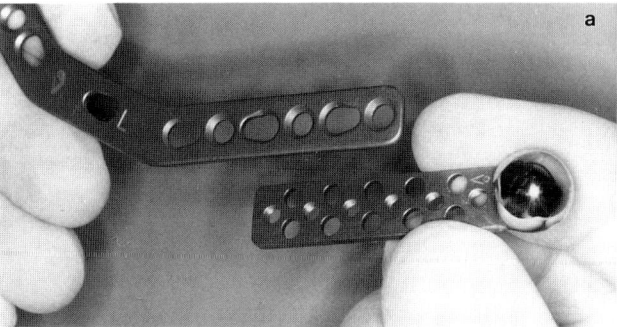

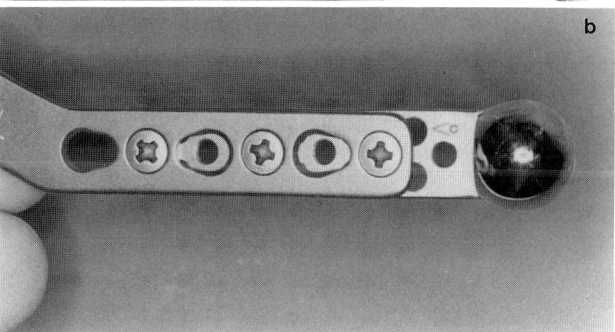

Figure 46.4 The ramus joint endoprosthesis is shown. (a) The shaft of the ramus joint shows three lines of holes. The holes of the middle line are prethreaded (metric threads). They serve for the special screws for the connection to one of the angled MRS plates. The outer holes are used when the ramus joint is fixed directly with common 2.7-millimeter bone screws to the ascending ramus (rare indication). (b) The angled MRS plate is fixed by three screws to the shaft of the underlying ramus joint. Variation in the position of the artificial condyle is possible within a range of 20 millimeters.

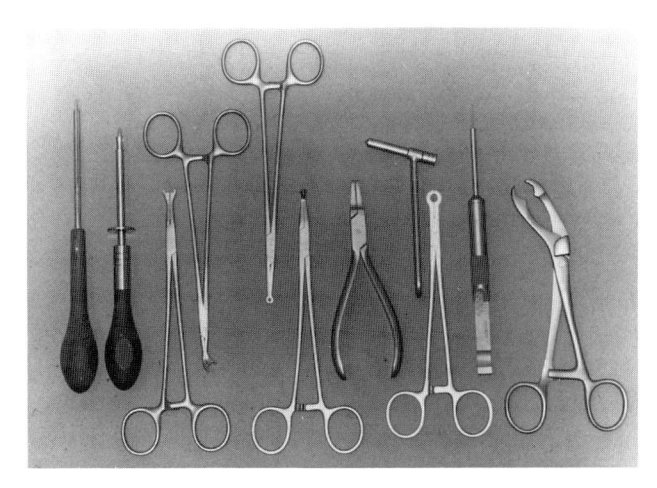

Figure 46.5 The instrumentation of the MRS is identical to that of the MCS System except for the bone-holding forceps (extreme right). It consists of (left to right) screwdrivers (self-retaining and standard), plate- and screw-holding clamps, pliers for contouring the plates out of plane, a protective sleeve with a holding clamp for the transbuccal approach, and a depth gauge.

---

[1]In cases where the glenoid fossa itself is affected by a tumor or infection, the application of the MRS condyle prosthesis is not indicated.

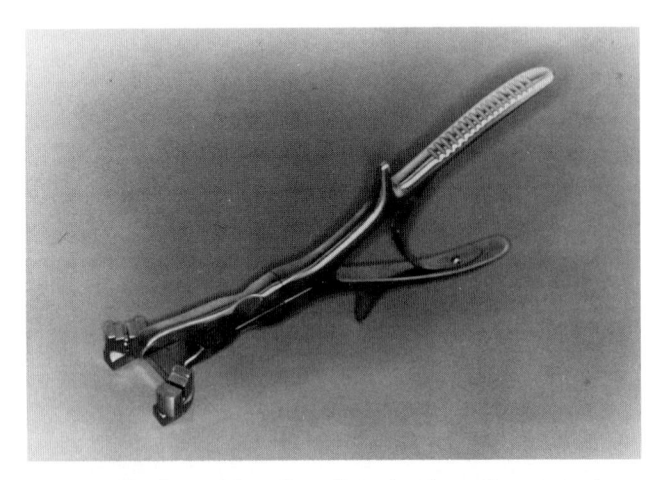

Figure 46.6 Special bending pliers for three-dimensional MRS plates are used for in-plane contouring of the plates.

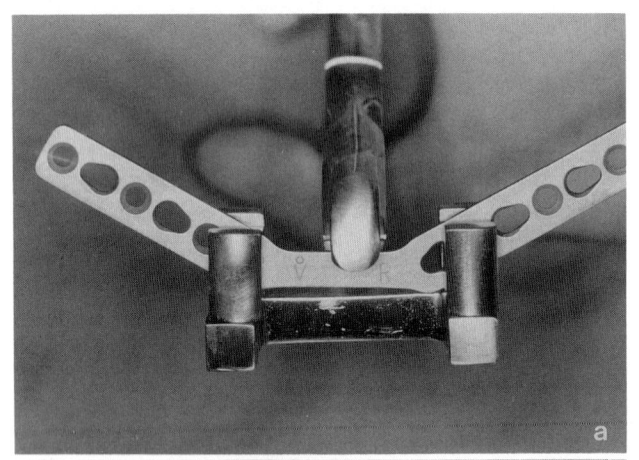

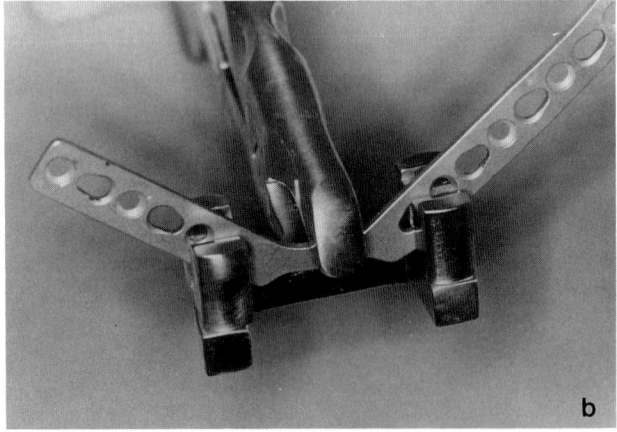

Figure 46.7 When in-plane contouring of the plate is required (for example, to change the angle of the plate), the bending section of the plate is inserted into the slotted support (a) and the branches of the instrument are closed until the desired angle is achieved (b). The plate should not be overstressed by repeated bending trials, and the change of the angle should be limited to 20° (in one direction or the other). In-plane contouring should be performed before the plate is contoured out of plane with common bending pliers. Templates made of a soft, malleable tin alloy facilitate the procedure of plate contouring.

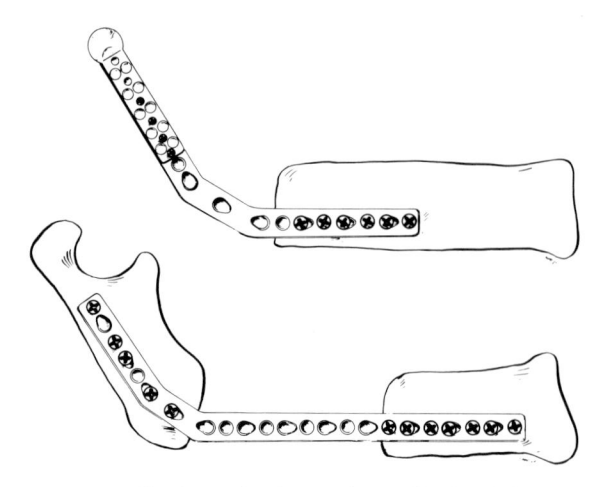

Figure 46.8 Alloplastic bridging of mandibular defects and joint replacement are shown. A minimum of four screws is required in each segment. In larger defects, more screws are necessary to withstand the greater leverage forces.

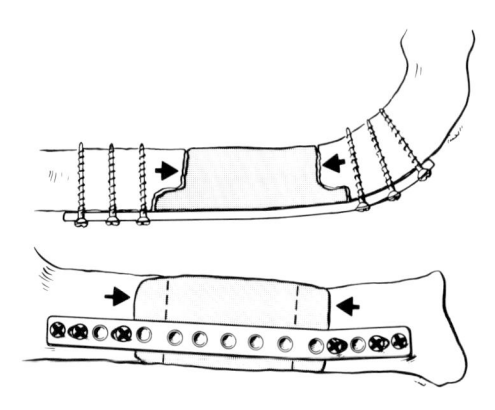

Figure 46.9 The technique of rigid fixation of bone grafts in bridging of major mandibular defects is shown. A steplike preparation of the resection stumps is recommended to enlarge the contact surfaces of the graft. Because the MRS plates are equipped with eccentric compression holes, the graft can be fixed by axial compression. A minimum of three screws is required in each resection stump when major defects are bridged by bone grafts.

ation of bone grafts to bridge major mandibular defects (see Figure 46.9). Because MRS plates are equipped with eccentric compression holes, the principle of axial compression can be applied to provide fast and economic bone healing.

Alloplastic Bridging of Mandibular Defects

The primary bridging of mandibular defects in ablative tumor surgery and the reconstruction of the mandibular arch is desirable to avoid a later displacement of the resection stumps due to scar traction and the deviation of the remaining mandible. This is particularly true when the resected area includes the mandibular symphysis. This is an absolute indication for

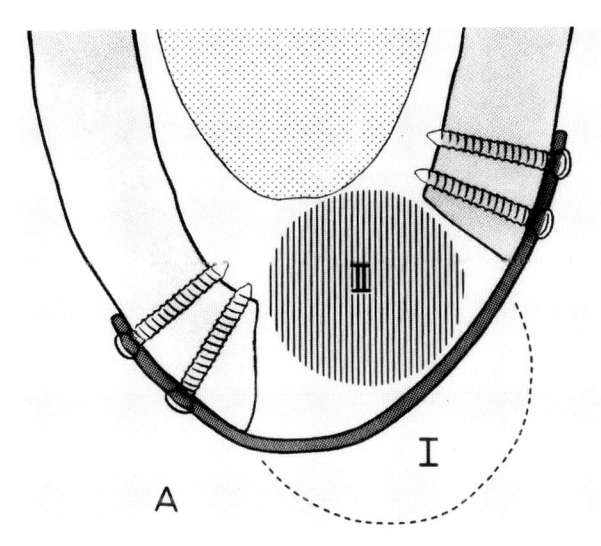

Figure 46.10 The principles of plate fixation and contouring in alloplastic bridging following radical tumor resection are demonstrated. (a) An unfavorable technique is shown. In alloplastic bridging of boxlike mandibular defects one should not contour the plate to the original outer mandibular contour. The subsequent plate prominence may result in soft-tissue breakdown (zone I) and plate exposure. It also makes it difficult to close the soft-tissue defect resulting from tumor resection in the floor of the mouth (zone II). Fixation with only two screws is wrong and frequently will result in loosening of the screws. (b) Contouring the plate to the lingual side relieves stress on the outer soft-tissue cover and simultaneously facilitates a tension-free closure of the oral soft tissues. This maneuver therefore decreases the problems in both zone I and II. A minimum of four screws in each fragment is required for prolonged stability in alloplastic bridging of mandibular defects.

primary bridging, because it re-establishes the suspension of the tongue and the larynx and avoids the need for a tracheostomy and a long-lasting tracheostoma.

In malignant tumor surgery an alloplastic bridging of mandibular defects is preferred over primary bone grafting, because alloplastic bridging is a fast and simple procedure that does not extend significantly the overall time of surgery. To withstand the muscle pull and scar traction acting on the resection stumps, a reasonable degree of rigidity is needed for alloplastic bridging appliances. This is best achieved by such screw and plate systems as the MRS.

Some basic principles must be closely observed if pitfalls and complications are to be minimized:

1. Plates must be contoured exactly to the resection stumps. Trial templates made of a soft, malleable tin alloy facilitate this procedure. The occlusion of the remaining teeth must be ensured during plate fixation by maxillomandibular fixation (MMF).
2. Low-speed drilling (less than 1000 revolutions per minute) of the bone and continuous cooling are critical.
3. Bicortical fixation of the self-tapping screws is mandatory.
4. In alloplastic bridging procedures, the plates must be anchored with at least four screws in each resection stump. In extensive defects, larger than 6 centimeters, the number of screws must be increased (up to eight screws per fragment) in order to absorb the greater leverage forces created by mandibular motion and mastication. The same applies to plate fixation in alloplastic replacement of the mandibular condyle (see Figure 46.8).
5. The implant should be covered by adequate soft-tissue bulk. Muscle or cutaneous flaps, which may be local or free flaps, are necessary to provide adequate cover. Close fixation of those tissues to the implant is accomplished with absorbable sutures through the plate holes.
6. In defects of the mandibular body, the plate can be contoured so that it is situated centrally (that is, between the lingual and buccal sides of the mandible) (see Figure 46.10b). This is to avoid undue stress on the surrounding soft tissues and later plate exposure at the outer skin or intraorally.

A patient example demonstrates the application of the MRS in alloplastic bridging of a defect following ablative tumor surgery (see Figure 46.11).

Alloplastic bridging appliances are temporary because they do not allow the patient to wear dentures. There is no alveolar ridge to allow the fit of any dental prosthesis; rather, there is a flat area, usually of thin mucosa and scar tissue, on top of the MRS plate. Any pressure of dentures soon would result in soft tissue

Figure 46.11 Alloplastic bridging of mandibular defect resulting from radical tumor resection combined with radical neck dissection is shown. (a) Carcinoma of the glosso-alveolar sulcus affected the mandible. (b) En-bloc resection specimen including the mandible (extreme left) and soft tissues of the neck is shown. (c) The mandibular defect is bridged by a long MRS plate. (d) Radiograph shows the patient five years after alloplastic bridging of the defect with a reconstruction plate. The patient refused a definitive reconstruction with a bone graft. (e and f) Frontal and profile view of the patient nine months following radical tumor resection and bridging of the alloplastic defect shows satisfactory symmetry and projection of the lower face.

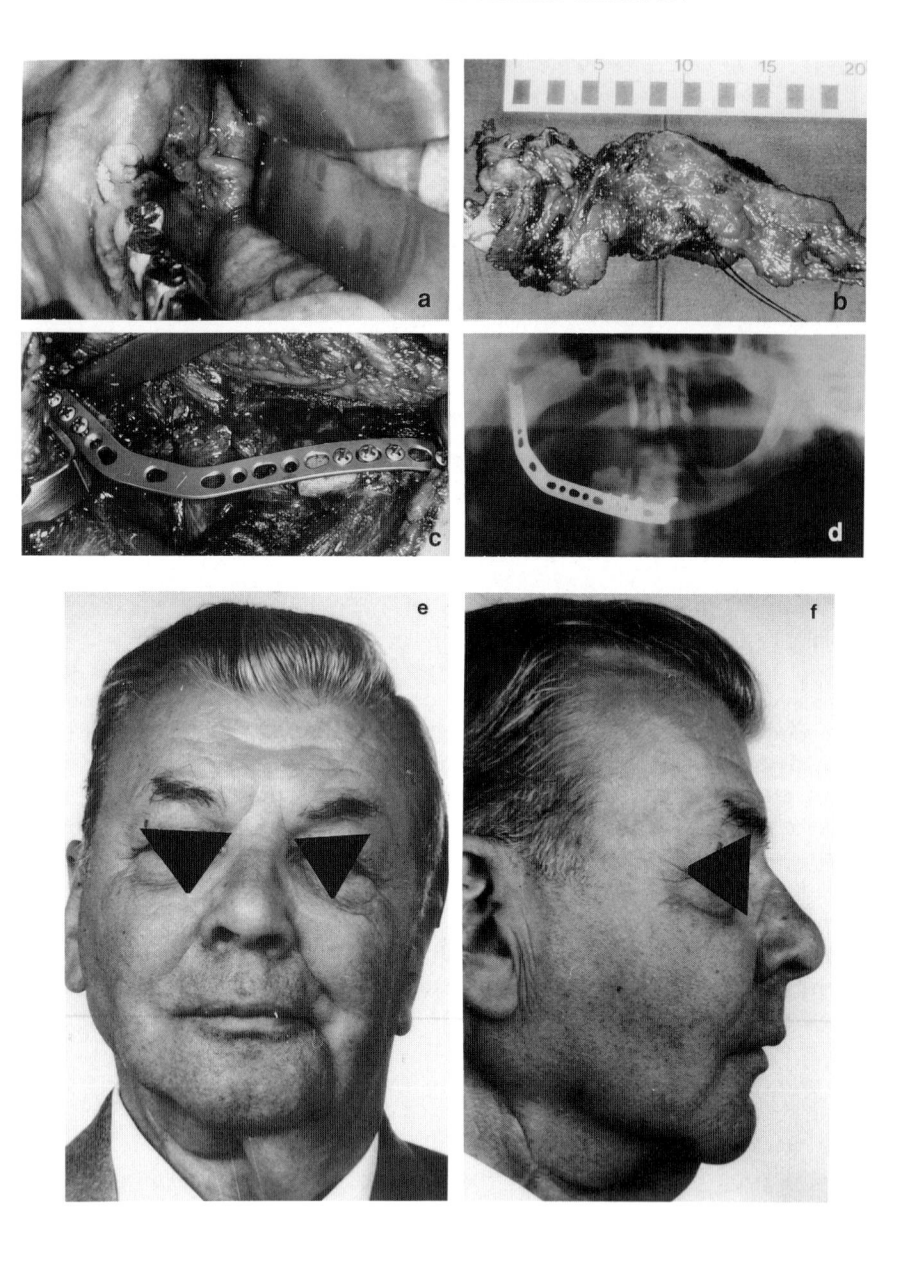

breakdown and exposure of the MRS plate to the oral cavity. Furthermore, plates may fracture due to the permanent stress of masticatory forces and muscle pull. A plate fracture, however, usually is not a disaster if it occur after the plate has been in place for six to eight months. By this time, sufficient scar often forms to maintain the position of the resection stumps. When plate fracture results in instability, the defect is bridged with a bone graft at the time of plate replacement.

Replacement of Mandibular Condyle by a TMJ Endoprosthesis

In cases of hemimandibulectomy including the mandibular condyle, the remaining part of the mandible needs support to avoid its deviation toward the affected side. Such deviation results in a severe malocclusion with masticatory insufficiency and an extreme asymmetry of the lower face and chin. The MRS endoprosthesis, usually used in combination with an angled MRS plate, can prevent these problems. The experience with costochondral grafts in condylar replacements, where a simple rounded cartilage end satisfactorily works as a condyle, led to the development of the MRS ramus joint with its highly polished hemispherical head 10 millimeters in diameter. Because in most cases of tumor surgery the glenoid fossa and the articular disc are not affected and will stay in situ, an additional fossa prosthesis is not needed.[2]

Figure 46.12 demonstrates the clinical application of the MRS endoprosthesis following hemimandibulectomy. After radical tumor resection, the intraoral soft-tissue defect should be closed with a double layer of

---
[2]The MRS ramus joint should not be used in those rare cases where the glenoid fossa itself is affected by tumor or infection!

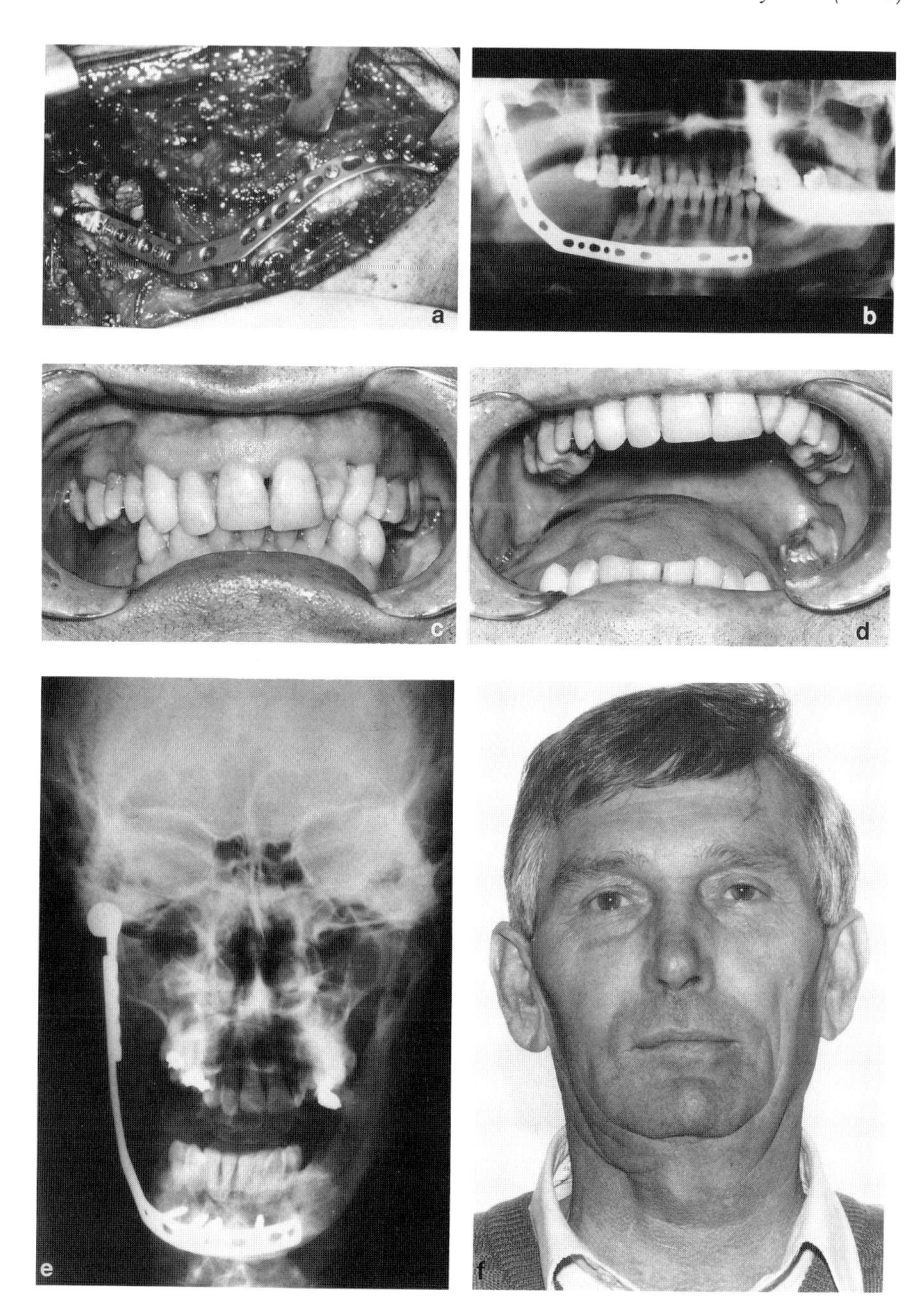

Figure 46.12 A sarcoma of the right mandible required hemimandibulectomy. Mandibular reconstruction was performed with an MRS plate and a TMJ endoprosthesis. (a) The ramus joint is positioned in the glenoid fossa and connected to the MRS angled plate by three special screws. The plate is contoured to the resection stump at the symphyseal area and fixed by five bicortical screws. (During plate fixation, the occlusion was ensured by MMF, which was released at the end of surgery.) (b) Postoperative radiograph demonstrates alloplastic mandibular reconstruction. Note the extension of the plate to the contralateral side of the mandible in order to absorb the great leverage forces. The artificial condyle shows a slight dislocation inferiorly and posteriorly. This sagging of the condyle is a common finding, particularly following radical tumor surgery where the suspending masseter and internal pterygoid muscles need to be resected. (c) Satisfactory occlusion was achieved after mandibular reconstruction. (d) With artificial condyle replacement, the mandible commonly deviates toward the affected side when the mouth is opened. This occurs because the artificial condyle is a rotation joint only. (e) Anterior-posterior radiograph demonstrates the position of the MRS plate and ramus joint. (f) Frontal view of the patient shows good symmetry of the lower face. The TMJ endoprosthesis is functioning without problems more than three years after the operation.

sutures. The occlusion of the maxilla to the residual teeth of the mandible is ensured by archbars and MMF. Only then are the ramus joint and plate inserted: the plate is exactly contoured to the resection stump followed by bicortical screw fixation (see Figure 46.12a). At the end of surgery, MMF is released and the mandible can be moved freely. The avoidance of any postoperative MMF is one of the major advantages of rigid mandibular reconstruction procedures.

Although a painfree function and a satisfactory mouth opening usually is achieved, the condyle endoprosthesis does not simulate the complex motion of a normal, healthy TMJ. Because the artificial condyle is a rotation joint only, a common finding after joint replacement is a deviation of the mandible toward the affected side when the mouth is opened (see Figure 46.12a). Later postoperative radiograms show that the condyle usually no longer sits in the glenoid fossa (although during surgery it was exactly positioned). Usually we found a sagging of the artificial condyle in a downward direction following hemimandibulectomy (see Figure 46.12b). This sagging, however, obviously does not affect function.

Bone Graft Fixation by the MRS in Mandibular Reconstruction

All MRS plates are equipped with eccentric plate holes to allow the fixation of bone grafts under axial compression. The principle of axial compression results

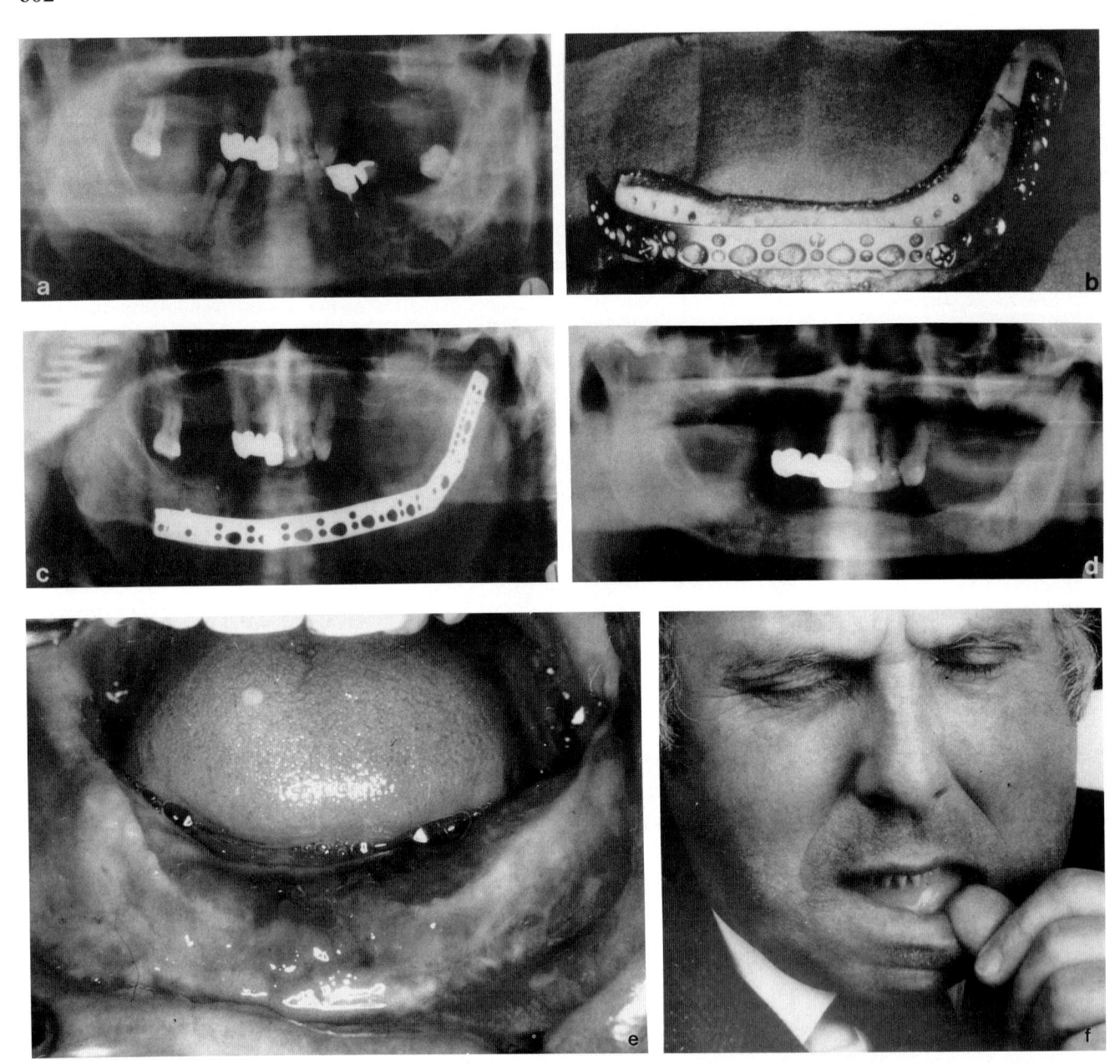

Figure 46.13 Primary mandibular reconstruction including the condyle following hemimandibulectomy by iliac bone grafts is shown. (a) An extensive myxofibroma of the left mandible required hemimandibulectomy. (b) A corticocancellous iliac bone graft was harvested and fixed to a contoured MRS plate (older type of plate) on the instrument table. A smaller piece of cortical iliac bone was inserted at the upper end of the large graft. This piece was shaped to serve as a condyle. The composite graft together with the MRS plate was transferred to the operative site and fixed to the residual mandibular segment. (c) Radiograph three weeks after surgery demonstrates the MRS plate and the composite bone graft. (The reconstruction plate was removed five months later to expose the graft to functional stress.) (d) Radiograph six years after mandibular reconstruction shows excellent remodeling of the graft with only a minor degree of graft atrophy. (e) Intraoral appearance is seen seven years after tumor resection and primary bony reconstruction. A vestibuloplasty had been performed four months after plate removal, resulting in an alveolar crest, which allows denture wearing. (f) The dentures are fitted so tightly that the patient can remove them only with strong finger pressure.

in an optimal impaction of the graft to the resection stumps and provides a maximum of rigidity during bone healing. Usually there is no need for MMF postoperatively. The preferred graft is the corticocancellous iliac bone block, which is precisely wedged between the mandibular resection stumps.

In fixation of larger bone grafts (greater than 3 centimeters in length) a minimum of three screws in each resection stump is required to absorb the leverage forces during the healing period. The graft is compressed between the resection stumps and thereby is sufficiently stabilized. Thus additional insertion of screws into the graft itself is rarely necessary. The resection stumps are prepared in a steplike configuration to increase the contact surface to the graft. The increased contact surface facilitates vascularization and bone healing in these contact areas.

Primary bone grafting is usually performed following resection of benign tumors such as ameloblastomas and dermatofibromas (see Figure 46.13). In ablative surgery of malignant tumors, however, we prefer alloplastic bridging of defects (see Alloplastic Bridging of Mandibular Defects). In these cases the definitive bony reconstruction (see Figure 46.14) is performed

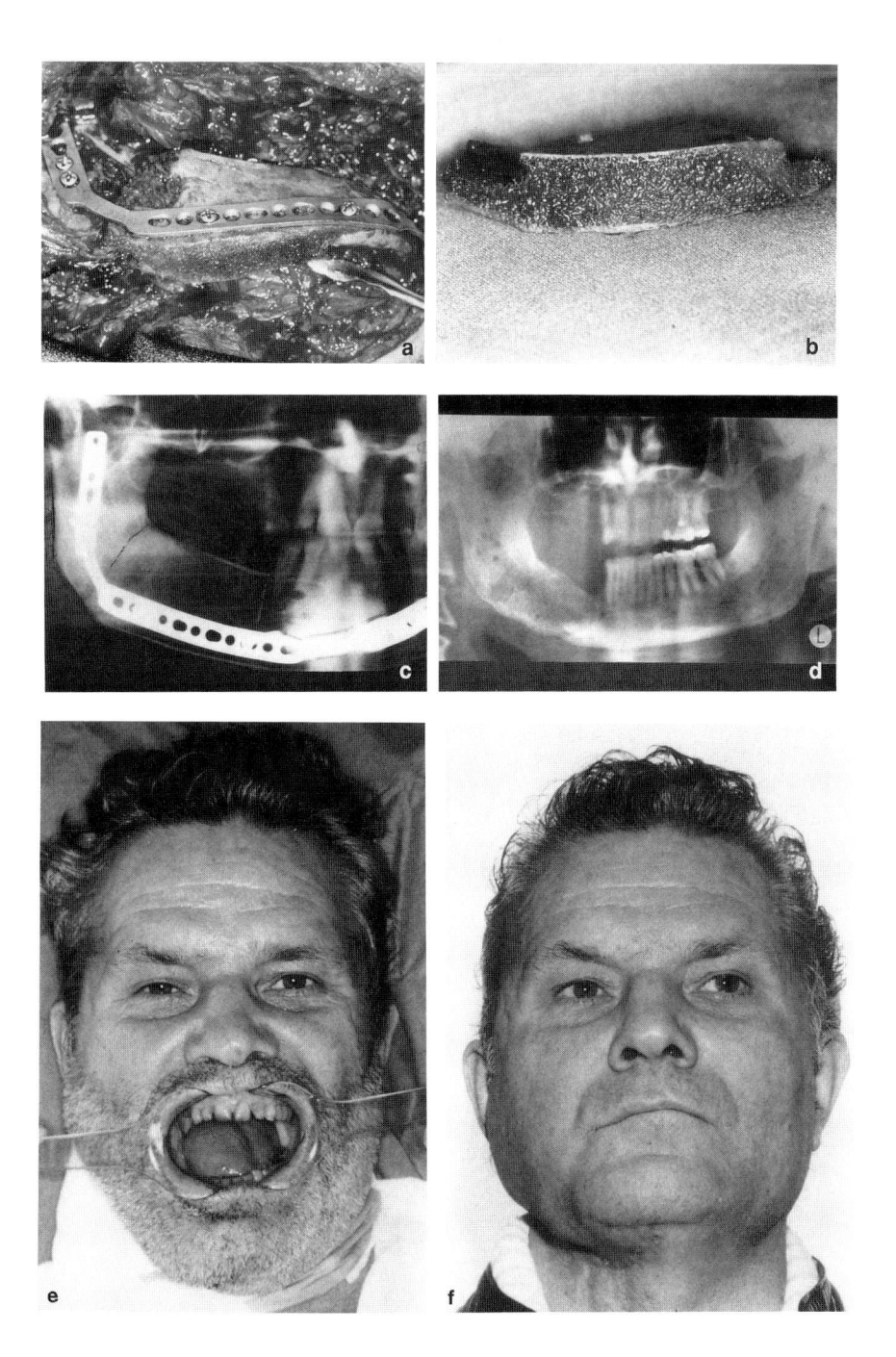

Figure 46.14 Reconstruction of the right mandible by an iliac bone graft was performed four years following the resection of a carcinoma. The mandibular defect had been bridged by an MRS plate without a graft for this period of time. (a) The graft is precisely wedged between the resection stumps and fixed with a three-dimensional MRS plate. Note that only two screws are placed into the bone graft. The anterior screw is used as a lag screw at the steplike anterior connection between graft and resection stump. (b) Detail of the corticocancellous graft shows the steplike configuration at both ends. These steps correspond to the steps prepared at the mandibular stumps. (c) In this postoperative x ray, the contours of the graft are outlined because the reduced density of the iliac bone does not show clearly on radiographs. (d) Radiograph shows the patient one year after bone grafting. The MRS plate was removed five months after grafting in order to expose the graft to functional stress during the period of remodeling. Some screw holes are still visible. Resorption is limited. (e) The patient is shown on the second day following mandibular reconstruction with an iliac bone graft. There is no MMF postoperatively (the arch bars and MMF, which had ensured the occlusion during surgery, were removed at the end of the operation). The free movement of the mandible immediately after surgery is one advantage of rigid fixation in bone grafting. (f) Frontal view shows the patient's fairly good symmetry of the lower face.

Figure 46.15 Mandibular reconstruction by a microvascular anastomosed osseocutaneous iliac bone graft is shown. The mandibular symphysis had to be resected previously because of a carcinoma of the floor of the mouth. Alloplastic bridging by an MRS plate was performed at that time. After the patient was without tumor recurrence for 2½ years, the definitive mandibular reconstruction was performed. (a) The vascularized bone graft is fixed to the resection stumps, and the vessels are ready to be anastomosed. (b) The vessels are anastomosed to the facial artery and vein. (c) Radiograph after the MRS plate was removed does not show any atrophy of the graft. (d) Dental implants are inserted into the graft.

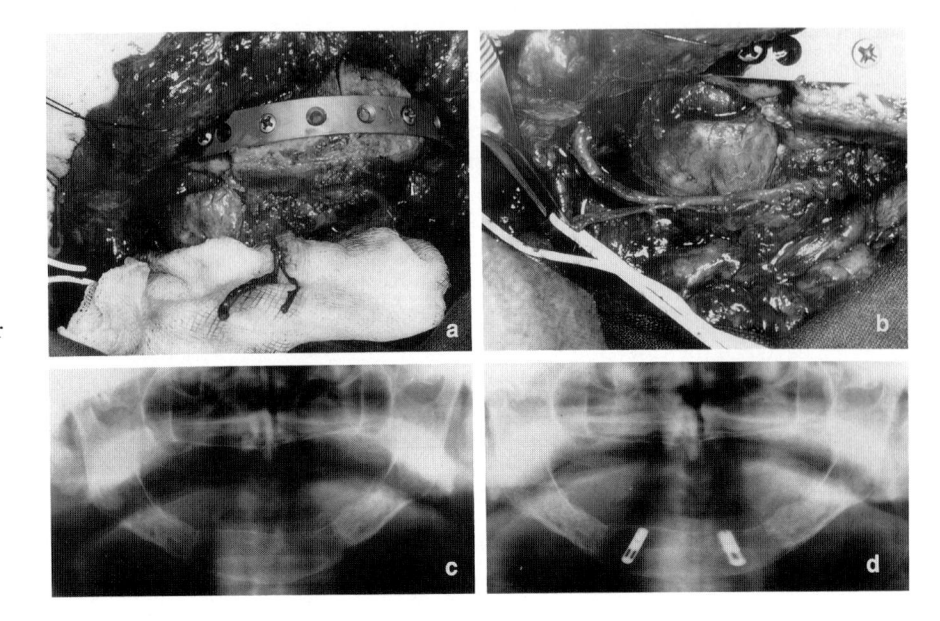

secondarily when the patient is without tumor recurrence and her or his general health condition allows this procedure.

In selected cases, immediate vascularization of the iliac crest transfer using microvascular techniques may be performed. This procedure prevents major resorption of the grafted bone (see Figure 46.15). However, we usually prefer the nonvascularized iliac bone graft which has much lower donor site morbidity. This procedure results in a high degree of success, as Lentrodt et al. (1985) have demonstrated. In a larger series of mandibular reconstructions by iliac bone grafts using the MRS and axial compression for graft fixation, these authors achieved graft healing without infection in 62 of 63 cases. However, nonvascularized free bone grafts are expected to undergo a certain degree of resorption during the process of remodeling. On average, a 30% decrease in the height of these bone grafts can be measured. To minimize the atrophy of the bone graft, the stabilizing MRS-plate should be removed after a period of three to five months following surgery. This will allow the bone graft to be exposed to functional stress during the later period of bone remodeling.

SUMMARY

The MRS has been used successfully for 15 years for alloplastic bridging of mandibular defects and for joint replacement as well as for bone graft fixation following tumor resection. The design of the Vitallium MRS results in a fast and simple surgical technique with a wide range of indications for mandibular reconstruction.

REFERENCES

Conley JJ: The use of Vitallium prosthesis and implants in the reconstruction of the mandibular arch. Plast Reconstr Surg 8:150, 1951.

Freeman FB: The use of Vitallium plates to maintain function following resection of the mandible. Plast Reconstr Surg 2:73, 1948.

Lentrodt J, Fritzemeier CU, Bethmann I: Beitrag zur osteoplastischen Rekonstruktion des Unterkiefers. Dtsch Z Mund-Kiefer Gesichts Chir 9:5, 1985.

Luhr HG: Ein Plattensystem zur Unterkieferrekonstruktion einschließlich des Gelenkersatzes. Dtsch Zahnärztl Z 31:747, 1976.

Luhr HG: Vitallium Luhr systems for reconstructive surgery of the facial skeleton. Otolaryngol Clin North Am 20:573, 1987.

CHAPTER 47

Mandible Reconstruction for Tumor Defects Using AO Plates and the THORP

Douglas Klotch

Restoration of mandibular function requires reconstruction of mandibular contour and maintenance of a full range of motion under a dynamic load. Theoretically, alloplasts serve only to provide function and contour without truly reconstructing the bone. However, this functional repair provides support of soft tissue, thus decreasing oral incompetence and potential collapse of the airway. Likewise, early return of function improves the ability to swallow and to rehabilitate speech. Ultimately, free vascularized bone and soft-tissue transfer can, in a single stage, provide the same benefits. Unfortunately the increased technical skills required and the need for two teams, thus doubling operative time, significantly detracts from these procedures. These are particular drawbacks for elderly patients of less than ideal medical status and in the presence of tumors that portend a relatively low survival. Certainly, for such patients, the more simply applied rigid internal fixation device affords an attractive alternative. AO/ASIF (Association for the Study of Internal Fixation) plates have been proven to be well tolerated in nonirradiated tissue, where they have an overall success rate of greater than 86% (Klotch 1987). Others (Papel 1986) have reported an exposure rate of 45% in patients receiving radiotherapy. Numerous other authors (Gullane 1986, Raveh 1984, Wenig 1988) have substantiated success using reconstruction plates with a variety of applications of plates and soft-tissue techniques. The best results have been reported by Raveh using his THORP (Titanium Hollow-Screw Reconstruction Plate) system. He recorded 100% success for reconstruction of mandibular defects in 49 patients. Although 7 of 49 patients had mucosal dehiscence, wounds healed spontaneously without plate removal. This group was not homogenous for size of defect, tumor type, or inclusion of radiotherapy. Raveh demonstrated, in one radiated patient, integration of the bone within the hollow screw. Raveh did not address the problem of postoperative radiotherapy for a homogenous group of patients (this is a failing of all authors to date).

The AO system has a variety of plates; some also have an attached condylar head prosthesis. Success with these prostheses has been reported (Klotch 1987, Lindquist 1986); however, application is tedious. Raveh and Sutter (1984) have designed an adjustable condylar head prosthesis with condyles of varying sizes. Although this device is not readily available, it solves several problems. The size of condyle can be chosen to better fit fossa variations, and the prothesis has a system of joints to allow easier and improved positioning of the prosthesis within the fossa. Theoretically, this decreases the risk for subluxation of the prosthesis and more easily allows for correct positioning without potential occlusal disturbance. Conversely, once positioned, the AO condylar head prosthesis may be altered only by in situ bending of the plate, which is often cumbersome and time consuming.

The following material will provide technique tips to assist the surgeon in appropriate application of the AO reconstruction plates; comparison will be made to the THORP system. These tips will help obviate the perils and pitfalls that accompany application of these plates.

APPLICATION

Patient selection is important because not all defects require reconstruction to achieve reasonable function. Although repair of lateral defects affords a high rate of success, nonrepair still allows the edentulous elderly patient reasonable function as long as the defect does not sacrifice the mental processes. A safe, quick, primary closure of the soft-tissue may be the patient's best alternative because the minimal contour defect accompanied by mandibular drift during mastication and the inability to wear dentures are a small price to pay for the patient with poor tissues and marginal tolerance for more extensive surgery. The patient with the anterior defect cries for repair, because this defect, if left unrepaired, will be functionally and aesthetically devastating.

Incision

A large, superiorly based cervical flap generally is preferable to a lip-splitting incision because it allows excellent exposure without compromising the aesthetics or the vascular supply to the lip. Care must be taken to preserve both the mandibular branches of the facial nerve, if not involved with tumor, because injury to these nerves will contribute to oral incompetence.

Plate Bending

Once the mandible is exposed, the length of the mandibular resection must be planned and marked on the mandibular surface. An aluminum template is fitted to the bone surface; at least four holes are planned for each potential mandibular stump. This helps to eliminate bending errors and allows for the selection of the correct plate length. It is better to err in selecting a longer plate because after the plate is bent extra length may be removed with a bolt cutter. A minimum of three screws (preferably four) should be placed in each stump, so at least four holes (better five) should be planned to avoid any inadvertent technical errors. The THORP system requires only three screws, and two screws may be adequate for situations where there is a lack of bone to accommodate greater plate length (such as in the condylar area). Although the use of only two screws has been suggested by Raveh, we caution this application for radiated bone because delayed bone healing and consequent delayed osseous integration may lead to instability and failure of the prosthesis. Fitting of the plate may be facilitated by smoothing irregular or angular surfaces of the mandible with a cutting burr. This technique is especially helpful in the region of the chin and angle of the mandible.

Plate Fitting

The adapted plate is then positioned on the mandible with the plate-bone-holding forceps. Holes are then drilled, measured, and tapped to accept the 2.7-millimeter screw (the THORP screw is 4.0 millimeters). Copious irrigation should be done while drilling to clean away debris and cool the bone. Irrigation after tapping clears away additional bone chips and so helps to decrease the potential for microfracture of the bone threads when screws are placed. Screws are inserted into the inner holes first. The entire procedure is repeated for each hole in sequence so that small contouring errors do not affect accurate screw placement. Drawing a diagram recording each screw length and position prevents screw and plate-positioning errors.

Resection

The plate is then removed, and the screws are saved. Osteotomies are performed at the previously marked sites, and the ablative surgery is completed. Careful planning is necessary prior to the plate fitting to ensure appropriate bone margins for the cancer being treated. Although one has some leeway if extra holes are planned, errors in planning require reapplication of a longer plate, which is tedious.

Reconstruction

When the surgeon has planned correctly, the mandibular reconstruction is virtually foolproof at this point. A decision needs to be made as to whether the soft tissue may be closed primarily or whether additional soft tissue is required. Occasionally lateral and rarely anterior defects may be closed primarily. Generally tumors invading the mandible also require extensive soft-tissue resection. These cases are in many instances planned for postoperative radiotherapy so that well vascularized tissue is needed without tension at the closure to prevent wound breakdown and to avoid tethering of the tongue or obliteration of the normal vestibules. A variety of flaps are available; however, the pectoralis flap can usually be applied with reasonable results. The extended pectoralis major myocutaneous flap occasionally is too fatty in females. For these cases, the muscle alone can be used and the skin and fat can be removed. The skin may be replaced as a full-thickness skin graft with good results. Although radial forearm flaps and other free flaps have been advocated for soft-tissue coverage, they require additional time and expertise, and if they do not carry vascularized bone the patient is committed to yet another procedure. A review of the possibilities is not the object of this presentation. Suffice it to say that a randomized trial comparing morbidities and success is presently not published.

For simplicity, we will discuss the placement of a pectoralis major myocutaneous flap (see Figures 47.1 and 47.2). The surgeon has the option to do the intraoral closure before placing the plate. This approach usually is easier and is most beneficial when the flap is bulky. If the surgeon is undecided, the plate can be placed and replaced because the screw holes are pretapped. Several key points are essential to remember to

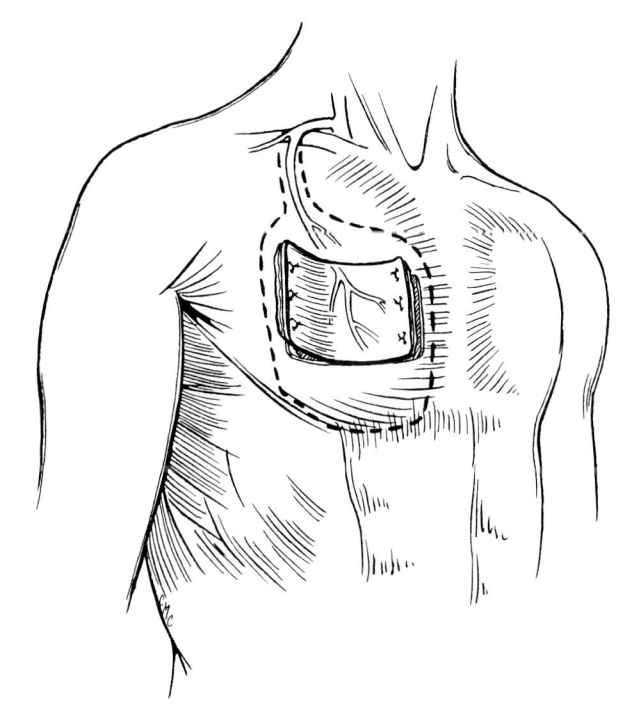

Figure 47.1 The flap is elevated with an excess of muscle relative to the skin to allow adequate muscle coverage of the plate. The skin paddle is sutured to the underlying muscle to avoid its shearing during transfer.

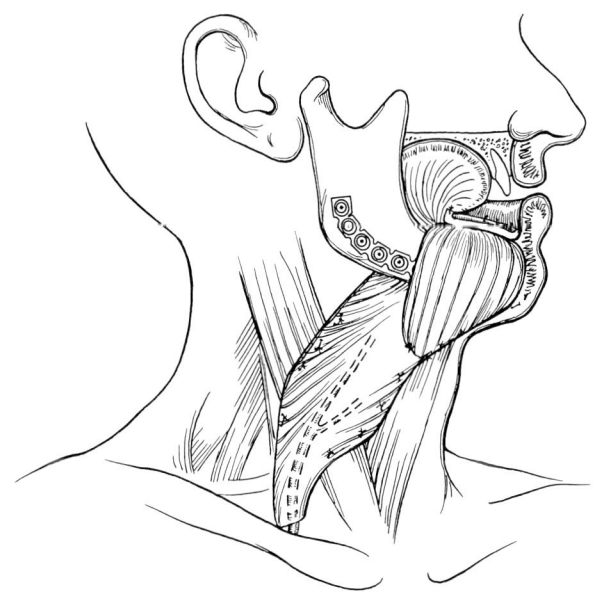

Figure 47.2 The muscle is used to obliterate dead space created by plate placement and to provide additional soft-tissue padding over the plate to avoid subsequent skin erosion. A cutaneous paddle may be used for the intraoral lining. It is useful to leave an extension of rectus fascia at the distal end of the flap to allow secure suturing of the flap around the plate.

minimize failures and errors. The muscle flap should be made oversized in width and length in relationship to the size of the skin paddle. Carrying the dissection a few centimeters inferiorly to include the superior rectus abdominis fascia is helpful. The dermis of the skin along the side of the paddle is sutured to the muscle immediately beneath the skin. One needs to preserve a few centimeters of free muscle to surround the plate and bone edges completely. Enough muscle width and length is preserved to protect the carotid artery, but only a thin muscle pedicle with fascia is used to carry the thoracoacromial artery. This produces better contour at the clavicle and gives extra length to prevent any tension. The edges of the muscle of the flap are sutured to the deep muscle of the neck, and the muscular flap is gradually advanced superiorly to prevent tension of the suture line or the vascular pedicle and to provide maximal length. If not well supported, the tongue is suspended anteriorly to the mandible—or even to the plate, if necessary—to prevent separation of the suture line. The flap must be positioned so that the muscle will rest loosely against the plate. The plate may be positioned in its predetermined screw holes at this point, if it is not already placed, or after closure of the intraoral defect. The lateral edge of the muscle is sutured to the posterior superior periosteum of the mandible. The superior edge of the mandible should be smoothed so that it does not protrude through the repair. The intraoral watertight closure is completed with interrupted absorbable suture. Because the skin paddle was not sutured to the superior and inferior muscle flap, the skin can be sutured into position so that the suture line does not rest above the plate. The inferior muscle and rectus fascia should be draped loosely over the plate. The fascia should be sewn superficially to the pectoralis muscle within the neck; the surgeon should be careful not to devascularize the flap.

Drains

At least two suction drains are placed to coapt soft tissues and to prevent hematoma collection. Drains are removed 24 hours after drainage has stopped.

Closure

The type of neck and skin closure are the surgeon's choice and will not affect the result of this system. Care should be taken that no constricting dressing or other fasteners for tubes or ventilating masks compresses the flap over the clavicle, the neck, or the reconstruction plate.

Antibiotics

Antibiotics are given in a preoperative bolus and in a postoperative prophylactic course. Protracted therapeutic antibiotics do not seem beneficial. Antibiotic coverage should be appropriate for aerobic and anaerobic bacteria. No randomized studies have been reported to substantiate the effectiveness of antibiotics for these procedures. This author uses a protocol of either Ancef (1 gram IV every six hours) with Flagyl (500 milligrams IV every six hours) or Cleocin (900 milligrams IV every eight hours); no difference is noticed between either schedule. The use of topical antibiotic irrigation and mouthwash has likewise not been studied but may prove beneficial as an adjunctive antimicrobial therapy.

Radiation

A high success rate has been reported by multiple authors (Klotch 1987, Raveh 1984, Wenig 1988) for nonhomogenous patient populations in whom reconstruction plates were used for a variety of defects due to both benign and malignant disease. The adverse effect of radiation for wound healing is especially critical in patients undergoing mandibular reconstruction with plates. The metals used for reconstruction plates are of high atomic weights, and they will induce back-scatter in front of the beam and reduce the dose delivered behind the plate. Higher energy sources tend to increase the back-scatter effect. Although some reports suggest this is negligible (Wenig 1988) for standard energy source of 6 megaelectron volts delivered by opposed ports, a zone of increased dosage appears at the plate interface. It is interesting to note that failures for reconstruction have largely been in soft tissue and not bone. Raveh (1984) has described osseous integration within hollow screws in a patient who received 7000 rads preoperatively. Theoretically, the THORP system offers an advantage over the AO reconstruction plate in that the bone may integrate with the screw and the screwhead is expanded into the plate hole and requires no plate–bone compression for stability. This serves to decrease the potential for devascularization of the bone beneath the plate, which is especially desirable in a radiated field. In a recent review of 31 patients reconstructed with the THORP prostheses (Klotch 1990), two plates removed at 8 and 28 weeks showed no osseous integration. The patient whose plate was removed at 8 weeks had failed preoperative radiotherapy. His recurrence was resected, and the defect was reconstructed with a plate and local tissue. The patient whose plate was removed at 28 weeks had postoperative radiotherapy and her plate extruded intraorally. She was nutritionally deficient and had a soft-tissue recurrence requiring resection and plate removal. Screws showed no loosening or bone integration at these intervals. Likewise, in no patient undergoing plate removal following bone repair at longer than 18 months from primary resection was osseous integration noted in all screws. Therefore it remains unclear to this author when predictable osseous integration will occur in tumor patients requiring postoperative radiotherapy.

Despite this, screw failure seems to be negligible for both systems.

Plate Failures

The surgeon must understand that, presently, no marketed prosthesis will function indefinitely under the functional load of the mandible. Five plate fractures were reported in sixty reconstructions done with the AO stainless steel plate (Klotch 1987). That study prompted design of a thicker plate in titanium with increased strength to meet load demands. No long-term data are available for this plate. Although plate reconstruction for the mandibular defect provides a relatively easy alternative for immediate restoration of mandibular function, it should not be considered a permanent reconstruction. Younger patients who have benign disease and can physically tolerate additional surgery should proceed to bony reconstruction.

Dental Implants

Patients who had previously radiated beds or nonradiated tissues have been shown in small series to tolerate osseous-integrated dental implants in nonvascularized grafts. Since the study reported in 1990 (Klotch) we have placed dental implants in two patients. It is interesting to note that the density and thickness of the secondary bone graft appeared better than those of the preexisting radiated mandible. No implant failures have presently been observed in this small series; however, failures in the range of 25% can be expected in irradiated bone. Further dental implants are planned where indicated following bony repair for the remainder of patients. Despite this reported success it appears that vascularized bone is more desirable to avoid potential implant failure. Larger series will shed more light on this problem.

Condyle

The condyle generally can be preserved, without causing an increase in local recurrence, in patients requiring resection of the mandible for intraoral cancers. Recurrence of these tumors is rare at the condyle or glenoid fossa, but more common at the skull base around the foramen ovale. The soft tissues medial to the mandible can be removed to the level of the skull base without removal of the head and neck of the condyle. For tumors located more anteriorly, the entire inferior alveolar nerve and the medullary compartment of the mandible can be removed, thus sparing the coronoid process and the condyle (see Figure 47.3). The present AO plate system can be applied with one screw in the condylar neck, one screw in the junction of the neck and head, and one screw in the condylar head. Screws placed into the condyle should be 2 millimeters shorter

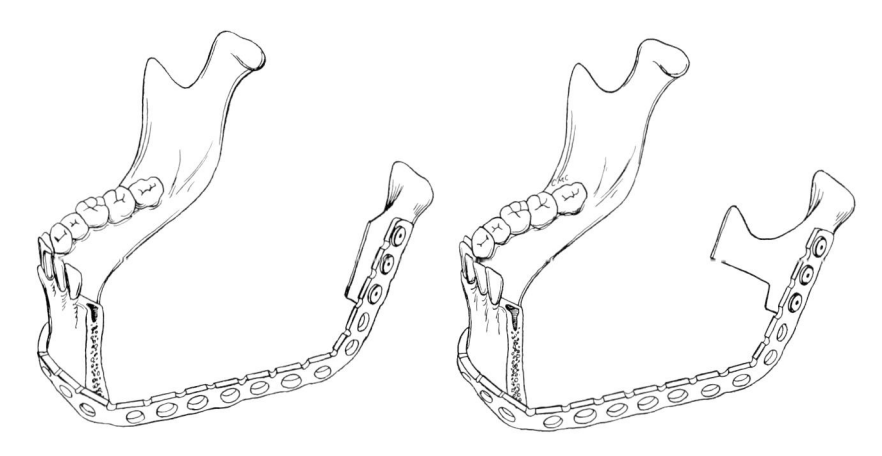

Figure 47.3 Radical resection of intraoral cancers can usually be performed with preservation of the condylar process alone or with the coronoid remnant. This allows adequate bone stock for reconstruction with plate and screw fixation. (a) A plate is fixed to the condylar remnant. (b) A plate is fixed to remnants with the condyle and coronoid.

than the actual measured hole length so as not to interfere with the joint space. The THORP system offers an advantage in that only two screws are necessary to support the functional load (Raveh 1984). From a purely mechanical point of view, two screws provide only a class I lever system, in which one of the screws becomes the fulcrum. Although this does not seem ideal biomechanically, this system appears to work in a clinical setting. More data are necessary to assess the success of two-screw fixation for the postoperatively radiated patient. For patients having resections extending to the condylar region, the surgeon must provide rigorous mandibular functional rehabilitation with exercises for the patient. The range of excursion must be followed. This will prevent trismus and potential ankylosis. This is especially mandated for radiated patients. Although the smaller segments of condyle and neck function largely as free grafts, they seem to function for years despite reported alterations of contour (Hadjtanghelou 1986). I have seen only one plate failure in this site. This occurred in a THORP fixed to the condyle region with two hollow screws. Despite the loosening of the plate, secondary bone repair with iliac crest resulted in a successful union of the bone graft; the plate eventually was removed and function was normal. This overall success leads me to preserve the condyle rather than use a condylar prosthesis as long as tumor resection is not jeopardized. This is even more important for radiated patients. The failure rate with this approach is low, and the surgeon always has the opportunity for secondary condylar prosthetic reconstruction for failures.

The surgeon should note that if a condylar prosthesis is employed the meniscus should be left in place. I do not advocate total joint replacement for tumor surgery. Any attempt to reconstruct a meniscus should be performed with autogenous materials. When using the AO condylar prosthesis, the surgeon must reconstruct the capsule around the prosthesis to avoid subluxation. Sufficient capsular tissue usually remains in the sphenomandibular and temporomandibular ligaments. It is also helpful to attach the newly reconstructed capsule to the uppermost plate hole for further stability (see Figure 47.4).

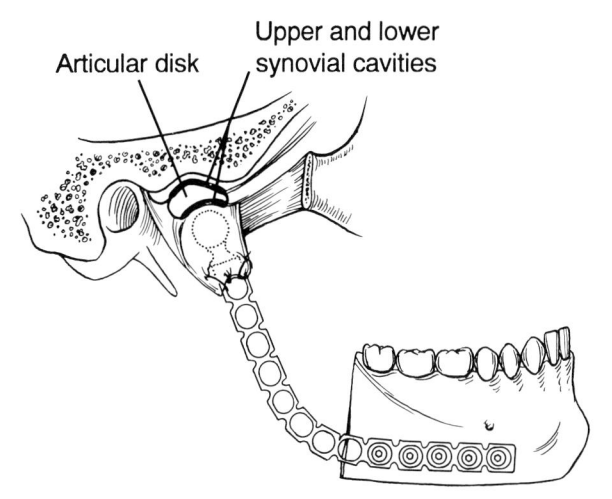

Figure 47.4 An AO reconstruction plate is shown with condylar prosthesis. If possible, the meniscus is left in place. The capsule is reconstructed around the condylar prosthesis to avoid its subluxation.

RESULTS

A review of data regarding use of the AO reconstruction plate through December 1986 shows that in 52 of 60 patients (86.7%) successful reconstruction was achieved without requiring plate removal to achieve soft-tissue healing (Klotch 1987). Of 8 plate removals, 6 occurred in the 15 radiated patients, and of 8 plate extrusions, 4 were found in these patients also. Other factors contributing to failure of repair included direct trauma over the reconstruction site, combining plate reconstruction with hydroxyapatite, and extensive soft-tissue resection. No screw-related plate failures were seen in this group of 60 patients.

A recent publication (Klotch 1990) evaluated 31 patients in whom mandibular reconstruction was achieved with the THORP system between August 1988 and December 1989. All patients had been treated for squamous cell cancers of the oral cavity. All patients had plates placed either in a field to be radiated or in a field that was previously radiated. Eleven patients had failed prior radiotherapy and surgery. Sixteen patients completed postoperative radiotherapy starting at four to six weeks after the surgical resection and repair. Three patients had repair of large defects secondary to osteoradionecrosis. Wounds healed in 61% of patients without further intervention. Major complications of plate exposure or fistula occurred in 39% of patients. Eight intraoral and 5 extraoral (one patient with both sites) plate exposures occurred in 12 patients. Fistulas occurred in 3 of these patients; all had plate exposure. Two of these healed spontaneously. One patient died of advanced pulmonary disease before repair. The most common cause for plate exposure was tumor recurrence (occurring in 5 of 12 patients). All patients with recurrence and plate exposure have died from their cancer. Three of the 12 patients had infection causing plate exposure, and 2 of the 12 patients repaired for osteoradionecrosis had plate exposure. In 1 patient the cause of intraoral plate exposure was eating solid food the second postoperative day. Only 4 patients required plate removal without available secondary repair. Only 1 of these patients, who is still surviving her cancer, has required secondary microvascular repair to repair a resultant bone and soft-tissue defect.

Multiple regression analysis demonstrated the following risk factors for plate exposure: Nutrition ($p < 0.04$) and recurrence ($p < 0.0005$). There was a strong suggestion that accelerated fraction radiotherapy led to greater mucosal separation ($p < 0.05$) and resultant plate exposure ($p < 0.03$). The small size of this group warrants further investigation to substantiate this association.

This prospective study supports a reasonable success applying the THORP for reconstruction of larger mandibular defects secondary to cancer ablative surgery in combination with radiotherapy. The unadjusted, uneventful healing was 61%. When patients dying of recurrence were excluded, the success was 73%. If patients with successful secondary repair are included, the overall success was 85%. Only one patient with severe pulmonary disease died within 30 days of surgery.

As of September 1990, 43 patients had been entered into the above prospective study. They are all evaluated for at least six months. Data has been reassessed as of March 1991, with the following results. Thirty-two patients remain disease free (NED), 1 remains alive with disease (AWD), 1 died of other cause with disease (DOCD), 2 died of other causes free of disease (DOC). Sixteen patients had the major complications of plate exposure and fistula. All 4 patients with fistulas had plate exposures; 1 patient had both intraoral and extraoral exposure. These complications occurred in 16 patients (37%), 63% of whom healed uneventfully. Recurrence occurred in 11 patients; six of these patients developed intraoral plate exposure ($p < 0.0027$). Extraoral plate exposure occurred in 7 patients; 5 of these were related to loose screws ($p < 0.0001$) with focal areas of osteitis. These patients largely had wound infections or were repaired for osteoradionecrosis. Likewise patients (3) with extreme malnutrition because of massive tumor growth were subject to delayed plate exposure. The tissue literally "melted away," allowing the plates to cut through very atrophic tissue in previously well-healed patients.

Nine of the 32 patients who remain NED have undergone reconstruction with nonvascularized iliac bone grafts. Grafts have been stabilized with a hollow screw fixing the graft to the plate. No graft or screw–graft failure has occurred. Grafts have healed despite being intraorally exposed in 2 patients and extraorally exposed in 1 patient. Likewise in 2 patients the grafts healed despite the fact that screws had become loose and the plate had become mobile. The grafts were fixed to buttress the instability in the defect.

CONCLUSION

An overview of the use of reconstruction plates for repair of large mandibular defects is presented. Technique tips, pitfalls, and perils were represented to help the surgeon make the appropriate reconstruction choice. Data were presented to compare plate usage in nonradiated fields to that in radiated fields. Comparisons between the older AO stainless steel reconstruction plate and the Raveh–Sutter THORP system were made. Further discussion of the latter system can be found in Chapter 49. The inevitable choice of metal is titanium or one of its alloys. Whether or not hollow or solid titanium screws will make a significant difference in outcome remains to be determined in a randomized trial. Likewise, comparative studies between the use of microvascular free flaps with or without plate reconstruction and plate reconstruction with local or axial flaps need to be undertaken. Reconstruction plates still remain a reasonable alternative for the management for large mandibular defects.

REFERENCES

Dutreix J, Bernard M: Dosimetry at interfaces for high energy X and gamma rays. Br J Radiol 39:205–210, 1966.

Gullane PH, Holmes H: Mandibular reconstruction: New concepts. Arch Otolaryngol Head and Neck Surg 112:714–719, 1986.

Hadjtanghelou O: Temporary reconstruction of the lower jaw by condylar reimplantation. J Maxillofac Surg 14:221–226, 1986.

Hellem S, Oloffson J: Titanium coated hollow screw and reconstruction plate system (THORP) in mandibular reconstruction. J Cranio Maxillofac Surg 16:173–183, 1988.

Klotch DW, Prein J: Mandibular reconstruction using AO plates. Am J Surg 154:384–388, 1987.

Klotch DW, Gump J: Reconstruction of mandibular defects in irradiated patients. Am J Surg 160:396–398, 1990.

Lindquist C, Santavirta S: Arthroplasty of the temporomandibular joint with condylar steel protheses. Proc Finn Dent Soc 82:9–14, 1986.

Mian TA, Van Putten MC Jr, Kramer DC, Jacob RF, Boyer AL: Backscatter radiation at bone-titanium interface from high energy X and gamma rays. Int J Radiat Oncol Biol Phys 13(12):1943–1947, 1987.

Papel ID, Price JC, Kashima HK, Johns ME: Compression plates in the treatment of advanced anterior floor of mouth carcinoma. Laryngoscope 96:722–725, 1986.

Raveh J, Rous M, Sutter F, et al: Use of titanium-coated hollow screw and reconstruction system in bridging of lower jaw defects. J Oral Maxillofac Surg 42:281–294, 1984.

Schmoker R, Spiessl B, Mathys R: A total mandibular plate to bridge large defects of the mandible. In New Concepts in Maxillo-Facial Bone Surgery. B. Spiessl, Berlin, Heidelberg, New York, Springer 1976.

Spiessl B: A new method of anatomical reconstruction of extensive defects of mandible with autogenous cancellous bone. J Maxillofac Surg 8:78, 1980.

Wenig BL, Keller AJ, Stern JR, et al: Anatomic reconstruction and functional rehabilitation of oromandibular defects with rigid internal fixation. Laryngoscope. 96:154–159, 1988.

CHAPTER 48

Use of the Reconstruction Plate in Complex Tumor Reconstruction

M. Jean Davidson
Patrick J. Gullane

Reconstruction of composite defects following resection of oral cavity and oropharyngeal malignancies continues to challenge the head and neck surgeon. Attention must be directed to both cosmesis and function (speech, deglutition, oral continence) without compromising oncologic extirpative principles. The ideal reconstruction should be reliable, achieved in one stage, and yet not technically difficult. It should provide rigid mandibular fixation, adaptable to a variety of bony defects, and it should permit adequate functional rehabilitation and cosmetic contour. A multitude of techniques have been proposed over the years, attesting to the fact that none of these methods fulfills all the criteria of the ideal reconstruction.

Primary mandibular reconstruction utilizing free cortical bone grafts were used in the middle 1960s, but high failure rates rendered them unsatisfactory, particularly for the rehabilitation of composite defects. Oral contamination leading to secondary infection, the limited osteogenic potential of cortical bone, and the poor vascularity of irradiated recipient beds all contributed to graft failure.

Autogenous trays packed with cancellous bone chips, used in the late 1960s, provided superior osteogenic activity. This method of reconstruction, however, was also associated with a high failure rate, again due primarily to secondary infection.

In 1918 Blair introduced the technique of pedicled bone transfer. This technique was reintroduced in the 1970s with the trapezius/scapula and pectoralis major/rib osteomyocutaneous flaps. The failure rate in irradiated fields reached 85%, with variable but somewhat better results in nonirradiated recipient beds (20% to 65% failure rate). The blood supply to such bone segments is via small periosteal vessels; and although the soft tissues often survived, the bone frequently resorbed, likely due to devascularization.

The AO mandibular reconstruction plate, introduced into clinical use in 1976, provided a strong, relatively quick method for reconstruction of the mandible. This technique was initially associated with a high extrusion rate, secondary to infection and soft-tissue necrosis. Results improved dramatically with the advent of myocutaneous flaps for intraoral soft-tissue reconstruction and the routine use of perioperative antibiotics. The addition of metronidazole to the antibiotic regimen, some eight years ago, also contributed significantly to the reduction of postoperative wound infection.

Metallic plates meet many of the ideal criteria for mandibular reconstruction. They are readily available, versatile, and require minimal additional operating time. They can be adapted to any bone defect to provide rigid fixation without postoperative maxillo-mandibular fixation (MMF). The plates are relatively inert but do elicit some degree of foreign-body reaction. The Titanium Hollow-Screw Reconstruction Plate (THORP) elicits minimal inflammatory reaction and provides superior osteointegration when compared to the stainless steel plate. As bone regenerates and grows into the hollow, perforated bone screw, the rigidity of fixation actually increases. The plate is anchored to the intraosseous screw with a conical expansion bolt, theoretically preventing compression of the cortical bone and subsequent pressure necrosis, which appears to contribute to the long-term loosening of stainless steel screws and plates. The THORP system also provides a lingual plating system which is valuable for anterior arch defects because it prevents iatrogenic prognathism and secondary soft-tissue pressure necrosis. The titanium system is, however, not yet commercially available.

The long-term stability of reconstruction plates is unknown, in part due to the poor survival of the population in which it is used. Our experience indicates that approximately 10% of AO reconstruction plates in situ for more than three years will fracture or loosen. For this reason, we suggest that consideration be given to secondary bone grafting in those surviving beyond two years. Bone grafting may also facilitate the successful wearing of lower dentures by adding stability to the mandibular reconstruction. We have, however, successfully fitted several patients with dentures following reconstruction with a metallic plate and myocutaneous flap alone.

Many have expressed concern regarding the perturbation of radiation beams by metallic prostheses. Recent studies have shown that if bilateral opposed ports are utilized (cobalt 60 or 6 megaelectron volts), the radiation dosage is increased by only approximately 15% at the bone–plate interface, with insignificant soft-tissue scatter. We have radiated 19 patients with reconstruction plates in situ without experiencing an increased complication rate—a finding consistent with other studies.

Microvascular transfer of bone segments was the most reliable method of mandibular reconstruction prior to the routine use of pedicled myocutaneous flaps with metallic plates. Myocutaneous flaps provide a reliable blood supply to the recipient bed, thereby reducing infection, fistulae and flap loss. This makes alloplastic reconstructions very acceptable. Both the short-term and long-term results of microvascular free bone reconstructions are excellent. Unfortunately, specialized expertise is mandatory and operating time is significantly prolonged. The associated increase in morbidity may not be warranted for patients with a poor prognosis; in these patients the simpler alloplastic reconstructive techniques may be more appropriate.

CLASSIFICATION OF DEFECTS

A defect is classified into one of three categories: bone, soft tissue, and recipient bed. With respect to the bone defect, the mandible is divided into three segments: Segment I extends from mental foramen to mental foramen; segment II extends from the mental foramen to the angle of the mandible; and segment III the ramus, which is further subdivided depending on whether (C+) or not (C−) the condyle is resected (see Figure 48.1). Any osseous defect may then be accurately described simply by summing the mandibular segments resected; for example, a resection from angle to angle would be described as II + I + II. The soft-tissue defect may involve the loss of lining, cover, both, or neither. The

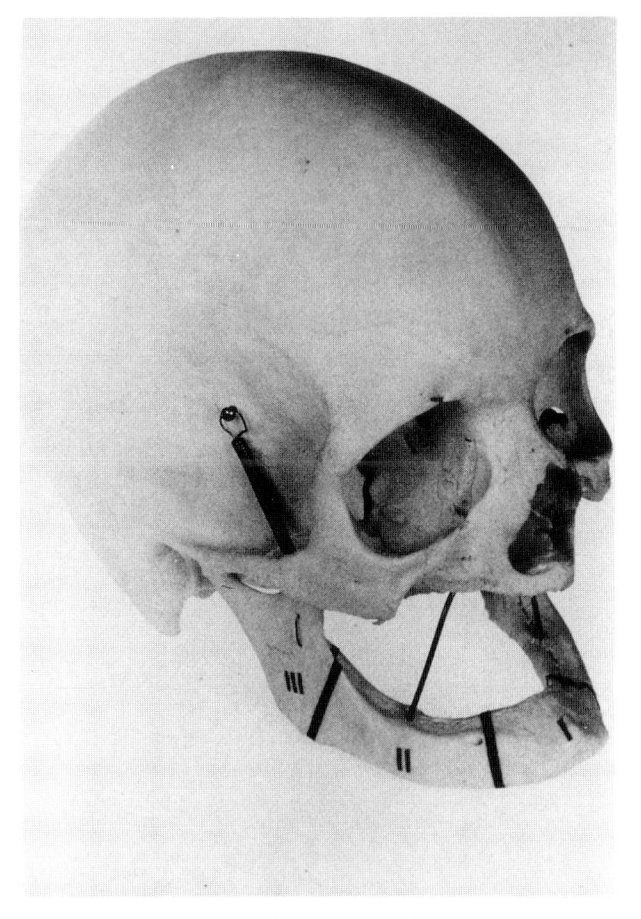

Figure 48.1 Defect classification is depicted on a skull: (I) mental foramen to mental foramen, (II) mental foramen to angle of mandible, (III) angle to condyle.

recipient bed may be healthy and clean; or it may be compromised, by prior radiation, tumor necrosis, or active infection.

The majority of oncologic defects are composed of both bone and soft-tissue lining. Primary osseous malignancies may, however, involve only bone; and some extensive tumors may cause through defects requiring reconstruction of intraoral lining, bony arch, and soft-tissue cover.

In the past, the majority of our patients were irradiated preoperatively. At our center, oropharyngeal malignancies are still usually managed with primary radiotherapy and surgery for salvage. Recently, however, we have been managing oral cavity malignancies with primary surgery; this is combined with postoperative radiotherapy for the more advanced neoplasms.

DIAGNOSIS

The diagnosis of most head and neck malignancies is made clinically and confirmed histologically with a biopsy. Endoscopic and radiologic assessment facilitate clinical staging. Radiologic evaluation provides valu-

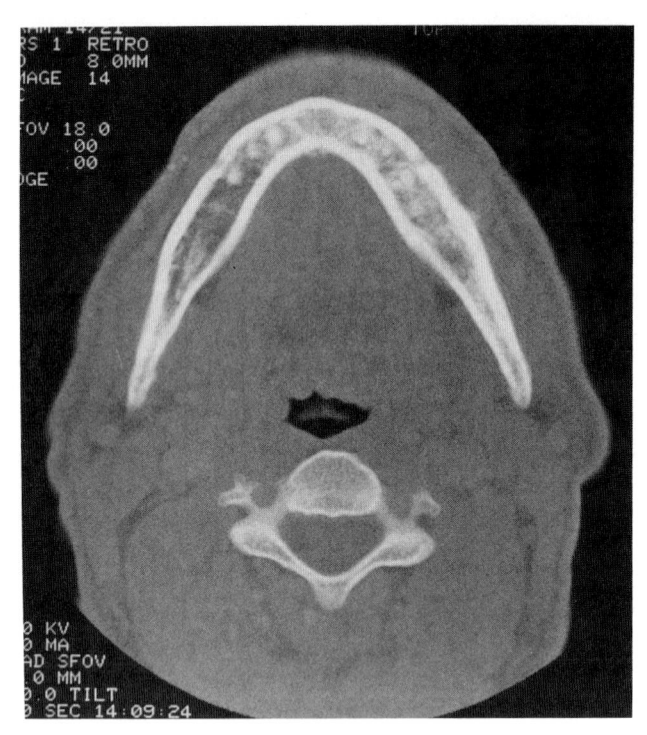

Figure 48.2 Axial CT shows a malignant fibrous histiocytoma involving the left hemimandible.

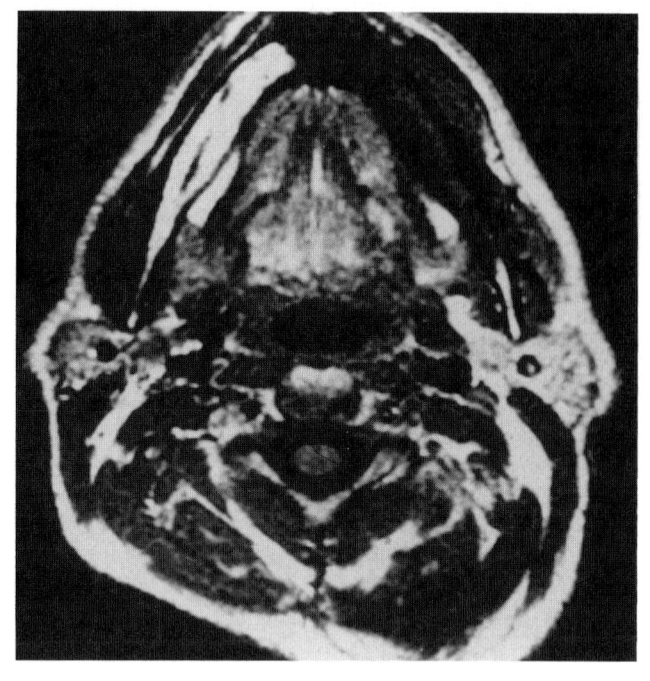

Figure 48.3 MRI scan of the same patient as in Figure 48.2. Note the destruction within the left hemimandible. MRI defines the lesion much more clearly than does CT.

able information pertaining to the extent of disease. Computerized tomography (CT) is the definitive method of diagnosis of osseous invasion as well as of delineating soft-tissue extension. Postradiation changes in soft tissue, particularly edema, can be difficult to distinguish from tumor. The exquisite capability of magnetic resonance imaging (MRI) to differentiate soft tissue makes it superior to CT for highlighting soft-tissue tumor involvement. Although inferior to CT for detecting bone erosion, MRI is superb for delineating the extent of disease within the bone marrow (see Figures 48.2 and 48.3). At our institution, MRI remains a rarely used diagnostic tool due in part to its limited availability.

OPTIONS FOR RECONSTRUCTION

Once the surgical resection has been completed, the decision regarding optimal reconstruction will be influenced by the extent of the surgical defect and the patient's general health and survival prognosis. Mandibular continuity can be restored with either a metallic mandibular reconstruction plate (AO or THORP) or a transfer of microvascular bone (iliac crest or radius). The majority of patients with extensive malignant disease involving bone have a poor prognosis for survival. In general, we feel that the prolonged operating time and higher morbidity associated with these microvascular procedures are often unwarranted. We therefore tend to reserve this form of reconstruction for younger patients and for those with a better prognosis—for example, those with primary osseous tumors. To date, we have used metallic reconstruction plates in over 70 patients.

The majority of oncologic resections result in defects of soft-tissue lining as well as of osseous support. Selection of the flap to be used for soft-tissue reconstruction is dictated largely by the bulk of tissue required. If bulk is necessary—for example, following near-total glossectomy—the pectoralis major myocutaneous flap is our first choice if the mandible is being plated, and iliac crest with the overlying cutaneous skin if microvascular transfer is utilized. If the pectoralis flap is unavailable, the latissimus dorsi or trapezius, in the form of free or pedicled myocutaneous flaps, are our options. If bulk is not required—for example, following resection of the anterior floor of the mouth—we prefer to use the radial forearm free cutaneous flap if possible, reserving myocutaneous flaps as second-line options. A two-team approach is employed, allowing simultaneous free flap elevation and tumor ablation and thus minimizing operative time. Through and through defects are especially difficult to reconstruct successfully; both the cosmetic and functional results are routinely suboptimal. Double paddle pectoralis major myocutaneous flaps have been used successfully for such defects; however, a large skin paddle is required and therefore a greater portion of it is random. The tendency to devascularize the distal portion, either when de-epithelializing or folding the flap to conform to the defect, has rendered them unpopular. Multiple flaps are more reliable but also more time-consuming. We usually use a combination of the pectoralis major myocutaneous and radial forearm cutaneous flaps, although almost any combination of myocutaneous and free flaps can and has been used.

AO TECHNIQUE

Although the technique for plate application following simple traumatic mandibular fractures is relatively straightforward, such is not the case following oncologic resection. The segmental defect makes alignment of the residual bone fragments more difficult, and a variety of approaches may be implemented in order to avoid malocclusion. The classic approach is to place the patient in MMF prior to mandibular resection, thus maintaining normal occlusion of the intact dentition. An additional advantage of this approach is that the plate is contoured following resection, and thus overprojection may be avoided. Following resection and plate application, the MMF is released. This technique is most appropriate for patients in whom the mandibular resection is within the confines of the existing dentition. The majority of our patients, however, are either edentulous or the resection extends into nondentigerous mandible; and in these patients this approach will not guarantee the position of both bone fragments.

Another option is to contour the plate prior to mandibular resection using the patient's mandible as a template. The proposed resection margins are identified, and the plate is contoured. At least four screw holes are allowed to overlap the planned bone stumps. At least two screws are then neutrally applied at each end of the plate; standard AO techniques are used. The plate is stabilized with plate-holding forceps; a neutral drill guide is positioned over a hole; and a 2.0-millimeter hole is drilled. Constant irrigation avoids overheating of the bone. The depth of the hole is then measured; the hole is tapped with a 2.7-millimeter tap; and a 2.7-millimeter screw is inserted. If the hole's measured length is between screw sizes, we advocate the use of the larger screw to ensure that both cortices are firmly engaged. At this point, the surgeon removes all screws, carefully documenting which screw was removed from each hole to ensure that the screws are later replaced in the appropriate order. The resection is then completed, and the intraoral soft-tissue reconstruction is executed. The plate is then reapplied, and additional screws are placed (again neutrally) one at a time. When a defect is bridged, at least four screws should be placed in each stump to ensure adequate fixation. Following most resections there is adequate room to orient the flap pedicle behind the plate. If space is limited and compression of the pedicle is excessive, the plate may be tunneled through the muscle pedicle or the pedicle may be draped over the plate. This plating technique is associated with the potential for iatrogenic prognathism, because the plate is contoured to the outer man-

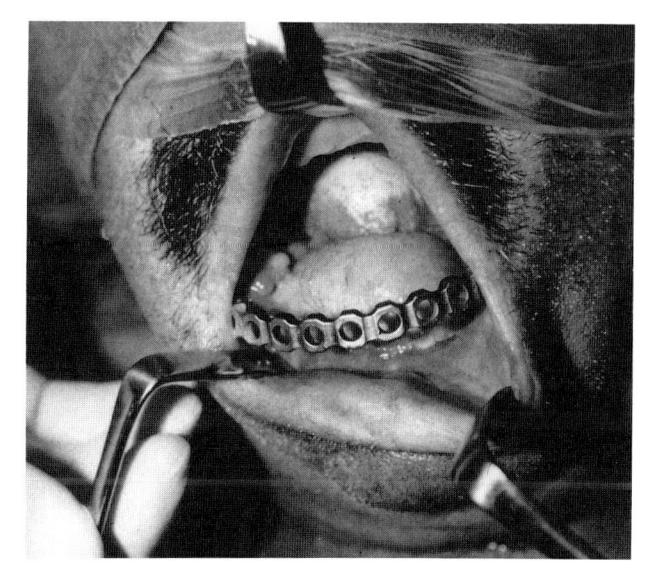

Figure 48.4 Extensive intraoral plate exposure is shown following suture line dehiscence secondary to plate overprojection.

dibular cortex. Also, the resulting increase in tension at the suture line, especially anteriorly, contributes to wound dehiscence, fistulae, and plate exposure (see Figure 48.4); and excessive pressure may be placed on the overlying skin flaps, thereby contributing to ischemic necrosis and extraoral fistulization. Draping the flap pedicle superficially to the plate will further compound such compression. In isolated cases, when the tumor has not extensively eroded the mandible, it is possible to bur down the outer cortex prior to contouring the plate, allowing plate contouring in a more lingual position.

A simpler, although less precise, approach is to complete the resection first, then contour the plate using the resected portion (now detached) to estimate the gap length. The advantage of this technique is twofold. First, it helps to prevent overprojection, because the plate can be contoured to lie more lingually than it would if the mandible were still intact. Second, it is faster because MMF is not used and strict replication of the shape of the resected segment is unnecessary, a gentle curve being adequate. However, care must be taken to avoid medialization of the bone fragments and subsequent temporomandibular joint (TMJ) dysfunction. Again, the intraoral reconstruction is executed prior to plate placement. With myocutaneous flaps it is of value to suture the muscle pedicle to the plate, through the free holes, to help prevent ptosis of the skin paddle and to supply muscle coverage for the plate.

Yet another alternative—one that will maintain precise positioning of the bone fragments, even in edentulous patients—is to apply an external fixation device prior to mandibular resection. The plate can then be contoured, avoiding overprojection, and the preliminary screws can be inserted as described above. The external fixator and plate are then removed, allowing

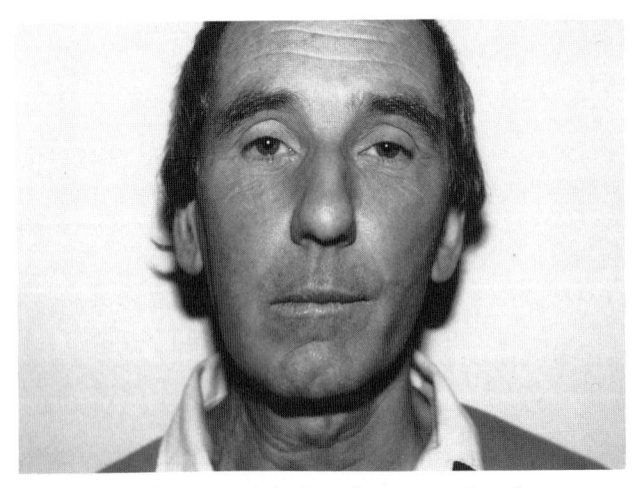

Figure 48.5 Postoperative view shows a patient four years after a composite defect was reconstructed with an AO condylar head prosthesis and pectoralis major myocutaneous flap.

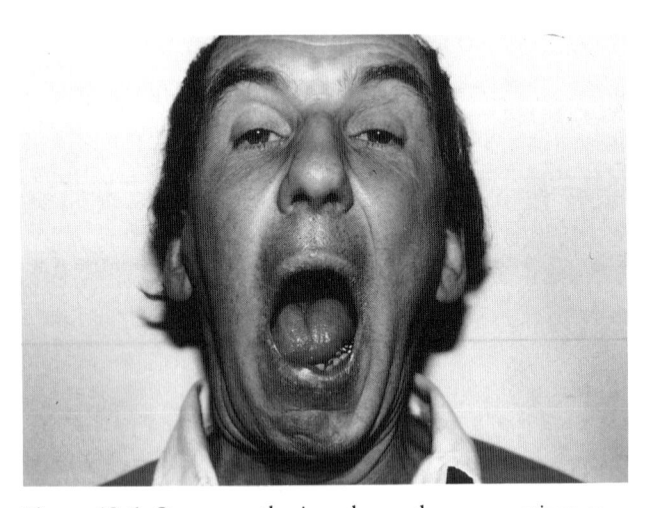

Figure 48.6 Open mouth view shows the same patient as Figure 48.5.

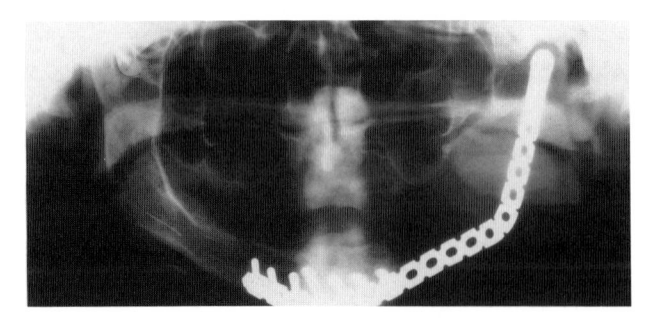

Figure 48.7 Panorex view shows the excellent position of the condylar head prosthesis within the glenoid fossa.

oral access for the soft-tissue reconstruction. The plate is then reapplied, and any additional stabilizing screws are placed. This approach, although precise, is very time-consuming.

If the mandibular resection extends to the TMJ, a condylar head prosthesis is used. The principles of application are similar to those already mentioned. It is, however, important to secure the proximal end of the plate to avoid subluxation. This may be accomplished either by plication of the regional soft tissues around the neck of the plate, or by passing a 26-gauge wire or a heavy nonresorbable suture through the first plate hole and around the zygomatic arch. Figures 48.5 and 48.6 show the excellent functional outcome that can be achieved. A postoperative panorex, Figure 48.7, shows that the plate is in good position.

THE TITANIUM HOLLOW-SCREW RECONSTRUCTION PLATE TECHNIQUE

Although many of the principles of reconstruction used by the THORP system mimic those used by stainless steel plates, there are a few important differences. The titanium system is designed to promote osseointegration, and its success in this respect has been proven histologically. With the stainless steel plate, the more screws properly placed, the stronger the stabilization. With the THORP, stability actually improves with time as new bone grows into the hollow screw. Historically, only two screws need be applied to each bone fragment, although we tend to place three screws when possible. At present, a condylar head prosthesis is not available; therefore this system is not appropriate for all defects.

The reconstruction of isolated defects of the anterior mandibular arch is perhaps the most challenging. Not uncommonly, overprojection, which is often associated with subsequent soft-tissue ischemic necrosis, complicates such reconstructions. The THORP lingual system circumvents this problem by allowing placement of the plate on the lingual cortex of the mandible (see Figure 48.8). The tumor is resected in the usual fashion before the plate is contoured, but the resected portion is measured in order to estimate the ideal gap length. The plate is then contoured to the inner table of the mandible and held in position with plate-holding forceps. While the plate is bent, cylindrical metallic plugs are placed in its holes to prevent distortion of these holes. A 4.0-millimeter hole is then drilled neutrally through both cortices, and its depth is measured. The hole is tapped with a 4.5-millimeter tap, and a 4.5-millimeter hollow, perforated screw of the appropriate length is inserted. A conical expansion bolt is then screwed into the hollow bone screw; this bolt, when tightened, compresses the bone screw to the plate rather than to the underlying bone, thus avoiding pressure necrosis of the bone cortex (see Figure 48.9). The lingual

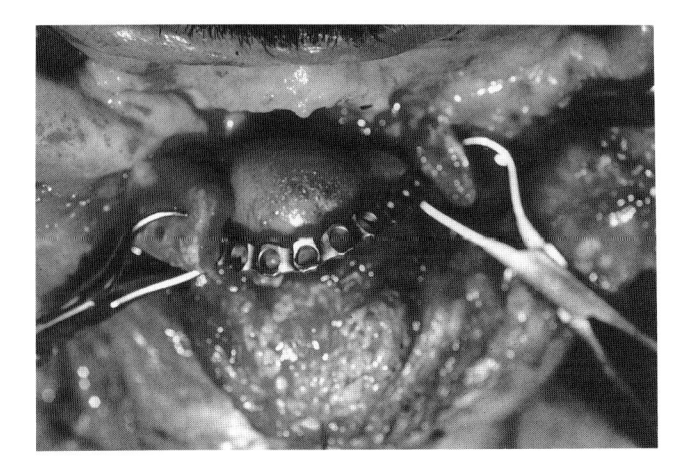

Figure 48.8 Intraoperative view shows the same patient as Figure 48.4 following removal of the failed plate/flap and positioning of a lingual THORP.

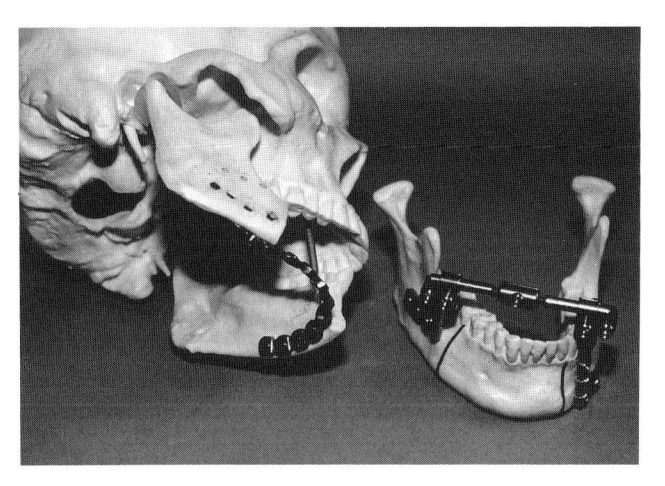

Figure 48.9 (right) A spacer maintains mandibular position during the application of the lingual THORP. (left) A lingual THORP is in position on a synthetic skull.

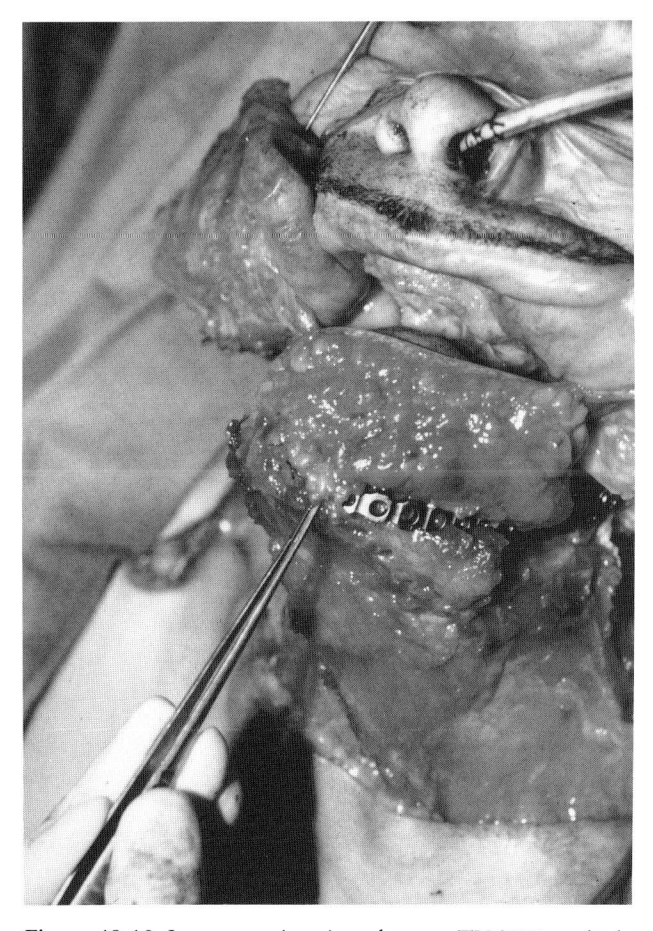

Figure 48.10 Intraoperative view shows a THORP applied to the buccal aspect of the mandible. A pectoralis major myocutaneous flap is in position; the flap pedicle passes behind the plate. The soft tissues of the flap pedicle are being wrapped around the plate to offer additional coverage and to help prevent extrusion.

system reliably avoids the problem of overprojection; however, its application is technically more difficult and thus more time-consuming. Because the plate sits more lingually, it reduces the space available for a soft-tissue pedicle (for example, a pectoralis major myocutaneous flap); however, this has not been a problem to date. Figure 48.10 shows an intraoperative view with a pectoralis major myocutaneous flap in position. The flap pedicle is passing behind a buccally applied titanium reconstruction plate, and the plate is being covered by plication of the soft tissue of the flap around it. In many patients the soft-tissue defect does not require a bulky reconstruction; we most commonly use a radial forearm cutaneous free flap. Because this flap does not have a bulky pedicle, we have not encountered the problem of vascular compression by the lingual plate. When a myocutaneous flap has been combined with a lingual plate, the intraoral resection has usually included a significant portion of the tongue as well as the floor of the mouth; and the resultant defect has permitted easy placement of the myocutaneous flap pedicle.

COMPLICATIONS

Early complications are generally related to the flap. Dehiscence at the suture line may be caused by too tight a closure or necrosis of the flap. Systemic vascular disease may contribute to flap necrosis, but necrosis is more commonly found secondary to infection or pedicle compromise—for example, compression by the osseous reconstruction (plate or bone) or external pressure (tight tracheotomy tube ties).

Of those patients rehabilitated with the AO reconstruction plate, over 45% experienced an uneventful recovery. An additional 35% developed minor wound complications, which were successfully managed without surgical intervention. Approximately 20% of these complex reconstructions will fail, half within the early postoperative period and half later. The patients at high risk for failure include those with diabetes, those with through and through defects, and those with heavily contaminated recipient beds. No statistically significant contribution to complication rate appears to be associated with either preoperative or postoperative irradiation. Significant aspiration, requiring nasogastric or gastrostomy tube feeding, is most strongly associated with the volume of intraoral soft-tissue loss than is the method of mandibular reconstruction. Plate fracture and/or screw loosening, particularly in the proximal bone segment, is a common cause of plate exposure/fracture. With the stainless steel system, if the proximal bone segment is too short to allow placement of at least three screws (stabilization will be inadequate with fewer screws), use of a condylar head prosthesis is advisable.

Experience is required to prevent complications referable to plate application. Overcontouring the plate may exert unnecessary—often excessive—pressure on the soft tissues and may promote the loosening of screws and subsequent plate exposure. Not every exposed plate requires removal; if the plate remains fixed, it may be left indefinitely or salvaged with local (or distant) flaps. We have had four plates fracture, and an additional three plates have become exposed. The fractured plates were removed; three were replaced, and the other needed no further reconstruction.

Although rarely significant, minor problems with temporomandibular joint (TMJ) dysfunction are common. In addition, a few patients complain of cold discomfort during the winter months.

We have successfully fitted several patients with lower dentures over their plate/flap reconstructions (see Figures 48.11, 48.12, and 48.13). Because of the unknown lifetime of the plate and to facilitate denture wearing, we recommend secondary onlay bone grafting following recurrence-free survival of two years. Not surprisingly, few patients are convinced that supplemental surgery is required.

Our experience with the THORP system includes 13 plates placed buccally and 3 lingually. Only 1 of these plates has fractured, at 11 months (see Figures 48.14 and 48.15); this plate was replaced with a new titanium plate and a free iliac crest bone graft. The superior osseointegration capability of the titanium system provides a theoretical advantage: the plate should actually become fixed more rigidly with time. Long-term follow-up studies are still required, however. The buccal application of the titanium plate is comparable to the AO system with respect to technical difficulty; however, application of the lingual plate is much more difficult and time-consuming. The lingual system remains superior for isolated defects of the anterior arch because less postoperative prognathism and flap necrosis are associated with its use in this select population.

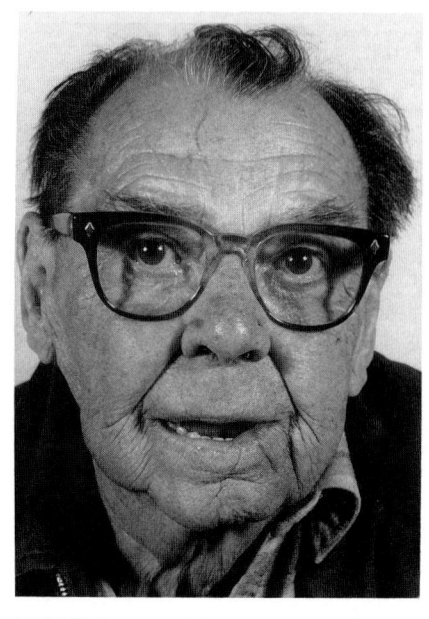

Figure 48.11 Full-face postoperative view shows a patient 18 months after a composite resection was reconstructed with a titanium plate and myocutaneous flap.

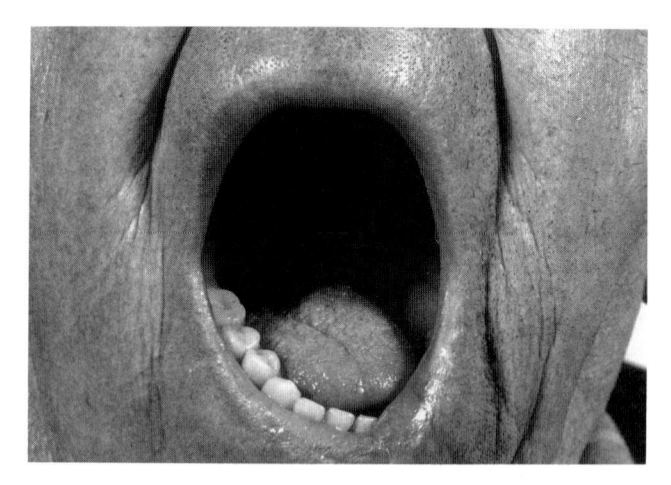

Figure 48.12 Open mouth view shows the same patient with a denture in place.

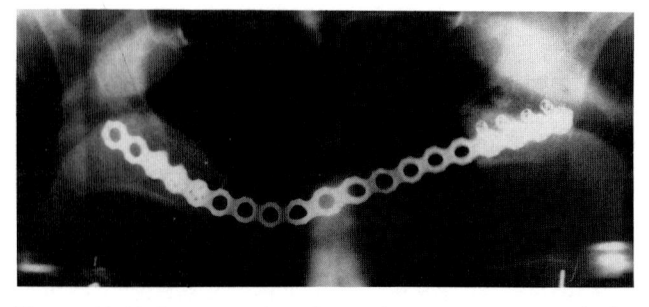

Figure 48.13 Panorex view shows the same patient with the lingual THORP in position. Note the hollow, perforated bone screws, particularly well seen on the left.

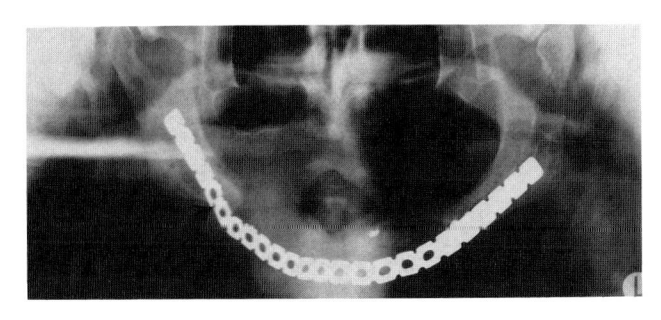

Figure 48.14 Panorex shows an AO plate fracture (arrow).

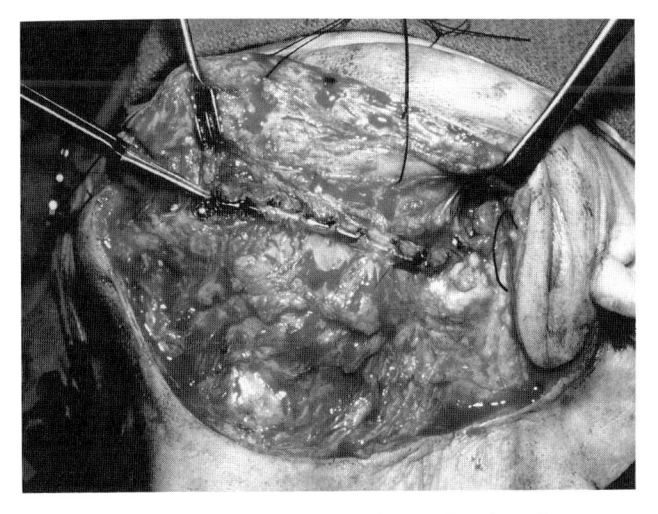

Figure 48.15 Intraoperative view shows the plate fracture at the tip of the forceps.

BIBLIOGRAPHY

Ariyan S: The viability of rib grafts transplanted with the periosteal blood supply. Plast Reconstr Surg 65:140–146, 1980.

Blair VP: Surgery and Disease of the Mouth and Jaws. St. Louis, C. V. Mosby, 269, 1918.

Boyne PJ, Zarem H: Osseous reconstruction of the resected mandible. Am J Surg 132:49–53, 1976.

Castigliame SG, Gross PP: Immediate prosthesis following radical resection in advanced primary malignant neoplasm of the mandible. J Oral Surg 9:31–38, 1951.

Chow JM, Hill JH: Primary mandibular reconstruction using the AO reconstruction plate. Laryngoscope 96:768–773, 1986.

Cuono CB, Ariyan S: Immediate reconstruction of a composite mandibular defect with a regional osteomusculocutaneous flap. Plast Reconstr Surg 65:477–483, 1980.

Gullane PJ, Holmes H: Mandibular reconstruction: New concepts. Arch Otolaryngol Head Neck Surg 112:714–719, 1986.

Gullane PJ: Primary mandibular reconstruction: Analysis of 64 cases and evaluation of interface radiation dosimetry on bridging plates. Laryngoscope 101: Supplement No. 54, 1991.

Jewer DD, Boyd JB, Manktelow RT, et al: Orofacial and mandibular reconstruction with the iliac crest free flap: A review of 60 cases and a new method of classification. Plast Reconstr Surg 83:391–402, 1989.

Klotch DW, Prein J: Mandibular reconstruction using AO plates. Am J Surg 54:384–388, 1987.

Leipzig B, Cummings CW: The current status of mandibular reconstruction using autogenous frozen mandibular grafts. Head Neck Surg 6:992–996, 1984.

Maisel RH, Adams GL: Osteomyocutaneous reconstruction of the oral cavity. Arch Otolaryngol 109:731–735, 1983.

Panje W, Cutting C: Trapezius osteomyocutaneous island flap for reconstruction of the anterior floor of the mouth and the mandible. Head Neck Surg 3:66–71, 1980.

Raveh Y, Stitch H, Sutter F: The use of titanium-coated hollow screw and reconstruction plate system in bridging of lower jaw defects. J Oral Maxillofac Surg 42:281–294, 1984.

Raveh J, Roux M, Sutter F: The lingual application of a reconstruction plate: A new method in bridging lower jaw defects. J Oral Maxillofac Surg 43:735–740, 1985.

Schwartz HC, Wollin M, Leak D, Kagan AR: Interface radiation dosimetry in mandibular reconstruction. Arch Otolaryngol 105:293–295, 1979.

Thatcher M, Kuten A, Helman J, Laufer D: Perturbation of cobalt-60 radiation doses by metal objects implanted during oral and maxillofacial surgery. J Oral Maxillofac Surg 42:108–110, 1984.

Vuillemin T, Raveh J, Sutter F: Mandibular reconstruction with the titanium hollow screw reconstruction plate (THRP) system: Evaluation of 62 cases. Plastic Reconstr Surg 82:804–814, 1988.

Wenig BL, Keller AJ, Shikowitz MJ, et al: Anatomic reconstruction and functional rehabilitation of oromandibular defects with rigid internal fixation. Laryngoscope 98:154–159, 1988.

CHAPTER 49

The Titanium Hollow-Screw Reconstruction Plate System (THORP)

Joram Raveh
Franz Sutter
Thierry Vuillemin

A feature of all conventional reconstruction systems for the bridging of mandibular defects is that the intraoperatively achieved primary stability and anchorage decrease with time. This weakness is most serious if the lower jaw has been irradiated. In contrast to simple fractures, in which bone consolidation may be expected within the relatively short period of three to five months, such defects often necessitate long-term stable bridging.

Because conventional systems do not fulfill the requirements for long-term functional stability, we strove to develop a completely new apparatus. Our previous experience in the years 1975 to 1980 with the AO (Association for Osteosynthesis) system convinced us that many of the already well-established and commonly accepted biomechanical principles and doctrines relating to conventional systems had to be altered.

In 1987, after successful experimental and clinical application of the Titanium Hollow-Screw Reconstruction Plate system (THORP) in maxillofacial departments (Hellem 1988, Raveh 1981, 1982a, 1982b, 1983, 1984a, 1984b, 1985a, 1985b, 1987a, 1987b, 1989, Sutter 1988, Vuillemin 1989a, 1989b) and in orthopedics (Morscher 1986), the THORP system was integrated into the AO program. We will highlight the various biomechanical and technical innovations, as well as the reconstructive methods, made possible by this system. Our experience and follow-up after the application of 141 plates will be discussed.

BIOMECHANICAL AND TECHNICAL ASPECTS

The THORP system (see Figure 49.1) was developed so as to fulfill the requirements of total osseointegration and long-term functional stability. These requirements are critical for the success of any implant device.

The Plate

Titanium IMI-160 (ISO Standard 5843/11, grade 4A) was chosen as the implant material because of its mechanical strength, resistance to fatigue, stiffness, crystal structure, and biocompatibility.

The titanium reconstruction plate is notched between the 4.0-millimeter-diameter holes (see Figure 49.2). These notches are designed to allow moments of inertia between the holes or on a plane lower than that of the holes. The plates can thus be easily bent in any direction, without deformation of the holes (see Figure 49.3a). The configuration of the notches is designed to spread the strain over a greater length on bending and to reduce the possibility of plate failure in this region. Comparative bend and fatigue tests have shown that titanium plates are more flexible but possess fatigue resistance similar to that of identical steel plates (see Figure 49.3b). Bending in the horizontal plane (see Figure

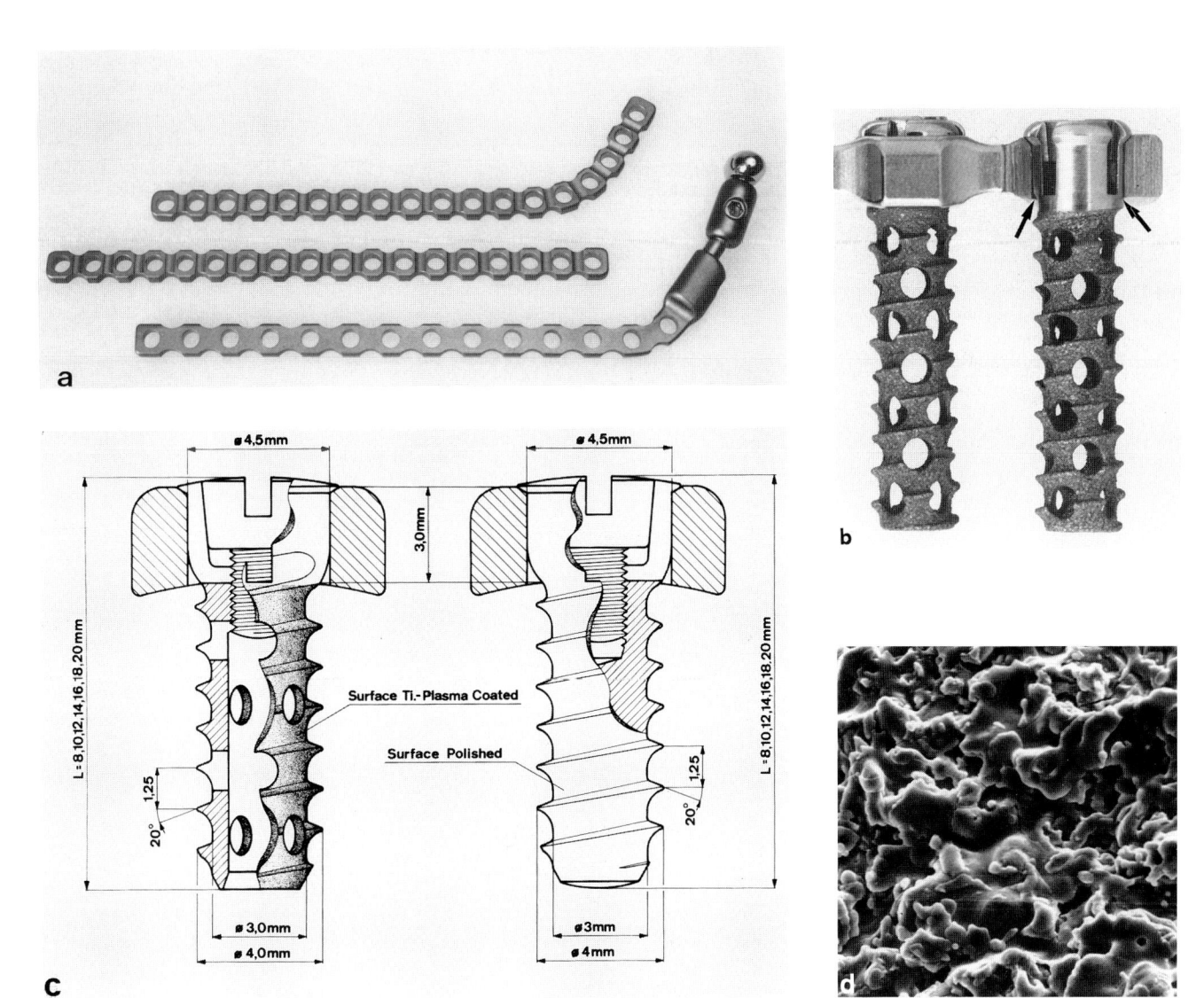

Figure 49.1 (a) THORP titanium reconstruction plates, straight, pre-bent, and with attachment for the three-dimensionally adjustable TMJ prosthesis are shown. The underside of these plates may be titanium plasma-spray coated. (b) Perforated hollow titanium screws are shown fixed to the plate. They are titanium plasma-spray coated. (c) The external diameter of the thread is 4.0 millimeters; thread depth is 0.5 millimeter; thread pitch is 1.50 millimeters. The section shows the exact fit of the expandable screwhead in the plate to form a rigid unit. (d) Scanning electron micrograph shows the titanium plasma-spray coated surface of a hollow screw.

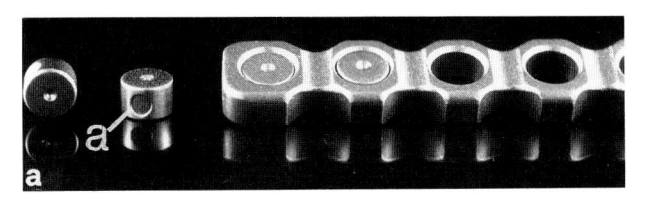

Figure 49.2 (a) Reconstruction plate designed to prevent deformation of the plate holes when the plate is bent, is shown. Plastic inserts (a) in the bolts are for retention. (b) The expansion bolt (E) is applied to the head screw, which has already been driven in.

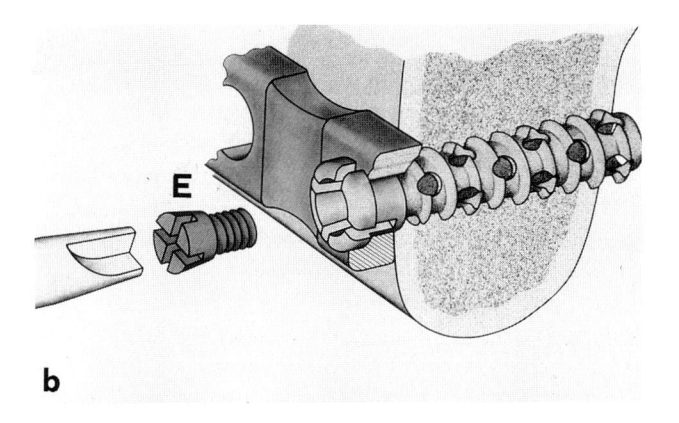

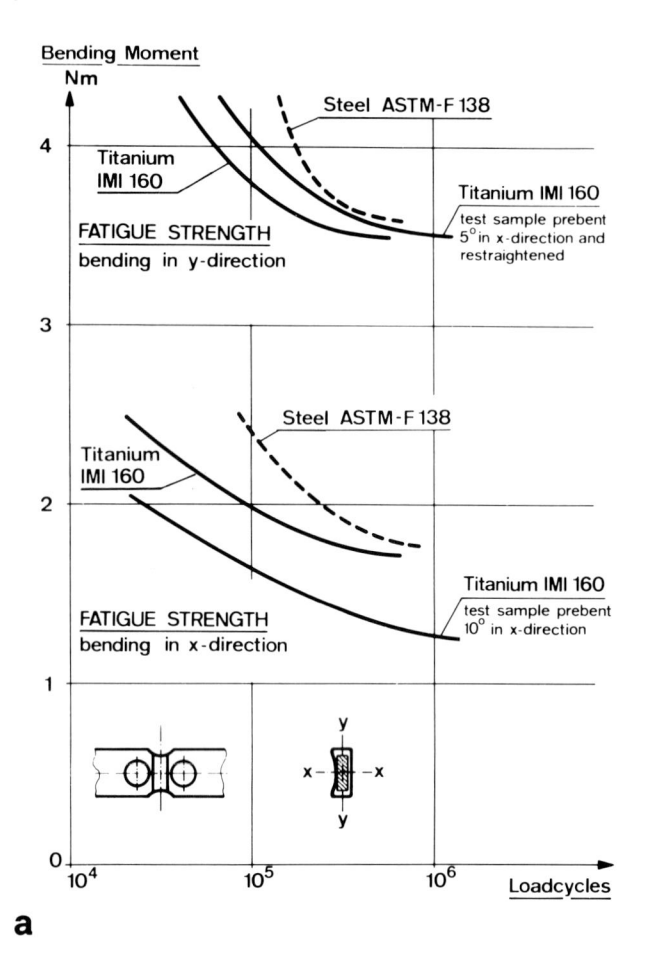

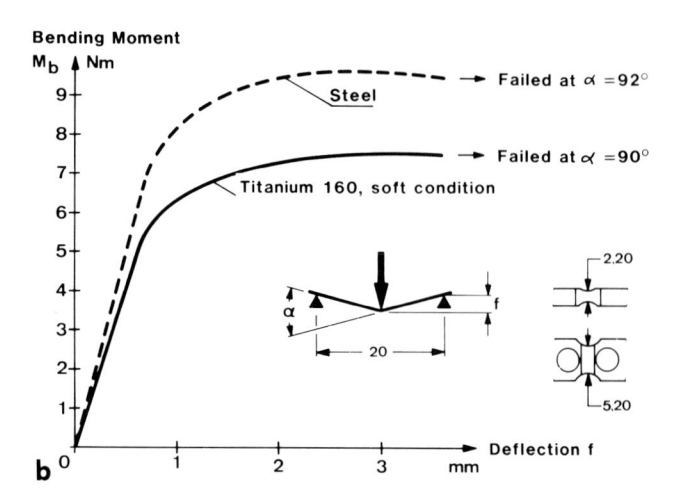

Figure 49.3 Steel and titanium are compared. (a) Fatigue curves are shown for the reconstruction plate for both vertical and lateral loads on the jaw. (b) Deflection of the plate on three-point loading; supports are 20 millimeters apart.

49.3a, top) does not affect the strength of the plate in the vertical plane. Under normal conditions, the direction of the load is primarily vertical.

In order to prevent any deformation of the precisely cylindrical plate holes, metal bolts are inserted before the plate is bent. The bolts have a plastic insert, which holds them in place while the plate is bent (see Figure 49.2a).

The Screw

Two types of titanium screws with expandable heads were designed:

1. the titanium plasma-coated, perforated hollow screw and
2. the titanium full-body screw.

The screwhead is cylindrical with an upper rim and is cross-split almost down to the start of the thread. A small screw with a tapered head is inserted into the expandable head, facilitating locking in the plate hole. The application procedure for the screw used in combination with a plate is shown in Figure 49.2b. In contrast to the conventional systems, this rigid fixation of the screwhead to the plate enabled us to integrate the advantages and characteristics of an external fixation device in an internally applied plate.

A further consideration in the design was to accommodate the high shear force on the screw. Thus a screw diameter of 4.5 millimeters for the hollow screw and 3.5 millimeters for the full-body screw and a thread depth of only 0.5 millimeter were chosen. With regard to our later experimental and clinical experience and so as to simplify the application, all screws in the new series have the same diameter, 4.0 millimeters (see Figure 49.1c). High local load peaks along the thread were avoided by maximizing the load-bearing area and by a design that favors the transmission of loads under physiological conditions. The implant volume was kept to a minimum so as to improve osseointegration. The regularly spaced lateral perforations in the hollow cylinder section enable new bone to penetrate into the screw lumen. The screw surface is coated to a thickness of 0.04 millimeter with an argon titanium plasma spray (see Figure 49.1d). The microtexture of this coating increases (six-fold) the effective surface area for bone attachment.

The decision as to the material and its surface properties are equally as important for the success of implantation as are the geometric and biomechanic design of the implant. The acceptance of the implant is primarily a function of the biocompatibility of the implant material.

Bone is an extremely heterogeneous material from the point of view of its structure and properties; the measurement of mechanical properties in bone under reproducible conditions is thus possible only by way of complicated experimental techniques. Because of this, our axial pull-out and side loading tests of screws were carried out using a porous (bonelike), homogenous plastic material instead of natural bone. Figure 49.4 il-

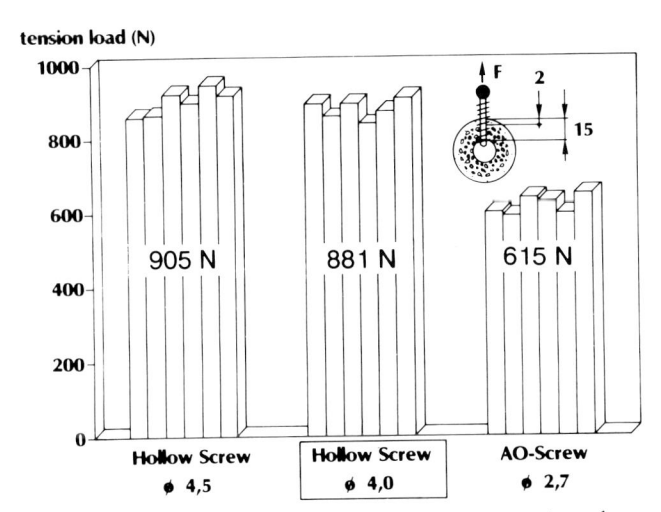

Figure 49.4 The results of axial pull-out tests are given for various screw types.

lustrates that the pull-out load is a function not only of the diameter of the screw but also of the pitch of the screw thread. In contrast to the AO screws, the reduced pitch of 1.25 millimeters (see Figure 49.5) is effective even if the compact bone is extremely thin. The 1.25-millimeter pitch supports a higher axial load and is more efficient in translating the applied torque into axial load; both of these factors contribute to the improvement in primary stability. The lower strength of bone than that of metal should be compensated for by a higher proportion of bone to metal in the longitudinal sections of the screw thread. Accordingly, the high bone–metal relation is maintained in the THORP screw, despite the small thread pitch, by its reduced thread depth.

Our experimental investigations showed that the attachment of bone to a titanium plasma surface is promoted by slight compression of the bone by the body of the screw. The thread tap for the hollow screws therefore is designed so as to cut a slightly smaller thread than the actual size of the screw (see Figure 49.5). The load-bearing surfaces of the thread are angled at 70°, which results in a more even spread of the compressive load over the complete surface of the screw thread at the expense of a slight increase in the radial forces. The force vectors transmitted to the screw are mainly perpendicular to the surface of the thread flank. In contrast to conventional screws, the compressive forces from the bearing surfaces of the 70° variant of our screws are thus directed toward the bone tissue lateral to the screw, thus improving the anchorage and stability.

Several variations of screws are possible with regard to size and the position and number of perforations in the cylinder walls. For example, the holes can be located entirely between the threads, thus preserving their continuity and further improving the axial-load bearing qualities.

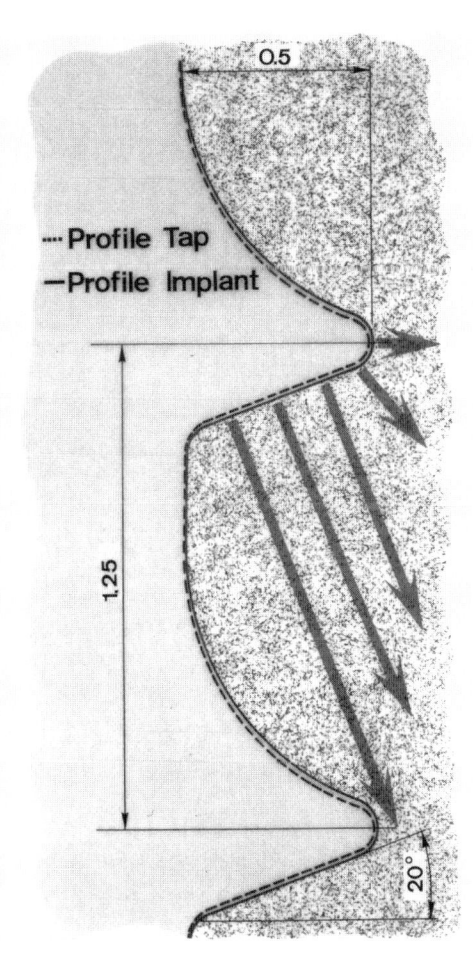

Figure 49.5 The 70° angled thread flanks result in a more even load distribution: The load is directly transmitted to the surface. The thread is cut 0.05 millimeter smaller to achieve an even pressure distribution on the screw profile.

If an early plate removal is indicated, full-body screws are used. The head of a full-body screw can be rigidly fixed to the plate just as can a hollow one (see Figure 49.6). Full-body screws are not titanium-plasma coated and are intended for fracture osteosynthesis or for bridging of defects following cyst or benign tumor resection or cystectomy. In these cases, normal bone reaction and consolidation are expected, making early removal of the plate possible.

One of the major innovations of this system is the rigid fixation of the head of the screw to the plate (see Figure 49.7). As with external fixation devices, the bone underneath the plate is not subject to compression or any other load. Indeed, the plate can be stably applied even if no contact points are established intraoperatively.

COMPARISON OF THE THORP AND CONVENTIONAL SYSTEMS

In our opinion, the major advantages of the THORP over conventional systems are as follows:

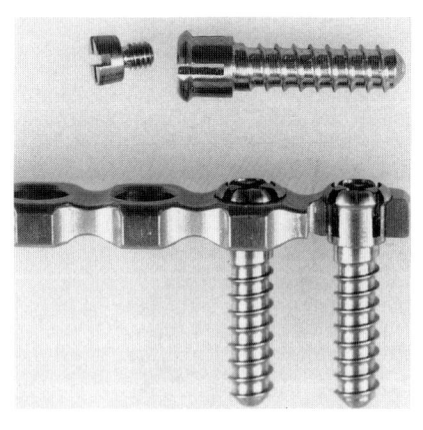

Figure 49.6 The full-body titanium screw has an expandable head, a diameter of 4.0 millimeters, and a smooth surface.

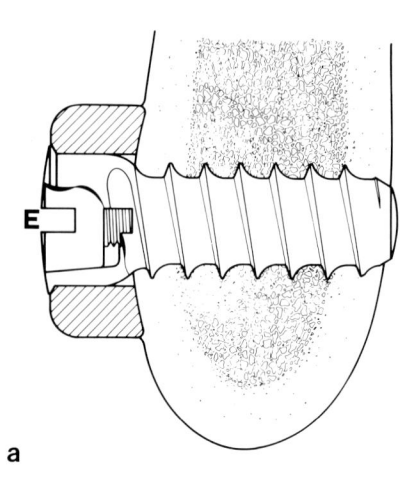

Figure 49.7 (a) Schematic view shows the definitive design of both full-body and hollow screws. (b) Note the direct compression of the screwhead to the plate. (E = expansion bolt.)

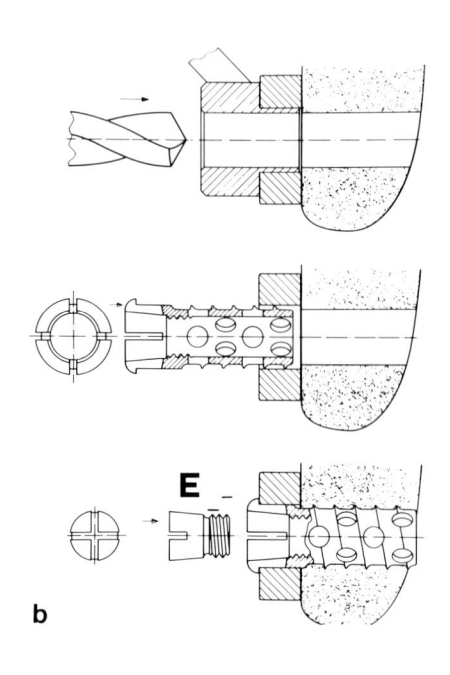

1. Unlike other systems, the THORP system provides rigid fixation of the head of the screw to the plate, and this fixation excludes all micromovements.
2. Compression of the plate to the bone is unnecessary for the THORP system to establish functional primary stability; thus the bone underneath the plate is spared unphysiologic loads. In the other systems, primary stability can be achieved only by pressing the plate to the bone surface with help of the thread of the screw. Micromovements between the loose head of the screw and the plate induce bone resorption along the body and thread of the screw as well as underneath the plate. Sinking of the plate into the compact bone and interpositioning of soft-tissue layers between the implant and bone represent the first signs of loosening.
3. Secondary osseointegration and new bone formation in the lumen and perforations of the body of the THORP system screw cause stability to increase during the implantation period. In conventional systems, not only is the establishment of secondary additional stability or osseointegration impossible, but also the primary intraoperatively achieved stability decreases with time. This means a competitive reaction between osteolysis and loosening of the plate on the one hand and consolidation of the bone on the other. Long-term or permanent bridging of defects with such a system cannot be expected to be successful.

An experimental study compared the AO conventional system and the THORP applied in irradiated and nonirradiated dog mandibles (see Figure 49.8) (Raveh 1982a, 1983, 1984b). In those series in which a dog's mandible was bridged on both sides, the THORP was fixed with only two screws, and the AO plate was fixed with three or four screws to each stump (as recommended by the AO) (see Figure 49.9 and Color Plate 22).

The histological results after three and six months confirmed the superior features of the THORP system. Even after three months the AO system revealed signs of loosening of the first screws nearest to the resection borders (Color Plate 22). In contrast, the THORP system showed increasing anchorage and osseointegration on the contralateral side (see Color Plate 23 and Figure 49.10). The longer the implantation period, the more evident was the loosening and osteolytic process along the AO screws. Thus, clearly the AO system does not fulfill the requirements for long-term bridging or permanent implantation, and this explains the necessity for as many screws as possible. This is a disadvantage in tumor surgery, particularly if irradiated bone or small fragments, such as the condylar process, should be integrated and preserved. The human histological results obtained several years after defect bridging with the THORP system and exposure to full loads, in spite of irradiation-damaged bone tissue, confirmed the stable anchorage (see Color Plates 24 and 25). The fact that the screws osseointegrate is crucial for a reliable functional bridging of the irradiated mandible and enables us to defer secondary bone transplantation for as long as necessary without being concerned about stability.

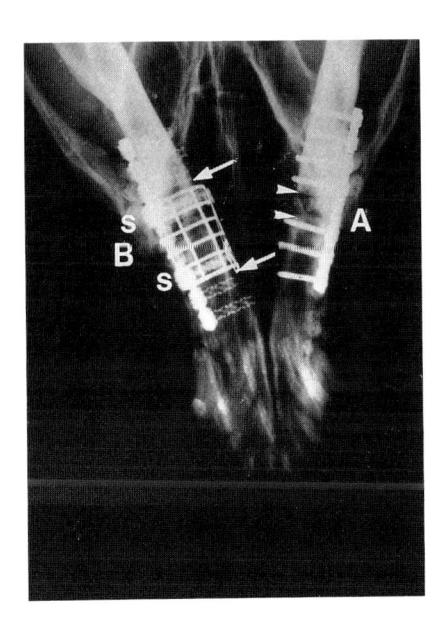

Figure 49.8 Experimental comparison of ASIF (A) and THORP (B) shows the systems bridging defects of the mandible in the same dog submitted to full loads for three and six months, respectively. Operative radiotherapy of 4000 to 7000 rads included only the THORP system. The ASIF reconstruction system (A) is fixed with three and four screws bridging the defect (arrowheads) with cancellous bone. The THORP system (B) is on the contralateral side bridging a larger defect (arrows) with only two or three screws to each stump. These screws (S) hold only a mesh with cancellous bone in place and have no function concerning anchorage.

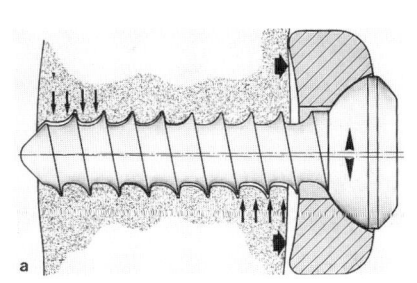

Figure 49.9 The histologic results of this experimental series after bridging of the defects for three and six months confirmed the biomechanical considerations. The staining was performed with fuchsin and light green in all slices. The ASIF system enables cyclic axial tilting movements of the screw (arrowheads) resulting in resorption underneath the plate (arrows) and along the thread. (See color plate 22.)

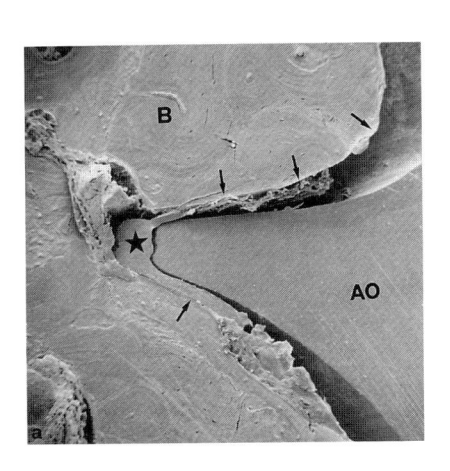

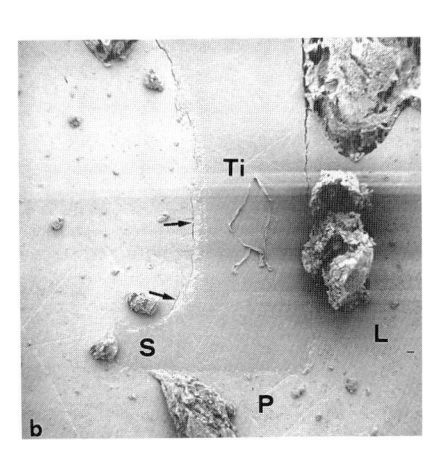

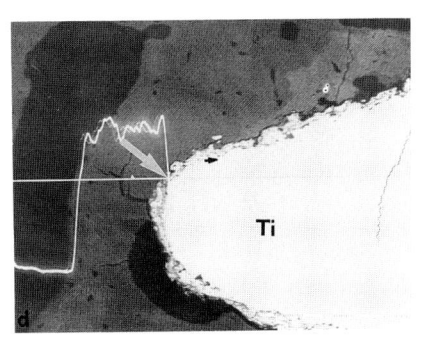

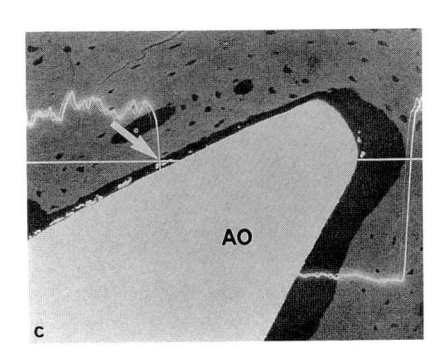

Figure 49.10 Scanning electron micrographs comprise the ASIF and THORP systems after the bridging of defects in a dog mandible for 3.5 months. (a) No bone surface contact is seen all over (arrows). Cement (star) has entered the space between the bone and the thread during preparation of the specimen. This is a nonirradiated specimen. (AO = thread shoulder, B = bone.) (b) The hollow shoulder of the screw thread (S), lumen (L), and perforation (P) are permeated and covered by bone. Direct bone contact is made with the titanium-sprayed surface. The fissures (arrow) lie within the bone itself, leaving intact the bone–plasma surface contact. (c) Energy dispersive X-ray analysis shows microprobe calcium-line analysis of the metal–bone interface of the thread of a conventional ASIF steel screw three months after fixation of a bridging plate in a nonirradiated dog mandible. The gap between the bone and the surface of the screw is clearly indicated by depression of the curve at the soft-tissue border (arrow). (d) The metal–bone interface of the thread of a hollow screw is shown three months after fixation of a bridging plate (irradiation 6000 rads). The presence of calcium in direct contact with the titanium plasma is indicated by the curve dropping at the borders of the thread surface (arrow).

The indication for the application of a bone transplant should be to provide the correct support for a denture or for dental implants and not, as in conventional systems, to stabilize the bone fragments in order to prevent loosening of the plate with time.

The innovative aspects of the THORP system differ in principle from the conventional systems and represent a different biomechanical understanding of the interaction between bone and plate in osteosynthesis. The variety of surgical advantages made possible by the THORP system will be described in relation to (1) tumor surgery and (2) osteosynthesis of fractures.

Reconstruction Following Tumor Surgery

Buccal Plate Application

For the bridging of angular and horizontal defects of the lower jaw, buccal application of the THORP is recommended. In contrast to the conventional systems, the fixation of the THORP system, performed with only two or three screws, is of crucial significance in resections that leave only a small stump of the condylar process (see Figure 49.11 a and b). The condyle thus can be preserved and functionally reintegrated, and a prosthetic substitution is avoided (see Figure 49.11b).

The biomechanical advantages and osseointegration of the anchoring elements provide permanent optimal stability, even after irradiation and in long-term implantation exposed to full loads. If such an attempt is made with the AO system and the plate is fixed with two screws (alio loco), loosening is inevitable, as shown in Figure 49.11d. Such a reconstruction is possible only with the THORP system.

The human histological examination of cases reconstructed in this manner provides further proof that only two screws are sufficient to guarantee optimal anchorage for the THORP system in bone (see Color Plate 26). The facts that there is no resorption of the bone

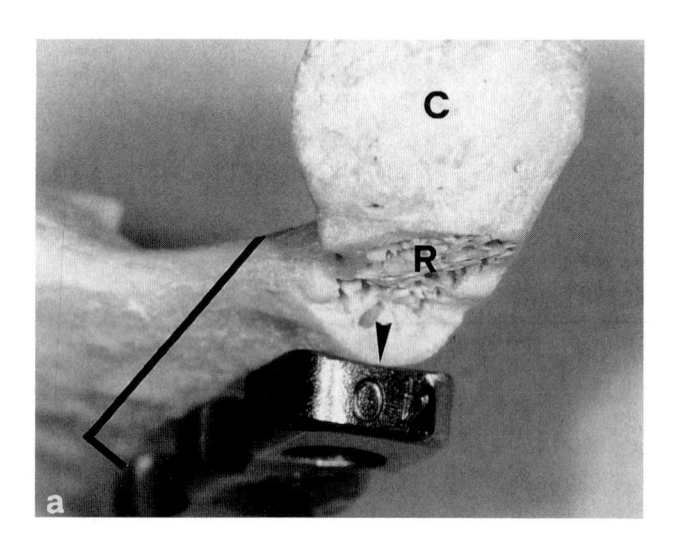

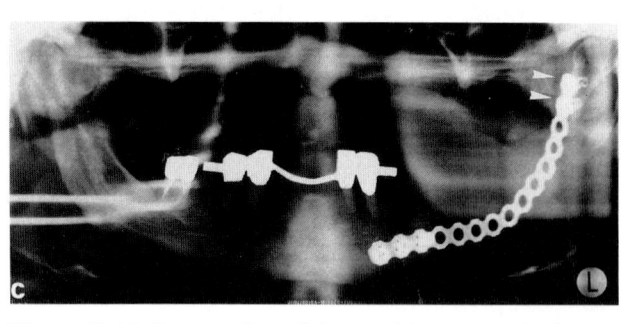

Figure 49.11 Preservation of the condylar process is demonstrated. (a) Extended resection (outline) leaves only the condylar process. The unfavorable anatomic configuration is visualized by the partially resected surface (R) of the condyle (C). Convexity of the neck enables only a limited point of contact between bone and plate. The bone is extremely thin in this region (arrowhead). (b) Intraoperative view shows the configuration following a high resection of the ascending ramus, including the coronoid part and horizontal portion of the mandible for carcinoma of the floor of the mouth and tonsillar fossa. Radiotherapy was 7000 rads. Retention of the condylar process is shown with only two hollow screws (arrow). (c) Radiograph of the same patient after three years shows perfect stability and position of both condyles. (d) This case was reconstructed elsewhere with an AO plate and two screws to the condylar process. Loosening is obvious and confirms the AO doctrine that two screws are insufficient for conventional plates. This is in contrast to the THORP system.

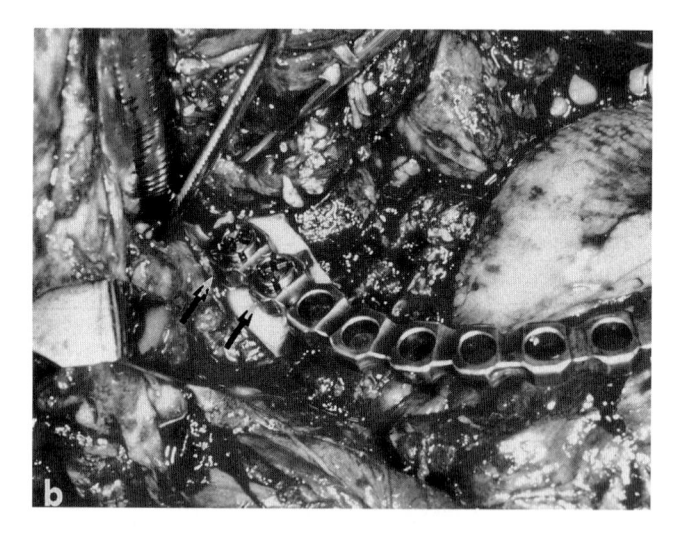

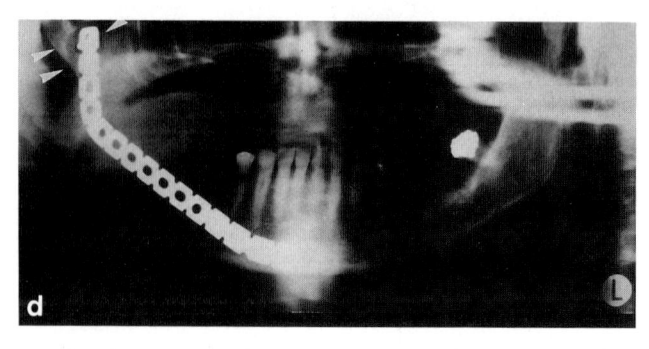

underneath the plate and that there is direct bone-to-thread contact as well as ingrowth of bone into the lumen and perforations of the screws establish confirmation of a physiologic distribution of stress to the bone.

Lingual Application of the THORP System

When bridging of defects is needed in the area of the mandibular symphysis, buccal application of a plate—particularly in irradiated cases or after extensive resection of the soft tissues—can result in pressure necrosis of the overlying skin. In a lingually applied plate the radius is reduced, leaving enough space for the local soft-tissue adaptation without any tension. Thus, the indication for skin flaps or grafts can be reduced. The lingual application (see Figure 49.12), possible only with the THORP system, is performed as described below.

After the mandible is exposed, two carrier plates for the fixation bar are placed distal to the intended resection site (see Figure 49.12b). The fixation bar,

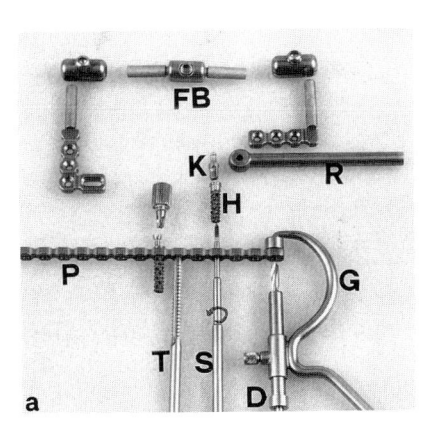

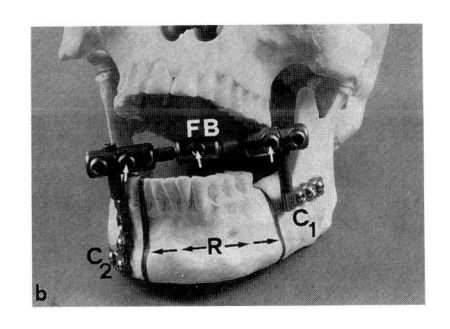

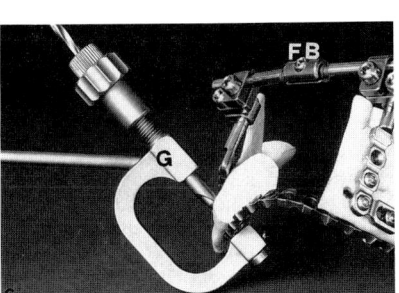

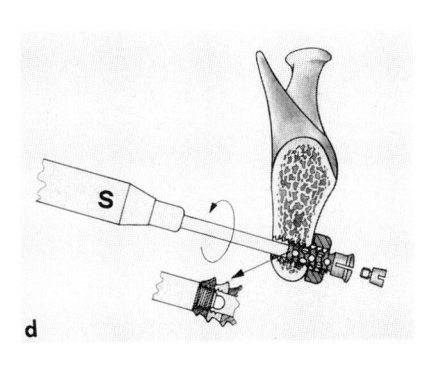

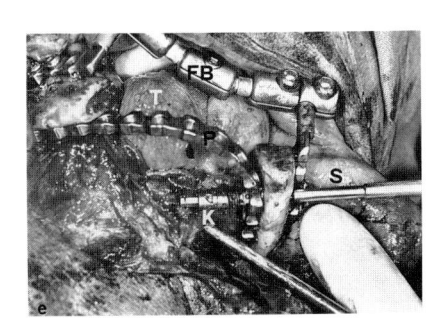

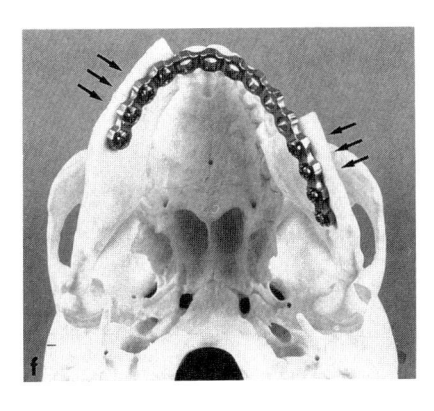

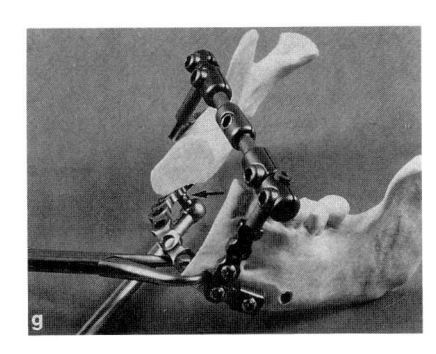

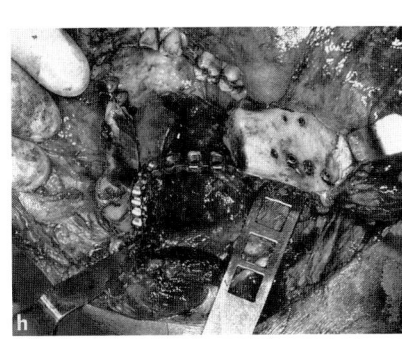

Figure 49.12 Lingual application is possible only with the THORP system. (a) The fixation bar (FB) is freely adjustable in all planes. The plate (P) is applied to the lingual cortex. Drilling (D) and tapping (T) the screw holes is performed with a drill guide (G). (H = hollow screw.) A screwdriver (S) is passed through the bone hole into the screw lumen to be fixed to the key (K) at the end of the screw. The screw is then driven counterclockwise from lingual to buccal (L). Final fixation of the head of the screw to the plate is accomplished with the ratchet (R). (b) The fixation bar (FB) is applied to the mandible prior to resection. (Arrows indicate ball joints and locking screws; C_1 and C_2 = carrier plates; R = area to be resected.) Note that an L-type carrier plate is to be applied so as to preserve the alveolar nerve. (c) Drill guide (G) for the bur holes is shown. (d) The screw is driven. The screwdriver (S) is inserted from the buccal approach through the lumen of the hollow screw and fixed to the key at the head of the screw. The screwdriver is turned counterclockwise. (e) Intraoperative view shows the technique described in Figure 49.12(d). The plate (P) is in situ. (T = tongue, S = screwdriver fixed to the key (K) at the head of the screw.) (f) The plate is shown in situ. (g) Tightening of the screw and application of the expansion bolt are performed with a ratchet. (h) The plate is in situ. Arrow indicates the apical end of the screws.

which is freely adjustable in three dimensions, can then be locked into position. The bar ensures that the original occlusion and the temporomandibular joint (TMJ) relation can be exactly reproduced after resection. A special drill guide is used to drill the screw holes (see Figure 49.12c), cut the thread, and measure the depth from the buccal access. The screws are then inserted from the lingual side and driven in with a special screwdriver from the buccal side (see Figures 49.12d and e). The screws are tightened with a ratchet driver (see Figure 49.12g). The intraoperative view and the radiographs illustrate the achieved reduction (see Figure 49.13).

The THORP Condylar Prosthesis

In order to avoid functional and aesthetic disadvantages as a result of hemimandibulectomy, a variety of condylar prosthetic devices have been developed over past years. Several different materials have been used, including chrome-cobalt-molybdenum alloy (Conley 1951, Hahn 1969), titanium (Hellem 1988, Raveh 1981, 1982a, 1982b, 1983, 1984a, 1984b, 1987a, 1987b, Vuillemin 1989a, 1989b), aluminium-oxide ceramics (Frenkel 1977) and proplast, ticonium (Kent 1983).

The currently available condylar prosthetic devices have a standardized, preformed articular head (spherical, elliptical, or cylindrical) that is rigidly fixed to a plate. Considering the fact that the fossa is of individual form and that the glenoidal relief of the condyle corresponds to the occlusion, the complexity of the anatomic and functional aspects is obvious. Such conventional prosthetic condyles can thus hardly be expected to fit exactly into the articular fossa and reproduce the original guidance and movements imposed by the dental occlusion. Consequently such prosthetic devices often lead to functional failures. Perforation and displacement into the middle cranial fossa, as well as abrasion of the tuberculum, anterior or distal luxation, and dysfunction, have already been described (Kent 1983, Sonnenburg 1985).

In order to eliminate these disadvantages, a three-dimensionally adaptable THORP was developed to include a three-dimensionally adjustable condylar prosthesis, which can itself be functionally adjusted intraoperatively (see Figure 49.14a and b). Thus the original articulation, including the rotatory and translatory movements, can be reproduced. The THORP condylar prosthesis consists of a carrier plate and a prosthetic condylar process. The titanium reconstruction carrier plate in Figure 49.14b and c corresponds to the plate developed for the bridging of bone defects and is part of the THORP system. The three-dimensionally malleable plate is segmented in notches. In consideration of anatomic variations, three sizes of titanium condyles are available. The condylar prosthesis is attached to the plate by two sand-blasted joints (see Figures 49.14a–c). These joints are freely adjustable in all planes and can be fixed by means of locking screws. This represents one of the major advantages of the THORP prosthesis.

In contrast to conventional systems, once adapted and fixed to the mandible (see Figure 49.14c), the condyle can be further functionally adjusted to the fossa by loosening the ball-joint locking screw. Such a meticulous adaptation of the condyle to the fossa in correct relation to the occlusion during rotatory and translatory passive movements is essential for the reproduction of the original joint function and to avoid interference along the glenoidal surface (see Figure 49.14d and e). Once the condyle is adapted, the ball-joint locking screws are finally tightened. Thus, in spite of an extensive bone resection and the necessarily long lever arm, the prosthesis can be stably fixed by only two or three screws and still guarantee optimal positioning and guidance of the condyle.

The radiographs presented in Figures 49.15 and 49.16 include most of the possible reconstruction varieties, having in common optimal positioning of the condyle and optimal function. We are of the opinion that the radiograms must include panorexes to demonstrate the correct relation of both condyles (see Figure 49.16), anterior–posterior radiographs to illustrate the correct angle toward the glenoid fossa and skull base and—in doubtful cases—tomograms. Only thus, we believe, can an objective proof of the correct relation be shown. Differing opinions are held by several others (Kellman 1987).

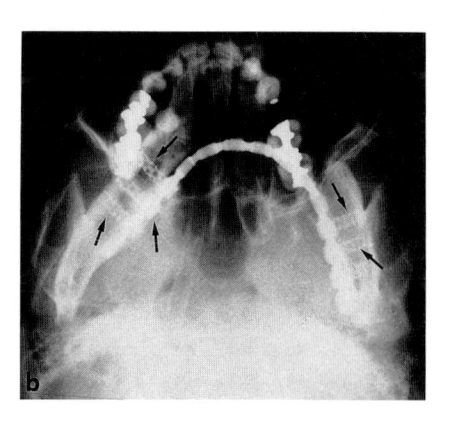

Figure 49.13 (a) The adapted lingual plate is shown. (b) Postoperative radiograph illustrates the significant reduction of the radius of the plate's curvature compared with buccal application.

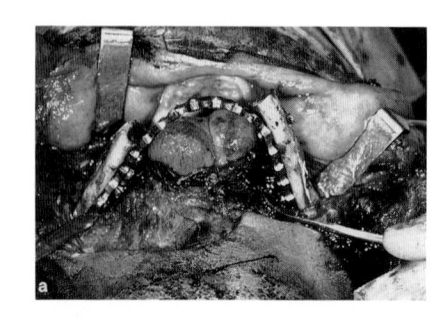

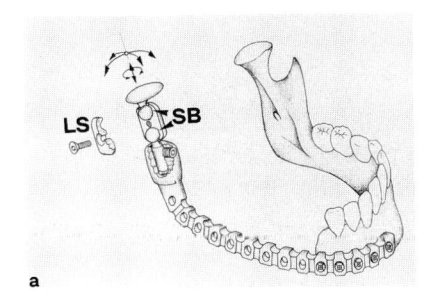

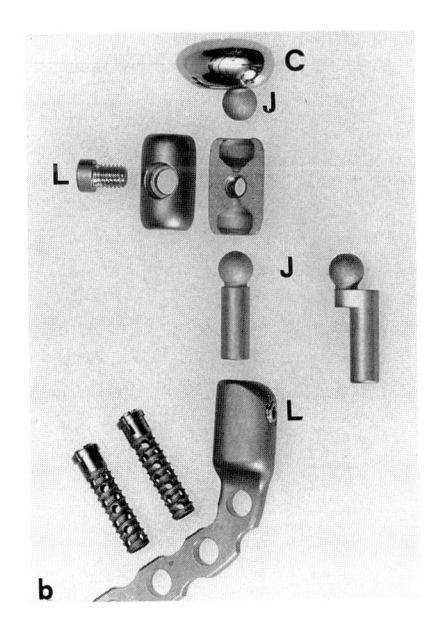

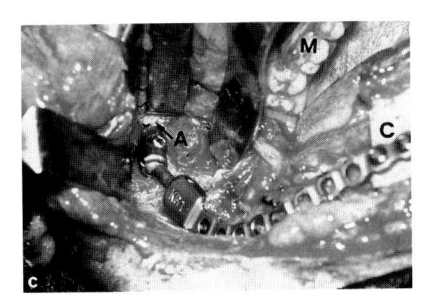

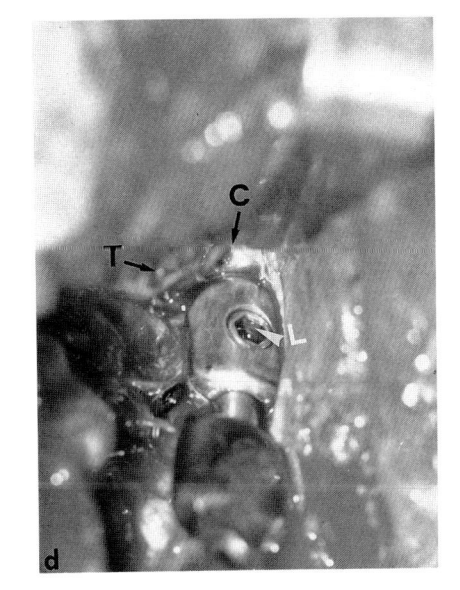

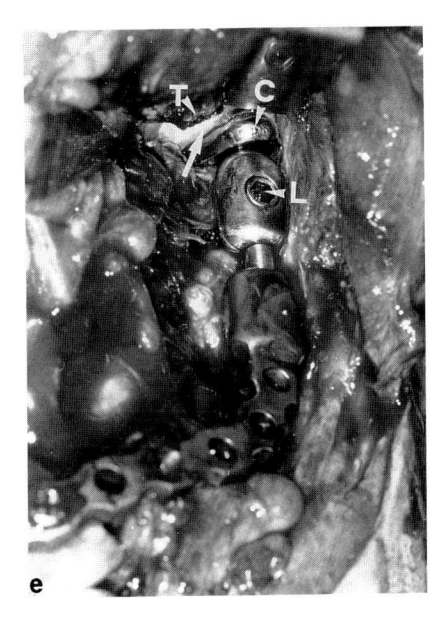

Figure 49.14 (a) The condylar prosthesis, freely adjustable in all directions, is fixed to the reconstruction plate by two sand-blasted joints (SB) and adjustment locking screws (LS). (b) The condylar head (C), sand-blasted joints (J), and locking screws (L) are shown. (c) Application of the THORP condylar prosthesis after hemimandibulectomy is demonstrated. The resection border (C) is fixed. The maxilla (M) and articular fossa with condylar prosthesis (A) are shown. (d) In contrast to conventional devices, the condylar head, once fixed to the mandible is subject to further functional adjustment. (T = tuberculum articulare, C = condyle in closed position, L = locking screws.) (e) Translatory movement is reproduced. At C, the condyle at its maximal opening (arrowhead). (T = tuberculum articulare, preserved disc (arrows), L = subsequent definite tightening of the locking screws.)

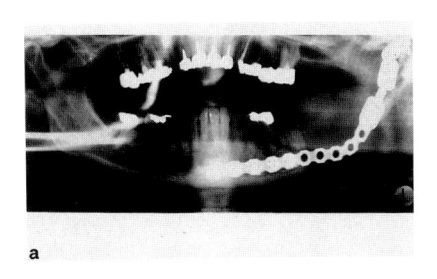

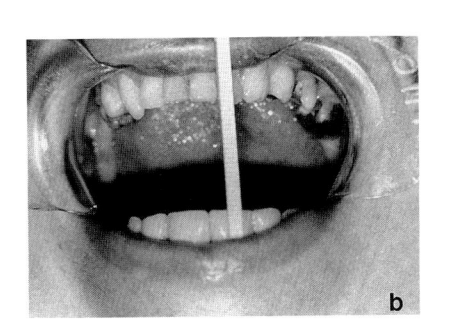

Figure 49.15 A condylar prosthesis seven years postoperatively shows optimal position and guidance.

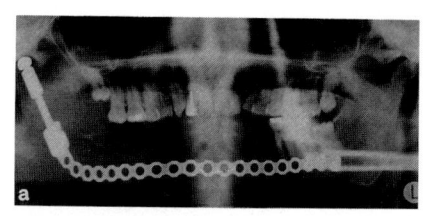

Figure 49.16 (a) Panorex and (b) lateral tomogram demonstrate the correct condylar adaptation.

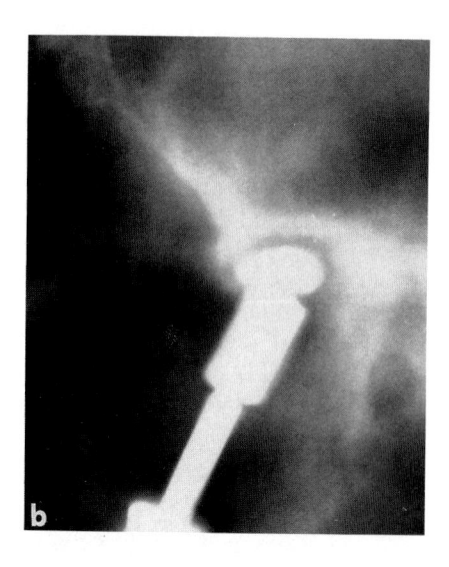

Figure 49.17 (a) Mandibular reconstruction with the condylar prosthesis and primary autologous iliac crest transplants (T) is shown. Fixation is achieved with hollow screws (large arrow) which is a cross-section through line A. The transplant is carried by the screws, which are rigidly fixed to the plate—loosening of a screw is impossible. (b) THORP reconstruction following exarticulation is shown in a young patient without irradiation. An L-shaped iliac crest bone transplant (T) is shaped to fit the articular fossa (triangle). (R = resection border.) (c) Postoperative radiograph after four years. (Lines show the resection border, heavy arrows, the angular area of the transplant, and arrows, the correct position of the reshaped transplant in the fossa.)

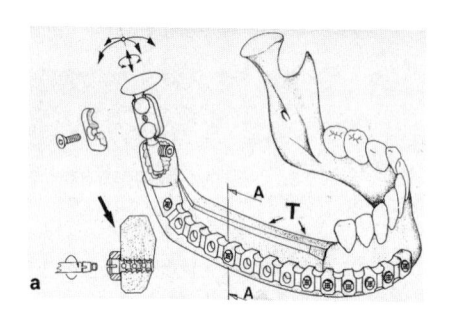

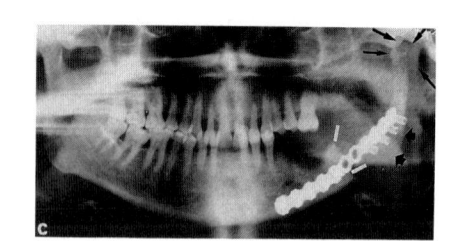

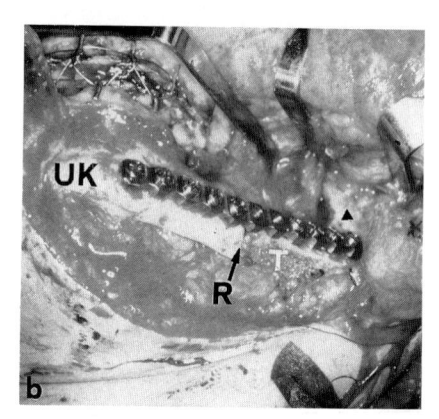

Primary and Secondary Bone Grafting with Simultaneous Application of Intraosseous Dental Implants

Because the THORP system provides long-term permanent stability, bone grafting is not necessary to avoid loosening of the plate and screws—as it is in conventional systems. Grafts are applied only in order to provide the necessary support for dentures or intraosseous dental implants. We usually perform primary grafting after the resection of benign tumors; we prefer a secondary procedure if malignant tumors are involved and extensive soft-tissue resection and irradiation are to be performed. In such cases, we prefer to wait for one or two years until the soft-tissue recipient bed has recovered and tumor recurrence has been excluded.

The specific advantage of the rigid fixation of the screws enables optimal fixation of the bone transplants without the risk of loosening of the screws (see Figure 49.17a). In conventional systems during the remodeling period of the bone transplant, the bone contact along the thread of the screw reduces. Thus the primary stability achieved by the screw's pressing the transplant to the plate decreases with time, and the incidence of loosening, as well as osteolysis, is higher. In contrast, the THORP screws carry and support the transplant; and being rigidly fixed to the plate, tilting, osteolysis, and loosening of the screws are avoided. Thus a reliable support for bone transplants is provided for various types of bone grafting (see Figure 49.17b and c). This optimal stability encouraged us to apply intraosseous dental implants simultaneously with transplantation (see Figures 49.18–49.20). This method was successfully practiced by us and by others (Raveh 1987b, Hellem 1988, Vuillemin 1989a, 1989b). The cases illustrated

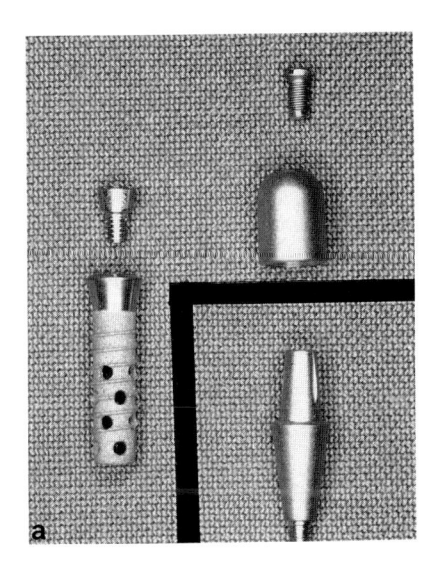

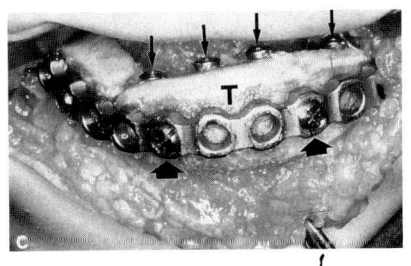

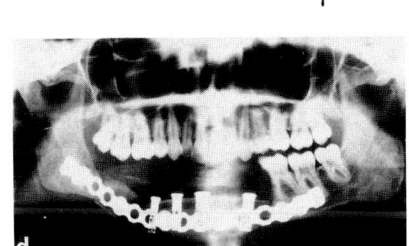

Figure 49.18 Bone grafting is shown with primary application of dental implants. (a) Abutment and ITI (International Team for Oral Implantology) dental implant are shown. (b) Implants are placed in the bone graft. (c) A transplant (T) with dental implants (→) is fixed to the THORP system with only two screws. (d) Postoperative radiograph after one year shows minimal resorption of the transplant and optimal stability of the dental implants. (e) Intraoral exposure shows the implants for application of the abutment. Optimally consolidated bone transplant is shown.

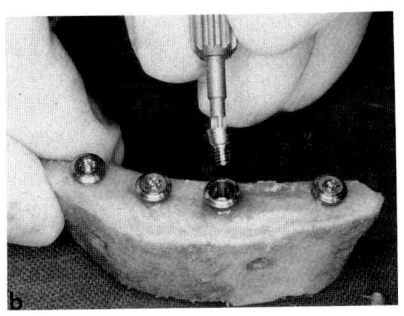

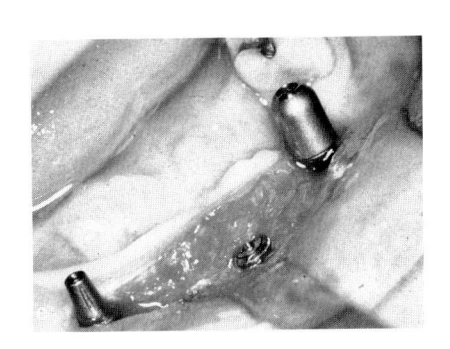

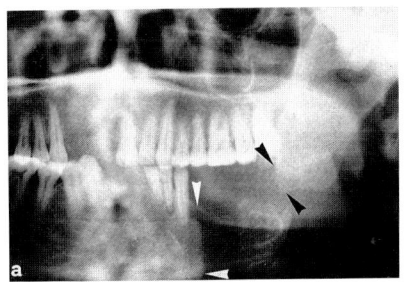

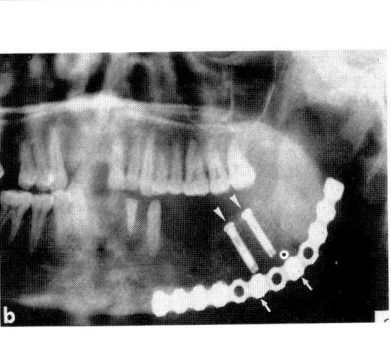

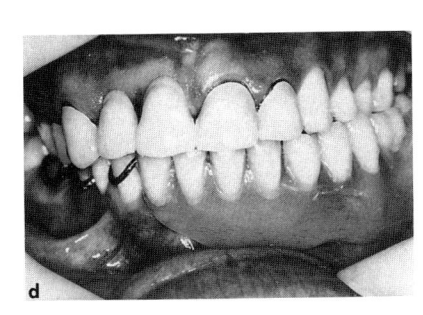

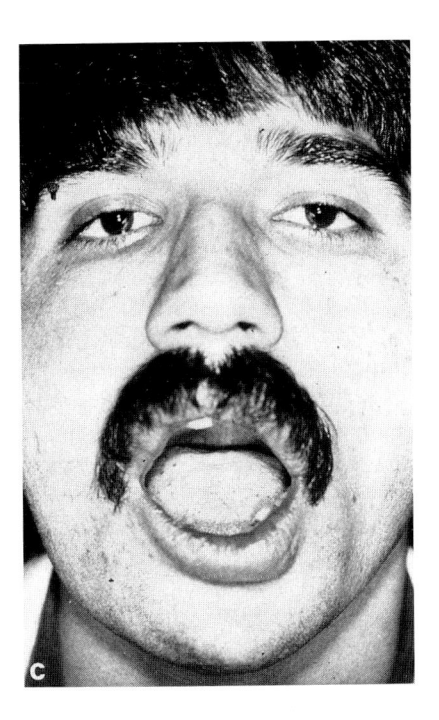

Figure 49.19 (a) This radiograph was produced one year after a gunshot wound. Defect angle of the left mandible (arrowheads) and mandibular deviation to the right side are shown. (b) The same patient is shown in a radiograph after reconstruction with the THORP. Bone grafting (iliac crest) was fixed with screws along with two Branemark implants (arrows). The TMJ (C) is in its correct position. (Operated in Sweden with Dr. S. Hellem (oral surgeon) and Prof. J. Olofsson (ENT).) (c and d) The patient is shown after four years with correctly reconstructed occlusion.

Figure 49.20 (a) Hemimandibulectomy up to the contralateral angle (R) for squamous cell carcinoma is shown. Reconstruction is achieved with the THORP prosthesis. Autologous iliac crest bone transplant and primary applied Branemark implants were used. Fixation was achieved with hollow screws (**HS**). (C = prosthetic condyle.) (b) The patient provided an intraoral radiograph after two years. Transplant consolidation is optimal, and dental implants are stable (arrows). (HS = hollow screws osseointegrated in the transplants.) (c) The patient's symmetrical opening is shown. (d) This intraoral view shows the patient six years postoperatively.

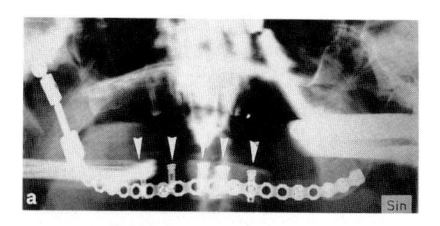

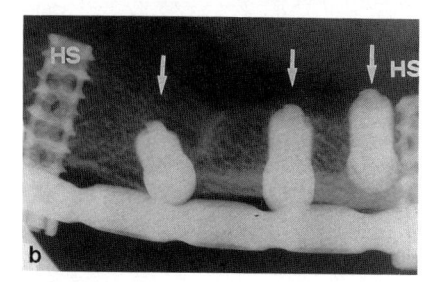

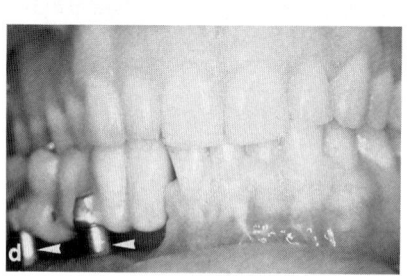

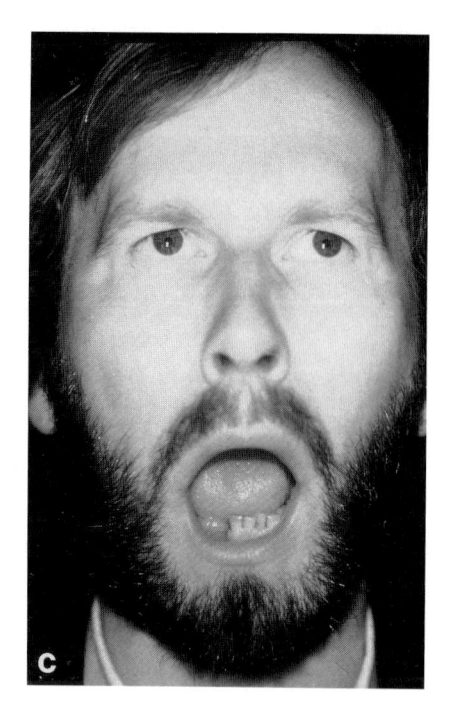

confirm the efficiency of this procedure. Particularly in extensive concomitant soft-tissue resection or irradiation, we prefer vascularized free composite osseomyocutaneous flap harvested from the iliac crest along with the deep circumflex iliac artery and vein. The anastomosis is performed with either the facial or superior thyroid vessels.

THORP Application in Traumatic Mandibular Defects and Fractures

Conventional fracture osteosynthesis is achieved by two types of plates: (1) the dynamic compression plate (DCP), and (2) the reconstruction plate. The latter is used for multifragmentary or defect fractures that make sufficient compression impossible.

In both types of plates, primary stability decreases. In fact, a competitive reaction establishes between loosening on the one hand and fracture healing and consolidation on the other. Thus reconstruction plates, particularly when applied to comminuted multifragmentary fractures and defects, are susceptible to instability. This instability leads to prolonged bone healing and a higher risk of loosening. The so-called primary bone healing is established only when all criteria for functional stability are fulfilled. Various screw types can be integrated in the THORP system (see Figure 49.21a) so as to achieve dynamic compression when indicated (see Figure 49.21b). Yet in multifragmentary, oblique, or defect fractures, the effect of a dynamic compression plate is in most cases reduced to a minimum and may even lead to distortion or incongruity of the intermediate fragments. This is the reason for the commonly recommended application of neutral reconstruction plates in such cases.

With regard to the limited stability of the conventional plates in such cases, we applied the THORP system using the full-body type of screw (see Figure 49.6). In those fracture types, in which an intermediate fragment can be compressed or an angulation of the screw is indicated, conventional screws can be interpositioned (see Figure 49.21). Thus the major advantages of the THORP system can be maintained. Even in those cases in which the AO conventional plates failed along with already established osteolysis and infection, optimal healing was achieved after replacing the AO plate with our system (see Figure 49.22b).

For simple fractures with an expected early consolidation, reconstruction or DC plates are quite sufficient, and the more expensive THORP system is not needed.

REMOVAL OF THE PLATE AND SCREWS

Any implant must be removable in a simple procedure that causes minimal trauma. THORP plates and full-body screws are easily removed, as in conventional

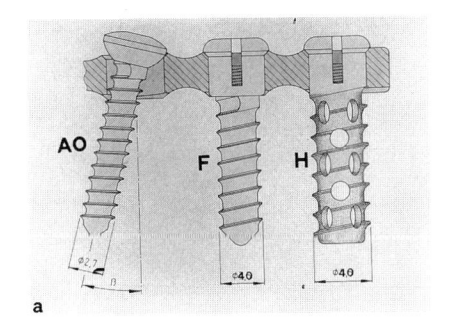

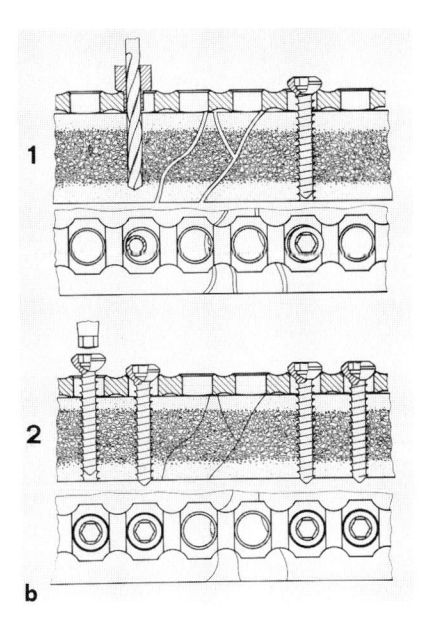

Figure 49.21 THORP application in traumatic cases is shown. (a) One possible screw combination in the THORP system is the conventional AO, THORP full-body (F), and hollow screws (H). The diameter of the THORP screws is 4.0 millimeters. (b) (1,2) Application of the THORP system in multifragmentary fractures is shown. Eccentric drilling enables compression. This is possible only in an ideal fracture configuration, as schematically indicated. Yet in most such cases compression is impossible, and neutral application is indicated. The THORP system is most advantageous in such cases.

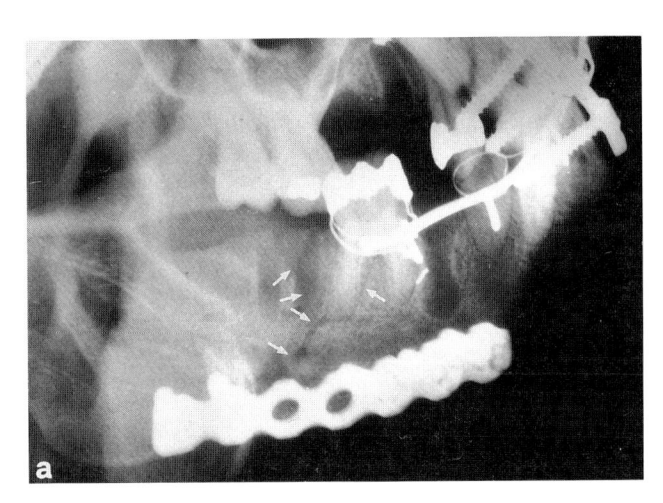

Figure 49.22 (a) Multifragmentary angular fracture (arrow) with concomitant alveolar defect is shown. Application of the THORP system is functionally stable. (b) This gunshot defect was primarily bridged with a conventional AO reconstruction plate fixed by four screws to each stump. Consequent loosening was accompanied by infection and osteolysis. Revision and reconstruction were achieved with the THORP system. After recovery of the recipient bed, grafting is planned.

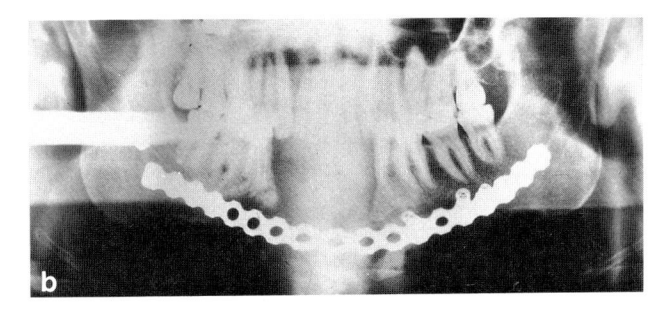

systems. The method for removal of the titanium plate and hollow screws is described below.

The heads can be broken off by a forcible twist of the screwdriver at a predetermined location (see Figure 49.23). The screwhead always breaks between the first perforation and the neck of the screwhead that is, flush with the outer surface of the bone (see Figures 49.23b–d). The plate can thus be removed, and the screw cyl-

inder is left in the bone. The torque required to sever the head is approximately 1.5 Newton meters. The cylinders being osseointegrated may be left in situ; no migration of the cylinders is to be expected.

The hollow cylinder can be removed even when it is fully incorporated. A thin-walled hollow mill is available to cut out the screw body without creating a large defect (see Figure 49.23e). The procedure is as follows:

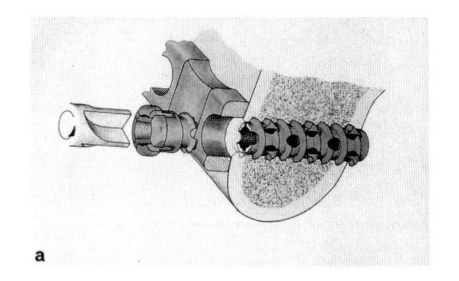

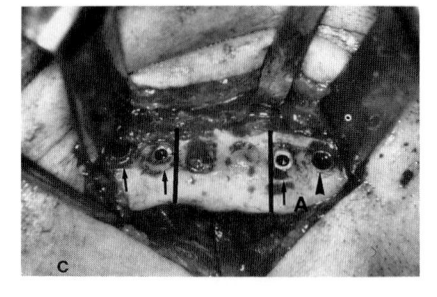

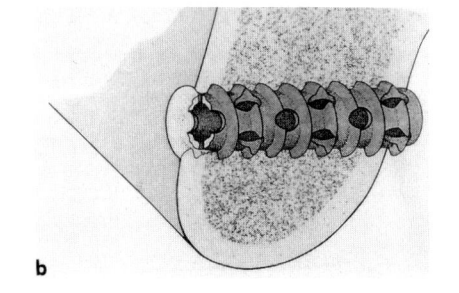

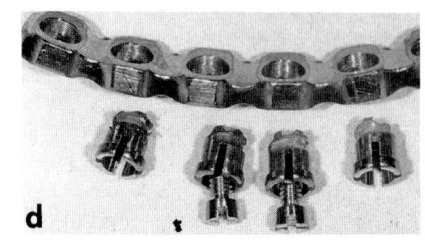

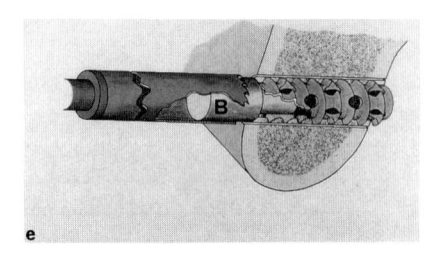

Figure 49.23 Removal of perforated titanium hollow screws is demonstrated. (a) The heads break off at a predetermined location—the first row of perforations flush to the bone surface—upon sudden twisting of the head with the cross-head screwdriver. (b) The cylinders are left behind. (c) Intraoperative view shows the situation after removal of the plate. Arrows indicate cylinders still in situ; arrowheads indicate cylinders already removed. Lines show the borders of the previous, now consolidated, bone graft. (A = angle of the mandible.) (d) Removed plate and broken-off screwheads are shown. (e) The cylinder is removed with a thin-walled trephine mill. The buccally protruding bolt (B) acts as a guide pin to maintain axial alignment of the trephine.

After the screwhead has been broken off and the plate has been removed, a special stepped bolt is inserted into the screw lumen. The buccally protruding bolt head (labeled B in Figure 49.23e), whose diameter is the same as the internal diameter of the thin-walled hollow mill (wall thickness approximately 0.15 millimeters) acts as a guide for the mill. This method may also be used to remove lingually adapted plates from the buccal side.

It must, however, be stressed, that the removal of the hollow cylinders is rarely necessary. Even if a second resection and bridging should become necessary, new hollow-cylinder screws can be inserted in direct contact with the already incorporated hollow cylinders.

The following reconstructive advantages are unique to the THORP system:

1. Increasing primary stability and optimal function as a long-term permanent implant.
2. Retention of the condylar process with only two screws.
3. Lingual plate application.
4. Stable bone transplant fixation excluding any loosening of the screws.
5. Functional adaptation of the THORP condylar prosthesis to the articular fossa.

RESULTS

The THORP system was clinically applied in 82 tumor and 59 traumatic cases. Tables 49.1 and 49.2 indicate the type and location of the plates utilized.

Table 49.1 Type of THORP device in 141 cases

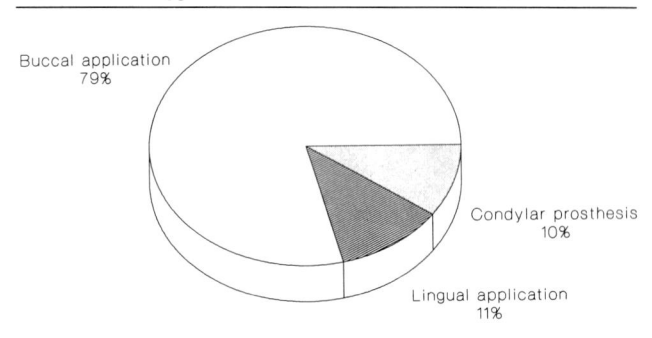

Buccal application 79%
Condylar prosthesis 10%
Lingual application 11%

The results and follow-up are indicated in Table 49.3, emphasizing the low rate of complications and the fact that only one plate fractured. One plate loosened in a comminuted fracture; the patient was undergoing immunosuppressive therapy during terminal renal insufficiency and already showed severe signs of general osteoporosis. In 4 transplants out of 18, resorption was manifest but the plates remained perfectly stable. These 4 cases were highly irradiated (6000 to 7000 rads), and the iliac crest transplants were nonvascularized free grafts. Thus, although the grafts were not rejected, a high degree of resorption occurred, making secondary grafting inevitable. In our opinion, only vascularized free grafts should be applied in such irradiated cases. In

Table 49.2 Mandibular reconstruction with the THORP system following tumor ablation and trauma

Defect Extent	Malignant Neoplastic Desease	Benign Neoplastic Desease	Osteomyelitis Osteoradionecrosis	TMJ Ankylosis	Fracture Defect	Complicated Fracture	Total
	14	-	1	-	7	-	22
	17	1	-	-	1	-	19
	15	1	1	-	4	-	21
	3	4	1	-	-	-	8
	2	2	-	-	-	-	4
	-	-	-	2	-	-	2
No Bone Defect	-	-	6	-	-	59	65
Total	51	7	9	2	12	59	141

Table 49.3 Complications of 141 THORP devices

	Number of cases
Loosening of plate	
Tumor	0
Traumatic	1
Plate fracture	1
Decubitus, skin perforation (closed by local flaps)	3
Mucosal dehiscence (local closure)	15
Loss of bone transplants	4
TMJ dysfunction	0

none of the cases in which small condylar fragments were fixed with only two screws did loosening or dysfunction occur. An exposure was manifest in 3 cases six to nine months postoperatively. In these cases the plate bridged the paramedian-horizontal part of the mandible and was applied to the buccal side. These cases are a further confirmation of the advantages of a lingual application. All prosthetic devices were successful, maintaining the correct intraoperatively set position and guidance during the follow-up period of up to eight years. The success rate in the traumatic cases confirms the indication for this system.

SUMMARY

The innovative biomechanical and technical aspects of the THORP system differ basically from, and even contradict, the principles and doctrine of conventional systems. In conventional systems, stability is achieved by compression of the bone fragments to the plate with the help of the thread of the screws. This primary, intraoperatively achieved stability is fully dependent on the anchorage of the thread in bone. Considering the physiology of bone reaction and remodeling, this intraoperatively achieved anchorage *must* reduce with time. As the head of the screw is not fixed to the plate, the loads cause micromovements between the head of the screw and the plate and consequently between the plate and the bone surface underneath. This results in axial tilting movements of the body of the screw, osteolysis, and the interpositioning of a soft-tissue layer between the thread and bone. Simultaneously, the plate sinks into the underlying compact bone. Thus loosening of the plate is inevitable and is only a question of time. In order to prolong stability of the plate, the only solution recommended is the application of as many screws as possible. Because conventional systems do not provide long-term stability, their success rate is dependent on reunion and consolidation of the fracture or defect borders.

These disadvantages were eliminated by the THORP system, which provides a reliable long-term or permanent implant. One of the THORP system's major innovative aspects is the rigid fixation of the screwhead to the plate, thus avoiding resorptive reactions along the body of the screw as well as unphysiologic pressure on the bone underneath the plate. This aspect corresponds to the principles of an external fixation device. Titanium allows osseointegration; and in those cases in which a long-term implantation is necessary, the titanium-sprayed hollow screws enable secondary increasing anchorage and stability. This is crucial for successful bridging of defects—particularly in irradiated, damaged bone tissue. As reported in this chapter, these advantages have enabled a broad variety of reconstructions.

Acknowledgment

The authors are very much indebted to the Bernese Cancer League and Stanley Thomas Johnson Foundation for the generous support of these projects and to Dr. H. C. H. Stich for the excellent histological preparations.

We are particularly grateful for the excellent secretarial work of Mrs. A. Zaugg.

REFERENCES

Conley JJ: The use of vitallium prosthesis and implants in the reconstruction of the mandibular arch. Plast Reconstr Surg 8:150–165, 1951.

Frenkel G, Niederdellman H: The possibilities afforded by the use of dense aluminium oxide ceramics in the reconstruction of the temporomandibular joint. Quintessence Int 8:19–26, 1977.

Hahn GW, Corgill DA: Chrome cobalt mesh mandibular prosthesis. J Oral Surg 27:5–11, 1969.

Hellem S, Olofsson J: Titanium-coated hollow screw and reconstruction plate system (THORP) in mandibular reconstruction. J Cranio Maxillofac Surg 4:173–183, 1988.

Kellman RM, Gullane PJ: Use of the AO mandibular reconstruction plate for bridging of mandibular defects. Otolaryngol Clin North Am 20:519–533, 1987.

Kent JN, Misiek DJ, Akin RK, Hinds EC, Homsy CA: Temporomandibular joint condylar prosthesis: A ten year report. J Oral Maxillofac Surg 41:245–254, 1983.

Morscher E, Sutter F, Jenny H, Olerud S: Die vordere Verplattung der Halswirbelsaeule mit dem Hohlschrauben-Plattensystem aus Titanium. Chirurg 57:702–707, 1986.

Raveh J, Stich H, Schawalder P, Sutter F, Straumann F: Konservative und chirurgische Massnahmen zur Wiederherstellung der Kiefergelenkfunktionen und neue Moeglichkeiten und Methoden zur Defektueberbrueckung am Unterkiefer. Schweiz Mschr Zahnheilk 90:920–932, 1981.

Raveh J, Stich H, Sutter F, Greiner R: Neue Rekonstruktionsmoeglichkeiten des Unterkiefers bei knoechernen Defekten nach Tumorresektionen. Tierexperimentelle und klinische Resultate. Der Chirurg 53:459–468, 1982a.

Raveh J, Geering AH, Sutter F, Stich H: Erste Erfahrungen mit einer neuen Kiefergelenkprothese. Schweiz Mschr Zahnheilk 97:681–689, 1982b.

Raveh J, Stich H, Sutter F, Greiner R: New concepts in the reconstruction of mandibular defects following tumor resection. J Maxillofac Surg 41:3–16, 1983.

Raveh J, Sutter F: Defektueberbrueckung unter lingualem Zugang und Knochentransplantatfixation am Unterkiefer mit dem THORP-System. Schweiz Mschr Zahnheilk 95:134–142, 1984a.

Raveh J, Stich H, Sutter F, Greiner R: Use of titanium-coated hollow screw and reconstruction system in bridging of lower jaw defects. J Oral Maxillofac Surg 42:281–294, 1984b.

Raveh J, Roux M, Sutter F: The lingual application of a reconstruction plate: A new method in bridging lower jaw defects. J Oral Maxillofac Surg 43:735–739, 1985a.

Raveh J, Roux M, Sutter F, Stich H: Erhaltung des Kiefergelenksfortsatzes und Anwendung von Titan-Vollkernschrauben bei Defektueberbrueckung. Schweiz Maschr Zahnheilk 95:925–936, 1985b.

Raveh J, Vuillemin T, Roux M, Laedrach K, Sutter F: Plate osteosynthesis of 367 mandibular fractures: The unrestricted indication for the intraoral approach. J Maxillofac Surg 15:244–253, 1987a.

Raveh J, Sutter F, Hellem S: Surgical procedures for reconstruction of the lower jaw using the titanium-coated hollow screw and reconstruction plate (THORP) system: Bridging of defects. Otolaryngol Clin North Am 20:535–572, 1987b.

Raveh J, Vuillemin T, Laedrach K, Sutter F: Temporomandibular joint ankylosis: Surgical treatment and long-term results. J Oral Maxillofac Surg 47:900–906, 1989.

Raveh J: Lower jaw reconstruction with the THORP system for bridging of lower jaw defects. Second International Conference on Head and Neck Cancer. July/August 1988, Boston (in press).

Sonnenburg I, Sonnenburg M: Total condylar prosthesis for alloplastic jaw articulation replacement. J Maxillofac Surg 13:131–136, 1985.

Sutter F, Raveh J: Titanium-coated hollow screw and reconstruction plate system for bridging of lower jaw defects: Biochemical aspects. Int J Oral Maxillofac Surg 17:267–274, 1988.

Vuillemin T, Raveh J, Sutter F: Mandibular reconstruction with the titanium hollow screw plate system (THORP): Evaluation of 62 cases. J Plast Reconstr Surg 82(5):804–814, 1989a.

Vuillemin T, Raveh J: Mandibular reconstruction with the THORP condylar prosthesis after hemimandibulectomy. J Cranio Maxillofac Surg 17:78–87, 1989b.

CHAPTER 50

Three-Dimensional Mandibular Reconstruction with Vascularized Bone Grafts

David A. Hidalgo

Free flap mandibular reconstruction is no longer a technical novelty. Since the early descriptions of the vascularized rib and ilium donor sites, a variety of flaps have been successfully used for this purpose. In addition to the ilium, current donor site options include the radius, metatarsal, scapula, and fibula. Although there is divergent opinion as to which donor site is best for a particular problem, all have proven reliable and capable of achieving excellent results.

Current efforts to improve function and aesthetic quality in mandible reconstruction focus on several areas. These include new methods of dental reconstruction and a more refined approach to reconstruction of the bone and soft-tissue defect. The latter is the subject of this discussion, with emphasis on the technique of shaping and fixing the bone with miniplates.

The contouring of bone free flaps for mandible reconstruction is now a very precise and sophisticated technique. Important factors in the evolution of the current method are improved donor site selection, the application of miniplate fixation techniques, and a systematic approach to contouring the graft with the aid of specially fabricated templates. A new aesthetic standard has been achieved in which each of these elements plays a vital role.

DONOR SITE SELECTION

Graft requirements for an optimal three-dimensional reconstruction of the mandible include adequate bone length, consistent shape throughout the length of the bone, and a hearty as well as anatomically predictable blood supply. It is often important for the bone to have sufficient associated soft tissue of the proper volume and insetting flexibility for reconstructing either the intraoral lining, the facial skin, or both.

Donor sites available for free flap mandible reconstruction include the ilium, radius, metatarsal, scapula, and fibula. Each site has inherent advantages and disadvantages. These include the amount and quality of bone available, the amount and quality of soft tissue that can be included for lining or skin replacement, and the practically of the donor site in terms of its location, ease of dissection, and associated morbidity.

The choice of donor site is usually influenced by the familiarity of the surgeon with a particular technique. However, if each donor site is critically evaluated in terms of its potential to provide the most anatomically correct reconstruction, some of the available options are clearly better than others.

Radius

Bone of limited length usually no more than 10 centimeters is available from the radius. The harvested bone contains only one cortex; the other is retained at the donor site to preserve function. The bone is therefore quite thin and not well suited for future placement of osseointegrated implants. Although it provides an ideal skin island for simultaneous soft-tissue reconstruction, this donor site can be associated with a major disability if a fracture occurs. The best indication for using the radius as a donor site is a defect that includes a large portion of oral mucosa and only a short lateral bone segment. It is not recommended for the elderly patient, particularly women, and should not be used for anterior mandible reconstruction. The amount of flap soft tissue available is insufficient to fill the large submental "dead space" that is characteristic of anterior defects.

Second Metatarsal

The second metatarsal is similar to the radius in terms of the tissue available for mandible reconstruction. Unlike the radius, the vascular anatomy can be variable and dissection quite tedious. In addition, donor site morbidity tends to be significant with skin graft healing problems and delayed ambulation. This donor site is not generally recommended for major defects of the mandible because other options provide both superior bone stock and fewer donor site problems.

Scapula

The major advantage of the scapula is that it offers abundant soft tissue as well as 14 centimeters of bone. The bone can be quite thin, and it has not yet been conclusively demonstrated that it can reliably accommodate osseointegrated implants. The bone can be shaped readily, although the blood supply to the more distally osteotomized segments may be questionable. The major disadvantage of the scapula donor site is that the flap cannot be raised during the time of resection due to its location on the back. This adds a significant amount of time to an already long operative procedure. The best indication for this donor site is for composite defects with an enormous combined internal and external soft-tissue component. In these patients the quality of the bony reconstruction is usually a secondary concern, however.

Ilium

The ilium offers an abundant amount of bone and readily accepts osseointegrated implants. This donor site was originally considered ideal because the shape of the bone resembled a hemimandible. Today, however, other alternatives allow a more accurate hemimandible reconstruction without the fixed-shape limitations of the ilium. The shape of the ilium is also difficult to work with in the case of anterior reconstructions that extend almost from angle to angle. Other disadvantages include bulky soft tissue that has an unpredictable blood supply and a formidable donor site closure that has a potential for significant morbidity. The internal oblique muscle can be raised with the bone to overcome some of the soft tissue limitations of this donor site. Despite its shortcomings, the ilium is currently the workhorse donor site for mandible reconstruction in most centers.

Fibula

The fibula provides as much as 25 centimeters of bone, more than any other donor site. Due to an abundant segmental periosteal blood supply, the bone can be osteotomized as many times as necessary to reproduce accurately the shape of the mandible. The fibula allows the most precise reconstruction of the mandible and consistently yields excellent aesthetic results. It is well suited to the placement of osseointegrated implants. The fibula can be raised with a skin island as large as that available with the scapula, although the blood supply may be unreliable in approximately 10% of patients. In addition, a substantial portion of muscle can be included with the bone. The muscle is ideal for replacement of the soft tissue loss in the submental area typically associated with resection of the mandible.

PLANNING THE RECONSTRUCTION

Two preoperative radiograph studies are needed for proper planning and execution of the reconstruction. These are the lateral cephalogram and a computerized tomographic (CT) scan transverse section of the mandible that shows its curve from angle to angle (see Figure 50.1). The CT study is magnified and reproduced as a 1:1 scale image. Templates of thin, clear acrylic plastic are then made on the basis of tracings of these two studies. This provides accurate models of the mandible in the lateral view and transverse plane; these models assist in shaping the bone. Of proven value, these templates provide an important reference for planning the angles of each osteotomy in the bone. They are the key reason that the graft can be shaped with a great deal of accuracy while still in place at the donor site.

The surgical specimen provides valuable information and should not be remove from the operating room until the bony reconstruction is complete. Besides providing precise measurements for graft length, the specimen gives the surgeon the opportunity to study subtle angles and nuances of contour that cannot be appreciated from the two-dimensional templates alone (see Figure 50.2). As a model, it also provides a means to estimate the amount and orientation of the soft-tissue component needed to reconstruct the defect. The tumor specimen should always be handled carefully, however.

Although they are an important reference in conventional aesthetic surgery, preoperative facial photographs contribute little to achieving a correct reconstruction of the mandible from an aesthetic viewpoint. They are not necessary except for documentation purposes. Three-dimensional CT scans, while providing interesting images of the mandible, have also proven superfluous for its reconstruction.

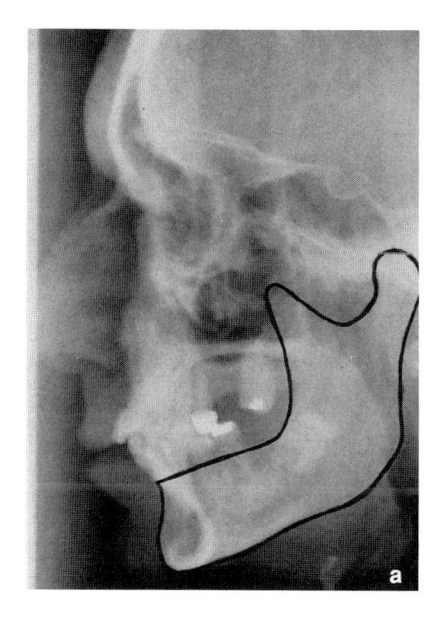

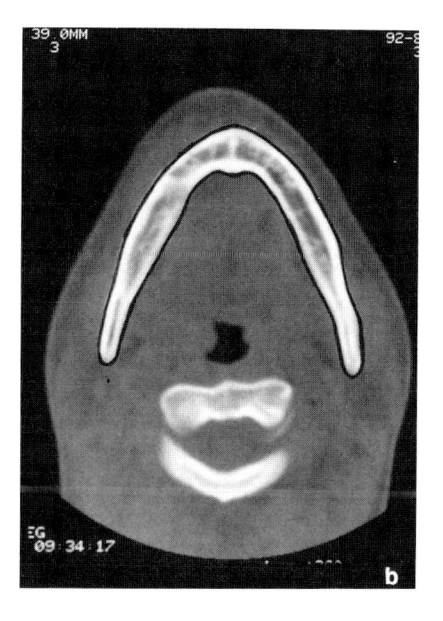

Figure 50.1 (a) The lateral cephalogram and (b) the 1:1 scale CT scan transverse section of the mandible are key preoperative studies for mandible reconstruction. Acrylic templates are fashioned from tracings of these studies for use during the graft-shaping process.

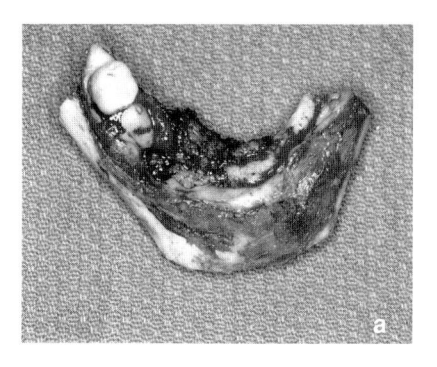

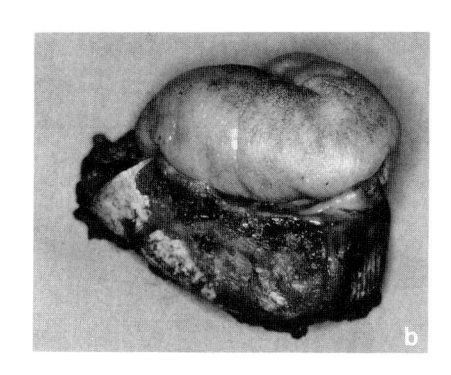

Figure 50.2 Anterior mandible specimens are shown. (a) Some have little associated soft tissue, (b) others a large amount. These specimens are important models and should be available for reference throughout the reconstruction process. (c and d) Lateral mandible specimens show varying amounts of contiguous soft tissue.

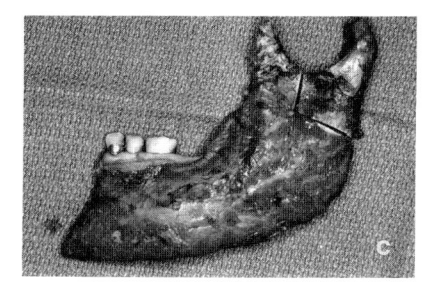

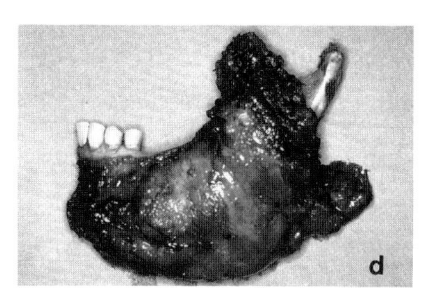

All patients should undergo preoperative pulmonary function tests and a stress cardiac radionuclide study. Mortality seen with resection and primary free flap mandible reconstruction is invariably cardiopulmonary in origin. Patients who do poorly on either of these tests should not be considered candidates for a free flap reconstruction.

MINIPLATE FIXATION

Interosseous wires are no longer preferred for graft fixation. They are tedious to apply, unstable when used in multiply osteotomized grafts, and subject to breakage and extrusion. Miniplates have replaced wires because of their versatility, rapid mounting, and great stability.

Miniplates are available from several manufacturers. The Würzburg Mini Bone Plate System (Walter Lorenz Surgical Instruments, Inc., Jacksonville, FL) is a representative type that has been used extensively for this application. These miniplates are made of titanium. Other types made of Vitallium (Luhr) and stainless steel (Champy) are also available and can be expected to give equally good results.

Miniplates need not be of the compression type because nonunion has proven to be rare in free flap mandible reconstruction. Newer, lighter versions of the

Wurzburg miniplates have been used but are not preferred. The standard miniplates are better able to withstand the high torsional stress present in the reconstructed mandible segment without giving way to flex and distortion. An essential feature of the miniplate system selected is that it has self-tapping screws. Self-tapping screws are very efficient to use and contribute to a reduction in the ischemic interval of the flap.

A wide variety of plates is not necessary for free flap mandible reconstruction (see Figure 50.3). Double-Y, single-Y, and L-shaped plates are needed for the external surface of the graft, and straight plates of several lengths are needed for the inferior border of the mandible. Other shapes are rarely used.

Screw lengths up to 15 millimeters are required. The graft is cross-drilled completely for screw placement. In the fibula, this requires great care on the second cortex because the blood supply is just behind it. The screw of appropriate length is selected after the hole is measured with a depth gauge; it should be long enough to traverse the second cortex completely.

Free flaps should never be stripped of periosteum during miniplate fixation. The plates are placed directly over the muscle cuff and periosteum without regard to exposing the bone. Removing the periosteum would no doubt devascularize the graft in most instances.

Most of the graft shaping process can be completed while the graft is still attached at the donor site (see Figure 50.4). This allows a significant reduction in the ischemic interval to which the flap is subjected. The plates are placed in two perpendicular planes at each osteotomy site, and, later, during insetting at the ends where the graft joins the mandible. This affords adequate resistance to the high deforming stresses experi-

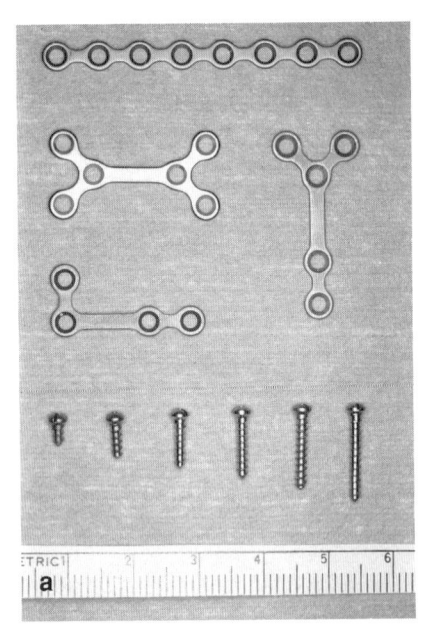

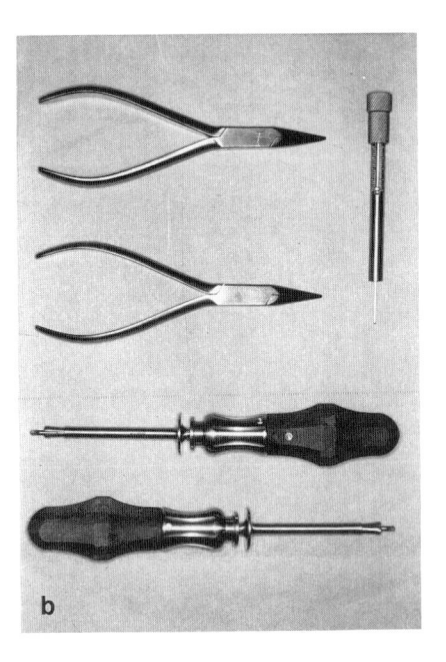

Figure 50.3 (a) The necessary plate shapes and screw lengths are shown. (b) The tools necessary for mounting the plates are few and simple.

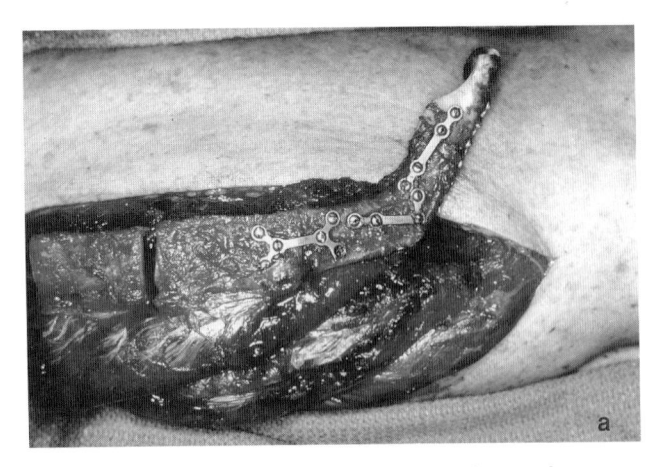

Figure 50.4 These hemimandible fibula grafts are shown following completion of shaping at the donor site. They are still attached to the leg by the vascular pedicle. Note that the condyle has been mounted on the ramus and that the opposite end of the grafts have been left long for final insetting at the recipient site. (a) The graft has been raised with muscle (flexor hallucis longus) attached to its lower border. (b) The graft has been raised with a skin island.

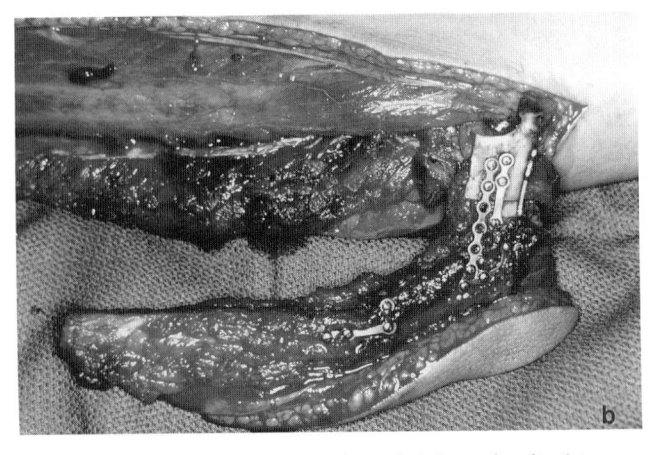

enced by a multiply osteotomized interposition graft. The plates are always placed on the outside surface of the graft, never on the inside. The remaining plates are placed along the inferior border of the mandible (see Figure 50.5).

Several patients have experienced fractures adjacent to an osteotomy site where two screws from two perpendicularly oriented plates are in close proximity. Fortunately, in clinical experience, this has not resulted in a nonunion. It is recommended, however, that only 5-millimeter or 7-millimeter screws be used in the plate placed along the inferior border of the mandible. In addition, it is safe to eliminate the screw from the limb of the Y-shaped plate that approaches the inferior border of the mandible on each side of the osteotomy. These two points will help avoid the potential for fracture associated with the use of miniplate fixation of the graft (see Figure 50.6).

Adjunctive forms of fixation are not necessary for purposes of graft stability when miniplates are used. Maxillo-mandibular fixation (MMF) is used only to maintain occlusion during final insetting of the bone graft. It is arbitrarily continued for two weeks postoperatively, particularly in those who undergo condyle transfer, in whom MMF helps to maintain the condyle in a properly seated position. External fixators provide poor support and are not recommended.

Some patients experience considerable pain, which appears directly related to the presence of the plates. Scatter or shielding may be associated with the plates, although this has not been well studied. Plate removal is not recommended prior to beginning radiation therapy because of concern regarding adequate bone healing. Delaying radiation therapy to allow complete bone healing and subsequent plate removal is also not recommended.

Miniplates are not routinely removed except in nonradiated patients who are believed to be free of disease and are candidates for the placement of osseointegrated implants. In these patients the plates are removed when it is convenient, usually 6 to 12 months after the initial procedure. The plates are removed as

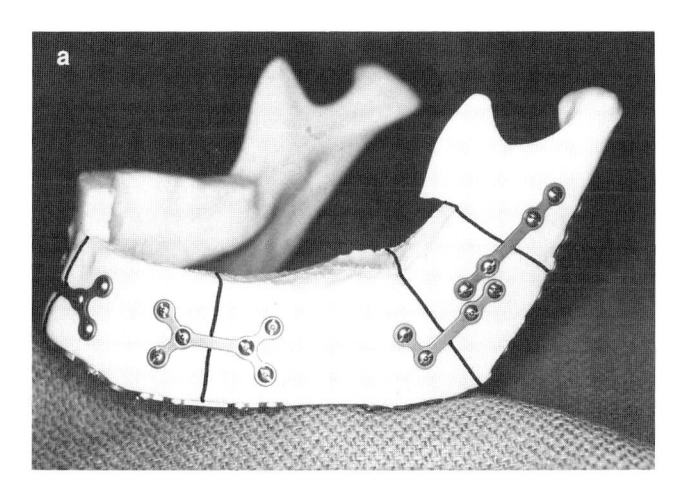

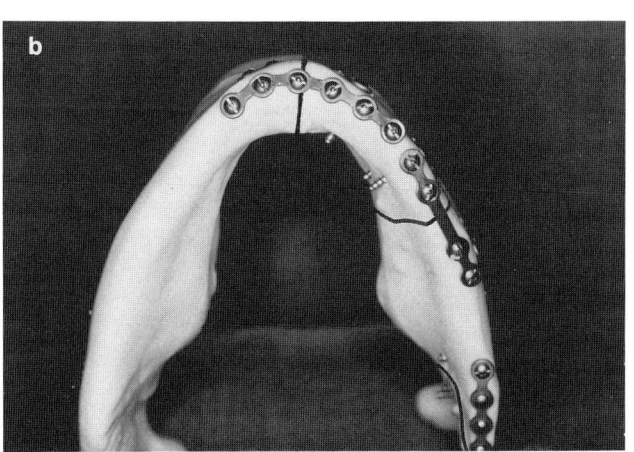

Figure 50.5 A simulated reconstruction is shown. The dark lines in the model represent osteotomies. The plates are placed both (a) on the outside surface and (b) along the inferior border of the graft and mandible.

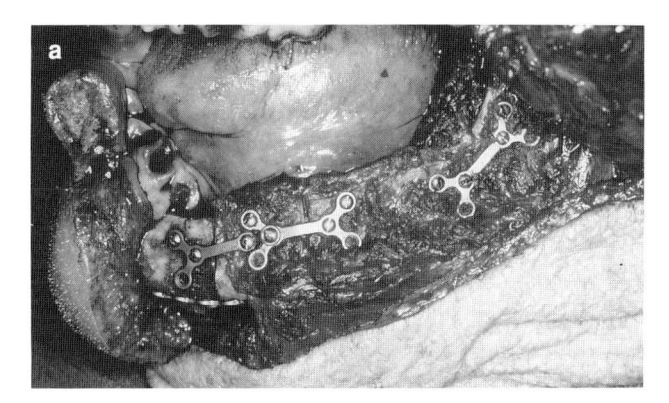

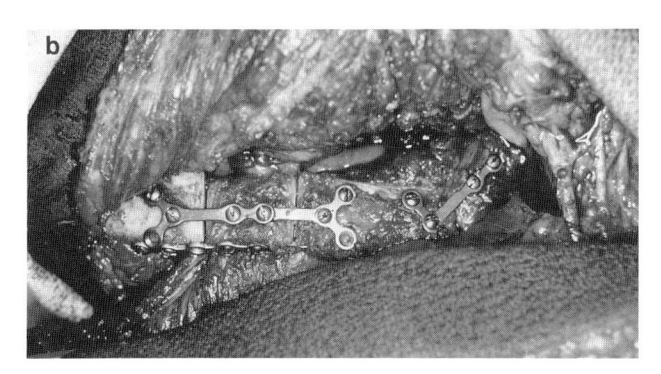

Figure 50.6 (a and b) Lateral mandible grafts are shown with completed fixation. In both patients the chin is to the left and a narrow skin island is seen below the graft. Note the proximity of the bottom holes of the Y-shaped plates to the plates along the inferior border. To reduce the chance of fracture, screws are not placed in these holes. Note that the plates on the outside surface of the graft are sometimes overlapped when this is convenient.

soon as the osteotomies are stable in patients in whom wound healing problems have resulted in plate contamination and infection. This is usually in six to eight weeks.

THREE-DIMENSIONAL RECONSTRUCTION

Shaping the Graft

The bone defect is usually one of two types. Either it is predominantly a hemimandible-type defect that contains a variable portion of the ramus and most of the body, or it is an anterior defect that contains the symphysis as well as an unequal portion of each adjacent body (see Figure 50.7). The type of defect influences the technique used for shaping the bone graft.

Anterior Reconstructions

Treatment of anterior defects begins with shaping the graft in the midline and working laterally to each side. Experience has shown that the segment of the graft corresponding to the anterior portion of the mandible usually should not measure more than 2 centimeters (see Figure 50.8). Cutting the anterior segment first facilitates fitting each body segment to the anterior piece in a symmetrical fashion.

The osteotomies at each end of the anterior segment must be angled correctly in two planes. The body diverges from the anterior segment both in a frontal plane, where it angles upward, and in a transverse plane, where it angles back from the anterior segment. Failure to appreciate the angle in the frontal plane will result in an abnormal rotation of the anterior mandible segment around its long axis. The relationship of the anterior segment to the body segments should not be considered rigid, as if the mandible were a bucket handle. Instead, the anterior segment lies in a plane independent of the lateral segments, much like the way the seat of a ferris wheel relates to its supporting spokes.

The anterior segment is fixed to the body segments with miniplates. The proper angle at each osteotomy site in both planes is checked with the aid of the lateral and transverse templates. This portion of the graft-shaping process is done at the donor site. Availability of the surgical specimen in primary reconstructions provides an important means of verifying the accuracy of the graft contour.

Lateral Reconstructions

Treatment of hemimandible defects begins with planning the location of the vascular pedicle so that it comes to lie at the angle of the mandible. The portion of the graft corresponding to the angle is therefore shaped first. In most cases the angle of the mandible is

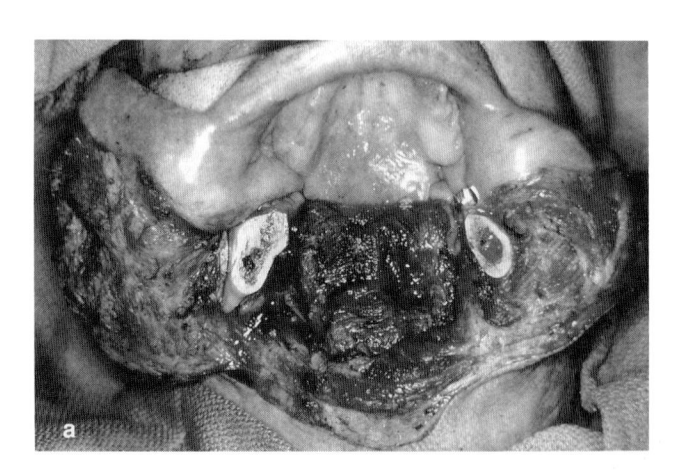

Figure 50.7 (a) A massive anterior defect is shown. The floor of the mouth, most of the tongue, and the submental soft tissues have been resected. The lateral mandible segments no longer have a stable relationship to each other or to the maxilla. Correct insetting of the graft is difficult when most of the normal landmarks are no longer available for reference. (b) A lateral mandible defect is shown. Placement of the contralateral dentition into MMF greatly enhances the accuracy of graft insetting.

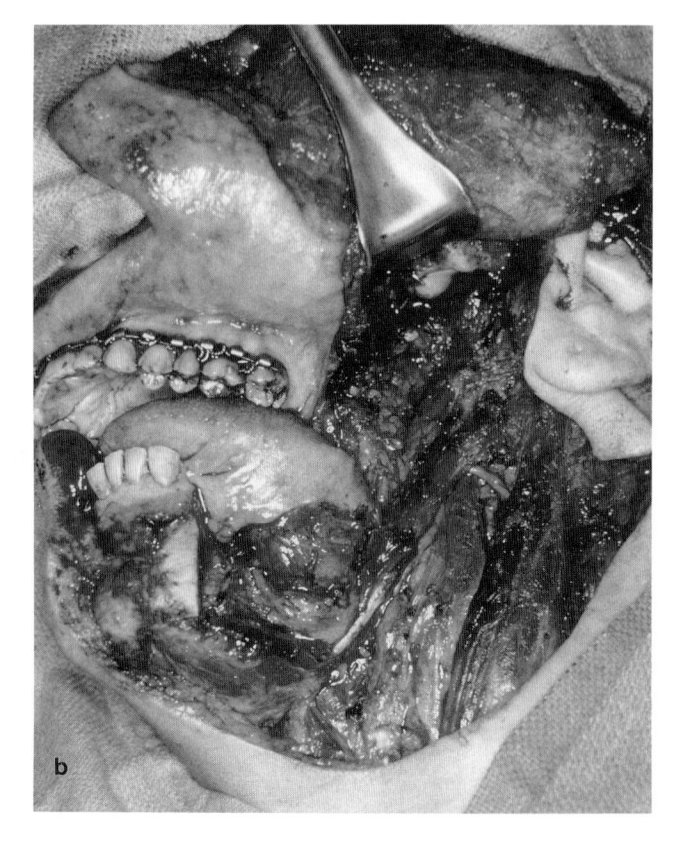

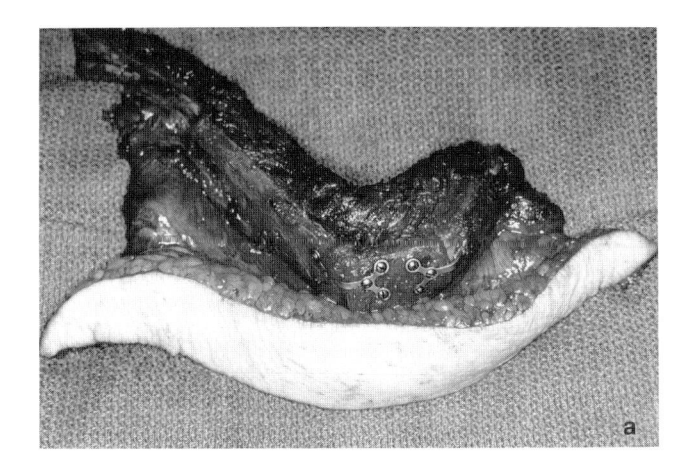

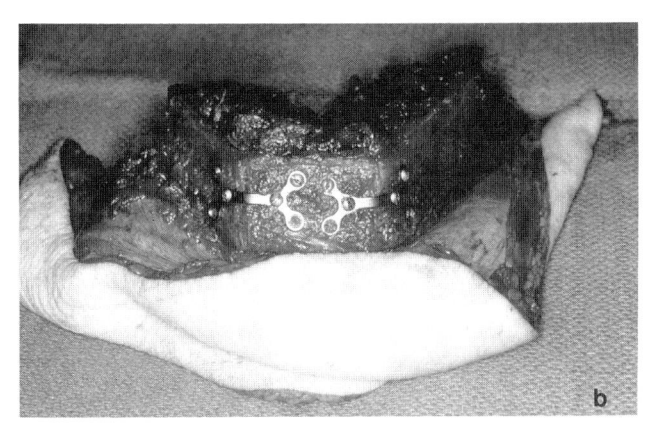

Figure 50.8 (a and b) Two fibula grafts for anterior reconstructions are shown immediately following division from the donor site. Skin islands have been included with the bone in each case. The anterior bone segment measures about 2 centimeters. Note the double-Y plates. The plates along the inferior border are not seen. The body segments on each side vary in length, but they are always left longer than estimated. Final length adjustments are made during insetting at the recipient site.

shaped with one osteotomy. However, in a few patients the angle has a gradual curve, and it is necessary to perform two osteotomies. This leaves a small pie-shaped segment of bone between the ramus and body. This interposed piece blunts the angle, giving it a gradual curve. In these cases, fixation is planned so that each plate spans all three segments. The angle made by the ramus and the body away from a sagittal plane is usually quite small. It is helpful to have the specimen available to confirm the appropriate angle because this information is not provided by either template.

The body is usually shaped with one or two osteotomies. Most commonly, one osteotomy in the midbody provides a means to curve the body in a transverse plane as well as to angle it slightly in the lateral view. In some patients an additional osteotomy is necessary to accurately reproduce the curve of the body. The angle of the mandible and the body usually can be shaped and fixed while the graft is in place at the donor site. The templates allow this to be done with great accuracy (see Figure 50.4). As in the case of anterior mandible reconstructions, both ends of the hemimandible graft are purposely left long. This allows the location of the final osteotomy at each end of the graft to be determined at the recipient site.

Insetting the Graft

Anterior Reconstructions

Precision in determining overall graft length is one of the most critical considerations in insetting the graft. Errors in graft length can result in prognathism, retrognathia, or shift of the midline if a length error occurs on one side only. MMF is usually not available as a means to help safeguard against length errors upon graft insetting because few teeth usually remain on the lateral mandibular segments.

The angle formed by the anterior segment and the body segments is critical. If this angle has been incorrectly set while the graft was contoured at the donor site, the lateral mandibular segments can be displaced either medially or laterally, or become internally or externally rotated, as the graft is inset.

An additional important consideration in the insetting of anterior grafts is that the intermaxillary distance in the midline be set correctly. This will avoid creating errors in lower facial height. Unfortunately, all reliable reference points for measurement on the mandible are lost as a result of resection. Therefore this distance is usually estimated by visual analysis alone.

After the final osteotomies are made on each end of the graft, it is joined to the lateral segments with miniplates placed in two planes. MMF is not necessary in the postoperative period.

Lateral Reconstructions

An error in length of a hemimandible graft will frequently result in noticeable facial asymmetry. Errors can be avoided by carefully measuring the surgical specimen and by avoiding displacement of the midline to either side as the graft is inset. MMF is routinely used during the insetting process to maintain the opposite (normal) side in occlusion and thereby prevent shift of the midline.

The transverse plane template derived from the CT scan is used to check the curve of the mandible as the graft is joined to the mandible medially. This may require exposing the inferior border of the normal side for a considerable distance in order to appreciate its curve as well as to fit the template. It is also important that the mandible angle on the reconstructed side is positioned at an equal distance from the midline as the angle on the normal side. The face may appear either "caved in" if the graft is too close to the midline relative to the normal side, or "bowed out" if too far away. Although it is not possible to set this distance by direct measurement, it can be estimated with considerable accuracy by palpating both sides simultaneously as the graft is inset.

The angle of the final osteotomy on the medial end of the hemimandible graft is fashioned with great care so that the fit is flush after the graft has been correctly positioned for symmetry. Miniplates are then placed in two planes in the manner previously described. The opposite end of the graft has been joined to the ramus with miniplates prior to this step. If the original condyle has been mounted onto the graft it is seated into the glenoid fossa. If possible, the capsule is repaired around the condyle to hold it in place. When there is difficulty securing the condyle in place the patient is maintained in MMF for two weeks postoperatively.

RESULTS AND COMPLICATIONS

Forty consecutive free flap mandible reconstructions requiring miniplate fixation have been followed from 3 to 36 months (Table 50.1). Thirteen reconstructions did not require a skin island, 14 required skin intraorally, 8 externally, and 5 both inside and outside. There were no flap failures. Bone defect length ranged from 5 to 16 cm (average 12.26 centimeters). The number of fixation sites in each patient ranged from 2 to 6 (average 4). The number of plates used ranged from 3 to 10 (average 6).

Table 50.1 Miniplate fixation in mandible reconstruction

Age/Sex	Donor Site	Length of Bone Defect	Number of Fixation Sites	Number of Plates (Screws)	Other Fixation	Plate Complication	Graft Status
53 F	Fibula	16 cm	4	4 (19)	None	None	Healed
43 M	Fibula	14.5 cm	4	5 (26)	None	None	Healed
60 M	Scapula	14 cm	3	4 (18)	None	None	Healed
32 M	Radius	10 cm	2	4 (14)	None	None	Healed
65 F	Radius	10 cm	4	4 (14)	None	None	Healed
43 M	Scapula	14 cm	3	4 (18)	None	None	Healed
36 M	Radius	7 cm	2	5 (22)	None	Intraoral exposure; plates removed	Nonunion at one site
61 M	Fibula	14 cm	4	5 (22)	None	None	Healed
34 M	Fibula	14.5 cm	4	7 (30)	MMF	None	Healed
44 F	Fibula	16 cm	4	7 (30)	None	None	Healed
41 F	Fibula	12 cm	4	5 (23)	None	None	Healed
53 M	Fibula	12 cm	5	6 (34)	MMF	None	Healed
52 F	Fibula	13 cm	5	6 (31)	None	None	Healed
37 F	Fibula	8 cm	4	5 (28)	MMF	None	Healed
61 M	Fibula	15 cm	5	7 (41)	MMF	None	Healed
60 M	Fibula	15 cm	6	10 (49)	MMF	None	Healed
41 M	Fibula	10 cm	4	6 (28)	MMF	None	Healed
61 M	Fibula	12 cm	4	7 (34)	None	None	Healed
64 F	Scapula	9 cm	4	5 (23)	None	None	Healed
14 M	Fibula	13 cm	5	8 (36)	None	None	Healed
71 F	Radius	6 cm	4	3 (14)	None	None	Healed
40 M	Fibula	5 cm	2	4 (18)	None	Orocutaneous fistula; plates removed	Healed
33 F	Fibula	9.5 cm	5	4 (24)	None	Plate fracture	Nonunion at one site

Aesthetic results were best in patients not requiring external skin replacement. Excellent results were clinically obvious but were also reflected in the degree of symmetry seen on the postoperative panorex study (see Figures 50.9 and 50.10). The overall quality of the result was compromised despite an accurate bony reconstruction in patients requiring either large anterior skin replacement or sacrifice of the facial nerve and adjacent deep soft tissues of the cheek.

There were four instances of orocutaneous fistula (10%). In each patient the miniplates were retained until bone healing was complete. They were removed 5 to 10 weeks after the initial procedure. Although this delayed healing of the fistula, all soft-tissue wounds healed quickly once the plates were removed. There were no nonunions or instances of osteomyelitis in these patients. In one other patient an external wound infection required plate removal at 16 weeks.

Nonunion was rare in this series. Bone healing was followed by serial panorex studies and clinical examination. In most patients evidence of bone healing was apparent on panorex by three months and at an advanced stage by six months. There were only two instances of nonunion in the entire series. This number is quite small considering that the average reconstruction included four fixation sites and required an average of six plates for solid fixation. The incidence of nonunion was therefore 2 sites out of 161, or 1.2%.

A superior functional and aesthetic mandible reconstruction can be consistently achieved by the methods described. The success of the procedure depends on selection of the proper donor site, the use of miniplate fixation, and appropriate preoperative studies to guide the bone contouring process. The incidence of primary wound healing is high, the complications are low, and the results are gratifying.

Table 50.1 Miniplate fixation in mandible reconstruction

Age/Sex	Donor Site	Length of Bone Defect	Number of Fixation Sites	Number of Plates (Screws)	Other Fixation	Plate Complication	Graft Status
27 F	Fibula	10.5 cm	4	5 (27)	None	Orocutaneous fistula; plates removed	Healed
60 F	Fibula	13.5 cm	4	7 (42)	None	Orocutaneous fistula; plates removed	Healed
33 F	Fibula	8 cm	4	6 (22)	None	None	Healed
53 M	Scapula	9 cm	4	6 (35)	None	None	Healed
57 M	Fibula	15 cm	5	6 (38)	None	None	Healed
57 M	Fibula	16.5 cm	5	7 (38)	MMF	None	Healed
57 M	Fibula	15 cm	5	7 (37)	MMF	Orocutaneous fistula; plates removed	Healed
53 M	Fibula	17.5 cm	6	9 (43)	None	None	Healed
15 F	Fibula	12 cm	5	8 (36)	None	None	Healed
55 F	Fibula	15 cm	3	6 (24)	MMF	None	Healed
53 F	Fibula	14 cm	6	9 (40)	MMF	None	Healed
43 M	Fibula	13 cm	4	7 (30)	MMF	None	Healed
36 M	Fibula	14 cm	5	5 (29)	None	None	Healed
54 M	Fibula	14 cm	4	8 (39)	None	None	Healed
51 M	Fibula	11 cm	4	4 (25)	MMF	None	Healed
65 M	Fibula	10 cm	3	7 (28)	MMF	None	Healed
32 M	Fibula	13.5 cm	4	6 (32)	MMF	None	Healed

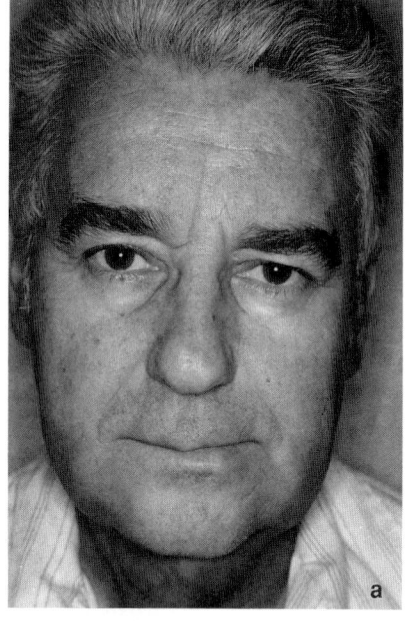

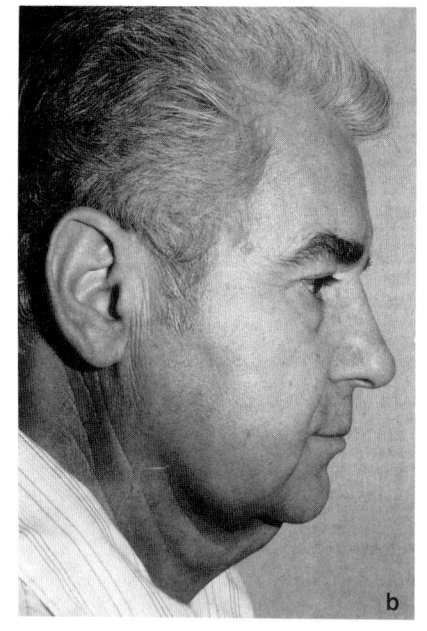

Figure 50.9 (a–f) Postoperative views of two patients who underwent left hemimandible reconstruction. (a) Frontal view of first patient. (b) Lateral view of first patient. (c) Panorex of first patient. (d) Frontal view of second patient. (e) Lateral view of second patient. (f) Panorex of second patient.

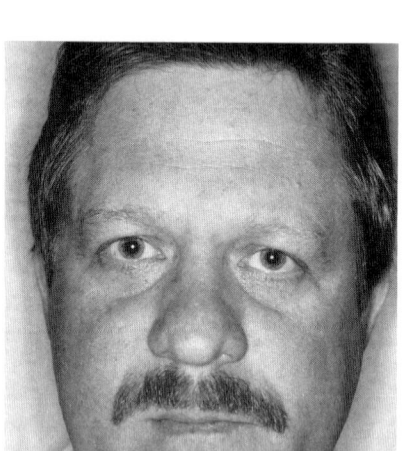

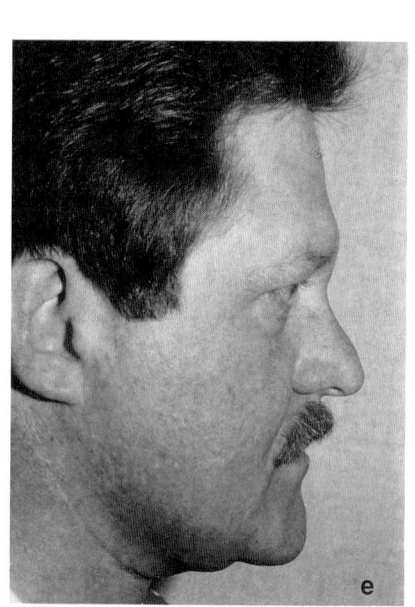

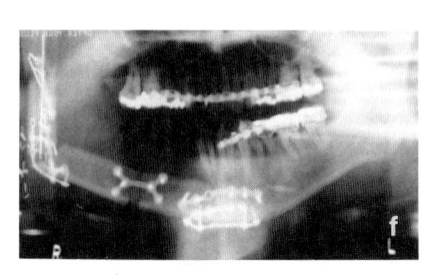

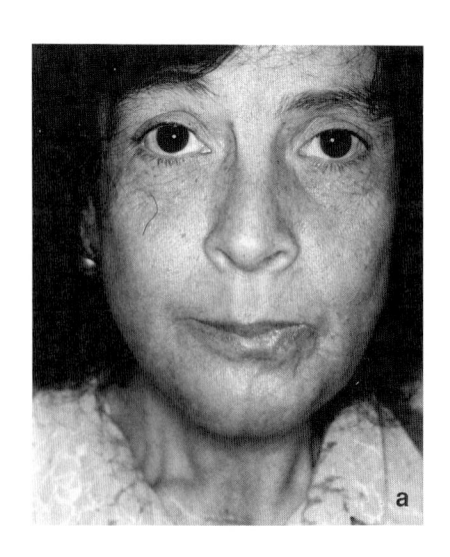

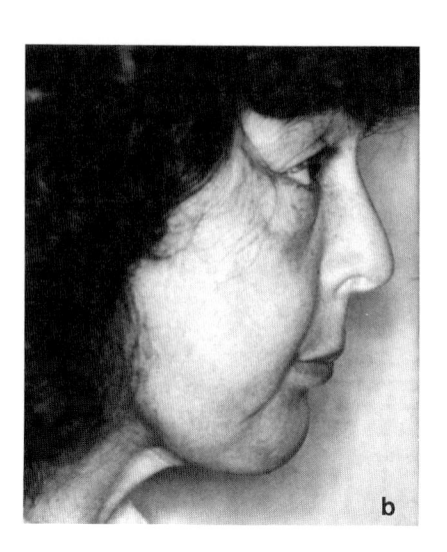

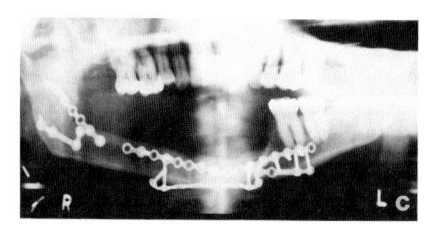

Figure 50.10 (a–c) Postoperative facial views and panorex study are given for a patient who underwent anterior mandible reconstruction. (a) Frontal view. (b) Lateral view. (c) Panorex.

BIBLIOGRAPHY

David DJ, Tan E, Katsaros J, Sheen R: Mandibular reconstruction with vascularized iliac crest: A 10-year experience. Plast Reconstr Surg 82:792–801, 1988.

Hidalgo DA: Fibula free flap: A new method of mandible reconstruction. Plast Reconstr Surg 84:71–79, 1989a.

Hidalgo DA: Titanium miniplate fixation in free flap mandible reconstruction. Ann Plast Surg 23:498–507, 1989b.

Hidalgo DA: Aesthetic improvements in free flap mandible reconstruction. Plast Reconstr Surg (in press).

MacLeod AM, Robinson DW: Reconstruction of defects involving the mandible and floor of the mouth by free osteo-cutaneous flaps derived from the foot. Brit J Plast Surg 35:239–246, 1982.

Marsh JL: The use of the Wurtzburg system to facilitate fixation in facial osteotomies. Clin Plast Surg 16:49–60, 1989.

Munro IR: The Luhr fixation system for the craniofacial skeleton. Clin Plast Surg 16:41–48, 1989.

Swartz WM, Banis JC, Newton ED, et al: The osteocutaneous scapular flap for mandibular and maxillary reconstruction. Plast Reconstr Surg 77:530–545, 1986.

Taylor GI: Reconstruction of the mandible with free composite iliac bone grafts. Ann Plast Surg 9:361–376, 1982.

CHAPTER 51

Total Functional Mandibular Reconstruction Using Vascularized Bone Grafts, Osteointegrated Implants, and Rigid Fixation

Frederick Lukash

Composite mandibular resection for malignancy leads to significant anatomical and functional difficulties with mastication and articulation. The resultant deformities caused by disruption of the mandibular arch and the loss of teeth can result in substantial psychological and social disabilities. To rehabilitate affected individuals successfully, the bony and dental arches must be reestablished. Although great strides have been made in replacement of hard and soft tissue, the insertion of a dental appliance and the return of function have always been problematic. Scarred intraoral tissues, thick insensate flaps, irregular bone contours, loss of vestibules, altered muscle function, and radiation changes to the mucosa have prevented successful fitting and maintenance of a removable denture. The fixed osseodental unit was conceived in order to overcome these obstacles. The unit consists of a dental prosthesis that is permanently secured to a vascularized bone graft, resting above the intraoral soft tissues in an occlusal plane.

PRINCIPLES

Functional reconstruction requires the close cooperation of the plastic surgeon, oral surgeon, prosthodontist, and oncologic surgeon. Careful presurgical planning is critical to a successful result. The surgical defect must be assessed preoperatively to determine the amount and location of bone necessary for replacement. Accurate radiologic studies are performed to assist in manufacturing templates and models of the graft. A hard acrylic replica of the graft is made as well as a soft template that will fit into the hip to aid in planning (see Figure 51.1).

Although there are many sources of hard tissue—such as the radius, fibula, and scapula—the iliac crest is my preference because of its size and contour. The deep circumflex iliac artery system nourishes almost the entire crest and also supplies a large soft-tissue paddle, if needed. The bone can be contoured to meet almost any criteria for reconstruction. With experience, the surgeon can dissect the iliac crest within two and one half hours with minimal morbidity (see Figure 51.2).

Miniplate osteosynthesis allows for precise placement and orientation of the graft. The ability to bend the plates allows for accuracy in overcoming contour irregularities between the mandible and the graft. Previous attempts with wires necessitated prolonged periods of maxillo-mandibular fixation (MMF). When wires were used, healing was slow and the graft often migrated inferiorly (see Figure 51.3).

The success of a vascularized bone graft depends on proper tissue isolation and patent anastomoses. To ensure these, a thermocouple monitoring system is applied to each buried transfer to provide continuous information as to the patency of the vascular anastomosis. In addition a technetium 99 bone scan is performed in the early postoperative period to confirm perfusion (see Figure 51.4).

Although many reconstructions have been successful to this point, it is here that function fails. Even the most skillfully crafted dental appliance becomes difficult to wear and use when dealing with dry, anesthetic, often bulky soft tissues and bone that is often contoured differently than its adjacent mandible (see Figure 51.5).

Previous attempts at placing dental implants, as with the Blade technique, have failed because of apical

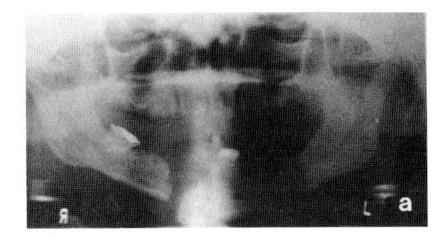

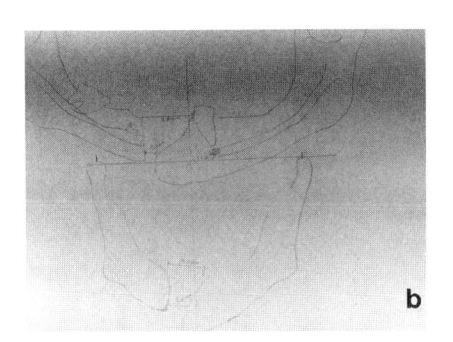

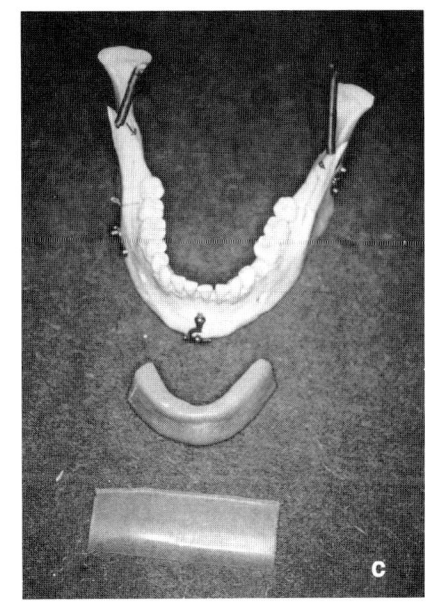

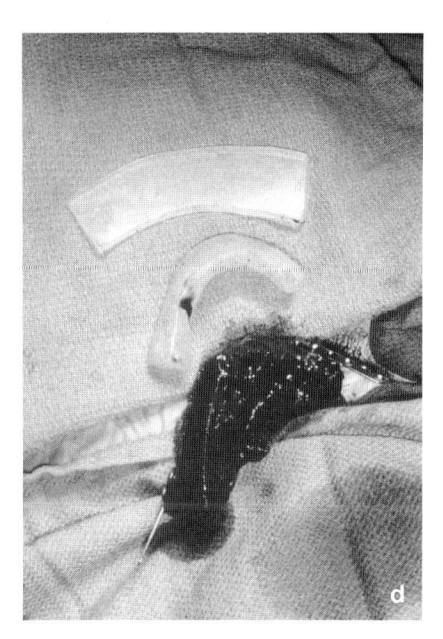

Figure 51.1 The steps of assessment and planning of mandibular reconstruction are shown. (a) A radiograph or panorex of the defect is taken. (b) Bone requirements are established. (c) Templates are fabricated. (d) Iliac crest bone graft is made by replicating the templates.

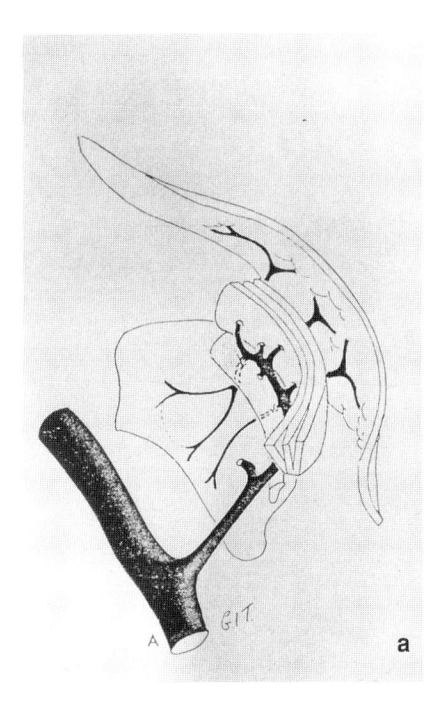

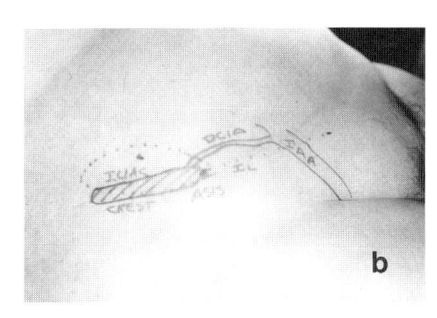

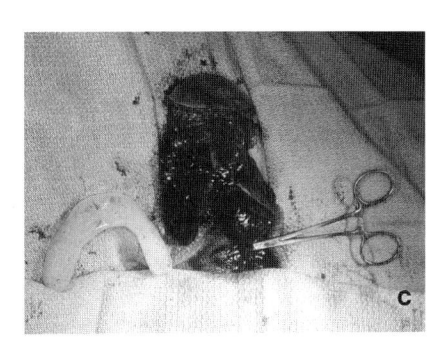

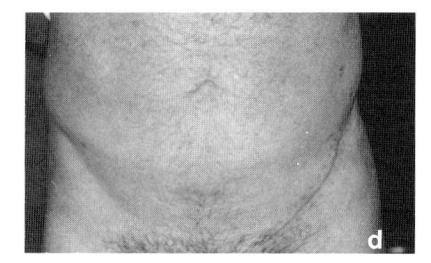

Figure 51.2 The iliac crest bone craft is shown. (a) This diagram shows the territory supplied by the deep circumflex iliac artery system. (b) Surgical site for bone harvesting is shown with available skin paddle. (c) Contoured iliac crest is shown with skin paddle. (Hemostat points to deep circumflex iliac artery) (d) The postoperative appearance of the hip donor site.

migration of connective tissue between the bone–implant interface. A breakdown results when forces of mastication are applied, resulting in infection and extrusion.

The Branemark (1977, 1982) technique succeeds because the titanium implant forms a ceramic bond with the implant (see Figure 51.6). This prevents contamination and responds well to mechanical loading forces.

After osseointegration is complete, the prosthodontist must take impressions and create a model that will successfully occlude with the upper denture or teeth. Once completed, the denture is permanently secured to the abutment posts.

The fixed bridge rests on implants permanently bonded to bone rather than on the bone itself or its soft tissues (as is true for the mandibular staple technique). Therefore, flap thinning procedures and skin graft vestibuloplasties are unnecessary. No frictional forces act on the bone or soft tissue; this eliminates ulceration, pain, and exposure of bone. It also prevents confusion as to whether an ulcer has been caused by the denture or is a neoplasia. The fixed unit provides a stable bite,

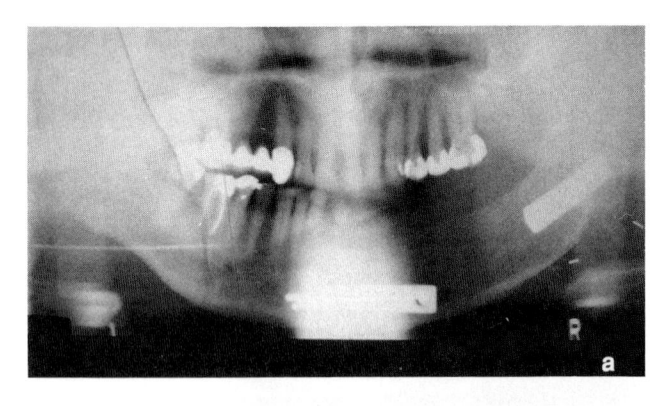

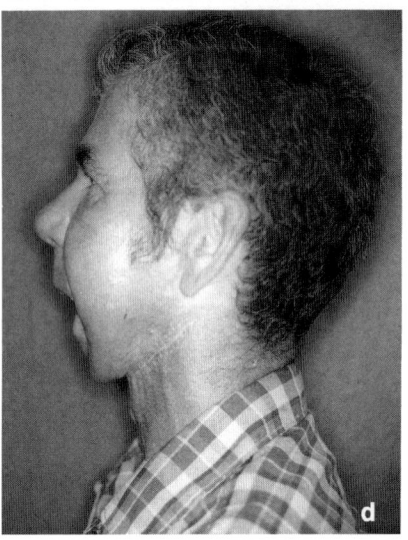

Figure 51.3 Plate fixation provides 3-dimensional stability of the graft. (a) Postoperative frontal Xray. (b) Postoperative lateral X-ray. Wire fixation is more likely to allow graft movement and change in mandibular contour. (c) Postoperative lateral shows loss of anterior projection due to posterior migration of graft. (d) Postoperative panorex of patient in 3-D.

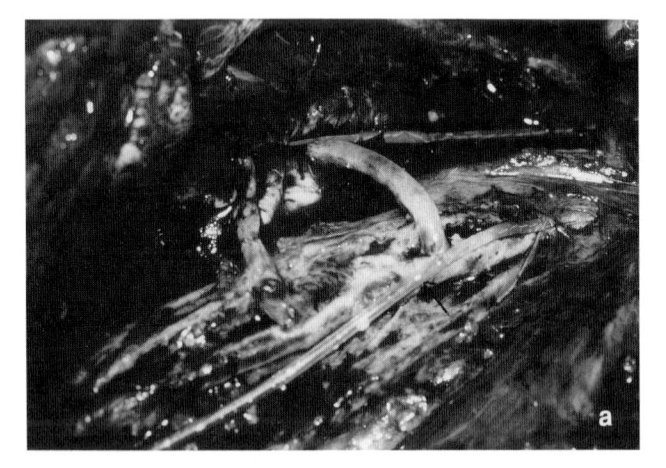

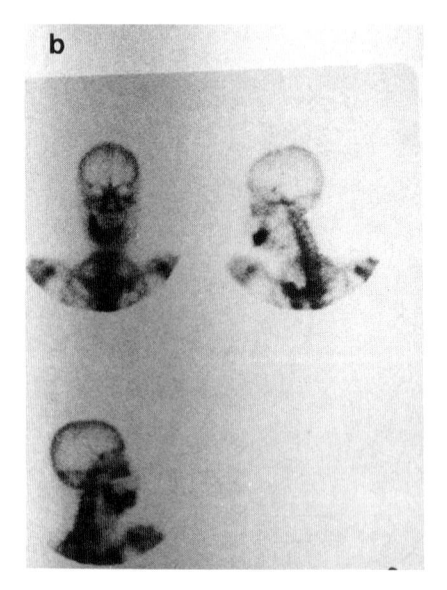

Figure 51.4 Methods of assessing viability of transfer are shown. (a) With the thermocouple monitoring system, probes (arrows) are placed to monitor flow through the vascular anastomosis. (b) Technetium 99 bone scan demonstrates the bone perfusion of the vascularized reconstruction.

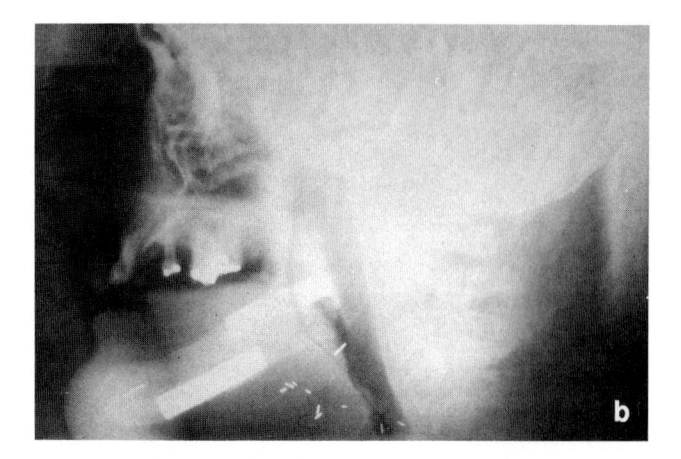

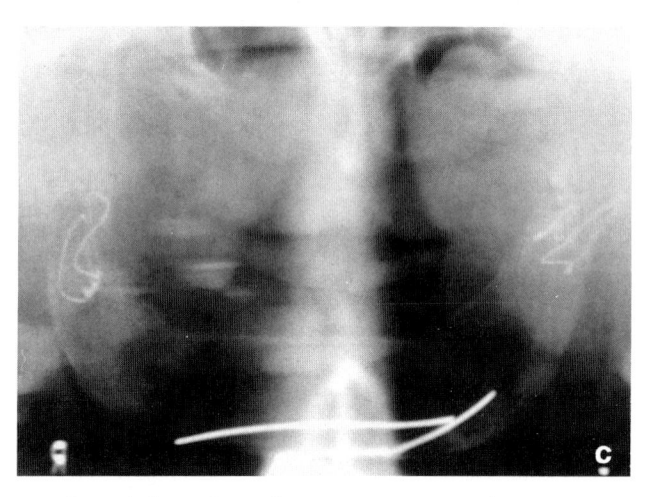

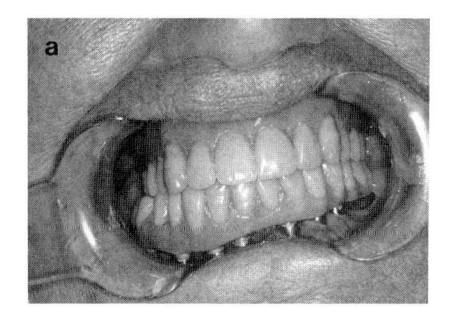

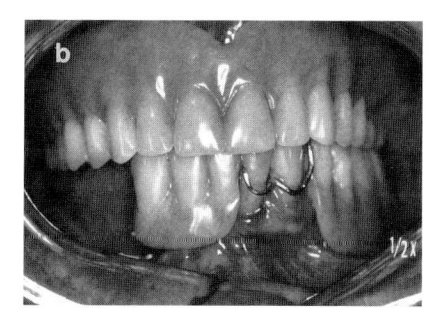

Figure 51.5 (a) A secured dental prosthesis fixed in occlusion to a vascularized iliac crest bone graft is compared to (b) a removable prosthesis.

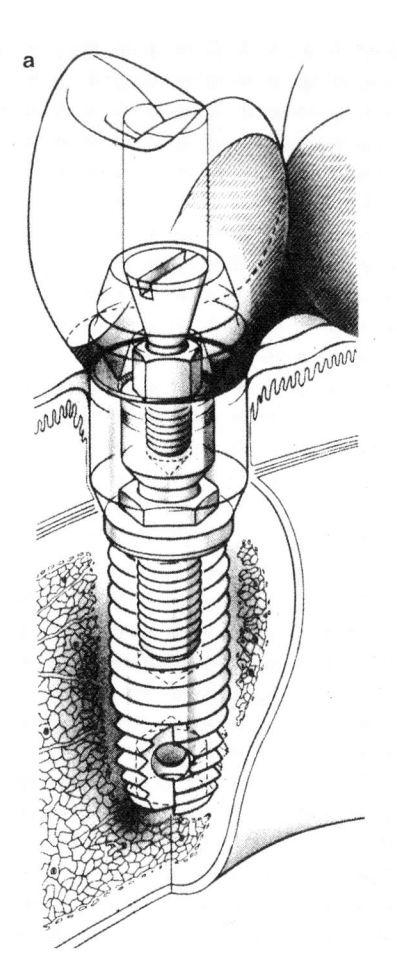

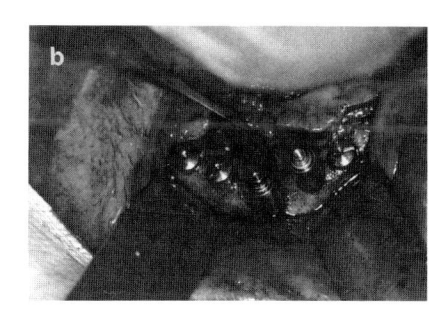

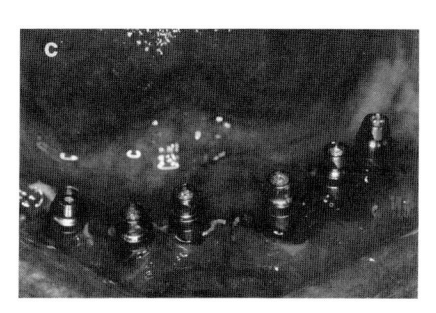

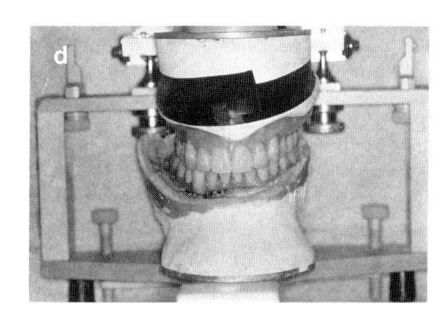

Figure 51.6 (a) Schematic representation shows how osteointegration is achieved. (b) Titanium implants are placed into bone. (c) The abutment post is screwed into osteointegrated implants. (d) The articulated fabrication of a secured denture is shown.

which is very helpful in those people who wear a removable upper denture. Additionally, the biomechanical forces from the implants enhance bone remodeling. This is in direct contrast to the bone atrophy known to occur with removable dentures.

TECHNIQUE: BONE GRAFT

A team approach is always used. The iliac crest graft is harvested at the same time that the head and neck surgeon is either extirpating the tumor (in immediate reconstructions) or recreating the anatomic defect and locating recipient vessels (2° reconstructions).

The dissection of the graft has been well described by Taylor (1982). In essence, the bone survives on the deep circumflex iliac artery system, which will vascularize most of the crest.

Once the bone and pedicle have been isolated, the prefabricated templates are placed into the hip area to locate the best place for the osteotomies. Before a cut is made, the templates are checked with the mandibular defect. The bone is then osteotomized with oscillating and reciprocating saws. The bone graft is delivered still attached to its vascular pedicle. Again the templates are utilized to determine size and shape. Segmental osteotomies can be performed in situ. The final preparatory

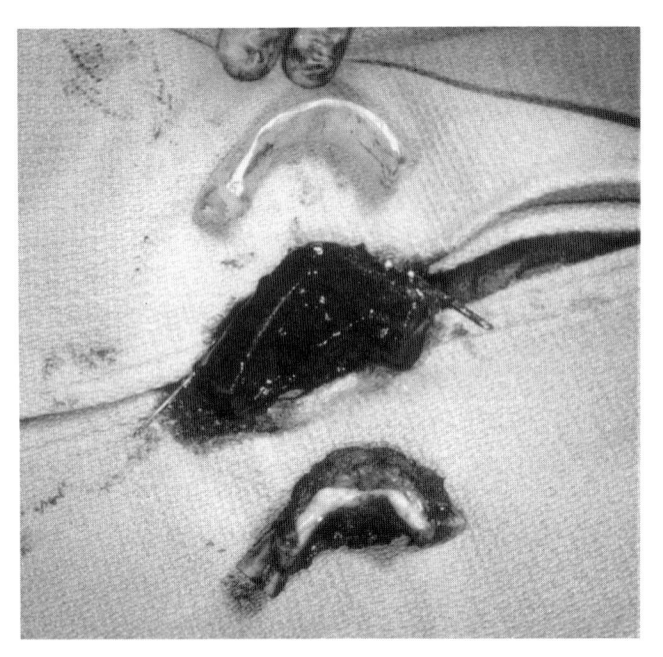

Figure 51.7 Vascularized iliac crest bone graft is shown with compression plates in place. The graft is identical to the extirpated bone and the presurgical template.

step prior to transfer is the placement of the miniplates to the graft. At this point there is no problem if the mandibular dissection is not completed; the contoured graft is vascularized and exists as an island system (see Figure 51.7).

When the recipient area is ready, the patient is placed into occlusion with temporary MMF. The pedicle is then divided; the remainder of the plate osteosynthesis is completed; and the microvascular anastomosis is performed. Once the bone is placed in an occlusal plane and fixed, the MMF is removed.

Because this is a buried transfer, there is no visible way to monitor the flap. The thermocouple monitoring system therefore is applied to provide moment-to-moment assessment of the anastomosis.

The neck and hip wounds are now closed simultaneously. All patients receive a temporary tracheostomy for airway protection.

At 72 hours postoperatively the patient receives a technetium 99 bone scan. With assurance of a patent anastomosis and good bone circulation, the monitors are removed and uneventful healing is expected.

TECHNIQUE: OSSEOINTEGRATION

Six months after bone graft reconstruction, scans are performed. With vascularity indirectly assured, the miniplates are removed, and bone biopsies are performed to assess viability directly.

At this point, the oral surgeon begins the preparation for placement of the implants. The bone graft and mandible are radiologically evaluated for size. A minimum of 7 to 10 mm of vertical height is required, and 6 millimeters of width is needed. This allows for 2 millimeters of bone on the lingual and buccal surfaces when accommodating the 3.25-millimeters titanium implants. The technique utilized is that developed by Branemark (see Chapter 13) for the treatment of the edentulous but otherwise normal jaw. The bone is exposed, leaving a healthy soft-tissue cuff for closure. Four to seven implant sites are spaced on the mandibular arch. Low-speed drills are used to create the bed for the implants, which are then secured into place. The cuff of tissue is replaced.

A minimum of three months of undisturbed healing passes before the implants are exposed. This is the period of osseointegration, when a ceramic bond occurs between the bone and implant.

Four implants must integrate successfully before a patient is able to tolerate a fixed prosthesis. Abutment posts are then placed through the soft tissues into the implants to "load" the jaw for the future appliance. At this point the patient sees a prosthodontist, who will take impressions and supply models to enable design of a prosthesis that will function in occlusion. Once the prosthesis is complete it is held in position by screws.

Case Reports

Case I

A 46-year-old female had a deviation deformity secondary to a segmental mandibulectomy. The deformity extended from the right angle to the midline (see Figure 51.8a and b). This was the result of treatment of a T_3, N_1, M_0 stage III gingival epidermoid carcinoma. Although successfully oncologically treated, she had great difficulty in chewing and speaking. This significantly interfered in her abilities to be socially and economically productive.

Reconstruction of the bony arch was performed with a vascularized deep circumflex iliac crest bone graft contoured and secured by plate fixation (see Figures 51.8c and d). A removable denture was fabricated and inserted. Although aesthetically pleasing, the denture failed to fit securely and provide a stable bite. The constant irritation of the prosthesis on the soft tissues led to mucosal ulcerations and pain (see Figure 51.8e). These ulcers were difficult to discern from recurrent disease, and multiple biopsies were required. To overcome the functional problems and diagnostic confusions caused by the onlay appliance, seven titanium implants were placed into the bone graft and adjacent mandible (see Figure 51.8 f, g, and h). Following a three-month period the implants were exposed. All seven were successfully osseointegrated, and the abutment posts were placed. The dental prosthesis was fashioned to meet the patient's occlusal needs and secured to the posts. She has functioned with the fixed bridge for over four years without any problems. She has a stable bite and has 3

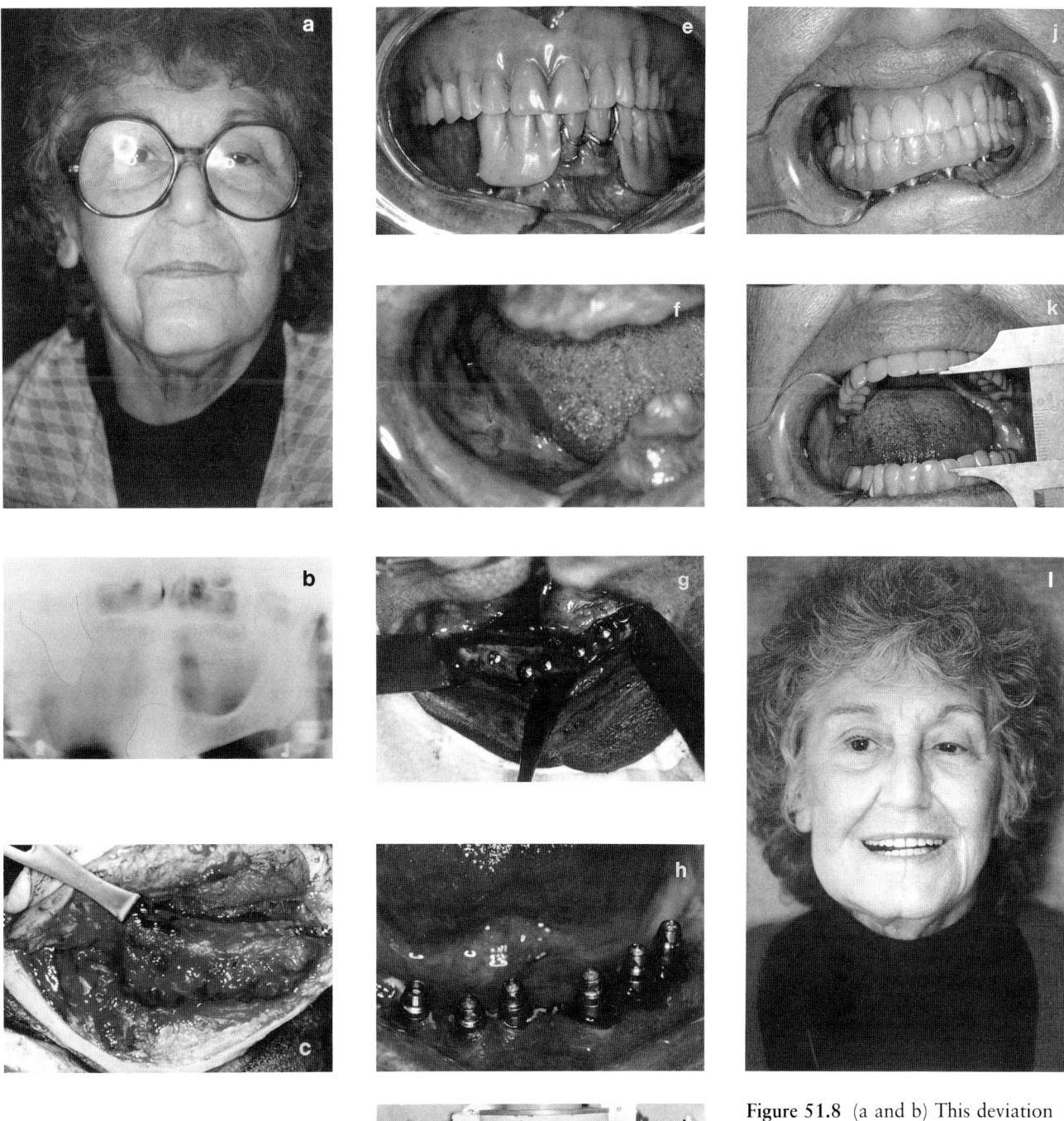

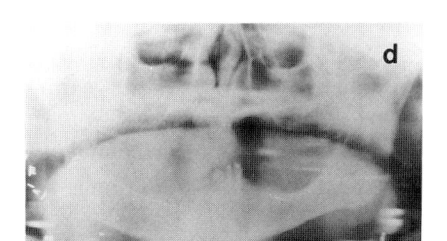

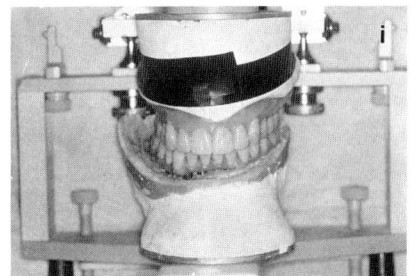

Functional Mandibular Reconstruction

Figure 51.8 (a and b) This deviation deformity is the result of a segmental mandibulectomy. (c and d) Osteosynthesis of iliac crest bone graft is shown. (e) The removable denture was the cause of ulceration. (f, g, and h) Osteointegration of titanium implants and abutment posts is shown. (i) Articulated functional prosthesis. (j, k, and l) The final functional result allows 3 centimeters of opening. The fixed osteodental unit is shown.

Figure 51.9 (a and b) This deviation deformity is the result of a large segmental mandibulectomy with atrophic mandible and loss of perioral muscle control. (c and d) Titanium implants are placed into vascularized iliac crest bone graft with rigid plate osteosynthesis. (e) The dental prosthesis is secured to osteointegrated implants. (f and g) The final functional result allows 3 centimeters of opening.

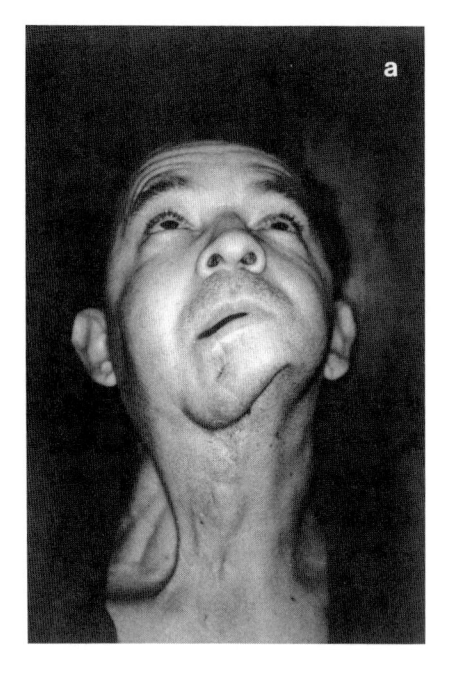

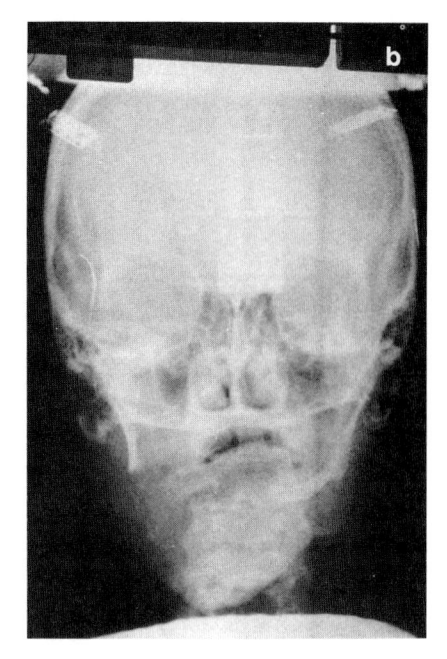

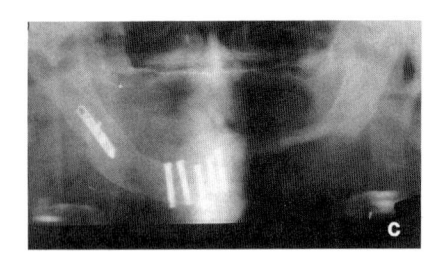

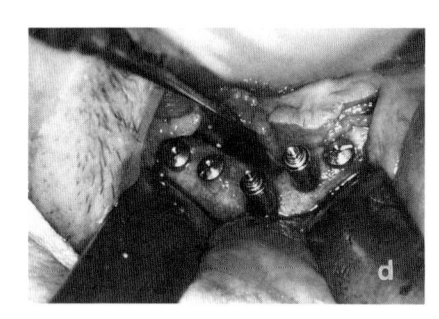

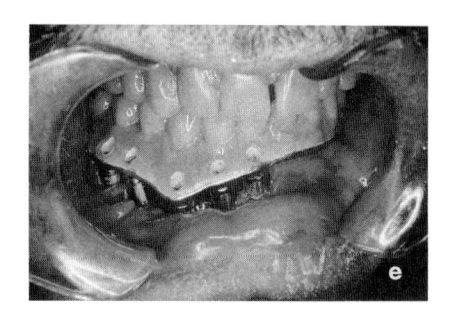

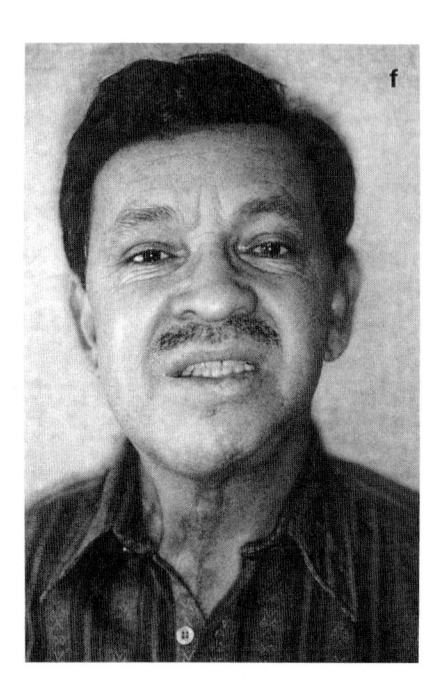

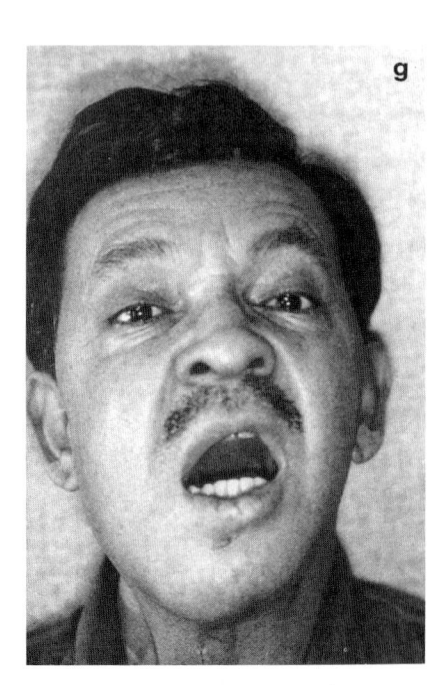

centimeters of opening. Because there is no pressure on the bone or mucosa, she has had no recurrent ulcers or pain.

Case II

A 50-year-old male had a significant deviation deformity as a result of a right segmental mandibulectomy extending from angle to midline (see Figure 51.9a and b). This was performed in conjunction with a radical neck dissection and floor of mouth excision of a T_3, N_1, M_0 epidermoid carcinoma. The loss of arch support contributed to poor control of his perioral musculature, causing difficulty in speaking and chewing. In addition, the years of edentulousness from the surgery led to significant atrophy of his remaining mandible. Initial reconstruction consisted of a vascularized iliac crest bone graft contoured to re-establish the bony arch. This was secured by plate fixation. A removable denture was not possible because of contour irregularities between the bone graft and atrophic mandible.

Five titanium implants were integrated into the bone graft (see Figure 51.9c and d). Three months later, following complete osteointegration, the abutment posts were loaded. The dental prosthesis was then constructed to span the entire arch but to bear load only on the graft (see Figure 51.9e). This patient has been followed for over three years. The implants have not weakened, and function remains excellent. There is 3 centimeters of opening (see Figure 51.9f and g).

CONCLUSION

In an editorial entitled "Logs vs. harpsichords, blobby flaps vs. finished results," the late Frank McDowell in 1979 made a plea to perform recognizable, functional, and aesthetic reconstructions—to create finished products.

"O-filling," a term coined by D. Ralph Millard, Jr., in his book, *The Principalization of Plastic Surgery,* refers to the importance of functional and aesthetic tissue transfers and emphasizes the need to avoid merely filling defects (holes).

The fixed osseodental unit utilizing vascularized iliac crest bone grafts, stabilized with plate and screw osteosynthesis, and a fixed dental prosthesis, secured with osseointegrated implants, together provide the patient with an anatomic and functional reconstruction. They enable accurate replacement of all the extirpated tissues and provide for psychological and social rehabilitation.

Acknowledgment

Special acknowledgment is given to Stephen A. Sachs, D.D.S., the oral and maxillofacial surgeon who has worked with me on all of my cases and provided invaluable service.

REFERENCES

Adell R, Lekholm, U, Rockler B, Branemark PI: A 15 year study of osseointegrated implants in the treatment of the edentulous jaw. Int J Oral Surg 10:387, 1981.

Ariyan S: The pectoralis major myocutaneous flap: A versatile flap for reconstruction of the head and neck. Plast Reconst Surg 63:73, 1973.

Bakamjian VY, Long M, Rigg B: Experience with medially based deltopectoral flap in reconstructive surgery of the head and neck. Br J Plast Surg 24:174, 1971.

Blomberg S: Rehabilitering Med Dakbensforankrad Bettersattning. 3. Kliniskt-Psykiatriska Aspekete Lakartidningen 69:4819–24, 1972.

Brånemark PI, Albrektsson T: Titanium implants permanently penetrating human skin. Scand J Plast Reconstr Surg 16:17, 1982.

Brånemark PI, Hansson BO, Adell R, et al: Osseointegrated implants in the treatment of the edentulous jaw. Scand J Plast Reconstr Surg Supp 16, 1977.

Franks AST, Hedeard B: Geriatric Dentistry. Oxford, London, Blackwell Scientific, 1973.

Hansson HA, Albrektsson T, Brånemark PI: Structural aspects of the interface between tissue and titanium implants. J Prosth Dent 50:108, 1983.

Hurst PS: Dental consideration in the management of head and neck cancer. Otolaryngol Clin North Am Aug. 18, 1985.

Linkow LI, Chercheve R: Theories and Techniques of Oral Implantology. St. Louis, C.V. Mosby, 1970.

Lukash FN, Sachs SA, Fischman B, Attie JN: Secured osseointegration denture in a vascularized bone transfer: Total functional jaw reconstruction. Ann Plast Surg 18, 12, Dec. 1987.

Lukash FN, Sachs SA: Functional mandibular reconstruction. Plast Reconstr Surg 83, 8, Aug. 1989.

Manchester WM: Immediate reconstruction of the mandible and temporomandibular joint. Br J Plast Surg 18:291, 1982.

May JW Jr, Lukash FN, Gallico GG III, Stirrat CR: Removable thermocouple probe microvascular patency monitor: An experimental and clinical study. Plast Reconstr Surg Sept. 1983.

McDowell F: Logs vs. harpsichords, blobby flaps vs. finished results. Plast Reconstr Surg 64:249, 1979.

Millard DR: The Principalization of Plastic Surgery. Little Brown, Boston, 1986.

Moskowitz GW, Lukash F: Evaluation of Bone Graft Viability, Semin Nucl Med XVIII, No. 3, July 1988.

Parel SM, Brånemark PI, Jansson T: Osseointegration in maxillofacial prosthetics. J Prosth Dent V55, B4, 1986.

Taylor GI: Reconstruction of the mandible with free composite iliac bone grafts. Ann Plast Surg 9:5, 1982.

CHAPTER 52

The Role of Plate and Screw Fixation in the Management of Pediatric Head and Neck Tumors

Jeffrey C. Posnick

Tumors of the head and neck are rare in children (Azey 1975, Batsakis 1979, Gaisford 1969, Jaffe 1973, Rapids 1988). In contrast to adults, in whom most head and neck tumors are either squamous cell carcinomas or salivary gland neoplasms, in children, head and neck tumors represent a heterogeneous group of conditions. Only 2% to 3% of all pediatric tumors are located in this area and range from neoplasms (both malignant and benign) to hamartomas and congenital growths.

The incidence of malignant tumors is higher during the first 5 years of life than during the subsequent 10 years (Azey 1975). This probably reflects the embryonal nature of the common tumors encountered in children.

Most malignant tumors of the head and neck that arise in infancy and childhood appear as a solid mass and may grow very quickly. Any rapidly progressive growth in an infant or child should therefore be considered malignant until proven otherwise. Malignant tumors of lymphoid tissue account for a high percentage of head and neck tumors in children. Treatment often involves biopsy followed by chemotherapy; major surgery is usually not needed.

Rhabdomyosarcomas account for almost one-third of malignancies of the head and neck in children. Others commonly diagnosed tumors are seen at an early age; they are often present at birth.

I divide pediatric head and neck tumors into two main categories: (1) congenital growths and benign tumors and (2) malignant tumors. Table 52.1 shows the distribution, and Table 52.2 shows the primary location of the tumors in patients I have managed surgically at The Hospital for Sick Children (HSC) in Toronto from 1986 to 1988.

Table 52.1 Pediatric head and neck tumors (1986–1988)

Congenital Growths and Benign Tumors	
Eosinophilic granuloma	2
Neurofibromatosis	9
Lipoma	1
Odontogenic	8
Fibro-osseous lesion	4
Fibrous dysplasia	5
Hemangioma	3
Vascular malformation	9
Dermoid	10
—midline	
—lateral	
Branchial cleft	5
Teratoma	3
Salivary gland	2
Malignant Tumors	
Sarcoma	9
Aggressive fibromatosis	4
Leukemic infiltrate	3
	N = 75

Table 52.2 Pediatric head and neck tumors: Resection and reconstruction, by primary location

Cranial vault	14
Orbit	12
Zygoma	6
Nose	7
Maxilla	7
Mandible	13
Soft tissue	18
	N = 75

Congenital growths and benign tumors often require immediate treatment at whatever age they present because of progressive deformation and immediate functional concerns affecting the brain, eyes, breathing, swallowing, speaking, and chewing as well as for psychosocial reasons. If immediate surgery is not indicated for functional reasons, and if the tumor proves to be a benign and nonprogressive lesion, an ideal time frame for surgery based on our current understanding of differential craniofacial growth patterns can be selected to maximize long-term reconstructive resistivity and limit permanent disability.

Patients with tumors that may be malignant should be assessed by an interdisciplinary team consisting of an oncologist, radiation therapist, and oncologic/reconstructive surgeons. In this way, maximum control of both local and systemic disease can be achieved if a malignancy is diagnosed.

Sarcomas, and in particular rhabdomyosarcomas, are among the most common malignant head and neck tumors in the pediatric population. Although each patient presents a unique set of circumstances, in general, the treatment protocol at HSC consists of a multidrug adjuvent chemotherapeutic regimen to control systemic disease and wide surgical excision with immediate reconstruction for management of local disease whenever feasible. This approach to treating local disease evolved gradually through experience in managing craniofacial congenital malformations and as a result of advances in reconstructive techniques. Because radiation therapy has a devastating effect on further growth of the facial bones and soft tissues in the treatment field, it is not used to control local disease except in the most extensive cases in which surgical free margins could not be expected.

Reconstruction of tumor resection defects is done immediately. Recent advances in techniques, including the use of internal plate and screw fixation for osteotomy and bone graft stabilization, calvarial bone grafts, pedicled flaps, microvascular free-tissue transfers, microneural repairs, and tissue-expansion techniques, have enabled us to achieve satisfactory results in the majority of patients.

CASE REPORTS

Case 1: Rhabdomyosarcoma of the Left Maxilla

An 18-month-old girl was noted to have swelling in her left cheek after she fell off her bicycle (see Figure 52.1). When the swelling did not subside, her parents took her to her general physician. He referred her to a surgeon, who diagnosed hemangioma of the left cheek. The swelling was progressive and distorted the nose, lower eyelid, and upper lip. She was referred to HSC, where a rock-hard fixed mass and an overlying flush to the skin was appreciated clinically and on computerized tomography (CT) scan. An intraoral biopsy confirmed the diagnosis of rhabdomyosarcoma.

In keeping with our interdisciplinary approach at HSC, this patient was reviewed by the hospital's Tumour Board. A decision was made to carry out tumor resection with immediate reconstruction and to provide a two-year course of combined chemotherapy to control systemic disease.

The patient underwent an en bloc resection of the involved cheek skin, underlying maxilla, floor and medial orbital wall, inferior orbital rim, left nasal bone, lateral nasal wall, and maxillary teeth on the affected side. The facial nerve, palatal mucosa, upper lip, eyelid, and nasal soft-tissue tip were preserved. Reconstruction was accomplished with full-thickness cranial bone grafts to reconstitute the orbital floor, medial orbital wall, orbital rim, nasal bone, anterior maxilla, and zygoma. Titanium miniplates were used to achieve fixation. The left temporalis muscle was rotated into the defect of the maxillary sinus. A radial forearm flap was harvested and transferred to the superficial temporal artery and vein as a free-tissue transfer. A portion of the radial forearm flap covered the soft-tissue defect in the cheek; the other portion was tucked into the soft-tissue defect of the lateral nasal wall for lining.

Chemotherapy, which had been initiated for two months before surgery, was resumed two weeks postoperatively. It has now been one year since this patient completed her two-year treatment course, and there is no evidence of tumor recurrence.

Critique

The use of rigid fixation, membranous bone graft, pedicled flaps, and free-tissue transfers performed by a multidisciplinary team allowed us to complete a major resection in the head and neck and leave the patient immediately rehabilitated. Furthermore, we were able to avoid any long delay in the necessary chemotherapy. Our only alternative for local disease control in this patient was radiation therapy, which would have severely impaired further growth and development in the radiated regions and would have damaged eye function. Deformities resulting from radiation can be almost impossible to correct later and may result in major psychosocial difficulties for the patient and family.

In a child of this age, the uncertainty of the skull thickness necessitates harvesting the cranial graft full thickness. In this case, once the craniotomy was completed and the graft was inspected, it was possible to split a portion of it.

Case 2: Ewing's Sarcoma of the Left Zygomatic Arch

A 12-year-old boy became aware of a hard, painless swelling in his left cheekbone (see Figure 52.2). He

Figure 52.1 This 18-month-old girl had biopsy-proven rhabdomyosarcoma of the left cheek extending into the bone. (a) Frontal view before treatment. (b) Frontal view after chemotherapy, surgical resection, and reconstruction. (c) Lateral view before treatment. (d) Lateral view after chemotherapy, surgical resection, and reconstruction. (e) Worm's eye view before treatment. (f) Worm's eye view after chemotherapy, surgical resection, and reconstruction. (g) Frontal view demonstrates good facial nerve function. (h) Illustration demonstrates en bloc resection and reconstruction. (i) Illustration demonstrates reconstruction. (j) The patient is shown after tumor resection, and before reconstruction. (k) The en bloc tumor specimen includes cheek skin, maxilla, lower orbit, and nasal bone. (l) Autogenous cranial bone is shown for orbital floor and medial wall reconstruction. Stabilization is achieved with titanium miniplates and screws before inset. (m) The temporalis muscle is elevated through the coronal incision before being inset in the maxillary sinus region. (n) Temporalis muscle within maxillary sinus region is shown. Bony reconstruction of orbit, maxilla, and anterior zygoma is complete. Stabilization is achieved with titanium bone plates and screws. (o) Full-thickness soft-tissue reconstruction is done with a radial forearm free-tissue transfer. (p) Anastomosis of radial forearm flap vessels with superficial temporal vessels is shown. (q) Elevated radial forearm is shown flap before transfer. (r) Skin-grafted radial forearm flap donor site is shown one year postoperatively. (s) Pretreatment CT scan demonstrates the extent of tumor spread. (t) Post-treatment CT scan demonstrates the symmetrical ocular globe positions and reconstructed maxilla.

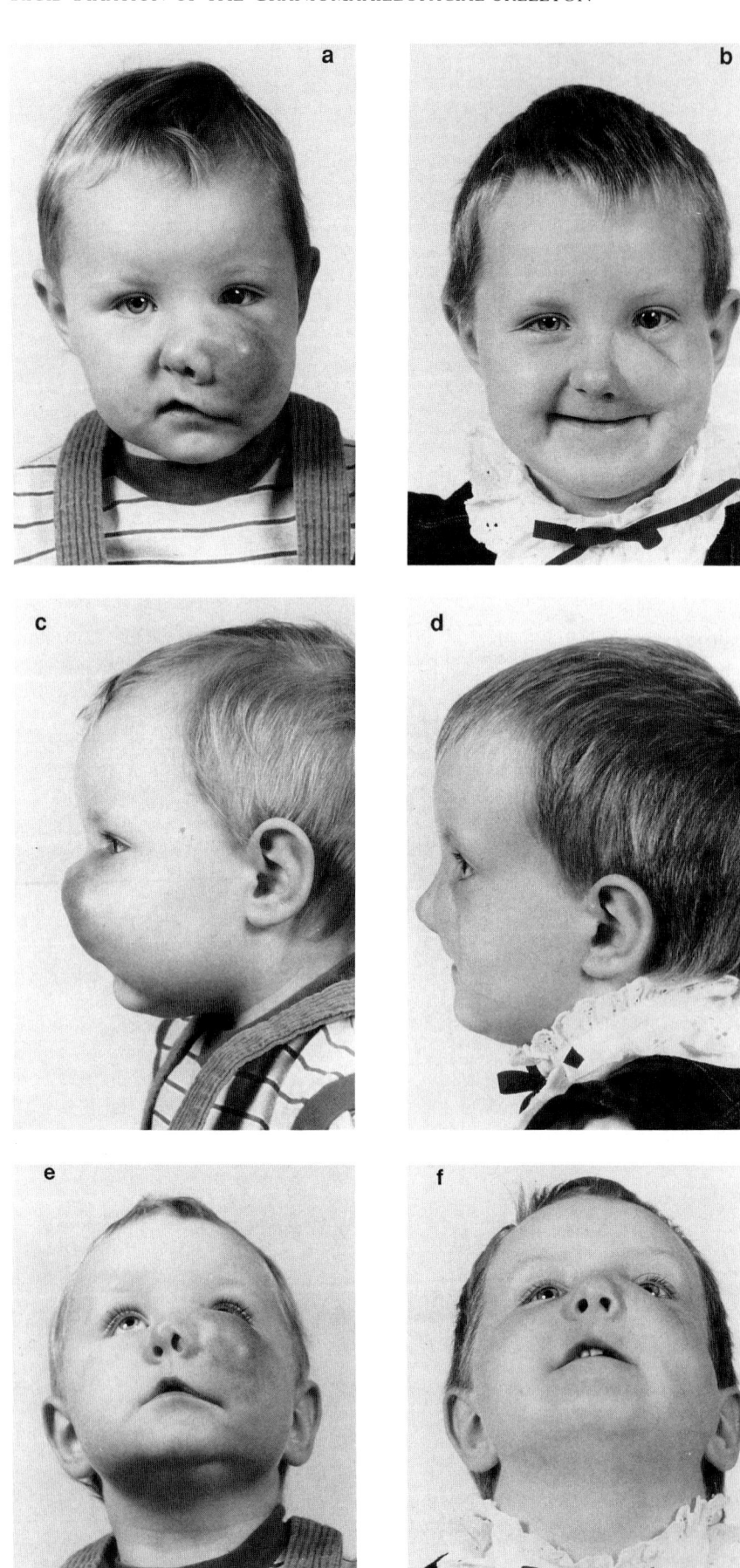

Pediatric Head and Neck Tumors 659

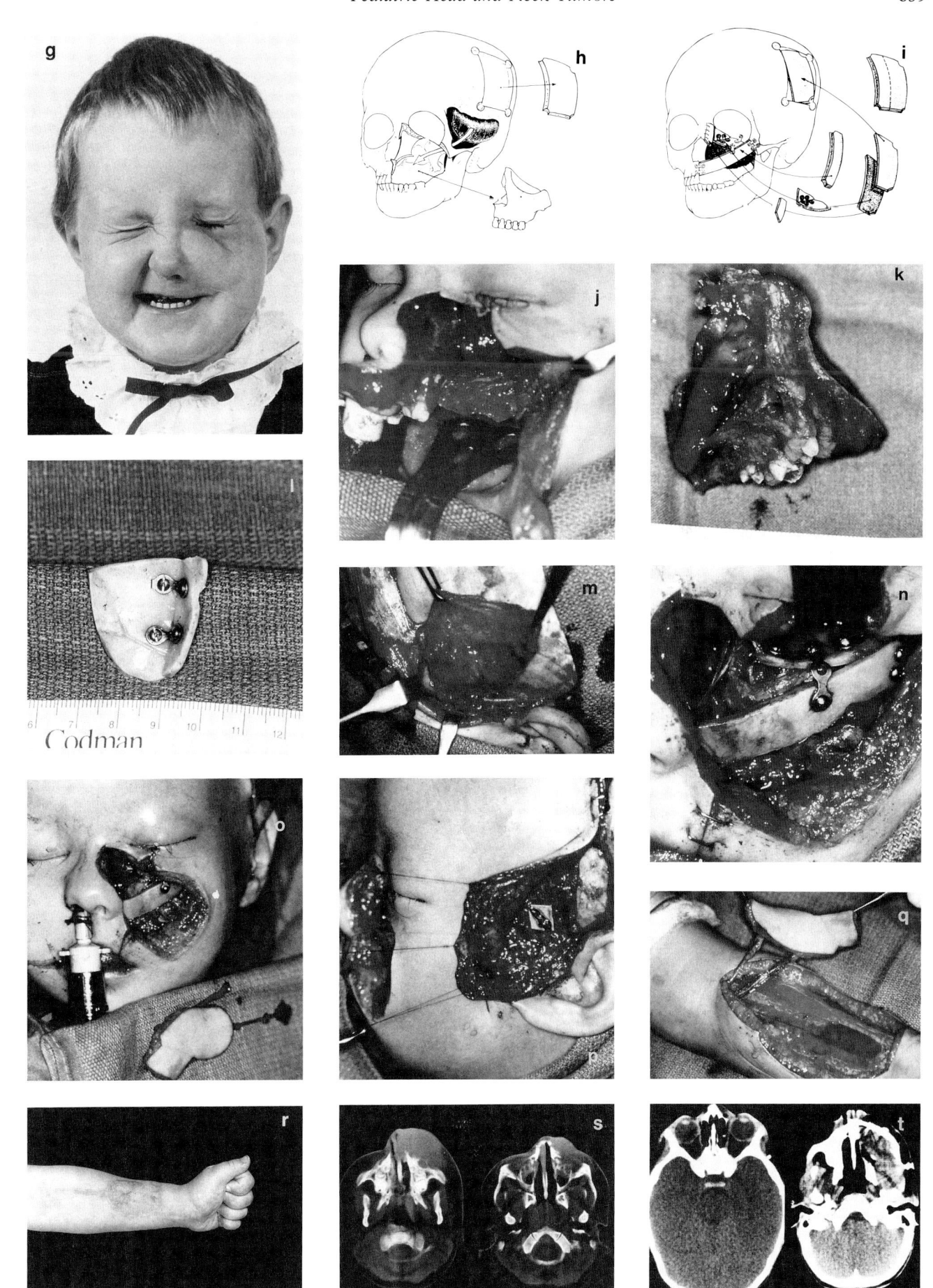

Figure 52.2 This 12-year-old boy had Ewing's sarcoma of the left zygomatic arch. (a) Lateral view two months after initiation of chemotherapy. The biopsy site of the temporal region is visible. (b) Pretreatment CT scan demonstrates the mass of the left zygomatic arch extending into the infratemporal fossa. (c) The coronal incision is completed; the biopsy tract is incised as part of the en bloc resection. (d) The coronal flap is elevated, and the en bloc specimen is in the process of removal. (e) En bloc specimen is shown. (f) The defect is visualized after tumor removal. (g) A full-thickness cranial bone graft has been crafted for zygomatic complex reconstruction. (h) The zygomatic complex is reconstructed with full-thickness cranial bone. Stabilization is achieved with titanium bone plates and screws. (i) The posterior half of the temporalis muscle is elevated. (j) The temporalis muscle is then inset to fill the soft-tissue defect over the reconstructed zygomatic complex. (k) Frontal view two years after completion of treatment. (l) Satisfactory return of facial nerve function is shown. (m) Full face lateral view. (n) Full face oblique view. (o) Two-year postoperative CT scan demonstrates reconstructed zygomatic complex compared to normal side. (p) Postoperative plain radiograph demonstrates the reconstructed zygomatic complex stabilized with titanium bone plates and screws.

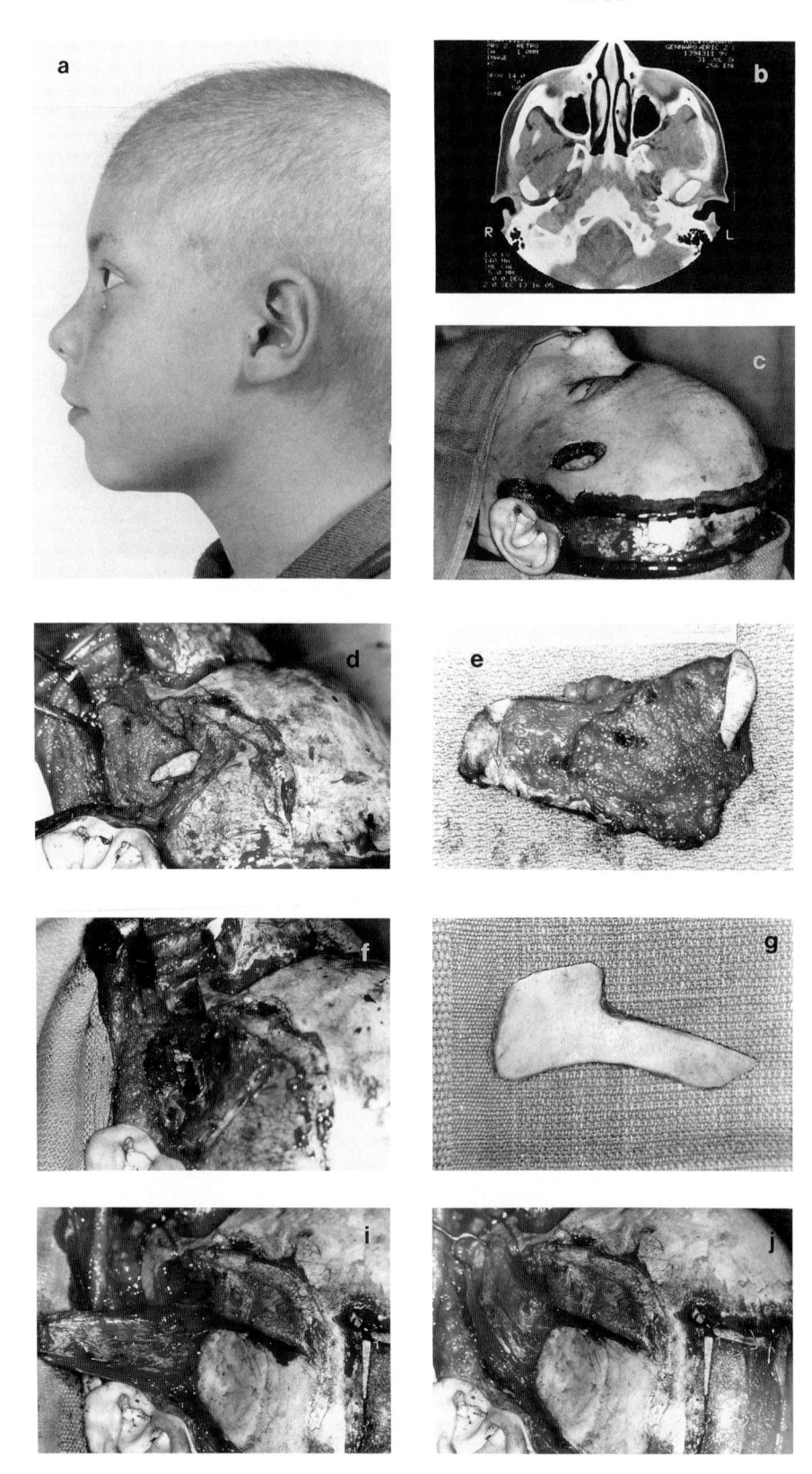

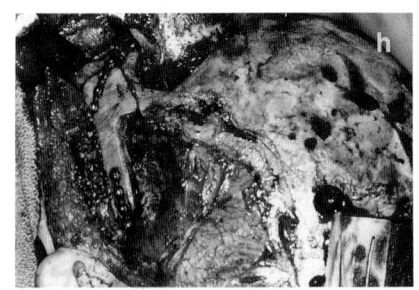

Pediatric Head and Neck Tumors 661

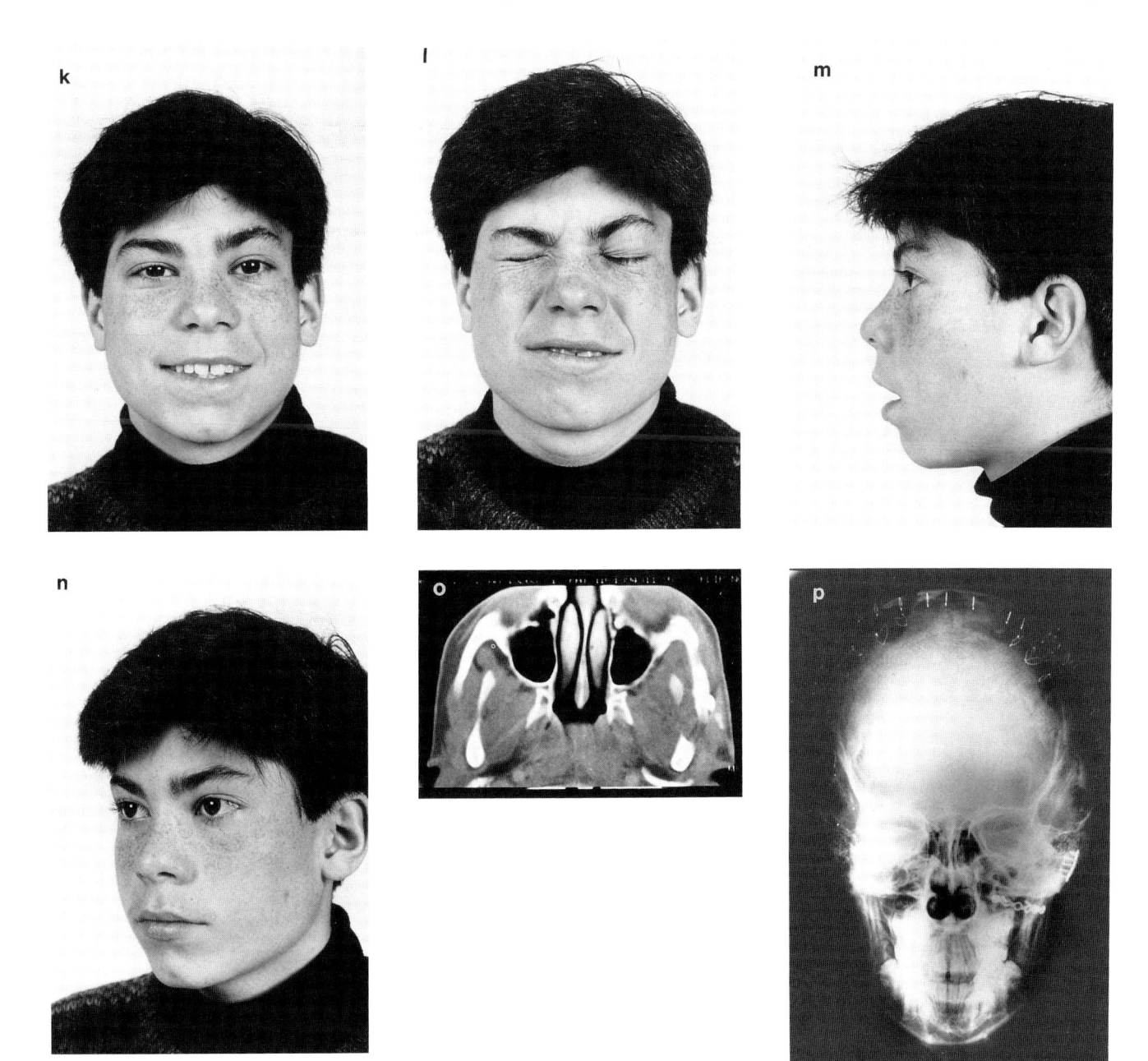

was taken to his internist and then referred to a surgeon, who completed an open biopsy through a left temporal incision. The pathology specimen showed Ewing's sarcoma. A systemic workup was negative for tumor spread, and therefore the left zygomatic arch was believed to be the primary tumor site.

The patient was presented to the Tumour Board at HSC who decided that he should undergo a multidrug chemotherapeutic regimen for two years to control systemic disease and surgery to manage local disease. The family agreed to the Tumour Board's recommendation of resection and immediate reconstruction for control of local disease.

At operation, the biopsy track was excised en bloc through a coronal incision together with the tumor of the zygoma. As part of the en bloc specimen, the superficial musculoaponeurotic system layer was taken superficially while the superficial layer of deep temporal fascia was the deep plane of dissection. After proximal dissection and identification of the upper branches of the facial nerve, the frontal and temporal branches were sacrificed as part of the en bloc resection.

Immediate reconstruction followed, including a full-thickness cranial bone graft to reconstruct the zygoma. This was fixed in place with titanium bone miniplates. The posterior half of the temporalis muscle was rotated down over the bone graft to fill in the soft-tissue deficiency. Using microsurgical techniques, the surgeon reconstructed the temporal branch of the facial nerve with a sural nerve graft.

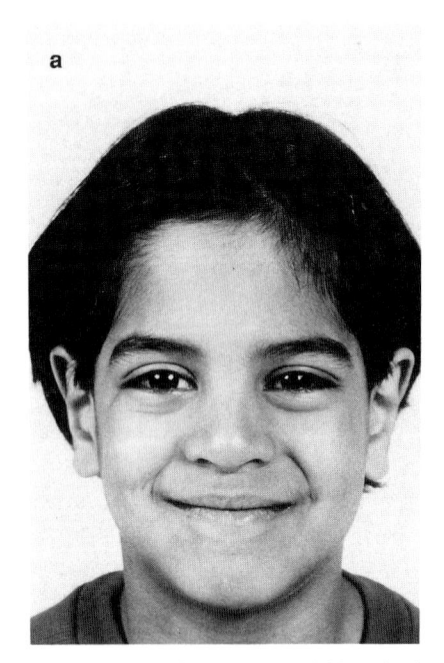

Figure 52.3 This six-year-old boy had recurrent aggressive fibromatosis involving the left mandible. (a) Frontal view before surgical resection. (b) Dental radiographs indicate left mandibular radiolucency and erosion of the roots of the teeth. (c) The en bloc resection includes the left mandible and overlying oral mucosa. (d) Full-thickness cranial bone graft is fixed to the mandibular Vitallium reconstruction plate before being inset. (e) The plate is inset and stabilized to the proximal and distal mandible through the intraoral approach. (f) The elevated temporoparietal fascia flap is visualized through a coronal incision based on the superficial temporal vessel. (g) The temporoparietal fascia flap is tunnelled through the coronal incision into the mouth or internal lining over the bone graft. (h) Plain radiograph demonstrates the mandibular reconstructive plate. (i) Breakdown of temporoparietal fascia flap with exposure of cranial bone graft, in the left body of the mandible region is shown. (j) The exposed cranial bone graft and reconstructive plate have been removed. Stabilization of the proximal and distal mandible is accomplished with an external pin fixator combined with MMF. (k) Secondary mandibular reconstruction is performed with a corticocancellous iliac graft. Stabilization is achieved with multiple titanium bone miniplates and screws. (l) The patient is seen in full face view after successfull iliac bone graft mandibular reconstruction. (m) Profile view after iliac bone graft reconstruction. (n) Satisfactory vertical opening of mandibular after reconstruction. (o) Occlusal view, three years after reconstruction with orthodontic brackets in place to upright mandibular anterior teeth. (p) Plain radiographs demonstrate the iliac graft mandibular reconstruction.

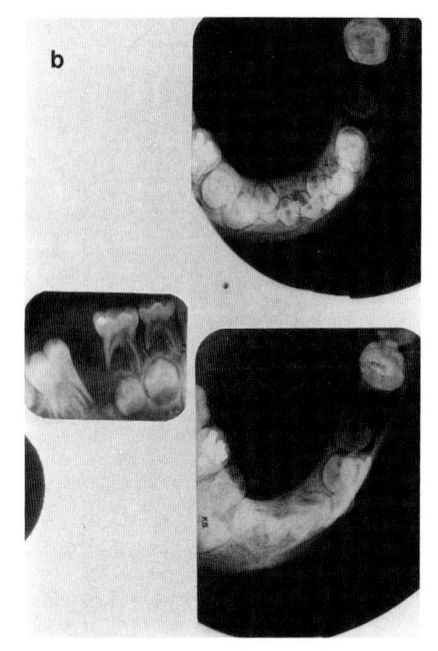

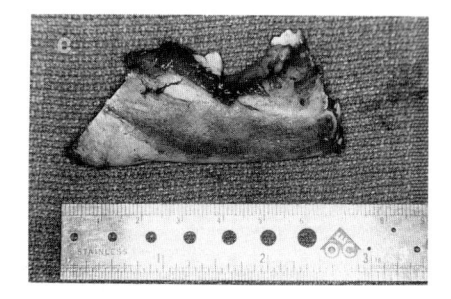

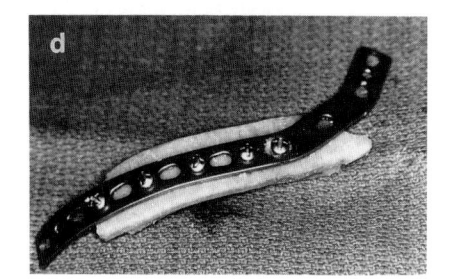

Chemotherapy resumed two weeks postoperatively, and the patient then completed a two-year chemotherapeutic regimen. Now two years later, he is free of disease.

Critique

To our knowledge, this is the first reported case of Ewing's sarcoma arising primarily in the cheekbone. Chemotherapeutic regimens have greatly improved the outlook for this previously incurable disease. When combined with good local disease control, the cure rate is about 70% to 80%. By using the techniques of cranial bone grafting, bone plate and screw internal fixation for bone graft stabilization, a pedicled muscle flap, and microsurgical reconstruction of the facial nerve, surgeons can offer improved management for this type of head and neck tumor. Thus, in this case, we were able to avoid the need for radiation therapy that might have severely damaged the boy's vision and temporomandibular joint (TMJ) function and prevented further growth of the facial bones in the radiation field.

Case 3: Aggressive Fibromatosis of the Left Mandible

A six-year-old boy, accompanied by his parents, complained to his dentist that an ulcer located in the left mandibular molar region refused to heal (see Figure 52.3). He was referred to a surgeon, and several primary teeth were removed and the sockets curetted. The pathology report revealed aggressive fibromatosis versus low-grade sarcoma.

He was presented to the Tumour Board at HSC, where a decision was made to resect the involved mandible and overlined mucosa en bloc. No systemic therapy was indicated for this locally aggressive tumor.

At operation, this patient underwent left hemimandibulectomy from the midramus of the mandible distally past the mental foramen. Reconstruction of the

Pediatric Head and Neck Tumors 663

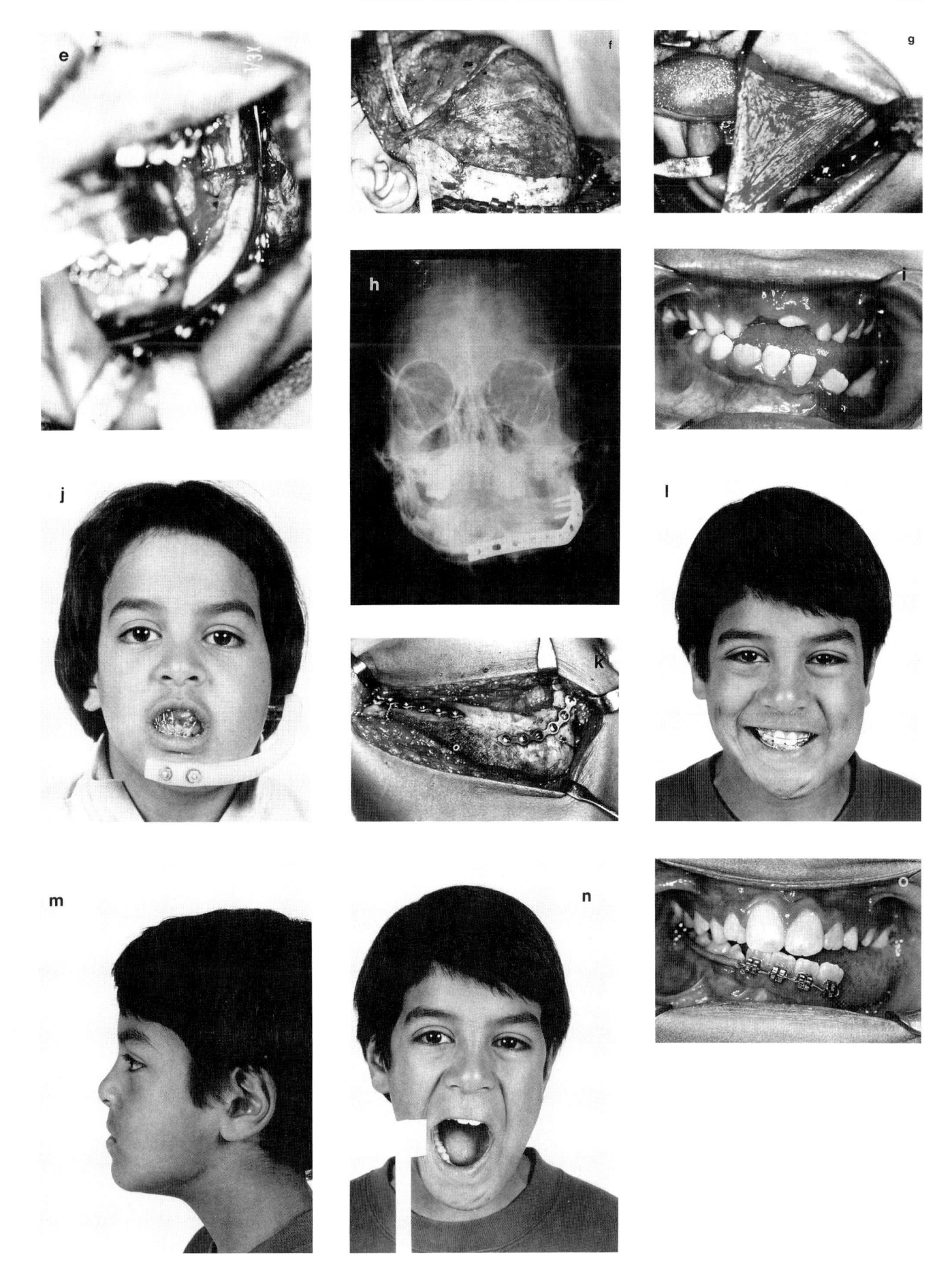

Figure 52.4 This eight-year-old girl had a left fronto-orbital and sphenoid wing monostatic fibrous dysplasia. (a) Frontal view shows mass of left fronto-temporal region. (b) Close up shows the left frontotemporal mass. (c) CT scans demonstrate bony lesion of the left fronto-orbital and sphenoid wing regions. (d) Three-dimensional CT scan reformation also demonstrates mass in left fronto-orbital sphenoid wing region. (e) Bone scan confirms the area of reactivity in the left fronto-orbital and sphenoid wing region. (f) View through the coronal incision demonstrates the left fronto-orbital and sphenoid wing mass. (g) The tumor mass is resected back to the optic foramen. (h) Cranial bone graft reconstruction. Stabilization is achieved with multiple titanium bone plates and screws. (i) Gross appearance of specimen. (j) Harvested cranial bone graft for reconstruction. (k) Frontal view shows the patient one year after resection and reconstruction. (l) Lateral view shows the patient one year after resection and reconstruction. (m) CT scan shows the reconstructed region. (n) Three-dimensional CT scan reformations are shown one year after resection and reconstruction.

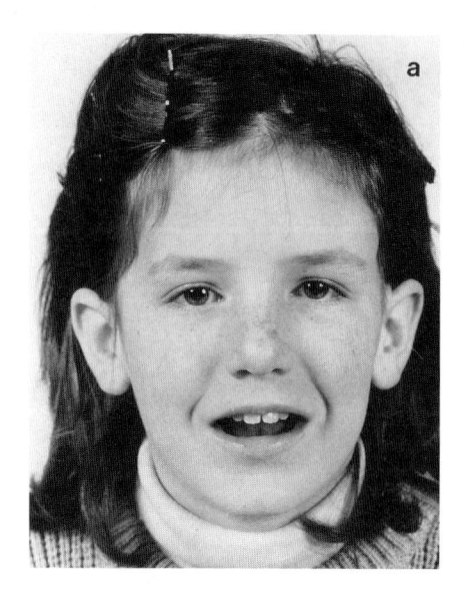

mandible was with full-thickness cranial bone grafts and a mandibular Vitallium reconstruction plate. The plate was secured proximally to the condyle ascending ramus unit and distally to the symphysis of the mandible. The deficit in the mucosa's internal lining was reconstructed with a pedicled temporoparietal fascia flap elevated on the superficial temporal artery and tunneled through the coronal incision intraorally.

Postoperatively, this patient did well initially with maintenance of a wide vertical opening of the mandible. However, after one year, the noninnervated, nonkeratinized temporoparietal fascial flap eroded through, exposing the bone graft. It was necessary to remove the reconstruction plate and bone graft while maintaining the space with an external pin fixator device until the wound was once again clean. At that point, an iliac corticocancellous graft was harvested and inset through a left neck incision. The graft was stabilized with miniplates and bicortical screws. The wound and bone graft healed uneventfully.

Further surgical orthodontic and prosthetic rehabilitation will likely be required later for the edentulous segment of the mandible.

Critique

The need for en bloc resection of the involved hard tissue and overlying soft tissue to remove the tumor and prevent local recurrence of the aggressive fibromatosis lesion cannot be disputed. However, several controversial reconstructive choices were made in this case. Although I initially selected autogenous cranial bone for the mandibular reconstruction, over time I have not had good success with cranial bone grafts placed in edentulous tooth-bearing regions, and this is a case in point. The bone is frequently thin, knife-edged, and much too cortical. Bone of this morphology cannot withstand the biting forces of normal mastication. I have also been disappointed with heavy reconstruction plates in the mandible because they have resulted in stress shielding and bone graft resorption. The use of a pedicled temporoparietal fascia flap rather than a free-tissue transfer was an attempt to limit the number of operated sites and the length of the surgical procedure. Perhaps a keratinized and innervated flap would have been a better choice. Once it became necessary to remove the initial bone graft and bone plate, the use of external pin fixation combined with maxillo-mandibular fixation (MMF) allowed the wound to heal while maintaining the gap in the region of the resected mandible. Other surgeons might prefer to use either MMF or an external pin fixation device alone or primary regrafting. This case demonstrates the need to remain versatile in all methods of reconstructive surgery and bone graft fixation.

Case 4: Left Fronto-Orbital Fibrous Dysplasia

An eight-year-old girl presented with a progressive, painless lump in the left forehead (see Figure 52.4). A CT scan revealed thickened bone in the region of the left frontal, orbital, and sphenoid wing. The orbital component showed involvement of the roof, lateral orbital wall, supraorbital ridge, and lateral orbital rim. On bone scan, the lesion showed increased uptake and was presumed to represent a mono-ostotic form of fibrous dysplasia.

After considering treatment options, it was decided to excise the involved bone and perform immediate reconstruction with autogenous cranial bone grafts. The procedure was carried out through a coronal incision and intracranial approach. The left orbital rims were reconstructed with full-thickness cranial bone graft, and split cranial grafts were utilized for the orbital roof, lateral orbital wall, and bone graft donor site. Bone miniplate and screw fixation was used for stable internal fixation of all grafts.

Pediatric Head and Neck Tumors 665

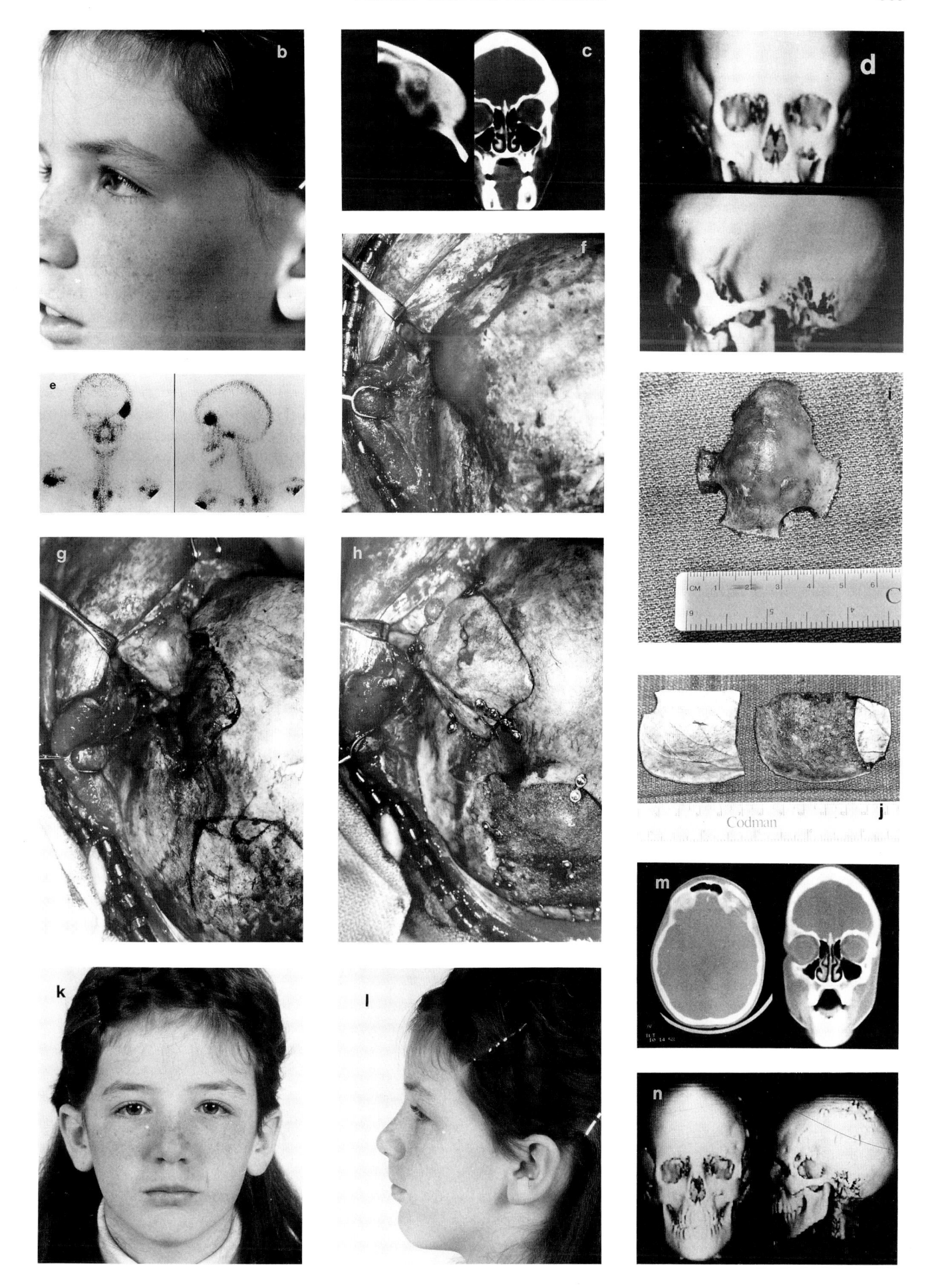

Figure 52.5 This 16-year-old girl underwent intracranial resection of an astrocytoma located in the frontal lobe, then radiation therapy. Loss of the bone flap with titantalum mesh methylmethacrylate cranioplasty resulted in recurrent cellulitis. A cranial bone cranioplasty was subsequently performed. (a) Frontal view before removal of methylmethacrylate and cranial bone cranioplasty. (b) Frontal view after reconstruction. (c) Oblique view before reconstruction. (d) Oblique view after reconstruction. (e) View of skull through coronal incision after subperiosteal dissection. (f) Removed methylmethacrylate mass. (g) The full-thickness cranial vault defect in frontotemporal region is shown. (h) Cranial vault, after reconstruction with split cranial grafts, is stabilized with multiple titanium miniplates and screws. (i) Plain radiographs demonstrate the methylmethacrylate mass over the frontotemporal bone defect before removal. (j) Three-dimensional CT scan reformation demonstrates the cranial bone cranioplasty stabilized with multiple titanium miniplates and screws.

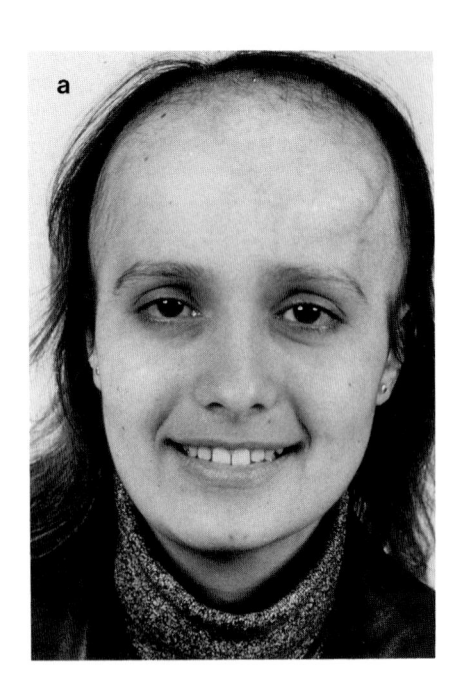

Critique

Our experience shows that cranio-orbital fibrous dysplastic lesions are usually progressive, do not involute over time, and may cause irreversible eye damage. Once the sphenoid wing is involved, with extension approaching the optic foramina, resection and immediate reconstruction are our choice. Others might watch these lesions from both a clinical and radiographic perspective, waiting for marked ocular compromise before a definitive resection. Our experience is that postponing resection until this time may limit the possibility of effective resection with functional and aesthetic reconstruction. If a major full-thickness segment of supraorbital ridge or lateral orbital rim must be reconstructed, a carved full-thickness cranial bone graft is required to achieve an aesthetic result rather than relying on a thin, brittle, and knife-edged external table graft. When bone miniplate and screw hardware is used for fixation, it may be palpable or even visible through the thin skin of the forehead and orbital rim regions. We now almost exclusively use microplates and screws that give adequate stability around the orbit but are not palpable or visible through the skin.

The advent of craniofacial techniques and the concepts of cranial bone graft reconstruction with plate and screw internal fixation permit the reconstruction of these defects with minimum morbidity and remarkably rapid convalescence. Patients are confined to the hospital or at home for a total of two weeks and then have six weeks of minimum physical activity. They are then allowed to return to all physical activities.

Case 5: Frontal Bone Defect Following Tumor Resection and Radiation Therapy

This 16-year-old girl underwent intracranial resection of an astrocytoma located in the frontal lobe followed by a full course of radiation therapy (see Figure 52.5). The frontal bone flap, which had been secured only with direct intraosseous wires, had become infected and required surgical removal. Eventually, the frontal bone defect was reconstructed with a titantalum mesh methylmethacrylate cranioplasty. This not only looked and felt unsightly but also was prone to cellulitis. Several hospitalizations were required for intravenous antibiotics, and oral antibiotics were used chronically.

The previously placed methylmethacrylate was removed. Immediate reconstruction of the defect followed, with cranial bone grafts fixed with bone miniplates and screws.

The cranioplasty was completed by first harvesting bilateral occipitoparietal full-thickness cranial bone through formal craniotomies. The grafts were then split on the bench, and the recipient site of the left frontotemporal region was reconstructed. The two bone graft donor sites were reconstructed with split cranial grafts, which were also fixed with miniplates. The wounds healed uneventfully.

Critique

Tissue expansion of the posterior scalp was suggested as a first stage of treatment so that the good scalp could be draped over the region undergoing cranio-

Pediatric Head and Neck Tumors   667

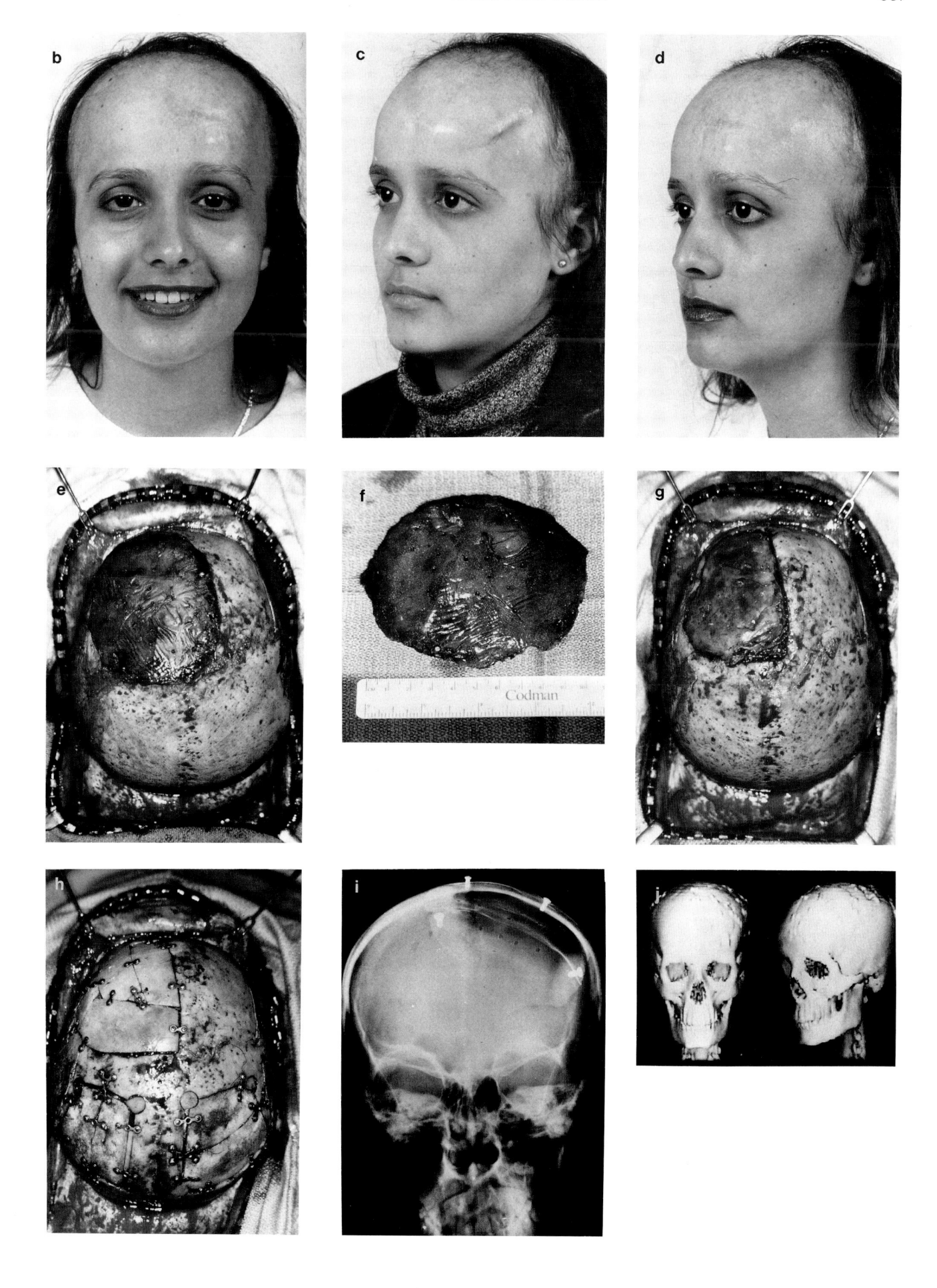

Figure 52.6 This girl had a biopsy-proven recurrent enchondrosarcoma of the maxilla, zygoma, and orbits. (a) Frontal view demonstrates left-eye proptosis and biopsy tract of left cheek. (b) MRI scan shows the tumor mass with encroachment into the orbit. (c) CT scan shows recurrent tumor mass of the left orbit, zygoma, and maxilla. (d) Intraoperative exposure shows the configuration after tumor resection is completed. (e) Tumor specimen is shown, including biopsy tract and eyeball. (f) The elevated rectus abdominus muscle is based on the inferior epigastric pedicle. (g) The orbital rims and zygoma are reconstructed with a full-thickness cranial bone graft. Stabilization is achieved with titanium bone plates and screws. The rectus abdominus muscle is inset into the defect. (h) Frontal view three months after tumor resection and reconstruction. (i) Lateral view three months after tumor resection and reconstruction. (j) Two- and three-dimensional CT scans six months after tumor resection and reconstruction.

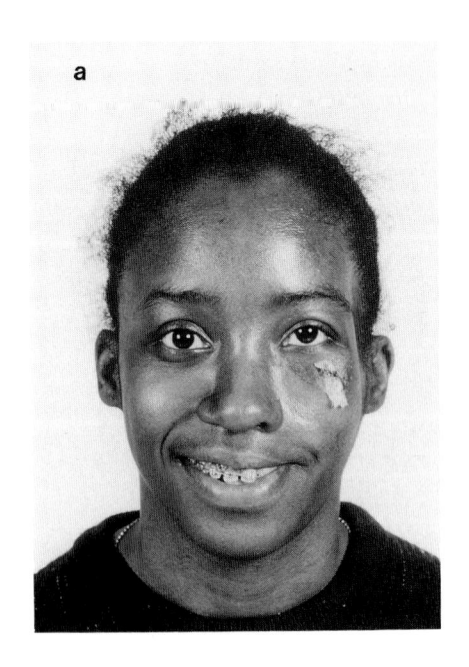

plasty. If the reconstruction had been staged in this way, the tissue expanders would probably have eroded the outer table of the posterior cranial vault, making it an unacceptable bone graft donor site.

Furthermore, it is doubtful whether one tissue-expansion sequence would have completely reconstructed the hair-bearing scalp. I believe that the use of rigid fixation was a major factor in the success of the bone graft in this case in which the skull defect followed radiation therapy. The bone miniplates and screws are palpable and in some places visible through the thin and radiated skin. In the future, I would use microplates and screws for fixation.

Case 6: Recurrent Enchondrosarcoma of the Left Maxilla, Orbit, and Zygoma

This unfortunate girl was originally thought to have fibrous dysplasia involving the left maxilla; biopsy later showed it to be an enchondrosarcoma (see Figure 52.6). She underwent left maxillary resection and reconstruction but refused chemotherapy. Six years later, a biopsy of a rapidly progressing mass that resulted in orbital proptosis proved this to be a recurrence of the enchondrosarcoma. Both CT scan and magnetic resonance imaging (MRI) showed extensive involvement of the residual maxilla and zygoma, and extension into the orbit, the pterygomaxillary space, and the infratemporal fossa.

This patient was presented to the Tumour Board at HSC, who decided that surgical resection was the best management for local disease control. Although there was no evidence of systemic spread, a multidrug chemotherapeutic regimen was suggested.

At operation, through an extended nasolabial incision, the tumor was resected en bloc, including the eyeball, zygomatic complex, residual maxilla, lower half of the bony orbit, and tissues within the pterygomaxillary and infratemporal spaces.

Immediate reconstruction followed, including full-thickness cranial bone grafts to reconstruct the orbital rims and zygoma. These were fixed in place with titanium bone miniplates and screws. A rectus abdominus muscle was elevated for free-tissue transfer and anastomosis to the superficial temporal vessels. The skin flaps were sutured and the intraoral raw muscle was left to re-epithelialize. Postoperatively, she was fitted with an ocular prosthesis.

The suggested chemotherapy was initiated but later refused by the family. She is followed closely because she is at high risk for tumor recurrence.

Critique

Wide surgical excision for this recurrent, radioresistant tumor offers the only hope for the patient's survival. Whether to reconstruct the defect simultaneously or leave the hole open for inspection is open to question. With the advent of CT scan and MRI, noninvasive monitoring for tumor recurrence can be an effective alternative. Furthermore, this patient would agree to tumor resection only if immediate reconstruction could follow.

DISCUSSION

The explosive advances in craniofacial surgery have had a major spin-off effect in the management of pediatric head and neck tumors. The degree of exposure possible through a coronal incision and the combination of an intracranial/extracranial approach coupled with other current techniques—including the use of cra-

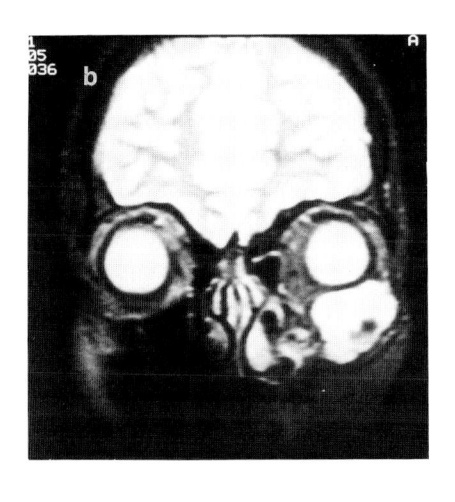

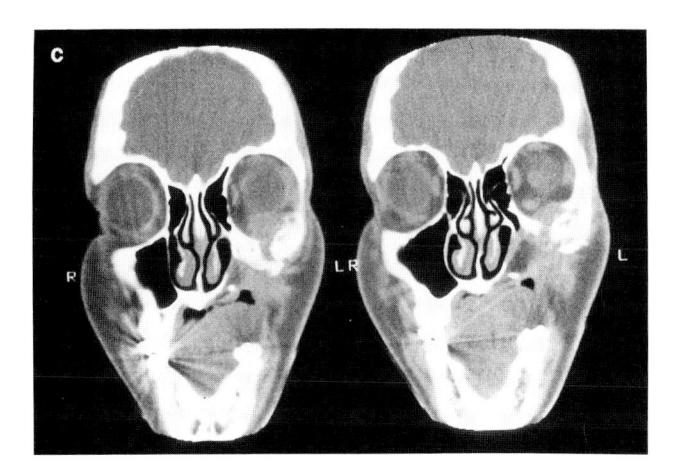

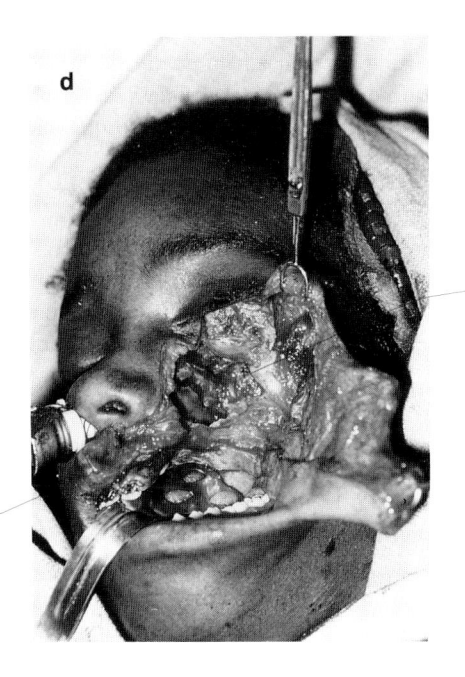

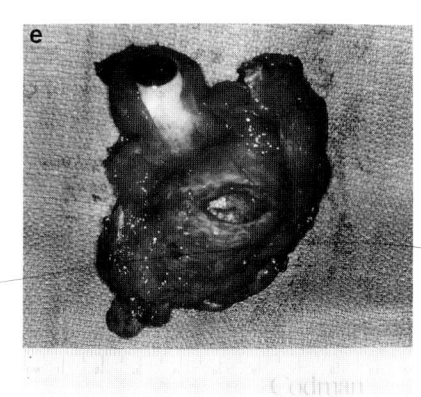

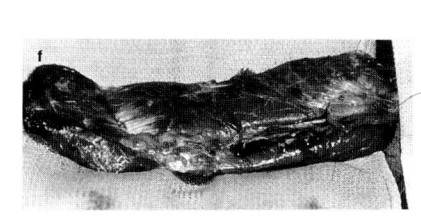

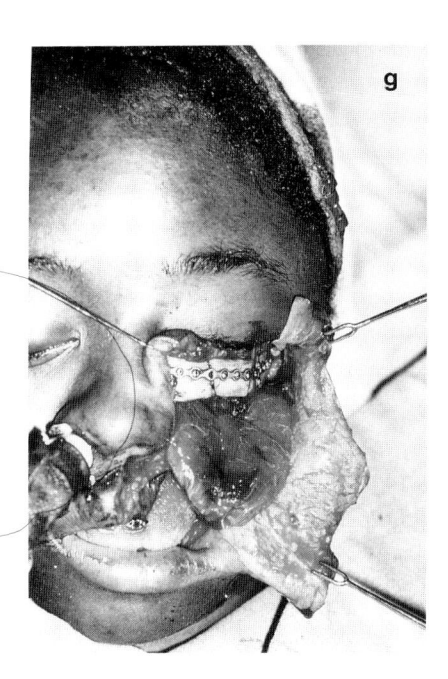

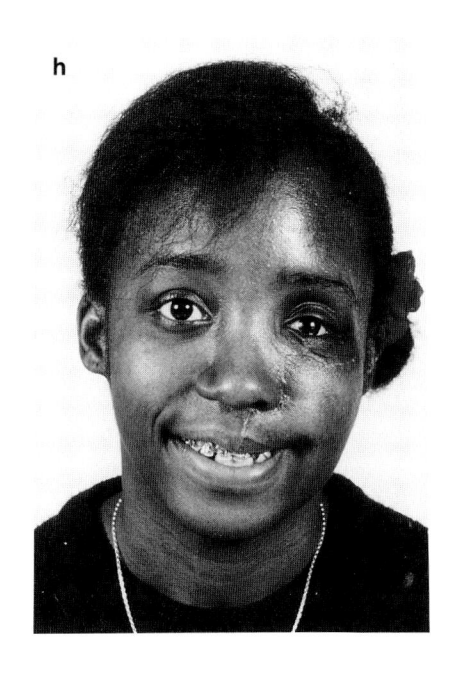

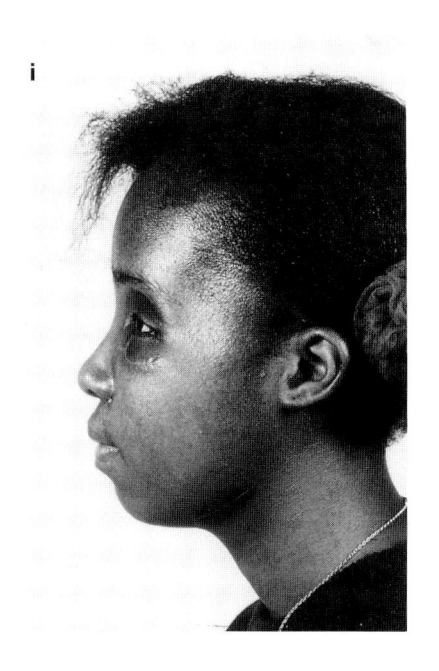

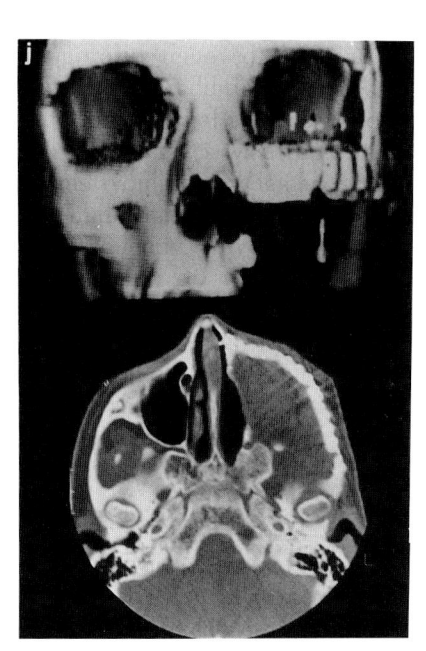

Pediatric Head and Neck Tumors 669

nal fixation for osteotomy and bone graft stabilization—have all been factors in allowing for aggressive surgical resection with acceptable immediate reconstruction (Donald 1984, Jackson 1983a, 1983b, Munro 1981, Tessier 1977).

The major advantage of stable miniplate and screw fixation for osteotomy and bone graft stabilization in the treatment of pediatric craniofacial tumors is that early, reliable bone and soft-tissue healing will occur (Phillips 1988, Rahn 1982, Perren 1979). This allows for early resumption of the chemotherapeutic regimen, which is so important to the patient's overall survival. It is also hoped that with the use of bone miniplates the overall three-dimensional shaping of the osteotomy units and bone grafts will improve the aesthetic results. In addition, skeletal relapse and bone graft resorption should be diminished. If radiation treatment is required, the application of bone plate fixation should not be a complicating factor in treatment decisions.

Once bone has healed, the bone plates and screws are no longer required. Whether they should be removed later to limit any restraint on further bone growth is not clear. Although we generally do not do it, additional basic science and clinical research is needed to clarify this issue.

SUMMARY

Pediatric head and neck tumors that involve the craniofacial skeleton are not common, but when they do occur, they require unique management. They are a heterogeneous group consisting of true neoplasms as well as hamartomas and congenital growths. The use of bone plate and screw internal fixation and a craniofacial approach have greatly improved the functional and aesthetic results we can now offer patients.

Acknowledgment

The author thanks Elizabeth Lang and the staff of Medical Publications, The Hospital for Sick Children, for editorial assistance in preparing this chapter.

REFERENCES

Azey JB: Tumors of the head and neck. In Textbook of Pediatrics. 10th ed. Vaughan R, Mackay J, Nelson WE (eds). Philadelphia, London, Toronto, Saunders, pp 1600–1606, 1975.

Batsakis JG: Tumors of the Head and Neck: Clinical and Pathological Considerations. 2nd ed. Baltimore, Williams and Wilkins, pp 269–279, 291–311, 1979.

Donald PJ: Pediatric malignancies. In Head and Neck Cancer: Management of the Difficult Case. Donald PJ. (ed). Philadelphia, Saunders, 330–339, 1984.

Gaisford JC: Tumors of the head and neck in children. In Symposium on Cancer of the Head and Neck. Gaisford JC (ed). St. Louis, Mosby, 162–172, 1969.

Jackson IT, Laws ER Jr, Martin RD: A craniofacial approach to advanced recurrent cancer of the central face. Head Neck Surg 5:474–488, 1983a.

Jackson IT, Marsh WR: Anterior cranial fossa tumors. Ann Plast Surg 11:479–489, 1983b.

Jaffe BF, Jaffe N: Head and neck tumors in children. Pediatrics 51:731, 1973.

Munro IR, Chen YR: Radical treatment for fronto-orbital fibrous dysplasia: The chain-link fence. Plast Reconstr Surg 67:719–729, 1981.

Perren SM: Physical and biological aspects of fracture healing with special reference to internal fixation. Clin Orthop 138:175, 1979.

Phillips JH, Rahn B: Fixation effects on membranous and enchondral onlay bone graft resorption. Plast Reconstr Surg 82:872–877, 1988.

Rahn BA: Bone. In Clinical Orthopedics. Summer-Smith G (ed). Philadelphia, Saunders, pp 346–347, 1982.

Rapids AD, Economidis J, Goumas PD, et al: Tumors of the head and neck in children: A clinico-pathological analysis of 1,007 cases. J Craniomaxillofac Surg 16:279–286, 1988.

Tessier P, Rougier J, Hervouet F, Wolliez M, Lekieffre M, Derome P (eds): Plastic Surgery of the Orbit and Eyelids. New York: Masson, 1977.

CHAPTER 53

Unusual Applications of Plating

Joseph S. Gruss

The use of plates and screws has been well defined in trauma, orthognathic, tumor, and craniofacial surgery. Plates and screws are often indicated for rigid internal fixation in the cranium, midface, and mandible. With experience, the surgeon can expand the role of plate and screw fixation to encompass other, more unusual, indications. These indications will expand further as surgeons become more familiar with plate and screw fixation. This chapter describes certain unusual indications where rigid internal fixation with plates and screws have been used.

MIDFACE

Reconstruction of the Inferior Orbital Rim

The inferior orbital rim is extremely important in providing support to the lower eyelid. Atrophy or loss of the rim usually causes sagging and ptosis of the lower eyelid (see Figure 53.1). This is clearly demonstrated following a total maxillectomy with resection of the orbital rim and floor but preservation of the ocular globe and periorbital contents. In this situation, the globe maintains its vertical position, being supported by Lockwood's ligament, but the eyelid sags, having lost its vital support.

Following full-thickness resection of the lower eyelid, reconstruction must provide cover, lining, and adequate support (see Figure 53.2). The support must be provided by reconstruction of the tarsal plate, usually with cartilage grafts. In order for the cartilaginous support of the lower eyelid to be adequate, the inferior aspect of the cartilage graft must be anchored to the inferior orbital rim.

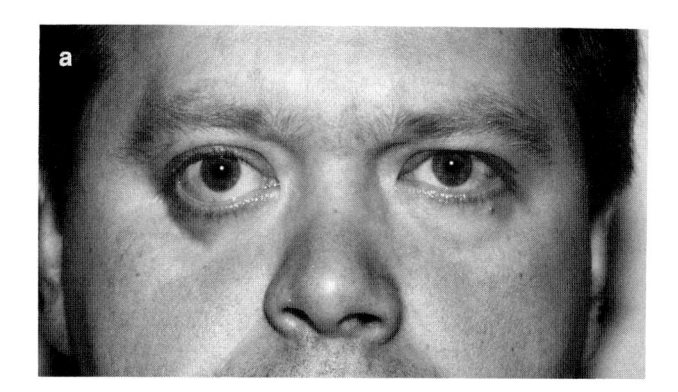

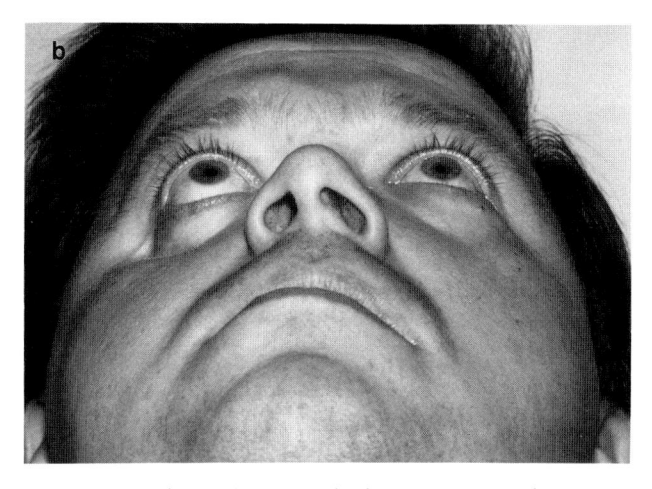

Figure 53.1 This male patient had osteomyelitis of the right inferior orbital rim as a child, resulting in severe hypoplasia of the rim. (a) The vertical position of the globe is maintained; but there is sagging and inferior displacement of the eyelid, which has lost its inferior support. (b) Inferior view shows maintenance of globe position. Obvious inferior and posterior displacement of the right lower eyelid can be seen.

Figure 53.2 This 60-year-old man had recurrent squamous cell carcinoma involving the right lower eyelid and anterior cheek and invading the underlying maxilla and inferior orbital margin. (a) Full thickness resection of two-thirds of the lower eyelid, the entire inferior orbital margin, the anterior half of the orbital floor, the anterior wall of the maxilla, and the cheek skin performed. A lateral suture is placed in the remaining eyelid. (b) Planned reconstruction is with a large cheek/neck rotation flap, combined with a lateral canthotomy and medial rotation of the remaining eyelid skin, tarsal plate, and conjunctiva. (c) Split calvarial bone grafts reconstruct the missing orbital rim (OR) and anterior wall of the maxilla (M). All bone grafts are carefully fixed in place with multiple lag screws. (d) Chondromucosal graft harvested from the nasal septum is now used to reconstruct the medial half of the eyelid. This is anchored inferiorly to the underlying bone graft (arrow). The lateral portion of the eyelid is brought across as a composite flap (E) and anchored to the chondromucosal graft medially. (e) The large cheek/neck rotation flap is now used to resurface the remaining eyelid and cheek in one large esthetic unit. (f) Result at three years shows good restoration of lower eyelid anatomy and support. There is a slight ectropion of the medial portion of the eyelid. Note the excellent contour restoration of the cheek and orbital rim and the support it provides to the lower eyelid. (g) Inferior view shows maintenance of ocular globe position. Position of the lower eyelid reconstruction can be seen as well as contour restoration of the anterior wall of the maxilla and inferior orbital rim.

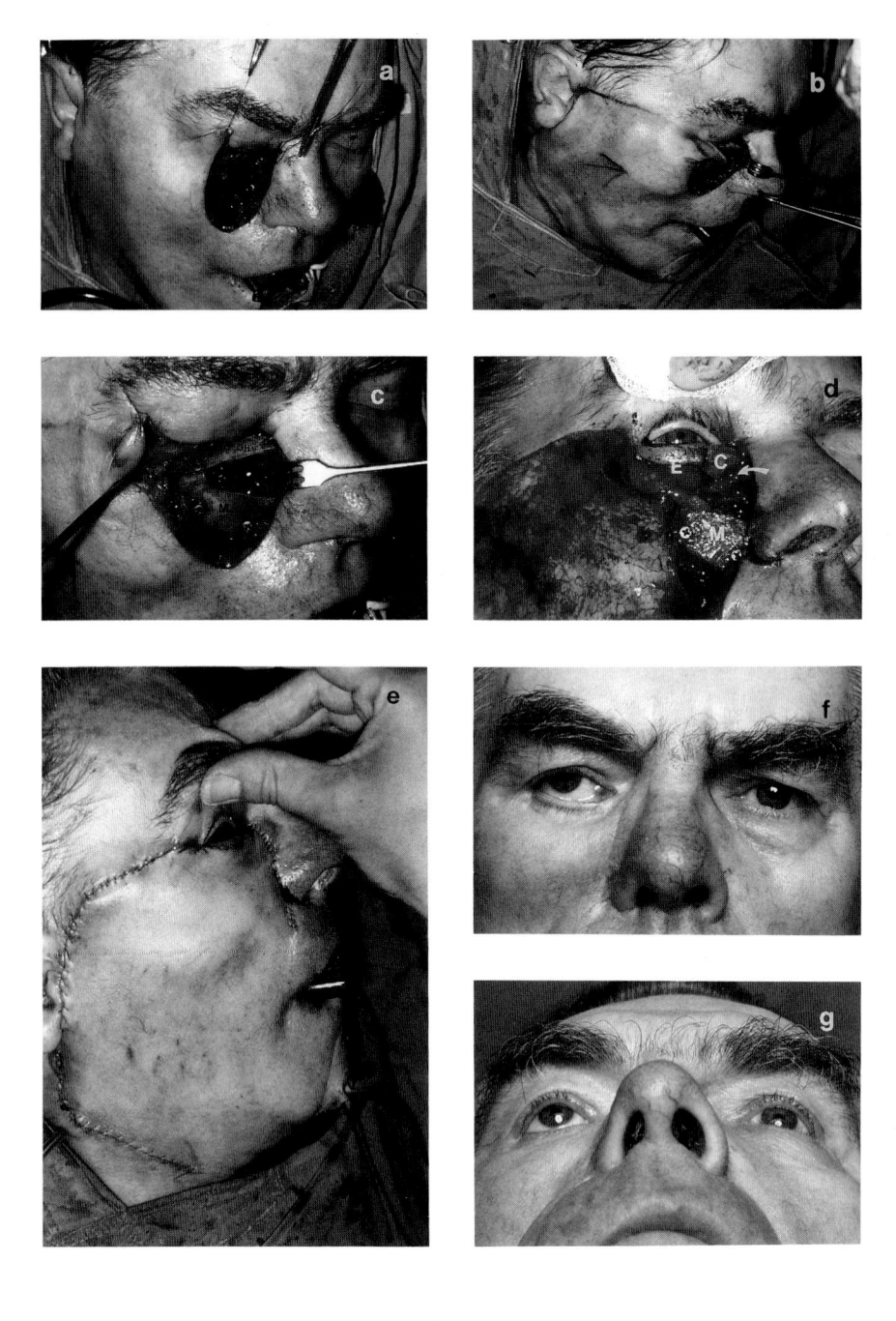

When the inferior orbital rim is lost or resected in combination with full-thickness loss or resection of the lower eyelid, then adequate reconstruction of the inferior orbital rim should precede reconstruction of the lower eyelid (see Figure 53.3).

Methods of Reconstruction

It is important first to delineate the extent of the defect of the orbital rim and wall. The defect may involve the inferior orbital rim alone, or it may also involve the lateral or medial orbital rim or walls, the floor of the orbit, and inferior wall of the maxilla.

In each situation, split calvarial bone grafts that are carefully shaped and contoured replace the defect in the inferior rim and any contiguous areas. The bone grafts used to reconstruct the orbital rim and anterior maxilla are rigidly fixed in position with lag screws and miniplates. Subsequent bone graft reconstruction of orbital wall defects can usually be performed by wedging the bone grafts into place. This can be done without fixation, or fixation with miniscrews or microscrews can be used when necessary. The bony reconstruction of the orbital rim now serves as a base for support of the lower eyelid or for subsequent reconstruction of the lower eyelid. The chondromucosal or conchal cartilage graft used for eyelid support is anchored to the underlying bone graft through multiple drill holes placed through the graft following its rigid fixation. In addition, the cheek soft tissues or flap can be suspended through the same drill holes with multiple 2-0 Dexon sutures. Rigid immobilization of the bone grafts with plate and screw fixation provides support to cartilaginous and soft tissue in the healing phase, without the risk of bone graft loss and subsequent soft-tissue displacement.

Nonunion of Midfacial Bones

Nonunion or fibrous union of the midfacial bones is frequently recognized at the time of exploration for secondary correction of post-traumatic deformities. Clinically, this situation is rarely symptomatic because the midfacial bones are under the influence of less muscular forces than the mandible, and their unique anatomical configuration usually ensures that they fracture at more than one site. Nonunion or fibrous union at one site may be accompanied by either relatively stable fibrous union or true bony union at another site. Bone segment displacement with gap formation, combined with inadequate fixation, allows micromovement that perpetuates the nonunion or fibrous union.

Clinical Case

A 40-year-old woman had an isolated depressed zygomatic arch fracture reduced by means of a Gillies' approach (see Figure 53.4). After initial uncomplicated healing she complained of severe and persistent pain in the region of the fracture site when chewing. A computerized tomography (CT) scan performed nine months after the injury revealed a bony nonunion. At exploration through a coronal incision, the displaced segmental fracture was identified with a dense fibrous union posteriorly and a fibrous union with gap formation anteriorly. The fibrous union was left intact; the segment was reduced; and a long miniadaptive plate was placed across the zygomatic arch, crossing and stabilizing both fracture sites. Resolution of symptoms was rapid following surgery.

Discussion

Nonunion of the midfacial bones may be infected or uninfected. Infected nonunion requires the control of infection and the subsequent application of rigid fixation with plates and screws. Uninfected nonunion may be displaced with gap formation, or the gap may contain fibrous tissue. When there is a fibrous union with minimal gap and the bone segments are not displaced enough to require mobilization and repositioning, then the fibrous union is left in situ and the plate is applied directly across the site of fibrous union. Axial compression can be used in selected cases, but care must be taken in midfacial repair because compression applied to occlusal segments will predispose to malocclusion. Bone grafts are not usually necessary; stability provided by the rigid fixation will encourage bony union.

When there is a bony gap, the plate bridges the gap, immobilizing the adjacent bone segments. Bone grafts need to be inserted into the bone gap to ensure bony continuity and healing.

Reconstruction of Anterior Nasal Spine

Deficiency of bone and cartilage in the region of the anterior nasal spine results in a typical deformity with an acute nasolabial angle (see Figure 53.5). Severe flatness may be seen in the region of the upper maxilla and columellar base. This deformity may arise following

1. midfacial fractures, particularly comminuted maxillary fractures;
2. rhinoplasty with overresection of the nasal spine;
3. septoplasty with superior displacement of the quadrangular cartilage; and
4. maxillary osteotomy.

In the past, restoration of the correct nasolabial angle has been achieved by the use of grafts of nonautogenous material or autogenous bone or cartilage. Fixation of grafts in this area is difficult.

Method

In relatively minor or moderate deficiencies, a square block of bone can be used to augment the region of the anterior nasal spine. The bone graft is fixed to the underlying maxilla with lag screws. The bone graft can now be contoured in situ with a dental bur.

In severe deficiencies, when additional projection is required, two separate grafts are placed in a tentlike configuration with the graft apices directly abutting. The graft bases are fixed to the underlying maxilla with lag screws.

MANDIBLE

Post-traumatic Bone Loss

Following post-traumatic mandibular bone loss, the gap can be bridged with a reconstruction plate. Then the bone gap can be replaced with a conventional bone graft, or a free-vascularized bone graft can be anchored at each end with compression plates.

When the gap is less than 4 centimeters in length, we prefer to pack conventional cancellous iliac bone grafts into the bony gap, which is rigidly maintained by

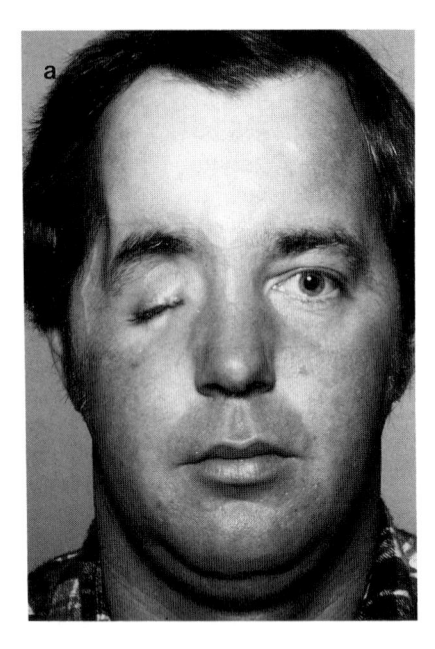

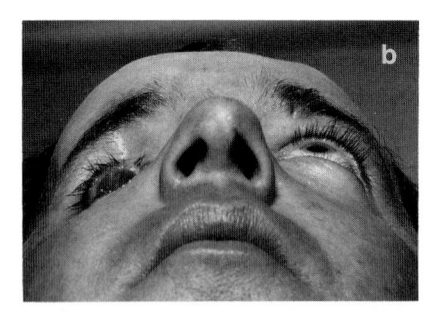

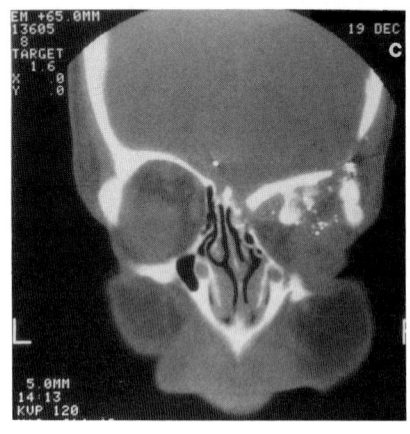

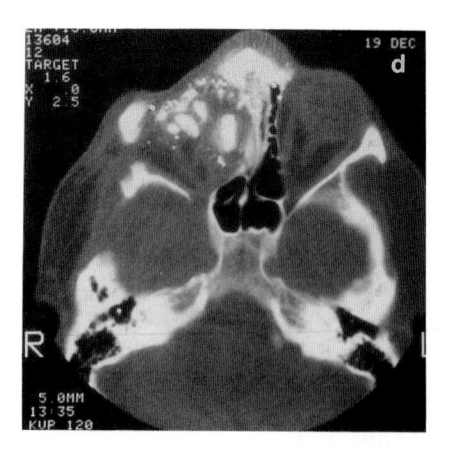

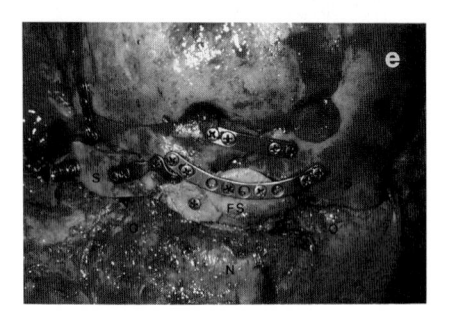

Figure 53.3 (a) Young man was seen two years after an extensive gunshot wound to the right orbit resulting in enucleation. Most of the bony socket is lost. Severe ptosis of the upper and lower eyelid is due to lack of support. This has prevented the fitting of an ocular prosthesis. (b) Inferior view demonstrates absence of the bony orbit, resulting in ptosis of the soft tissue. (c) Coronal CT scan shows massive destruction of the bony orbit with almost total absence of the inferior orbital rim and the lower portion of the lateral rim and wall. (d) Axial CT scan shows severe bony destruction in the region of the right orbit. (e) View from above through the coronal incision shows reconstruction of the anterior wall of the frontal sinus (FS) and right superior orbital rim and walls. Multiple bone grafts are held in place with miniplates and screws. (O = orbits, N = nose.) Bur holes from previous craniotomy can be seen. (f) Lateral view through the coronal incision shows the reconstruction of the superior orbital rim and roof of the orbit (S), the lateral orbital rim (LR), and the lateral orbital wall with bone graft (W), which is held in place with a miniplate. (T = temporal muscle.) (g) Initial result shows restoration of the bony orbit. Note that even with restoration of the bony orbit, there is insufficient support to the lower eyelid, which is still inferiorly displaced. (h) Close-up view shows the inferior positioning of the soft tissue support of the cheek and the lower eyelid. (i) Re-exploration at six months shows good healing of the previous split calvarial bone grafts, which were used to reconstruct the infraorbital margin and orbit floor. No resorption is seen. Previously used lag screws, which were necessary to fix the bone grafts, can be seen. A pocket has now been created underneath the residual soft tissue of the lower eyelid. (j) The complete concha is harvested from the right ear. This is going to be used to provide complete support to the lower eyelid. (k) The conchal cartilage graft (black arrow) has now been placed into the pocket in the eyelid and anchored inferiorly to the reconstructed inferior orbital rim. Multiple drill holes were used. The soft tissue of the cheek is now extensively mobilized right down to the upper buccal sulcus. The deep periosteum and muscle of the cheek soft tissue is now suspended upward through multiple drill holes in the inferior orbital margin and zygomatic body (white arrows). This results in correction of the ptotic soft tissues of the right cheek, as well as improving the support to the lower eyelid. (l) Result at six months shows restoration of the position of the right lower eyelid, almost exactly the same as the opposite, normal, side. Note the excellent support of the lower eyelid that is provided by the conchal cartilage graft. This graft is, in turn, supported on the reconstructed inferior orbital rim. In addition, note the restoration of a normal contour of the soft tissues of the right cheek following resuspension to bone. (m) Close-up view of the eyelid shows the excellent support of the reconstructed lower eyelid. This has resulted in deepening of the inferior fornix, which makes later insertion of an orbital prosthesis much easier. (n) Inferior view shows restoration of right cheek and orbital bony contour, which in turn supports the correction of the lower eyelid.

Unusual Applications of Plating   675

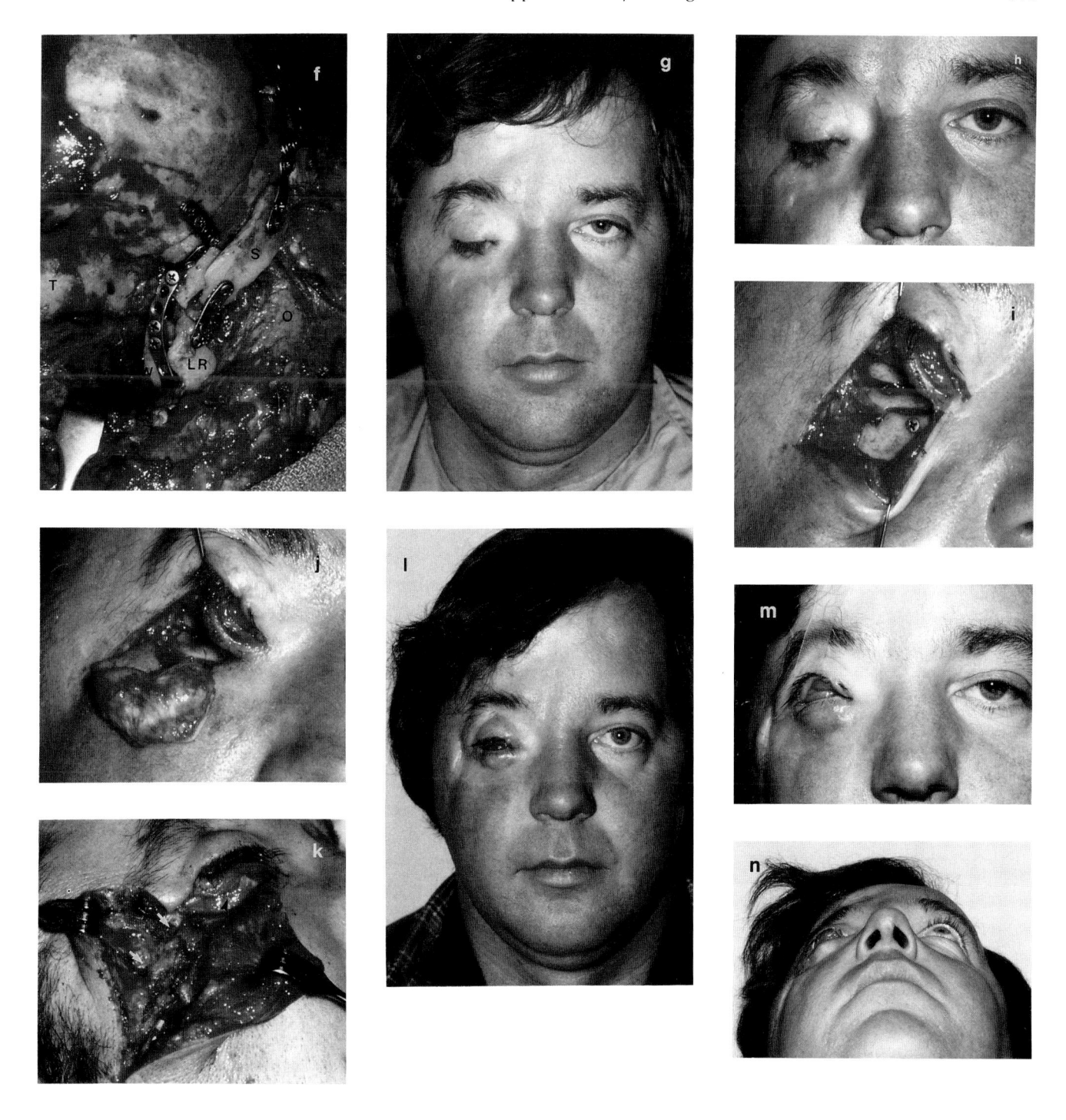

Figure 53.4 (a) This patient has a nonunion of the left zygomatic arch. Axial CT scan demonstrates area of bony nonunion. (b) Exposure of the zygomatic arch through the coronal incision demonstrates the depressed segment of the zygomatic arch. The posterior fracture site demonstrates a dense fibrous nonunion with minimal displacement. The anterior fracture site (solid arrow) demonstrates a dense fibrous union with some displacement. (c) The anterior fracture site is mobilized, and the fragment is repositioned. A miniplate is now placed across the entire displaced segment to hold it carefully in place. No bone grafting was needed because there was no bony gap. (d) X ray demonstrates position of miniplate. Healing was uneventful following rigid fixation, and painful symptoms disappeared.

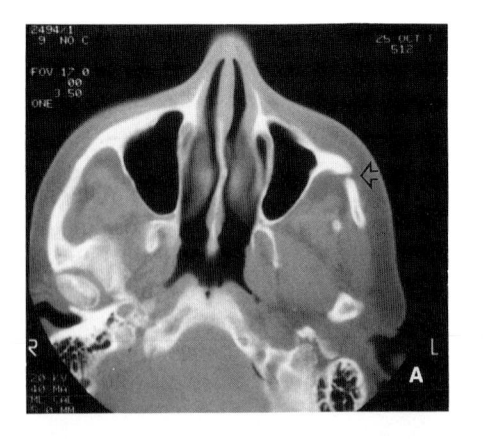

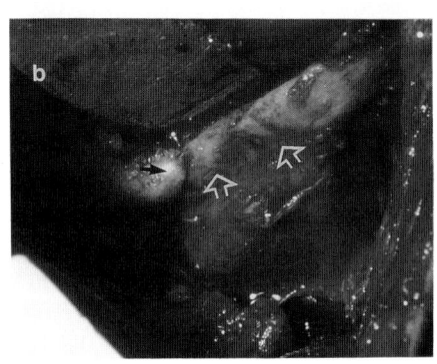

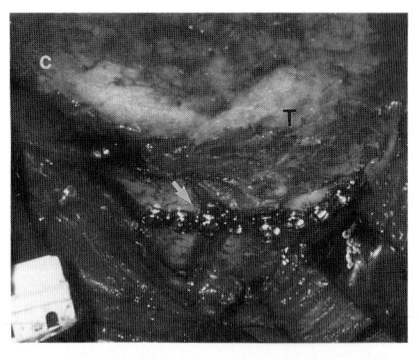

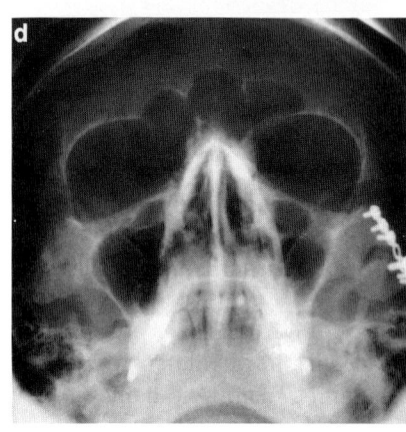

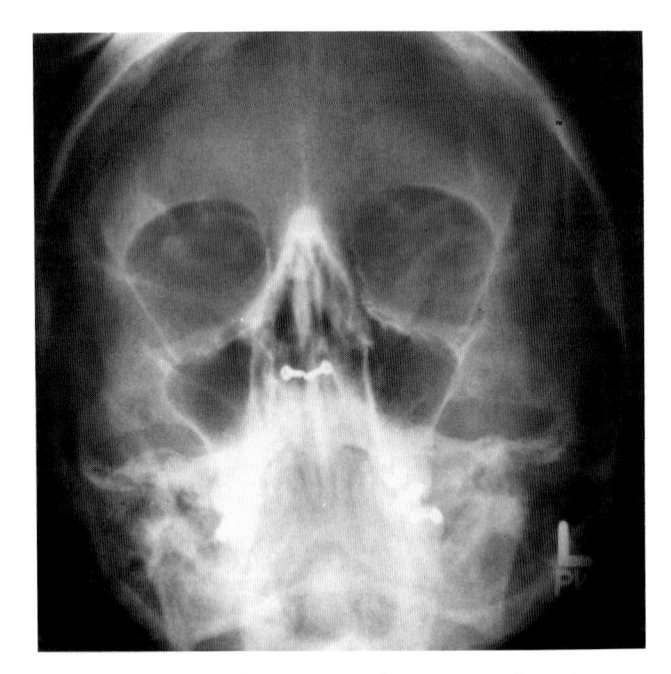

Figure 53.5 X ray demonstrates the position of two lag screws used to reconstruct the anterior nasal spine with split calvarial bone grafts used in a tentlike fashion. Lag screws are placed directly through the bone grafts into the anterior maxilla.

a reconstruction plate. With gaps larger than 4 centimeters, conventional bone grafts have proven unreliable in our hands, and we prefer to use free-vascularized bone grafts.

Case Report

A 21-year-old male presented 10 years ago with very complex craniofacial deformities following a gunshot wound suffered two years previously (see Figure 53.6). He had already undergone 14 procedures in attempts to reconstruct his deformity. The mandible was missing from the right angle to the left ramus. Both residual mandibular segments were displaced medially and superiorly into the oral cavity. Multiple previous attempts at mandibular reconstruction with iliac bone grafts had failed; thus both anterior iliac crests were absent.

An extensive craniofacial reconstruction was undertaken. Extensive midfacial bone grafting was compromised by the shrunken and scarred soft tissue. The mandibular segments were released, and the gap was bridged by a long reconstruction plate. The plate was deliberately overcontoured slightly to maintain internal soft-tissue expansion following the extensive dissection. The bone gap was replaced with multiple rib grafts. Ten years later, the patient remains fully rehabilitated. The mandibular reconstruction remains stable with bony union across the gap. The patient has declined to have the mandibular plate removed.

Unusual Applications of Plating 677

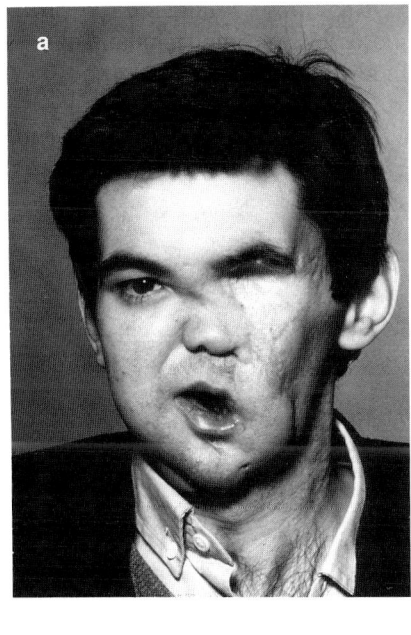

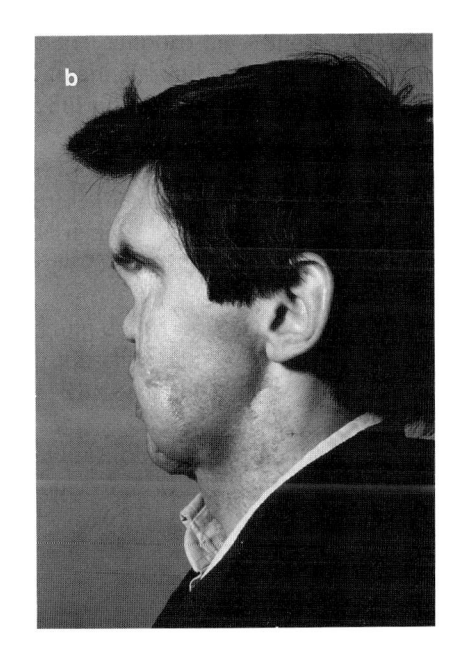

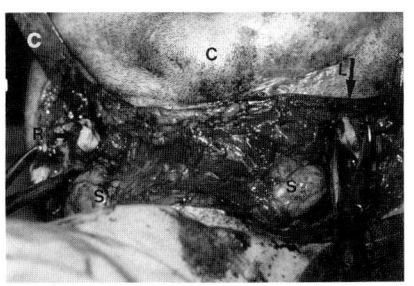

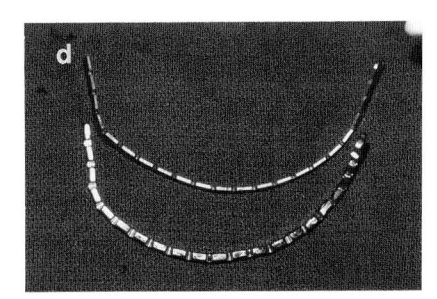

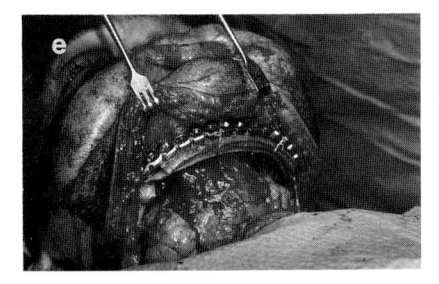

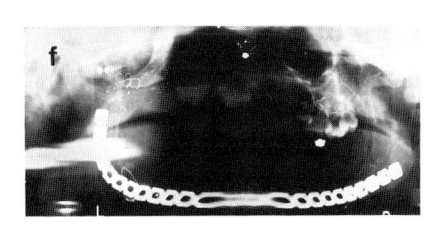

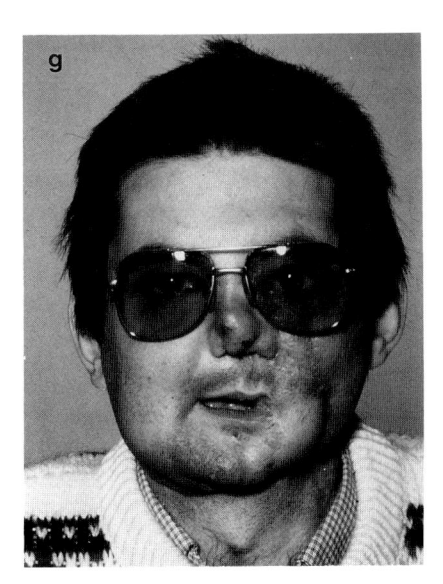

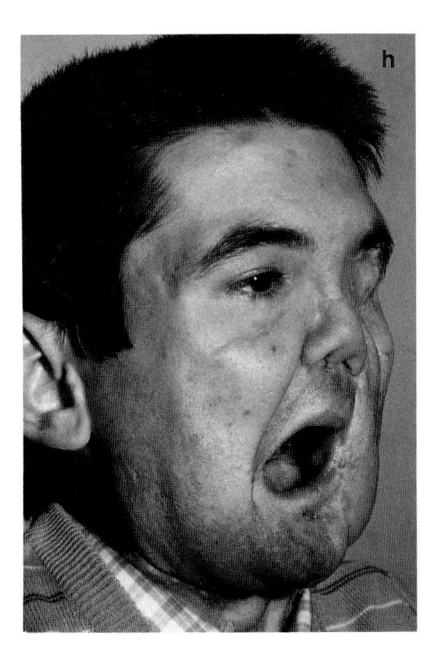

Figure 53.6 (a) This young man experienced severe gunshot wounds to the face, which resulted in massive loss of midfacial and mandibular bone. Note the severe shrinkage of soft tissue, which is stuck and scarred into the bony gaps. There is severe loss of mandibular function accompanied by loss of lip support and constant drooling. (b) Lateral view shows extensive bony loss and shrinkage of soft tissue. Note missing support of the lower third of the face due to extensive mandibular bone loss. (c) Exposure through an upper neck incision identifies the ends of the mandible (R = right, L = left). The displaced submandibular glands (S) can be seen. (C = chin.) (d) A template is taken of the defect and transferred to a reconstruction plate, which is overbent slightly to increase the internal expansion of the contracted soft tissues. (e) The reconstruction plate is firmly anchored to either end. Multiple stacks of split rib grafts are now anchored underneath the plate by multiple circumferential wires. (f) Panorex x ray at three years shows the reconstruction plate in place. Good bony continuity has been restored with the rib grafts across the bony gap. This is difficult to see in the panorex. (g) Anteroposterior view shows the patient at three years, following recent secondary nasal bone grafting. Note good contour restoration of lower third of the face and excellent lip support. There is no more drooling. (h) Excellent restoration of mandibular function and good lip support are shown.

Figure 53.7 (a) This young boy has an extensive, malignant, congenital form of osteopetrosis with massive involvement including osteomyelitis of the mandible. Note severe erosion of the skin with multiple sinuses. (b) An intraoral view demonstrates complete erosion of the mandible into the oral cavity with loss of the superior portion of the mandible and mucosa. Note the large abscess cavity (arrows). (c) Preoperative panorex demonstrates the moth-eaten appearance of the entire mandible and the enormous cavity in the symphyseal region. (d) Inferior view of the chin and upper neck demonstrates multiple areas of skin erosion and actively draining sinuses. Planned excision of skin and sinuses to approach the underlying mandible is visualized. (e) Total resection of the involved mandible is seen. Through and through defect from the neck into the oral cavity can be seen. The tongue (T) can be seen lying freely in the wound. (f) Resected specimen shows the total mandibular resection. Note the markedly deformed and osteomyelitic mandible. (g) A template is now taken of the missing mandible. (h) This template is now sent to the factory, where a total mandibular prosthesis containing bilateral condylar heads is manufactured. (i) At six weeks, the inferior incision is reopened and a pocket is created for the mandibular prosthesis. Care is taken to avoid entering the oral cavity. (j) Surrounding soft tissue and muscle are mobilized as soft-tissue flaps, and the plate is completely wrapped with these flaps. (k) Postoperative panorex at five years demonstrates good position of the mandibular prosthesis. Note total reconstruction of the mandible with one of the condylar heads placed in each glenoid fossa. (l) Appearance at six years demonstrates good restoration of mandibular contour and support. There has been no recurrence of infection following resection and reconstruction of the total mandible. (m) Lateral view demonstrates good contour and restoration of the lower third of the face. All sinuses have remained healed.

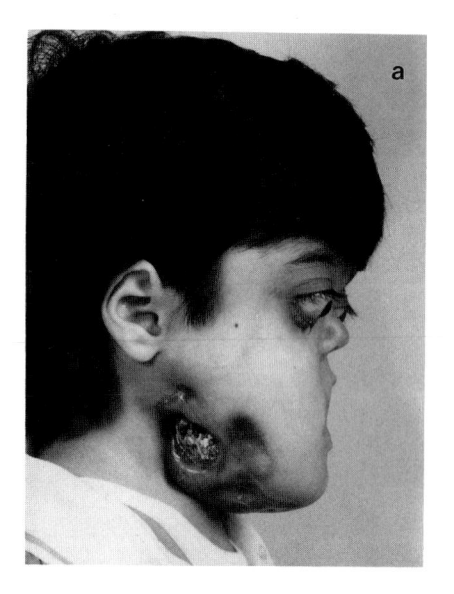

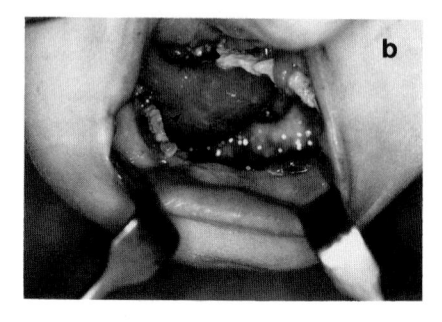

Ideally today, this mandibular gap would be bridged by a free-vascularized bone graft, considering the recent advances in this field. However, the use of plate and screw fixation and conventional bone grafting in this case has provided a long-term, stable reconstruction and is an option to consider if free-vascularized techniques are unavailable.

Osteopetrosis of the Mandible

Osteopetrosis (marble bone disease of Albers-Schönberg) is an uncommon genetic disorder characterized by a symmetric and progressive increase in density of bone throughout the skeletal system. Normal cortical and cancellous bone is replaced by excessively dense (but paradoxically weak) bone that is susceptible to pathological fractures. The production of osteopetrotic bone appears due either to a lack of physiologic bone resorption or to a disturbance in the timing of bone apposition and resorption. Both mechanisms may be related to a qualitative or quantitative deficiency in osteoelastic activity.

Fractures of the mandible have been reported following dental extractions in patients with osteopetrosis, and both the upper and lower jaws are thought to be more susceptible to osteomyelitis secondary to dental disease.

Bone involved with osteopetrosis is thought to have compromised vascular nutrition. Thus, local infection is more likely to lead to osteomyelitis, with death of the osteocytes and subsequent sequestrum formation. Osteomyelitis presents a problem equal to that of osteoradionecrosis. In the mandible, long-term antibiotic therapy, as well as multiple debridements, sequestrectomies, or even radical resection, may be required to control the infection.

Albers-Schönberg disease is found in patients of all ages. The most common classification recognizes two clinical types: the malignant variety and the benign adult variety. The clinically malignant "congenital" variety, the most severe form of the disease, is usually present at birth or is diagnosed by the time of early childhood. Patients in this group rarely survive adolescence, and death usually results from secondary infection or anemia.

Case Report

An 8-year-old boy, who had the malignant "congenital" variety of osteopetrosis, presented with generalized osteomyelitic involvement of the mandible (see Figure 53.7). The symphyseal region of the mandible demonstrated an enormous abscess cavity that had eroded into the oral cavity. The remainder of the mandible was extensively involved with osteomyelitis, ac-

Unusual Applications of Plating 679

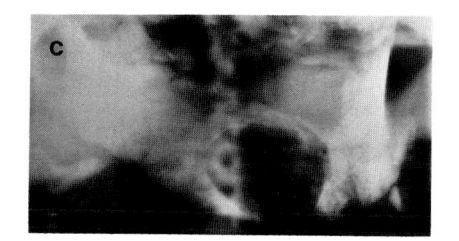

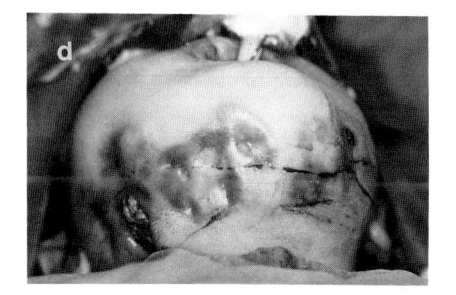

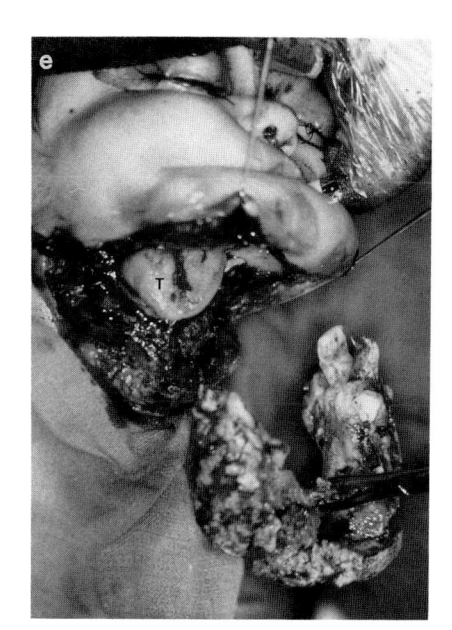

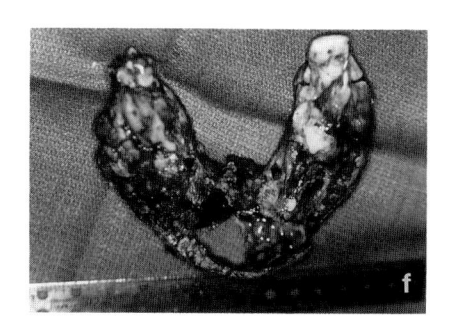

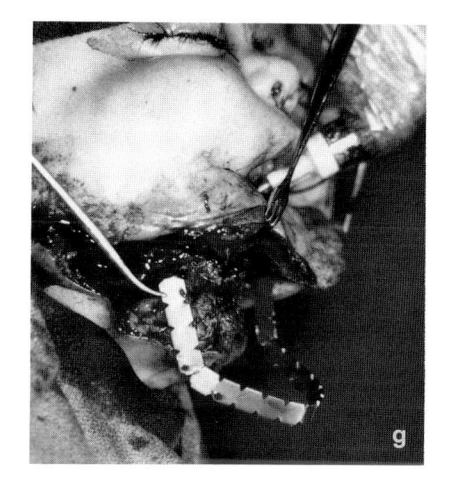

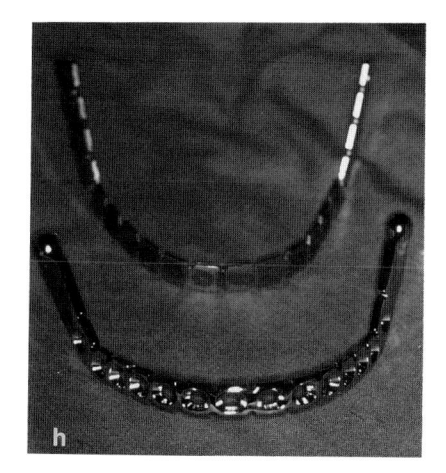

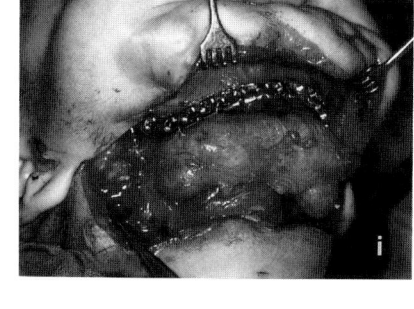

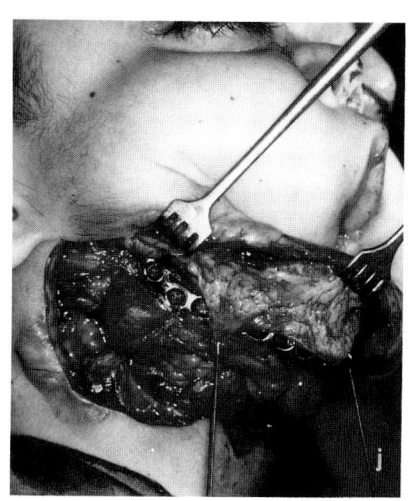

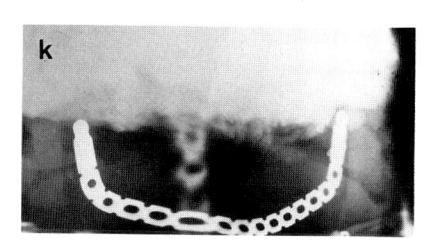

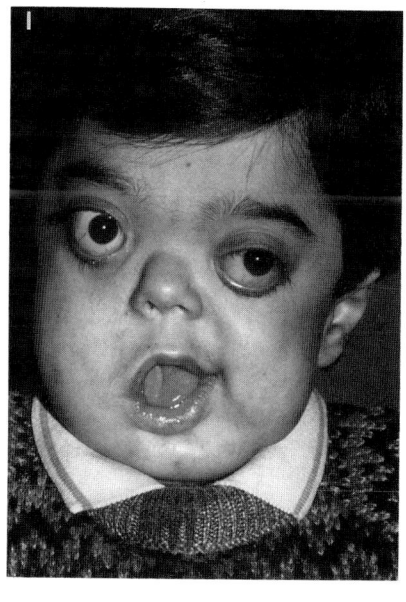

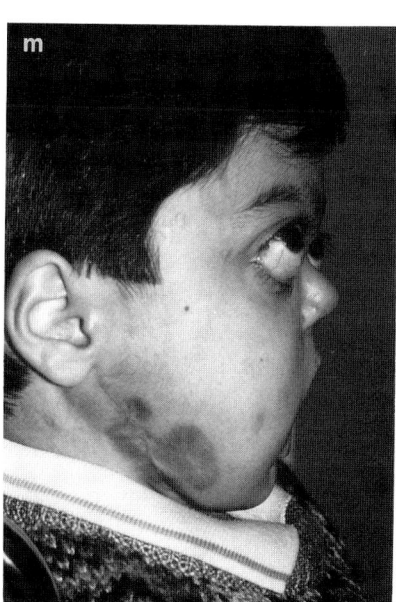

companied by multiple external sinus tracts in the cheeks and neck. The patient had failed to respond to antibiotic and local bone treatment over a prolonged period. The chronic infection, anemia, and nutritional deficiency had become life-threatening, necessitating radical surgical intervention.

A total resection of the entire mandible was performed in combination with careful repair of the intraoral lining. A template was taken of the missing mandible, and the external soft tissue was closed. The mandibular template was then used to construct a custom stainless steel total mandibular prosthesis with bilateral condylar heads.

At six weeks, the patient was returned to the operating room. The external incision was reopened and the pocket recreated for the mandibular prosthesis. Care was taken not to breach the intraoral lining. The prosthesis was inserted and wrapped with adjacent muscle and soft-tissue flaps. Primary healing occurred without infection. Six years later, the prosthesis has remained in situ with no infection and satisfactory function. Soft-tissue expansion of the lower third of the face has been maintained, and the nutritional and hematological abnormalities have remained corrected.

SUMMARY

With the experience gained from use in trauma, orthognathic, tumor and craniofacial surgery, the surgeon can use plate and screw techniques for the treatment of more unusual problems. The principles and techniques of rigid fixation allow him to significantly expand his reconstructive armamentarium.

Index

Absolute stability, in fracture fixation, 5
Albers-Schönberg disease, unusual applications of plates and, 678–680
  case study of, 678–680
Alloplastic bridging, in ablative tumor surgery with Mandibular Reconstruction System, 598–600
Alloy, of implant material, 33
Angle fractures, lag screws in mandibular fractures and, 189–191
  biomechanics of, 189–190
  surgical technique for, 190–191
Animal studies, infection and, 52–53
Anisotropic materials, for medical devices, 34
Annealing, for medical devices, 34
Anterior nasal spine of midface, unusual applications of plates, 673
Antibiotics
  for mandibular fractures, 186
  in mandibular reconstruction for tumor defects using AO plates and THORP, 607–608
  as therapy for infections of mandibular fractures, 233
  as therapy for nonunions of mandibular fractures, 233
Antigens, biocompatibility and, 49–50
AO Mandibular System
  AO Maxillofacial Implant System and, tenets of, 125–127
  dynamic compression plate for, 126
  eccentric dynamic compression plate for, 126
  reconstruction plate for, 126
AO Maxillofacial Implant System, 124–133
  AO Mandibular System and, tenets of, 125–127
  craniofacial instrumentation for, 131–133
    orbital-floor plates for, 132–133
    plates for, 132
    templates for, 132
  history of, 124–125
  instrumentation for, 127–133
    materials for, 127–128
    mandibular implants for, 128–133

    plates for, 128
AO plates
  for complex tumor reconstruction, 615–616
  with THORP
    in mandibular reconstruction for tumor defects. See Mandibular reconstruction, for tumor defects using AO plates
Apert syndrome
  block orbitalfacial advancement with facial bipartition osteotomies and, 553, 556, 558
  as craniofacial deformity, in subcraniofacial approach to craniofacial surgery, 573, 575
  craniomaxillofacial surgery and, 528
  Le Fort III osteotomy and, case study of, 550–551
  plates and screws in craniofacial deformities and case study of, 513, 516–517
Arbeitsgemeinschaft fur Osteosynthesefragen, 124
Arch bars
  for mandibular fractures, 181
  tension banding and, as complication in mandibular fractures, 226
Articular cartilage, repair of, 69–70
Association of Osteosynthesis/Association for the Study of Internal Fixation, 124
Asymmetries. *See* specific types of asymmetries

Binder's syndrome, midfacial and maxillary fractures in craniomaxillofacial surgery and, 540
Biocompatibility
  biologic response of, 48
  definition of, 48
  immunology and, 49–51
  of implant materials, 48–53
  infection and, 52–53
  testing methods for, 48–49
Biodegradable materials, as implant materials, 28–29
Biofunctionality of implant materials, 38
Bipartition osteotomies, facial. *See* Facial bipartition oste-

otomies
Block hydroxypatite. *See* Hydroxypatite
Block orbitofacial advancement, facial bipartition osteotomies and, 553–560
  Apert's syndrome and, 556, 558
  exposure in, 554
  frontal shortening in, 556
  surgical procedure for, 554–556
    exposure in, 554
Blowout fractures, treatment of pediatric facial fractures and, 399–400
Bone. *See also* Facial bone; Fracture(s)
  consistency of, 3
  continuity of, as complication in mandibular fractures, 229–230
  definition of, 3
  fragments of, plates and screws for
    in nasoethmoid-orbital fractures, 294
  frontal. *See also* Frontal bone fractures
  functions of, 4
  grafts of
    in ablative tumor surgery with Mandibular Reconstruction System, 601–604
    in congenital craniofacial surgery, 507–508
    in gunshot wounds, 340
    for maxillary and mandibular asymmetry, 590
    with mesh plates, craniomaxillofacial surgery and, 533, 538–539
    for orbital fractures, 309
    in post-traumatic maxillary and mandibular reconstruction, 385–386
    for reconstruction following tumor surgery with THORP, 630–632
    in superior division of panfacial injuries, 335
    three-dimensional mandibular reconstruction with vascularized bone grafts and, 642–644
    in total functional mandibular reconstruction, 651–652
      case studies of, 652–655
    vascularized, three-dimensional mandibular reconstruction and. *See* Mandibular reconstruction, three-dimensional
  healing of, 3–6
    with absolute stability, 5–6
    biomechanical aspects of, 4–5
    direct, 5–6
    indirect, 4–5
    plate-induced porosis in, 6
    problems in, 6
  immobilization of, effecting masticatory system, 63–64
  loose segments of, in maxillomandibular fixation for complex mandibular fractures, 197
  loss of
    nasoethmoid-orbital fractures with, 290
      plates and screws for, 292, 294
  microanatomy of, 3
  nonunion of in midface, unusual applications of plates and case study of, 673
  pathological, as complication of rigid internal fixation of mandibular fractures, 224
  segments of, in congenital craniofacial surgery, 508
  structure of, 3

Bony region, isolated nasoethmoid-orbital fractures in, 286–287
Brachycephaly, plates and screws in craniofacial deformities and case study of, 521, 524–525
Buccal plate application, for reconstruction following tumor surgery with THORP, 626–627
Bulk material testing of implant materials, 38

Canthal ligament, medial
  in nasoethmoid-orbital fractures, 284–286
    plates and screws for, 298
  orbital fractures and, 316
Canthopexy, medial
  orbital fractures and, 314–315
Canthoplasty, lateral
  orbital fractures and, 315
Cantilever action as biomechanical consideration in osteointegration, 173–174
Carcinogenicity, immunology and, 51–52
Cartilage, articular
  repair of, 69–70
Cast materials for medical devices, 33–34
Cells, of bone, 3
Central zone concept
  in inferior division of panfacial injuries, 332–333
  of panfacial injuries, 331–332
  in superior division of panfacial injuries, 334
Cephalometric analysis
  in diagnosis of single-segment osteotomies, 546
  of midface fractures, 353
Ceramics, as implant materials, 28–29
Champy's system, 116–122
  equipment for, 117–118
  history of, 116
  mandibular fracture and, 118–122, 120
    complications in, 120–121
  osteosynthesis material for
    biophysical characteristics of, 116–117
    miniplates and, 117
  technique for, 118–122
Cheek, orbital fractures and, 315
Chin asymmetry, 586
Chin surgery, plates and screws in cleft lip deformities and, 469
Cleaning, of medical devices, 34
Cleft, midline cranio-orbital with orbital hypertelorism, case study of, 517
Clefting syndromes, midfacial and maxillary fractures in craniomaxillofacial surgery and, 540
Cleft lip deformities, 486–499
  anatomy of, 486–487
  bilateral
    plates and screws in, 467–468
    case studies of, 474
  cephalometric analysis of, 487–495
    architectural analysis and, 488–495
    structural analysis and, 495
  clinical examination of, 487
  diagnosis of, 487–495
  isolated
    plates and screws in, 468

case studies of, 474, 482
plates and screws in, 466–484
  analysis of occlusion in, 467
  case studies of, 469–481
  chin surgery and, 469
  complications of, 482
  diagnosis of, 466–467
  long-term results and, 482–484
  residual deformities and, 467–468
  surgical techniques for, 468–469
    mandibular, 468–469
    maxillary, 468
  treatment of, 466–467
surgery for, 495–498
  functional genioplasty and, 495–496
  incisions in, 496–497
  maxillary osteotomy and, 497
  nasolabial muscles and, 497–498
unilateral
  plates and screws in, 467
  case studies of, 469–474
unilateral labiomaxillopalatine, 487
Closure, in mandibular reconstruction for tumor defects using AO plates and THORP, 607
Cobalt-chromium alloys
  as corrosion property of metal, 47
  as mechanical property of metal, 43
  as metal implant material, 36–37
  history of, 30–31
Cold working, for medical devices, 34
Collagen, in connective tissues, 72
Comminuted fractures
  lag screws in mandibular fractures and, 192–193
  plates and screw for, in nasoethmoid-orbital fractures, 291–294
  selection of plates for, 184
Compression
  eccentric dynamic plate for, 12
  in fracture fixation, 5
  for fractures, 9–11
  principles of, 7–14
  tension band and, 11
Compression osteosynthesis, as complication of rigid internal fixation of mandibular fractures, 227–228
Computed tomography, effects of implant materials on, 37
Condylar fractures, lag screws in mandibular fractures and, 191–192
Condylar neck fractures, surgical technique for in Mandibular Compression Screw System, 88–89
Condylar positioning, in combined surgery with maxilla and mandible, 455
Condylar process, of mandibular fractures
  treatment of pediatric facial fractures and, 400–402
Condylar prosthesis, for reconstruction following tumor surgery with THORP, 628
Condyles
  positioning of, as complication in mandibular fractures, 218
  for tumor defects using AO plates and THORP, 608–609
Congenital clefts, midfacial and maxillary fractures in craniomaxillofacial surgery and, 540
Congenital disorders, craniomaxillofacial surgery and, 528

Congenital maxillary hypoplasia, midfacial and maxillary fractures in craniomaxillofacial surgery and, 540
Connective tissues
  immobilization of, on masticatory system, 70–74
  periarticular. See Periarticular connective tissues
Contact healing, in direct bone healing, 5–6
Coronal flap, eyebrow and
  in subcranial approach to craniofacial surgery and craniofacial traumatology, 563
Coronal plane, ocular position in
  orbital fractures and, 316
Coronal synostosis
  bilateral, case study of, 521, 524–525
  unilateral, craniomaxillofacial surgery and, 528
Corrosion
  cracking, 46
  forms of, 45
  galvanic, 45
  general, 45
  localized, 46
  passivation methods of, 46–47
  properties of implant materials, 44–48
  stress, 46
  systemic considerations of, 47–48
  testing of, 46
Corrosion fatigue, 46
Cranial analysis, in cephalometric analysis of cleft lip deformities, 488–490
Cranial fractures
  anatomy of, in post-traumatic cranio-orbital reconstruction, 371
  plates and screws for nasoethmoid-orbital fractures in, 297
  treatment of in post-traumatic cranio-orbital reconstruction, 372–373
Cranial vault
  craniotomy of, with three-quarter orbital osteotomies
    for bilateral coronal stenosis, case study of, 521, 524–525
    for brachycephaly, case study of, 521, 524–525
    for trigonocephaly, case study of, 517
  osteotomy of, with monobloc bipartition osteotomy
    for midline cranio-orbital cleft with orbital hypertelorism, case study of, 517
  reshaping of
    with monobloc bipartition osteotomy for Apert syndrome, case study of, 513, 516–517
    with monobloc osteotomy for Crouzon's disease, case study of, 513
Cranial vault fractures
  in superior division of panfacial injuries, 334
  treatment of pediatric facial fractures and, 398–399
Craniofacial deformit(y)ies, 357–370
  combined nasoethmoid-orbital and Le Fort deformities as, 363, 366
  enophthalmos as, 360–361
  exposure in, 358
  fixation in, 358–359
  management of, 359
  orbitozygomatic deformity as, 361–363
  plates and screws in, 512–525
    Apert syndrome and, case studies of, 513, 516–517

bilateral coronal synostosis and case study of, 521, 524–525
Crouzon's disease and case study of, 513, 517, 520–521
midline cranio-orbital cleft with orbital hypertelorism and case study of, 517
Treacher Collins syndrome and case study of, 521
trigonocephaly and case study of, 517
in subcraniofacial approach to craniofacial surgery, 571, 573–575
results of, 575, 577–578
surgical technique for, 571, 573
treatment of, 358–369
Craniofacial injuries, extended nasoethmoid-orbital fractures with, 288
Craniofacial malformations. See Craniofacial deformit(y)ies
Craniofacial osteotomies, for post-traumatic craniofacial deformities. See Craniofacial deformit(y)ies
Craniofacial region, upper
craniomaxillofacial surgery and, 525–533
Craniofacial surgery
for congenital deformities, 507–508, 507–511
bone segments in, 508
craniofaciostenosis and, 509
craniosynotosis and, 508
hemifacial microsomia and, 509
orbital hypertelorism and, 509
stabilization in, 508–510
Treacher Collins syndrome and, 509–510
in infants, Micro-System for, 100
subcranial approach to, 561–579
craniofacial deformities and, 571, 573–575
results of, 575, 577–578
surgical technique for, 571, 573
craniofacial traumatology and, 561–571
case studies in, 569–575
nonsurgical conservative treatment of, 562
subcranial approach to, 563–571
surgical treatment of, 562–563
treatment modalities in, 562–571
Craniofacial suspension devices, 245–246
Craniofacial traumatology, subcranial approach to craniofacial surgery and, 561–571
case studies in, 569–575
nonsurgical conservative treatment and, 562
subcranial approach and, 563–571
surgical treatment and, 562–563
treatment modalities in, 562–571
Craniofaciostenosis, congenital craniofacial deformities and, 509
Craniomaxillofacial region, clinical applications of implant material for, 28
Craniomaxillofacial surgery
bone grafting in, with mesh plates, 533, 538–539
goal of, 525–526
Luhr Vitallium Maxillofacial Systems for, 105, 107–115
mandibular fractures and, 542
maxillary fractures and, 539–542
midfacial fractures and, 539–542
osteotomy design for, 527–543
upper craniofacial region and, 525–533
Craniomaxillofacial trauma, Vitallium Mini-System for, 95

Cranio-orbital reconstruction, post-traumatic, 371–378
anatomy of, 371–372
cranial fractures in, 371
glabellar fractures in, 371
nasoethmoid-orbital fractures in, 371
orbital fractures in, 372
orbitozygomatic fractures in, 371
supraorbital fractures in, 371
complications in, 376
diagnosis in, 372
long-term results and, 377
radiography in, 372
technique in, 377–378
treatment for, 372–377
cranial fractures and, 372–373
glabellar fractures and, 373–375
nasoethmoid-orbital fractures and, 375
orbital fractures and, 377
orbitozygomatic fractures and, 375–376
supraorbital fractures and, 373
Craniosynostosis
congenital craniofacial surgery and, 508
craniomaxillofacial surgery and, 528, 530
Cranium
anatomical considerations of monocortical miniplate, osteosynthesis in, 16–17
biomechanical principles of monocortical miniplate, osteosynthesis on, 20
Crouzon's disease
block orbitalfacial advancement with facial bipartition, osteotomies and, 553, 556
craniomaxillofacial surgery and, 528
midfacial and maxillary fractures in craniomaxillofacial, surgery and, 540
plates and screws in craniofacial deformities and case study of, 513, 517, 520–521
Cutting cones, in Haversian remodeling, 6

Deformities, residual
plates and screws in cleft lip deformities and, 467–468
Delayed unions
aseptic, 234
infected, 234
Demineralization, 53
Dental alveolar fracture, treatment of pediatric facial fractures and, 402
Dental analysis, in cephalometric analysis of cleft lip deformities, 494–495
Dental casts, in post-traumatic maxillary and mandibular reconstruction, 385
Dental compensations, spontaneous
in orthodontic surgery, 501
Dental implants
intraosseous, for reconstruction following tumor surgery with THORP, 630–632
for tumor defects using AO plates and THORP, 608
Würzburg Titanium System for, 148–149
Dental occlusion, 353–356
as complication in midface fractures, 351
Dental Osteointegration System. See ITI-Bonefit Dental Osteointegration System

Dentistry, osteointegration in, 167–169
Direct bone healing, 5–6
Dolichocephaly, craniomaxillofacial surgery and, 528
Double-jaw surgery, in orthodontic surgery, 502
Downsliding technique, in Le Fort osteotomies, 434–435
Drainage, for osteitis of mandibular fractures, 237
Drains
　in mandibular reconstruction for tumor defects, 6
　in mandibular reconstruction for tumor defects using AO plates and THORP, 607
Dural repair and fracture reduction in subcranial approach to craniofacial surgery and traumatology, 566–569
Dynamic compression plate (DCP)
　for AO Mandibular System, 126
　for nonunion of mandibular fractures, 238
Dysplasia
　fronto-orbital fibrous, case study of pediatric head and neck tumors and, 664–666
　skeletal. See Cleft lip deformities
Dystopia, orbital, 587

Eccentric dynamic compression plate (EDCP), 12
　for AO Mandibular System, 126
　for nonunion of mandibular fractures, 238–239
　tension banding and, as complication of rigid internal fixation of mandibular fractures, 226–227
Elastic modulus of implant materials, 39–40
Enchondrosarcoma of maxilla, orbit, and zygoma
　case study of pediatric head and neck tumors and, 668
Enophthalmos
　as craniofacial deformity, 360–361
　orbital fractures and, 315–316
Ewing's sarcoma of zygomatic arch
　case study of pediatric head and neck tumors and, 657, 660–662
Exposure
　in block orbitalfacial advancement with facial bipartition osteotomies, 554
　in complex mandibular fractures, 195–196
　as complication in mandibular fractures, 217–218
　in craniofacial deformities, 358
　frontal bone fractures and, 324
　in Le Fort osteotomies, 427–428
　in mandibular fractures, 181
　nasoethmoid-orbital fractures and, 290
　optic nerve decompression and, in subcranial approach to craniofacial surgery and craniofacial traumatology, 564–566
　orbital fractures and, 310
　in post-traumatic maxillary and mandibular reconstruction, 385
　in sagittal split ramus osteotomies, 435–437
　of zygomatic arch, 269
Extracellular fluid volume, changes in
　in protoglycens, 72
Eyebrow, coronal flap and
　in subcranial approach to craniofacial surgery and craniofacial traumatology, 563

Fabrication for medical devices, 34
Face, upper
　dimensions of, 352
　　anatomical considerations of monocortical miniplate osteosynthesis in, 16–17
　　biomechanical principles of monocortical miniplate osteosynthesis on, 20
Facial aesthetics, plates and screws in cleft lip deformities and, 466–467
Facial analysis
　anteroposterior relationships of, in cephalometric analysis of cleft lip deformities, 490–493
　in cephalometric analysis of cleft lip deformities, 490–495
　dental analysis of, in cephalometric analysis of cleft lip deformities, 494–495
　vertical relationships of, in cephalometric analysis of cleft lip deformities, 493–494
Facial asymmetries, 582–590
　acquired, 582–583
　classification of, 582–583
　congenital, 582–583
　diagnosis of, 584–586
　etiology of, 582–583
　indications for surgery of, 584
　patient assessment and, 583–584
　pediatric, 587
　surgical planning for, 584–586
　surgical techniques for, 587–590
Facial bipartition osteotomies, block orbitofacial advancement and, 553–560
　Apert's syndrome and, 556, 558
　frontal shortening in, 556
　surgical procedure for, 554–556
Facial bone, structural characteristics of, 3–4
Facial clefting syndromes, midfacial and maxillary fractures in craniomaxillofacial surgery and, 540
Facial deformities. See Craniofacial deformit(y)ies
Facial fractures, pediatric, 396–417
　airway management of, 398
　anatomy of, 397–398
　classification of, 397
　retrospective chart review of, 396–398
　surgical anatomy of, 397–398
　treatment of, 398–402
　　blowout fractures and, 399
　　case reports of, 402–417
　　cranial vault fractures and, 398–399
　　dental alveolar fractures and, 402
　　lateral orbital rim fractures and, 398–399
　　Le Fort fractures and, 399
　　mandibular fractures and, 400–402
　　maxillomandibular fixation and, 402
　　nasal fractures and, 399–400
　　nasofrontoethmoid fractures, 399
　　parasymphyseal fractures and, 402
　　supraorbital rim fractures and, 398–399
　　symphyseal fractures and, 397
　　zygomatic fractures and, 399
Facial projection, in panfacial injuries, 331
Facial skeleton, expansion of, 461–465
　anatomy of, 461–462
　gross findings of, 463
　histologic findings of, 463

patient selection for, 461
radiographic findings of, 463–464
results of, 462–464
technique for, 461–462
Fatigue versus stress, of implant materials, 42
Fibromatosis of mandible
case study of pediatric head and neck tumors and, 662–664
Fissures, palpebral, orbital fractures and, 316
Fistula, donor site and
three-dimensional mandibular reconstruction with vascularized bone grafts and, 638
Fistulectomy for infections of mandibular fractures, 237–238
Fixation, rigid
history of, 79–81
Fixation osteosynthesis
biomechanics of, 9
principles of, 7–14
screws used in, 7–9. *See also* specific types of screws
Fixation screw, 13–14
Fixture(s)
force distribution to, as biomechanical considerations in osteointegration, 172–174
single, in osteointegration, 174
Flexible prosthesis as biomechanical consideration in osteointegration, 173
Force of implant materials, 39
Forehead asymmetry, 587
Foreign bodies, infection and, 52–53
Fracture-line osteitis
definition of, 233–234
diagnosis of, 233–234
Fracture reduction
dural repair and, in subcranial approach to craniofacial surgery and craniofacial traumatology, 566–569
in maxillomandibular fixation for complex mandibular fractures, 197
Fracture(s). *See also* Bone; specific types of fracture
acute, incorrect placement of screws as complication in mandibular fractures, 222–223
aim of treatment of, 4
with bone defects, complex mandibular fractures and, 202, 204, 207
compression for, 9–11
defect, selection of plates for, 184
fixation of, 5
open, mandibular fractures and, 186
panfacial, Le Fort fractures and, 257, 260–261
plate selection
by location of, 182
by type of, 182
reduction of, in mandibular fractures, 182
Fracture segment, malalignment of
as complications in midface fractures, 351
Free flap mandibular reconstruction. *See* Mandibular reconstruction, three-dimensional
Frontal bone defect, following tumor resection and radiation therapy
case study of pediatric head and neck tumors and, 666–668
Frontal bone fractures, 323–329

anatomy of, 323–324
complications of, 326–329
diagnosis of, 324
exposure and, 324
frontal bone and, 325–326
frontal sinus fractures and, 324–325
indications for surgery of, 324–326
results and, 326–329
surgical technique for, 324–326
Frontal plane analysis, in post-traumatic maxillary reconstruction, 382
Frontal shortening, in block orbitalfacial advancement with facial bipartition osteotomies, 556
Frontal sinus, Micro-System for, 110
Frontal sinus fractures
frontal bone fractures and, 324–325
plates and screws for nasoethmoid-orbital fractures in, 297
Frontobasilar injuries, with extended nasoethmoid-orbital injuries, 288
Frontonasal buttress fixation, plates and screws for nasoethmoid-orbital fractures, 290–291
Fronto-orbital fibrous dysplasia
case study of pediatric head and neck tumors and, 664–666
Fronto-zygomatic suture line
in anatomy of zygomatic fractures, 273–274
of zygomatic fractures, 271

Gap healing, 6
Genioplasty
functional, surgery for cleft lip deformities, 495–496
for maxillary and mandibular asymmetry, 590
Vitallium Mini-System for, 103, 105
Glabellar fractures
anatomy of, in post-traumatic cranio-orbital reconstruction, 371
treatment of, in post-traumatic cranio-orbital reconstruction, 373–375
Globe, projection of
orbital fractures and, 315–316
Glycosaminoglycan, changes in
in protoglycens, 72–73
Grafts, bone. *See* Bone, grafts of
Gunshot wounds, 338–349
mandible in, 340
midface bone in, 339–340
reconstruction and, 338–349
soft tissue in, 340, 347–349

Haversian remodeling, in fracture healing, 6
Head and neck tumors, pediatric, 656–670
aggressive fibromatosis of mandible and case study of, 662–664
benign, 656–657
case studies of, 657–668
congenital, 656–657
enchondrosarcoma of maxilla, orbit, and zygoma, case study of, 668
Ewing's sarcoma of zygomatic arch, case study of, 657, 660–662
frontal bone defect following tumor resection and radiation

therapy, case study of, 666–668
fronto-orbital fibrous dysplasia, case study of, 664–666
malignant, 656–657
rhabdomyosarcoma of maxilla, case study of, 657
Healing. *See* Bone, healing of
Hemifacial microsomia, congenital craniofacial deformities and, 509
Hemorrhage, in subcondylar fractures, 210
Hollow-cylinder implants, in ITI-Bonefit Dental Osteointegration System, 156–157
Hollow-screw implants, in ITI-Bonefit Dental Osteointegration System, 157–158
Hot working for medical devices, 34
Hydoxypatite, 461–465
    anatomy for, 461–462
    gross findings of, 463
    histologic findings of, 463
    patient selection for, 461
    radiologic findings of, 463–464
    results of, 462–464
    technique for, 461–462
Hypersensitivity, immunology and, 50–51
Hypertelorism
    midfacial and maxillary fractures in craniomaxillofacial surgery and, 540
    orbital
        congenital craniofacial deformities and, 509
        midline cranio-orbital cleft, case study of, 517

Ilium, donor site and
    three-dimensional mandibular reconstruction with vascularized bone grafts and, 638
Immobilization, mandibular
    effects of on masticatory system. *See* Masticatory system
Immune response
    biocompatibility and, 49
    types of, 49–50
Immunology
    biocompatibility and, 49–51
    carcinogenicity and, 51–52
    hypersensitivity and, 50–51
Implant materials, 28–53
    anatomic considerations for, 31–32
    annealing and, 34
    biocompatibility of, 48–53
    biodegradable materials as, 28–29
    ceramics as, 28–29
    clinical applications in craniomaxillofacial region of, 28
    corrosion properties of, 44–48. *See also* Corrosion
    effects of on medical imaging, 37–38
    effects of on radiation therapy, 38
    material modification and manufacturing for, 33–34
    mechanical properties of, 38–44
    mechanical properties of metals as, 42–44
    metallic structure of, 32–38
    metals as, 28–31. *See also* Metals
    physical properties of metals as, 36–37
    polymers as, 28–29
    principles of, 28–53
    requirements of, 28
    working and, 34–35

Implant systems. *See* specific types of implant systems
Incisions
    as complication in mandibular fractures, 217–218
    in mandibular fractures, 181
    in mandibular reconstruction for tumor defects using AO plates and THORP, 606
    for osteitis of mandibular fractures, 237
    surgery for, in cleft lip deformities, 496–497
Indirect bone healing, 4, 5
Infection
    biocompatibility and, 52–53
    in bone healing, 6
    of mandibular fractures. *See* Mandibular fractures, infections of
        combination therapy for, 241–243
        fistulectomy of, 237–238
Intermaxillary fixation (IMF). *See* Maxillomandibular fixation (MMF)
Intraoral approach for mandibular fractures, 85–88
Intraorbital fractures, Micro-System for, 110
Isotropic materials for medical devices, 34
ITI-Bonefit Dental Osteointegration System, 152–162
    bone reactions and, 153
    characteristics of, 154–159
    for distal extension in mandible, 160–161
    for edentulous mandible, 160
    epithelium and, 153
    gingival collar and, 153
    hollow-cylinder implants in, 156–157
    hollow-screw implants in, 157–158
    implant material for, 152
    implant surface of, 152
    indications for, 160–162
    as integrated system, 159
    packaging of, 158–159
    presentation of, 158–159
    properties of, 154–159
    screw implants in, 158
    for single tooth replacement in maxilla, 161
    soft tissues reactions and, 153
    subepithelial connective tissue and, 153
    tissue reactions and, 152–154

Jaw asymmetry, 586
Jaw deformities. *See* Cleft lip deformities
Joints, synovial
    immobilization of effecting masticatory system, 67–70

Kitayama lag screw technique, 192

Lag screw(s), 12–13. *See also* Screw(s)
    compression osteosynthesis and, as complication in mandibular fractures, 228
    Kitayama technique of, 192
    in mandibular fractures, 181. *See also* Mandibular fractures, lag screws in
    for nonunion of mandibular fractures, 239
    Petzel technique of, 192
    through plate compression osteosynthesis and, as complication in mandibular fractures, 228
Lag screw osteosynthesis

definition of, 22
indications for, 23–24
principles of, 22–23
technique of, 24–27
Lag screw principle, in surgical technique in Mandibular Compression Screw System, 88
Lateral-load experiments in osteointegration, 169–170
Lateral zone concept
in inferior division of panfacial injuries, 333–334
in superior division of panfacial injuries, 334–336
Lattice defects in metallic structure, 32–33
Le Fort deformities
combined with nasoethmoid-orbital deformity, 363, 366
maxillary reconstruction and, 387–392
Le Fort downfracture technique, in Le Fort osteotomies, 423
Le Fort downsliding technique, in Le Fort osteotomies, 426
Le Fort fractures, 245–261. See also Midface fractures
anatomical considerations of, 247–248
displaced zygomatic arch in, 255–257
with extended nasoethmoid-orbital fractures, 289–290
history of, 249–250
mandibular condylar positioning for, 254–255
mandibular plates for, 254
maxillary sinus drainage in, 261
miniplates for, 250–261
buttress plating for, 250–253
panfacial fractures and, 257, 260–261
sagittal maxillary fractures and, 257
in superior division of panfacial injuries, 335
surgical technique for, 248–249
treatment of pediatric facial fractures and, 399
Vitallium Mini-System for, 97–100
Würzburg Titanium System for, 145
Le Fort osteotomies. See also Cleft lip deformities; Le Fort I osteotomies; Le Fort III osteotomies
case studies of, 443–449
Le Fort I osteotomies, 423–435. See also Le Fort osteotomies; Le Fort III osteotomies
biological foundation of, 423–424
complications in, 435
design of, 424–427
disadvantages of, 435
downsliding technique in, 434–435
exposure of site of, 427–428
high-level, design of, 426–427
inferior repositioning of maxilla in, 434
Le Fort downfracture technique in, 423
Le Fort downsliding technique in, 426
low-level, design of, 425
maxillary step osteotomies as, design of, 425–426
osteotomy design in, 428
plates and screws in, 430–434
sectioning maxilla for, 428–430
segmentation of maxilla in, 433–434
stabilization in, 430–434
traditional, design of, 425
Le Fort III osteotomies, 545–551. See also Le Fort osteotomies; Le Fort I osteotomies
anatomy of, 545
case study of, 500–501, 550–551
complications of, 549

for Crouzon's disease, case study of, 517, 520–521
diagnosis of, 545–547
multiple-segment osteotomies and, 546–547
single-segment osteotomies and, 546–547
long-term follow-up and, 549–550
technique of, 547–549
Lingual plate application, for reconstruction following tumor surgery with THORP, 627–628
Luhr Vitallium Maxillofacial Systems
for craniomaxillofacial surgery, 105, 107–115
history of rigid fixation and, 79–115
Mandibular Compression Screw System of, 81–91
Micro-System of, 105, 107–115
Vitallium Mini-System of, 91–105

Magnetic resonance imaging, effects of implant materials on, 37–38
Malunion, in post-traumatic maxillary and mandibular reconstruction, 380–381
Mandible
anatomical considerations of monocortical miniplate, osteosynthesis in, 15–16
atrophic fractures of, surgical technique for in Mandibular Compression Screw System, 89–90
combined surgery with maxilla, 451–459
anatomy of, 451
case study of, 458–459
complications of, 458
diagnosis of, 451–452
long-term follow-up and, 459
technique of, 452, 455–457
condylar positioning and, 455
osteotomies and, 455–457
rigid fixation and, 457–458
definition of osteosynthesis line on, 19
distal extension in, ITI-Bonefit Dental Osteointegration System for, 160–161
edentulous, ITI-Bonefit Dental Osteointegration System for, 160
fibromatosis of, case study of pediatric head and neck tumors and, 662–664
in gunshot wounds, 340
masticatory stress distribution into, 17–20
osteoporosis of, case study of unusual applications of plates and, 678–680
post-traumatic bone loss in, case study of unusual applications of plates and, 673, 676–678
in post-traumatic maxillary and mandibular reconstruction, 380
sagittal split ramus osteotomy of, 101–103
unusual applications of plates and, 673, 676–680
vertical portion of, in inferior division of panfacial injuries, 333–334
Mandibular asymmetry, 587–590
Mandibular Compression Screw System (MSC)
indications for, 84
of Luhr Vitallium Maxillofacial Systems for mandibular fractures, 81–91
for mandibular fractures, 113
mandibular fractures and, compressed plating in, 90–91
screws used in, 81–82

specifications of, 81–83
surgical technique for, 84–86, 84–90
lag screw principle in, 88
Mandibular condylar positioning, for Le Fort fractures, 254–255
Mandibular condyle, replacement of by TMJ endoprosthesis in ablative tumor surgery with Mandibular Reconstruction System, 600–601
Mandibular fractures, 179–186
alignment in, 181–182
antibiotics for, 186
Champy's system and, 118–122
in children, 120
complications in, 120–121
in children, surgical technique for Mandibular Compression Screw System, 90
complex, 195–207
diagnosis of, 195
exposure in, 195–196
fractures with bone defects and, 202, 204, 207
maxillomandibular fixation for, 196–197
segmental fractures and, 198–202
complications of, 217–231
bone continuity and, 229–230
compression osteosynthesis and, 227–228
exposure and, 217–218
improper plate placement and, 221–222
incisions as, 217–218
incorrect plate and, 220–221
incorrect screw placement and, 222–223
maxillomandibular fixation and, 218
pathological bone and, 224
plate contouring and, 218
plate length and, 218–220
positioning condyles and, 218
soft-tissue cover and, 228–229
tension banding and, 224, 226–227
compressed plating in Mandibular Compression Screw System and, 90–91
craniomaxillofacial surgery and, 542
fracture-line osteitis of, diagnosis of, 234–235
goal of therapy for, 179
infections of, 233–244
pathogenesis of, 234
treatment of, 235–246
intraoral approach for, 85–88
lag screws in, 181, 187–194
angle fractures and, 189–191
biomechanics of, 187
comminuted fractures and, 192–193
condylar fractures and, 191–192
fixation of, 187
graft fixation and, 193
radiographs for, 187
sagittal fractures and, 188–189
Mandibular Compression Screw System for, 113
Mandibular Compression Screw System of Luhr Vitallium Maxillofacial Systems for, 81–91
method of treatment of, 17
nonunions of, 233–244
diagnosis of, 234–235

pathogenesis of, 234
treatment of, 235–246
open fractures, 186
operative sequence in, 181–186
plate adaptation for, 184–185
plate fixation for, 185–186
plates for, 179–181
post-traumatic maxillary reconstruction and, 392–394
screws for, 179–181
selection of plates for, 182–184
traumatic, THORP for, 632
treatment of pediatric facial fractures and, 400–402
Mandibular immobilization, effects on masticatory system of. See Masticatory system
Mandibular implants for AO Maxillofacial Implant System, 128–130
plates for, 128
reconstruction plates for, 128–133
screws for, 130–131
Mandibular osteotomies
in combined surgery with maxilla and mandible, 455–457
sagittal split ramus, Vitallium Mini-System for, 101–103
Mandibular reconstruction
complications in, 394
free flap. See Mandibular reconstruction, three-dimensional
long-term results of, 395
post-traumatic, 379–395
anatomy of, 379–382
bone grafts in, 385–386
clinical assessment in, 382–385
dental casts in, 385
diagnosis in, 382–385
exposure in, 385
frontal plane analysis in, 382
malunion in, 380–381
nonunion in, 380–381
occlusal analysis in, 385
pediatrics and, 381–382
profile analysis in, 383–384
treatment in, 385–392
three-dimensional, with vascularized bone grafts, 637–646
complications in, 644–646
donor site and, 637–638
fistula and, 638
ilium and, 638
metatarsal and, 638
radius and, 637–638
scapula and, 638
miniplates and, 639–642
planning of, 638–639
results and, 644–646
total functional, 648–655
bone grafts in, 651–652
case studies of, 652–655
osteointegration in, 652–655
case studies in, 652–655
for tumor defects using AO plates and THORP, 605–610
antibiotics in, 607–608
application of, 605–610
closure in, 607
condyle in, 608–609

dental implants in, 608
drains in, 607
incisions in, 606
plate bending in, 606
plate failures in, 608
plate fitting in, 606
radiation in, 608
reconstruction in, 606–607
resection in, 606
results of, 609–610
Mandibular Reconstruction System (MRS)
in ablative tumor surgery, 595–604
alloplastic bridging for, 598–600
bone grafts in, 601–604
indications for, 597–604
instrumentation for, 597
MRS ramus joint in, 596–597
plates for, 596–597
replacement of mandibular condyle by TMJ endoprosthesis, 600–601
screws for, 595–596
specifications of, 595–597
for TMJ, 113–114
Mini-System for, 114–115
of Würzburg Titanium System, 136–138
equipment for, 136
Mandibular teeth, in orthodontic surgery, 502
Masticatory stress distribution, into mandible, 17–20
Masticatory system
effect of immobilization of bone on, 63–64
effect of immobilization of muscles on, 64–67
effect of immobilization of periarticular connective tissues on, 70–74
effects of immobilization of synovial joints on, 67–70
effects of mandibular immobilization on, 63–74
Material refinement for medical devices, 33
Materials
bioresorbable, 57–60
resorbable, potential of, 57–60
Material testing of implant materials, 41–42
Maxilla
combined surgery with mandible, 451–459
anatomy of, 451
case study of, 458–459
complications in, 458
diagnosis of, 451–452
long-term follow-up and, 458
technique of, 452, 455–458
condylar positioning and, 457
osteotomies and, 455–457
rigid fixation and, 457–458
echondrosarcoma of, case study of pediatric head and neck tumors and, 668
expansion of. See Facial skeleton
inferior repositioning of, in Le Fort osteotomies, 434
in post-traumatic maxillary and mandibular reconstruction, 379–380
rhabdomyosarcoma of, case study of pediatric head and neck tumors and, 657
sectioning for, in Le Fort osteotomies, 428–430
segmentation of, in Le Fort osteotomies, 433–434

single tooth replacement in, ITI-Bonefit Dental Osteointegration System for, 161
Maxillary asymmetry, 587–590
Maxillary bone, loss of in gunshot wounds, 339–340
Maxillary fractures. See also Le Fort fractures
central, nasoethmoid-orbital fractures with, 287–288
craniomaxillofacial surgery and, 539–542
post-traumatic maxillary reconstruction and, 386–392
Maxillary hypoplasia, congenital
midfacial and maxillary fractures in craniomaxillofacial surgery and, 540
Maxillary osteotomies, 103–105
in combined surgery with maxilla and mandible, 455–457
in surgery for cleft lip deformities, 497
Vitallium Mini-System for, 103–105
Maxillary reconstruction, post-traumatic, 379–395
anatomy of, 379–382
bone grafts in, 385–386
clinical assessment in, 382–385
complications in, 394
dental casts in, 385
diagnosis in, 382–385
exposure and, 385
frontal plane analysis in, 382
Le Fort deformities and, 387–392
long-term results of, 395
malunion in, 380–381
mandibular fractures and, 392–394
maxillary fractures and, 386–392
nonunion in, 380–381
occlusal analysis in, 385
pediatrics and, 381–382
profile analysis in, 383–384
treatment in, 385–392
Maxillary sinus drainage, in Le Fort fractures, 261
Maxillary step osteotomies, as Le Fort osteotomies
design of, 425–426
Maxillary teeth, in orthodontic surgery, 501
Maxillomandibular fixation (MMF), 63
for complex mandibular fractures, 196–197
as complication in mandibular fractures, 218
for mandibular fractures, 181
treatment of pediatric facial fractures and, 402
Measurement, units of, of implant materials, 38–39
Medical devices, material modification and manufacturing for, 33–34
Metallic bond in metallic structure, 32
Metallic structure of implant materials, 32–33
Metals
as implant materials, 28–31
as mechanical properties of implant materials, 42–44
as physical properties of implant materials, 36–37
Metatarsal, donor site and
three-dimensional mandibular reconstruction with vascularized bone grafts and, 638
Micromesh, used in Micro-System, 107–108
Microplates, used in Micro-System, 107–108
Microsomia, hemifacial
congenital craniofacial deformities and, 509
Micro-System in craniomaxillofacial surgery
drill bits used in, 109

indications for, 110–112
instrumentation for, 109
of Luhr Vitallium Maxillofacial Systems, 105, 107–115
for Mandibular Reconstruction System for TMJ, 115
micromesh used in, 107–108
microplates used in, 107–108
screws used in, 108–109
specifications of, 107–109
surgical technique for, 110–112
Midface
anterior nasal spine of, case study of unusual applications of plates and, 673
inferior orbital rim of, unusual applications of plates and, 671–673
nonunion of bones in, case study of unusual applications of plates and, 673
unusual applications of plates and, 671–673
Midface bone, in gunshot wounds, 339–340
Midface dislocation
and concomitant dislocation of skull base midline structures, case study of subcranial approach to craniofacial surgery, 569, 571
Midface fractures. *See also* Le Fort fractures
complications in, 351–356
dimensions of face in, 352
etiology of, 351–353
improper fixation technique in, 353
inadequate reduction as, 351–353
management of, 353–356
recognition of, 353
treatment of, 353–356
craniomaxillofacial surgery and, 539–542
restoration of width in, 352
Vitallium Mini-System for, 100
Würzburg Titanium System for, 143–145
Midfacial injuries, zygomatic arch and, 265
Midline cranio-orbital cleft with orbital hypotelorism, case study of, 517
Miniplate osteosynthesis. *See* Monocortical miniplate osteosynthesis
Miniplates, three-dimensional mandibular reconstruction with vascularized bone grafts and, 639–642
Miniplate system of Würzburg Titanium System, 138–141
biological considerations of, 138–139
instrumentation for, 140–141
mechanical considerations of, 138–139
plates for, 140
screws for, 139–140
Mini-System for Mandibular Reconstruction System for TMJ, 114
MMF. *See* Maxillomandibular fixation (MMF)
Modulus of elasticity of implant materials, 39–40
Moment of implant materials, 39
Monobloc bipartition osteotomy
with cranial vault osteotomy for midline cranio-orbital cleft with orbital hypertelorism, case study of, 517
with cranial vault reshaping for Apert syndrome, case study of, 513, 516–517
Monobloc osteotomy with cranial vault reshaping for Crouzon's disease, case study of, 513
Monocortical miniplate osteosynthesis, 15–20

anatomical considerations of, 15–17
biomechanical principles of, 17–20
in cranium, 20
definition of osteosynthesis line on mandible and, 19
goals of treatment and, 17
masticatory stress distribution into mandible and, 17–20
in upper face, 20
MRS ramus joint in ablative tumor surgery with Mandibular Reconstruction System, 596–597
Multiple-segment osteotomies, diagnosis of Le Fort III osteotomies and, 547
Muscles
immobilization of effecting masticatory system, 64–67
nasolabial, in surgery for cleft lip deformities, 497–498

Nasal bone graft fixation, plates and screws for nasoethmoid-orbital fractures in, 294–297
Nasal fractures, treatment of pediatric facial fractures and, 400
Nasal spine, anterior, unusual applications of plates and, 673
Nasal surgery, sagittal split ramus osteotomies, 448–449
Nasoethmoidal fractures, Micro-System for, 110
Nasoethmoid-orbital deformity combined with Le Fort deformity, 363, 366
Nasoethmoid-orbital fractures, 283–301
anatomy of in post-traumatic cranio-orbital reconstruction, 371
bone fragments in, 294
with bone loss, 290
with central maxilla fractures, 287–288
classification of, 286–290
closed reduction for, 283
comminuted fractures with, 291–294
confined space and, 297–298
cranial fractures and, 297
exposure and, 290
extended, 288
frontal sinus fractures and, 297
frontonasal buttress fixation in, 290–291
isolated, in bony region, 286–287
loss of bone with, 292, 294
management of, 286–290
medial canthal ligament and, 284–286, 296, 298
nasal bone graft fixation in, 294–297
nasolacrimal system in, 298, 300
with oculo-orbital displacement, 290
pathological anatomy of, 284
plates and, 290–300
problems in, 300
screws and, 290–300
treatment of in post-traumatic cranio-orbital reconstruction, 375
unilateral, in zygomatic arch fractures, 280–281. *See* Nasoethmoid-orbital fractures
Naso-fronto-ethmoid fractures, treatment of pediatric facial fractures and, 399
Nasolabial muscles in surgery for cleft lip deformities, 497–498
Nasolacrimal drainage, orbital fractures and, 316
Nasolacrimal system, plates and screws for in nasoethmoid-orbital fractures, 298, 300

Neck tumors. *See* Head and neck tumors, pediatric
Nonunions
   aseptic, 234–235
   with bone defect, 235
   in bone healing, 6
   diagnosis of, 234–235
   incorrect placement of screws for, as complication in mandibular fractures, 223
   infected, 234
   of mandibular fractures
      compression plating for, 238–239
      corrective osteotomy for, 239–240
      reconstruction plates for, 239–240
   in post-traumatic maxillary and mandibular reconstruction, 380–381

Oblique fractures, selection of plates for, 183
Occlusal evaluation in post-traumatic maxillary and mandibular reconstruction, 385
Occlusion
   analysis of plates and screws in cleft lip deformities and, 467
   in inferior division of panfacial injuries, 332–333
Ocular function, orbital fractures and, 315
Ocular position in coronal plane, orbital fractures and, 316
Oculo-orbital displacement, nasoethmoid-orbital fractures with, 290
Open reduction of subcondylar fractures. *See* Subcondylar fractures, open reduction of
Optic nerve decompression, exposure and in subcranial approach to craniofacial surgery and traumatology, 546–566
Orbit
   enchondrosarcoma of, case study of pediatric head and neck tumors and, 668
   internal, 317–322
      anatomy of, 317–318
      complications of, 320
      diagnosis of, 318–320
      results and, 320
      treatment of, 318–320
Orbital cavity, orbital fractures and, 312–314
Orbital dystopia, 587
Orbital-floor plates for craniofacial instrumentation for AO Maxillofacial Implant System, 132–133
Orbital fractures, 302–316
   anatomy of, 302–305
      in post-traumatic cranio-orbital reconstruction, 372
   anterior segment of, 302–304
   characteristics of, 302–307
   clinical features of, 306–307
   enophthalmos and, 315–316
   etiology of, 305
   fixation of, 307–309
      with bone grafts, 309
      with interosseous wire, 308
      with miniplates, 308–309
   globe projection and, 315–316
   management of, 307
   medial canthus and, 316
   nasolacrimal drainage and, 316
   ocular function and, 315
   ocular position in coronal plane and, 316
   orbital cavity and, 312–314
   orbital rim and, 310–312
   palpebral fissures and, 316
   pathology of, 305–306
   periorbital soft tissue and, 314–315
   posterior segment of, 304–305
   surgery for, 310–315
      exposure and, 310
   treatment of in post-traumatic cranio-orbital reconstruction, 377
Orbital hypertelorism
   congenital craniofacial deformities and, 509
   midline cranio-orbital cleft with, case study of plates and screws in craniofacial deformities and, 517
Orbital osteotomies
   cranial vault craniotomy for bilateral coronal stenosis, case study of, 521, 524–525
   with cranial vault craniotomy for trigonocephaly, case study of, 517
Orbital rim
   in gunshot wounds, 339
   inferior
      of midface, unusual applications of plates and, 671–673
      orbital fractures and, 312
      in zygomatic arch fractures, 274
   lateral
      orbital fractures and, 310–311
      in zygomatic arch fractures, 274, 280
   medial, orbital fractures and, 311–312
   orbital fractures and, 310
   supraorbital, orbital fractures and, 310
Orbital rim fractures, lateral, treatment of pediatric facial fractures and, 398–399
Orbitofacial advancement, block. *See* Block orbitofacial advancement
Orbitozygomatic deformity, 361–363
Orbitozygomatic fractures, treatment of in post-traumatic cranio-orbital reconstruction, 375–376
Orbitozygomatic injuries, zygomatic arch and, 265
Orbitozygomatic-orbital fractures, anatomy of in post-traumatic cranio-orbital reconstruction, 371
Orthodontic appliances in orthodontic surgery, 501–502
Orthodontic surgery, 500–504
   intraoperative steps in, 503
   maxillary and mandibular teeth in, 501
   plates and screws in, 500
   postoperative steps in, 503–504
   preoperative steps in, 500–503
Orthognathic surgery. *See also* Orthodontic surgery
   Vitallium Mini-System for, 100–105
Osseodental unit, fixed, in total functional mandibular reconstruction, 648
Osteitis
   fracture-line. *See* Fracture-line osteitis
   of mandibular fractures, incision and drainage of, 237
Osteoblasts of bone, 3
Osteoclasts of bone, 3
Osteocytes of bone, 3
Osteointegration, 163–174

biomechanical considerations in, 171–174
   cantilever action as, 173–174
   flexible prosthesis, 174
   force distribution to fixtures as, 172–174
   rigid prosthesis, 172–173
   screw form in, 171
   single screw as, 171–172
definition of, 164
in dentistry, 167–169
experimental investigations in, 169–171
fixtures in, 174
history of, 163–164
natural teeth in, 174
single fixture in, 174
system of, for craniomaxillofacial region, 164–167
in total functional mandibular reconstruction, 652–655
   case studies of, 652–655
Osteon of bone, 3
Osteosynthesis. *See* Lag screw osteosynthesis
   fixation. *See* Fixation osteosynthesis
   monocortical miniplate. *See* Monocortical miniplate osteosynthesis
Osteosynthesis line, ideal, on mandible, 19
Osteotomies. *See* specific types of osteotomies
   corrective, for nonunion of mandibular fractures, 240–241
   in sagittal split ramus osteotomies, 437–440
Oxycephaly, 528

Palate jaw deformities. *See* Cleft lip deformities
Panfacial injuries, 330–337
   anatomy of, 330–331
   central zone concept of, 331–332
   complications of, 337
   definition of, 330
   diagnosis of, 331
   long-term results and, 337
   treatment of, 331–332
   treatment sequence of, 332–336
      inferior division and, 331–334
      in superior division of, 334–337
Parasymphyseal fractures, treatment of pediatric facial fractures and, 402
Passivation for medical devices, 34–35
Periarticular connective tissues, immobilization of on masticatory system, 70–74
Periodontal ligament in dental occlusion, as complications in midface fractures, 351
Pretzel lag screw technique, 192
Phase, of implant material, 33
Photography in post-traumatic maxillary and mandibular reconstruction, 384
Plagiocephaly, craniomaxillofacial surgery and, 528
Plate-induced porosis in bone healing, 6
Plates
   for ablative tumor surgery with Mandibular Reconstruction System, 596–597
   adaptation of, for mandibular fractures, 184–185
   bending of, in mandibular reconstruction for tumor defects using AO plates and THORP, 606
   buttress, for Le Fort fractures, 250–253
   in cleft lip and palate jaw deformities. *See* Cleft lip deformities
   compression, for nonunion of mandibular fractures, 238–239
   contouring of as complication of rigid internal fixation of mandibular fractures, 218
   in craniofacial deformities. *See* Craniofacial deformities, plates and screws in
   for craniofacial instrumentation for AO Maxillofacial Implant System, 132
   failures in, for tumor defects using AO plates and THORP, 608
   fitting of, in mandibular reconstruction for tumor defects using AO plates and THORP, 606
   fixation of, for mandibular fractures, 185–186
   improper placement of, as complication in mandibular fractures, 221–222
   incorrect, as complication in mandibular fractures, 220–221
   in Le Fort osteotomies, 430–434
   length of, as complication in mandibular fractures, 218–220
   longer, compression osteosynthesis and, as complication in mandibular fractures, 227–228
   mandibular, for Le Fort fractures, 254
   for mandibular fractures, 179–181
   for mandibular implants for AO Maxillofacial Implant System, 128
   mesh, for bone grafting, 533, 538–539
   for miniplate system of Würzburg Titanium System, 140
   nasoethmoid-orbital fractures and, 290–300
   neutralization, compression osteosynthesis and as complication in mandibular fractures, 227–228
   in orthodontic surgery, 500
   in pediatric facial features. *See* Facial fractures, pediatric
   in pediatric head and neck tumors. *See* Head and neck tumors, pediatric
   reconstruction
      in complex tumor reconstruction. *See* Tumor reconstruction, complex
      for nonunion of mandibular fractures, 239–240
   removal of, in THORP, 632–634
   resorbable, 58–60
   selection of, for mandibular fractures, 182–184
   stabilization, compression osteosynthesis and, as complication in mandibular fractures, 227–228
   THORP and, 620–622
   unusual applications of, 671–680
      Albers-Schönberg disease and, case study of, 678–680
      in mandible, 673, 676–680
      in midface, 671–673
         case study of anterior nasal spine and, 673
         inferior orbital rim and, 671–673
         nonunion of bones and, case study of, 673
      osteoporosis of mandible and, 678–680
         case study of, 678–680
      in post-traumatic bone lone in mandible, 673, 676
         case study of, 676–678
   upper border, tension banding and, as complication in mandibular fractures, 227
   used in Mandibular Compression Screw System, 81–82, 82–83, 83–84

used in Vitallium Mini-System, 92–93, 94–95
Polymers
　bioresorbable, 57–58
　as implant materials, 28–29
Porosis under plates, 6
Profile analysis in post-traumatic maxillary and mandibular reconstruction, 383–384
Projection
　facial, in panfacial injuries, 331
　of globe, orbital fractures and, 315–316
Prosthesis
　flexible, as biomechanical consideration in osteointegration, 173
　rigid, as biomechanical consideration in osteointegration, 172–173
Proteoglycans in connective tissues, 72–73
Psesudoarthrosis, in bone healing, 6
Pull-out experiments, in osteointegration, 169

Radiation therapy, effects of implant materials on, 38
Radiographs, effects of implant materials on, 37
Radiology, in post-traumatic maxillary and mandibular reconstruction, 384–385
Radius, donor site and
　three-dimensional mandibular reconstruction with vascularized bone grafts and, 637–638
Reconstruction plates
　for AO Mandibular System, 126
　for mandibular implants for AO Maxillofacial Implant System, 128–130
Reduction
　closed, for nasoethmoid-orbital fractures, 283
　fracture
　　dental repair and, in subcranial approach to craniofacial surgery and traumatology, 566–569
　　in maxillomandibular fixation for complex mandibular fractures, 197
　inadequate, as complication in midface fracture, 351–353
　open, of subcondylar fractures. See Subcondylar fractures, open reduction of
Residual deformities, plates and screws in cleft lip deformities and, 467–468
Rhabdomyosarcoma of maxilla
　case study of pediatric head and neck tumors and, 657
　pediatric, 656, 657
Rigid fixation, history of, 79–81
Rigid prosthesis as biomechanical consideration in osteointegration, 172–173

Sagittal fractures
　lag screws in mandibular fractures and, 188–189
　selection of plates for, 183
Sagittal maxillary fractures, Le Fort fractures and, 257
Sagittal split ramus osteotomies (SSRO), 435–443
　case studies of, 443–449
　exposure in, 435–437
　of mandible, 101–103
　nasal surgery and, 448–449
　neuromuscular rehabilitation in, 443
　osteotomy in, 437–440

screws in, 440–442
stabilization in, 440–442
techniques of, 435–443
Sarcoma, Ewing's, of zygomatic arch
　case studies of pediatric head and neck tumors and, 657, 660–662
Scaphocephaly, craniomaxillofacial surgery and, 528, 530, 532–533
Scapula, donor site and
　three-dimensional mandibular reconstruction with vascularized bone grafts and, 638
Screw(s). See also Lag screw
　for ablative tumor surgery with Mandibular Reconstruction System, 595–596
　in craniofacial deformities. See Craniofacial deformities, plates and screws in
　for craniofacial instrumentation for AO Maxillofacial Implant System, 131–132
　fixation type of, 13–14
　form of, as biomechanical consideration in osteointegration, 171
　as implants in ITI-Bonefit Dental Osteointegration System, 159
　incorrect placement of, as complication in mandibular fractures, 222–223
　lag type of, 13–14
　in Le Fort osteotomies, 430–434
　for mandibular fractures, 179–181
　for mandibular implants for AO Maxillofacial Implant System, 130–131
　for miniplate system of Würzburg Titanium System, 139–140
　nasoethmoid-orbital fractures and, 290–300
　in orthodontic surgery, 500
　in pediatric facial fractures. See Facial fractures, pediatric
　in pediatric head and neck tumors. See Head and neck tumors, pediatric
　removal of, in THORP, 632–634
　resorbable, 58–60
　in sagittal split ramus osteotomies, 440–442
　single, as biomechanical consideration in osteointegration, 171
　THORP and, 622–623
　used in fixation osteosynthesis, 7–9
　used in Mandibular Compression Screw System, 81–82, 83–84
　used in Micro-System, 108–109
　used in Vitallium Mini-System, 92
Segmental fractures,
　butterfly, 199–200
　comminution, 201–202
　complex mandibular fractures and, 198–202
　edentulous, 200–201
　horizontal splitting, 201
　large, 198–199
　multiple, 201–202
　sagittal splitting, 201
　selection of plates for, 184
Sequestrectomy
　as therapy for infections of mandibular fractures, 233

as therapy for nonunions of mandibular fractures, 233
Single-segment osteotomies, Le Fort III osteotomies and, 546–547
Sinus
  frontal, Micro-System for, 110
  frontal fractures of
    frontal bone fractures and, 324–325
    plates and screws for nasoethmoid-orbital fractures in, 297
Sinus drainage, maxillary
  in Le Fort fractures, 261
Skeletal dysplasia. *See* Cleft lip deformities
Skull, reconstruction of
  Micro-System for, 110
Skull base
  dislocation of bone fragments in, case study of, 569, 571
  midline structures and concomitant dislocation, in subcranial approach to craniofacial surgery, 569
Soft tissue
  in gunshot wounds, 340, 347–349
  periorbital fractures and, 314–315
  in superior division of panfacial injuries, 335
Soft-tissue cover as complication of rigid internal fixation of mandibular fractures, 228–229
Splint fixation, external, for nasoethmoid-orbital fractures, 283
Spontaneous dental compensations in orthodontic surgery, 501
Stability, absolute, 6
Stabilization in maxillomandibular fixation for complex mandibular fractures, 197
Stainless steel
  as corrosion property of metal, 47
  as mechanical property of metal, 43
  as metal implant material, 36
  history of, 30
Sterilization of medical devices, 35
Strain
  in bone healing, 4–5
  of implant materials, 40
Stress
  versus fatigue, of implant materials, 42
  of implant materials, 39–40, 41–42
  material testing and, 41–42
Stress protection in plate-induced porosis, 6
Stress shielding, infection and, 53
Subcondylar fractures
  anatomy of, 209–210
  bilateral, 211
  diagnosis of, 210–212
  long-term results and, 216
  mandibular motion in, 211
  open reduction of, 209–216
    anatomy of, 209–210
    in children, 209
    complications in, 215–216
    extraoral approach for, 215
    indications for, 212
    intraoral approach for, 213–215
    surgical technique for, 212–213
    treatment of, 212–215
  radiographs of, 211–212
Supraorbital fractures
  anatomy of, in post-traumatic cranio-orbital reconstruction, 371
  treatment of, in post-traumatic cranio-orbital reconstruction, 373
Supraorbital rim fractures, treatment of pediatric facial fractures and, 398–399
Surface properties of medical devices, 35–36
Surgical handling of medical devices, 35
Symphyseal fractures, treatment of pediatric facial fractures and, 402
Synostosis
  bilateral coronal
    case study of plates and screws in craniofacial deformities and, 521, 524–525
  unilateral coronal, craniomaxillofacial surgery and, 528
Synovial joints
  articular surfaces in, nutrition and, 69
  immobilization of, effecting masticatory system, 67–70

Teeth
  malalignment of, as complications in midface fractures, 351–352
  maxillary and mandibular, in orthodontic surgery, 501
  natural, in osteointegration, 174
Temporomandibular bone, in subcondylar fractures, 209–210
Temporomandibular joint
  immobilization of, 68–69
  Mandibular Reconstruction System for, 113–114
    Mini-System for, 114–115
Temporomandibular joint endoprosthesis
  in ablative tumor surgery with Mandibular Reconstruction System, 596–597
  replacing mandibular condyle in ablative tumor surgery with Mandibular Reconstruction System, 600–601
Tension band, compression and, 11
Tension banding
  as complication in mandibular fractures, 224, 226–227
  in maxillomandibular fixation for complex mandibular fractures, 197
THORP, 620–636
  with AO plates, in mandibular reconstruction for tumor defects. *See also* Mandibular reconstruction, for tumor defects using AO plates and THORP
  biomechanical aspects of, 620–623
  comparison with conventional systems and, 623–632
    reconstruction following tumor surgery and, 626–632
  for complex tumor reconstruction, 616–617
  in complex tumor reconstruction, 612
  plates and, 620–622
  removal of plates and screws in, 632–634
  results and, 634–635
  screws and, 622–623
  technical aspects of, 620–623
  for traumatic mandibular fractures, 632
Three-dimensionally bendable reconstruction plates (3-DBRP) for nonunion of mandibular fractures, 239–240
Tissue
  in bone healing, 4–5
  periarticular connective. *See* Periarticular connective tissues
Titanium
  as corrosion property of metal, 47

as mechanical property of metal, 43–44
as metal implant material, 37
history of, 31
Titanium Hollow-Screw Reconstruction plate (THORP). See THORP
TMJ. See Temporomandibular joint
Tooth, replacement of single in maxilla, ITI-Bonefit Dental Osteointegration System for, 161
Torque experiments in osteointegration, 169
Transition temperature of implant materials, 33
Transverse fracture(s), selection of plates for, 182–183
Treacher Collins syndrome
　congenital craniofacial deformities and, 509–510
　case study of plates and screws in craniofacial deformities and, 521
Trigonocephaly
　craniomaxillofacial surgery and, 530, 532–533
　case study of plates and screws in craniofacial deformities and, 517
Tumor reconstruction, complex, 595–604, 612–619
　AO plates for, 614, 615–616
　classification of defects in, 613
　complications in, 616–619
　diagnosis of, 613–614
　Mandibular Reconstruction System, 595–604
　options for, 614–615
　THORP for, 614, 616–617
Tumor resection, frontal bone defect following
　case study of pediatric head and neck tumors and, 666–668
Tumors. See Head and neck tumors, pediatric
Tumor surgery, ablative, Mandibular Reconstruction System in. See Mandibular Reconstruction System, in ablative tumor surgery
Turricephaly, 528

Unit cell, in metallic structure, 32

Vitallium Mini-System
　indications for, 95–97
　instruments used in, 92
　for Le Fort fractures, 97–100
　of Luhr Vitallium Maxillofacial Systems, 91–105
　for orthognathic surgery, 100–105
　plates used in, 94–95
　screws used in, 92
　specifications of, 91
　surgical technique for, 95

Working, for medical devices, 34
Wrought materials, for medical devices, 33–34
Würzburg Compression-Plate System of Würzburg Titanium System
　history of, 134–135
　indications for, 135
Würzburg Titanium System, 134–149
　complications in, 143
　for craniofacial surgery, 145–148
　for dental implants, 148–149
　for Le Fort fractures, 145
　Mandibular Reconstruction System of, 136–138
　　equipment for, 136
　material for, 141
　for midface fractures, 143–145
　miniplate system of, 138–141
　　biological considerations of, 138–139
　　instrumentation for, 140–141
　　mechanical considerations of, 138–139
　　plates for, 140
　　screws for, 139–140
　for orthognathic surgery, 145–148
　for trauma, 141–142
　Würzburg Compression-Plate System of
　　history of, 134–135
　　indications for, 135

Young's modulus, of implant materials, 40

Zone concept, central. See Central zone concept
Zygoma, enchondrosarcoma of
　case study of pediatric head and neck tumors and, 668
Zygomatic arch, 263, 265
　in anatomy of zygomatic fractures, 274
　in craniofacial deformities, 358
　displaced, 269
　in Le Fort fractures, 255–257
　exposure of, 269, 271
　fractures of
　　interior orbital rim in, 274
　　lateral orbital rim in, 274, 280
　　pattern of, 274, 280–281
　　unilateral nasoethmoid-orbital fractures in, 280–281
　　zygomaticomaxillary buttress in, 274
　in gunshot wounds, 339
Zygomatic bone, reconstruction of
　case study for Treacher Collins syndrome, 521
Zygomatic fractures, 263–281
　anatomy of, 271, 273–274
　classification of, 265, 267
　in craniofacial deformit(y)ies, 358
　diagnosis of, 265
　displaced, 267
　surgical anatomy of, 265
　surgical repair of, 267–271
　treatment of pediatric facial fractures and, 399
　Vitallium Mini-System for, 96–97
Zygomaticomaxillary buttress in zygomatic arch fractures, 274
Zygomatic orbital complex in superior division of panfacial injuries, 334–335